Dental Caries

Dental Caries

The Disease and its Clinical Management

Second Edition

Edited by

Ole Fejerskov and Edwina Kidd

with

Bente Nyvad and Vibeke Baelum

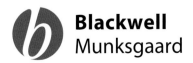

Blackwell
Munksgaard

Blackwell Munksgaard, a Blackwell Publishing Company,
Blackwell Publishing Ltd, 9600 Garsington Road, Oxford OX4 2DQ, UK
  Tel: +44 (0)1865 776868
Blackwell Publishing Professional, 2121 State Avenue, Ames, Iowa 50014-8300, USA
  Tel: +1 515 292 0140
Blackwell Publishing Asia Pty Ltd, 550 Swanston Street, Carlton, Victoria 3053, Australia
  Tel: +61 (0)3 8359 1011

First published 2003 by Blackwell Munksgaard Ltd
Second edition published 2008

ISBN: 9781405138895

Library of Congress Cataloging-in-Publication Data
Dental caries: the disease and its clinical management/edited by Ole Fejerskov and Edwina A.M. Kidd, with Bente Nyvad and Vibeke Baelum. -- 2nd ed.
p. XX; cm.
Includes bibliographical references and index.
ISBN-13: 978-1-4051-3889-5 (hardback : alk. paper)
ISBN-10: 1-4051-3889-0 (hardback : alk. paper)
1. Dental caries--Diagnosis. 2. Dental caries--Treatment. I. Fejerskov, Ole. II. Kidd, Edwina A. M.
[DNLM: 1. Dental Caries--diagnosis. 2. Dental Caries--therapy. 3. Dental Restoration, Permanent. WU 270 D4145 2008]

RK331.D465 2008
617.6'7--dc22
   2007021650

A catalogue record for this title is available from the British Library

Set in Minion and Frutiger
by Gray Publishing, Tunbridge Wells, UK
Printed and bound in Singapore
by Markono Print Media Pte Ltd

The publisher's policy is to use permanent paper from mills that operate a sustainable forestry policy, and which has been manufactured from pulp processed using acid-free and elementary chlorine-free practices. Furthermore, the publisher ensures that the text paper and cover board used have met acceptable environmental accreditation standards.

For further information on Blackwell Munksgaard, visit our website:
www.dentistry.blackwellmunksgaard.com

Contents

Preface: an Editors' guide to reading the book

To our immense pleasure, the first edition of this book has found its way all over the world. In the genesis of this second edition we have enlisted the help of two associate editors, Vibeke Baelum and Bente Nyvad, who have helped us at the planning stage and by contributing extensively to the book. Most of the old text has been updated and there are 10 new chapters. Our band of 30 international authors has grown to 49.

A textbook reflects the way in which the authors interpret scientific data on a given subject, but we do not pretend that this is the 'truth' about the complex disease called 'dental caries'. There are extensive data available on today's internet and the stream of information will continue to grow. This is an enormous challenge to clinical students and practitioners. How can sense be made of the bombardment of information? The authors have been asked to present their respective subtopics carefully, so that it is not just a compilation of data, but selected data critically brought together in order to explain why dental caries presents itself in the individual and in populations in the way it does in today's world.

This preface aims to give a sequential, bird's-eye view of our efforts and map your journey through these pages by highlighting features that we, the editors, consider important. The aim of this book is to present the dental student and the dental practitioner with an update on the available knowledge about dental caries, and the consequences of this to its diagnosis, and how most appropriately and cost-effectively to control caries progression. Clinical decision-making and the balance between non-operative and operative treatments become even more important parts of daily life in clinical practice. An understanding of the caries process is needed to estimate the prognosis of treatment procedures and the possibility of assessing the risk of disease development in individuals and populations.

This book will demonstrate that in real life the processes involved in dental caries are highly complex. In an ideal world there would be a perfect model that could relate all the potential determinants to caries outcome. It will appear throughout the book that most of the determinants that influence caries can, at best, be measured only as proxy variables. The most we can hope for, therefore, is to develop probabilistic models that relate determinants to risk of caries progression. However, even under such circumstances, caries would remain unpredictable. Such inputs as:

- variable exposure to fluoride
- times, lengths, frequencies and types of sugar consumption
- quality of tooth cleaning
- fluctuations in salivary flow rates and composition

- quality and composition of biofilms
- the behavior of the individual
- the societal context of the individual

are themselves highly variable. It is likely that this variability and unpredictability of the inputs may play a crucial role in the way in which the caries process develops. But all these factors make up the fascination and challenge of our profession.

It is our hope that this book will prepare the reader to become a less dogmatic and more knowledgeable health professional who strives to control dental caries in the most cost-effective way.

Part I. The disease and its diagnosis

Chapter 1 defines caries as a localized chemical dissolution of a tooth surface resulting from metabolic events taking place in a biofilm (dental plaque) covering the affected area. These metabolic events are the *carious process*. The interaction between the microbial deposits and the hard tissues of the teeth may result in the *caries lesion* that is the sign or symptom of the process. Most of the components of the caries process, such as biofilm, diet and saliva, can be interfered with. They act at the tooth surface, but another set of determinants acts at the level of the individual. These include the person's behavior, knowledge, attitudes and education, and they may be much more difficult to modify.

Dental caries can be considered on a number of levels: the tooth surface, the individual and the population. This should be remembered throughout the book. There is a section on terminology, introducing the student to ways of classifying lesions, by their site on the tooth and their activity. This activity concept is critical to this book that is about *controlling lesion progression*, so that the ubiquitous natural process that is caries does not result in progressive tooth destruction.

Chapter 2 shows the student what caries lesions look like clinically on various tooth surfaces. In the past we thought that the clinical appearance of dental caries was known to every student, but teachers from around the world have asked us to show the spectrum which we consider to be important. So make yourselves familiar with the extensive variations in the clinical features. The theme of caries control is carried forward by showing lesions that are designated as 'active' and 'progressing' as well as those that are 'arrested'. There are also pictures of 'active lesions' being converted to 'inactive lesions' by non-operative treatments such as improved oral hygiene and fluoride application.

Having described the clinical manifestations of caries in Chapter 2, Chapter 3 goes on to describe histological manifestations. Lesions manifest themselves in different ways, depending on variations in anatomical structures. Understanding how anatomy influences clinical presentation is important in the diagnosis of caries. It is also important in appreciating how lesions progress and when a restoration might be required. It is anatomical features that influence when and how the tooth surface breaks to form a cavity and whether this hole can be cleaned by the patient. If the biofilm cannot be disturbed, the lesion cannot be controlled and is likely to progress.

The following four chapters all concern diagnosis, which is an essential resting place for the mind before making a treatment decision. Chapter 4 concentrates on what the eyes can see (visual), aided by gentle use of a probe (tactile). The chapter starts by warning the student that the lesion is the consequence of the metabolic activity of the biofilm. Thus, the dentist is looking at the reflection of the caries process, not the process itself. The authors then stress that the purpose of diagnosis is to direct the clinician to appropriate management. This explains why features such as cavitation and lesion activity are so important. A hole in a tooth may require repair if the patient cannot keep it clean; active lesions require active management, whereas arrested lesions do not. The student is warned that a good diagnostic test will be valid (measure what it claims to measure) and reliable (the measurement can be repeated and give the same result). Commonly used visual–tactile criteria are described and a systematic clinical approach is suggested and, very importantly, the results of this are linked to clinical management.

Sometimes vision is obscured, perhaps by an adjacent tooth, and radiographs may be needed to detect lesions. It should be noted, however, that a radiograph taken on a single occasion cannot determine lesion activity and it cannot say whether there is a hole in the tooth. Moreover, ionizing radiation should not be used as an excuse for slovenly clinical examination. Chapter 5 describes the use, indications and limitations of radiography in caries diagnosis, suggesting when radiographs are indicated.

In Chapter 6 several additional diagnostic measures are described. These methods are often quantitative and seek to improve on clinical–visual and radiographic examination. However, the methods will often involve expensive kit and must still be interpreted by the dentist, who must never pass the responsibility for diagnosis to a machine. The authors conclude that of the measures described only laser fluorescence and digital radiography are currently used in practice. The chapter is a salutary read for the geeks among us!

Part I concludes with a most thoughtful Chapter 7 that considers the foundations or building blocks for good diagnostic practice. What are we looking for and why? To what use will we put this information and what will be the consequences of error? We are warned that diagnosis is an error-prone exercise and that decisions are inevitably made under uncertainty. This is a chapter that should be read more than once! It argues for diagnostic methods that link directly to appropriate management options (for instance cavitation versus non-cavitation), an appreciation of error and a bias towards a less invasive management approach. This is probably the most important consideration in caries management.

Part II. Clinical caries epidemiology

Epidemiology is the study of health and disease in populations. Chapter 8 begins by explaining how caries is measured in these studies and questions whether such measures can be used to assess treatment needs at the population level. There would seem to be considerable difficulties in this approach. The chapter goes on to consider the distribution of caries and the influence of environment, particularly the social environment. Caries is just as much a disease of social deprivation as it is a problem of bad diet. These are critical concepts because they show the limitations within which a dental profession operates. The key to disease control lies in improving the broad social environment as well as the intraoral environment.

Chapter 9 expands on measurement issues in caries epidemiology. Examples demonstrate how different diagnostic thresholds influence just how much or how little of the total caries experience of an individual or population is captured. In particular, the term 'caries free' should be interpreted with caution because sometimes it may just mean 'cavity free', but certainly not free of a spectrum of early signs of caries lesions.

Part III. Dental caries in a biological context

Part III of the book focusses on the biofilm, saliva, and chemical interactions between the tooth and the oral fluids. Not only is this a part of the book that looks into the conditions prevailing in the oral cavity, but in most of the examples the authors deal with events taking place at the single tooth surface.

Chapter 10 concerns the biofilm, a community of resident microorganisms that grow on a surface and function together and whose ecology is influenced by saliva and diet. The development and structure of the biofilm are described and the importance of the microbial community is stressed; these organisms function in concert, not as individuals. The microbiology of caries is described and it is emphasized that no single organism, or group of organisms, may be held solely responsible for the initiation or progression of caries. Lesion progression is a result of a shift in the balance of the resident microflora driven by a change in the local environmental conditions. Thus, changes in diet, saliva and oral hygiene are of extreme relevance to caries, and identifying what is driving deleterious changes is the key to control strategies, tailored to the individual patient.

Chapter 11 explores the very complex secretion, saliva, from a cariological point of view. This oral lubricant is not fully appreciated until its flow is diminished. It is a unique fluid film covering all mucous membranes of the oral cavity as well as tooth surfaces. Hence, its composition and relative velocity (flow rate) are of decisive importance for the microenvironment throughout all niches in the oral cavity.

The chemical interactions between the tooth and saliva (or rather the oral fluids) are considered in Chapter 12. The caries lesion is the result of loss of mineral from the dental tissues and this occurs over months and years. The metabolism in the biofilm results in fluctuating pH values at the interface between the apatite crystals and their immediate fluid surroundings. Thus, the equilibrium between the tooth mineral and the plaque fluid is constantly interfered with. This chapter explains the basic chemical reactions behind caries dissolution and the way the fluoride ion plays a role in lesion progression.

Erosion is a surface loss of tooth tissue in the absence of biofilm. The key to understanding whether we end up with a mineral loss beneath an apparently intact enamel surface (a caries lesion) or end up with a so-called erosion (surface etching) lies in understanding the concept of saturation of the oral fluids with respect to the minerals comprising the bulk of mineralized dental tissues. Chapter 13 explains the basic chemical differences between erosion and caries. Of particular importance, the chapter explains why fluoride should not be expected to be helpful in controlling this type of chemical dissolution of teeth. The chapter briefly describes causes of erosion, clinical appearances and management options.

Part IV. Non-operative therapy

Part IV of the book is about caries control using non-operative means or treatments. Chapter 14 questions what is meant by the word 'treatment'. Many interpret this word to be synonomous with filling teeth, but the biological thrust of the text thus far has been the concept of *caries control*, and thus the phrase non-operative treatment emerges.

For decades it has been claimed that a clean tooth never decays. Despite this, the relative role of oral hygiene in caries control is hotly debated and questioned by many as playing a key role. Chapter 15 therefore presents the evidence of the importance of mechanical plaque control at the level of the individual surface, the patient and the population.

Since the caries process takes place in the microbial biofilm, caries control by chemical or antimicrobial means may at first seem an attractive prospect. Chapter 16 reviews various antimicrobial approaches, but concludes that the ideal chemical agent for dental biofilm control is not yet available and, apart from fluoride, there is little evidence for a prophylactic effect in humans. This is due to the fact that the causative microorganisms are organized in complex biofilms. The organisms within biofilms communicate with each other and this communication may regulate pathogenic traits. Further understanding of these communication systems may lead to developments in antimicrobial therapy.

Chapter 17 follows a discussion of this antimicrobial approach by questioning whether caries control might involve immunization and gene therapy. In a nutshell, the answer is 'no, not at the moment'. Although work on vaccines goes back 50 years and much has been learnt, there are some significant problems in the approach. The multitude of microorganisms involved and the fact that they are commensals are particularly important. It seems doubtful whether vaccines will ever go to human clinical trials. Similarly, there has been much work on an immune response-based approach, but although much has been learnt about cariogenic bacteria, translation to a practical therapy in humans seems unlikely.

The presence of fluoride in the oral environment, together with the mother's educational background, explains about 50% of the caries reduction in contemporary child populations. Every dentist must have a profound knowledge about how fluoride acts in the control of caries lesion development and progression. Chapter 18 introduces the reader to how fluoride came into dentistry and how it may be used most appropriately today based on our current understanding of cariostatic mechanisms. Fluoride from any source ingested during tooth formation results in varying degrees of hypomineralization in enamel, the severity of which is a direct result of the fluoride dose. Therefore, the chapter also includes sections on this dose–response relationship, as well as how dental fluorosis manifests itself clinically and histologically. The chapter gradually reveals how the spectrum of various topical fluoride measures work together so as to obtain the most effective caries control.

Chapter 19 distills a vast literature on diet and caries and also includes a section on diet and erosion. Much of the evidence on diet and caries is now old history, and some of the experimental protocols would not stand up to contemporary scrutiny. Despite this, the volume of effort argues strongly for the importance of the relationship. That said, some aspects of the evidence are conflicting or maybe a little confusing; for instance, can starch be dismissed as blameless in the story? One of the most important questions addressed in this chapter is the relative role of dietary control in the postfluoride era. Another relevant question is what matters more, the total amount of sugar consumed or the frequency of intake. Fortunately, frequency and amount are linked, so if we advise in this way, we may be covering both options. It is salutary to realize that human experiments on diet and caries are virtually impossible to design ethically. Thus, we must take every opportunity to evaluate current eating patterns and their likely role in dental health.

Part V. Operative intervention

Part V consists of chapters on operative treatment. Chapter 20 is entitled 'The role of operative treatment in caries control' and to some this very title will be an anathema because they contend that operative dentistry has no role in caries control; all it can do is replace, rather inadequately perhaps, damaged tooth tissue. Perhaps this attitude comes as an overreaction to an unfortunate attitude that appeared prevalent in operative dentistry in the middle of the twentieth century. The Editors were at dental school during this period, and cariology and the management of caries seemed to have no place in the departments of adult dentistry when we were students. Caries was presented as a disease of children, managed preventively in this age group, but in adults caries was 'treated' by filling holes in teeth. This attitude, once inculcated, dies hard and there will still be departments of operative dentistry where the science of disease processes is not the bedrock of the teaching.

Chapter 21 is about caries removal. It was challenging to write because the evidence for the current operative paradigm of removing infected tissue before tooth restoration seems scant. Indeed, what evidence there is seems to indicate that current practice may even be detrimental to the pulp–dentin complex by interfering too soon and too vigorously in active lesions before the natural defense reactions of sclerotic and reparative dentin have had a chance to work.

The argument presented is that it may not be necessary to remove 'infected' demineralized tissue to arrest the caries process. This argument makes total sense if it is accepted that the process takes place in the biomass and the infected caries lesion is merely a reflection of this process. Perhaps the bacteria in the demineralized tissue are merely opportunistic squatters rather than major players in the game once the overlying biomass, designated as plaque, has been removed.

However, this suggestion, although possibly logical biologically, is contentious. At present there is too little research on which to base decisions. In other words, an evidence base for practice is missing. The practitioner must therefore rely on 'current practice' as the only evidence available. There is an urgent need to design randomized clinical trials where varying amounts of infected tissue are removed and the results followed longitudinally.

Chapter 22 deals with tooth restoration and puts the emphasis on achieving cavity seal to protect the pulp–dentin complex. Materials science has made enormous strides since G.V. Black spent time working on amalgam. This remarkable dentist addressed the problems of operative dentistry with total logic. First, he studied the disease, clinically and microscopically. Then he applied this knowledge to preventing the problem by plaque removal and designing cavities to try to place their margins in areas where plaque did not stagnate. He then made restorations to the highest technical standards possible, given the limitations of the equipment and materials of the day. The approach is exemplary and it is the approach taken in this chapter 100 years later.

The available materials are described and the emphasis is placed firmly on adhesive materials that support tooth tissue, give a good cavity seal when handled correctly and are tooth colored.

The fastidious clinicians take up the story, showing, mainly pictorially, ways in which restorations may be placed. Notice the concentration on technical perfection. After all, if the aim of restoration is to make the tooth cleanable, perfect junctions between tooth and filling are important. The dental student should be inspired by the technical prowess demonstrated here. You too can achieve this provided you demand that your teachers are constructively critical and prepared to pick up a handpiece, an instrument, and show how your efforts can be improved. So only those who can achieve the highest quality should be allowed to teach restorative care.

Chapter 23 is about the atraumatic restorative technique (ART). This was originally developed in response to the need to find a method of preserving decayed teeth in people of all ages, in developing countries. The restorative material is generally a chemically polymerized, adhesive, glass-ionomer cement. Evidence is presented to show the success of the technique in occlusal restorations, but a somewhat lower success rate in the load bearing approximal situation. The technique is used alongside non-operative treatment. The chapter demystifies the subject. ART is not a second rate restorative technique for low-income countries, but a biologically based and rational approach to caries removal and restoration that is applicable anywhere.

The part ends with Chapter 24, considering the longevity of restorations. It is stressed that restorations have a limited lifetime and many fail owing to clinically diagnosed recurrent caries. Longitudinal randomized clinical trials and cross-sectional studies noting dentists' pragmatic decisions to replace restorations can both be used to assess longevity. Once a tooth has been restored, the filling is likely to be replaced several times in the patient's life and this repeated restoration can compromise the survival of the tooth. A tooth surface should not be restored unless it is unlikely that the lesion can be arrested. The durability of restorations should be maximized by optimal choice and use of restorative materials, prevention of recurrent disease and judicious refurbishment to postpone replacement for as long as possible. The perspicacious student will notice the authors of Chapters 23 and 24 disagree on their interpretation of the literature on the longevity of glass ionomer relative to analgam restorations.

Part VI. Caries control and prediction

The part of the book that concerns caries control and prediction starts with Chapter 25, that summarizes the thought processes and ethics behind the concept of caries control. It emphasizes the need to base caries management decisions on biological knowledge rather than technical solutions. The Editors winced at the quote of the long-standing joke around science centers that 'the dental students are the only professional students on campus that can't locate the library'. We are uncomfortable because we know they can't locate the library at our schools because the dedicated dental libraries have been closed! The chapter emphasizes again the limited role of technical dentistry in the control of the biological process that is caries. It also argues that diagnosis should be linked to relevant treatment strategies and these should be based on the best evidence available; hence the need for a library.

Chapter 26 concerns health education and behavior, a subject of enormous importance in caries control because many non-operative treatments rely on patient compliance. The chapter outlines the theory of oral health promotion and education. There are useful practical tips for influencing behavior. However, the Editors are struck by the lack of research available in this field related to dentistry and therefore the lack of evidence base in this area. This seems surprising because studies of behavior, and its possible modification, seem salient to health in general, let alone the narrow field of caries control.

Chapter 27 on caries control for the individual patient is written by three dentists who relished the challenge of writing down what they actually do for patients based on the evidence presented in this book. We hope this chapter will be useful and understandable to ancillary dental workers and junior students as well as dentists. The authors argue it is important to identify patients at risk to caries progression and itemize important biological factors. They also caution that social factors, which may be impossible for the dentist to modify, can have an overriding influence. The non-operative treatments of plaque control, use of fluoride and dietary modification are dealt with in a practical way. Caries control in children and adolescents, patients with dry mouths and people who cannot care for themselves, is covered individually.

The reader may emerge from Chapter 27 with a warm, rosy glow at the thought of what might be achieved in the surgery setting, but beware the blast of cold reality that follows in Chapter 28. Now a group of community dentists considers caries control for populations and this chapter is uncomfortable reading for the wet-fingered dentist. We are reminded of the recent caries decline, but any self-congratulatory smile is wiped off our faces by the evidence showing chairside dentistry can take little credit for this success. To bring about a reduction in caries levels in populations a focus beyond the purely biological to the societal setting is required. A focus on making healthier choices easier and unhealthy ones more difficult is required (e.g. it should be usual for toothpaste to be fluoridated).

Two fundamentally different approaches to prevention are discussed: a high-risk strategy that targets efforts at those considered to be high risk, versus a whole-population strategy that targets everyone. The arguments for the whole population approach are persuasive. Finally, and perhaps most interesting and persuasive of all, is the common risk factor approach to prevention. Hygiene, diet and tobacco cessation are relevant to many diseases, so that in future dentists may find themselves promoting health in general, rather than dental health in particular.

Over the years the Editors have noticed some apathy from students studying dental public health. It can be seen as a waste of time, a distraction from the clinic. We can only conclude that in some schools the subject may be badly taught. We hope that students will be inspired by this chapter and its links to Chapters 8, 26, 29, 30 and 32.

Chapter 29 concerns caries prediction. Is it possible, on an individual patient basis, to predict who will and who will not develop progressing caries lesions? The answer to the question is intensely practical. If it is possible to predict, caries control strategies should be targeted at those at risk (the high-risk strategy). If it is not possible to predict, and the problem is still a common one, a whole-population strategy should be adopted. The chapter presents the evidence showing that clinical examination, together with a proper dental history, are the most important sources of information on which to base the decision. However, prediction prior to lesion formation is not reliable. Thus caries control should be based on a whole population or a directed population strategy. Clinical dentists, in focussing on the control of lesions currently present with self-care strategies, will also help to prevent the onset of future caries. This chapter links with the previous two showing how an individual patient and a population approach can combine to facilitate health.

This section on caries control and prediction ends with Chapter 30, considering economic issues. Economics is defined as a set of principles that allow decisions to be based on the efficient allocation of resources. One of the difficulties in writing this chapter is thrown into sharp relief in the opening sentences. The authors claim that the USA spends on health nearly half of what the whole world spends on health care. Read that sentence again please and consider for a moment. How can one possibly compare the economic issues pertaining to such a high-income country with those in a low-income economy? A few themes emerge, however. The cost of restorative treatment seems almost obscene when considered against the average wage of some populations. Indeed, any dentist-delivered program, in economic terms, may be unacceptable. In contrast, community water fluoridation schemes are cheap, but to run them a central water supply is required. Fluoridated toothpaste may be no more expensive than its non-fluoride counterpart, so efforts to encourage improved oral hygiene using fluoridated dentifrices would seem the obvious way to go. However, it is not just as simple as providing 'free' paste and brushes. This also has a cost. Caries lesions are concentrated in socially deprived people. These economic considerations should make uncomfortable reading for the socially aware dental student.

Part VII. Dentistry in the twenty-first century

The final two chapters are very challenging and a must for any student because they lift the essentials from the minute details of the preceding chapters into a global view on:

- clinical decision making and
- the consequences of our knowledge for the future of dentistry if we are to serve the interest of the population.

Chapter 31 squares up to the variation in clinical decision making related to caries. It meticulously unpicks the problem to explain the reasons behind variation in both lesion detection and management options. It then lays out the consequences of the variation, and by this time the reader could be forgiven for being somewhat depressed. Fortunately, the cavalry comes over the hill in the last part of the chapter. There are real possibilities to reduce the variation by using systematically reviewed, scientific evidence. But how often are these reviews available?

Chapter 32 reflects on the role of chairside dentistry in the management of caries and periodontal diseases. It examines epidemiological data from high-income, middle income and low-income populations. It shows, uncomfortably, that the traditional chairside, dentist-to-patient approach to oral health-care delivery is both very expensive and inefficient. More scaling, more fillings, do not result in more functioning teeth. For a low-income society to follow the example of the high-income nations and devote resources to training dentists would be as unproductive as it is impractical. Furthermore, for high-income nations to train more dentists would be an expensive mistake. The key to oral health is desperately simple: a whole-population approach to improve oral hygiene with a fluoride dentifrice and encouraging abstinence from tobacco use. This chapter will raise the blood pressure of many but, when they have calmed down, they should reflect that the authors used the evidence available to reach these conclusions. The chapter ends with recommending how the dental team might be composed in the future if we are to serve the majority of this world's populations as cost-effectively as can be done based on the available evidence.

O. Fejerskov & E.A.M. Kidd
December 2007

Contributors

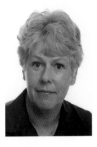

Birgit Angmar-Månsson
Department of Cariology and Endodontology
Institute of Odontology
Karolinska Institutet, Huddinge
Huddinge, Sweden

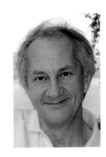

Dowen Birkhed
Sahlgrenska Academy
Department of Cariology
University of Göteborg
Goteborg, Sweden

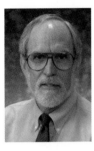

James D. Bader
Operative Dentistry
University of North Carolina, School of
Dentistry
Chapel Hill, North Carolina, USA

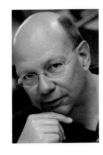

Dirk Bittermann
Giessenburg, The Netherlands

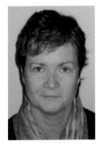

Vibeke Baelum
Department of Community Oral Health and
Paediatric Dentistry
School of Dentistry
Faculty of Health Sciences
University of Aarhus
Aarhus, Denmark

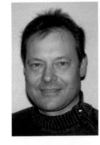

Lars Bjørndal
School of Dentistry
Faculty of Health Sciences
University of Copenhagen
Copenhagen, Denmark

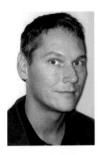

Allan Bardow
Department of Oral Medicine
Institute of Odontology
Faculty of Health Sciences
University of Copenhagen
Copenhagen, Denmark

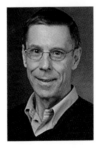

Brian A. Burt
School of Public Health
Epidemiology
University of Michigan
Ann Arbor, Michigan, USA

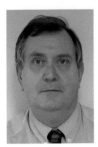

David Beighton
Oral Microbiology
Dental School, King's College London
Guy's Tower, London Bridge
London, UK

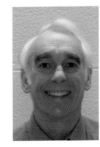

Brian H. Clarkson
University of Michigan School of Dentistry,
1011, N. University,
Ann Arbor, Michigan, USA

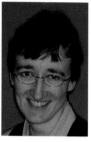

Rebecca Craven
School of Dentistry
The University of Manchester
Manchester, UK

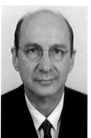

Jaime A. Cury
Faculty of Dentistry of Piracicaba
Piracicaba, Brazil

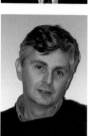

Roger P. Ellwood
Dental Health Unit
University of Manchester
Manchester, UK

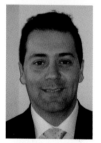

Shahrokh Esfandiari
Oral Health and Society Research Unit
Department of Epidemiology and Biostatistics
Faculty of Dentistry
McGill University
Montreal, Quebec, Canada

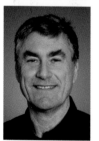

Ivar Espelid
Faculty of Dentistry
University of Oslo
Oslo, Norway

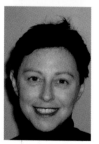

Jocelyne Feine
Oral Health and Society Research Unit
Department of Epidemiology and Biostatistics
Faculty of Dentistry and Faculty of Medicine
McGill University
Montreal, Quebec, Canada

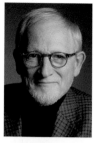

Ole Fejerskov
Department of Anatomy
Faculty of Health Sciences
University of Aarhus
Aarhus, Denmark

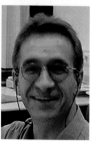

Jo E. Frencken
WHO Collaborating Centre for Oral Health
Care Planning and Future Scenarios
College of Dental Sciences
Radboud University Medical Centre
Nijmegen, The Netherlands

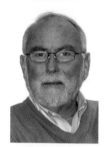

Hans-Göran Gröndahl
Department of Oral and Maxillofacial
Radiology
Institute of Odontology
Sahlgrenska Academy
University of Göteborg
Göteborg, Sweden

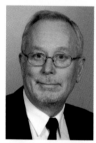

Hannu Hausen
Institute of Dentistry
University of Oulu
Oulu, Finland

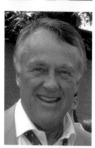

Anders Hugoson
School of Health Sciences
Department of Natural Science and
Biomedicine
Jönköping, Sweden

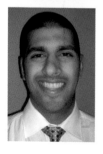

Nekky Jamal
Faculty of Dentistry
University of Saskatchewan
Saskatoon, Saskatchewan, Canada

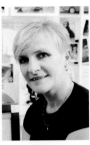

Elizabeth Kay
Peninsula Dental School
Plymouth, UK

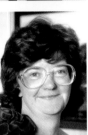

Edwina Kidd
Dental School
King's College London
London, UK

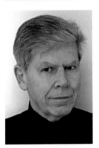

Folke Lagerlöf
Department of Cariology and Endodontology
Institute of Odontology
Karolinska Institutet
Huddinge, Sweden

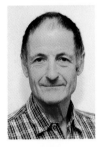

Mogens Joost Larsen
Department of Dental Pathology
Operative Dentistry and Endodontics
School of Dentistry
Faculty of Health Sciences
University of Aarhus
Aarhus, Denmark

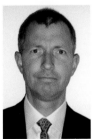

Peter Lingström
Department of Health Sciences
Kristianstad University
Kristianstad, Sweden
and
Department of Cariology
Institute of Odontology
Sahlgrenska Academy at Göteborg University
Göteborg, Sweden

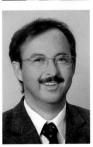

Adrian Lussi
Department of Preventive, Restorative and
Pediatric Dentistry
School of Dental Medicine
University of Bern
Bern, Switzerland

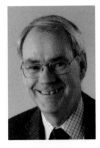

Philip D. Marsh
Centre for Emergency Preparedness
and Response
Health Protection Agency
Salisbury, UK
and Leeds Dental Institute, Leeds, UK

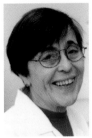

Ingegerd Mejàre
Faculty of Odontology
Malmö University
Malmö, Sweden

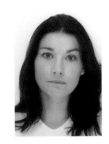

Paula Moynihan
Child Dental Health
School of Dental Sciences
University of Newcastle upon Tyne
Newcastle upon Tyne, UK

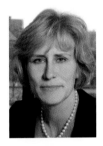

Birgitte Nauntofte
Department of Oral Medicine
Institute of Odontology
Faculty of Health Sciences
University of Copenhagen
Copenhagen, Denmark

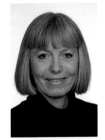

Bente Nyvad
Department of Dental Pathology Operative
Dentistry and Endodontics
School of Dentistry
Faculty of Health Sciences
University of Aarhus
Aarhus, Denmark

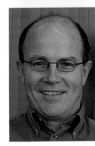

Niek J.M. Opdam
University of Nijmegen Medical Centre
Department of Cariology and Endodontology
Nijmegen, The Netherlands

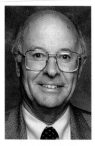

E.I.F. Pearce
Dental Research Group
Department of Pathology and Molecular
Medicine
Wellington School of Medicine
Wellington South, New Zealand

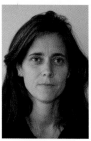

Fernanda Cristina Petersen
Department of Oral Biology
Faculty of Dentistry
University of Oslo
Oslo, Norway

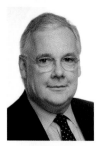

Nigel Pitts
Dental Health Services Research Unit and
Centre for Clinical Innovations
University of Dundee
Dundee, UK

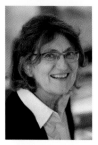

Vibeke Qvist
Department of Cariology and Endodontics
School of Dentistry
Copenhagen, Denmark

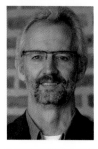

F. Joost M. Roeters
University of Nijmegen Medical Centre
Department of Cariology and Endodontology
Nijmegen, The Netherlands

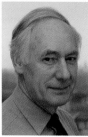

Roy Russell
Oral Biology
School of Dental Sciences
Newcastle University
Newcastle upon Tyne, UK

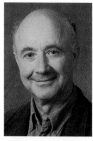

Anne Aamdal Scheie
Department of Oral Biology
Faculty of Dentistry
University of Oslo
Oslo, Norway

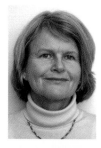

Aubrey Sheiham
Department of Epidemiology and Public
Health
University College London
London, UK

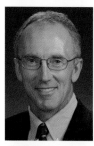

Daniel A. Shugars
Operative Dentistry
University of North Carolina, School of
Dentistry
Chapel Hill, North Carolina, USA

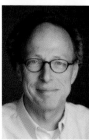

Bob ten Cate
Department of Cariology, Endodontology and
Pedodontology
ACTA–Vrije Universiteit
Amsterdam, The Netherlands

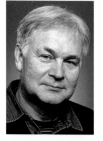

Jorma Tenovuo
Department of Cariology
Institute of Dentistry
University of Turku
Turku, Finland

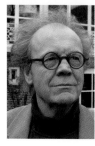

J. Peter van Amerongen
Department of Cariology, Endodontology,
Pedodontology
ACTA
Amsterdam, The Netherlands

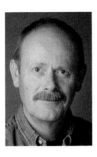

W. Evert van Amerongen
Department of Cariology, Endodontology and
Pedodontology
ACTA
Amsterdam, The Netherlands

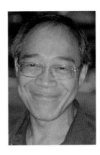

Robert Yee
Dentaid
Salisbury, UK

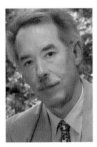

Wim van Palenstein Helderman
WHO Collaborating Centre for Oral Health
Care Planning and Future Scenarios
Radboud University Medical Centre
Nijmegen, The Netherlands

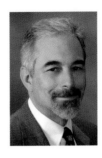

Domenick T. Zero
Department of Preventive and Community
Dentistry
Indiana University School of Dentistry
Oral Health Research Institute
Indianapolis, Indiana, USA

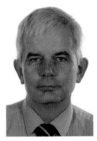

Timothy Watson
Department of Conservative Dentistry
Dental School
King's College London
London, UK

Part I
The disease and its diagnosis

1 Defining the disease: an introduction

2 Clinical appearances of caries lesions

3 Pathology of dental caries

4 Visual–tactile caries diagnosis

5 Radiography for caries diagnosis

6 Additional diagnostic measures

7 The foundations of good diagnostic practice

1

Defining the disease: an introduction

O. Fejerskov, E.A.M. Kidd, B. Nyvad and V. Baelum

Introduction

Terminology

Background literature

References

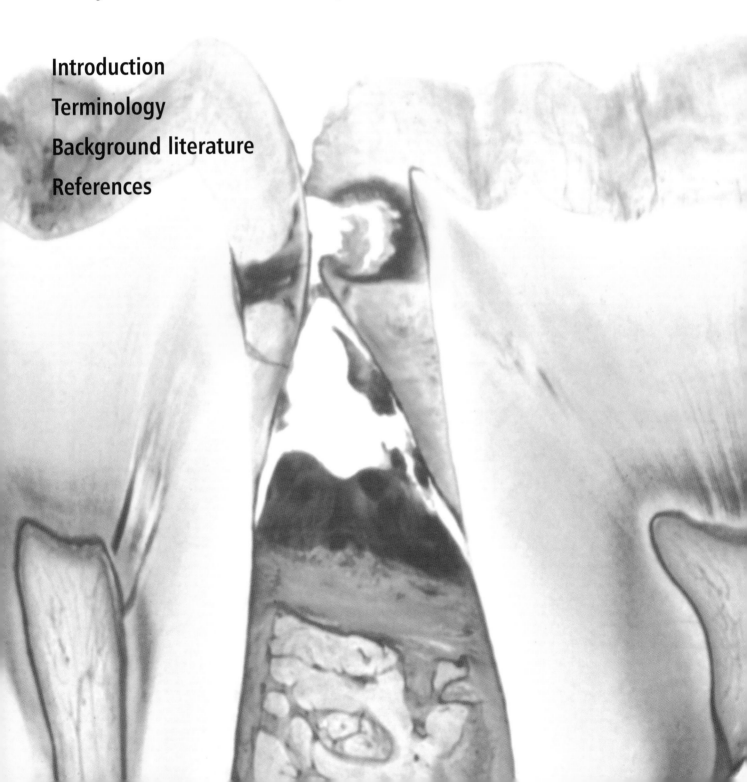

Introduction

The term dental caries is used to describe the results – the signs and symptoms – of a localized chemical dissolution of the tooth surface caused by metabolic events taking place in the biofilm (dental plaque) covering the affected area. The destruction can affect enamel, dentin and cementum. The lesions may manifest themselves clinically in a variety of ways, as will be dealt with in the next chapter.

In principle, dental caries lesions may develop at any tooth site in the oral cavity where a biofilm develops and remains for a period of time. It is therefore a misconception to talk about more or less susceptible surfaces as this may erroneously give rise to the belief that certain parts of a tooth are more 'resistant' or 'less susceptible' to developing caries lesions owing to variations in the chemical and structural composition (Black, 1914; Weatherell *et al.*, 1984).

This is not to say that all tooth surfaces within the oral cavity of an individual develop caries lesions at the same rate. Dental caries lesions develop at relatively protected sites in the dentition where biofilms (dental plaque) are allowed to accumulate and mature over time. Such sites include pits, grooves and fissures in occlusal surfaces, especially during eruption, approximal surfaces cervical to the contact point/area and along the gingival margin. Insertion of foreign bodies to the dentition (e.g. fillings with inappropriate margins, dentures, orthodontic bands) may also result in such 'protected' sites. These areas are relatively protected from mechanical influence from the tongue, the cheeks, abrasive foods and, not least, tooth brushing. Thus, these are the sites where lesion development is more likely to occur because the biofilm is allowed to stagnate there for prolonged periods.

This knowledge is very important and it is nearly 100 years ago that Black (1914) stated:

> … the beginning of caries of the teeth occurs at such points as will favour such lodgement or attachment in which the microorganisms will not be subject to such frequent dislodgement as would prevent a fairly continuous growth. This is the cause of the localisation of the beginnings of caries on particular parts of the surface of the tooth.

Dental caries lesions result from a shift in the ecology and metabolic activity of the biofilm (Chapter 10), whereby an imbalance in the equilibrium between tooth mineral and biofilm fluid has developed. It is important to appreciate that a biofilm (dental plaque) which forms and grows ubiquitously on solid surfaces does not necessarily result in the development of *clinically visible* caries lesions. However, the biofilm is a prerequisite for caries lesions to occur. The biofilm is characterized by continued microbial activity resulting in continued metabolic events in the form of minute pH fluctuations. The metabolism may be dramatically enhanced by changing the nutritional conditions, e.g.

by adding fermentable carbohydrates, and the results of the metabolism can be recorded as pH fluctuations. Any shift in pH will influence the chemical composition of the biofilm fluid and the relative degree of saturation of this fluid with respect to the minerals that are important for maintaining the chemical composition of the tooth surface (see Chapter 12). From the very moment of eruption into the oral cavity, the tooth surface apatite will continue to be subject to such chemical modifications on innumerable occasions. Most of these modifications are so subtle that they can only be recorded at nanolevel. Surfaces that are frequently covered by biofilm (such as a cervical enamel surface) will gradually accumulate fluoride in the very surface layers (outermost 100 μm) (see Figure 18.10). Thus, the enamel surface is in a state of dynamic equilibrium with its surrounding environment. When the cumulative result of the numerous pH fluctuations over months or years is a net loss of calcium and phosphate of an extent that makes the enamel sufficiently porous to be seen in the clinic, we may diagnose it as 'a white spot' lesion (see Chapters 2–4). It is important to appreciate, however, that although the metabolic events may result in detectable caries lesion formation, most sequences of metabolic events tend to cancel each other out, which is why the metabolic events should be considered intrinsic to biofilm physiology. The caries lesions arise when there is a drift in the metabolic events, that is when the pH drops result in a net loss of mineral. *Thereby, the dental caries lesions are a result of an imbalance in physiological equilibrium between tooth mineral and biofilm fluid.*

These considerations lead to some important points.

- The dissolution (demineralization) when pH drops below a certain level in the biofilm and the redeposition (remineralization) of minerals when pH goes up (see Chapter 12) take place in the enamel surface at the interface between the biofilm and the tooth surface. These processes occur numerous times during a day and can be modified extensively. If, for example, the biofilm is partly or totally removed mineral loss may be arrested or even reversed towards mineral gain because saliva is supersaturated with respect to the enamel apatite (see Chapters 10–12). This will result in arrest of disease progression, and may even result in some redeposition of minerals in the very surface of the tooth.
- Any factor that influences the metabolic processes, such as the composition and thickness of the biofilm, the salivary secretion rate and composition (Chapters 10 and 11), the diet (Chapter 19) and the fluoride ion concentration in the oral fluids (Chapters 12 and 18), will contribute to determine the likelihood of a net loss of mineral, and the rate at which this occurs. Figure 1.1 indicates how the many determinants of the caries process may act at the level of the individual tooth

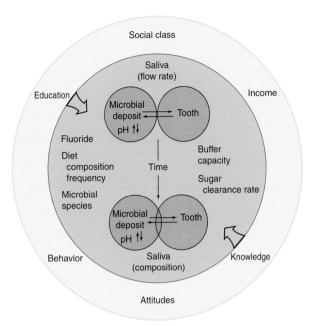

Figure 1.1 Schematic illustration of the determinants of the carious process. Those that act at the tooth-surface level are found in the inner (green) circle. With time an ecological shift in the composition and metabolic activity of the biofilm (microbial deposit) may result in an imbalance in the equilibrium between biofilm fluid and the mineral of the tooth. Thus, a net loss of mineral results in formation of a caries lesion (overlap of the two small circles). In the outer (yellow) ring are listed more distant determinants which influence these processes at individual and population level. (Adapted from Fejerskov & Manji, 1990.)

surface (inner circle) – the strictly biological determinants – or at the individual/population level (outer circle) in the form of behavior, education, knowledge and attitudes – the determinants of the strictly biological determinants.

- At any given point in time the net mineral loss or gain is part of a continuous spectrum of events. The absence of a clinically detectable caries lesion does not necessarily mean that no mineral loss has occurred (Chapter 3), it only means that it could not be discerned clinically. If this concept of a continuum is appreciated it will immediately be understood why diagnosis of various stages of lesion progression is a question of defining certain cut-off points (Chapter 4).

Terminology

Caries lesions may be classified in a number of ways. Unless the student is familiar with this terminology it can be difficult to understand what is written. The following section introduces and defines various terms that will trip off the writers' pens in subsequent chapters.

Caries lesions can be classified according to their *anatomical site*. Remember there is nothing chemically special about these sites. Thus, lesions may commonly be found in *pits and fissures* or on *smooth surfaces*. Smooth-surface lesions may start on enamel (*enamel caries*) or on the exposed root cementum and dentin (*root caries*).

Primary caries is used to differentiate lesions on natural, intact tooth surfaces from those that develop adjacent to a filling, which are commonly referred to as *recurrent* or *secondary caries*. These two latter terms are synonyms, but in this textbook we will use the term recurrent caries throughout. Recurrent caries is simply a lesion developing at a tooth surface adjacent to a filling. As such, its etiology is similar to that of primary caries.

Residual caries, as the term implies, is demineralized tissue that has been left behind before a filling is placed.

An important classification is whether a lesion is *cavitated* or *non-cavitated*, as it impinges directly on the management of the lesion (Chapter 4).

Caries lesions may also be classified according to their activity. This is a very important concept and one that impinges directly on management, although it will be evident from the text that the clinical distinction between *active* and *inactive* (arrested) lesions is sometimes difficult (for details see Chapters 3 and 4).

A lesion considered to be progressing (the lesion would have developed further at a subsequent examination if not interfered with) would be described as an *active caries lesion*. This distinction is based on a judgment of the features of the lesion in question in combination with an assessment of the oral health status of the patient. In contrast to this is a lesion that may have formed years previously and then stopped further progression. Such lesions are referred to as *arrested caries lesions* or *inactive caries lesions*.

The terms *remineralized* or *chronic lesions* may also be used to signify arrested lesion, but the term remineralization should be used with caution (Chapters 3 and 12). The distinction between active and inactive/arrested lesions may not be totally straightforward. Thus, there will be a continuum of transient changes from active to inactive/arrested and vice versa. A lesion (or occasionally part of a lesion) may be rapidly progressing, slowly progressing or not progressing at all. This will be entirely dependent on the ecological balance in the biofilm covering the site and the environmental challenge. Clinically, if in doubt the dentist should always react as though he or she is dealing with an active lesion.

Despite the diagnostic difficulties these distinctions are very important to the clinician because if a lesion is not active, no action is needed to control further progression. If a lesion is considered active, steps should be taken to influence the metabolic activities and possibly the ecological balance in the biofilm in favor of arrest rather than further demineralization.

At this point it is also sensible to discuss a possible confusion in terminology. The first sign of a carious lesion on enamel that can be detected with the naked eye is often called a *white-spot lesion*. This appearance has also been described as an early, *initial* or *incipient lesion*. These terms are meant to say something about the stage of lesion development. However, a white-spot lesion may have been present for many years in an arrested state and to describe such a lesion as early would be inaccurate. A dictionary definition of incipient is 'beginning'; an initial stage. In other words, an initial lesion appears as a white, opaque change (a white spot), but any white-spot lesion is not incipient!

Rampant caries is the name given to multiple active carious lesions occurring in the same patient. This frequently involves surfaces of teeth that do not usually experience dental caries. These patients with rampant caries can be classified according to the assumed causality, e.g. *bottle or nursing caries, early childhood caries, radiation caries* or *drug-induced caries*.

Hidden caries is a term used to describe lesions in dentin that are missed on a visual examination but are large enough and demineralized enough to be detected radiographically. It should be noted that whether a lesion is actually hidden from vision depends on how carefully the area has been cleaned and dried and whether an appropriate clinical examination has been performed.

Background literature

Baelum V, Fejerskov O. Caries diagnosis: 'a mental resting place on the way to intervention'? In: Fejerskov O, Kidd EAM, eds. *Dental caries. The disease and its clinical management*, 1st edn. Oxford: Blackwell Munksgaard, 2003: 101–10.

Fejerskov O. Changing paradigms in concepts on dental caries: consequences for oral health care. *Caries Res* 2004; **38**: 182–91.

References

Black GV. *Operative dentistry*, Vol. 1, *Pathology of the hard tissues of the teeth*. London: Claudius Ash, 1914.

Fejerskov O, Manji F. Risk assessment in dental caries. In: Bader J, ed. *Risk assessment in dentistry*. Chapel Hill, NC: University of North Carolina Dental Ecology, 1990: 215–17.

Weatherell JA, Robinson C, Hallsworth AS. The concept of enamel resistance – a critical review. In: Guggenheim B, ed. *Cariology today*. Basel: Karger, 1984: 223–30.

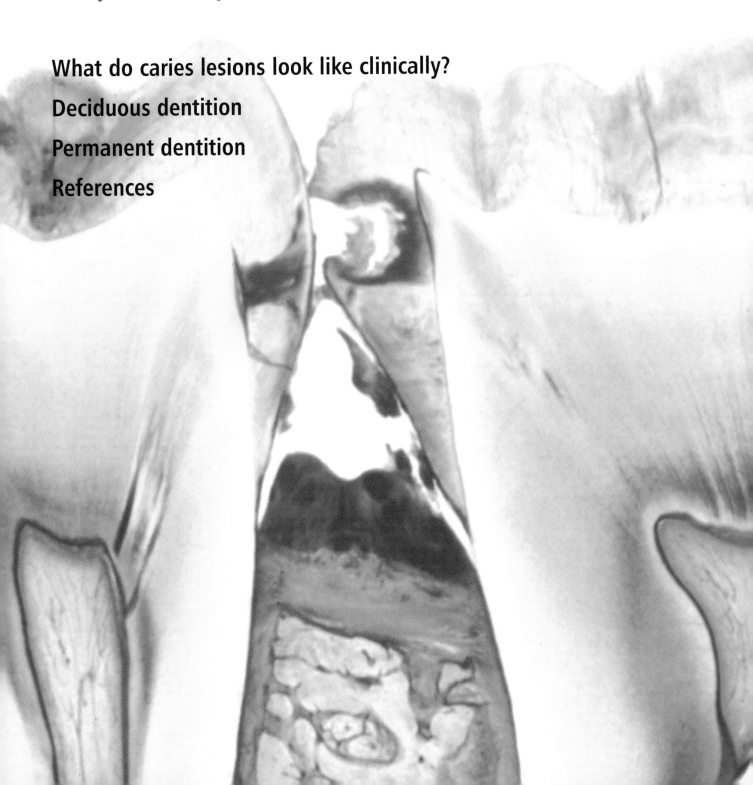

2

Clinical appearances of caries lesions

O. Fejerskov, B. Nyvad and E.A.M. Kidd

What do caries lesions look like clinically?
Deciduous dentition
Permanent dentition
References

What do caries lesions look like clinically?

As was stressed in the previous chapter, dental caries lesions are the outcome, or symptoms, of innumerable metabolic events in biofilms which have covered a tooth surface. When this outcome results in a cumulative loss of mineral from the tooth of such a magnitude that the porosity in the enamel (see Chapter 3) gives rise to a decrease in enamel translucency, we can diagnose white opaque lesions. Early stages in enamel lesion formation will therefore manifest themselves as white-spot lesions. Because these are indicative of increased porosity of the enamel it is to be expected that food stain will sieve into the enamel and hence a white-spot lesion may, over time, change color to brown and even almost black.

The shape of the lesion reflects where the biofilm has been allowed to grow and remain for prolonged periods. In the days – not long ago – where children had no or very poor oral hygiene it was common to see kidney-shaped lesions beneath contact facets approximally extending onto buccal and lingual surfaces as a band of dull, chalky white enamel along the gingival margin. With the much better oral hygiene in today's populations the extent of lesions is much reduced, and the shape will be determined by the particular shape of the stagnation area.

The following will demonstrate a spectrum of manifestations of caries lesions in children, adults and elderly people. Be aware that what you see here is photographed and magnified and reproduced at high quality. In the clinic visual inspection is much more difficult. Therefore, several chapters in this book are devoted to covering various aspects of diagnosis of dental caries lesions (Chapters 4–6), and Chapter 7 focusses on what it means to learn good diagnostic practice.

Deciduous dentition

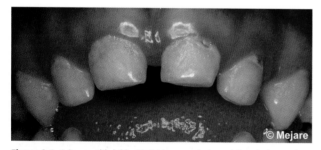

Figure 2.1 A 3-year-old child with thick accumulations of dental plaque along the gingival margin of the buccal surfaces covering active caries lesions, some of which present with distinct cavities

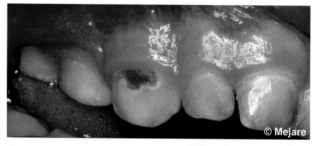

Figure 2.3 Upper deciduous canine from a 5-year-old with an active, cavitated lesion along the gingival margin. On probing it would be soft, but there is no reason to probe such a lesion unless you wish to provoke a pain reaction!

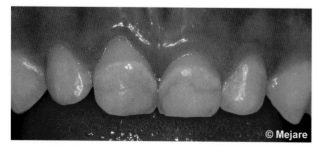

Figure 2.2 Inactive or arrested caries lesions on buccal surfaces of upper central incisor teeth in a 5-year-old child. Note that the shape of the lesions indicates where the gingival margin was located at the time when these lesions developed. The oral hygiene is now improved and the surfaces of these non-cavitated opaque lesions are smooth and shiny.

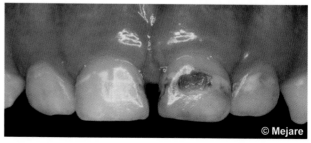

Figure 2.4 Upper incisors in a 5-year-old child. Several narrow, white, opaque inactive caries lesions are located 1–2 mm from the gingival margins. One of the lesions exhibits a large cavity which on probing is hard. This is an example of an inactive, cavitated lesion.

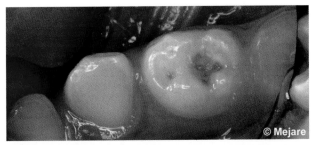

Figure 2.5 Deciduous first lower molar in a 2½-year-old child with two cavitated active caries lesions.

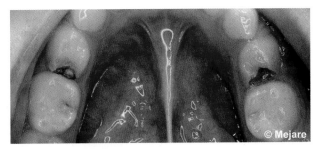

Figure 2.6 Lower first deciduous molars with active, cavitated lesions in the distal and disto-occlusal surfaces of a 6-year-old child.

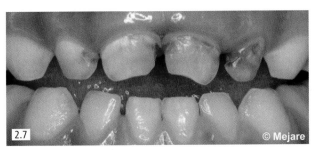

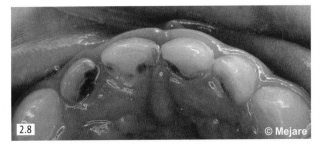

Figures 2.7, 2.8 A case of a 2-year-old child with extensive, active, partly cavitated caries lesions encircling the teeth. This is an example of bottle nursing caries, or bottle caries. (All figures on deciduous teeth courtesy of I. Mejàre.)

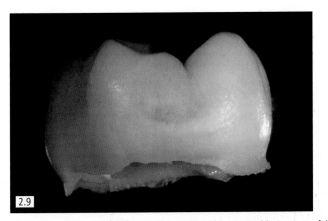

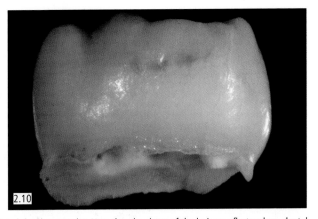

Figures 2.9, 2.10 Slightly discolored non-cavitated approximal lesions on exfoliated deciduous molar. Note that the shape of the lesions reflects where dental plaque has been retained above the position of the gingival margin.

Permanent dentition

Free smooth surfaces

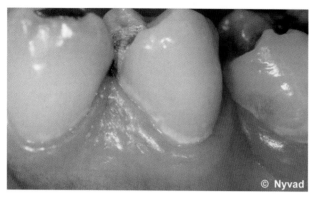

Figure 2.11 Active, non-cavitated carious lesion (lower second premolar). The shape is typical as it follows the curvature of the marginal gingiva and corresponds to where a narrow band of dental plaque has been located in a stagnant area. The surface is dull and chalky. It is called a white-spot lesion, although it extends from the approximal amalgam filling all along the gingival margin. On the mesiobuccal surface of the lower first molar another non-cavitated lesion has taken up brown stain. Note also the very thin lesion on the buccal surface of the first premolar along the gingival margin.

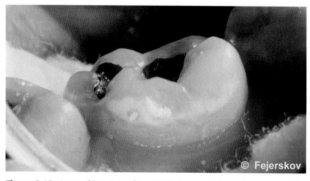

Figure 2.13 Arrested/inactive, white-spot lesion on the lower first molar which is non-cavitated except for a localized circular surface defect. The position of this lesion corresponds to where the marginal gingiva would have been during part of the eruption of this tooth 30 years earlier. When viewing the lesion from different angles it is apparent that the surface is shiny and smooth, although a probe tip moved along the surface will clearly fall into the defect (which is also hard).

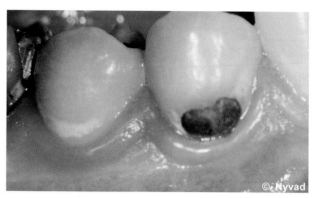

Figure 2.12 Active, non-cavitated carious lesion at lower second premolar with a typical banana shape of the white, opaque lesion with the cervical border following the shape of the slightly inflamed marginal gingiva. A 1 mm rim of normal enamel between the lesion and gingiva indicates that the gingivitis, with swelling of the tissue, has been reduced as a result of attempts to control the oral hygiene. Note also the remains of a white, opaque lesion on the lower first premolar along the mesial and distal margin of the amalgam filling. On the lower first molar a band of partly discolored, non-cavitated lesion extends between the two amalgam fillings. Along the margins of the fillings this could be classified as recurrent caries (secondary caries), but is obviously the remains of primary lesions.

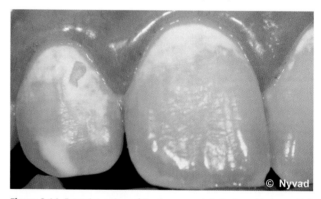

Figure 2.14 Extensive active, white, opaque and chalky buccal lesions which are non-cavitated on the upper central incisors. A large superficial defect is seen on the upper right lateral incisor. Notice the obvious difference between the chalky, dull appearance of the carious lesion and the creamy appearance of the white, opaque hypomineralized lesions of developmental origin (impaired enamel maturation) located at the incisal third of this tooth. If a probe tip is moved gently across the surface an obvious difference in surface texture is felt between the smooth (and shiny) surface of the developmental defect and the chalky texture of the carious lesion. (From Nyvad *et al.*, 1999.)

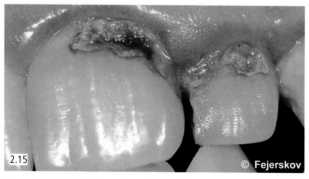
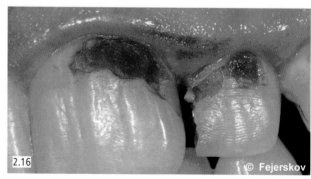

Figures 2.15, 2.16 Active cavitated lesions filled with microbial deposits. The dark brown appearance of the lesion is the result of discoloration of the softened dentin. This is obvious when most of the dental plaque is removed with a toothbrush, as in Fig. 2.16. Even these buccal lesions can be converted into arrested lesions by non-operative intervention with use of a fluoride-containing toothpaste. The dentin becomes hard as a result of mineral deposition (see details in Chapter 3). In this patient, after 2–3 weeks of proper plaque control, the lesions were no longer sensitive to hot, cold and sweet, and 4 months later they were very hard on probing.

Approximal smooth surfaces

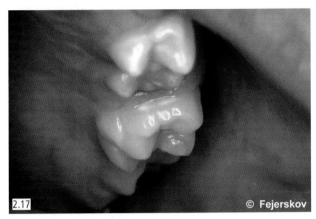
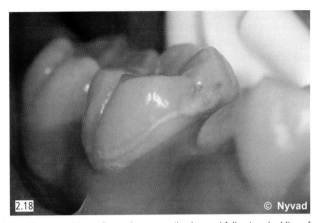

Figures 2.17, 2.18 Active, non-cavitated early white-spot lesions on mesial surfaces of upper and lower first molars are easily observed following shedding of primary teeth. The shape of each lesion indicates the stagnant areas where the biofilm (dental plaque) remained undisturbed. In the most demineralized areas in the center of the lesions, the porous enamel has taken up stain. The lesion in Fig. 2.17 was treated non-operatively and has remained as an inactive, non-cavitated lesion for 25 years. (Figures 2.18 and 2.19 from Nyvad *et al.*, 1999.)

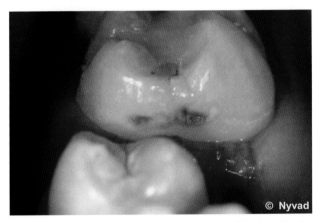

Figure 2.19 Active, discolored lesion on first molar with obvious small cavity. Note that the cavity contains microbial deposits (dental plaque).

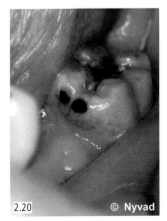
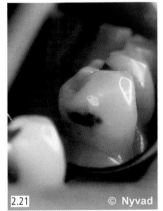
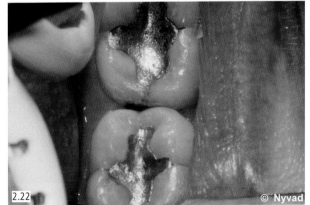

Figures 2.20–2.22 Approximal lesions are difficult to detect by direct visual inspection (Fig. 2.22), but inactive, severely discolored lesions can easily be diagnosed once the neighboring tooth is extracted (Figs 2.20, 2.21).

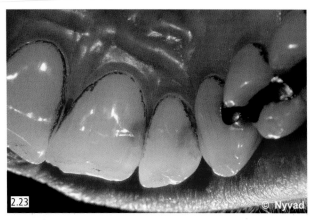

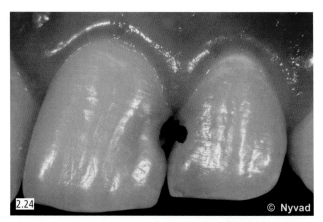

Figures 2.23, 2.24 In incisors approximal lesions are easily discerned either directly or by reflected light. The cervical black rim of discoloration is a result of cigarette smoking and can be removed. (Figure 2.24 from Nyvad *et al*.,1999.)

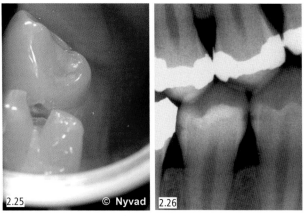

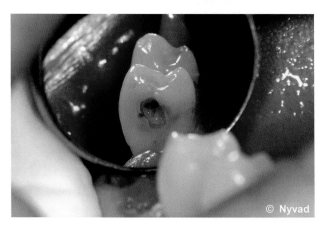

Figures 2.25, 2.26 In the premolar and molar regions it is much more difficult to see approximal lesions by direct inspection, even with careful training and experience. This is where bitewing radiographs can be of diagnostic help (see Chapter 5). In this example the cavity seen could have been the unfortunate result of removal of the carious lesion in the second premolar, whereby the bur due to uncontrolled movement could have destroyed the neighboring enamel surface which was severely porous, but not yet cavitated, before the bur hit it (iatrogenic damage).

Figure 2.27 Even extensive active, cavitated lesions can remain difficult to detect until the adjacent tooth is lost. Such lesions may, however, reveal themselves by a bluish discoloration of the undermined occlusal enamel ridge.

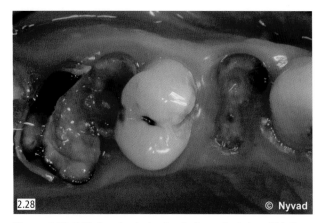

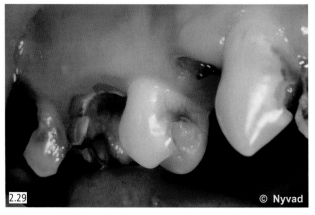

Figures 2.28, 2.29 Dental caries is a locally destructive lesion which, if not controlled or operatively treated, will continue to progress until the entire crown is destroyed. If left uncontrolled the lesion will penetrate further into the root dentin.

Occlusal caries

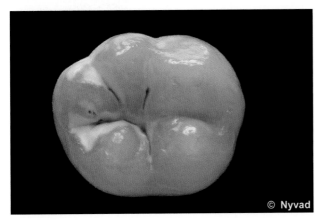

Figure 2.30 Parts of the irregular occlusal surface, particularly in molars, invite plaque stagnation and hence active, non-cavitated lesions appear as chalky white, opaque lesions along the groove, fossa, pits and fissure systems.

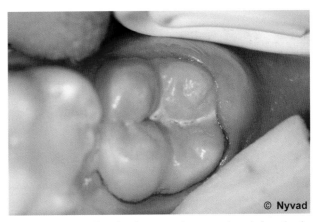

Figure 2.31 In the clinic the plaque must be removed gently from the the occlusal surface with the explorer as otherwise this active, non-cavitated lesion may not be seen. (From Nyvad *et al.*, 1999.)

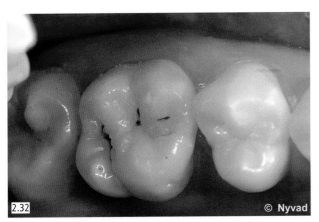

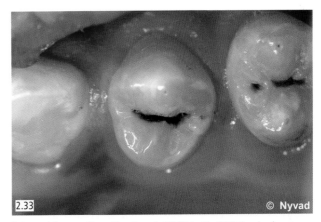

Figures 2.32, 2.33 Arrested, non-cavitated lesions often present as darkly stained pits and fissures. (From Nyvad *et al.*, 1999.) In Fig. 2.33 the cloudy, opaque areas with a shiny enamel surface on cusps and enamel ridge represent dental fluorosis.

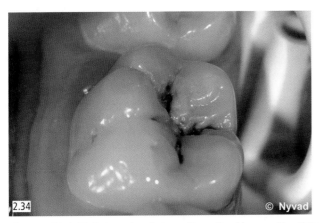

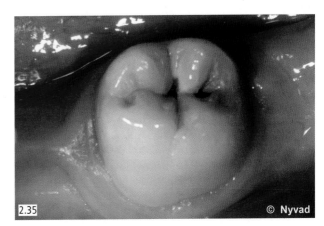

Figures 2.34, 2.35 Active carious lesions with small and large cavities. Note how the enamel appears bluish along the fissures as a result of the undermining nature of the occlusal caries lesions. In Fig. 2.35 the distal part of the occlusal surface will exhibit substantial destruction when opened with a bur.

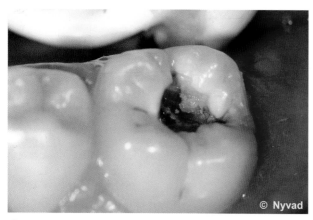

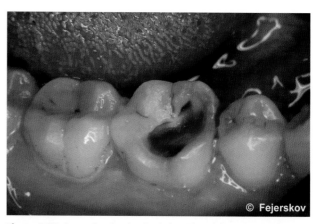

Figure 2.36 Active carious lesion with large cavity extending deep into dentin. (From Nyvad *et al.*, 1999.)

Figure 2.37 Arrested occlusal caries lesion. The partly undermined enamel margins have been fractured and abraded away by mastication and the dental plaque in the dentin cavity has been removed because the surface is in functional occlusion. The dark brown dentin is hard and painless.

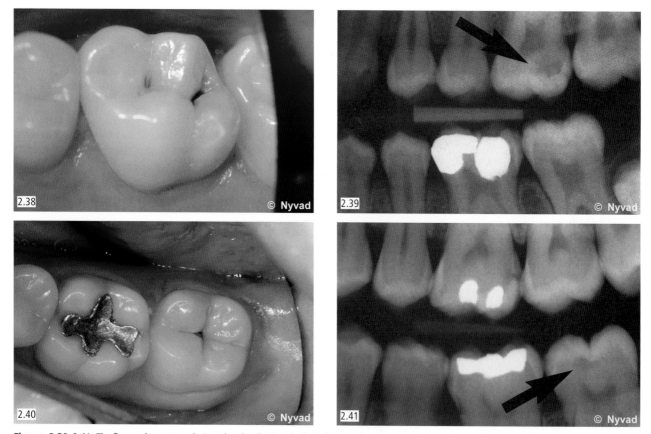

Figures 2.38–2.41 The figures demonstrate lesions that the clinicians had misdiagnosed as an arrested lesion (Fig. 2.38) and sound (Fig. 2.40). The lesions may be easy to miss unless the tooth surface is absolutely clean and dry. The radiographs in both cases demonstrate extensive radiolucent lesions in the occlusal dentin (arrows) indicative of rather deep carious lesions (Figs 2.39 and 2.41). The bluish appearance of the distolingual cusp in Fig. 2.38 should make the clinician aware of a possible undermining larger lesion. Likewise, there is an obvious cavity in the central fossa in Fig. 2.40. These cases represent examples of 'hidden' caries because the dentist clinically had overlooked the signs of lesions and the patient had not complained of any symptoms. The fact that these patients have otherwise very few fillings, and no other signs of active or arrested carious lesions despite being 18–20 years old, probably makes the dentist perform a quicker and more superficial regular dental examination in such patients.

Root-surface caries

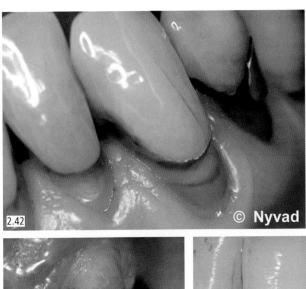

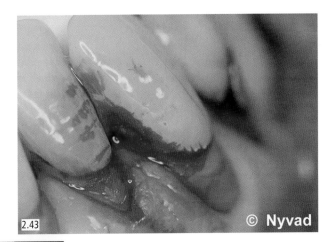

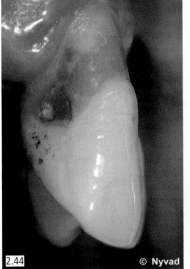

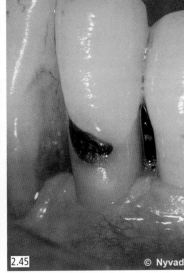

Figures 2.42–2.45 Anywhere on root surfaces where dental plaque accumulates (along the cervical margin at the enamel–cementum junction and along the gingival margin) active root surface lesions may develop with or without distinct cavities. Cavities may be soft (Fig. 2.44) or leathery (Fig. 2.45) and partly filled with microbial deposits. The color of the lesions may vary from yellowish to brownish or black.

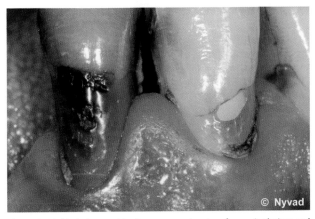

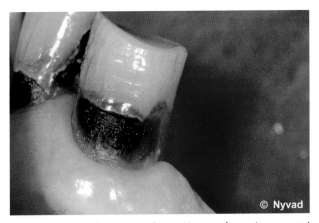

Figure 2.46 Meticulous oral hygiene can arrest root-surface caries lesions and make the root surface appear shiny and polished, although small surface cavities may remain. Arrested root surface lesions feel hard on gentle probing and are very dark or even black discolored.

Figure 2.47 Root-surface lesions in the transition stage from active to arrested often exhibit a dull, leathery appearance. Lesion arrest is often a slow process that continues over years. The changes comprise surface abrasion and polishing as well as mineral uptake (see Chapter 3). For examples of transition stages, see case reports on Figs 2.48–2.57.

Examples of non-operative treatment of root-surface caries

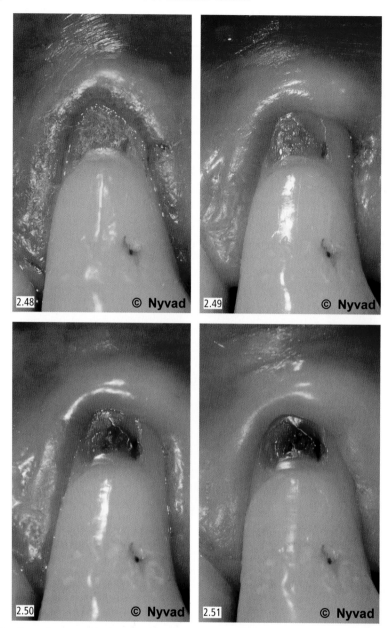

Figures 2.48–2.51 Consecutive stages of non-operative treatment of an active non-cavitated root-surface caries lesion on the buccal surface of the upper left canine. The figures show changes in the clinical appearance of the lesion after 3, 6 and 18 months, respectively. Note that within the observation period improved oral hygiene leads to gradual changes in the color and surface structure of the lesion, from soft and yellowish to hard and darkly discolored. Also note changes in the topography of the marginal gingiva. (From Nyvad and Fejerskov, 1986.)

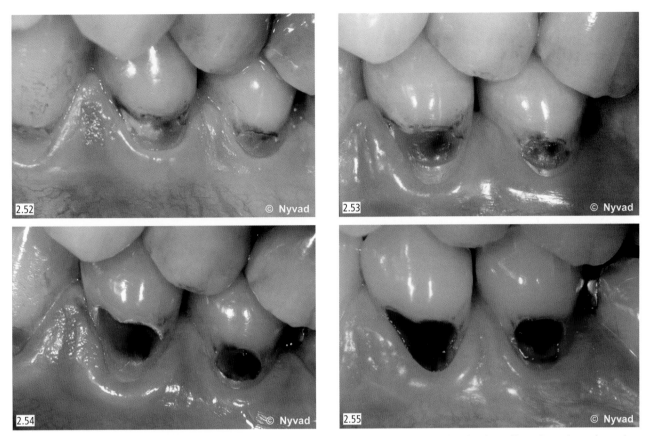

Figures 2.52–2.55 Consecutive changes of non-operative treatment of active cavitated root-caries lesions on the buccal surfaces of lower first and second premolars. The illustrations show the clinical appearance of the lesions after 2, 4 and 10 years, respectively. The successful treatment was achieved through careful daily plaque removal with a fluoride toothpaste. After 4 years an overhanging rim of unsupported enamel at the occlusal aspect of the lesion was removed to facilitate cleaning. Although cosmetically a problem to most patients these lesions do not need operative treatment, which may weaken the teeth substantially and in the long run reduce their survival. (From Nyvad & Fejerskov, 1997.)

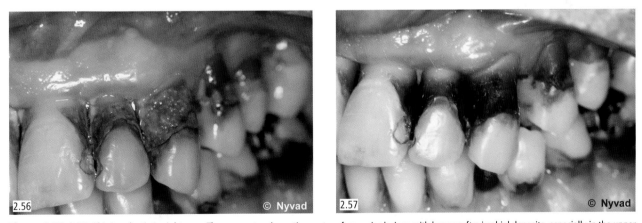

Figures 2.56, 2.57 This is a dentist's nightmare. There are extensive active root-surface caries lesions with heavy soft microbial deposits, especially in the upper left canine. These teeth are very difficult or impossible to restore. Figure 2.57 shows the patient 4 months later. All that was done was plaque control. The lesions are now mostly arrested. The previously soft surface is leathery to hard, and from a biological point of view restorative dentistry has no role to play. However, if the patient required improvement in appearance, restorations could achieve this, but they would still be difficult to place, even using contemporary adhesive materials. The restorations would not contribute to tooth survival, rather the opposite.

References

Nyvad B, Fejerskov O. Active root surface caries converted into inactive caries as a response of oral hygiene. *Scand J Dent Res* 1986; **94**: 281–4.

Nyvad B, Fejerskov O. Assessing the stage of lesion activity on the basis of clinical and microbiological examination. *Community Dent Oral Epidemiol* 1997; **25**: 69–75.

Nyvad B, Machiulskiene V, Baelum V. Reliability of a new caries diagnostic system differentiating between active and inactive caries lesions. *Caries Res* 1999; **33**: 252–60.

3

Pathology of dental caries

O. Fejerskov, B. Nyvad and E.A.M. Kidd

Introduction

Dental caries is the localized destruction of the tooth (see Chapter 1), but is often also described as a chronic disease or process that progresses very slowly in most individuals. What progresses is the gradual demineralization of the involved tissues kept active because of a disturbance in the physiological equilibrium in the biofilm or dental plaque (see Chapter 10) covering the affected site. The disease can affect enamel, dentin and cementum. The disease is seldom self-limiting unless the dental plaque covering the site is removed and, in the absence of treatment, dental caries progresses until the tooth is destroyed (see Figs 2.28, 2.29). The localized destruction of the hard tissues, often referred to as the *lesion*, is the *sign or symptom* of the disease.

The lesions can be arranged on a scale ranging from initial loss of mineral at the ultrastructural or nanoscale level to total tooth destruction (Fig. 3.1a). Even though many scientists consider caries initiation and progression to be a result of multiple interrelated factors, it is a prerequisite for caries destruction to develop, that oral bacteria form a

biofilm (dental plaque) on the tooth surface. However, teeth may be covered by dental biofilm (plaque) without visible signs of caries, and we can therefore conclude that, while microbial deposits are necessary, they are not sufficient to cause caries. As described in Chapter 1, the metabolic events in the biofilm result in multiple fluctuations in pH in the plaque fluid. Thus, the tooth surface minerals will constantly be in a dynamic equilibrium with the oral fluids. Changes in pH and degree of saturation of minerals in the fluid phase will influence this equilibrium over time. This is presented schematically in Fig. 3.1b. As pH fluctuates (the upper line) within minutes, hours, days and months, dissolution and redeposition of minerals occur. The three curves illustrate three different scenarios in terms of net loss or gain of minerals at the tooth surface. When (and if) the net loss of mineral reaches a certain level (indicated by the dotted horizontal line) the increased pore volume (see later in this chapter) results in a clinically visible white, opaque change in the affected enamel: a 'lesion'. Each of the lines represents what may happen at a given tooth surface. If

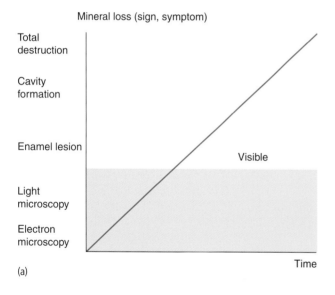

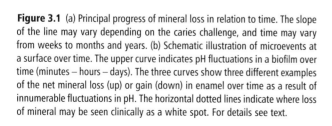

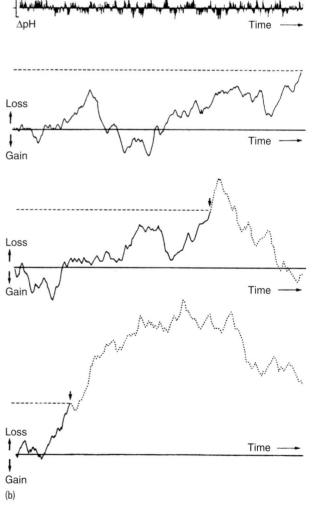

Figure 3.1 (a) Principal progress of mineral loss in relation to time. The slope of the line may vary depending on the caries challenge, and time may vary from weeks to months and years. (b) Schematic illustration of microevents at a surface over time. The upper curve indicates pH fluctuations in a biofilm over time (minutes – hours – days). The three curves show three different examples of the net mineral loss (up) or gain (down) in enamel over time as a result of innumerable fluctuations in pH. The horizontal dotted lines indicate where loss of mineral may be seen clinically as a white spot. For details see text.

averaged they give straight lines of different inclination reflecting, arbitrarily, the rate of lesion progression at the given surface.

To provide relevant information for diagnosis and treatment of the disease, chapters on pathology of dental caries conventionally focus on clinical, histological and ultrastructural changes characterizing different stages of tissue destruction. Since any caries lesion is a result of past or present metabolic activities in microbial plaque, it is preferable to combine information on intraoral plaque accumulation with corresponding tissue reactions. This approach is followed here for two reasons: first, because diagnosis and treatment decisions cannot be made on the basis of clinical signs only, but require appreciation of the local environment (the oral cavity of the patient) in its broader sense; and secondly, because examination of the interplay between dental plaque and the tooth gives important information which is useful for an understanding of intraoral mechanisms for caries initiation, progression and arrest. The ultimate objective of this chapter is to improve the intellectual tools for clinical examination.

Although dentists cannot use electron microscopes or sectioning techniques in their clinical examinations, these techniques will be referred to widely in this chapter. However, what we see and perceive depends to a large extent on what we know. Thus, a freshman looking into the mouth of a patient observes only two arches of teeth, but a trained dentist recognizes teeth of specific types, different kinds of treatment and past diseases. This book cannot provide experience, but seeks to supply biological information on which observations may be based.

This chapter will deal with:

- how the enamel structure in principle interacts with the oral environment, and possible prerequisites for caries initiation, progression and arrest.
- On the basis of the fundamental structural characteristics of the white spot lesion, it will then deal with:
  - caries lesion development in approximal and occlusal surfaces
  - the gradual lesion progression involving the pulpodentinal organ.
- The final section will consider root caries.

Enamel reactions during eruption

When a tooth erupts into the oral cavity the enamel is, in principle, fully mineralized. At eruption the enamel has attained its final concentrations of 95% mineral and 5% water and organic matrix by weight. The corresponding figures on volume basis are 86% mineral, 2% organic material and 12% water.

Normal and sound enamel consists of hydroxyapatite crystals so tightly packed that the enamel has a glass-like appearance; the enamel is translucent. The yellow–white color of teeth is therefore the result of dentin shining through the translucent enamel cover. The enamel crystals are not haphazardly packed, but are arranged in rod and interrod enamel. The packing of crystals is slightly looser along the rod periphery than in the rod and interrod enamel. Even though crystal packing is very tight at the microscopic level, each crystal is separated from its neighbors by tiny intercrystalline spaces (Fig. 3.4) (Boyde, 1976). These spaces are not empty, but filled with water and organic material. The intercrystalline spaces together form a fine network of diffusion pathways which are often referred to as micropores, or simply pores, in the enamel. Their size can be estimated in a number of ways.

There is no doubt that the very outermost enamel is rather porous, as demonstrated by the openings of the striae of Retzius at the surface (Figs 3.2, 3.3); the perikymata grooves act as larger diffusion pathways. Similarly, the numerous pits of Tomes' processes are partly encircled by the openings of the arcade-shaped spaces that, throughout the enamel, partly separate the rod (or prism) from the interrod enamel (Johnson, 1967; Fejerskov et al., 1984). Moreover, a varying number of developmental defects, designated focal holes, small irregular fissures and microholes less than 1 μm in diameter, is observed in the enamel.

Although these potential diffusion pathways may be seen in the scanning electron microscope (SEM) following deproteinisation and dehydration, it is important to appreciate that under in vivo conditions all spaces within the enamel, irrespective of their size, will contain protein of developmental origin, lipid and water. The presence of this organic component will naturally modify the diffusion processes into and out of enamel, as well as modify the reaction of the mineral phase to the environmental factors in the oral cavity. It is therefore reasonable to consider dental enamel, including the external microsurface, as a microporous solid composed of tightly packed crystals. In the enamel and at the surface, however, there are variations in crystal packing related to different anatomical structures.

Once the enamel has erupted into the oral cavity, its surface constantly undergoes modification and, therefore, it must be regarded as being in dynamic transformation at all times.

Because of the surface porosity, it has been suggested that the enamel undergoes a period of posteruptive maturation subsequent to eruption. Nobody has fully explained the nature of such a maturation, but it is thought that during this period mineral ions and fluoride in the oral environment diffuse into the surface enamel. Evidence for such a process is suggested by the fact that the fluoride concentration in surface enamel increases after eruption. However, from a chemical point of view it is difficult to appreciate how such a process is mediated as there does not seem to be a true driving force existing under natural (neutral) pH conditions. So let us consider what may happen during eruption that may explain this phenomenon.

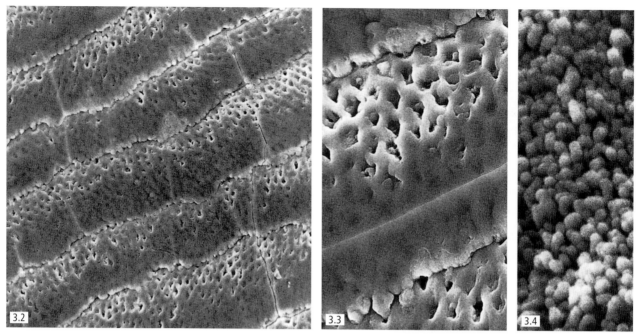

Figures 3.2–3.4 Scanning electron micrographs showing an unerupted enamel surface at different levels of examination. Figure 3.2 shows an overview of perikymata and Tomes' processes pits which is detailed in Figure 3.3. Figure 3.4 shows the ends of rounded crystals separated by distinct intercrystalline spaces. The surface is examined after removal of organic films. (Courtesy of IRL Press.)

Teeth, unlike mushrooms, do not erupt overnight! When a tooth gradually emerges, the partially erupted tooth does not participate in mastication. For this reason, such teeth offer more favorable conditions for bacterial accumulation (Fig. 3.5) than fully erupted teeth (Thylstrup & Fredebo, 1982; Holmen & Thylstrup, 1984; Carvalho *et al.*, 1989, 1991, 1992). Microbial accumulation may, furthermore, be even further enhanced because children frequently avoid tooth brushing of erupting teeth as eruption is accompanied by gingival bleeding, and the area may be sore to touch. Erupting teeth are consequently exposed to microbial plaque several months before functional occlusion is obtained. During this period, innumerable minute processes of mineral dissolution and redeposition occur at the enamel–plaque interface, and it is therefore not surprising

that the enamel surface at the subclinical level exhibits a variety of microsurface destructions, as seen in Figs 3.6 and 3.7. These changes are not clinically visible, but correspond to those observed after 1 week of exposure to cariogenic challenge of dental plaque in a clinical controlled experiment (Thylstrup *et al.*, 1994).

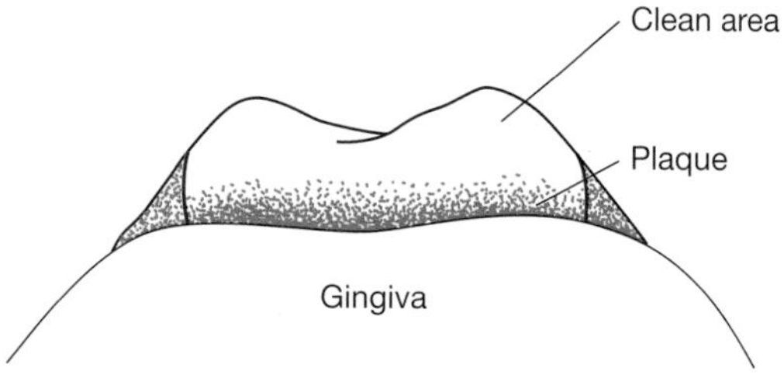

The changes represent active enamel lesions at the subclinical level. As the tooth approaches complete occlusion, shear forces from functional chewing will modify microbial accumulation, and hence cusps are often devoid of dental plaque.

Enamel surfaces free of microbial deposits, once fully erupted, are always covered by the proteinaceous pellicle. Beneath this coating, signs of minor attrition may be observed in the form of scratches. Furthermore, larger irregular defects may represent scars as a result of previous surface dissolution.

These macroscopically invisible changes can be understood as inactive enamel lesions at the subclinical level. On this basis it can be concluded that subclinical active lesions can be turned into inactive lesions when microbial accumulations are removed at regular intervals. This means that further progression of the lesion has ceased owing to control of the unfavorable environmental conditions.

Since these changes from active to inactive lesions have taken place at the subclinical level, and hence are not recognized clinically, it is easy to understand that the factors that have promoted the transition (e.g. tooth brushing)

Clean area

Plaque

Gingiva

Figure 3.5 Drawing illustrating partly erupted premolar with microbial accumulations predominantly located along the gingival margin.

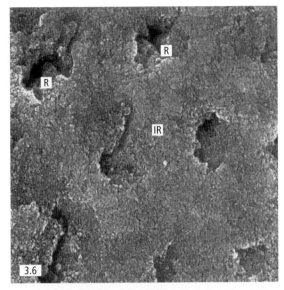

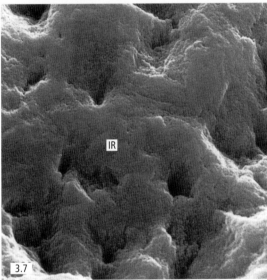

Figure 3.6 Enamel surface beneath the microbial plaque showing distinct signs of dissolution of rod (R) and interrod (IR) areas. These features are characteristic of active lesions at the subclinical level.

Figure 3.7 Enamel surface from the 'clean' cuspal region showing marked wear particularly corresponding to the interrod areas (IR). These features are characteristic of inactive lesions at the subclinical level. (Courtesy of INSERM.)

have most commonly been regarded as prevention of caries. It might, however, be more appropriate to see the transition from active to inactive lesion, even at the subclinical level, as a result of treatment aiming at arrest of further lesion progression.

As the occlusal surfaces of posterior teeth approach full eruption, bacterial deposits are still relatively protected against removal forces in the deeper parts of the occlusal groove–fossa system corresponding to sites where visible

signs of caries may occur (Holmen & Thylstrup, 1984; Carvalho *et al.*, 1989). Hence, it is reasonable to conclude that visible signs of caries develop where bacterial deposits remain for the longest period, and a similar situation pertains to the approximal lesion.

Thus, establishment of the approximal contact leads to arrest of active subclinical caries in the facet areas, owing to approximal wear and removal of bacterial deposits (Thylstrup & Fredebo, 1982; Thylstrup *et al.*, 1983). Beneath the proximal facet, bacteria are still protected and, in conjunction with a gingival reaction, may be the focus from which later clinically detectable lesions may develop (compare the shape of the lesion in Figs 2.17–2.19). It is therefore important to appreciate that the development of posterior approximal caries implies the existence of simultaneous gingivitis, since the interdental papilla normally fits snugly under the contact area of adjoining teeth. After this long explanation, it should be understandable that probably the most important period for any tooth is between its eruption through the mucous membrane until it is in functional mastication.

At this stage three aspects are important to bear in mind:

- First, it will be understood that what we commonly refer to in the clinic as sound or normal enamel is really enamel which, once the tooth is fully erupted into functional occlusion, has been subjected to substantial chemical and minor mechanical modifications.
- Secondly, what is referred to as secondary maturation is more likely to reflect the outcome of these chemical events, which have occurred at a subclinical level and have been described, perhaps incorrectly, as the period of passive mineral uptake.
- Finally, to understand how fluoride may modify the caries lesion development and the rate of lesion progression, it should, therefore, be remembered that the entire enamel surface must be regarded as being in a dynamic equilibrium with its surrounding oral fluid at all times.

Enamel changes during early caries lesion development

There is no such thing as caries-susceptible sites (see Chapter 1), although this is a commonly used phrase. Carious lesions occur within the dentition in a very characteristic pattern both in the primary and permanent dentition, but this does not reflect differences in chemical composition of the enamel between parts of the dentition where caries lesions rarely or never develop, and sites where lesions frequently appear (Weatherell *et al.*, 1984). Dental caries develops where microbial deposits are allowed to form biofilms that are not frequently removed or disturbed by mechanical wear (mastication, attrition, abrasion from brushing, flossing or toothpicks).

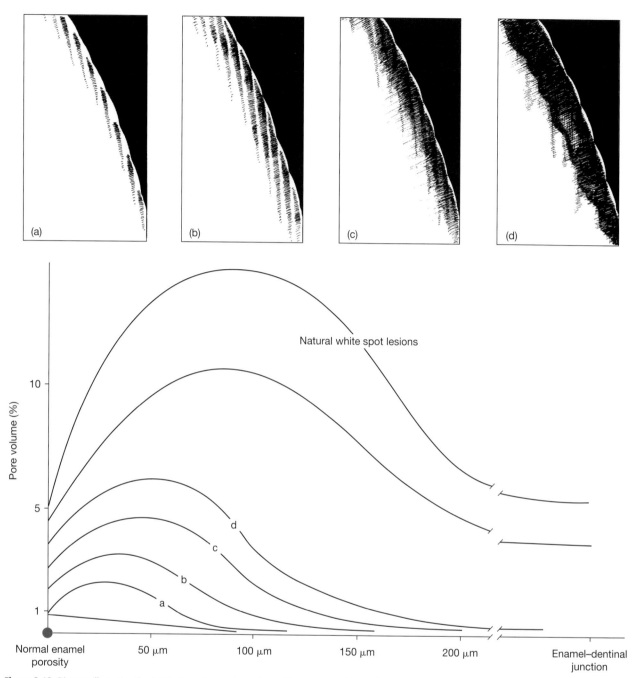

Figure 3.12 Diagram illustrating the distributions of enamel porosity at different stages of caries dissolution from the surface towards the enamel–dentinal junction. Parts (a)–(d) illustrate the gradual increase in pore volume after (a) 1 week to (d) 4 weeks of experimental caries *in vivo*.

How do such early lesions change when dental plaque is removed?

After 4 weeks an active enamel lesion, the white-spot lesion, has a characteristic chalky surface (Figs 3.13 and 3.15). This is partly because an increase in the internal enamel porosity, due to demineralization, causes a loss of translucency and this makes the enamel appear opaque. It is also partly caused by the direct surface erosion. The enamel loses its shiny appearance because the irregular surface generated by the erosion of the very outermost surface gives rise to a diffuse reflection of light.

Owing to the surface erosion it is also possible to make small scratches with a probe in the surface of active lesions. When such lesions created experimentally were re-exposed to the oral environment none of them continued to progress (Holmen *et al.*, 1987b; Nyvad & Fejerskov, 1987a). After only 1 week they showed signs of clinical regression,

Pathology of dental caries 27

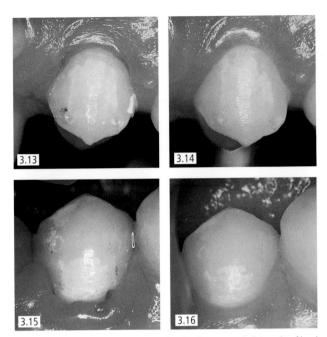

Figure 3.13 Experimental tooth immediately after removal of 4 weeks of local protection by an orthodontic band. Note the typical appearance of an active enamel white-spot lesion.

Figure 3.14 The same tooth 1 week after re-exposure to wear in the oral environment. The inactive or arrested lesion appears less whitish due to wear and polishing of the external partly dissolved surface.

Figure 3.15 Experimental tooth immediately after cessation of 4 weeks of local protection. The active enamel lesion is less opaque than that seen in Figure 3.13, indicating a less advanced stage.

Figure 3.16 The same tooth 2 weeks after re-exposure to wear in the oral environment. The arrested lesion is not readily visible in the clinic. Note the more shiny appearance of the surface. (Courtesy of Karger.)

i.e. the whitish appearance had diminished (Figs 3.14, 3.16). After 2 and 3 weeks where the surfaces were brushed, these surfaces had almost resumed the hardness as well as the shiny appearance of normal enamel. How can the clinical observation of arrest of lesion progression, and even regression, be interpreted?

Examination of the surfaces in relation to time after re-exposure to the oral environment showed a rapid and gradual increase in wear of the eroded surface. This indicates that mechanical brushing and removal of the cariogenic and acid-producing plaque is the dominating factor for lesion arrest *in vivo*. The clinical impression of the surface of the arrested lesion as shiny and hard is therefore the result of abrasion or polishing of the dull, partly dissolved surface of the active lesion (Figs 3.17–3.20). The mechanical removal of the outermost, partly dissolved, crystals (polishing) results in exposure of more tightly packed crystals, explaining the clinical impression of resumed surface hardness. The polarized light examinations revealed that the porosity of the deeper parts of lesions was reduced after removal of the acid-producing plaque. The complete end of acid production at the surface results in a gradual return to

neutral pH in the inner part of the lesion. For this reason there is an outward diffusion of protons. The reduced enamel porosity in the inner lesion part is therefore probably the result of a gradual return of enamel fluids to a stage of supersaturation with respect to apatites, causing a shift in equilibrium and reprecipitation of minerals in the sites of demineralization (see also Chapter 12). Detailed histological examination, particularly at the surface, suggests, however, that the repair of the inner lesion part is not fully completed even 3 weeks after cessation of cariogenic challenge (Holmen *et al.*, 1987a).

Occasionally, orthodontic treatment with fixed appliances gives rise to side-effects in terms of gingivally located caries lesions because the patients are not instructed in proper oral hygiene (Fig. 3.21). After removal of the appliance and professional plaque removal, further lesion progression ceases, and after 3 months (Fig. 3.22) the lesion show features of a typical arrested lesion, with a hard and shiny surface but still with a maintained interior opacity (Årtun & Thylstrup, 1986, 1989). Low-magnification SEM images of replica models clearly show that the transition from an active to an inactive stage is associated with wear, as the mark made in the sound enamel has almost been worn away during a period of 3 months (Figs 3.23, 3.24). The active lesion was a result of a prolonged period with partly undisturbed plaque accumulation, and the marked distinct border between sound enamel and the surface of the active lesion is therefore a clear indication of the degree of surface erosion during caries progression.

The approximal white-spot lesion

The shape of the white-spot lesion is determined by the distribution of the microbial deposits between the contact facet and the gingival margin, which results in a kidney-shaped appearance. On the proximal smooth surface there will typically be an interdental facet area surrounded by an opaque area extending in the cervical direction. The cervical border of the lesion is formed according to the shape of the gingival margin (Figs 2.17, 2.18). It is often possible in such surfaces to see thin extensions of the opaque area, in buccal and lingual directions, running in parallel with the gingival margin. Some of these lesions will be active and others inactive owing to different efforts to control the microbial accumulations, for example with dental floss.

Surface features of the clinical white-spot lesion

When examining the surface of an active white-spot lesion (Fig. 3.25) characteristic changes can be observed on interproximal surfaces, in principle corresponding to those described previously. The contact facet has a smooth appearance without the perikymata pattern, but along the periphery of the facet, irregular fissures and other small defects can be observed. In the opaque surface enamel

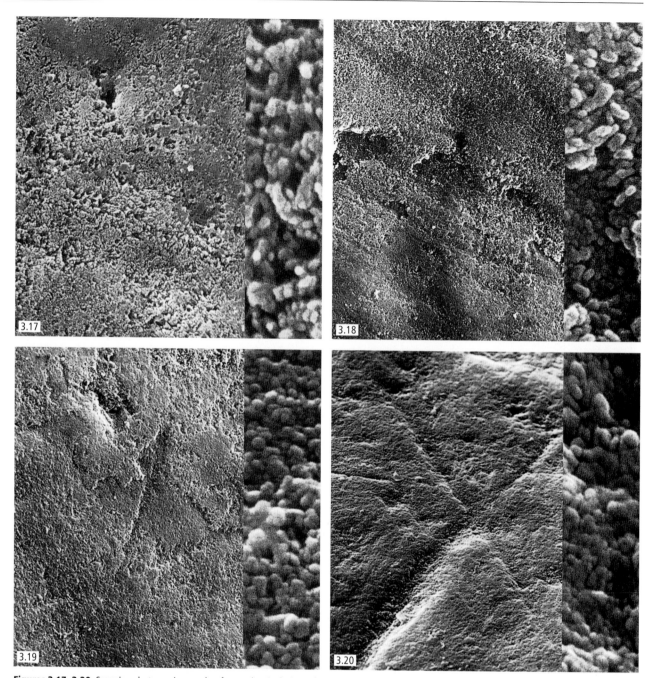

Figures 3.17–3.20 Scanning electron micrographs of enamel caries lesions after removal of local protection. Overview (left) and high-magnification detail (right).
Figure 3.17 Typical features of active enamel lesion with partial and complete dissolution of outermost crystals immediately after removal of 4 weeks of local protection.
Figure 3.18 After 1 week of exposure to the oral environment multiple microscratches can be seen in the outermost partly dissolved crystal layer. Loosely bound crystals have been worn away (right).
Figure 3.19 Microwear after 2 weeks. Parts of the porous external microsurface have been removed by wear. The exposed underlying crystals appear more tightly packed (right).
Figure 3.20 After 3 weeks, the surface appears smoother with classical wear striation patterns due to more complete removal of the eroded microsurface. The complete removal of loosely bound and partly dissolved crystals has exposed tightly packed crystals separated by a distinct network of intercrystalline spaces. (Courtesy of Scandinavian University Press.)

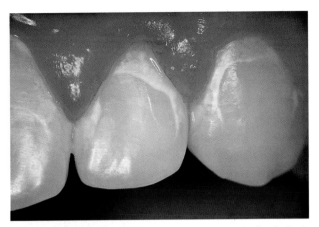

Figure 3.21 Clinical features immediately after removal of orthodontic appliances and cleaning. The orthodontic treatment had lasted for 2 years. Note the marked gingival reaction and the characteristic chalky surface appearance of the active enamel lesion.

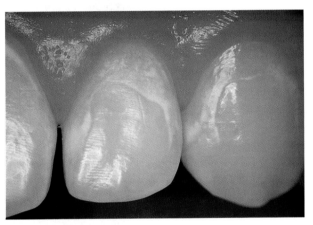

Figure 3.22 After 3 months with careful oral hygiene the gingival tissues have recovered and the active lesion has been completely arrested. The white appearance of the lesion has diminished markedly due to polishing away of the eroded outermost enamel surface.

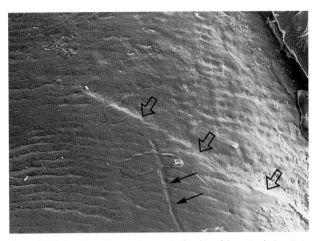

Figure 3.23 Scanning electron micrograph of replica of the active lesion. Note the distinct step between the eroded surface of the active lesion and the adjacent sound enamel (open arrows). A furrow has been made in the sound enamel area (arrows).

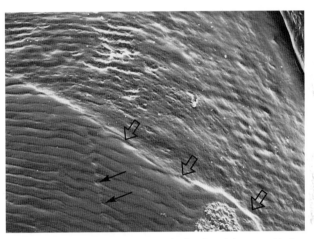

Figure 3.24 Scanning electron micrograph of replica of the arrested lesion. After 3 months, the furrow (arrow) has almost disappeared, and the step between the sound and arrested surface is slightly enhanced (open arrows). (Courtesy of A. Thylstrup and J. Årtun.)

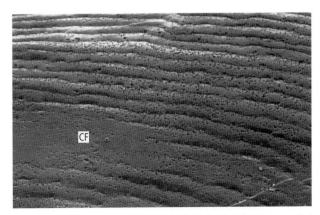

Figure 3.25 Scanning electron micrograph of initial surface dissolution cervical to contact facet (CF) in an active enamel lesion. (Courtesy of IRL Press.)

cervical to the facet, innumerable irregular holes are seen. These are deepened and more irregular pits of Tomes' processes and also an increased number of eroded focal holes. In other areas the deepened pits of Tomes' processes appear to merge together, forming larger areas of irregular cracks or fissures (Figs 3.26–3.28). The final enamel exhibits distinct patterns of dissolution with widened inter-crystalline spaces, and minor fractures of the perikymata edge are frequently found.

In other lesions these fractures may be so extensive that they involve two, three or more perikymata whereby micro-cavities are formed. At the bottom of such microcavities, the classical honeycomb pattern of enamel rods is seen. The overlapping character of the enamel in these defects is evident, with the opening of striae of Retzius corresponding to the bottom of each 'step'.

When examining inactive, arrested lesions, which still clinically appear as white-spot lesions, some of these may also comprise microcavities (Figs 2.13, 3.29). The surface enamel surrounding such cavities exhibits marked abrasion with irregular scratches, but in between rows of pits of Tomes' processes, irregular deeper holes may be seen. The rod and interrod enamel in such areas is, however, also smooth (Fig. 3.30). In contrast, the enamel surface in sheltered areas such as the bottom of the microcavities appears densely granular (Fig. 3.31), indicative of merging ends of the individual crystals.

In conclusion, the early stages in enamel dissolution involve a distinct disintegration of the actual enamel surface, even leading to microcavities. It is also evident that approximal attrition and attrition, caused by mechanical oral hygiene, significantly interfere with the surface features, because the outermost enamel surface, only a few micrometers thick, is soft as a result of demineralization.

Histology of the white-spot lesion

By sectioning the enamel perpendicular to the surface, it is possible to produce 80–100-μm-thick ground sections and examine these by microradiography and polarized light microscopy. When examining air-dried sections (air has a refractive index, RI, of 1.0) in the polarized light microscope the porous lesion (area in the tissue where pore volume exceeds 1%) appears as a wedge-shaped defect with the base at the enamel surface. When examining the same section with the intercrystalline spaces filled with water (RI 1.33), areas where there is more than 5% pore volume in the tissue are observed mainly beneath the enamel surface, but still extending in a triangular shape into the tissue (Figs 3.32, 3.33). In this way, it is possible to distinguish between the apparently relatively intact surface zone which varies in width from 20 to 50 μm and the body of the lesion where the pore volume exceeds 5%. The principal distribution of pore volume in an enamel lesion is illustrated in Fig. 3.34.

Two other histological zones are of interest in enamel carious lesions. These zones are only visible when the ground sections are examined imbibed in a clearing agent such as Canada balsam or quinoline. The latter, in particu-

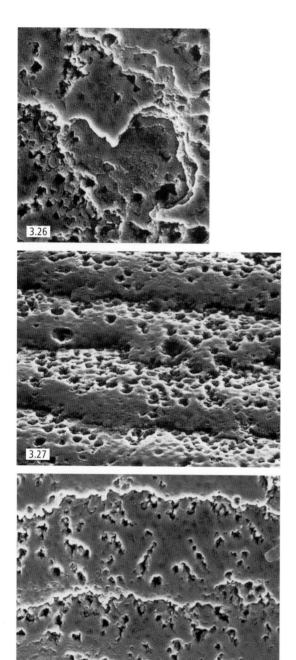

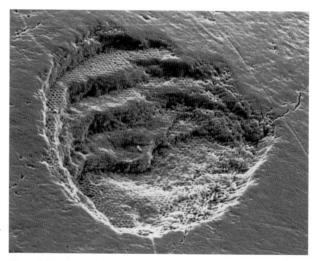

Figure 3.29 Scanning electron micrograph of part of an inactive enamel lesion with a microcavity. At the bottom of the cavity openings of striae of Retzius are seen. The rod pattern is clearly seen in the exposed enamel in contrast to the abraded surface enamel.

Figures 3.26–3.28 Details of surface dissolution patterns seen in Figure 3.25.

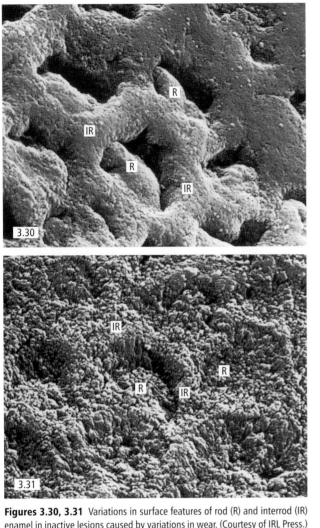

Figures 3.30, 3.31 Variations in surface features of rod (R) and interrod (IR) enamel in inactive lesions caused by variations in wear. (Courtesy of IRL Press.)

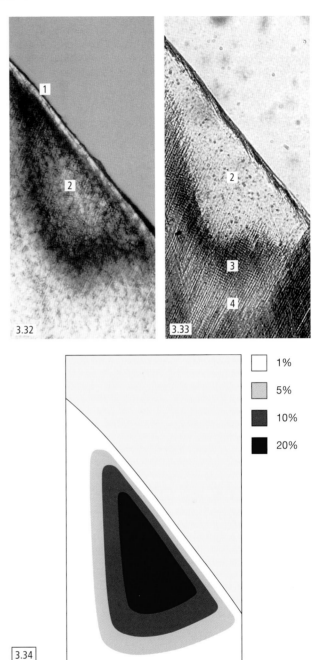

Figures 3.32, 3.33 Ground section cut through the center of a small enamel lesion examined in polarized light after imbibition in water (Figure 3.32) and quinoline (Figure 3.33). 1: Surface zone; 2: body of the lesion; 3: dark zone; 4: translucent zone.

Figure 3.34 The principal pore volume distribution in the section.

lar, is very suitable since its refractive index is identical to that of enamel. When a ground section is examined in transmitted light after imbibition with quinoline, an apparently structureless translucent zone may be seen at the advancing front of the lesion (Fig. 3.33). This zone may vary from 5 to 100 μm in width and is located corresponding to that part of the lesion with a pore volume of slightly more than 1% when examined in dry air. Detailed microdensitometry studies of microradiograms have shown that there is a slight loss of mineral in this zone. The explanation for the translucent appearance of this zone with the enamel structures being less evident appears to be that initial dissolution of the enamel mainly occurs along the gaps between rod and the interrod enamel in the tissue. For this reason the quinoline is assumed to penetrate more easily into these enlarged pores, and as the medium has the same refractive index as that of the enamel crystals (RI = 1.62), the final result will look like a structureless zone.

The dark zone is a more constant feature of the advancing front of carious lesions than is the translucent zone. Thus, the dark zone occurs in 90–95% of lesions, and if the translucent zone is present, the dark zone is located between this and the body of the lesion (Fig. 3.33). Polarized light studies of the dark zone indicate a pore volume between 2 and 4% and, based on extensive *in vitro* studies, this zone possibly represents the results of a multitude of demineralization and reprecipitation processes. The designation 'dark zone' originates from early studies showing that the zone appears dark brown in ground sections when examined in transmitted light after imbibition with quinoline. The dark appearance of the zone indicates that large quinoline molecules have not penetrated all micropores. The fact that quinoline is unable to penetrate the dark zone indicates that this contains very small pores in addition to the relatively large ones that were present in the previous stage, the translucent zone. The occurrence of micropores impermeable to the large quinoline molecule is thought to be a result of precipitation of minerals in the sites of previous demineralization within the lesion, whereby parts of the large pores may be reduced by deposition of material. Supporting this concept is the observation that *in vivo* caries lesions with a long history, i.e. slowly progressing or inactive lesions, frequently exhibit very wide dark zones.

Microradiographically, the increased pore volume as observed in the polarized light microscope is reflected as a loss of mineral deep to the relatively unaffected surface zone (Fig. 3.35). In principle, the loss of mineral is most pronounced corresponding to the body of the lesion, with a gradual decrease in loss towards the advancing front. However, the distribution of minerals within the enamel lesion varies greatly. Frequently, very thick surface zones are found. Similarly, deep within the body of the lesion a laminated appearance of the mineral distribution may be observed, indicative of periods with lesion arrest followed by new periods with active caries. This phenomenon is often particularly evident in the occlusal part of approximal lesions corresponding to where the interproximal attrition facet gradually develops.

Within the enamel the spread of dissolution takes place particularly along the rod boundaries, as seen in the electron microscope (Figs 3.36, 3.37). At higher magnifications larger rhomboid, irregular crystals, 'caries crystals', may be found along these diffusion pathways. These crystals are interpreted as being a result of redeposition of minerals. In actively ongoing lesions, however, the apatite crystals exhibit various degrees of peripheral dissolution. Central dissolution along the *c*-axis of the crystals may also occasionally occur in the central lesion part.

It is just apparent that, assuming a constant but high cariogenic challenge, there will be gradual subsurface dissolution of enamel, being most pronounced deep to the enamel surface and spreading into the enamel following the rod directions. If, however, the cariogenic challenge varies as a result of, for instance, improved oral hygiene or topical fluoride application, such phases of remission and recurrences may result in a much more irregular pattern of mineral distribution within the lesion.

Progression of the enamel lesion

The classical description of enamel lesion histology has been based on the incipient lesion positioned at the cervical margin of the interdental facet on the proximal surfaces. Typically, as described in the previous section, the lesion appears triangular in sections cut through the central lesion part. Carious dissolution follows the direction of the rods. Systematic measurements of enamel porosity along traverses following the rod direction make it possible to understand the morphogenesis of the conically shaped approximal lesion (Bjørndal, 1991). Figure 3.38 shows a typical lesion. A line is drawn which has been designated the central traverse (CT), in the rod direction from the deepest point of lesion penetration to the surface. The highest degree of tissue porosity is always observed along this line, irrespective of lesion depth. Measurements of the surface-layer thickness where the CT crosses the surface disclose a gradual increase in surface-layer thickness in relation to lesion depth. Comparisons of surface-layer thickness within lesions showed that the peripheral part of the surface layer was always thinner than the central part, thus probably reflecting a less advanced stage of lesion progress in the lesion periphery.

Initiation, spread and progress of the approximal lesion are simple reflections of the specific environment created by the microbial communities (the biofilm) on the enamel surface in the approximal space. Conversely, if bacteria are offered similar growth conditions anywhere in the dentition by allowing biofilms to become established, for example beneath an orthodontic band positioned so that a space is created between the band and the enamel surface, then the metabolism in this biofilm produces lesions with the advancing front of the lesion running parallel to the outer enamel surface.

Arrest of the caries lesion

For several years it has been common to use the word 'remineralization' synonymously with arrest of caries lesion progression. This is misleading, however, for several reasons. Most important is the fact that the first step in arrest of further lesion progress is removal of the acid-producing origin of the disease, the cariogenic plaque. Secondly, clinical changes associated with lesion arrest are partly explainable in terms of wear and polishing of the partly dissolved external microsurface of the active lesion. Thus, there is no sign of salivary surface repair of the arrested surface lesion in accordance with surface alterations *in vivo* after artificial etching with acid. Collectively, these studies demonstrate that the clinical impression of repair after acid etching is not due to mineral deposition, but instead is the result of salivary deposits (the pellicle) masking the characteristic etch pattern. In 1960, Mannerberg demonstrated in a series

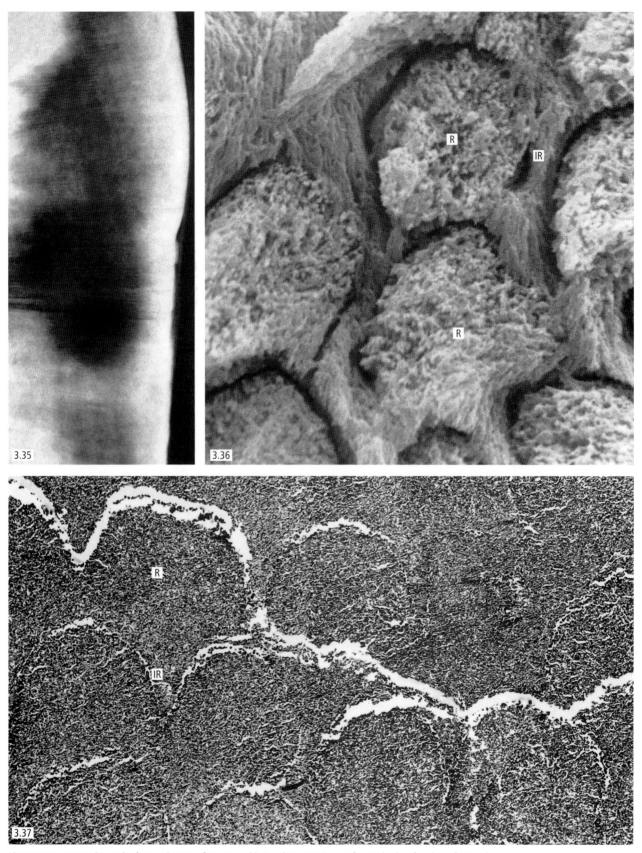

Figure 3.35 Microradiograph of ground section from enamel lesion demonstrating preferential subsurface loss of mineral.
Figures 3.36, 3.37 Scanning and transmission electron micrographs from body of the lesion showing partly dissolved enamel with enlarged gaps between rod (R) and interrod (IR) enamel. (Figure 3.37 courtesy of *Arch Oral Biol*.)

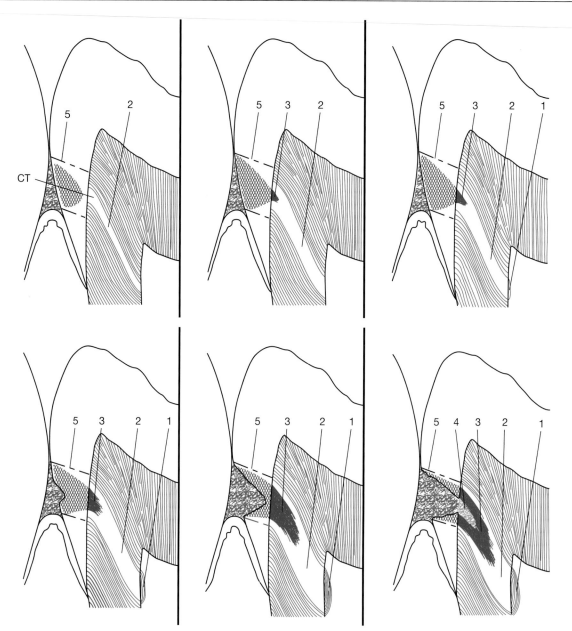

Figure 3.38 Schematic illustration of progressive stages of lesion formation. 1: Reactive dentin; 2: sclerotic reaction or translucent (transparent) zone; 3: zone of demineralization; 4: zone of bacterial invasion and destruction; 5: peripheral rod direction. (Modified from Bjørndal, 1991.)

of studies that changes in surface enamel micromorphology after etching were a result of abrasion, and not precipitation of salivary minerals. *In vivo*, the enamel surfaces are not restored by salivary repair mechanisms after direct loss of surface minerals. This is likely to be a result of the aforementioned salivary inhibitors, which prevent spontaneous and selective precipitation of calcium phosphate or crystal growth of these salts onto the enamel surface.

Concerning redeposition of mineral through the surface layer into the internal (subsurface) lesion *in vivo*, available data suggest that the surface layer in itself forms a diffusion barrier against subsurface uptake of mineral (Larsen &

Fejerskov, 1989). For this reason it is a well-known clinical phenomenon that arrested lesions with an intact surface layer remain as scars in the tissue (Fig. 2.13). This does not preclude that there are subtle alterations at the crystal level between oral fluids supersaturated with respect to dental apatites (see Chapter 12) and enamel crystals. It is worthwhile, however, briefly to consider the clinical elements of the most oft-cited study on lesion arrest, because this study conventionally has been taken as proof of the 'remineralization phenomenon'.

Backer Dirks (1966) studied 184 buccal surfaces of maxillary first molars in the same children at 8 years of age and

Table 3.1 Distribution of buccal surfaces of maxillary first permanent molars in three diagnostic categories at 8 and 15 years of age; the same surfaces are examined

Diagnosis	Age (years)		Total
	8	15	
Sound	93	74	111
		37	
White-spot lesion	72	15	41
		26	
		4	
Caries with cavitation	19	9	32
		19	
			84

From Backer Dirks (1966).

again at 15 years. Table 3.1 indicates the clinical diagnoses. The last column shows the diagnoses at age 15. The arrows point to the changes that have taken place with the individual lesion during the study period. Of the 72 surfaces with white-spot lesions at 8 years of age, 37 (51%) were sound at age 15, while 26 (36%) remained unchanged and nine had progressed to cavitation stage. To understand these results it is important to remember that the gingival level at the buccal surface of the maxillary first molars undergoes a marked change between the ages of 8 and 15 years. During this period there is a gradual recession of the gingival margin along the surface of the tooth and a continuing exposure of the clinical crown. Also during this period the second maxillary molar erupts, leading to a further repositioning of the gingival attachment on the distal part of the first molar. Thus, the physiological passive exposure of the tooth leads to a change in local conditions for plaque accumulation. For this reason, in his original report Backer Dirks considered the lesion arrest and lesion regression to be mainly a result of the altered environmental conditions owing to better use of the fully erupted teeth, which promoted natural removal of bacterial accumulations, and hence lesion arrest. Prolonged wear of particularly superficial enamel lesions eventually leads to a complete wearing away of opaque enamel giving the impression of a repaired lesion (as seen corresponding to the wear facet approximally).

In short, this means that lesion arrest *in vivo* is always the result of mechanical removal of cariogenic plaque. Tooth brushing and professional plaque removal result not only in arrest of further progression, but also in enamel lesions often regressing to an extent where they are not readily recognized in the clinic. The subtle rearrangement of crystals that is likely to occur after exposure to saliva or the redeposition of dissolved minerals in the subsurface lesion parts, which has often been designated 'remineralization', does not, however, play any causal role in the arrest, but is

entirely an accompanying phenomenon to the removal of the acid-producing plaque.

The use of the word remineralization as being synonymous with lesion arrest is particularly unfortunate because it is often stated that remineralization only occurs in cases with an intact surface layer. However, as will be seen later in this chapter, cavitated lesions can still arrest when plaque accumulation is sufficiently controlled (Levine, 1974). Because the surface layer acts as a diffusion barrier against subsurface uptake of mineral, its removal may promote mineral deposition in the exposed porous enamel.

Careful clinical examination, particularly of adults, often reveals several arrested lesions at various stages. Most often, the arrested approximal lesion is seen on teeth where the adjacent tooth has been extracted, whereby the local environmental conditions have been changed completely (Figs 2.18, 2.20, 2.21). Opaque bands can often be discerned on the labial surface of incisor teeth, indicating arrested lesions that developed during eruption of the teeth. Inactive lesions with a long history are often discolored through the uptake of dyes. Classically, such lesions are designated as chronic lesions, arrested lesions or brown-spot lesions. Typically, gentle probing will reveal that they have the same hardness as normal enamel, in contrast to the softer surface of the active lesion. Therefore, they are often described as remineralized lesions as well. However, as previously mentioned, remineralization is not the cause of the arrest of further progress of the lesion, although reprecipitation of mineral from oral fluids may be a consequence of lesion arrest.

Occlusal caries

Numerous epidemiological data and common clinical experience have repeatedly shown that occlusal surfaces of posterior teeth are the most vulnerable sites for dental caries. Conventionally, the high incidence of caries on these surfaces has been directly related to the narrow and inaccessible pits and fissures on occlusal surfaces, and for that reason it has been natural in the past simply to refer to occlusal caries as 'fissure caries'. Recent clinical and structural studies combined with accepted knowledge have made it possible, however, to dismiss the narrow fissures as being per se the focus for caries initiation on posterior surfaces, and for that reason the term occlusal caries is preferred in this chapter (Carvalho *et al.*, 1989, 1991, 1992; Ekstrand *et al.*, 1991).

It is a common clinical experience that caries on occlusal surfaces does not involve the entire fissure system with the same intensity, but merely occurs as a localized phenomenon. This can be understood when looking at a permanent molar occlusal surface in a stereomicroscope, where it presents itself as an elaborate landscape, with high mountains separated by a variety of valleys, some of which are deep rifts and others appear like open river valleys (see Figs 2.30–2.37, 3.39a–g). Each tooth type in the dentition has its own specific occlusal surface anatomy, and caries is usually detected in relation to the same specific anatomical configuration in identical tooth types. In the maxillary molar, for example, the central and the distal fossae are sites that typically accumulate plaque and hence are also sites where caries most often occurs. In general terms, occlusal caries initiation takes place in locations where bacterial accumulations are best protected against functional wear (Carvalho *et al.*, 1989). Thus, two factors have been considered of importance for plaque accumulation and caries initiation on occlusal surfaces: stage of eruption or functional usage of teeth, and tooth-specific anatomy (Carvalho *et al.*, 1989, 1991, 1992). Progressive destruction of the occlusal surface is therefore initiated by a local process either in the deepest

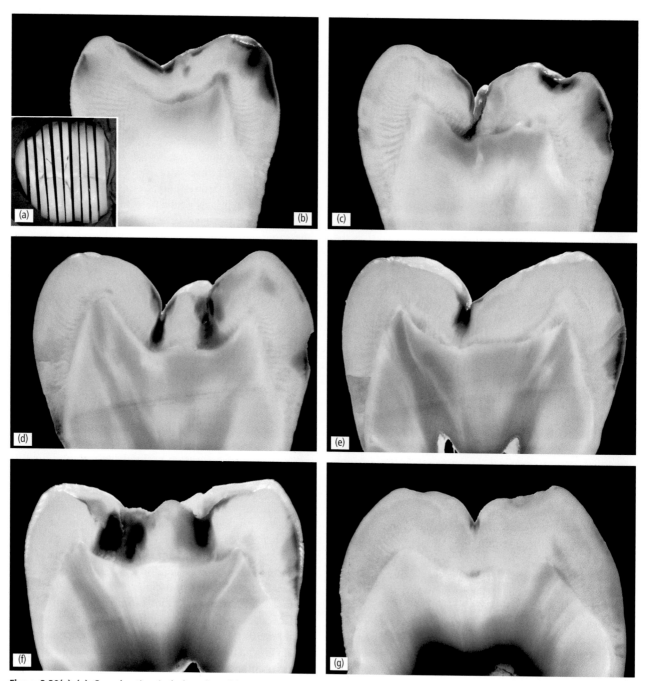

Figure 3.39(a)–(g) Ground sections in the buccolingual direction through a lower first molar, where the occlusal surface exhibits different stages of early caries lesion development. See the intact occlusal surface of the tooth in Figure 2.30.

part of the groove–fossa system owing to accumulation of bacterial deposits or along the entrance to deep fissures (Fig. 3.39a–g), or both. In such areas, which already offer protection against physical wear (Figs 3.40, 3.41) the formation of microcavities (e.g. resulting from vigorous probing) further improves local conditions for the lodgment and growth of oral bacteria. This accelerates demineralization and destruction, which again improves local conditions for bacterial growth (Figs 3.41–3.45).

To understand the rapid progression of occlusal caries under natural conditions, i.e. in people living in communities without provision of dental health care, it is necessary to appreciate the particular anatomical configuration of the occlusal surface where caries is initiated (Figs 3.40, 3.46). First, it is important to understand the process in three dimensions, as caries on occlusal surfaces most often is ini-

tiated in fossae, which are the depressions where two or more interlobal grooves meet. For this reason several surfaces are involved in the initial dissolution. Because enamel demineralization always follows the rods, it is natural that the enamel lesion initiated in a fossa gradually assumes the shape of a cone with its base towards the enamel–dentinal junction (compare Figs 3.41–3.43 and the schematic drawings in Fig. 3.46). The dentin reaction reflects the rod direction in the involved enamel. Sections cut through such a lesion thus give the two-dimensional impression of two separated and independent lesions. In a fossa, however, where several surfaces are involved, the lesion entity is, in reality, shaped as a cone in three dimensions. It is no wonder, then, that textbooks during the years have paid special attention to the 'undermining' character of occlusal caries (Figs 3.43, 3.44). However, in the light of the structural

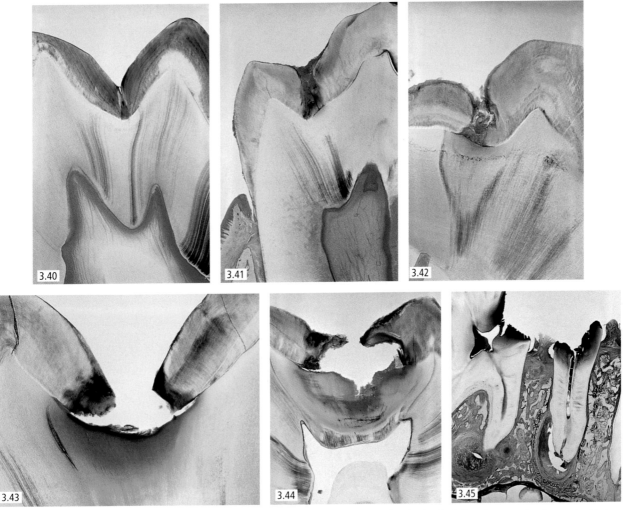

Figures 3.40–3.45 Histological sections through teeth exhibiting different stages of progression of occlusal caries lesions. By comparing these natural lesions with the diagram in Fig. 3.46, it will be appreciated why occlusal caries presents itself as undermining the enamel. If left untreated, a caries lesion stimulates the pulpo-dentinal organ to carry out reparative processes, but the final outcome will be necrosis and periapical inflammatory reactions (Fig. 3.45) if not treated. (Courtesy of Professor T. Yanagizawa from the Hanagawa collection.)

arrangement in rods in the occlusal groove–fossa system, the mode of lesion growth in these areas is not particularly surprising. With progressing enamel destruction, a proper cavity is formed and again the outlines of the cavity reflect the arrangement of rods in the area. The cavity is thus shaped as a truncated cone. The particular anatomical configuration of that part of the occlusal surface where caries begins explains why the openings of occlusal cavities are always smaller than the base. The 'closed' nature of the process obviously favors undisturbed growth of bacteria and hence accelerated destruction of the tissue. Occlusal enamel breakdown is the result of further demineralization from an initially established focus, rather than being a general demineralization involving the entire fissure system.

As previously mentioned, the major part of clinical and scientific concern with regard to occlusal caries has been

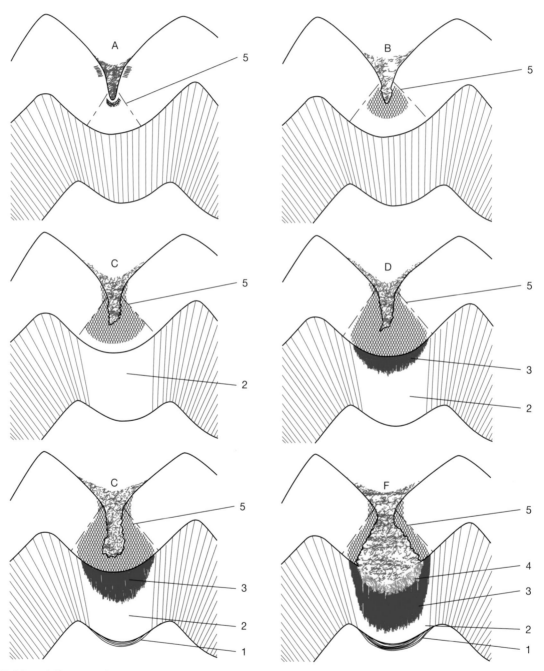

Figure 3.46 Schematic illustration of progressive stages of occlusal lesion formation in an occlusal fossa. 1: Reactive dentin; 2: sclerotic reaction or translucent (transparent) zone; 3: zone of demineralization; 4: zone of bacterial invasion and destruction; 5: peripheral rod direction. (Modified from Ekstrand *et al.*, 1991.)

devoted to the possible events taking place in the deep and inaccessible fissures. However, caries destruction is almost always initiated at the entrance owing to metabolic activities in bacterial accumulations on the surface. It is interesting in this context that the structural organization of dental plaque in a distinct biofilm is observed not in the fissures, but along the entrance of fissures.

Dentin reactions to caries progression

Conventionally, enamel caries and dentin caries are described as two independent entities. This convention is to some extent explainable, as the two tissues differ markedly from each other in terms of both developmental origin and structure. The enamel is derived from the ectodermal component of the tooth germ, while the pulpo-dentinal organ is developed from the mesenchymal component. The enamel is avascular and acellular and cannot respond to injuries, whereas the dentin and the dentinal cells, the odontoblasts, are integral parts of the pulpo-dentinal organ and thus considered to be a vital tissue possessing specific defense reactions to external insults. As will be remembered, the enamel is a microporous solid and hence it is under-

standable that stimuli from the oral cavity pass through the tissue into the pulpo-dentinal organ, even in intact enamel. With increasing porosity as a result of enamel demineralization it is to be expected that the underlying pulpo-dentinal organ reacts (Figs 3.40, 3.47–3.49).

Changes in dentin during caries progression cannot be understood, therefore, without taking the spread of the enamel lesion into account. The most common defense reaction by the pulpo-dentinal organ is tubular sclerosis, which is deposition of mineral along and within the dentinal tubules, resulting in their gradual occlusion (Figs 3.50–3.56) (Massler, 1967; Johnson *et al.*, 1969; Levine, 1974; Mjør, 1983; Stanley *et al.*, 1983).

Age changes in the dentin are commonly described as a gradual mineralization of the peritubular dentin, eventually resulting in complete obturation of the tubules or tubular sclerosis. Attrition of teeth accelerates tubular sclerosis. It is reasonable, therefore, to consider age-related tubular sclerosis as being the result of mild stimuli from the oral environment mediated through the enamel. Caries is another stimulus that accelerates tubular sclerosis, a process which requires the presence of a vital odontoblast (Figs 3.48, 3.49). The tubular sclerosis observed in conjunction with

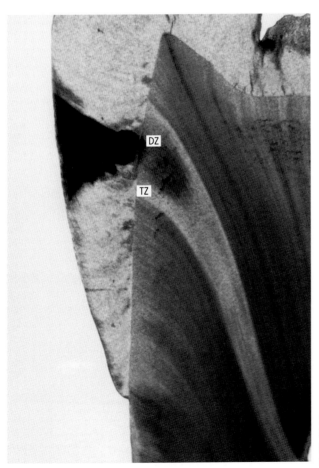

Figure 3.47 Ground section of active approximal lesion examined in transmitted light. The triangular enamel lesion reaches the enamel–dentin junction with demineralization of the outer dentin (DZ) and sclerotic reactions (TZ) corresponding to the less advanced peripheral parts of the enamel lesion.

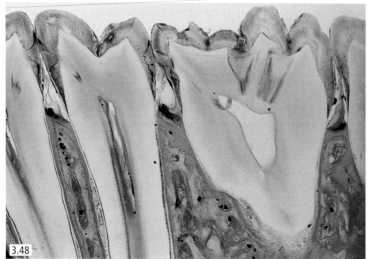

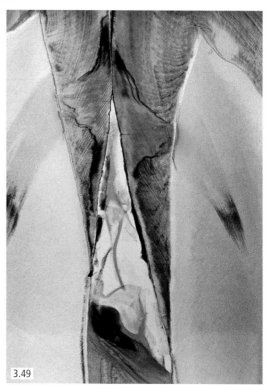

Figures 3.48, 3.49 Histological ground sections in the mesiodistal direction through human mandibular premolars and molars. In the approximal surfaces caries lesions extend at a varying depth towards the dentin. Note how reactions in dentin (the translucent zone) and pulp may appear even at these stages of lesion development, which may not be recorded in a rapid clinical examination, and may also be missed in a bitewing radiograph. Figure 3.49 is a higher magnification of the approximal space between the premolars. Note how the lesions penetrate in depth below the contact area. The approximal space appears partly empty because substantial shrinkage occurs during tissue preparation (the gingiva is edematous and swollen) and some of the microbial deposits are lost. (Courtesy of Professor T. Yanagizawa from the Hanagawa collection.)

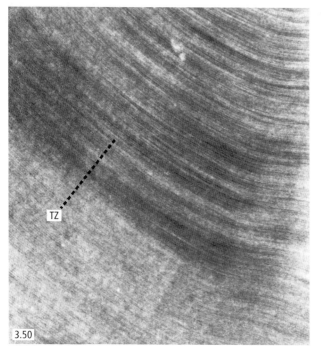

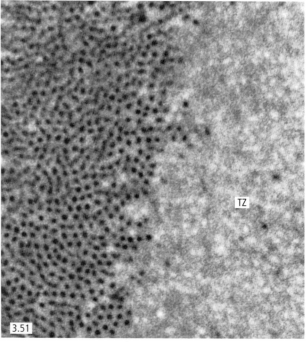

Figures 3.50, 3.51 Microradiographs of the border between the translucent zone (TZ) and normal dentin, with open dentinal tubules seen as dark lines. The dotted line in Fig. 3.50 indicates the plane of view in Fig. 3.51.

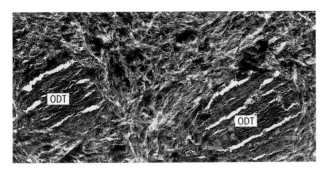

Figure 3.52 Transmission electron micrograph from the translucent zone showing two completely occluded dentinal tubules (ODT). (Courtesy of Karger.)

caries has been described as being a result of either initial mineralization of the peritubular space followed by calcification of the odontoblast process, or an initial intracytoplasmic calcification followed by a secondary periodontoblastic mineralization (Frank & Voegel, 1980). In addition to the presence of intratubular hydroxyapatite crystals, large rhombohedral crystals have often been observed and identified as whitlockite crystals (Frank & Voegel, 1980; Daculci *et al.*, 1987). At the light-microscopic level it is not possible to distinguish between the different form of sclerosis, and in sections the obturated dentinal tubules appear translucent because the mineral in the tubules makes the tissue more homogeneous, reducing the scattering of light passing through the affected tissue. Sclerotic dentin is therefore often referred to as translucent (transparent) dentin or a translucent zone (Fig. 3.47).

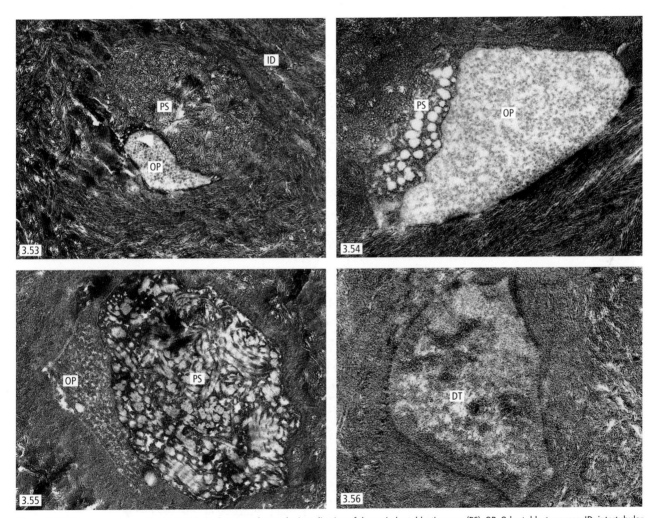

Figure 3.53 Transverse section of a dentin tubule showing advanced mineralization of the periodontoblastic space (PS). OP: Odontoblast process; ID: intertubular dentin.
Figure 3.54 Transverse section of odontoblast process (OP) and partly mineralizaed periodontoblastic space (PS).
Figure 3.55 Transverse section of mineralized odontoblast process (OP) and large, periodontoblastic space (PS) in which the majority of collagen fibers are mineralized.
Figure 3.56 Completely mineralized dentinal tubule (DT). (Figures 3.53–3.56 courtesy of Karger.)

Pulpo-dentinal reactions

Pulpo-dentinal reactions before bacterial invasion into the dentin

The first signs of dentin reactions to the enamel lesion that can be seen in the light microscope are tubular sclerosis which forms corresponding to the deepest part of the progressing enamel lesion (Figs 3.38, 3.47, 3.49). Enamel demineralization increases enamel porosity and hence also the permeability of the enamel, and it is therefore no wonder that the first mild stimuli initiating the defense reaction reach the dentin corresponding to the most porous part of the enamel lesion. Because the light microscope is a relatively coarse level of examination, much earlier dentin reactions have been noted at the biochemical and histochemical level. Initial tubular sclerosis is seen before the advancing front of the enamel lesion reaches the enamel–dentinal junction. When contact between the enamel lesion and the enamel–dentinal junction is established the first sign of dentin demineralization can be seen along the junction in terms of brownish discoloration (Figs 3.41 and 3.49). For many years it has been common in textbooks to read that the dentin demineralization is spreading in a lateral direction along the enamel–dentinal junction because it has been implicitly assumed that the anatomical discontinuity between the two tissues favors penetration of destructive agents.

However, the first systematic studies performed to examine this issue concluded that brownish dentin demineralizations never extend beyond the limits of the enamel lesion contact area with the enamel–dentinal junction (Bjørndal, 1991). In continuation of the orthodox concept of lateral spread along the enamel–dentinal junction it has been natural to see the tubular sclerosis around the central demineralization as an attempt to wall off the lesion. It seems more logical to interpret the dentinal sclerosis lateral to the demineralization as a reaction to stimuli in the direction of the rods from the less advanced parts of the enamel lesion approaching the enamel–dentinal junction. At this stage of lesion progression, the dentin lesion should therefore not be considered as an entity in itself with a 'central and spreading focus of destruction', as conventionally assumed. The dentinal changes merely represent a continuum of pulpo-dentinal reactions to variations in acid challenge at the enamel surface with transmission of the stimulus through the enamel in the directions of the rods (Bjørndal, 1991). The implication of this understanding is that when acid production ends at the surface owing to regular disturbance or removal of the cariogenic microbial biomass then further demineralization also ends, thus arresting further lesion progression. As previously mentioned, the mineral uptake in the enamel and in the dentin from the saliva is very limited after arrest of the disease, and for that reason demineralized enamel as well as demineralized dentin remain as scars in the tissue. Conventionally, dentin involvement has been assumed to be a stage in caries progression that required operative treatment to arrest further destruction, and many studies have therefore focussed on possibilities to detect this stage on radiographs. The common use of dentin involvement is, however, too vaguely defined to cover the continuum of changes occurring in the pulpo-dentinal organ during caries progression, and therefore is useless as an indicator for operative treatment (see Chapter 20).

The next section looks at the gradual destruction of the enamel and the eventual exposure of the pulpo-dentinal organ to the oral environment.

Enamel destruction and bacterial invasion

To understand the gradual exposure of the pulpo-dentinal organ during progressive lesion formation it is important to appreciate that even though minerals have been removed from the enamel and the lesion is thus characterized as porous, the remaining mineral still preserves the structural composition of the enamel (Figs 3.47, 3.49, 3.57). Rather than an empty space beneath the surface zone, there is a certain degree of mineral loss in a still highly mineralized tissue. The first signs of surface breakdown are therefore limited to the outermost enamel and presumably created by mechanical injuries during mastication, microtraumas during interdental wear or careless probing. If such areas are not kept relatively free of dental plaque, the process will continue because the bacteria harbored in the microcavity, all other matters being equal, will receive more protection than those on the surface, which again will favor the ecological shift toward anaerobic and acid-producing bacteria, as described in Chapter 10. The progressive destruction of the enamel or the gradual enlargement of the cavity is therefore the combined result of continued acid production in the protected microbial biomass and mechanical microtraumas.

Considering the role played by bacteria and their metabolic products in inflammatory reactions, it is no wonder that questions about the time for 'bacterial invasion' have been the focus of attention for many clinicians in order to define more precisely the time for operative intervention. Because major interest has been devoted to initial caries and to advanced stages with dentin destruction, little is known about the events taking place during the progressive destruction of the enamel before exposure of the dentin. It is therefore relevant to distinguish between the limited (if any) destructive capacity of isolated groups of bacteria in the tissue and that of the protected microbial biomass in the enamel cavity growing with direct access to the nutrient-rich oral environment (Thylstrup & Qvist, 1987). Occasionally, bacteria may be found within the porous enamel and some may penetrate along the organic meshwork in the enamel, e.g. the lamellae. Proper superficial tubular invasion of bacteria in coronal dentin has not been noted before direct exposure of the dentin to the bacterial biomass in the cavity.

In principle, similar conditions occur when bacteria accumulate directly on exposed root surfaces, leading to active root-surface caries. Since such initial lesions can be arrested by proper non-operative treatment, it is possible to conclude that superficial bacterial invasion into the dentinal tubules cannot per se be used as an indication for operative treatment. It is relevant therefore to raise the question: What is the possible harmful effect of these brave but lonesome invaders into an environment showing little evidence of hospitality compared with the masses of acid-producing surface bacteria? There is no doubt that the microbiota in the dentinal tubules are able to excrete metabolic endproducts that may be associated with destruction (see Chapter 10). However, their relative contribution to the destruction compared with bacteria in the necrotic dentin and bacteria harbored in the cavity may be extremely limited. It is therefore reasonable to assume that bacterial invasion also into the dentinal tubules is merely a sign of lesion progress, rather than being an integrated and significant part of the destruction (Thylstrup & Qvist, 1987).

Following exposure of the dentin to the masses of bacteria in the cavity, the most superficial part of the dentin will soon be decomposed through the action of acids and proteolytic enzymes. This zone is referred to as the zone of destruction (Figs 3.38, 3.58). Beneath this zone, tubular invasion of bacteria is frequently seen (Figs 3.58, 3.59). If the lesion progression is very rapid it is not uncommon to see 'dead tracts' in the dentin, which means that the odontoblast processes are destroyed without having produced tubular sclerosis. Such empty tubules are particularly invaded by bacteria, and occasionally groups of tubules coalesce, forming liquefaction foci (Fig. 3.60). Between the zone of bacterial penetration and the sclerotic dentin, the translucent zone, there is a zone of demineralization resulting from acids produced in the biomass of anaerobic and aciduric bacteria in the cavity.

The first reaction in the pulpo-dentinal organ is tubular sclerosis. When the enamel lesion reaches the enamel–dentinal junction, the superficial part of the dentin

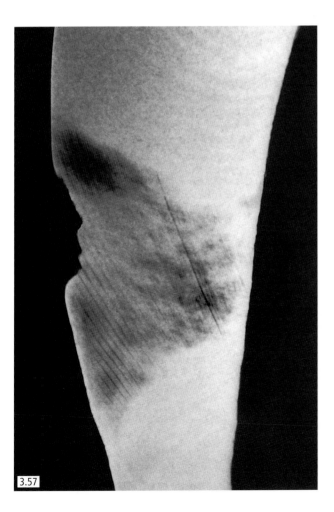

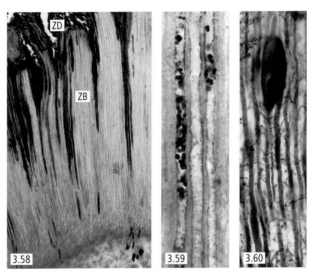

Figure 3.57 Microradiograph of ground section through inactive approximal lesion which has been arrested for several years. In the enamel redeposition of some mineral can be seen, corresponding to the bottom of the cavity, whereas the peripheral dentin demineralization remains unchanged after lesion arrest.
Figure 3.58 Histological section of dentin in a lesion with cavitation into the dentin, with superficial zone of destruction (ZD) and zone of bacterial invasion (ZB).
Figures 3.59, 3.60 Clusters of bacteria penetrating dentinal tubules and forming liquefaction foci.

undergoes demineralization which clinically can be seen as a yellow-brownish discoloration of the soft tissue. The discoloration may be a result of the biochemical changes of the collagenous dentin due to the demineralization. As the process continues, the defense mechanism in terms of tubular sclerosis will proceed. It is clear then that the demineralization will take place in dentin with partly obturated tubules, explaining why the superficial part of the translucent zone is softer than the sound dentin (Fig. 3.61).

Pulp reaction

There is still some uncertainty in the literature concerning the degree of pulp reactions to various stages of caries development. It is known that reactionary (reparative or tertiary dentin) may form even before bacterial invasion into the dentin (Bjørndal, 1991). The reactionary dentin is less well mineralized and contains irregular dentinal tubules. When the demineralization of the dentin approaches the pulp at a distance between 0.5 and 1 mm, inflammatory reactions may be seen in the subodontoblastic region (see Chapter 21). It is important to realize that there is no infection of the pulp, and the inflammatory cell reactions are therefore believed to be a result of bacterial products (Reeves & Stanley, 1966; Massler, 1967; Shovelton, 1972).

Root-surface caries

Clinical appearance of root caries lesions

Recession of the gingival margin is an inevitable result of poor oral hygiene and loss of periodontal attachment with age (Baelum et al., 1991; Baelum, 1998). Even in populations with regular oral hygiene some recession occurs, and its pattern of distribution within elderly populations is very characteristic (Fejerskov et al., 1993). In today's populations it is frequent that even adolescents experience some exposure of the cervical root surfaces in several teeth owing to inappropriate plaque control procedures.

As the gingival margin recedes the enamel–cementum junction becomes exposed. This region of the tooth is highly irregular and represents a particular bacterial retention site (Figs 2.42–2.45). Therefore, a majority of root caries lesions develop at this site.

It is occasionally claimed that root-surface caries may occur within a deep periodontal pocket. From a biological point of view this is not very likely, as the pH of the gingival exudate flushing the pocket is above 7. It seems more likely that in such cases the carious process has originated along the gingival margin. Gingival inflammation and swelling of gingiva may subsequently lead to the impression that the lesion is 'hidden in the pocket'.

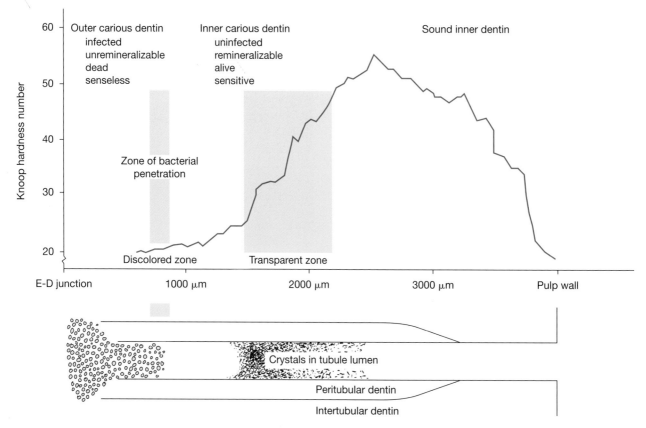

Figure 3.61 Schematic drawing of relationship between a Knoop hardness curve, the outer carious dentin, the translucent zone and the inner sound dentin. Below is shown the relation to bacterial invasion, and mineralization phenomena in the dentinal tubules. (Modified from Ogawa et al., 1983.)

Root-surface caries comprises a continuum of clinical manifestations ranging from small, slightly softened and discolored areas to extensive, yellow–brown soft or hard areas, which may eventually encircle the entire root surface (see Figs 2.42–2.57). The lesions may or may not be cavitated. However, even in the case of rather extensive lesions, cavitation does not necessarily involve the pulp.

As for enamel lesions, root-surface caries lesions may be classified as active or arrested (inactive) according to the following diagnostic criteria:

An *active root-surface lesion* is a well-defined, softened area on the root surface that shows a yellowish or light-brown discoloration. The lesion is likely to be covered by visible plaque. Some slowly progressing lesions may be brownish or black and reveal a leathery consistency on probing with moderate pressure.

An *arrested (inactive) root-surface lesion* appears shiny and is relatively smooth and hard on probing with moderate pressure. The color may vary from yellowish to brownish or black. In both active and inactive lesions, cavity formation may be observed, but in the latter case the margins appear smooth. No visible microbial deposits are seen to cover such lesions.

Although characteristic in their classical manifestations, there will be a range of transitory stages between active and arrested lesions. Thus, it is important to appreciate that when using the diagnosis arrested (or inactive), this is a reflection of a clinical judgment that no further progression of that lesion is expected to take place. This does not imply that there may not be minute niches within certain areas of the lesion that, if examined for example in a microscope, will show bacteria and very localized demineralization. However, if at the time of examination a lesion is judged to be arrested, the lesion is considered to remain clinically unchanged unless the patient's oral hygiene deteriorates at that particular site.

If there is doubt over whether to assign a lesion into the active or the inactive category, the surface texture of the lesion (soft/leathery or hard) is a more valid criterion than is the mere color of the lesion.

It is clinically important to distinguish between active and inactive lesions because root surfaces also respond to the dynamic metabolic processes in the plaque. Thus, if these processes are interfered with, for example by regular plaque removal, active lesions may become arrested, with associated changes in surface texture and color of the lesions (see Figs 2.42–2.57).

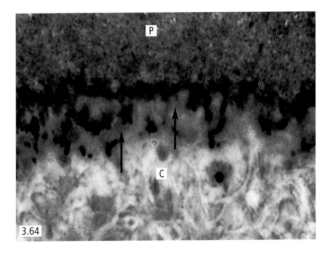

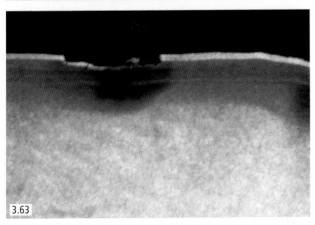

Figures 3.62, 3.63 Microradiograms of early stages of root-surface caries. Distinct demineralization is observed throughout the cementum, but also extending into the underlying dentin deep to a relatively well-mineralized cementum zone. Note the laminated appearance of the cementum in Fig. 3.63, which reflects variations in the mineral content of the imbrication lines.

Figure 3.64 One-micrometer-thick section through the surface layer of an active root-surface caries lesion covered by microbial deposits. At this early stage, the microorganisms penetrate into the superficial layer of the cementum (arrows), which explains why the active root-surface caries lesion appears soft on probing. P: microbial plaque; C: cementum.

From a differential diagnostic point of view a root surface caries lesion is easy to distinguish from other root surface discolorations because the latter usually are widespread and ill-defined.

Histopathological features of root caries lesions

The early root-surface caries lesion appears as a radiolucent zone in the root cementum (Figs 3.62, 3.63). Improper tooth brushing or scaling of root surfaces often damages or removes the cementum, thus exposing the dentin. Therefore, root-surface caries often develops in the exposed dentin.

Microradiographically, mineral loss occurs deep to a relatively well-mineralized surface zone (Figs 3.65–3.67), which frequently exhibits a mineral content that is higher than that of the unaffected dentin. As in enamel lesions, the surface zone varies in thickness and mineral content depending on the cariogenic challenge of the covering microbial plaque. Experimental studies have shown that under suitable conditions, the surface zone forms within a relatively short period (Ogawa *et al.*, 1983). Thus, if root surfaces are covered by undisturbed plaque for 1–3 months in the oral cavity, a progressive subsurface loss of mineral occurs in the dentin concomitant with the build-up of a surface zone (Figs 3.65–3.67). The high mineral content of the surface zone may reflect a selective redeposition of minerals in this region, as it has been shown that the size of the apatite crystals in the surface zone is significantly larger than in normal cementum (Tohda *et al.*, 1996) (see Chapter 12, Fig. 12.16).

Very different from the early enamel lesions, however, is the finding that, at an early stage of root-surface caries development, the surface may appear softened. This is due to the fact that microorganisms penetrate the surface zone of the lesion between partly demineralized collagen fibers

(Fig. 3.64). Therefore, probing of the vulnerable surface zone should be avoided, as destruction of the surface may facilitate further penetration of bacteria into the dentin and impair the possibility of proper plaque control. In any case, vigorous scaling of root surfaces in caries-active patients should not be performed before it is ascertained that active carious lesions have been arrested.

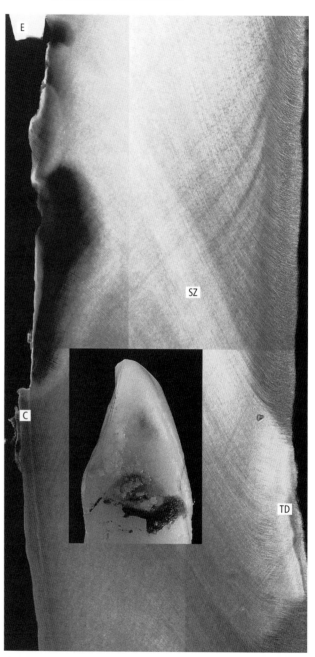

Figure 3.68 Approximal active root-surface caries lesion covered by dental plaque (inset). A microradiogram of a section through the center of the lesions shows loss of cementum (C) corresponding to the part of the surface where extensive loss of mineral has occurred. The body of the lesion is located deep to a surface zone which varies in mineral content. The dentinal tubules affected by the carious attack show sclerosis (SZ), and towards the pulp tertiary dentin has formed (TD). E: enamel (Nyvad & Fejerskov, 1987b).

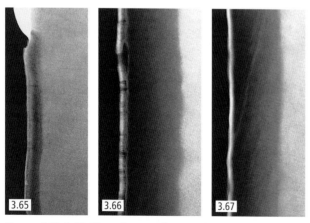

Figures 3.65–3.67 Microradiograms of sections through root caries lesions which have been developed experimentally in the oral cavity during 1, 2 and 3 months, respectively. Note how the mineral content in the surface zone increases with increased duration of the cariogenic challenge while there is a progressive subsurface loss of mineral in the dentin (Nyvad *et al.*, 1989).

At more advanced stages of destruction, the demineralization spreads into the underlying dentin, often extending several hundred micrometers below the surface (Fig. 3.68). However, even when shallow cavities are observed the exposed dentin surface may exhibit a relatively well-mineralized surface layer below which the demineralization takes place. The dentin response is similar to that described for coronal caries, i.e. the pulpo-dentinal organ responds with a zone of increased mineral deep within the tissue corresponding to the width of the carious lesion at the surface. Likewise, tertiary (reactive) dentin may be formed towards the pulp, corresponding to the involved tubules.

Arrested lesions (Fig. 3.69a–c) demonstrate that a pronounced surface abrasion has taken place. Furthermore, redeposition of mineral may have occurred deep within the

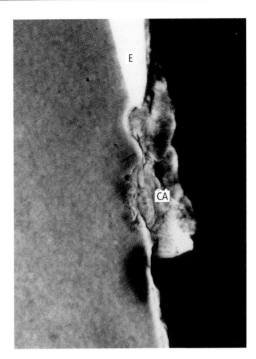

Figure 3.70 Section through an arrested root-surface lesion where the microradiographic picture demonstrates extensive calculus formation extending into microcavities. Note the subsurface lesion cervical to the rim of calculus. E: Enamel; CA: calculus.

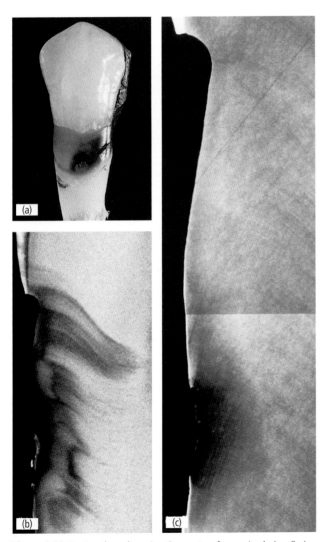

Figure 3.69 Section through an inactive root surface caries lesion (lesion shown in a). When examined in transmitted light (b) and by microradiography (c), it is apparent that a considerable surface abrasion has occurred. Part of the lesion has been abraded away, but a localized radiolucent area remains, possibly reflecting a caries active site (Nyvad & Fejerskov, 1987b).

dentin. In such lesions it may be possible to identify localized radiolucencies which apparently, at the time of examination, have been 'active sites'. In view of the knowledge presented above, it is clear that regular plaque removal from the surface of active root-surface caries lesions is not likely to eliminate the microorganisms that have penetrated deep into the dentin. However, based on the clinical experience that root caries lesions can be converted from active into inactive stages by non-operative treatment (Nyvad & Fejerskov, 1987a) see Figs 2.48–2.55, it may be appreciated that neither antimicrobial nor operative treatment is required to control the microorganisms within the root dentin. In fact, a change in the environmental condition prevailing in the dental plaque covering a root caries lesion may result in mineral deposition within the microbial mass (calculus formation). Thus, calculus may be found partially occluding root-surface defects corresponding to the arrested caries lesions (Fig. 3.70).

Background literature

Fejerskov O, Nyvad B. Dental caries in the aging individual. In: Holm-Pedersen P, Löe H, eds. *Textbook of geriatric dentistry*, 2nd ed. Copenhagen: Munksgaard, 1996: 338–72.

Fejerskov O, Thylstrup A. Dental enamel. In: Mjør I, Fejerskov O, eds. *Human oral embryology and histology*. Copenhagen: Munksgaard, 1986: 50–89.

Frank RM. Structural events in the caries process in enamel, cementum and dentin. *J Dent Res* 1990; **69** (Special Issue): 559–66.

Holmen L, Thylstrup A, Øgaard B, Kragh F. A polarized light microscopic study of progressive stages of enamel caries *in vivo*. *Caries Res* 1985; **19**: 348–54.

Nyvad B, Fejerskov O. Active root surface caries converted into inactive caries as a response to oral hygiene. *Scand J Dent Res* 1986; **94**: 281–4.

Nyvad B, Fejerskov O. An ultrastructural study of bacterial invasion and tissue breakdown in human experimental root surface caries. *J Dent Res* 1990; **69**: 2218–25.

Schmidt WJ, Keil A. *Polarizing microscopy of dental tissues*. Oxford: Pergamon Press, 1971.

Silverstone LM. Structure of carious enamel including the early lesion. *Oral Sci Rev* 1973; **3**: 100–60.

Silverstone LM. Remineralization phenomena. *Caries Res* 1977; **11**: 59–84.

Theilade E, Fejerskov O, Hørsted M. A transmission electron microscopic study of 7-day old bacterial plaque in human tooth fissures. *Arch Oral Biol* 1976; **21**: 587–98.

References

Årtun J, Thylstrup A. Clinical and scanning electron microscopic study of surface changes of incipient enamel caries lesions after debonding. *Scand J Dent Res* 1986; **94**: 193–210.

Årtun J, Thylstrup A. A three-year clinical and SEM study of surface changes of carious enamel lesions after inactivation. *Am J Dentofac Orthop* 1989; **95**: 27–33.

Backer Dirks O. Posteruptive changes in dental enamel. *J Dent Res* 1966; **45**: 503–11.

Baelum V. The epidemiology of destructive periodontal disease. Thesis. Aarhus: Aarhus University, Royal Dental College, 1998.

Baelum V, Manji F, Fejerskov O. The distribution of periodontal destruction in populations in non-industrialized countries: evidence for the existence of high risk groups and individuals. In: Johnson NW, ed. *Risk markers for oral diseases*, Vol. 3, *Periodontal diseases. Markers of disease susceptibility and activity*. Cambridge: Cambridge University Press, 1991: 27–74.

Bjørndal L. Carieslæsionens tidlige udvikling i emalje og pulpa-dentinor-ganet. Dissertation. Copenhagen: University of Copenhagen, 1991.

Black GV. *Operative dentistry*, Vol. 1, *Pathology of the hard tissues of the teeth*. London: Claudius Ash, 1914.

Boyde A. Amelogenesis and the structure of enamel. In: Cohen B, Kramer IRH, eds. *Scientific foundations of dentistry*. London: Heinemann Medical Books, 1976: 335–52.

Carvalho JC, Ekstrand KR, Thylstrup A. Dental plaque and caries on occlusal surfaces of first permanent molars in relation to stage of eruption. *J Dent Res* 1989; **68**: 773–9.

Carvalho JC, Ekstrand KR, Thylstrup A. Results of 1 year of non-operative occlusal caries treatment of emptying permanent first molars. *Community Dent Oral Epidemiol* 1991; **19**: 23–8.

Carvalho JC, Ekstrand KR, Thylstrup A. Results of 3 years of non-operative occlusal caries treatment of erupting permanent first molars. *Community Dent Oral Epidemiol* 1992; **20**: 187–92.

Daculci G, Legeros RZ, Jean A, Kerebel B. Possible physico-chemical processes in human dentin caries. *J Dent Res* 1987; **66**: 1356–9.

Ekstrand K, Carlsen O, Thylstrup A. Morphometric analysis of occlusal groove–fossa-system in mandibular third molar. *Scand J Dent Res* 1991; **99**: 196–204.

Fejerskov O, Josephsen K, Nyvad B. Surface ultrastructure of unerupted mature human enamel. *Caries Res* 1984; **18**: 302–14.

Fejerskov O, Baelum V, Østergaard ES. Root caries in Scandinavia in the 1980s – and future trends to be expected in dental caries experience in adults. *Adv Dent Res* 1993; **7**: 4–14.

Frank RM, Voegel JC. Ultrastructure of the human odontoblast process and its mineralization during dental caries. *Caries Res* 1980; **14**: 367–80.

Haikel Y, Frank RM, Voegel JC. Scanning electron microscopy of human enamel surface layers of incipient carious lesion. *Caries Res* 1983; **17**: 1–13.

Hay DI. Specific functional salivary protein. In: Guggenheim B, ed. *Cariology today*. Basel: Karger, 1984: 98–108.

Holmen L, Thylstrup A. Variations in 'normal' enamel surface as visualized in the SEM. In: Ruch JV, Belcourt A, eds. *Tooth morphogenesis and differentiation* II. Paris: INSERM, 1984: 283–94.

Holmen L, Thylstrup A, Øgaard B, Kragh F. A scanning electron microscopic study of progressive stages of enamel caries *in vivo*. *Caries Res* 1985; **19**: 355–67.

Holmen L, Thylstrup A, Årtun J. Clinical and histological features observed during arrestment of active enamel carious lesions *in vivo*. *Caries Res* 1987a; **21**: 546–54.

Holmen L, Thylstrup A, Årtun J. Surface changes during the arrest of active enamel carious lesions *in vivo*. A scanning electron microscope study. *Acta Odontol Scand* 1987b; **45**: 383–90.

Johnson NW. Some aspects of the ultrastructure of early human enamel caries seen with the electron microscope. *Arch Oral Biol* 1967; **12**: 1505–21.

Johnson NW, Taylor BR, Berman DS. The response of deciduous dentine to caries studied by correlated light and electron microscopy. *Caries Res* 1969; **3**: 348–68.

Larsen MJ, Fejerskov O. Chemical and structural challenges in remineralization of dental enamel lesions. *Scand J Dent Res* 1989; **97**: 285–96.

Levine RS. The microradiographic features of dentine caries. *Br Dent J* 1974; **137**: 301–6.

Mannerberg F. Appearance of tooth surface as observed in shadowed replicas. *Odontol Rev* 1960; **11** (Suppl 6).

Massler M. Pulpal reactions to dental caries. *Int Dent J* 1967; **17**: 441–60.

Mjør IA. Dentine and the pulp. In: Mjør IA, ed. *Reaction patterns in human teeth*. Boca Raton, FL: CRC Press, 1983: 63–156.

Nyvad B, Fejerskov O. Transmission electron microscopy of early microbial colonization of human enamel and root surface *in vivo*. *Scand J Dent Res* 1987a; **95**: 297–307.

Nyvad B, Fejerskov O. Active and inactive root surface caries – structural entities? In: Thylstrup A, Leach SA, Qvist V, eds. *Dentine and dentine reactions in the oral cavity*. Oxford: IRL Press, 1987b: 165–79.

Nyvad B, ten Cate JM, Fejerskov O. Microradiography of experimental root surface caries in man. *Caries Res* 1989; **23**: 218–23.

Ogawa K, Yamashita Y, Ischij T, Fusayama T. The ultrastructure and hardness of the transparent layer of human carious dentin. *J Dent Res* 1983; **62**: 7–10.

Reeves R, Stanley HR. The relationship of bacterial penetration and pulpal pathosis in carious teeth. *Oral Surg* 1966; **22**:59–65.

Shovelton DS. The maintenance of pulp vitality. *Br Dent J* 1972; **133**: 95–107.

Stanley HR, Pemeira JC, Spiegel E, Broom C, Schultz M. The detection and prevalence of reactive and physiologic sclerotic dentin, reparative dentin and dead tracts beneath various types of dentinal lesions according to tooth surface and age. *J Pathol* 1983; **12**: 257–89.

Thylstrup A, Fejerskov O. Surface features of early carious enamel at various stages of activity. In: Rølla G, Sønju T, Embery G, eds. *Proceedings of a workshop on tooth surface interactions and preventive dentistry*. London: IRL Press, 1981: 193–205.

Thylstrup A, Fredebo L. A method for studying surface coatings and the underlying enamel features in the scanning electron microscope. In: Frank R, Leach S, eds. *Surface colloid phenomena in the oral cavity: methodological aspects*. London: IRL Press, 1982: 169–84.

Thylstrup A, Qvist V. Principal enamel and dentine reactions during caries progressions. In: Thylstrup A, Leach SA, Qvist V, eds. *Dentine and dentine reactions in the oral cavity*. Oxford: IRL Press, 1987: 3–16.

Thylstrup A, Featherstone JDB, Fredebo L. Surface morphology and dynamics of early enamel caries development. In: Leach SA, Edgar WM, eds. *Demineralization and remineralization of the teeth*. London: IRL Press, 1983: 165–84.

Thylstrup A, Bruun C, Holmen L. *In vivo* caries models – mechanisms for caries initiation and arrestment. *Adv Dent Res* 1994; **8**: 144–57.

Tohda H, Fejerskov O, Yanagisawa T. Transmission electron microscopy of cementum crystals correlated with Ca and F distribution in normal and carious human root surface. *J Dent Res* 1996; **75**: 949–54.

Weatherell JA, Robinson C, Hallsworth AS. The concept of enamel resistance – a critical review. In: Guggenheim B, ed. *Cariology today*. Basel: Karger, 1984: 223–30.

4

Visual–tactile caries diagnosis

B. Nyvad, O. Fejerskov and V. Baelum

Introduction

This chapter on visual–tactile caries diagnosis discusses the very basics of clinical cariology. Dentists diagnose caries every day of their practicing lives – or do they? Consider for a moment the description of caries in Chapter 1: Caries is a result of metabolic activities in the microbial deposits covering the tooth surface at any given site. Clearly, clinical inspection of the teeth at the chairside does not allow the dentist to observe the caries process itself. What dentists can do is to examine the consequences of microbial metabolic activity when looking for signs of lesions that have formed as a result of it. This is what caries diagnosis is about: *detection of signs and symptoms of caries*.

The history of visual–tactile caries examination goes back to antiquity. However, the caries diagnostic criteria used and the means and methods employed have changed over time. Until the 1920s, when bitewing radiography was introduced (Raper, 1925), clinical caries diagnosis completely relied on a combined visual and tactile examination of the teeth using a probe to search for caries lesions. This practice still prevails, especially in countries where dentists do not have easy access to dental radiography or other 'advanced' diagnostic methods. However, concurrently with the spread of bitewing radiography, generations of dentists seem to have lost reliance on the classical visual–tactile caries examination. Many explanations may be offered for the success of bitewing radiography over the visual–tactile examination, including the general fascination with technology and striving for documentation. However, the risk of underdiagnosis (Raper, 1925) (Chapter 7) is probably the main reason why most cariology courses continue to stress the importance of repeated bitewing examinations. This concept is still haunting the profession, in spite of an overall lower rate of lesion progression in many populations today. As a consequence, in some parts of the world it is now considered inappropriate to screen a patient for caries without at the same time performing a radiographic examination (Deery, 2004). There are several reasons why this belief and the resulting clinical practice are very unfortunate, and this chapter will demonstrate that the large majority of initial caries lesions can indeed be diagnosed by visual–tactile methods only, even in difficult-to-reach areas such as approximal surfaces. However, to do this, dentists must acquire the necessary knowledge and skills.

The aim of this chapter is to discuss the theoretical foundation and the practical implementation of visual–tactile caries examination, and to show that the visual–tactile caries examination is the only clinical method that provides the information necessary for the choice of appropriate treatment.

The diagnostic process

In dentistry, we have often turned to medicine when searching for clarification of concepts and methods, and caries diagnosis is no exception. In medicine, diagnosis is defined as the "art or act of identifying a disease from its signs and symptoms" (Merriam-Webster, 2003).

The medical perspective on diagnosis

Medical diagnostic reasoning is thought to be a complex process that involves elements of simple pattern recognition (pathognomonic signs and symptoms), considerations about the probability of various differential diagnostic alternatives, and the generation of hypotheses about the underlying disease, followed by diagnostic tests, the results of which may be used to disprove the hypothesis in favor of an alternative diagnosis (hypotheticodeductive thinking) (Wulff & Gøtzsche, 2000). Basically, a patient presents with complaints (symptoms), e.g. abdominal pain. The clinician makes a mental list of the diseases most likely to cause the symptoms (a list of tentative diagnoses). Using the most probable tentative diagnosis as a starting point, he or she begins a deductive process which involves taking a patient history, performing a physical examination and prescribing diagnostic tests to obtain information that will allow him or her to confirm or refute this tentative diagnosis. This process of pattern recognition and testing of alternative hypotheses concerning the diagnosis is continued until a final diagnosis is reached, which is consistent with the results of the various tests carried out. When the diagnosis has been established, the treatment selection process begins. This is usually rather straightforward once the diagnosis is clear. If, for unforeseen reasons, the patient does not respond to the treatment, the physician may ultimately have to reconsider and revise the diagnosis.

The dental perspective

However, the medical and the dental diagnostic universe differ in important aspects (Baelum *et al.*, 2006). Most of the patients seen in general dental practice in high-income countries are asymptomatic and come for routine check-ups in the belief that by doing so they achieve better oral health outcomes. This implies a screening examination for caries, periodontal diseases and other forms of oral pathology. The dentist should not overlook oral disease/pathology in need of treatment and, at the same time, should avoid unjustified diagnoses leading to overtreatment. Therefore, the main task for the dentist is not to find out what disease the patient has, but whether the patient has caries, periodontal disease or other forms of oral pathology and, not least, whether the patient would benefit from treatment. The logic behind this strategy is that the course of these diseases may be changed for the better if they are detected and treated before they reach a stage at which they elicit symptoms or require more invasive intervention. Therefore, in dental practice, diagnosis is closely linked with the management options.

Caries scripts

When screening for oral pathology, the dentist does not use the differential diagnostic approach described for the medical situation. Dentists know that they are examining for a relatively limited number of oral diseases (caries, periodontitis, mucosal lesions). Moreover, the major oral diseases affect different anatomical locations (e.g. the oral mucosa, the periodontium or the dental hard tissues), and these are examined separately. Even though the number of dental pathologies of differential diagnostic relevance is limited, differential diagnostic reasoning is too difficult to repeat for each tooth surface present in each patient. A caries examination of a patient with a full dentition of 32 teeth would thus involve going through 148 differential diagnostic processes (20 molar and premolar teeth with five surfaces plus 12 incisor and canine teeth with four surfaces). Clearly, this does not happen. When dentists diagnose caries they use preconceived 'caries scripts' to identify particular clinical manifestations of interest. All the differential diagnostic considerations that are relevant for examination of the dental hard tissues, as well as all the management considerations, are incorporated in these caries scripts. Caries diagnostic reasoning predominantly consists of a 'this-clinical-manifestation-needs-this-kind-of-treatment' classification of the tooth surfaces (Bader & Shugars, 1997). However, as will be shown in this chapter, the clinical manifestations looked for, and the caries scripts used, have varied over time, as a function of changing knowledge about the caries processes and the management options available.

Why do we diagnose caries?

The medical literature on diagnosis cites at least five reasons why diagnosis is important (Knottnerus & van Weel, 2001). These include:

- detecting and excluding disease
- assessing prognosis
- contributing to the decision-making process with regard to further diagnostic and therapeutic management
- informing the patient
- monitoring the clinical course of the disease.

As discussed before, this list applies well to the medical situation owing to the medical focus on differential diagnosis. However, the situation is different in dentistry, and tends to be the opposite. In caries diagnosis, dentists know what disease they are looking for, namely the signs and symptoms that can be attributed to dental caries. They do not perform classical differential diagnosis in the medical sense, but seek to differentiate between 'caries-free' and 'caries-affected' tooth surfaces, just as doctors try to classify lesions into categories. When selecting a lesion classification it should always be acknowledged that caries examinations are carried out to influence the patient's oral health outcome for the better. A lesion classification must therefore reflect the best caries management options available. When caries management options change as a function of increasing evidence, lesion classifications should change accordingly to ensure that the best possible health outcomes are achieved for the patient.

Diagnosis in a dental caries perspective

On the basis of this discussion the list of reasons for diagnosis provided by Knottnerus and van Weel (2001) can be revised to suit caries diagnosis. Caries lesions can be diagnosed , or perhaps more correctly, classified to be able:

- to achieve the best health outcome for the patient by classifying caries lesions corresponding to the best management options for each lesion type
- to inform the patient
- to monitor the clinical course of the disease.

Achieve the best health outcome for the patient by classifying caries lesions corresponding to the best management options for each lesion type

It should now be clear that the best diagnostic classification of caries lesions cannot be discussed without due reference to the management options available. As explained in detail in Chapters 10–12, a caries lesion may result when the metabolic activity of bacteria in the biofilm shifts the physiological equilibrium at the biofilm–tooth interface towards a net mineral loss. If not interfered with, this mineral loss may continue until the entire crown of the tooth has been destroyed, leaving only a relic root (the word 'caries' originates in Latin and means 'rot'). The classification of caries should reflect the best management options for the different stages of lesions.

Cavitated caries lesions

A distinctive stage in the caries process is the stage of cavity formation. When a carious cavity has formed it is much more difficult to control the biofilm by oral hygiene procedures. As explained in Chapters 20–24, the treatment of choice for such cavitated lesions usually involves operative intervention in the form of restorations. This intervention will not manage the causes of caries, but restoring the tooth makes it easier to perform proper oral hygiene.

Non-cavitated caries lesions

Non-cavitated lesions can be managed by non-operative means (Chapters 14–19). Like clinically sound surfaces, all non-cavitated lesions should as a minimum be subjected to basic prevention, such as daily tooth brushing with fluoride toothpaste. This regimen is a simple but highly effective method of non-operative caries control when performed properly (Chapter 15). However, depending on the activity state of the lesions and the risk factors of the patient, some non-cavitated lesions may need professional non-operative treatments (Chapter 27).

Active lesions

Caries lesions that reflect ongoing mineral loss due to metabolic activity in the biofilm are designated 'active lesions'. Active non-cavitated lesions always require professional non-operative management as otherwise such lesions are likely to progress (Nyvad *et al.*, 2003) (Fig. 4.1). By means of such professionally applied treatment, progressive (active) non-cavitated caries lesions may be turned into arrested (inactive) non-cavitated caries lesions. Lesion-specific instruction in improved oral hygiene procedures is a must, since the most effective management for an active non-cavitated caries lesion involves daily removal of the biofilm in conjunction with the use of fluoride toothpaste. Occasionally, the dentist may need to help the patient in achieving this goal by performing regular professional cleaning of the teeth. Topical fluoride application is another professional management option that may be applied in patients with numerous active non-cavitated lesions. Moreover, in some patients caries control cannot be obtained without instruc-

tions in proper dietary control. This highlights the important fact that the general treatment philosophy for active lesions advocated in the decision tree in Fig. 4.1 ('active caries lesions need professional management') should be tailored to the particular needs of the patient (see Chapter 27).

Inactive lesions

By contrast, inactive or arrested lesions do not require professional intervention because the metabolic activity in the biofilm is unlikely to result in mineral loss (Fig. 4.1). Indeed, such professional intervention would be a waste of time and money. It is important to note that inactive non-cavitated caries lesions may also be seen in patients who have never received professional non-operative interventions, as lesion arrest could happen in response to tooth eruption and salient changes in oral health behavior.

As will be shown later in this chapter, active and inactive non-cavitated caries lesions have clinically distinct features. The ideal caries diagnostic method is therefore one that allows a distinction between cavitated and non-cavitated caries lesions, as well as between active and inactive non-cavitated caries lesions. The visual–tactile clinical examination is the only method so far available that can fulfill this purpose.

Informing the patient

The patient is central to the management of the carious process. It is the patient who will control the process, not

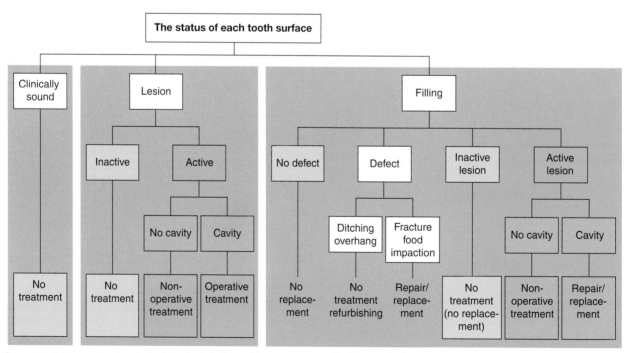

Figure 4.1 Decision-making tree for dental caries including activity assessment as a key factor in the decision process. The flow diagram promotes the concept that active lesions (cavitated and non-cavitated as well as recurrent lesions) need professional management, whereas inactive lesions do not need treatment besides self-performed tooth brushing with fluoride toothpaste. The flow diagram does not consider individual factors that may influence the modality or intensity of the professional treatment. See text for further explanation. (Modified after Nyvad & Fejerskov, 1997.)

the dental professional. The dentist's role is to inform the patient of the diagnosis and prognosis, and whether any action is required.

Many patients still expect the dentist to 'take care of their mouths' and think that caries control can be obtained by merely visiting a dentist at regular intervals. If the dentist does not share the diagnosis with the patients and inform them of their crucial role for the control and management of their caries lesions, this may lead to disappointment at best or legal action at worst.

Longitudinal assessment of the caries process

Once it has been decided to intervene with an active caries lesion the dentist should monitor the fate of the lesion over time and record any changes in surface integrity and activity status. An active lesion that converts into an inactive lesion or regresses to a sound surface is considered a positive outcome. Active lesions that remain active most often reflect a lack of compliance. Alternatively, it should be considered whether the chosen intervention is suitable.

Longitudinal monitoring of caries lesions is also relevant at the population level. Health service planners organize epidemiological studies for surveillance of the caries status in selected populations. Such reports are used to identify possible trends in the caries profile in given populations over time in an attempt to allocate limited economic resources in the most appropriate way.

How early should caries lesions be detected?

The signs and symptoms of caries form a whole continuum of changes ranging from barely discernible at the ultrastructural level to overt cavities. This raises the question of which (lower) threshold to use to distinguish between caries and no caries. So far, this lower threshold has predominantly been determined by the limits of detection of the traditional diagnostic methods, i.e. what we are able to detect based on the visual–tactile examination or in bitewing radiographs. The low prevalence of dental caries observed in many countries today has prompted researchers to look for more refined diagnostic tools that can detect carious lesions before the stage at which they may be observed by the naked eye (Chapter 6). This development has essentially been driven by the belief that the earlier a lesion is detected, the better the possibility for successful non-operative intervention. However, there are several reasons why this philosophy of earlier detection may be questioned. First of all, lowering of the diagnostic threshold results not only in the detection of more small lesions, but also in more false-positive diagnoses, because caries diagnosis, like any other measurement process, is prone to error (Chapter 7). One consequence of lowering the detection threshold is therefore more unnecessary non-operative treatment. Secondly, many subclinical lesions will arrest or

regress without active professional intervention as a result of natural physiological processes in the biofilm (Fejerskov, 1997). Thus, lowering of the diagnostic threshold may not be cost-effective. Finally, there is currently no advanced caries diagnostic alternative to the visual–tactile clinical examination that allows a distinction between active and inactive non-cavitated lesions. Use of advanced diagnostic methods with a better resolution than that provided by the visual and tactile examination will therefore add to the aforementioned problem of unnecessary non-operative treatment, primarily because such methods cannot distinguish between active lesions in need of treatment and inactive lesions for which treatment has no effect.

Numerous studies have shown that clinically detectable carious lesions can be arrested by non-operative interventions at any stage of lesion development when plaque control is adequate (for review, see Nyvad & Fejerskov, 1997), particularly when lesions are easily accessible to cleaning (Backer Dirks, 1966; Nyvad & Fejerskov, 1986, Årtun & Thylstrup, 1986). It thus remains to be demonstrated that lowering of the diagnostic threshold by means of more refined caries diagnostic methods can bring about a health benefit to the patients that outweighs the additional costs that will be incurred due to unnecessary treatments. Until such evidence has been presented, we cannot recommend lowering of the diagnostic threshold below that which can be obtained by the visual–tactile examination for practical clinical purposes. However, this does not preclude the use of more advanced methods for research purposes (see Chapter 6).

What are the best visual–tactile caries diagnostic criteria?

As shown in Chapter 2, carious lesions come in various sizes, surface features and colors. This may explain why the literature has described a large spectrum of visual or visual–tactile classifications of carious lesions (Ismail, 2004a). Each of these classifications has been developed to serve specific purposes of individual researchers, and it may therefore be difficult for the clinician to appraise their usefulness critically. Some classifications focus specifically on the presence of cavitated lesions, while others seek to include both cavitated and non-cavitated lesions. Some are mainly concerned about estimation of lesion depth, while others classify lesions according to the dental tissues involved.

In recent years a new dimension has been added to the classical visual–tactile caries examination; the concept of lesion activity assessment (Nyvad et al., 1999). It has thus been shown that in addition to determining the surface integrity of a lesion (cavitated or non-cavitated), it may be sensible to classify lesions according to their activity state on the basis of surface characteristics (Nyvad et al., 2003). These observations hold great promise for clinical cariology as such simple recordings have prognostic value and may assist in treatment planning as well as monitoring individual lesions over time.

It is important to stress that there is no universal set of diagnostic criteria or diagnostic threshold that can be recommended for all purposes. It is up to the clinician or researcher to choose the classification that is best suited for the purpose. For some epidemiological surveys, where reliability and comparability with previous surveys may be key issues, a classification that records cavities only may occasionally be advised. However, in clinical settings and research it is now mandatory that both cavitated and non-cavitated lesions are recorded (Pitts, 2004; Ismail, 2004b). When a clinician or researcher wants to monitor changes in the activity state of lesions over time it is essential to apply a diagnostic method that has proved its suitability for such purposes.

Caries diagnostic methods are frequently introduced without much prior scientific evaluation. This is highly unfortunate as it may later turn out that a diagnostic technique cannot deliver what it promises. It is often stated that the fundamental requirement for a good diagnostic method is that it is valid and reliable. However, no pre-determined bounds have been agreed for the validity and reliability of caries diagnostic tests. It is therefore important to have some understanding of these concepts.

The concept of validity

A valid method results in measurements that measure what they purport to measure (Last, 2001). For example, whenever a carious cavity is clinically recorded in an approximal surface, the clinical recordings should represent the true state of this condition. In the case of approximal carious cavities the truth could (theoretically) be established by extracting the teeth and verifying the presence of cavities by means of meticulous inspection in the laboratory. This is referred to as the 'gold-standard truth'. This experiment may generate a 2 × 2 table as shown in Table 4.1. For the

perfectly valid test, the test results would show a perfect match with the gold-standard truth. However, only rarely have tests been described that are perfectly valid, and researchers are usually faced with a situation where they have to consider the consequences of the errors made. In the hypothetical example in Table 4.1, 15 true-positive (TP) cavity diagnoses were made, i.e. a cavity was found in 15 cases where a cavity was indeed present. Ten false-negative (FN) cavity diagnoses were made, i.e. 10 cavities were overlooked. Thereby, the ability of the test to find cavities (test sensitivity) = 15/(15+10) = 0.60 (Table 4.1). Five false-positive (FP) diagnoses and 170 true-negative (TN) diagnoses were also made. These numbers can be used to express the ability of the test to exclude cavities where there are no cavities (test specificity) = TN/(TN+FP) = 170/(170+5) = 0.97. Apparently, in this case the clinical diagnostic test was better suited to rule out cavities (specificity) than to rule them in (sensitivity), but the trade-off also involves balancing the health consequences of 10 overlooked cavities against five diagnoses of non-existent cavities (see Chapter 7).

The validity concept just described is a form of criterion validity that is termed concurrent validity. This necessitates a gold-standard reference of truth. However, as discussed in much greater detail in Chapter 7, it is usually not possible to identify a real reference of truth. An example that illustrates this is the diagnosis of active caries, as no gold standard exists for caries activity assessment. In such circumstances, a different form of criterion validity is used, namely predictive validity. Predictive validity makes use of the fact that a truly active lesion, if not interfered with, will progress, whereas this will not happen if the lesion is truly inactive. In other words, a higher probability of lesion progression is predicted for a caries lesion judged to be active than for one judged to be inactive. This approach was used by Nyvad et al. (2003) to determine whether certain diagnostic categories were better than others in predicting particular outcomes (e.g. cavity formation). This method of validity assessment is particularly meaningful because it has direct clinical implications for prognosis and treatment decisions (Nyvad et al., 2003) (see later in this chapter).

From the patient perspective, however, information about validity is relatively uninteresting. What matters to the patient is not a precise judgment of the true or predicted state of affairs, but rather the prognosis of his or her condition under different treatment alternatives (Wulff, 1979). Patients will only benefit from a diagnostic test if the information generated by the test can be used to alter the subsequent treatment decision in the direction of a better health outcome (Lijmer & Bossuyt, 2002). The clinical relevance of a caries diagnostic method is therefore closely linked with its ability to alter the treatment towards interventions that achieve better long-term health outcomes (Chapter 7).

Table 4.1 The 2 × 2 table that might arise from an attempt to verify approximal cavity diagnoses in 200 consecutively examined first molars by means of subsequent extraction and inspection of the teeth

		Gold standard (the truth)		
		Cavity	No cavity	Total
Result of clinical examination	Cavity	15 = TP	5 = FP	20
(our test)	No cavity	10 = FN	170 = TN	180
	Total	25	175	200

TP: true-positive diagnoses = 15; FP: false-positive diagnoses = 5;
FN, false-negative diagnoses = 10; TN: true-negative diagnoses = 170.
Sensitivity = ability of test to detect cavity, when cavity is truly present = TP/(TP+FN) = 15/25 = 0.60.
Specificity = ability of test to exclude cavity, where there is truly no cavity = 170/175 = TN/(TN+FP) = 0.97.

The concept of reliability

A reliable diagnostic method is a method that can be used by the same or by different examiners so that they obtain identical results. The reliability of a diagnostic method can easily be evaluated, for example by repeat (but independent) examinations of a number of patients carried out within a time interval sufficiently short to ensure that no real change in the disease situation has occurred. Examinations may be repeated by a single examiner, in which case we talk about intraexaminer reliability, or by different examiners (interexaminer reliability). In the simplest scenario, where the diagnostic method distinguishes between presence and absence of disease (e.g. cavity or not), the results of such repeat examinations can be presented in a 2 × 2 table (Table 4.2). If the reliability is calculated as the observed proportion of agreement, it is high, amounting to 0.99. However, the observed proportion of agreement may be misinterpreted if it is not taken into account that when most surfaces are cavity free there is a substantial risk that some of the agreement reflects chance. The analogy is that if a person who is completely ignorant of a subject takes a multiple-choice test, he or she will by chance check some correct answers. For this reason, it has become customary in dental diagnostic research to express the reliability in the form of kappa, which is a chance-corrected measure of agreement. The kappa value for the data shown in Table 4.2 is 0.74, showing that the agreement between the two examiners was 74% of the maximum obtainable beyond chance agreement. As discussed in Chapter 7, this kappa value is usually interpreted in the caries diagnostic literature as indicative of a high reliability. Unfortunately, neither the observed nor the chance-corrected agreement (kappa) can be used to judge whether the diagnostic test is good for clinical practice. The two dentists, AA and BB (Table 4.2), have diagnosed a similar number of cavities, 162 and 158, respectively. While this may seem fine, it is indeed problematic from a clinical perspective that the two dentists only agreed on 140 (64%) of the total of 220 cavities diagnosed by one or the other dentist. The practical consequence of such observations of less than

perfect reliability should be obvious if it is assumed that the patients first visited dentist AA, where the 'necessary' 158 restorations were made, and then visited dentist BB, only to have an additional 42 cavities filled. With this level of reliability one might advise patients never to change dentist, and in any case not to go too often, as the intraexaminer reliability of caries diagnostic methods is typically only marginally better than the interexaminer reliability. The discussion on how to act clinically in such circumstances is expanded in Chapter 7.

Commonly used visual–tactile criteria

The following diagnostic classifications represent selected examples of commonly applied strategies of visual–tactile caries diagnosis. Note that the methods differ by their clinical approach. Furthermore, the examples illustrate how differences in the diagnostic criteria may influence the clinical outcome with regard to total numbers of lesions, cavitated and non-cavitated lesions, and active and inactive lesions (Fig. 4.2).

Recording of cavities only (WHO 1997)

The World Health Organization (WHO) recommends that carious lesions be diagnosed at the level of cavitation. A community periodontal index (CPI) probe should be used to verify the diagnosis when a lesion has "an unmistakable cavity, undermined enamel, or a detectably softened floor or wall". This approach is still advocated owing to the belief that it is not possible to obtain a reliable diagnosis of the non-cavitated stages of caries (WHO, 1997). Even so, several studies have shown that this assumption does not hold when examiners are thoroughly trained and calibrated (e.g. Pitts & Fyffe, 1988; Manji et al., 1989; Ismail et al., 1992; Nyvad et al., 1999). By focussing on frank cavities only, the WHO approach to caries diagnosis ignores the opportunity for non-operative interventions and therefore cannot be recommended in modern caries management.

Recording of cavitated and non-cavitated lesions (Pitts & Fyffe, 1988)

As mentioned before, caries recording in surveys and in clinical studies requires that lesions be assessed at the non-cavitated level. Pitts and Fyffe (1988) presented a classification in which non-cavitated lesions were included along with cavitated stages of caries. A plane mouth mirror and a sickle probe were used by the examiners, and the following diagnostic levels were applied:

- D_1 (enamel lesions, no cavity)
- D_2 (enamel lesions, cavity)
- D_3 (dentin lesions, cavity)
- D_4 (dentin lesions, cavity to the pulp).

A major advantage of including non-cavitated lesions in the classification is that it gives a more realistic picture of

Table 4.2 The hypothetical 2 × 2 table that might arise from an evaluation of the interexaminer reliability of cavity diagnoses in 6000 surfaces in 50 consecutively examined patients

		Examiner BB		
		Cavity	No cavity	Total
Examiner AA	Cavity	120	38	158
	No cavity	42	5800	5842
	Total	162	5838	6000

Observed proportion of agreement = (120 + 5800) / 6000 = 0.99.
Chance-corrected proportion of agreement: kappa = 0.74.

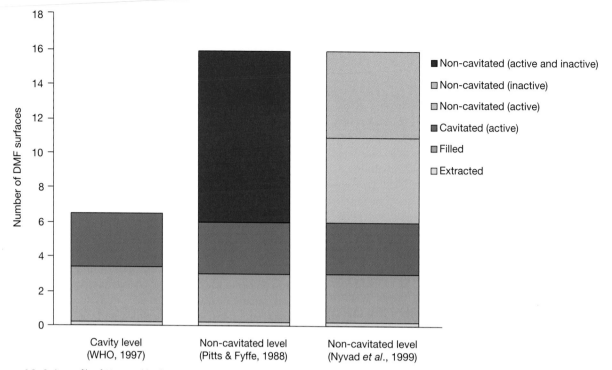

Figure 4.2 Caries profile of 12-year-old Lithuanian children according to three different visual–tactile classifications. Note differences in the clinical outcome with regard to total number of lesions, cavitated and non-cavitated lesions, and active and inactive lesions. (Data from Machiulskiene *et al.*, 1998.)

the total caries experience in individuals or populations. Caries recording including non-cavitated diagnoses typically increases the diagnostic yield by more than 100% compared with counting cavities only (Pitts & Fyffe, 1988; Manji *et al.*, 1989, 1991; Amarante *et al.*, 1998; Machiulskiene *et al.*, 1998) (Fig. 4.2). Diagnosis of non-cavitated level lesions can be performed reliably by trained examiners, and the approach is compatible with the philosophy of non-operative caries control. However, the method does not inform about the activity status of lesions.

Lesion depth assessment (Ekstrand et al., 1995, 1997)

Ekstrand *et al.* (1995) presented a visual ranked scoring system for assessment of the depth of lesion penetration, including non-cavitated stages of caries. The authors performed visual examination (without the use of a probe) of cleaned occlusal surfaces on extracted teeth and demonstrated that distinct macroscopic changes on the occlusal surface were related to the histological depth of the lesion (Ekstrand *et al.*, 1997):

- no or slight change in enamel translucency after prolonged air-drying (5 s)
- opacity or discoloration hardly visible on the wet surfaces, but distinctly visible after air-drying
- opacity or discoloration distinctly visible without air-drying

- localized enamel breakdown in opaque or discolored enamel and/or grayish discoloration from the underlying dentin
- cavitation in opaque or discolored enamel exposing dentin.

This method is based on the well-known phenomenon that white spot lesions may change their optical properties, depending on whether the lesion is examined in the wet or dry stage (Thylstrup & Fejerskov, 1994). When a wet enamel lesion is dried it becomes more opaque because of increased light scattering in the tissue. This phenomenon also explains why a lesion that is distinctly visible in the wet stage penetrates more deeply into the tissue than a lesion that can only be seen when it is examined dry. A non-cavitated lesion that is only visible after thorough drying may have penetrated halfway into the enamel. However, when a non-cavitated lesion is visible on a wet tooth the demineralization may extend into the outer dentin (Ekstrand *et al.*, 1997).

Lesion depth assessments have been reported to be reliable when extracted teeth are dried and examined under laboratory conditions. However, it has not been evaluated whether this particular method of visual caries diagnosis of occlusal surfaces has prognostic value in clinical settings.

Lesion activity assessment (Nyvad et al., 1999)

Increasing knowledge about the dynamic chemical processes in caries has prompted the development of a new refined visual–tactile caries diagnostic method based on assessment of lesion activity. Rather than concentrating on lesion depth, this diagnostic method focusses on the surface characteristics of lesions. Two discrete surface features are addressed: activity, as reflected by the surface texture of the lesion, and surface integrity, as expressed by the presence or absence of a cavity or microcavity in the surface. The pathobiological rationale of the method is based on the observation that the surface characteristics of enamel change in response to changes of the activity of the biofilm covering the tooth surface (for review, see Thylstrup *et al.*, 1994) (Chapter 3).

According to the criteria (Nyvad *et al.*, 1999), lesions should be assigned to one of the following diagnostic categories:

- active non-cavitated
- active cavitated
- inactive non-cavitated
- inactive cavitated
- filling
- filling with active caries
- filling with inactive caries.

The typical characteristics of an active non-cavitated enamel caries lesion are those of a whitish/yellowish opaque surface with loss of luster, exhibiting a chalky or neon-white appearance. The surface feels rough when the tip of a sharp probe is moved gently across it (Fig. 4.3a, b). By contrast, inactive enamel caries lesions are generally shiny and feel smooth on gentle probing (Fig. 4.3c, d). The color of an inactive lesion may vary from whitish to brownish or black, but color is not a reliable differential diagnostic characteristic. For cavitated lesions, the diagnostic criteria mimic those applied for dentin/root caries (Fejerskov *et al.*, 1991); active lesions are soft or leathery, while inactive lesions may be shiny and feel hard on gentle probing (Fig. 4.3e, f).

The chalky opacity of an active enamel caries lesion relates to two discrete phenomena. First, the opacity is explained by the previously discussed increase in the internal porosity of the lesion due to subsurface demineralization. The second phenomenon is caused by dissolution of the outermost intercrystalline enamel spaces (surface erosion). When the surface is eroded the enamel loses its shiny appearance owing to diffuse back-scattering of light (Thylstrup *et al.*, 1994). This is the very reason why an active enamel caries lesion may appear whiter, almost neon-like, than an inactive enamel lesion. If an active lesion is exposed to mechanical disturbances in the oral cavity the lesion gradually assumes a smooth surface; however, the internal opacity often persists. Therefore, in most cases the inactive lesion is seen as an opaque 'scar' in the enamel (see Chapter 3).

When diagnosing activity it is also important to distinguish between the general surface roughness resulting from dissolution of the outermost enamel crystals and shallow

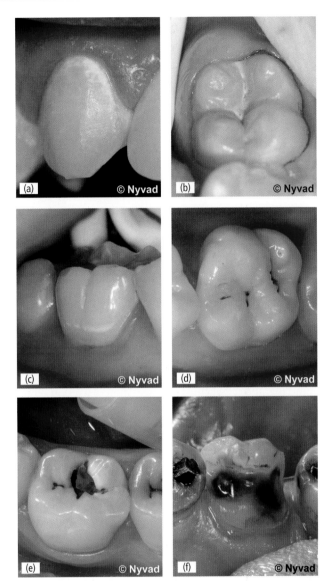

Figures 4.3 a–f Caries lesion activity assessment according to Nyvad *et al.* (1999). (a, b) Typical active non-cavitated lesion on smooth surface and occlusal surface, respectively. (c, d) Typical inactive non-cavitated lesion on smooth surface and occlusal surface, respectively. (e, f) Active and inactive cavitated lesions, respectively. See text for further explanation. (a, b, and d from Nyvad *et al.*, 1999.)

surface defects, such as microfractures in the very surface zone of the lesion, which may arise as a response to wear and tear in the oral cavity (Årtun & Thylstrup, 1986, Carvalho *et al.*, 2004); (Fig. 4.4). When the local environment changes, e.g. as a result of tooth eruption, such shallow surface defects may become inactivated. Hence, enamel lesions with an overall smooth topography should be recorded as inactive, in spite of the presence of several microcavities (Fig. 4.5).

Such a refined scoring system necessitates clean and dry teeth. Active non-cavitated lesions are normally covered by tacky bacterial deposits, which are physically interrelated with the eroded enamel surface (Frank & Brendel, 1970),

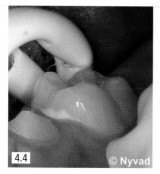
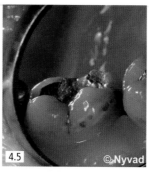

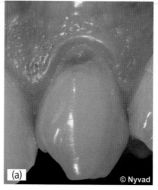
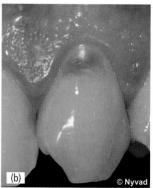

Figures 4.4, 4.5 Active (Fig. 4.4) and inactive (Fig. 4.5) smooth-surface caries lesions presenting microfractures in the surface.

Figure 4.6 (a) Active root-surface caries lesion in upper canine presenting a softened surface. (b) Same lesion after 1 year of non-operative caries control by improved toothbrushing with fluoride toothpaste. The lesion has turned into an inactive stage, as evidenced by the hard and shiny surface. Note also inactive lesion in the gingival part of the enamel.

and removal of this biofilm (using the side of the probe or a brush) is an integral part of the diagnostic process. The probe should never be used to poke vigorously into the tissues, but rather serve as a highly refined tactile tool. Rough and careless probing can force the probe through the surface zone of the lesion and create a cavity. In fact, poking with the probe requires a firm grip, which precludes the tactile approach proposed with the Nyvad criteria.

When using activity assessment it has to be borne in mind that the actual clinical presentation of a lesion represents the cumulated result of numerous demineralization and remineralization episodes that have occurred over a longer period (Fejerskov, 1997) (Chapter 3). For some lesions it may therefore be difficult to decide whether a lesion should be scored as active or inactive. Furthermore, lesions may contain elements of both active and inactive sites. A lesion is scored as active only when the predominant part of the lesion reveals the classical signs of activity (dullness and roughness) and the examiner concludes that overall the lesion is considered to be progressing. When adopting such decision rules, these criteria have been shown to be reliable when used under epidemiological conditions by trained examiners (Nyvad *et al.*, 1999).

As previously discussed, lesion activity assessments cannot be validated by the classical gold-standard approach because there is no gold standard for caries activity. However, it has been shown that activity assessments have predictive validity for lesion activity when used in a clinical trial of the effect of daily supervised brushing with fluoride toothpaste (Nyvad *et al.*, 2003). It was thus demonstrated that active non-cavitated lesions had a higher risk of progressing to a cavity than inactive non-cavitated lesions which, in turn, had a higher risk of progressing to a cavity than sound surfaces. The important implications of these predictions are that activity assessments have prognostic value and therefore may help to guide the subsequent course of treatment.

Root-surface caries (Fejerskov et al., 1991)

Fejerskov and co-workers introduced a classification for diagnosing root-surface lesions which integrates activity

assessment as well as assessment of surface integrity. The criteria were developed on the basis of empirical observations of experimental non-operative treatments of root-surface caries (Nyvad & Fejerskov, 1986) (see Chapter 2, Figs 2.48–2.51). Active lesions were described as soft or leathery (Fig. 4.6a) and were usually found at plaque-retention sites next to the gingival margin or along the cementoenamel junction. Inactive lesions were typically located at some distance from the gingival margin, felt hard on gentle probing and often presented with a shiny appearance (Fig. 4.6b). The color of the lesion was not helpful in distinguishing between active and inactive stages. The following diagnostic categories were identified:

- inactive lesion without surface destruction
- inactive lesion with cavity formation
- active lesion without definitive surface destruction
- active lesion with surface destruction (cavitation), but cavity is estimated not to exceed 1 mm in depth (visually)
- active lesion with a cavity depth exceeding 1 mm, but not involving the pulp
- lesion expected to penetrate into the pulp
- filling confined to the root surface or extending from a coronal surface onto the root surface
- filling with an active (secondary) lesion along the margin
- filling with an inactive lesion (secondary) confined to the margin.

Recurrent (secondary) caries

The term recurrent (secondary) caries refers to caries at the margin of restorations (Mjör 2005). Hence, recurrent caries reflects the result of unsuccessful plaque control. Recurrent carious lesions are most often located on the gingival margins of class II–V restorations. Recurrent caries is rarely diagnosed on class I restorations.

Diagnosis of recurrent caries may be accomplished according to the Nyvad criteria by differentiating between

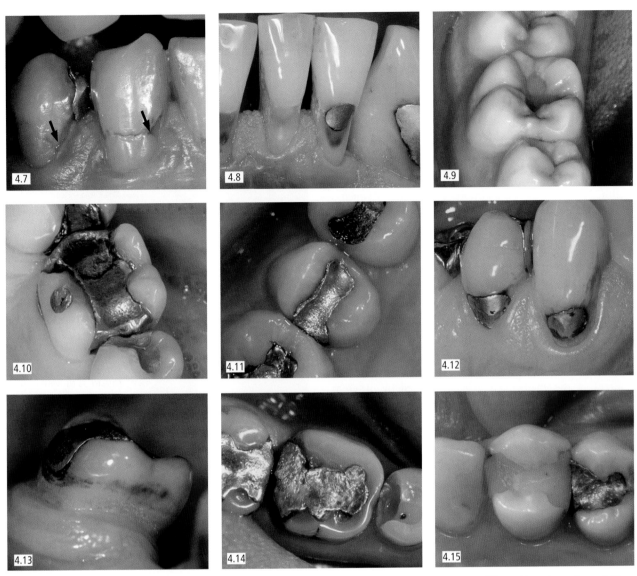

Figures 4.7–4.15 Figure 4.7: Active recurrent root-surface caries lesions on lower canine and premolar next to composite fillings with overhangs (arrows). These lesions should be treated by non-operative intervention (site-specific improved hygiene and application of topical fluoride) in conjunction with refurbishing of the lesions to facilitate biofilm removal. Note also dark shadow on the buccal surface of the premolar, reflecting an underlying amalgam filling; Figure 4.8: Inactive recurrent root-surface lesion next to an amalgam filling on a lower incisor. No treatment is needed; Figure 4.9: Active recurrent caries lesion next to composite filling on the occlusal surface. The lesion needs operative treatment because the cavity cannot be cleaned properly. The cavity is soft on probing; Figure 4.10 This filling has fractured across the isthmus and part of the restoration is loose. Biofilm forms beneath the loose amalgam, resulting in an active recurrent caries lesion that needs operative treatment. The cavity is soft on probing; Figure 4.11: Ditching along margins of amalgam restoration which probably developed because of overfilling. No caries is detected. No treatment is needed; Figure 4.12: Gingival amalgam fillings with stained margins and inactive recurrent caries. Refurbishing of the fillings may facilitate oral hygiene; Figure 4.13: Buccal amalgam with overhang and inactive recurrent caries. The filling should be refurbished to make cleaning easier; Figure 4.14: Old amalgam fillings in patient with erosion. Note that the normal anatomy of the teeth has gone and that the fillings are elevated above the eroded enamel/dentin surface. In spite of defective margins no caries is present. No treatment is advocated. Filling in neighboring premolar was lost owing to progression of erosion; Figure 4.15: Stained margins of composite filling in upper premolar. The stain may be due to incomplete removal of previous amalgam filling. No need for replacement if the margins of the filling are clinically intact and food impaction does not occur.

cavitated and non-cavitated as well as active and inactive stages of caries (see p. 57). This approach automatically guides the subsequent treatment (Fig. 4.1). Hence, non-cavitated active recurrent lesions that are amenable to plaque removal should principally be managed by non-operative procedures (Fig. 4.7), while non-cavitated in-

active recurrent lesions need no further treatment apart from daily tooth brushing (Fig. 4.8). By contrast, active lesions with cavity formation (soft on probing) that cannot be cleaned properly should be repaired or replaced (Figs 4.9, 4.10). Diagnosis of caries at the margins of restoration is sometimes difficult, but it is imperative to distinguish recurrent lesions from ditching (Fig. 4.11) and minor defects, as some defects such as overhangs (Figs 4.12–4.13) may be managed adequately by refurbishing (Mjör, 2005). Furthermore, dark shadows reflecting an underlying amalgam filling (Fig. 4.7) or staining of composite fillings due to residual amalgam (Fig. 4.15) may confuse the diagnosis. Some dentists routinely replace fillings with staining and minor defects (Figs 4.11–4.15) in the belief that such clinical signs are indicative of microleakage that leads to caries. However, recurrent caries does not develop as a result of microleakage along the tooth–restoration interface (Mjör, 2005). Bacteria may invade larger gaps between a filling and a tooth (>0.4 mm) (Kidd *et al.*, 1995; Kidd & Beighton, 1996), but the presence of bacteria in this location should not be confused with recurrent caries, which develops as a surface lesion similar to primary caries lesions (Chapter 3).

Differential diagnosis

When performing a caries diagnosis it should be appreciated that not all opaque lesions on the tooth surface represent dental caries. All opacities reflect a decreased mineral content in the enamel, but may be caused by different mechanisms, either during enamel, formation or posteruptively. Differential diagnostic considerations of white opaque lesions are particularly relevant in populations showing evidence of dental fluorosis. Because of its developmental origin, dental fluorosis has a symmetric distribution on homologous teeth (Dean *et al.*, 1942; Thylstrup & Fejerskov, 1978). In mild cases (TF1), fluorosis appears as fine white horizontal striae reflecting the perichymatal pattern of enamel. When such white lines merge (TF2) in the gingival part of a tooth they are suggestive of inactive non-cavitated caries lesions (smooth on probing) (Fig. 4.16). By contrast, the typical non-cavitated enamel caries lesion is arch, banana or kidney shaped, reflecting the retention of plaque along the curvature of the present (or former) gingival margin (Figs 4.3a, 4.3c, 4.4, 4.5, 4.17). Therefore, in populations with dental fluorosis, to facilitate diagnosis the dentist should quickly check for signs of dental fluorosis before performing a visual–tactile caries examination.

Opacities of non-fluoride origin rarely represent a differential diagnostic problem as they are mostly round or oval and clearly defined from the adjacent enamel. They appear on single teeth, especially incisors (Fig. 4.18), and predominantly in the incisal two-thirds of the crown. Occasionally, patches of whitish, yellowish or brownish enamel opacities occur on several molars and/or incisors in the same individual (molar–incisor hypomineralization) (Weerheim, 2004). Depending on the severity of the hypomineralization such developmental defects may exhibit a softened surface with or without posteruptive loss of enamel.

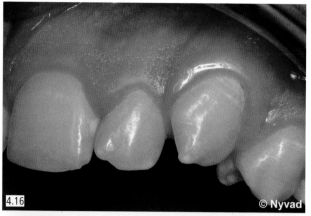

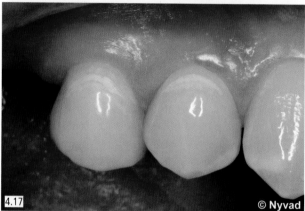

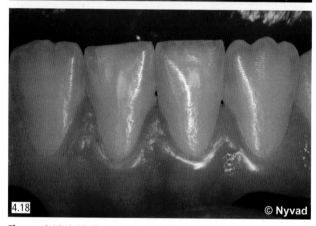

Figures 4.16–4.18 Figure 4.16: Dental fluorosis (TF1) in the gingival part of upper canine and premolar. Note the fine white horizontal lines, which reflect the perichymatal pattern of enamel. This clinical manifestation is distinctly different from the arch-shaped inactive non-cavitated caries lesions shown in Fig. 4.17, reflecting the retention of plaque along the former gingival margin. Figure 4.18: well-demarcated opacities of non-fluoride origin in the incisal part of lower incisors (Nyvad *et al.*, 2007).

Table 4.3 gives a summary of the differential diagnostic characteristics that should be considered when distinguishing among carious lesions, dental fluorosis and enamel opacities of non-fluoride origin (Nyvad *et al.*, 2007).

Table 4.3 Differential diagnostic characitstics of dental caries, dental fluorosis and developmental defects of non-fluoride origin (Nyvad et al., 2007)

	Dental caries (Nyvad et al., 1999)	Dental fluorosis (Thylstrup & Fejerskov 1978)	Developmental defects of non-fluoride origin (Fejerskov et al., 1988)
	Non-cavitated	*TF 1–4*	*Opacity/hypomineralization*
Surface characteristics	Active lesion: 'chalky'/dull; rough on probing. Inactive lesion: glossy; smooth on probing	Smooth/glossy (pearl like)	Smooth/glossy
Color	Active lesion: whitish to light brown. Inactive lesion: whitish to brownish/black	Whitish (opaque) TF 3–4 may be stained secondarily	Whitish (opaque) or creamy yellowish to brownish
Demarcation characteristics	Active lesion: most often sharply demarcated (corresponding to plaque-retention sites). Inactive lesion: well demarcated, or with diffuse borders	White striae reflect perichymatal pattern. In mild cases 'snow capping' on the cuspal/incisal and marginal ridges may appear	Well demarcated (often spherical). May be bordered by a narrow, translucent halo
Distribution in dentition	Active lesion occurs on plaque-retention sites: • occlusal pits and fissures • approximal surfaces below the contact point (kidney shaped) • smooth surfaces reflecting position of gingival margin (arch and banana shaped). Inactive lesion is often located further away from gingival margin	Occurs symmetrically on homologous teeth, with almost the same level of severity. The tooth surface is affected according to duration of systemic exposure	Occurs on single teeth (most commonly incisors). Occasionally a symmetrical distribution may be observed
Histopathological characteristics	Subsurface demineralization (bacterial origin)	Subsurface hypomineralization due to disturbance of enamel maturation	Subsurface hypomineralization due to localized (traumatic) disturbance of mineralization
	Cavitated	*TF 5–9*	*Hypoplasia*
Surface characteristics	Active lesion: cavity with exposed dentin; soft or leathery on probing. Inactive lesion: cavity with exposed dentin; hard on probing	Surface defects vary from focal loss of enamel (pit formation) to loss of most of the outer enamel. Hard on probing (enamel may chip off on probing)	Surface defect with smooth rounded margins varying in depth and shape (spherical or irregular). Hard or rough on probing
Color	Yellowish to brownish-black	May be secondarily discolored	Yellowish or brownish
Demarcation characteristics	Active lesion: sharply demarcated. Inactive lesion: no sharp demarcation of lesion margins	Pit formation	No sharp demarcation of lesion margins. Often follows perichymatal pattern
Distribution in dentition	Lesion occurs on plaque-retention sites: • occlusal pits and fissures • approximal surfaces below the contact point • smooth surfaces next to gingival margin	Occurs symmetrically on homologous teeth. Tooth surface is affected according to duration of systemic exposure	Localized or generalized. Lesion may vary from a grooved fine line across the tooth surface to a wider band of faulty deformed enamel
Histopathological characteristics	Demineralization with loss of surface zone. Breakdown of enamel and possibly bacterial invasion into dentin	Subsurface hypomineralization with loss of surface zone corresponding to pit formation	Developmental disturbance of enamel resulting in disturbed surface contour. Mineralization of enamel may be unaffected

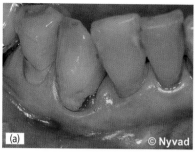
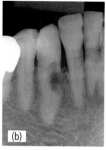

Figure 4.19 (a) Clinical manifestation of invasive cervical root resorption on lower canine. Note the sharp occlusal border of the lesion and the presence of reddish granulation tissue. (b) It is obvious from the radiograph that the lesion is subgingival. There is a small opening to the periodontal membrane (Zubzevic & Nyvad, 2007).

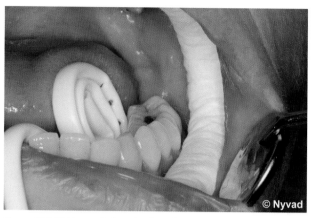

Figure 4.20 Making ready for a visual–tactile caries examination after isolation of the teeth with cotton rolls and a suction device.

In recent years dentists have noted an apparent increase in the occurrence of subgingival lesions in otherwise caries-inactive patients (Fig. 4.19a). Some researchers claim that such cavitated lesions may represent root caries lesions (Katz, 1995), but in most cases the subgingival location makes it is more plausible that they are external cervical root resorptions. First, the biofilm in this econiche is deprived of dietary carbohydrates that could shift the ecological balance (Chapter 10), and secondly, the alkaline pH of the gingival fluid precludes the preservation of an acid environment for longer periods (Bickel & Cimasoni 1985). Therefore, external cervical root resorption should always be considered a possible differential diagnosis when root defects are observed subgingivally (Gold & Hasselgreen, 1992). Root-surface caries lesions may occasionally appear in a subgingival location owing to secondary swelling of the gingival tissues. However, root caries lesions are relatively easy to distinguish from cervical root resorptions as the latter are hard on probing and present with sharp undermined borders (Fig. 4.19b). Furthermore, root resorptions may be associated with granulation tissue, which is redder in colour than the surrounding gingiva and bleeds freely on probing. Finally, most cervical root resorptions are asymptomatic until a very advanced stage of development (Gold & Hasselgreen, 1992).

Visual–tactile caries examination: a systematic clinical approach

The clinical caries examination should be carried out in a systematic manner after each quadrant of the mouth has been isolated with cotton rolls and a suction device to prevent saliva from wetting the teeth once they have been dried (Fig. 4.20). For practical purposes, begin with the upper right molars and move tooth by tooth and surface by surface to the upper left molars, then jump to the lower left molars and finish up with the lower right molars. A consistent examination pattern ensures that no teeth or surfaces are missed.

Good lighting and clean, dry teeth

Visual–tactile caries examination requires good lighting and clean, dry teeth. Thorough drying is performed with a gentle blast of air from a three-in-one syringe. An initial non-cavitated enamel lesion is more easily disclosed when the tooth is dry, since the difference in the refractive index between carious and sound enamel is greater when water is removed from the porous tissue. It is not feasible to give a standardized drying time, as the humidity and salivary flow in the oral cavity may vary considerably from site to site and from patient to patient.

The teeth are examined by the aid of a dental mouth mirror and a sharp probe (see later). The mouth mirror is used to displace the cheeks and lips and to facilitate vision in difficult to reach areas on the teeth. Reflected light from the mouth mirror can be applied to search for dark shadows, which may be suggestive of dentinal lesions (Fig. 4.21). Transmitted light from the operating lamp is particularly helpful for examining the approximal surfaces of anterior teeth (Fig. 4.22). Many dentists do not look for non-cavitated lesions on approximal surfaces. However, even if direct access to an approximal surface is limited, careful inspection may reveal a non-cavitated lesion that extends onto the buccal or lingual surfaces (Fig. 4.23).

Sensible use of the probe

If the teeth are heavily covered by plaque, it may be necessary to clean the dentition before a proper caries diagnosis can be performed (Fig. 4.24a, b). However, it should be appreciated that the presence of plaque covering a lesion may be of diagnostic value when assessing lesion activity (see pp. 57–58). Sticky adhering plaque covering a chalky/opaque enamel lesion is strongly indicative of activity. Therefore, in most situations it is more sensible to remove the plaque concurrent with performing a caries examination rather than just removing it before looking. In any case, for plaque-removal purposes as well as for assessment

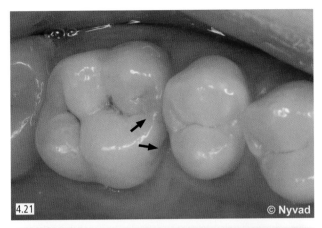

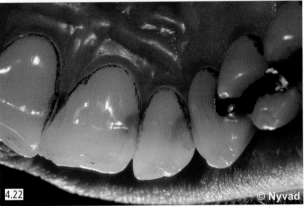

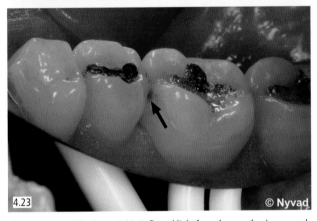

Figures 4.21–4.23 Figure 4.21: Reflected light from the mouth mirror reveals a dark shadow on the mesial approximal surface of upper first molar (arrow). Note also the presence of a non-cavitated lesion on the mesio-palatal part of the same surface (arrow); Figure 4.22: Transmitted light from the operating lamp allows detection of approximal lesions in upper anterior teeth; Figure 4.23: Inactive non-cavitated lesion on the mesial surface of lower molar detected after careful inspection using a mouth mirror (arrow).

of surface roughness the use of a sharp metal probe is recommended. The probe serves two purposes: first, to remove the biofilm (using the side of the probe) to check for signs of demineralization and surface break and, secondly, to 'feel' the surface texture of a lesion, as sensed through minute vibrations of the instrument by the supporting fingers when moving the tip of the probe at an angle of 20–40 degrees across the surface (Fig. 4.25). It may take some training to learn this tactile skill, but once it has been acquired it is an important adjunct to the visual assessment. One should definitely abstain from poking vigorously into the tissue, thereby running the risk of causing irreversible damage to the surface layer of an incipient lesion (Ekstrand *et al.*, 1987) (Fig. 4.26), which may potentially accelerate localized lesion progression. Histological evaluation has shown that gentle probing does not disrupt the surface integrity of non-cavitated lesions (Lussi, 1993). A clinical caries examination performed according to these principles takes about 5–10 min, depending on the caries status of the patient (Nyvad *et al.*, 1999).

Some researchers are concerned that probing of suspected carious lesions may serve to spread infective plaque (i.e. mutans streptococci) to other teeth in the same mouth (Loeche *et al.*, 1979), thereby facilitating caries lesion development. However, this concern has not been confirmed by longitudinal studies of second molars in which probing of fissures was repeated at regular intervals (Hujoel *et al.*, 1995). Furthermore, such a hypothesis is incompatible with the ecological concept of caries. Transferred microorganisms would not survive unless their new econiche favored their existence (see Chapter 10).

Caries predilection sites

In every dentition there are sites that are at increased risk of lesion development. These sites reflect the stagnation areas for dental plaque, mainly the areas along the gingival margin, occlusal fissures and gingival margins of restorations. Furthermore, caries predilection sites vary distinctly according to the age of the patient. In preschool children the distal surface of the first primary molar is the most caries prone, followed by the mesial surface of the second primary molar. Children with erupting first and second permanent molars require special attention. Because of a relatively long eruption period, permanent molars run an increased risk of lesion development, particularly on occlusal surfaces (Carvalho *et al.*, 1989). In teenagers, the distal surfaces of the second premolars and the mesial surfaces of the second molars are particularly prone to lesion development (Mejáre *et al.*, 1999). In elderly patients with gingival recession, root caries may become a problem. Root caries lesions are confined to stagnation sites, such as the area along the gingival margin, the cementoenamel junction and other difficult-to-clean irregularities on the root surface.

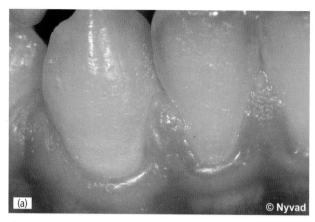
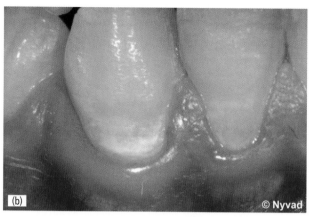

Figure 4.24 Lower canine and incisor (a) before and (b) after plaque removal. Note the presence of typical active non-cavitated lesions after plaque has been removed with the side of a probe.

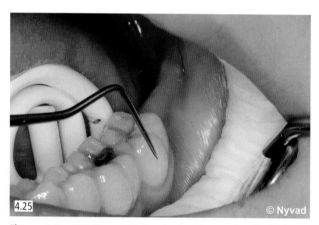
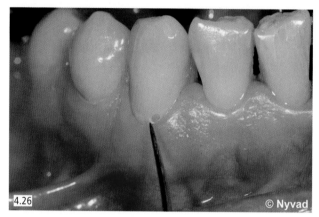

Figures 4.25, 4.26 Figure 4.25: Examination of non-cavitated caries lesion using the tip of a sharp probe that is moved gently across the surface of the lesion at an angle of 20–40 degrees to assess lesion texture; Figure 4.26: Forceful poking with the probe perpendicular to the lesion should be avoided in order not to cause irreversible damage to the surface of the lesion.

Additional aids in visual–tactile caries diagnosis

Fiber-optic transillumination

Fiber-optic transillumination (FOTI) is a diagnostic method by which visible light is transmitted through the tooth from an intense light source, e.g. from a fine probe with an exit diameter of 0.3–0.5 mm. If the transmitted light reveals a shadow when the tooth is observed from the occlusal surface this may be associated with the presence of a carious lesion. The narrow beam of light is of crucial importance when the technique is used in the premolar and molar region. For optimal performance the probe should be brought in from the buccal or lingual aspect at an angle of about 45 degrees to the approximal surfaces pointing apically, while looking for dark shadows in the enamel or dentin (Fig. 4.27). Shadows are best noticed when the office light is switched off.

Although transillumination is a simple, fast and cheap supplementary method well known to most practitioners for diagnosing approximal caries in the anterior teeth (Fig. 4.22), the fiber-optic method has never become broadly accepted for detection of lesions in approximal surfaces in the premolar and molar regions. One of the reasons for this may be that the sensitivity of the method is rather low when using radiography as the gold standard. Hence, the sensitivity has been shown to vary between 50 and 85% (Verdonschot *et al.*, 1991; Vaarkamp *et al.*, 2000), with higher values for dentin lesions than for enamel lesions (Wright & Simon, 1972; Purdell-Lewis & Pot, 1973; Mitropoulos, 1985a, b; Holt & Azevedo, 1989). Although the specificity of the method has also been reported to be high, over 95%, it remains to be documented that FOTI adds substantially to the clinical caries examination for detecting lesions with dentin involvement.

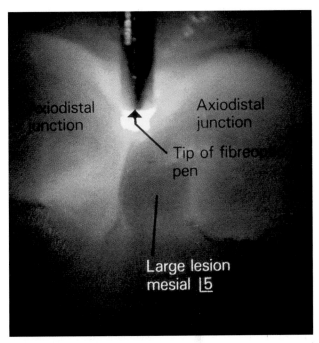

Figure 4.27 Caries lesion detected by fiber-optic transillumination on the mesial aspect of upper second premolar (arrow). The lesion is seen as a dark shadow. (Reproduced courtesy of Dr C. Pine.)

Tooth separation

It is anticipated that the presence of a cavity, if not interfered with, increases the rate of progression of a caries lesion. Neither radiographs nor FOTI can help to identify the presence of a cavity on contacting approximal surfaces. Therefore, other methods such as tooth separation have been introduced. With this technique orthodontic elastic separators are applied for 2–3 days around the contact areas of surfaces to be diagnosed, after which access to inspection and probing is improved (Fig. 4.28a, b).

Most studies that have applied tooth separation have detected more non-cavitated enamel lesions than visual–tactile examination without separation or bitewing examination (Pitts & Rimmer, 1992; Hintze *et al.*, 1998). However, accessibility for inspection after tooth separation is not always improved as much as needed, and the use of the technique may create some discomfort, especially in patients with established dentitions. Furthermore, it requires an extra visit. Therefore, at present the technique is not recommended for routine use in general practice. In the past, however, the technique has generated important knowledge about the relationship between radiographic lesion depth and the presence or absence of cavity formation on contacting approximal surfaces (Pitts & Rimmer, 1992; Hintze *et al.*, 1998). Such information is highly useful when deciding whether to treat a dentin lesion operatively or non-operatively (see Chapter 20).

Magnification

Some contemporary textbooks advocate the use of magnification in caries diagnosis. Indeed, most dentists above the age of 40 should be concerned with potential eyesight difficulties and wear glasses. However, it should be pointed out that there is no scientific evidence that magnification per se improves caries detection in clinical settings. On the contrary, there is a risk that magnification may raise the diagnostic threshold with an associated unnecessary increase in treatment needs. Any dentist who has used a digital camera for high-magnification imaging of teeth would be familiar with this problem.

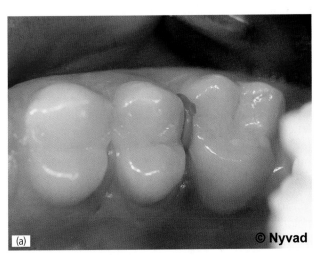
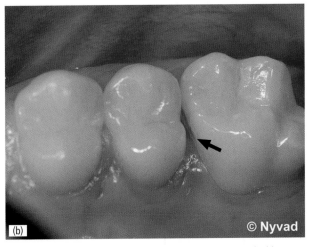

Figure 4.28 (a) An orthodontic elastic separator has been placed between upper premolar and molar. To insert the separator the elastic is stretched between two surgical forceps and one half of the elastic is worked down through the contact point. (b) After 2–3 days the separator is removed. It is now possible to see and 'feel' the surface texture of the lesion with the tip of a probe.

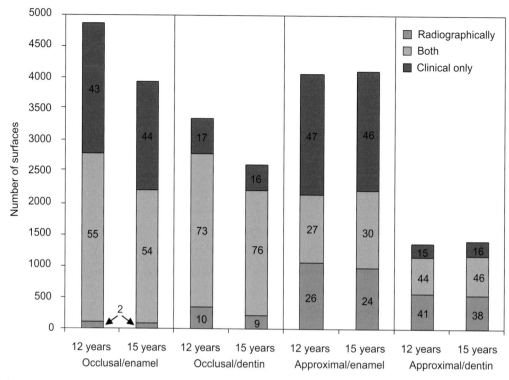

Figure 4.29 Relative diagnostic yields of clinical and radiographic examinations of approximal and occlusal surfaces at the cavitated and non-cavitated levels, respectively. The data were obtained from children examined at 12 and 15 years of age. Note that at the non-cavitated/enamel level of diagnosis, the clinical examination revealed a higher number of lesions than did the radiographic method. Only for approximal lesions at the cavity/dentin level of diagnosis did the radiographic method perform better than the clinical examination. Age of the individuals did not influence the results (Machiulskiene *et al.*, 1999, 2004).

Benefits and limitations of visual–tactile caries diagnosis

This chapter has reviewed the clinical application of visual–tactile caries examination. A visual–tactile caries examination incorporating activity assessment according to the criteria suggested by Nyvad *et al.* (1999) is presently the best choice for performing a caries diagnosis. These criteria are the only criteria that reflect the current evidence-based management options for different stages of caries lesion formation. Importantly, the criteria have predictive value for lesion activity, which means that they are highly relevant for clinical decision making. The criteria can be applied for all entities of caries, including root-surface caries and recurrent caries. Last, but not least, a visual–tactile caries examination is quick and easy to perform, it does not require expensive equipment and unwarranted radiation is prevented.

It should be appreciated that the effectiveness of a visual–tactile caries examination depends strongly on the caries diagnostic level used (Machiulskiene *et al.*, 1998, 2004). When non-cavitated diagnoses are included in the classification, the diagnostic yield of the visual–tactile caries examination is greater than that of radiographic examination (Fig. 4.29). This observation may seem surprising as it is often postulated that radiography is superior to clinical caries examination in lesion detection, particularly on approximal surfaces (Kidd & Pitts, 1990; Pitts, 1996). However, minor mineral losses cannot be detected on radiographs, and the additional diagnostic yield of bitewing radiography is confined to lesions diagnosed at the cavity/dentin level (Fig. 4.29). Furthermore, the radiographic examination is unable to determine lesion activity and cavity formation, and suffers from a high number of false-positive diagnoses (see Chapter 7). Not every dentinal lesion that appears on a radiograph needs a filling, and too much reliance on radiographic diagnosis inevitably leads to overtreatment. Visual–tactile caries examination and activity assessment circumvents this problem by identifying most of the lesions that are indicated for professional treatment. Certainly, clinical signs such as dark occlusal or approximal shadows call for supplementary analyses. However, only after having exploited the full potential of the visual–tactile examination is it time to consider whether additional caries diagnostic tools should be employed.

References

Årtun J, Thylstrup A. Clinical and scanning electron microscopic study of surface changes of incipient caries lesions after debonding. *Scand J Dent Res* 1986; **94**: 193–201.

Amarante E, Raadal M, Espelid I. Impact of diagnostic criteria on the prevalence of dental caries in Norwegian children aged 5, 12, and 18 years. *Community Dent Oral Epidemiol* 1998; **26**: 87–94.

Backer Dirks O. Posteruptive changes in dental enamel. *J Dent Res* 1966; **104**: 480–5.

Bader JD, Shugars DA. What do we know about how dentists make caries-related treatment decisions? *Community Dent Oral Epidemiol* 1997; **25**: 97–103.

Baelum V, Fejerskov O. Caries diagnosis: 'a mental resting place on the way to intervention'? In: Fejerskov O, Kidd A, eds. *Dental caries: the disease and its clinical management.* Oxford; Blackwell Munksgaard, 2003: 101–10.

Baelum V, Heidmann J, Nyvad B. Dental caries paradigms in diagnosis and diagnostic research. *Eur J Oral Sci* 2006; **114**: 999.

Bickel M, Cimasoni G. The pH of human crevicular fluid measured by a new microanalytical technique. *J Periodontol Res* 1985; **20**: 35–40.

Carvalho JC, Ekstrand KR, Thylstrup A. Dental plaque and caries on occlusal surfaces of first permanent molars in relation to stage of eruption. *J Dent Res* 1989; **68**: 773–9.

Carvalho JC, van Neeuwenhuysen J-P, Maltz M. Traitement non opératoire de la carie dentaire. *Realites Cliniques* 2004; **15**: 235–48.

Dean HT, Arnold FA, Elvove E. Domestic water and dental caries. *Public Health Rep* 1942; **57**: 1155–79.

Deery C, Hosey MT, Waterhouse P. *Paediatric cariology.* London: Quintessence Publishing, 2004; pp. 9–30.

Ekstrand KR, Qvist V, Thylstrup A. Light microscope study of the effect of probing in occlusal fissures. *Caries Res* 1987; **21**: 368–74.

Ekstrand KR, Kuzmina I, Bjørndal L, Thylstrup A. Relationship between external and histological features of progressive stages of caries in the occlusal fossa. *Caries Res* 1995; **29**: 243–50.

Ekstrand KR, Ricketts DNJ, Kidd EAM. Reproducibility and accuracy of three methods for assessment of demineralization depth on the occlusal surface. *Caries Res* 1997; **31**: 224–31.

Fejerskov O. Concepts of dental caries and their consequences for understanding the disease. *Community Dent Oral Epidemiol* 1997; **25**: 3–12.

Fejerskov O, Manji F, Baelum V, Møller IJ. *Dental fluorosis. A handbook for health workers.* Copenhagen: Munksgaard, 1988.

Fejerskov O, Luan W-M, Nyvad B, Budtz-Jørgensen E, Holm-Pedersen P. Active and inactive root surface caries lesions in a selected group of 60- to 80-year-old Danes. *Caries Res* 1991; **25**: 385–91.

Frank RM, Brendel A. Ultrastructure of the approximal dental plaque and the underlying normal and carious enamel. *Arch Oral Biol* 1966; **11**: 883–912.

Gold SI, Hasselgreen G. Peripheral inflammatory root resorption. A review of the literature with case reports. *J Clin Periodontol* 1992; **19**: 523–34.

Hintze H, Wenzel A, Danielsen B, Nyvad B. Reliability of visual examination, fibre optic transillumination, and bitewing radiography, and reproducibility of direct visual examination following tooth separation for the identification of cavitated carious lesions in contacting approximal surfaces. *Caries Res* 1998; **32**: 204–9.

Holt ED, Azevedo MR. Fibre optic transillumination and radiographs in diagnosis of approximal caries in primary teeth. *Community Dent Oral Epidemiol* 1989; **6**: 239–47.

Hujoel PP, Mäkinen KK, Bennett CB, *et al.* Do caries explorers transmit infections within persons? An evaluation of second molar caries onsets. *Caries Res* 1995; **29**: 461–6.

Ismail AI. Visual and visual–tactile detection of dental caries. *J Dent Res* 2004a; **83** (Special Issue C): C56–66.

Ismail A. Diagnostic levels in dental public health planning. *Caries Res* 2004b; **38**: 199–203.

Ismail AI, Brodeur J-M, Gagnon P, *et al.* Prevalence of non-cavitated and cavitated carious lesions in a random sample of 7–9-year-old schoolchildren in Montreal, Quebec. *Community Dent Oral Epidemiol* 1992; **20**: 250–5.

Katz RV. The clinical diagnosis of root caries: issues for the clinician and the researcher. *Am J Dent* 1995; **8**: 335–41.

Kidd EAM, Beighton D. Prediction of secondary caries around tooth-colored restorations. *J Dent Res* 1996; **75**: 1942–6.

Kidd EA, Pitts NB. A reappraisal of the value of the bitewing radiograph in the diagnosis of posterior approximal caries. *Br Dent J* 1990; **6**: 195–200.

Kidd EAM, Joyston-Bechal S, Beighton D. Marginal ditching and staining as a predictor of secondary caries around amalgam restorations: a clinical and microbiological study. *J Dent Res* 1995; **74**: 1206–11.

Knottnerus JA, van Weel C. General introduction: evaluation of diagnostic procedures. In: Knottnerus JA, ed. *The evidence base of clinical diagnosis.* London; BMJ Books, 2001; 1–17.

Last JM. *A dictionary of epidemiology*, 4th edn. Oxford: Oxford University Press, 2001.

Lijmer JG, Bossuyt PM. Diagnostic testing and prognosis: the randomised controlled trial. In: Knottnerus AJ, ed. *The evidence base of clinical diagnosis.* London: BMJ Books, 2002: 61–80.

Loeche WJ, Svanberg ML, Pape HR. Intraoral transmission of *Streptococcus mutans* by a dental explorer. *J Dent Res* 1979; **58**: 1765–70.

Lussi A. Comparison of different methods for the diagnsis of fissure caries without cavitation. *Caries Res* 1993; **27**: 409–16.

Machiulskiene V, Nyvad B, Baelum V. Prevalence and severity of dental caries in 12-year-old children in Kaunas, Lithuania. *Caries Res* 1998; **32**: 175–80.

Machiulskiene V, Nyvad B, Baelum V. A comparison of clinical and radiographic caries diagnoses in posterior teeth of 12-year-old Lithuanian children. *Caries Res* 1999; **33**: 340–48.

Machiulskiene V, Nyvad B, Baelum V. Comparison of diagnostic yields of clinical and radiographic caries examinations in children of different age. *Eur J Paediatric Dent* 2004; **3**: 157–62.

Manji F, Fejerskov O, Baelum V. The pattern of dental caries in adult rural population. *Caries Res* 1989; **23**: 55–62.

Manji F, Fejerskov O, Baelum V, Luan W-M, Chen X. The epidemiological features of dental caries in African and Chinese populations: implications for risk assessment. In: Johnson NW, ed. *Dental caries. Markers of high and low risk groups and individuals*, Vol. I. Cambridge: Cambridge University Press, 1991; 62–99.

Mejáre I, Källestål C, Stenlund H. Incidence and progression of approximal caries from 11 to 22 years of age in Sweden: a prospective radiographic study. *Caries Res* 1999; **33**: 93–100.

Merriam-Webster 2003: www2.Merriam-webster.com/cgi-bin/mwmednlm

Mitropoulos CM. The use of fibre-optic transillumination in the diagnosis of posterior approximal caries in clinical trials. *Caries Res* 1985a; **19**: 370–84.

Mitropoulos CM. A comparison of fibre-optic transillumination with bitewing radiographs. *Br Dent J* 1985b; **159**: 21–3.

Mjör I. Clinical diagnosis of recurrent caries. *J Am Dent Assoc* 2005; **136**: 1426–33.

Nyvad B, Fejerskov O. Active root surface caries converted into inactive caries as a response to oral hygiene. *Scand J Dent Res* 1986; **94**: 281–4.

Nyvad B, Fejerskov O. Assessing the stage of caries lesion activity on the basis of clinical and microbiological examination. *Community Dent Oral Epidemiol* 1997; **25**: 69–75.

Nyvad B, Machiulskiene V, Baelum V. Reliability of a new caries diagnostic system differentiating between active and inactive caries lesions. *Caries Res* 1999; **33**: 252–60.

Nyvad B, Machiulskiene V, Baelum V. Construct and predicitve validity of clinical caries diagnostic criteria assessing lesion activity. *J Dent Res* 2003; **82**: 117–22.

Nyvad B, Machiulskiene V, Fejerskov O, Baelum V. Differential diagnosis of dental caries, dental fluorosis and localized opacities of non-fluoride origin. 2007 (personal communication).

Pitts NB. The use of bitewing radiographs in the management of dental caries: scientific and practical considerations. *Dentmaxillofac Radiol* 1996; **25**: 5–16.

Pitts NB. Modern concepts of caries measurement. *J Dent Res* 2004; **83**: (Special Issue C): C43–7.

Pitts NB, Fyffe HE. The effect of varying diagnostic thresholds upon clinical caries data for a low prevalence group. *J Dent Res* 1988; **67**: 591–6.

Pitts NB, Rimmer PA. An *in vivo* comparison of radiographic and directly assessed caries status of posterior approximal surfaces in primary and permanent teeth. *Caries Res* 1992; **26**: 146–52.

Purdell-Lewis DJ, Pot T. A comparison of radiographic and fibre-optic diagnoses of approximal caries lesions. *J Dent* 1973; **2**: 143–8.

Raper HR. Practical clinical preventive dentistry based upon periodic roentgen–ray examinations. *J Am Dent Assoc* 1925; (Sept): 1084–100.

Thylstrup A, Fejerskov O. Clinical appearance of dental fluorosis in permanent teeth in relation to histological changes. *Community Dent Oral Epidemiol* 1978; **6**: 315–28.

Thylstrup A, Fejerskov O. Clinical and pathological features of dental caries. In: Thylstrup A, Fejerskov O, eds. *Textbook of clinical cariology*. Copenhagen, Munksgaard, 1994: 111–57.

Thylstrup A, Bruun C, Holmen L. *In vivo* caries models – mechanisms for caries initiation and arrestment. *Adv Dent Res* 1994; **8**: 144–57.

Vaarkamp J, ten Bosch JJ, Verdonschot EH, Bronkhorst EM. The real performance of bitewing radiography and fiber-optic transillumination in approximal caries diagnosis. *J Dent Res* 2000; **79**: 1747–51.

Verdonschot EH, Bronkhorst EM, Wenzel A. Approximal caries diagnosis using fiber-optic transillumination: a mathematical adjustment to improve validity. *Community Dent Oral Epidemiol* 1991: **19**: 329–32.

Weerheim KL. Molar incisor hypomineralization (MIH): clinical presentation, aetiology and management. *Dent Update* 2004; **331**: 9–12.

World Health Organization. *Oral health surveys: basic methods*, 4th edn. Geneva: WHO, 1997.

Wright GZ, Simon I. An evaluation of transillumination for caries detection in primary molars. *J Dent Child* 1972; **39**: 199–202.

Wulff HR. What is understood by a disease entity. *J R Coll Physicians Lond* 1979; **13**: 219–20.

Wulff HR, Gøtzsche PC. *Rational diagnosis and treatment: evidence-based clinical decision making*, 3rd edn. Oxford; Blackwell Science, 2000.

Zubcevic M, Nyvad B.. Invasiv cervikal rodresorption – et overset klinisk problem? In: Holmstrup P, ed. *Odontologi 2007*. Copenhagen: Munksgaard Danmark, 2007: 127–40 (in Danish).

5

Radiography for caries diagnosis

I. Mejàre and E.A.M. Kidd

Introduction

Technical and quality aspects

Prescription and timing of bitewing radiography

References

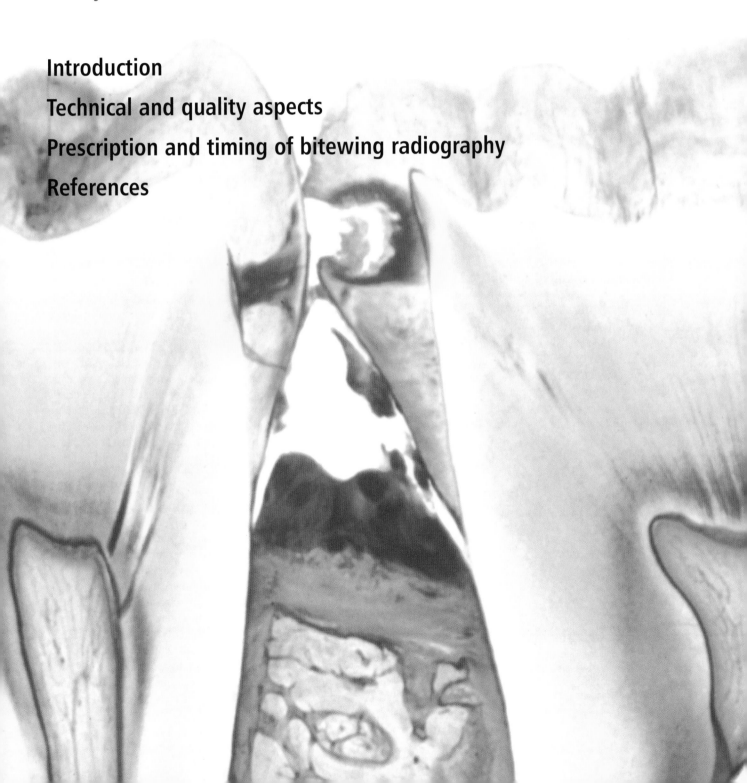

Introduction

The most commonly used radiographic method for detecting caries is the bitewing technique. The purpose of bitewing examination is to detect lesions that are clinically 'hidden' from a careful clinical–visual examination, such as when an adjacent tooth prevents the dentist from seeing an approximal lesion. The radiograph will also help to estimate the depth of this lesion. Furthermore, bitewing radiographs should always be examined for occlusal caries in dentin. It is very important to realize that this examination serves as an aid to caries diagnosis and that there are limitations to its benefits. Thus, for example, this examination will not determine whether a cavity is present. As with any diagnostic method, there are also inherent errors. In addition, the risks of exposing a person to ionizing radiation have to be considered and balanced against the benefits of bitewing examination. This is equally important for digital radiography, even if the radiation dose is reduced with this system.

The first part of this chapter will discuss technical aspects, benefits, risks and validity of bitewing radiography as an aid to diagnosis of caries. The second part deals with prescription and timing of bitewing examinations in relation to the expected rate of caries incidence and lesion progression.

Technical and quality aspects

How is the radiograph taken?

The central beam of X-rays is positioned to pass at right angles to the long axis of the tooth, and tangentially through the contact area. When film is used, a beam-aiming device on the film holder guides the position of the tube (Fig. 5.1). This directs the beam at right angles to the film. This predictably produces a good radiograph. In addition, it allows the operator to take subsequent films with almost identical

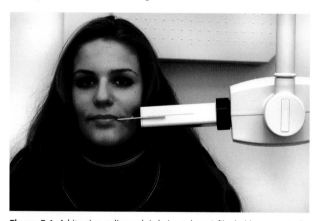

Figure 5.1 A bitewing radiograph is being taken. A film holder supports the film lingually and the patient closes together on a part of this holder. A beam-aiming device helps the operator to position the tube so that the beam is directed at right angles to the film.

geometry. This is very important when radiographs are compared for disease progression or arrest. In the fully dentate patient the central beam should be directed at the contact between the second premolar and first molar. In teenage populations with low caries prevalence, one radiograph on each side is sufficient, while in adults two films on each side are recommended.

Bitewing with film and with digital receptors

Digital radiography is now increasingly used in clinical practice and radiography based on film may therefore not be relevant in the near future. Current digital intraoral radiography systems and recently developed fast dental films have been reported to be as accurate as traditional films for the detection of caries (Wenzel, 1998). The potential advantages of digital radiography are as follows:

- The facilities for density and contrast enhancement can optimize the diagnostic quality and reduce retakes.
- The radiation dose is lower.
- No wet chemicals are involved in processing.
- The technique is less time consuming.

The effectiveness of digital radiography systems has usually been investigated in university settings. However, several issues regarding the use and effectiveness of digital radiography in clinical practice deserve attention. Thus, there is no evidence that the number of retakes has been reduced. Rather, surveys from Scandinavia indicate that the number of retakes increases, one major reason being difficulties in positioning the film when using the charge-coupled device (CCD), where a cord connects the receptor and the computer (Wenzel & Gotfredsen, 2000; Wenzel & Moystad, 2001). For bitewing radiography these sensors are suboptimal since the effective radiation field is smaller than the 2×2 film size, and in a study recording positioning errors the CCD sensors usually failed to show approximal canine and first premolar surfaces (Bahrami *et al.*, 2003). The thickness of the sensor and the cable that must come out of the mouth also make the system bulky, resulting in positioning problems, particularly in children. For these reasons dentists use digital radiography in parallel with the conventional film technique (Wenzel & Gotfredsen, 2000; Wenzel & Moystad, 2001). In a Dutch survey (Berkhout *et al.*, 2003), the total number of radiographs increased after conversion to digital radiography, and the authors conclude that the effective dose reduction may be less than 25% owing to the greater number of radiographs taken. Furthermore, there is sparse evidence that the facilities for density and contrast enhancement have changed clinical practice including improved diagnostic effectiveness. Possible economic benefits for the patient, the dentist and the society also remain to be established (Wenzel, 1998).

Another issue related to image quality of digital radiography that has received comparatively little attention is the quality of the digital hardware and software, along with the need for developing standards to ensure high quality in digital dental radiographs (Hellén-Halme *et al.*, 2005). Thus, adjustments of brightness and contrast of the monitor may have a considerable impact on image quality and observer performance (Hellén-Halme *et al.*, 2007).

No doubt, digital dental radiography will replace film radiography. Technical improvements are ongoing and include the development of a CCD that allows use of a beam-aiming device so that comparable geometry can be achieved.

Tools to facilitate detection of caries lesions such as computer-automated programs have been marketed but, at the time of writing, no accurate and objective system seems to be available for clinical practice (Wenzel, 2004). Subtraction image for monitoring lesion progression is another technique that may serve as an aid in the future. This technique requires that two radiographs are recorded in a standardized way with at least partly controlled projection angles. The information from the most recent radiograph can then be digitally subtracted from that of the former. Unchanged anatomical structures will cancel, and unchanged areas will be displayed in a neutral gray shade in the subtraction image. Areas with mineral loss during the follow-up time will be displayed in darker shades of gray (Wenzel, 1991). An example is shown in Fig. 5.2. It has to be appreciated, however, that this technique still only gives a two-dimensional picture of three-dimensional structures.

Radiographic diagnostic criteria

The most commonly used criteria for assessing the depth of approximal caries lesions are given in Fig. 5.3.

Balancing risks and benefit

A number of factors have caused the profession to re-evaluate the need for radiographic dental examinations. These factors are:

- the decrease in caries prevalence
- the relatively slow rate of progression of most carious lesions in populations regularly exposed to fluoride
- a revision of the estimates of health detriment caused by exposure to low-dose ionizing radiation, particularly for children.

Questions have been brought into focus such as when bitewing radiography for caries diagnosis is justified and how long the intervals between radiographic examinations should be (Pitts & Kidd, 1992; Smith, 1992). It is important to have appropriate selection criteria for radiography in order to arrive at the best diagnosis and treatment of the individual patient.

The balance between benefits and putative harmful effects is, however, a complex and delicate issue. Regarding possible health risks due to exposure to low-dose ionizing radiation, children are more sensitive than adults, the major risk being the induction of malignant disease, mainly parotid, thyroid and bone marrow cancer (ICRP, 1991). There is, however, no conclusive evidence that dental radiographs taken during childhood increase the risk of malignant disease (Preston-Martin & White, 1990; Rohlin & White, 1992). At present, the best available evidence, based on estimates of the lifetime risk from a single small dose of radiation, has been expressed as 'a small, difficult to quantify risk' of cancer from dental diagnostic exposures. Accordingly, the recommendations from the International

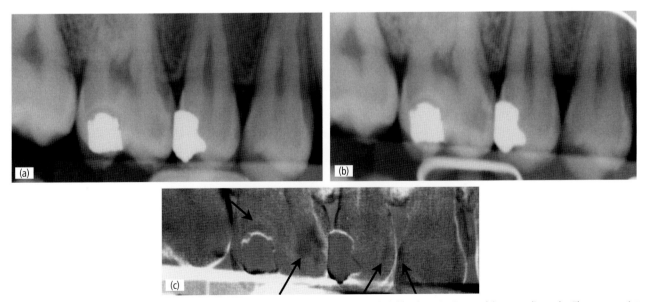

Figure 5.2 (a, b) Two digital bitewing radiographs taken 21 months apart in the same individual. (c) Subtraction image of the two radiographs. The arrows point to dark gray areas corresponding to the difference in radiolucency between baseline and follow-up after 21 months. (Courtesy of Roger Ellwood.)

R0 = no radiolucency
R1 = radiolucency confined to the outer
half of the enamel

 R2 = radiolucency in the inner half of the enamel
including lesions extending up to but not beyond
the enamel–dentin junction

 3 = radiolucency in the dentin;
broken enamel–dentin junction but without
obvious spread in the dentin

 R3 = radiolucency with obvious spread
in the outer half of the dentin
(< halfway through to the pulp)

 R4 = radiolucency with obvious spread
in the inner half of the dentin
(> halfway through to the pulp)

Figure 5.3 Radiographic scores used to classify depth of approximal carious lesions. Score 3 (in parentheses) was used by Mejàre *et al.* (1985) for assessing rate of progression in the dentin.

Commission on Radiological Protection (ICRP) are based on the following principles: 'No practice involving exposure to radiation should be adopted unless it produces sufficient benefit to the exposed individuals' and 'the magnitude of individual doses should be kept as low as reasonably achievable, economic and social factors being taken into account' (ICRP, 1991). It also says that it is necessary to make sound value judgments about the relative importance of different kinds of risk and about the balancing of risk and benefits.

It follows that unnecessary radiation to the patient should be avoided, implying that radiography for detecting caries must not be routinely used for all patients. Consequently, systematic and periodic radiographic examinations (screening) are not justified and, likewise, radiography for the diagnosis of dental caries in surveys is unethical. Instead, the decision to take radiographs should be based on individual grounds and there should be a clinical indication for every radiograph taken.

However, considering this element of risk should not become a fetish. It is important not to refrain from necessary radiography, or relevant information about the patient may be lost. One may put it like this: if a careful clinical examination has been performed with or without the use of additional diagnostic measures, such as fiber-optic transillumination (FOTI) or tooth separation, and a carious lesion is still suspected, then bitewing radiography is indicated to arrive at a proper caries diagnosis and treatment decision.

Technical quality of the radiographic examination

According to the recommendations of ICRP, it is the responsibility of the dental professional to reduce the radiation dose as much as possible, and unnecessary radiation

can be avoided to a very large extent if the examination is performed in a technically correct way. There are several simple ways to achieve this:

- use of a thyroid shield
- use of rectangular collimation, limiting the shape of the X-ray beam and reducing the patient exposure by up to 50% (Rohlin & White, 1992); this procedure also improves the quality of the image by reducing scattering of the X-ray beam
- use of digital radiography or the fastest film type, the F-type
- use of a film holder, for example Kwik-bite (Hawe Neos Dental, Bioggio, Switzerland), facilitating correct positioning of the film; this would give a good quality of the radiographic image and prevent retakes.

A radiograph with optimal contrast and exposure is best for an adequate interpretation while, for example, underdevelopment makes it difficult to detect a carious lesion. For caries diagnosis, the radiographs need to be relatively dark and with good contrast and sharpness. Film properties, exposure and film processing influence the film contrast. Of these, correct film processing is the most important. The radiation pattern transferred to the radiographic film is dependent on film properties, but the handling in the darkroom is critical to the quality of the image. Increase in film density (darkness) is achieved by increasing radiation dose.

The radiographic imaging of mineral loss caused by the carious process in the hard tissues also depends on the following:

- *A certain amount of mineral must be lost* before it can be detected in the radiograph. This minimum amount of mineral loss is determined by technical and physical factors such as film contrast, film processing and viewing conditions, but also by how the interpreter perceives the image.
- *The shape, extent and location of the carious lesion* and the anatomy of the tooth influence the radiographic depiction. As an example, a shallow but relatively widespread lesion along the proximal surface may create an image of being deeper than a relatively deep lesion, whose spread along the surface is comparatively narrow (Fig. 5.4).
- *Direction of the X-rays* has an important bearing on the image; they should pass in such a way that overlapping is avoided. If the projection deviates in either the vertical or the horizontal plane, the radiation has to travel a longer way through the tooth, resulting in a lower exposure than ideal, causing a decreased image contrast. Also, and perhaps more importantly, the lesion will be depicted in the wrong way, resulting in underestimation or overestimation of its extent. Such an example is given in Fig. 5.5. This figure emphasizes the importance of beam-aiming devices so that comparable geometry is achieved when

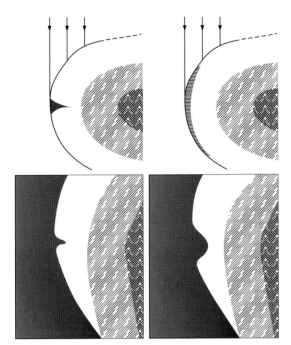

Figure 5.4 The shape and extent of a lesion influence its radiographic depiction. A superficial lesion with a great extent along a proximal surface may seem both deeper and darker than a lesion that is smaller in the direction of the X-rays but actually deeper.

films taken on different occasions are compared. These devices are very important when lesions are to be monitored radiographically.

Quality of interpretation of the radiographic image

Good diagnostic quality is not only good technical image quality. The perception and interpretation of the image

play an equally important role in the diagnostic process. Knowledge, experience, interest and expectations about what might be present in the image are factors that should be emphasized. With the decreasing caries prevalence in combination with reduced expectations, carious lesions may be overlooked. Figure 5.6 illustrates how too light an image, probably combined with no expectation to detect any carious lesions, resulted in neglected diagnosis and less than optimum treatment. It may also illustrate the ineffectiveness of bitewing radiography when it becomes a routine, rather than being based on individual judgment for the best individual treatment decision.

The opposite situation, the possibility of overdiagnosis and overtreatment, is equally important. As caries prevalence decreases, the risk of false-positive diagnoses increases (Gröndahl, 1994). Thus, it is important to have knowledge about the caries prevalence of the population under treatment. It also means that not all populations should be handled in the same way. In other words, the caries activity of the individual patient and the possibilities to reverse a high caries activity must be considered when making treatment decisions. In clinical practice, caries activity in children and adolescents is best assessed in terms of present carious lesions and restorations (see Chapter 29). Progression of lesions since the last examination also indicates that the patient is caries active. When radiographic images are to be compared in this way the use of film holders and beam-aiming devices is very important, so that comparable geometry is achieved (Fig. 5.5).

Detection of approximal caries: the bitewing technique

The value of the bitewing radiographic technique for detecting and assessing the depth of approximal caries

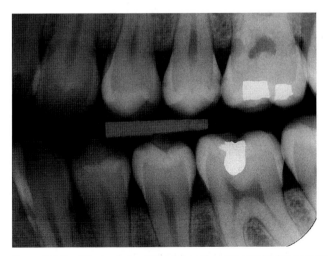
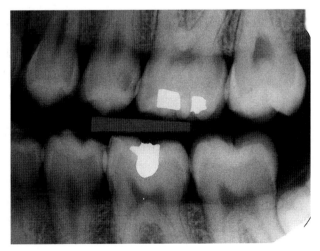

Figure 5.5 Two bitewing radiographs taken on the same occasion in a 14-year-old. Owing to different horizontal angulations of the X-ray beam, the radiograph on the left gives an image of the lesion of the distal surface of the upper left second premolar that is less extensive than what is seen in the radiograph on the right.

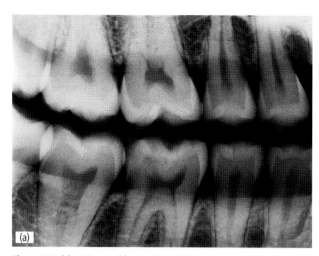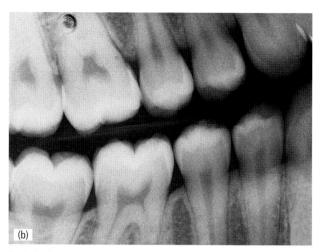

Figure 5.6 (a) A 25-year-old presenting with toothache in the lower right first molar (46). The bitewing radiograph reveals a deep occlusal dentin lesion in 46; (b) bitewing radiograph taken less than 2 years previously. It is far too light, without contrast and useless for caries diagnosis.

lesions is indisputable. It might be expected that the bitewing examination will become needed less as caries incidence has decreased. In fact, the opposite may be the case; perhaps it is increasingly important. The apparent decrease in caries prevalence reflects a slower rate of lesion progression and fewer fillings, but the disease has not disappeared. This particularly concerns approximal caries. Recent studies in Scandinavia show that at the age of 18–19 years, the mean number of approximal enamel lesions amounts to six or seven, while the mean number of restorations is low (Wang, 1995; Edblad *et al.*, 1998; Mejàre *et al.*, 1998). The strict philosophy towards limiting restorations in favor of other measures for preventing lesion progression does not negate the importance of assessing lesion progression through bitewing radiography.

The advantages of the bitewing technique are as follows.

- Surfaces that are inaccessible to clinical–visual inspection can be studied. More carious lesions are usually found when bitewing radiography is added to the clinical visual inspection. However, this depends on the thoroughness of the clinical examination. This will be discussed again later in this chapter.
- The depth of an approximal lesion can be assessed and the relation to the pulp estimated.
- Bitewing radiography is a non-invasive method; it does not mechanically harm possible demineralized tissues, unlike the probe, which has the potential to do so if not handled with care.
- The radiograph can be filed and re-examined. Thus, it can be used at a later date and compared with a more recent radiograph to decide whether a lesion is progressing or not.

However, the bitewing also suffers from shortcomings that have to be balanced against the advantages. Besides putative risks with low-dose radiation, the main disadvantages are as follows.

- The validity in diagnosing early lesions is rather low; that is, the early stages of the enamel lesion cannot be detected accurately.
- The bitewing radiograph is not unambiguous and cannot always distinguish between sound surfaces, surfaces with initial caries and cavitated lesions or non-carious demineralizations (hypoplasia). Judgments about cavitation have to rely on clinical inspection or the probability of a cavity in relation to the depth of the lesion as judged radiographically.
- The bitewing radiograph usually underestimates the depth of the lesion and lesions apparently confined to the inner enamel on radiograph are in dentin histologically. Owing to projection errors, overestimation can also occur.
- At least two consecutive bitewing radiographs, with similar projections, are necessary for assessing the caries activity of a lesion. This means that just one radiograph cannot determine whether a lesion is arrested or in a stage of lesion progression.
- The interpretation of the radiograph is subject to variations both between and within investigators.
- Bitewing radiography can only serve as a part of the necessary information that forms a diagnosis. The information from the radiographic image adds to other clinical data to facilitate diagnosis.

The advantages and disadvantages have to be balanced. So, when should bitewing radiographs be taken to detect possible approximal lesions and at what intervals should lesions be monitored for possible progression? Before discussing this, the accuracy, that is the validity and reliability of the radiographic diagnosis, has to be mentioned.

Validity

All diagnostic methods have inherent errors. Thus, even the most skilled interpreter analyzing radiographic images of the best quality will not separate perfectly sound from diseased surfaces. Results from a study by Mejàre *et al.* (1985) will be used to illustrate this. In that study, the radiographic diagnoses from bitewing radiographs were compared with the clinical–visual diagnoses in premolars and molars in 14–15-year-old children. Bitewing radiographs of high quality were taken and examined by trained observers before the premolars were extracted for orthodontic reasons. After extraction, the surfaces of the premolars and their neighboring surfaces in the mouth were inspected and diagnosed with the unaided eye. The results are shown in Table 5.1. It can be seen that almost half (203/463) of the approximal surfaces judged as sound from the bitewing radiograph had obvious white-spot lesions on visual inspection and five out of 463 (1%) had cavitated surfaces. Of surfaces judged to have radiolucencies confined to the outer two-thirds of the enamel, 93/116 (80%) had white-spot lesions and 13/116 (11%) had a cavity, whereas 10/116 (9%) were clinically sound. Of surfaces judged radiographically to have reached the inner third of the enamel and up to the enamel–dentin border, all had carious lesions on direct visual inspection; nine out of 13 had white-spot lesions and four out of 13 had a cavity. Only six surfaces were diagnosed as having radiolucencies in the dentin, and they all had cavities.

The imperfection of the radiographic examination can be further analyzed by entering the data from the study into a diagnostic decision matrix as illustrated in Table 5.2. A cavitated lesion was used as the cut-off point between sound and diseased surfaces. According to the data, 28/598 = 4.7% of the surfaces had clinical cavities. With such a low disease prevalence (clinical cavitation), the proportion of false-positive diagnoses will be high if any radiolucency is considered as a positive test value (112/135 = 0.83). If the cut-off point was changed, so that only radiolucencies that had reached at least the inner third of the enamel were chosen, the outcome changed (represented by figures in parentheses) and the proportion of false-positive diagnoses decreased from 112/135 = 0.83 to 9/19 = 0.47. The prevalence of cavities also influences the proportion of false-

positive diagnoses. The lower the prevalence, the higher the proportion of false-positive diagnoses.

When comparing the accuracy (the proportion of correctly diagnosed surfaces), it will be seen that with the less strict criteria for disease presence, the true-positive and true-negative diagnoses amounted to (23 + 458)/598 = 80%. With the more strict criteria for disease presence, the accuracy was 95% (10 + 561/598). There are more missed cavities with the latter method. Unless this is a decisive drawback, it seems reasonable to choose the stricter diagnostic criteria when the prevalence of cavities in a population is low. If it is considered important to reduce the proportion of false-positive diagnoses further, the cut-off point should be moved further into the dentin (see p. 80). In this material this was not possible, because the number of radiolucencies in the dentin was too small. How different cut-off levels influence the percentage of true-positive and false positive findings is illustrated in Fig. 5.7. It is obvious that no single cut-off point or diagnostic criterion exists that completely separates surfaces with cavities from those without.

Strictly, the validity of radiographic diagnosis of carious lesions can be assessed only using histology as the reference standard. Such *in vivo* studies are mostly performed on third molars. Their location and anatomy, however, make it difficult to generalize the results to clinical practice. Studies where visual–tactile examination has been used as the reference standard report wide ranges of sensitivities and/or specificities; owing to varying diagnostic criteria, sampling of teeth and types of lesions, sensitivity from 0.34 to 0.87 was found for cavitated lesions, whereas in general the specificity was high (AHRQ, 2001; Bader *et al.*, 2002). Thus, the validity in general was difficult to determine. Even so, bitewing examination is still the best available method for diagnosing caries on surfaces not available for direct visual inspection. It is important, however, to be aware of the shortcomings of the technique when interpreting the radiographic image and to realize that the information provided by it is just the start of a diagnostic process. The outcome in terms of treatment decision relies on sound judgment.

Table 5.2 Agreement between radiological findings and diagnoses upon direct inspection

Direct inspection	Radiolucency present	Radiolucency absent	Total
Cavity present	TP 23 (10)	FN 5 (18)	28
No cavity	FP 112 (9)	TN 458 (561)	570
Total	135 (19)	463 (579)	598

From Mejàre *et al.* (1985).
The figures represent two different extents of the radiolucencies considered positive for cavity presence. The numbers to the left represent surfaces where any radiolucency was considered positive, while the numbers in parentheses represent surfaces where only radiolucencies extending to at least the inner one-third of the enamel were regarded as positive for cavity presence.
TP: true positive; FN: false negative; FP: false positive; TN: true negative.

Table 5.1 Distribution of caries diagnoses upon direct inspection in relation to radiographic state

Bitewing examination	Visual inspection			
	Sound	White spot	Cavity	Total
Sound	255	203	5	463
Outer two-thirds of enamel	10	93	13	116
Inner one-third of enamel	0	9	4	13
In dentin	0	0	6	6
Total	265	305	28	598

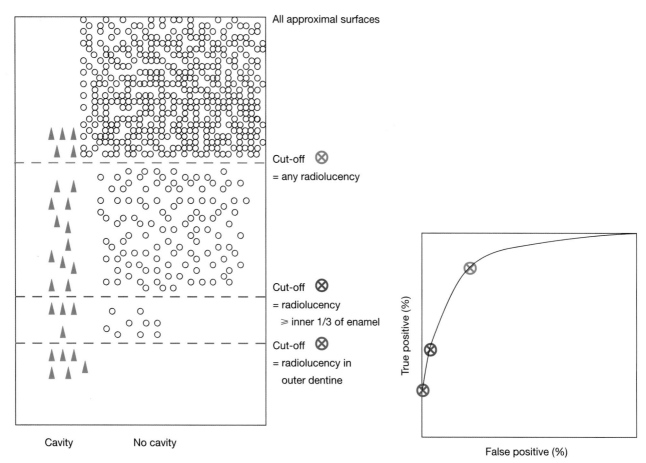

Figure 5.7 Illustration of the effect of using different cut-off levels on the number of true-positive findings (sensitivity) and the number of false-positive findings (1 – specificity). Three cut-off levels are shown in the figure to the left, where the red triangles represent approximal surfaces with a cavity and the circles surfaces without a clinical cavity. In the figure to the right, the results from using the three cut-off levels are depicted on a receiver operating characteristic (ROC) curve. For example, if lesions reaching outer dentin were chosen as cut-off, 21% (6/28) of the cavities would be correctly diagnosed without any false-positive findings. This value is represented by the green cross on the ROC curve. If the cut-off were set at lesions reaching at least to the inner third of the enamel, 10/28 cavities would be correctly diagnosed, but at the cost of nine false-positive findings. This cut-off level is represented by the blue cross on the ROC curve. If any radiolucency were used as cut-off, all but five cavities would be correctly diagnosed, but at the expense of a large number of false-positive findings corresponding to the red cross on the ROC. The data originate from a study on the accuracy of radiographic diagnosis of approximal surfaces (n = 598) using visual inspection as the reference standard (Mejàre et al., 1985).

It is important to realize that to avoid having to restore every approximal surface, some false-negative diagnoses must be accepted. Figure 5.8 shows a radiographic image of an approximal premolar surface without any obvious radiolucency, but a cavity is present. The entrance to the cavity was narrow, but it extended into the dentin; if left undisturbed, this carious lesion would probably have progressed fairly quickly. The relatively small amount of mineral loss in the direction of the X-ray beam probably explains why it was overlooked in the radiograph.

Detection of occlusal caries

The difficulties in correctly diagnosing occlusal caries by visual examination only, particularly in young permanent molars, have been highlighted in the literature since the mid-1990s. Bitewing radiographs should therefore complement the clinical–visual diagnosis, and this raises the sensi-

tivity of the diagnosis. However, this is only valid if obvious dentin caries is to be detected. For diagnosing occlusal enamel caries, bitewing radiography is inaccurate. Thus, fewer than half of occlusal lesions were detected radiographically compared with histological sectioning as the reference standard (Wenzel & Fejerskov, 1992).

As with approximal caries diagnosis, the film density has an impact on the diagnostic quality and relatively dark radiographs are preferable. It is particularly important to be aware of the Mach-band effect. This is a perceptual phenomenon where the contrast between a dark and a relatively light area is sharply demarcated, giving rise to a dark band (Fig. 5.9). This effect may result in false-positive diagnoses because there is a tendency to see radiolucency in the dentin at the enamel–dentin junction even though no dentin caries may be present. Therefore, the radiograph should be interpreted with caution, bearing in mind the

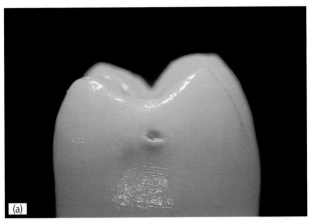
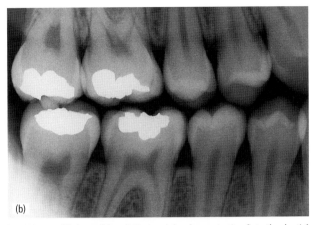

Figure 5.8 (a) Lower right second premolar (45) extracted for orthodontic reasons in a 14-year-old. A small but distinct and deeply penetrating (into the dentin) cavity is present on the distal surface; (b) a bitewing radiograph taken just before extraction shows no obvious radiolucency on the distal surface of 45.

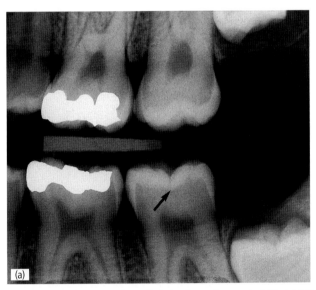
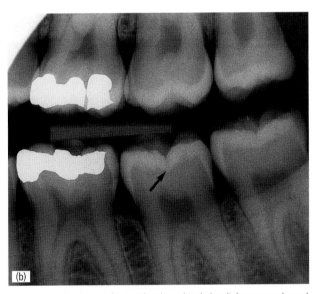

Figure 5.9 Two bitewing radiographs belonging to the same individual. (a) At 13 years of age: in the lower left second molar, a thin dark radiolucent area (arrow) can be detected at the occlusal enamel–dentin junction; (b) 8 years later (at 21 years of age), the same thin dark radiolucency can be seen, most probably representing the Mach band effect.

possibility of false-positive diagnosis in the enamel–dentin area.

Other diagnostic techniques such as FOTI and electrical resistance have higher sensitivity and lower specificity than bitewing radiography (Verdonshot *et al.*, 1992). FOTI seems to be as inaccurate as radiography for detecting occlusal enamel caries, but inferior to radiography for detecting obvious dentin lesions. The relatively new laser-fluorescence technique as an adjunct for occlusal caries diagnosis is discussed in Chapter 6.

Relative diagnostic yields of clinical and radiographic caries examination

It has been estimated that clinical examination alone detects less than 50% of the total approximal lesions found when clinical and radiographic diagnoses are combined, while bitewing examination used alone generally detects more than 90% of the total number of detected approximal lesions (Pitts, 1996). This has led to the common opinion that clinical–visual caries examination is a much poorer diagnostic tool than radiographic caries examination and that if clinical caries examination is not followed up by bitewing examination, a substantial number of caries lesions will be overlooked.

Two recent studies have demonstrated that the efficacy of bitewing examination strongly depends on the refinement of the clinical caries diagnostic criteria (Machiulskiene *et al.*, 1999, 2004). Figure 5.10 shows the results from the latter study, in which the relative diagnostic yields of independent clinical and radiographic caries recordings of the perma-

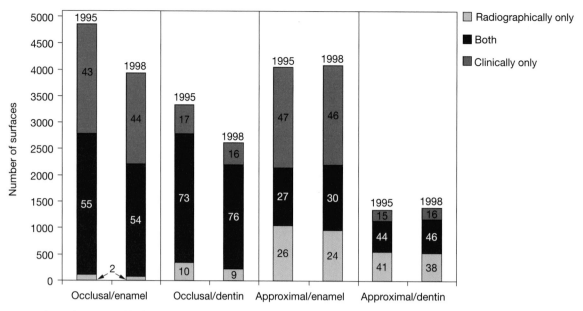

Figure 5.10 Relative diagnostic yield of clinical and radiographic methods in occlusal and approximal surfaces at the non-cavitated/enamel level and the cavitated/dentin level, respectively, in 12- and 15-year-old Lithuanian children with high caries prevalence. Numbers in the bars represent percentages. (From Machiulskiene *et al.*, 2004.)

nent posterior teeth in 12- and 15-year-old children were compared. The figure shows that the relative diagnostic yield of the two examination methods remained essentially the same for the two age groups. The results suggest that the radiograph was relatively unimportant for diagnosing non-cavitated enamel lesions, but of considerable importance at the approximal cavity/dentin level. It is important to appreciate that this study was carried out by one highly trained examiner. It is likely that the radiographic diagnostic yield would be higher in clinical practice. These two studies are important, however, because they emphasize the importance of careful visual examination of approximal sites so that early active enamel lesions are not overlooked.

Detection of caries in deciduous teeth

Radiographic examination of deciduous teeth has received comparatively little attention. Apart from their smaller dimensions and being set in comparatively small mouths, there are no differences between deciduous and permanent teeth. Thus, as with permanent teeth, the clinical–visual examination alone fails to detect a number of both occlusal and approximal carious lesions in primary molars. At the age of 5–6 years, for example, only 9% of approximal carious lesions could be detected without bitewing radiography (Stecksén-Blicks & Wahlin, 1983).

At the age of 5 years a majority of children present with contacting molars. From that age, most children can also co-operate with bitewing radiography and the sensitivity of detecting both occlusal and approximal caries increases with the use of this method compared with a visual examination alone. In a study by Ketley and Holt (1993), using

clinical–visual examination and bitewing radiography for diagnosing occlusal caries in second primary molars and first permanent molars, the accuracy for the permanent molars was 82% and for the primary molars 91%, suggesting somewhat better results for the deciduous teeth.

The use of FOTI for diagnosing approximal caries in deciduous teeth was investigated by Holt and Azevedo (1989). Using radiography as the validating criterion, the sensitivity for FOTI was 0.67–0.74 and the specificity was 0.95–0.97 (enamel and dentin caries were not separated). The reliability was, however, inferior to that of radiography and the authors concluded that in terms of accuracy and reliability, the use of FOTI offered no advantage over radiography. For children not accepting bitewing radiography and for radiographically overlapping surfaces, however, FOTI can serve as an alternative and/or complement to radiography for caries diagnoses in deciduous teeth.

Detection of recurrent and residual caries

Bitewing radiographs are important in the diagnosis of recurrent caries because this usually occurs cervically in the area of plaque stagnation (Fig. 5.11a). Sometimes a radiolucent area indicates that residual caries was left behind when the restoration was placed. Figure 5.11b shows a radiolucent area adjacent to an occlusal glass-ionomer cement restoration. The clinical picture taken after removal of the filling confirmed the presence of residual caries (Fig. 5.11c). As for interpreting occlusal caries at the enamel–dentin border, one has to be aware of the Mach-band effect and the possibility of false-positive diagnosis at the border between a filling and the adjacent dentin.

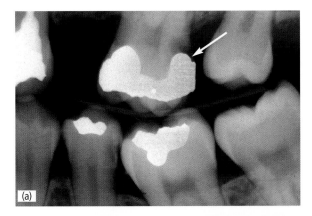

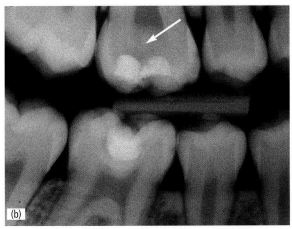

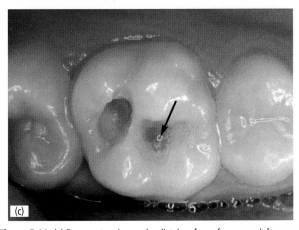

Figure 5.11 (a) Recurrent caries on the distal surface of an upper left second molar (arrow); (b) a radiolucent area adjacent to an occlusal glass-ionomer cement filling in the upper first molar (arrow); (c) soft dentin caries is present after removal of the filling (arrow).

Prescription and timing of bitewing radiography

For populations with low caries prevalence, annual bitewing radiographs are no longer justified. Instead, the decision to take radiographs should be based on the benefit to the individual patient in relation to the risks associated with low-dose radiation exposure and the costs. Prolonged

intervals up to 2.5–3 years between bitewing examinations for populations with generally low caries prevalence were suggested in 1986 (Shwartz et al., 1986), and more recent reports have confirmed that the intervals can be prolonged without jeopardizing the dental health of populations (Lith & Gröndahl, 1992). The expected benefits of bitewing examination depend on several factors, such as:

- the extent to which caries lesions can be detected from visual–tactile examination or by other means
- at what stage of lesion development the professional wants to detect lesions
- the expected rate of lesion progression
- at what stage the lesions are restored
- the amount of risk that the dentist is willing to take
- the quality of the radiographs and the diagnosis.

Key ages for bitewing examination in children and adolescents

Based on epidemiological data on caries risk at different ages, and the rate of lesion progression in children and teenagers with a generally low caries prevalence, four key ages have been identified when bitewing examination would be beneficial: 5, 8–9, 12–14 and 15–16 years (Mejàre, 2005). The rationale is to facilitate non-operative treatment by identifying lesions that are hidden from visual–tactile examination at an early stage and avoid arbitrary and 'just in case' radiographs.

Age 5

Even in populations with supposedly low caries prevalence, several studies have shown that bitewing radiographs at 5 years of age give a considerable diagnostic yield regarding otherwise undetected approximal lesions in primary molars for the majority of the children (Sköld et al., 1997; Boman et al., 1999; Raadal et al., 2000; Anderson et al., 2005). The diagnostic gain from bitewing examination compared with visual–tactile examination was 1.2–1.8 lesions (Sköld et al., 1997; Anderson et al., 2005). It would be useful to exclude children with negligible risk of approximal caries detected only by bitewing radiography. However, recent work has shown this is difficult (Anderson et al., 2005). An average accuracy of 73% was the best obtained when several clinical predictors were tested. The average sensitivity for the presence of enamel and dentin lesions was 0.48 and for the presence of dentin lesions it was 0.66. This implies that every second enamel lesion and every third dentin lesion was overlooked if the examination did not include bitewing radiography. Wide contact points are probably the major reason for the difficulties in the visual diagnosis of primary molars. Figure 5.12 shows the difference in the number of detected lesions without and with bitewing examination in a group of 5-year-olds with generally low caries prevalence. Twelve per cent of the children had at least one dentin lesion and 33% had at least one

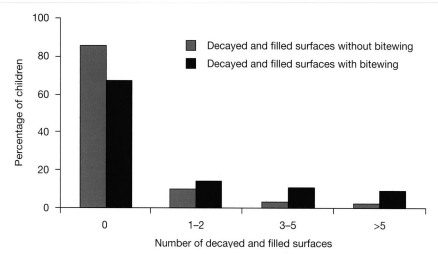

Figure 5.12 Percentage distribution of decayed and filled posterior surfaces without and with bitewing examination in Swedish 5-year-olds ($n = 267$). (From Anderson *et al.*, 2005.)

enamel lesion that could be detected from bitewing radiography only. The mean gain from adding bitewing examination was 1.2 lesions.

Age 8–9

The rationale behind age 8–9 as a second key age for bitewing examination is that the first permanent molar has been in contact with the second primary molar for about 2 years and therefore this surface is at risk of approximal caries. The image of the occlusal surface of the first permanent molar is also important to look for the presence of a dentin lesion that might have been overlooked at the clinical visual–tactile inspection. The mean diagnostic yield from bitewing radiography at age 8–9 was 1.43 enamel and dentin lesions including primary molars and mesial surfaces of permanent first molars (Lillehagen *et al.*, 2007). Altogether, 48% of the children benefited from bitewing examination. There is also benefit from identifying caries-free 8–9-year-olds; these children run a comparatively small risk of developing new approximal lesions during the next 2–3 years (unless other relevant risk factors or indicators are identified).

Age 12–14

The next key age is 12–14 years. Even in low caries prevalence populations, about 20% of the children have at least one approximal carious lesion that will be overlooked without bitewing radiography. The loss of information when excluding bitewing radiography in a population with low caries prevalence in young permanent teeth in Dutch children at the ages of 12 and 14 has been estimated (de Vries *et al.*, 1990; Flinck *et al.*, 1999). At the age of 12, 10.3% of the approximal surfaces were incorrectly judged as sound by clinical examination only and this number increased to 14.6% at the age of 14. The DMFS (decayed, missing and filled surfaces) values of approximal surfaces from the clin-

ical and radiographic examinations are shown in Table 5.3. It can be seen that if radiography was used as the validation criterion, a mean of 2.8 (4.1–1.3) enamel lesions would be left undiagnosed without radiography, while only a mean of 0.4 (1.1–0.7) dentin lesions was left undiagnosed without radiography. Likewise, regarding dentin caries, in a study of 14-year-old Danish children with low caries prevalence, only 1.6% of the approximal surfaces were incorrectly classified as sound through clinical examination only (Hintze & Wentzel, 1994).

So, if only dentin lesions are considered of interest, very small numbers will be overlooked by clinical examination alone at these ages. However, it is equally important to target children with active enamel lesions of approximal surfaces. It therefore seems reasonable to conclude that, even in a population with low caries prevalence, a majority of children will benefit from bitewing examination at the age of 12–14 years. The choice of age should be adjusted individually with respect to the time of eruption of permanent premolars and second molars. Figure 5.13 illustrates how the stage of tooth eruption may differ in 12-year-olds.

Table 5.3 Approximal caries lesions in premolars and molars in 14-year-old Dutch children: mean (SD) of decayed (D), missing (M) and filled (F) approximal surfaces per child according to clinical and radiographic criteria

Diagnosis	Approximal surfaces ($n = 24$)		All surfaces
	D2MFS	D3MFS	DMFS
Clinical	1.3 (2.2)	0.7 (1.5)	5.0 (5.1)
Radiographic	4.1 (5.0)	1.1 (2.1)	5.4 (5.5)

From de Vries *et al.* (1990).
D2MFS: including enamel lesions; D3MFS: excluding enamel lesions. Number of children: 317.

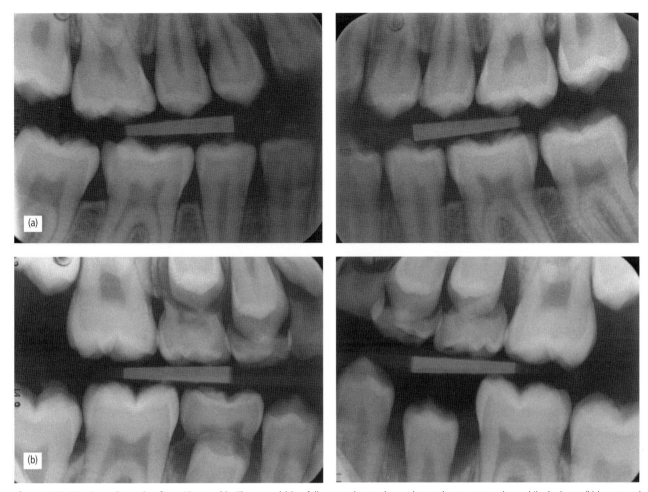

Figure 5.13 Bitewing radiographs of two 12-year-olds. The upper (a) has fully erupted premolars and second permanent molars, while the lower (b) has several primary molars still in place and only partly erupted second permanent molars. In (b), bitewing examination is not be needed because a visual inspection of approximal sites would reveal any lesion.

Children judged as having negligible caries risk (good oral hygiene and dietary habits and no previous caries experience) may be excluded from bitewing radiography at these ages, since the diagnostic yield from bitewing radiography may be minimal. Age 12–14 is also useful for risk assessment; individuals who are caries free (including approximal surfaces) at this age run a small risk of developing approximal lesions, whereas those with several approximal lesions run a high risk of developing one or more new approximal lesions up to the age of 22 years (Table 5.4).

Age 15–16

Age 15–16 is the fourth key age. The first 3–4 years after tooth eruption and establishment of approximal contacts constitute a period of particular risk of new approximal carious lesions (Mejàre *et al.*, 2004) and age 15–16 is therefore a key age for considering bitewing examination. As for the other key ages, a caries-free 15–16-year-old runs a very small risk of developing new lesions during the next

3 years, assuming no other relevant risk indicators. Further intervals between radiographic examinations should be scheduled individually and risk assessment should include the number and extent of approximal carious lesions found at baseline (see below). It should be remembered that intervals between clinical and radiographic examination do not have to be identical.

Diagnostic yield from bitewing examination in adults

There is comparatively little evidence concerning diagnostic yield of bitewing radiography for caries in adults. Since the caries process and caries activity are dependent on the same factors as in children and adolescents, it seems reasonable to assume that the information available from studies of children and young adults can be used for adults. In general, the caries process is comparatively slow, but rapid behavior and lifestyle changes can have a significant impact on both caries incidence and lesion progression. Special attention should also be paid to the third molar and

Table 5.4 Relative risk (RR) of new approximal lesions up to age 21 in relation to caries experience at age 12–13

No. of approximal lesions at age 12–13[a]	Incidence	RR
0	3.1[b]	1.0
1–2	5.0	1.5
3	7.7	1.9
4–8	10.8	2.3
>8	21.1	3.2

From Stenlund *et al.* (2002).
[a] Including enamel lesions.
[b] Interpreting incidence: if 100 surfaces at risk are followed for 1 year, 3.1 new carious lesions can be expected.

the distal surface of the second molar, since the location may imply difficulties in plaque removal (Fig. 5.14).

Rate of lesion progression

Monitoring lesion progression (or arrest) of approximal enamel and dentin lesions and occlusal dentin lesions requires repeated bitewing examinations. It is important to remember that the good quality of radiographs and caries diagnosis is more important than frequent intervals between examinations. However, even with radiographs of good quality, small differences in projection, darkness and/or contrast can make it difficult to assess whether the lesion has diminished, progressed or become arrested.

The rate of lesion progression varies from patient to patient. In assessing the risk for further caries development, dentists use mainly the number of lesions with which the patient presents. However, other information about the patient such as oral hygiene, dietary habits, attitudes and sociological factors, medical and salivary status may also be relevant. This package of information provides the best

basis for treatment decision related to the caries risk of patients. The dentist will, however, rarely have all the necessary information available to be able to predict what is going to happen to a particular lesion. In fact, the clinical decision is often made on rather uncertain foundations. Based on the clinician's knowledge and experience, caries diagnoses may be looked upon as educated guesses. Importantly, these educated guesses should be based on the best available information.

Factors related to lesion progression in children, adolescents and young adults

Caries rates and survival times of approximal enamel caries in permanent posterior teeth

In populations with generally low caries risk, the rate of progression of approximal enamel lesions in young permanent teeth is slow (Shwartz *et al.*, 1984; Lervik *et al.*, 1990; Mejàre *et al.*, 1999), e.g. the mean annual caries rate from 11 to 22 years was 3.9 new approximal enamel lesions (reaching at least the inner half of enamel) per 100 tooth surfaces at risk (Mejàre *et al.*, 1999). The annual caries rate was 5.4 from the inner half of the enamel to the outer half of the dentin and the median survival time for these lesions was more than 8 years. It should be noted that not all enamel lesions progressed slowly; 10% progressed from enamel to dentin within 2.5 years.

Caries rates and survival times of approximal dentin caries in permanent posterior teeth

There are very few studies reporting on the rate of progression in the dentin. The following is based on a radiographic prospective longitudinal study of Swedish individuals from 12 (DMFT = 3.2 at this age) to 22 years of age where restorative treatment was performed only for lesions that showed

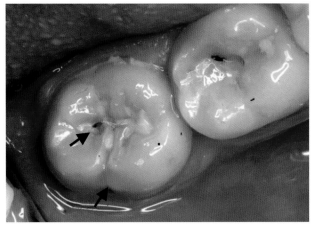 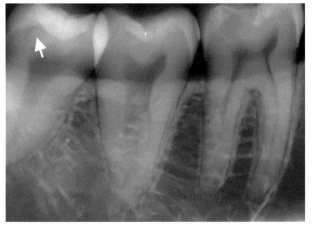

Figure 5.14 A 27-year-old patient previously classified as low caries risk because of no approximal lesions or fillings and few occlusal lesions. The clinical picture shows a lower right third molar with visible plaque on the lingual surface and cavities on the occlusal and buccal surfaces (arrows). A radiolucency in the dentin is shown in the radiograph (arrow). Note that the relative positions of the second and third molars resulted in an overlapping contact point so, in this case, it was not possible to check whether or not there were approximal lesions on the distal surface of the second molar and the mesial surface of the third molar.

obvious progression in the outer half of the dentin (Mejàre *et al.*, 1998, 1999). The population was exposed to regular dental care and prophylactic programs. The rate of progression in dentin was almost four times higher than from inner enamel to dentin, and 20.3 new lesions per 100 surfaces at risk progressed into the outer half of the dentin each year (Fig. 5.15). The corresponding medial survival time was 3.1 years (Fig. 5.16). This means that of the approximal lesions that had reached and just passed the enamel–dentin border but revealed no obvious radiolucency in the dentin (edj-lesions, score 3; see Fig. 5.3), 50% progressed into the dentin within 3 years as judged radiographically, while 50% did not. Again, these figures are median values, implying that there were considerable variations both between surfaces and between individuals. Thus, for example, out of those 50% that had progressed into the dentin, 20% did so within 1.2 years. The above-mentioned population lived in an area where the fluoride

content in the drinking water was 0.3 ppm. A slightly higher median survival time of lesions in the outer dentin of 3.4 years was reported by Lith *et al.* (2002), who studied a population living in an area with 1.2 ppm fluoride in the drinking water.

Considerable differences in the caries rates have been reported between the different surfaces (Mejàre *et al.*, 1999). Figure 5.17 shows the median time for progression in the dentin (from the edj to progression in the outer half of the dentin) for different posterior surfaces between 11 and 22 years of age. The distal surface of the lower first molar and the distal surface of the upper second premolar are surfaces at risk for relatively fast progression in both enamel and dentin. It should be noted that the values of the rates of caries progression come from carefully performed studies with high demands on the technical quality of the radiographs. If radiographs with poorer quality are used, the values may not correspond.

Most of the above-mentioned figures are median values, and their relevance to the individual patient in the clinic depends on a number of factors:

- cavitation
- depth of the lesion as judged radiographically
- caries activity (previous caries experience; number of active enamel lesions)
- posteruptive age of the tooth (until young adulthood)
- specific tooth surface (e.g. distal of upper second premolar versus distal of lower first premolar)
- status of the neighboring surface
- iatrogenic preparation damage of the surface.

Lesion progression related to cavitation

Irrespective of the radiographic extension of the lesion, cavitation is the crucial turning-point for the rate of lesion progression. Now lesion progression will speed up (Fig. 5.18). The radiographic image cannot help the dentist to decide

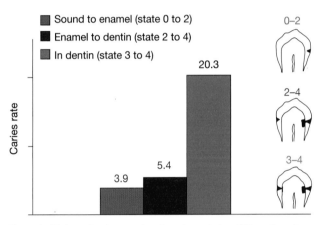

Figure 5.15 Annual caries rates (number of new lesions/100 tooth surface-years) of posterior approximal surfaces from 12 to 22 years of age. Median values of all surfaces. (From Mejàre *et al.*, 1999.)

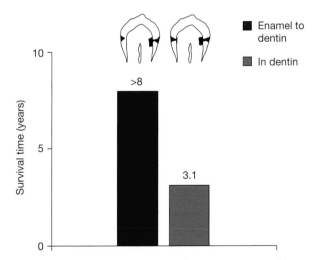

Figure 5.16 Median survival time in years for posterior approximal lesions from 11 to 22 years of age. (From Mejàre *et al.*, 1999.)

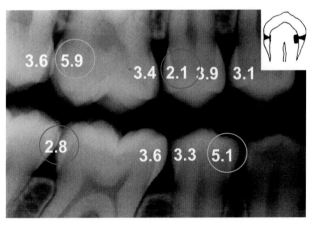

Figure 5.17 Median time for progression (50% survival) in years from state 3 to state 4 for the different approximal surfaces in a Swedish cohort from 11 to 22 years of age. (From Mejàre *et al.*, 1999.)

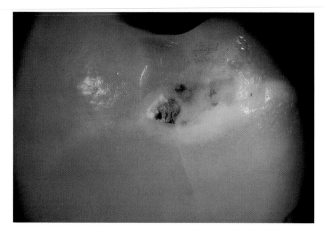

Figure 5.18 A cavity on an approximal surface of a premolar extracted for orthodontics reasons. The cavity is limited in extent, but with deep penetration into enamel and dentin. Supposing the premolar had been left in place and unrestored at this stage, this lesion would have progressed fairly rapidly.

whether or not there is a cavity. One way to confirm the presence or absence of a cavity is to use the tooth separation technique. There are, however, no comprehensive studies reporting on the efficiency of such risk-assessment procedures. The depth of the lesion as judged radiographically is related to the presence of a cavity; the deeper the lesion the higher the risk of cavitation (Mejàre & Malmgren, 1986). Table 20.1 summarizes the clinical studies that have linked radiographic appearance and cavitations in permanent teeth.

Lesion progression related to caries experience

Based on the number of lesions at baseline, Shwartz *et al.* (1984) found a higher rate of caries progression through the enamel in high- versus low-risk children and adolescents. Thus, individuals with a high number of approximal lesions run a greater risk than individuals with few lesions. Moreover, several studies have shown that children with one or more approximal dentin lesions or restorations at the age of 12–13 years run a higher risk of developing new approximal lesions than those without such lesions (Gröndahl *et al.*, 1984; Lith & Gröndahl, 1992; Mejàre *et al.*, 1999). A corresponding influence on the rate of caries progression of the number of decayed and filled surfaces at baseline has been observed in older adults (Berkey *et al.*, 1988). Therefore, the previous history of restorations is a valuable indicator in risk assessment.

Lesion progression related to posteruptive age

Only a few studies have compared the rate of progression as a function of the posteruptive age of the surface. According to Shwartz *et al.* (1984), the rate of progression through the enamel in permanent teeth is relatively fast in young children; in a group of Swedish and US children and young adults, the median time for progression through the enamel was about 4 years for 10–11-year-olds and >7 years for 17–22-year-olds (the ages at the end of study). In another study (Mejàre & Stenlund, 2000), the caries rate for the mesial surface of the first permanent molars was compared in two age groups, 6–11 and 12–22 years of age, in the same individuals. While the rate of progression into the inner half of the enamel was non-significantly higher in the younger age group, the rate from the inner half of the enamel to the outer half of the dentin was almost four times faster in the younger age group. Thus, progression through the enamel is comparatively fast in newly erupted young permanent teeth, particularly for the mesial surface of the first permanent molar, while it is slower in older adolescents and young adults. Since older children, in general, clean their teeth better than younger children, it cannot be ruled out that plaque stagnation plays an important role in explaining the faster progression of caries in young children.

In a longitudinal study, the rates of lesion progression expressed as survival times were compared for three age groups: 12–15, 16–19 and 20–27 years of age (Fig. 5.19). It can be seen that the survival time of both sound surfaces and progression of enamel and dentin lesions depended on age; the older the individual, the longer the survival times.

Limited data exist on the effect on lesion development of caries on neighboring approximal tooth surfaces. A Swedish study of 6–12-year-olds showed that the mesial surface of the first permanent molar had a negligible risk for developing caries when adjacent to a sound approximal surface of a primary second molar. If the primary molar had a carious lesion, the rate was almost 15 times higher (Mejàre *et al.*, 2001).

Lesion progression due to iatrogenic damage

Preparation damage of neighboring approximal surfaces when preparing class II cavities seems to occur embarrassingly frequently (Medeiros & Seddon, 2000; Qvist *et al.*, 1992). It has been shown that the bur had damaged almost 70% of all surfaces neighboring a class II restoration during cavity preparation (Qvist *et al.*, 1992). This damage resulted in a four-fold increase in restorative treatment compared with those without a restored neighboring surface. Therefore, a proximal protector should be used for the adjacent tooth when preparing class II and class III restorations. Explorers must also be used with care.

Caries rates and survival times of occlusal caries in permanent teeth

For occlusal surfaces, particularly permanent molars, progression rates were still high in the 1980s, with 50–60% of occlusal surfaces of first permanent molars being decayed or restored at the age of 11–12 years (Abernathy *et al.*, 1986; Dummer *et al.*, 1988). More recent studies on the incidence of occlusal dentin caries are scarce, but for premolars and

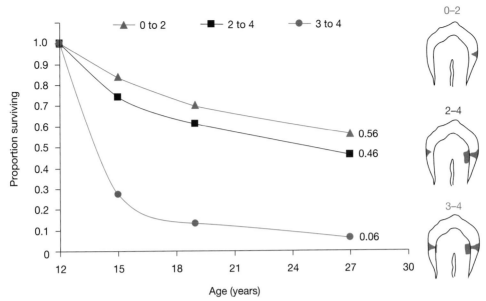

Figure 5.19 Survival curves (cumulative proportion surviving) of posterior approximal surfaces from 12 to 27 years of age; from radiographically sound to the inner half of the enamel (0–2), from inner enamel to outer dentin (2–4) and from enamel–dentin border to outer dentin (3–4). (From Mejàre *et al.*, 2004.)

second molars, longitudinal data suggest that lesion progression is rather slow in populations with low caries risk (Mejàre *et al.*, 2004). The frequent use of fissure sealants for first permanent molars in contemporary child populations makes it difficult to assess the natural history of progression of this surface.

The initiation and rate of progression of caries in permanent molars are highest during the first few years after eruption (Abernathy *et al.*, 1986), and the time immediately after eruption appears to be the most critical (Carvalho *et al.*, 1992). Survival curves on the incidence of occlusal dentin caries in a population where fissure sealing was not used illustrate this (Fig. 5.20). The slope of the curve shows that most new dentin lesions occurred between 12 and 15 years of age. It should be noted that, for the first molar, the data show only those who were radiographically sound at the age of 12 (when the study started at the age of 12, first molars that were already filled or had dentin caries were

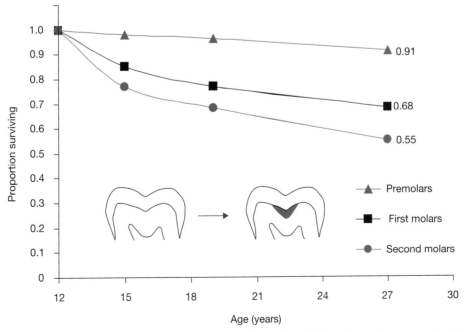

Figure 5.20 Survival curves (cumulative proportion surviving) of occlusal surfaces of premolars and first and second permanent molars from 12 to 27 years of age; from radiographically sound to obvious radiolucency in dentin. (From Mejàre *et al.*, 2004.)

excluded from the analysis). The figure also shows that the incidence of dentin caries of premolars is considerably lower than for molars. Perhaps this is explained by the premolar being easier to clean because it is farther forward in the mouth and less likely to be missed by the brush.

When examining bitewing radiographs, it is important not to forget the occlusal surfaces. This may seem obvious, but occlusal surfaces are easily forgotten when one is focussing on approximal sites (Kidd *et al.*, 1992). Fissure sealed occlusal surfaces should be analyzed carefully, since recent reports indicate that decay under sealants in young adults may be a frequent finding. Thus, in 20-year-olds, radiolucencies in bitewing radiographs were observed underneath one-quarter of the sealants applied (Poorterman *et al.*, 2000). It is not yet known whether these lesions will progress.

Rate of caries progression in primary teeth

Available data suggest that the progression of enamel lesions in primary teeth is about twice that of young permanent teeth, possibly because the approximal enamel of primary teeth is considerably thinner than that in permanent teeth. In one study, the median time for progression through the enamel was about 2.5 years (Shwartz *et al.*, 1984). However, neither the different surfaces nor the age of the children were specified in that study.

In children aged 6–12 years, the caries rates for the distal surface of the second primary molar and the mesial surface of the first permanent molar have been estimated between two stages: from sound surfaces to inner enamel lesions and from inner enamel to dentin lesions (Mejàre & Stenlund, 2000) (Fig. 5.21). The caries rate (caries rate = incidence = number of surfaces expected to progress in 1 year out of 100 surfaces at risk) in the enamel of the primary molar was more than twice that of the permanent molar, while the

rates into the dentin were relatively high for both surfaces and not statistically significant from each other. To date, there are no other data on the caries rates for the different approximal surfaces of primary molars. This different progression time should be considered when deciding on the interval between radiographic examinations.

Lesion progression in older adults

Data on the rate of progression in older adults are scarce. In the USA, two cohorts of men, 41 and 51 years of age at baseline, were followed for 10 years (Berkey *et al.*, 1988). Because of the different analytical design, comparisons are hardly justified, but the results indicate a median time for progression through the enamel of about 6 years. The rate of progression was slightly higher for the younger group. Using direct measurements, the rate of progression in the dentin was estimated in 19–79-year-olds. After 3 years, 50% of the lesions that had just penetrated the edj (radiolucency in the dentin <0.5 mm) at baseline had progressed, while almost 90% of deeper lesions (radiolucency in the dentin ≥0.5–1 mm) had progressed within 20 months (Foster, 1998). These data indicate that there are no major differences in the rate of progression between younger and older adults.

Implications for the prescription of bitewing examination

Since treatment philosophies have changed and operative treatment is usually no longer advocated for approximal caries until the lesion has progressed in the dentin, the depth of the approximal lesion should be taken into account when deciding on the interval before the next radiographic examination. Traditionally, radiographic examinations have been carried out at yearly intervals

	Enamel			Dentin		
	Radiographic scores: 0–2			2–4		
Tooth surface	Caries rate	Relative risk		Caries rate	Relative risk	
16m+26m+36m+46m	4.6			20.5		
55d+65d+75d+85d	11.3	2.5		32.6	1.6*	

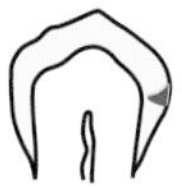

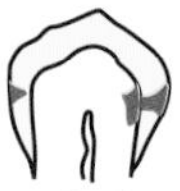

*Difference not statistically significant

Figure 5.21 Caries rates for the mesial surface of the first permanent molar and the distal surface of the second primary molar, and relative caries rate risks of the two neighboring tooth surfaces from 6 to 12 years of age; from radiographically sound to enamel caries and from enamel caries to dentin caries. (From Mejàre & Stenlund, 2000.)

when any approximal lesion is present. However, as the median survival time of lesions from inner enamel to outer dentin is more than 8 years in populations with low caries risk, occasional inner enamel lesions do not require radiographs at yearly intervals. The caries activity of the individual must, however, be taken into consideration and in this respect, the number of lesions is an important factor. The presence of several lesions increases the risk that at least one of them will progress relatively quickly, compared with one single lesion.

Regarding approximal lesions that have reached the enamel–dentin border (edj lesions), the rate of progression is markedly higher. Assuming that it is important to detect the 20% edj lesions that progress into the outer half of the dentin within about a year and avoid further progression in the dentin, edj lesions should be monitored at yearly intervals. Notably, it is not only the depth of the dentin lesion that is important; the risk of undermining of the cusps also has to be considered when caries progresses in the dentin. Preferably, an individually based risk assessment for edj lesions should be performed. As with enamel lesions, the number of lesions is an important risk factor; the more edj lesions, the higher the risk that at least one will progress relatively quickly. An example of this is shown in Fig. 5.22.

To summarize, intervals between bitewing examinations should be based on individual risk assessment. According to available data on expected rates of caries incidence and lesion progression, annual examinations should be considered in the following situations:

- age 5–7: one or more approximal dentin lesion or several approximal enamel lesions in primary molars
- age 7–12 (mixed dentition): a permanent first molar with approximal caries, half through the enamel or several approximal lesions in primary molars

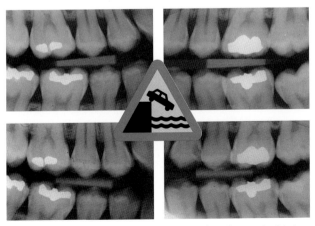

Figure 5.22 A 19-year-old appears with a number of approximal lesions radiographically judged as being at the enamel–dentin border. After 1 year, one of these lesions (the distal surface of the upper left first premolar) has progressed to a deep dentin lesion.

- age 12–13:
  - one or more approximal dentin lesion or restored approximal surface
  - three or more approximal enamel lesions
  - any unrestored approximal dentin lesion
  - a recently restored approximal neighboring surface.

The degree of caries risk should be reassessed individually by considering the number of new lesions, and progression of existing lesions, as well as other relevant risk factors. The interval to the next bitewing examination is adjusted accordingly. Intervals shorter than 1 year are seldom indicated. A 6-month interval is, however, advocated if several approximal dentin lesions are left unrestored. This applies to children and young adults. Evidence for the need for 6-month intervals in adults is at present lacking.

References

Abernathy JR, Graves RC, Greenberg BG, Bohannan HM, Disney JA. Application of life table methodology in determining dental caries rates. *Community Dent Oral Epidemiol* 1986; **14**: 261–4.

AHRQ. *Diagnosis and management of dental caries.* Evidence Report/Technology Assessment, No. 36. AHRQ Publications No. 01–E056, 2001.

Anderson M, Stecksen-Blicks C, Stenlund H, Ranggård L, Tsilingaridis G, Mejàre I. Detection of approximal caries in 5-year-old Swedish children. *Caries Res* 2005; **39**: 92–9.

Bader JD, Shugars DA, Bonito AJ. A systematic review of the performance of methods for identifying carious lesions. *J Public Health Dent* 2002; **62**: 201–13.

Bahrami G, Hagström C, Wenzel A. Bitewing examination with four digital receptors. *Dentomaxillofac Radiol* 2003; **32**: 317–21.

Berkey CS, Douglass CW, Valachovic RW, Chauncey HH. Longitudinal radiographic analysis of carious lesion progression. *Community Dent Oral Epidemiol* 1988; **16**: 83–90.

Berkhout WE, Sanderink GC, Van der Stelt PF. Does digital radiography increase the number of intraoral radiographs? A questionnaire study of Dutch dental practices. *Dentomaxillofac Radiol* 2003; **32**: 124–7.

Boman R, Enochsson B, Mejàre I. Should we take bitewing radiographs in 5-year-olds showing no clinical signs of approximal caries? *Tandläkartidningen* 1999; **91**: 37–40. (English summary.)

Carvalho JC, Thylstrup A, Ekstrand KR. Results after 3 years of non-operative occlusal caries treatment of erupting permanent first molars. *Community Dent Oral Epidemiol* 1992; **20**: 187–92.

Dummer PM, Addy M, Oliver SJ, Hicks R, Kingdon A, Shaw WC. Changes in the distribution of decayed and filled tooth surfaces and the progression of approximal caries in children between the ages of 11–12 years and 15–16 years. *Br Dent J* 1988; **164**: 277–82.

Edblad E, Gustafsson A, Svenson B, Jansson L. Number and frequency of bitewing radiographs and assessment of approximal caries in 14- to -19-year-old Swedish adolescents. *Swed Dent J* 1998; **22**: 157–64.

Flinck A, Källestål C, Holm AK, Allebeck P, Wall S. Distribution of caries in 12-year-old children in Sweden. Social and oral health-related behavioural patterns. *Community Dent Health* 1999; **16**: 160–5.

Foster LV. Three year *in vivo* investigation to determine the progression of approximal primary carious lesions extending into dentine. *Br Dent J* 1998; **185**: 353–7.

Gröndahl H-G. Radiographic diagnosis in caries management. In: Thylstrup AFO, ed. *Textbook of clinical cariology*, 2nd ed. Copenhagen: Munksgaard, 1994: 367–82.

Gröndahl HG, Andersson B, Torstensson T. Caries increment and progression in teenagers when using a prevention- rather than restoration-oriented treatment strategy. *Swed Dent J* 1984; **8**: 237–42.

Hellén-Halme K, Rohlin M, Petersson A. Dental digital radiography: a survey of quality aspects. *Swed Dent J* 2005; **29**: 81–7.

Hellén-Halme K, Nilsson M, Petersson A. Digital radiography in general dental practice: a field study. *Dentomaxillofac Radiol* 2007; **36**: 249–55.

Hintze H, Wenzel A. Clinically undetected dental caries assessed by bitewing screening in children with little caries experience. *Dentomaxillofac Radiol* 1994; **23**: 19–23.

Holt RD, Azevedo MR. Fibre optic transillumination and radiographs in diagnosis of approximal caries in primary teeth. *Community Dent Health* 1989; **6**: 239–47.

ICRP Publication 60. 1990 Recommendations of the International Commission on Radiological Protection. *Ann ICRP* 1991; **21**: 1–201.

Ketley CE, Holt RD. Visual and radiographic diagnosis of occlusal caries in first permanent molars and in second primary molars. *Br Dent J* 1993; **174**: 364–70.

Kidd EA, Naylor MN, Wilson RF. Prevalence of clinically undetected and untreated molar occlusal dentine caries in adolescents on the Isle of Wight. *Caries Res* 1992; **26**: 397–401.

Lervik T, Haugejorden O, Aas C. Progression of posterior approximal carious lesions in Norwegian teenagers from 1982 to 1986. *Acta Odontol Scand* 1990; **48**: 223–7.

Lillehagen M, Grindefjord M, Mejàre I. Detection of approximal caries by clinical and radiographic examination in 9-year-old Swedish children. *Caries Res* 2007; **41**: 177–85.

Lith A, Gröndahl HG. Intervals between bitewing examinations in young patients when applying a radiologic algorithm. *Community Dent Oral Epidemiol* 1992; **20**: 181–6.

Lith A, Lindstrand C, Gröndahl HG. Caries development in a young population managed by a restrictive attitude to radiography and operative intervention: II. A study at the surface level. *Dentomaxillofac Radiol* 2002; **31**: 232–9.

Machiulskiene V, Nyvad B, Baelum V. A comparison of clinical and radiographic caries diagnoses in posterior teeth of 12-year-old Lithuanian children. *Caries Res* 1999; **33**: 340–8.

Machiulskiene V, Nyvad B, Baelum V. Comparison of diagnostic yields of clinical and radiographic caries examinations in children of different age. *Eur J Paediatr Dent* 2004; **5**: 157–62.

Medeiros VA, Seddon RP. Iatrogenic damage to approximal surfaces in contact with class II restorations. *J Dent* 2000; **28**: 103–10.

Mejàre I. Bitewing examination to detect caries in children and adolescents – when and how often? *Dent Update* 2005; **32**: 588–90, 593–4, 596–7.

Mejàre I, Malmgren B. Clinical and radiographic appearance of proximal carious lesions at the time of operative treatment in young permanent teeth. *Scand J Dent Res* 1986; **94**: 19–26.

Mejàre I, Stenlund H. Caries rates for the mesial surface of the first permanent molar and the distal surface of the second primary molar from 6 to 12 years of age in Sweden. *Caries Res* 2000; **34**: 454–61.

Mejàre I, Gröndahl HG, Carlstedt K, Grevér AC, Ottosson E. Accuracy at radiography and probing for the diagnosis of proximal caries. *Scand J Dent Res* 1985; **93**: 178–84.

Mejàre I, Källestål C, Stenlund H, Johansson H. Caries development from 11 to 22 years of age: a prospective radiographic study. Prevalence and distribution. *Caries Res* 1998; **32**: 10–16.

Mejàre I, Källestål C, Stenlund H. Incidence and progression of approximal caries from 11 to 22 years of age in Sweden: a prospective radiographic study. *Caries Res* 1999; **33**: 93–100.

Mejàre I, Stenlund H, Julihn A, Larsson I, Permert L. Influence of approximal caries in primary molars on caries rate for the mesial surface of the first permanent molar in swedish children from 6 to 12 years of age. *Caries Res* 2001; **35**: 178–85.

Mejàre I, Stenlund H, Zelezny-Holmlund C. Caries incidence and lesion progression from adolescence to young adulthood: a prospective 15-year cohort study in Sweden. *Caries Res* 2004; **38**: 130–41.

Pitts NB. The use of bitewing radiographs in the management of dental caries: scientific and practical considerations. *Dentomaxillofac Radiol* 1996; **25**: 5–16.

Pitts NB, Kidd EA. Some of the factors to be considered in the prescription and timing of bitewing radiography in the diagnosis and management of dental caries. *J Dent* 1992; **20**: 74–84.

Poorterman JH, Weerheijm KL, Groen HJ, Kalsbeek H. Clinical and radiographic judgement of occlusal caries in adolescents. *Eur J Oral Sci* 2000; **108**: 93–8.

Preston-Martin S, White SC. Brain and salivary gland tumors related to prior dental radiography: implications for current practice. *J Am Dent Assoc* 1990; **120**: 151–8.

Qvist V, Johannessen L, Bruun M. Progression of approximal caries in relation to iatrogenic preparation damage. *J Dent Res* 1992; **71**: 1370–3.

Raadal M, Amarante E, Espelid I. Prevalence, severity and distribution of caries in a group of 5-year-old Norwegian children. *Eur J Paediatr Dent* 2000; **1**: 13–20.

Rohlin M, White SC. Comparative means of dose reduction in dental radiography. *Curr Opin Dent* 1992; **2**: 1–9.

Shwartz M, Pliskin JS, Gröndahl H, Boffa J. The frequency of bitewing radiographs. *Oral Surg Oral Med Oral Pathol* 1986; **61**: 300–5.

Shwartz M, Gröndahl H-G, Pliskin JS, Boffa J. A longitudinal analysis from bite-wing radiographs of the rate of progression of approximal carious lesions through human dental enamel. *Arch Oral Biol* 1984; **29**: 529–36.

Sköld UM, Klock B, Lindvall AM. Differences in caries recording with and without bitewing radiographs. A study on 5-year old children in the County of Bohuslan, Sweden. *Swed Dent J* 1997; **21**: 69–75.

Smith NJ. Selection criteria for dental radiography. *Br Dent J* 1992; **173**: 120–1.

Stecksén-Blicks C, Wahlin YB. Diagnosis of approximal caries in pre-school children. *Swed Dent J* 1983; **7**: 179–84.

Stenlund H, Mejàre I, Källestål C. Caries rates related to approximal caries at ages 11–13: a 10-year follow-up study in Sweden. *J Dent Res* 2002; **81**: 455–8.

Verdonschot EH, Bronkhorst EM, Burgersdijk RC, Konig KG, Schaeken MJ, Truin GJ. Performance of some diagnostic systems in examinations for small occlusal carious lesions. *Caries Res* 1992; **26**: 59–64.

de Vries HC, Ruiken HM, Konig KG, van't Hof MA. Radiographic versus clinical diagnosis of approximal carious lesions. *Caries Res* 1990; **24**: 364–70.

Wang N. Approximal caries lesions and restorative treatment strategies in adolescents. *Caries Res* 1995; **29**: 317. Abstract no. 87.

Wenzel A. Influence of computerized information technologies on image quality in dental radiographs. *Tandlaegebladet* 1991; **95**: 527–9.

Wenzel A. Digital radiography and caries diagnosis. *Dentomaxillofac Radiol* 1998; **27**: 3–11.

Wenzel A. Bitewing and digital bitewing radiography for detection of caries lesions. *J Dent Res* 2004; **83** (Spec. No. C): C72–5.

Wenzel A, Fejerskov O. Validity of diagnosis of questionable caries lesions in occlusal surfaces of extracted third molars. *Caries Res* 1992; **26**: 188–94.

Wenzel A, Gotfredsen E. An interview study with Danish dentists who work with direct digital radiography. *Tandlegebladet.* 2000; **3**: 130–6. (In Danish with English summary.)

Wenzel A, Moystad A. Experience of Norwegian general dental practitioners with solid state and storage phosphor detectors. *Dentomaxillofac Radiol* 2001; **30**: 203–8.

6

Additional diagnostic measures

A. Lussi and B. Angmar-Månsson

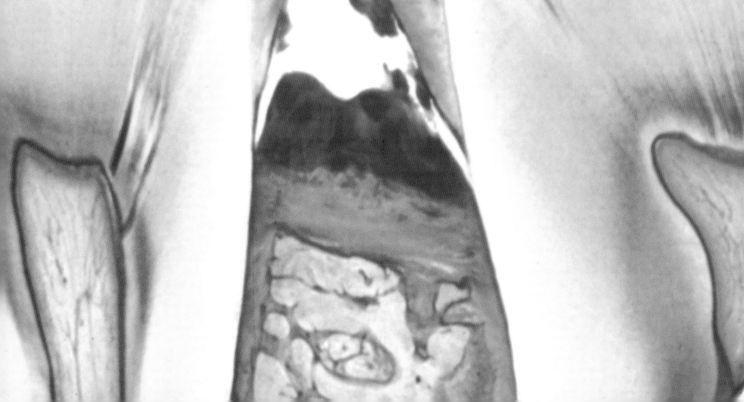

Introduction

Caries diagnosis implies more than just detecting lesions. Since diagnosis is a mental resting place on the way to a treatment decision, it is intimately linked with that treatment plan. Thus, diagnosis must include an assessment of activity because active lesions require active management (non-operative and operative treatment), whereas arrested lesions do not. Herein lies a problem. How can activity be assessed? The clinical–visual features of active and arrested lesions were described in Chapter 5. But is it really that simple? After all, there are pitfalls along the way. The detection process may miss lesions (false negatives) or say lesions are present when they are not (false positives). The assessment of activity may be similarly wrong.

It seems logical to suggest that attempting this at a single point in time simply adds to the problem. Would it not be easier to be able to monitor lesion progression or arrest over time? It was shown in Chapter 5 that clinical–visual diagnosis may be amenable to longitudinal monitoring even though the assessment is qualitative. Would it not be easier, and maybe even foolproof, to have a device that would not only detect demineralization but also quantify it? Then monitoring progression or arrest would be simple: use the device again and see in what direction the numbers change. The concept is hugely appealing, so no wonder researchers have made such efforts to develop, test and perfect such devices.

This chapter concerns these devices and seeks to answer, for each method, the following questions.

- What has been developed and how are the techniques meant to work?
- Are the methods valid and reproducible?
- Are the methods suitable for use in clinical practice or only useful for research?
- Can the methods stand alone or are they only adjuncts to a clinical–visual examination?

All quantitative methods for caries detection are based on the interpretation of physical signals. These are causally related to one or more features of a caries lesion. Table 6.1 shows the types of physical principle that may be used and the corresponding diagnostic methods that are going to be described.

Methods based on X-ray

Digital radiography

To appreciate the value of digital radiographic diagnosis it is imperative to understand what a digital radiograph is. The explanation starts with an ordinary intraoral film radiograph (Fig. 6.1a). This image contains information, i.e. varying optical density, which represents details of the human anatomy, disease (designated 'signal') and 'noise'. In

Table 6.1 Overview of additional diagnostic methods

Physical principle	Method
X-rays (digital radiography)	Digital image enhancement*
	Digital subtraction radiography
	Tuned aperture computed tomography (TACT)
Light	Laser-fluorescence measurement (DIAGNOdent)*
	Quantitative light-induced fluorescence (QLF)
	Digital imaging fiber-optic transillumination (DIFOTI)
Electrical current	Electrical conductance measurement (ECM)
	Electrical impedance measurement

Only applications marked with an asterisk are widely used in clinical practice. The others are currently being researched or are only used for research

digital radiography the image is divided into a number of rectangular areas with respective gray scales. These shades are digitized and displayed on the computer monitor as shades of gray (Fig. 6.1). The smaller the area of the rectangles, the better the resolution. It is generally not necessary to attain the resolution of radiographic film to use the full diagnostic range. Moreover, it is senseless to increase the resolution of a digital radiograph beyond the resolution of the monitor screen. The most important advantage of digital radiographs is the fact that they are easy to manipulate. The numbers in a digital radiograph, as they are stored in a computer's working memory, can be modified. Special computer algorithms (filters) have been designed to change the values such that specific features within the image are enhanced. The numbers of the enhanced image are converted in gray values and shown on the computer monitor, where the dentist may interpret the enhanced image. Up to now the majority of studies on current digital intraoral radiography systems have reported them to be as accurate as traditional films for the detection of caries (for review, see Wenzel, 2000, 2004).

Digital image enhancement

The advantages of digital versus film radiographs are numerous, but only the quantitative diagnostic aspects will be delineated in this chapter. One of the aims of contemporary cariology is to find initial, small lesions as well as obvious cavities, and it is essential that caries diagnosis from digital radiographs is at least as valid as from film radiographs. The spatial resolution of digital images and the range of gray shades are lower than that of conventional radiographic films. From this it has been hypothesized that the diagnostic performance of unenhanced digital images will not exceed that of radiographic films. The diagnostic performance of dentists in diagnosing small carious lesions from film radiographs and digital radiographs was investigated by Verdonschot et al. (1992a). It was demonstrated that the diagnostic performance from film radiographs exceeded that from unenhanced digital radiographs. Apparently, the somewhat lower spatial resolution in

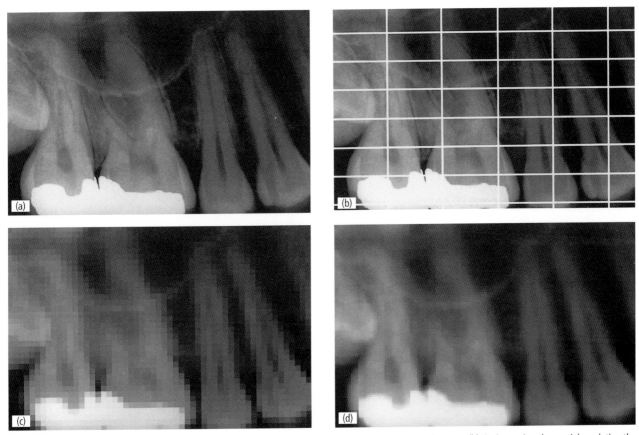

Figure 6.1 The quintessence of digital radiology. A regular intraoral radiograph (a) is divided into rectangular areas (b). By increasing the spatial resolution the amount of detail displayed in the image can be increased (c, d).

digital images led to more incorrect diagnoses. The dentists were subsequently shown the same radiographs after the images had been digitally enhanced. When the diagnostic task was to discriminate between 'caries' and 'no caries', enhanced radiographs performed equally well. With the decision cut-off between 'dentinal caries' and 'no dentinal caries', the sensitivity was statistically significantly superior to that of radiographs, but this enhancement was also associated with a statistically significant reduction in specificity. Figure 6.2a shows an unenhanced bitewing radiograph. In Fig. 6.2b the contrast has been digitally enhanced using an algorithm.

Digital subtraction radiography

By subtracting the gray values for each coordinate of the first radiograph from the equivalent coordinate of a second radiograph a subtraction image is obtained. If no changes have occurred the result of a subtraction is zero. A non-zero result will be obtained in the case of changes such as the progression of demineralization. These sites can be found easily by the observers on the subtraction images. To date, subtraction has been used mostly in laboratory studies, which have shown that the method could be a powerful tool in the diagnosis of primary and recurrent caries

(Nummikoski *et al.*, 1992; Wenzel & Halse, 1992; Halse *et al.*, 1994; Minah *et al.*, 1998). However, although commonly used in clinical dental research, the method has not yet routinely been applied in the clinic, mainly because of the difficulty of image registration, i.e. aligning the second radiograph with the first (Fig. 6.3).

Tuned aperture computed tomography

Recently introduced diagnostic methods based on digital radiography are tuned aperture computed tomography (TACT) and limited cone beam computed tomography. Both methods construct radiographic slices of different thickness of teeth. The slices can be viewed for the presence of radiolucencies. In addition, the slices can be brought together in a three-dimensional computer model called a pseudohologram. These slices and pseudoholograms perform adequately in the detection of small primary and recurrent carious lesions (Webber *et al.*, 1997; Shi *et al.*, 2001a), although their performance in occlusal and approximal caries diagnosis is not significantly better than film radiography and digital radiography (Webber *et al.*, 1997; Tyndall *et al.*, 1997; Abreu *et al.*, 1999a, b, 2004; Shi *et al.*, 2001b; Harase *et al.*, 2006). Other studies concluded that the application of TACT showed markedly improved

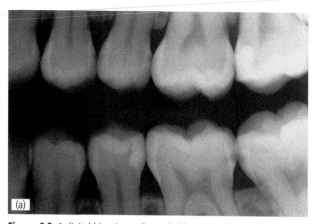
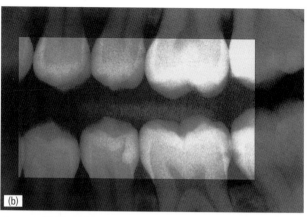

Figure 6.2 A digital bitewing radiograph (a) can be enhanced to facilitate caries diagnosis (b). The enhancement was applied within the window to increase local contrasts.

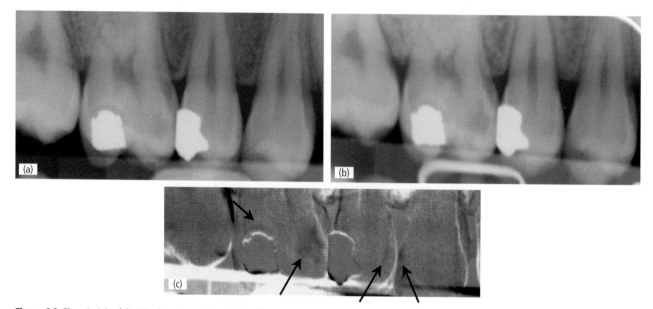

Figure 6.3 The principle of digital subtraction radiography. (a, b) Two digital bitewing radiographs taken 21 months apart in the same individual; (c) the subtraction image of the two radiographs. The arrows point at dark gray areas corresponding to the difference in radiolucency between baseline and follow-up after 21 months. (Courtesy of R. Ellwood.)

diagnostic accuracy on caries detection (Nair *et al.*, 1998a,b; Akdeniz *et al.*, 2006). However, the device is currently too expensive to be used in a small clinical practice.

Methods based on light

Light transmission

Sound enamel consists mainly of carbonate-rich and calcium-deficient hydroxyapatite crystals which are very densely packed, giving the enamel a glass-like, translucent appearance. The yellow–white color of teeth is the result of the dentin shining through the translucent enamel layer. Light that shines on a tooth will, in part, penetrate the tooth and is scattered or absorbed inside. Scattering is the process in which the direction of a photon is changed

without loss of energy. Absorption is the process in which photons lose their energy, mostly by conversion into heat. Since scattering does not cause the light to be lost, scattering may occur many times consecutively along the path, a phenomenon called multiple scattering. After one or more scatter events, a photon may reach the tooth surface again and leave the tooth. Back-scatter is the phenomenon where photons leave through the surface by which they entered. When photons leave through another surface, the phenomenon is called diffuse transmission.

In a sound tooth, scattering is much more probable than absorption. In dentin, both scattering and absorption occur more frequently along the light path than either occurs in the enamel. The whitish appearance of teeth is due to the fact that absorption is much lower than scattering (ten Bosch, 1996). Primary teeth show more scattering and therefore have a whiter appearance than permanent teeth.

In a white-spot carious lesion, scattering is stronger than in sound enamel. The penetrating photons change direction more often in carious enamel than in sound enamel and are generally back-scattered before they reach the dentin. Therefore, such a lesion appears whiter than the surrounding sound parts of the tooth. Brown lesions are due to the presence of light-absorbing material in the lesion and/or exogenous stain.

A slight increase in enamel porosity leads to a change in the optical properties of enamel in such a way that light is increasingly scattered. This is presumed to be primarily due to the fact that the remaining small mineral particles in the lesion are embedded in water rather than in mineral-rich sound enamel (Angmar-Månsson & ten Bosch, 1987), thereby increasing the difference in refractive index (RI) between the scattering photon and its environment. The RI of enamel apatite is 1.62, and the RIs of water and air are 1.33 and 1.0, respectively. Thus, when the pores of a white spot enamel lesion are filled with water, the light scattering is less than when the lesion is dry and the pores are filled with air. After dehydration of enamel it looks whiter, as a result of more scattered light.

Laser light-induced fluorescence

Laser light is composed of electromagnetic waves with equal wavelengths and equal phases. Some materials possess the characteristic of fluorescence when illuminated with (laser) light. Fluorescence is a phenomenon by which the wavelength of the emitted light (coming from the light source) is changed into a larger wavelength as it travels back for detection. The larger wavelength is caused by some loss of energy to the surrounding tissue and therefore will have a different color from the emitting light. By using a filter through which only the fluorescent light may pass, the intensity of the fluorescent light can be measured. The intensity of the fluorescent light is proportional to the amount of material that causes the fluorescence. The fluorescence of dental hard tissues has been known for a very long time (Benedict, 1928). Spectra have been presented by several authors (Armstrong, 1963; Spitzer & ten Bosch, 1976; Alfano & Yao, 1981; Hibst et al., 2001). Three types of fluorescence can be distinguished: blue fluorescence is excited in the near ultraviolet, yellow and orange fluorescence is excited in the blue and green, and red fluorescence in the far red and near infrared.

The chromophores causing the fluorescence of dental hard tissues are not clearly identified. (A chromophore is a molecule that gives an object color by selectively absorbing light at particular wavelengths.) The blue fluorescence was assigned to dityrosine (Booij & ten Bosch, 1982). It seems likely that most of the yellow fluorescence stems from proteinic chromophores, probably cross-links between chains

of structural proteins (Scharf, 1971). It has also been discussed whether or not the apatite of dental hard tissues would contribute as well (Spitzer & ten Bosch, 1976; Hafström-Björkman et al., 1991). The red–infrared fluorescence has been assigned to a protoporphyrin, which is present as a bacterial breakdown product (König et al., 1998). Dental enamel and dentin possess the characteristic of fluorescence and this natural fluorescence is called autofluorescence. Caries lesions, plaque and microorganisms also contain fluorescent substances. The difference between the fluorescence of sound tooth tissues and that of a caries lesion can be made visible by the quantitative laser- or light-induced fluorescence (QLF) and by the DIAGNOdent method.

DIAGNOdent

When red light with a wavelength of 655 nm is applied, caries-induced changes in teeth lead to increased fluorescence (Hibst et al., 2001). The DIAGNOdent (KaVo Biberach, Germany) is based on this principle. The fluorescent light is measured and its intensity is an indication of the depth of the caries lesion. The intensity of the fluorescent light is displayed as a number ranging from 0 to 99, with 0 indicating a minimum and 99 a maximum of fluorescent light (Figs 6.4, 6.5).

Since its first presentation many studies have extensively investigated this laser fluorescence device for occlusal and smooth surface caries detection. The threshold between occlusal caries limited to enamel and caries into dentin was found to be around 18 under humid conditions (Lussi et al., 1999, 2001; Shi et al., 2000). Clinically visible white-spot lesions are measurable with this device. However, very initial lesions, with no fluorophores from bacteria present, are not captured by the DIAGNOdent. The same registration under dry conditions led to higher cut-off points (Shi et al., 2000; Lussi et al., 2005). Thus, it would be important

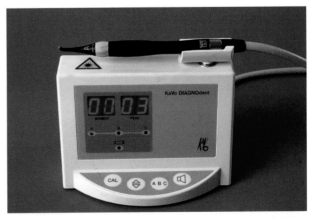

Figure 6.4 DIAGNOdent showing real-time and maximum (peak) digital display. The device consists of a probe, a fiber-optic lead, and a unit containing the electronics and the laser diode.

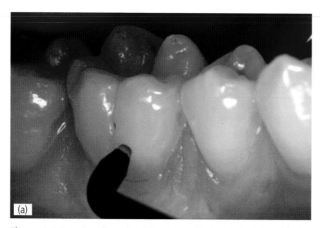
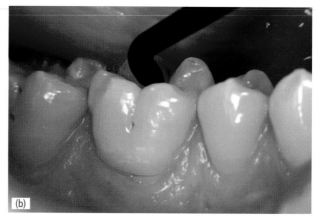

Figure 6.5 Procedure for occlusal detection with the DIAGNOdent. (a) After calibration is accomplished the zero value is measured on a sound tooth surface. (b) The tip of the laser device has to be carefully rotated around the vertical axis until the maximum fluorescence value of the site under study is found.

to standardize hydration conditions for longitudinal measurements. Based on systematic reviews of the performance of DIAGNOdent for detecting caries it was concluded that DIAGNOdent is more sensitive than traditional diagnostic methods (Bader & Shugars, 2004; Lussi *et al.*, 2004; Ricketts, 2005). However, the increased likelihood of false-positive diagnoses when using the DIAGNOdent means that it should not be relied on as a clinician's primary diagnostic method.

DIAGNOdent has also been tested *in vitro* and *in vivo* for measurement of carious lesions adjacent to fixed orthodontic appliances (Aljehani *et al.*, 2004, 2006; Staudt *et al.*, 2004). Other studies have addressed further possible clinical applications: the detection of recurrent caries (Boston, 2003; Ando *et al.*, 2004; Bamzahim *et al.*, 2004, 2005), residual caries (Lennon *et al.*, 2002), caries under sealants (Takamori *et al.*, 2001; Deery *et al.*, 2006), root caries (Wicht *et al.*, 2002, 2003) and detection of subgingival calculus (Krause *et al.*, 2003).

Recently, a new laser device (DIAGNOdent*pen*, DD*pen*, KaVo Biberach, Germany) was introduced, which allows fluorescence from the approximal surfaces of teeth, in addition to occlusal surfaces, to be captured (Lussi *et al.*, 2006) (Fig. 6.6). When an adjacent tooth is present, it is not possible for the original designed tip (Fig. 6.5) to access the lesion. Because of the different architecture, new tips for the detection of occlusal and approximal surfaces had to be developed. Comparison of the DIAGNOdent*pen* with the DIAGNOdent on occlusal surfaces revealed a similar detection performance of the two devices (Lussi & Hellwig, 2006). For both DIAGNOdent devices, careful tilting on occlusal surfaces around the spot to be measured is crucial for adequate detection (Fig. 6.7).

The tip is placed against the tooth surface and the laser light penetrates the tooth. Further, the tip for approximal surfaces is constructed in a way that it is able to reflect the light of excitation and detection laterally. When using the instrument approximally it is important to apply it on the oral and facial side of the surface under detection and to move the tip underneath the contact point (Fig. 6.8). This allows the dentist to search for the spot with the highest fluorescence. However, owing to the thickness of the tip (0.4 mm), access to the approximal surface may still be difficult or sometimes hardly possible. The advantage of the laser-based system could probably be a decrease in the number of bitewing radiographs taken, using laser fluorescence measurements more frequently at times between taking bitewing radiographs for monitoring caries regression or progression.

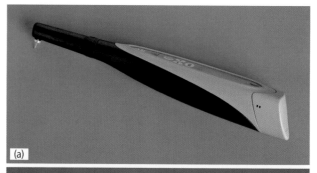
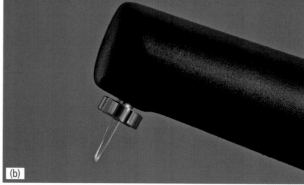

Figure 6.6 (a) The DIAGNOdent*pen* with the tip for detection of occlusal caries. (b) Close-up of the tip for approximal detection and the knob for turning it around.

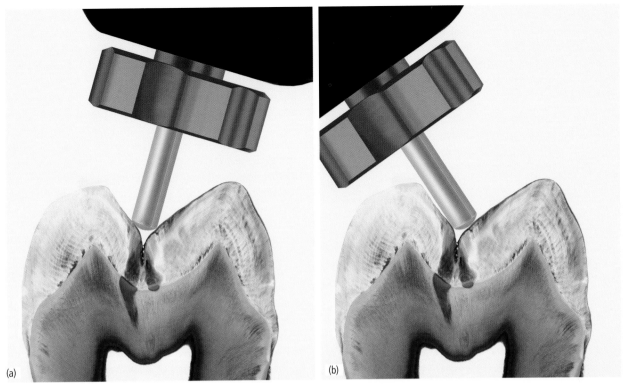

Figure 6.7 Procedure for occlusal detection with the DIAGNOdentPen. As with the first device, the tip has to be rotated around the vertical axis (a, b). This ensures that the tip picks up fluorescence from the slopes of the fissure walls where the carious process may start. The position shown in (b) gives no signal.

The devices have shown good intraexaminer reproducibility *in vitro* and *in vivo*, indicating that the equipment measured consistently (Lussi *et al.*, 2001, 2006; Tranaeus *et al.*, 2004). This means that the DIAGNOdent can be used for monitoring the carious process. However, it has to be taken into account that monitored differences of 4 units and below are not clinically relevant.

Quantitative light-induced fluorescence

Demineralization of a dental hard tissue results in loss of its autofluorescence, the natural fluorescence. As early as the 1920s this phenomenon was suggested to be useful as a tool for diagnosing dental caries (Benedict, 1929). More recently, laser light was used to induce fluorescence of enamel in a sensitive, non-destructive diagnostic method for detection of caries (Bjelkhagen & Sundström, 1981; Bjelkhagen *et al.*, 1982). The tooth was illuminated with a broad beam of blue–green light from an argon laser, producing diffuse monochromatic light with a wavelength (λ) of 488 nm. The fluorescence of the enamel occurring in the yellow region was observed through a yellow high-pass filter ($\lambda = 520$ nm), which filters out all reflected and

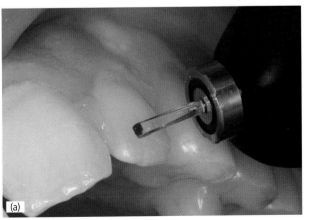

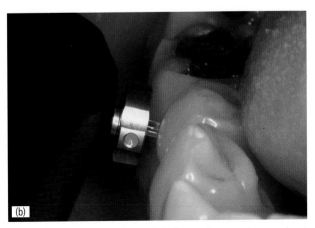

Figure 6.8 Procedure for approximal detection with the DIAGNOdentPen. (a) Measurement of the fluorescence (zero value) of a sound spot on the coronal part of the facial surface. (b) Measurement at the approximal site. The proximal space is carefully penetrated.

back-scattered light. Demineralized areas appeared as dark areas because the fluorescence of a caries lesion viewed by QLF is lower than that of sound enamel.

Several effects may contribute to the decreased fluorescence of white-spot carious lesions and the most probable ones are as follows.

- The light scattering in the lesion, which is much stronger than in sound enamel (ten Bosch, 1996), causes the light path in the lesion to be much shorter than in sound enamel; thus, the absorption per unit of volume is much smaller in the lesion and the fluorescence is less strong.
- The light scattering in the lesion acts as a barrier for excitation light to reach the underlying fluorescent sound tooth tissues, and as a barrier for fluorescent light from the layers below the lesion to reach the tooth surface. This is one of the reasons for limited depth detection with QLF (up to 400 μm).

The laser fluorescence method was developed further for *in vivo* quantification of mineral loss in natural enamel

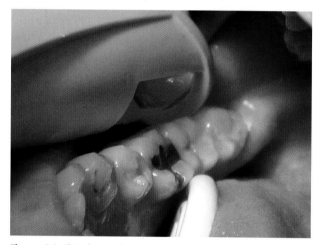

Figure 6.9 Clinical use of quantitative light-induced fluorescence (QLF). (Courtesy of S. Tranaeus.)

lesions using a color microvideo charge-coupled device (CCD) camera and computed image analysis (de Josselin de Jong *et al.*, 1995) (Fig. 6.9). To enable calculation of fluorescence loss in the caries lesion, the fluorescence of the lesion is subtracted from the fluorescence of the surrounding sound tissue. The difference between the actual values and the reconstructed ones gives the resulting fluorescence loss, as demonstrated in Fig. 6.10. Figure 6.10a shows the actual fluorescence image of a caries lesion; Fig. 6.10b shows the reconstructed image in which the fluorescence of the original sound enamel at the lesion site was taken from the fluorescence of the sound enamel around the lesion. The difference between the measured and the reconstructed values gave the resulting fluorescence loss in the lesion (Fig. 6.10c). From this, three lesion quantities may be obtained: mean fluorescence loss over the lesion (in per cent), maximum fluorescence loss in the lesion (in per cent) and area of the lesion (in square millimeters). To facilitate clinical studies at different locations, a small, portable system for intraoral use was developed with a regular, i.e. non-coherent, light source and filter system to replace the laser source (Al-Khateeb *et al.*, 1997b). The illumination system consists of a 50 W xenon microdischarge arc lamp provided with an optical bandpass filter with a maximum wavelength of 370 nm to produce blue light. The light illuminating the tooth is transported through a liquid-filled light guide. The resulting fluorescence from the tooth is collected by the video camera. A highpass optical filter with $\lambda = 540$ nm prevents any excitation light reaching the detector. Data are collected, stored and analyzed by custom-made software. The portable QLF device was validated against chemical analysis and microradiography for the assessment of mineral changes in enamel and compared with results from measurements with the laser light equipment (Al-Khateeb *et al.*, 1997b). It was concluded that QLF was a sensitive, reproducible method for quantification of enamel lesions limited to a depth of about 400 μm.

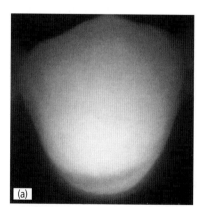 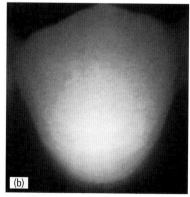 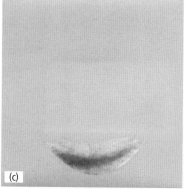

Figure 6.10 Principles of the quantitative light-induced fluorescence (QLF) method for quantification of an enamel caries lesion. (a) The actual fluorescence image of a caries lesion; (b) the reconstructed image, in which fluorescence radiance of the original sound enamel at the lesion site was reconstructed by interpolation of values indicating sound enamel around the lesion. (c) The difference between the measured and the reconstructed values gave the resulting fluorescence loss in the lesion.

A relationship between mineral loss and fluorescence has been found for artificial and natural caries lesions with correlation coefficients of $r = 0.73–0.86$ (Hafström-Björkman *et al.*, 1991, 1992; Emami *et al.*, 1996; Al-Khateeb *et al.*, 1997a). Thus, a measure of fluorescence may indicate the amount of mineral loss.

The intraexaminer and interexaminer reliability of the analytical stage of the QLF procedure was tested on artificial lesions produced *in vitro*, and the researchers concluded that the reliability was good for experienced examiners, while novices needed sufficient training before practice, as with most methods (Pretty *et al.*, 2002). The *in vivo* repeatability and reproducibility of QLF are excellent for the quantification of smooth-surface caries, with interclass correlation coefficients for interexaminer reliability of $r = 0.95–0.99$ (Tranæus *et al.*, 2002). The QLF method has been applied in a few clinical studies, on orthodontic patients (Al-Khateeb *et al.*, 1998) and on caries-active adolescents (Tranæus *et al.*, 2001; Heinrich-Weltzien *et al.*, 2005).

Attempts to adapt the QLF method for occlusal caries diagnosis have been made. Preliminary results comparing the QLF method with other diagnostic methods showed that QLF was more sensitive than electrical conductance for measurements of shallow occlusal lesions (Tranæus *et al.*, 1997a, Ando *et al.*, 2000; Pretty *et al.*, 2003a). Discrimination of deeper lesions, however, was limited. The QLF method has been further modified for the detection and quantification of recurrent caries (Tranæus *et al.*, 1997b; Gonzales-Cabezas *et al.*, 2003; Pretty *et al.*, 2003b), but this application has yet to be tested clinically.

Digital imaging fiber-optic transillumination

Fiber-optic transillumination (FOTI) has been introduced as a qualitative diagnostic method by which teeth are transilluminated. The observation of 'shadows' has been associated with the presence of carious lesions. The method is described in Chapter 4. The major problem associated with the validity of FOTI is the low sensitivity (Verdonschot *et al.*, 1991; Vaarkamp *et al.*, 2000).

The technique of digital imaging fiber-optic transillumination (DIFOTI) was introduced to improve this sensitivity by replacing the human eye with a CCD receptor (Keem & Elbaum, 1997) (Fig. 6.11). A clinical validation study determined the ability of DIFOTI to detect primary caries (Ando, 2006). Deciduous molars of 119 children (aged 8–12 years) were examined at 6-month intervals throughout a 2-year study period. Exfoliated teeth were collected for the validation of lesion presence and depth using polarized light microscopy as the gold standard. Results indicated that lesions involving over half of the enamel were better detected than lesions restricted to only the outer half of enamel for both smooth and occlusal surfaces. In other words, DIFOTI may not be able to detect small lesions, such as lesions within half of enamel thickness, and this is not as good as a visual examination (see Chapter 4). Occlusal caries detection was better than smooth-surface caries detection.

Methods based on electrical current

Electrical conductance and electrical impedance

When an electrical current passes through a material the electrical properties of this material determine the extent to which the current is conducted. Biomaterials with high concentrations of fluids and electrolytes are more conductive than materials with low concentrations. It follows that immature, porous enamel is more conductive than mature enamel, and dentin is more conductive than enamel. When a current is applied by placing an electrode onto a tooth surface, the electrical conductance of all material between this electrode and the contraelectrode, which is generally held in the hand, can be measured. Since all of these materials have high concentrations of electrolytes except for dental enamel, the measurement of the conductance is mainly that of enamel. Demineralized sites in enamel, sites with a high pore volume and cavities can be detected by measuring the conductance.

Impedance is the measure of the degree to which an electric circuit resists electric current flow when a voltage is impressed across two electrodes. Impedance, like electrical resistance expressed in ohms, is the ratio of the voltage impressed across a pair of terminals to the current flow between those electrodes. In direct current (d.c.) circuits, impedance corresponds to resistance. In alternating current (a.c.) circuits, impedance is a function of resistance, inductance and capacitance. Every material has different electrical impedance determined by its molecular composition: some materials have high electrical impedance, while others have low electrical impedance. Carious tissues have

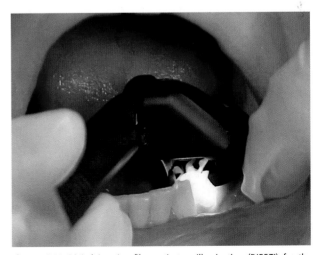

Figure 6.11 Digital imaging fiber-optic transillumination (DIFOTI) for the detection of occlusal caries. (Courtesy of M. Ando.)

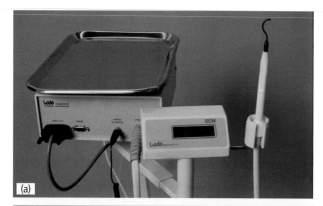

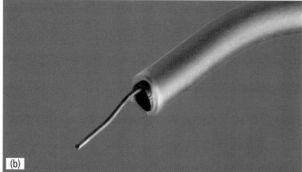

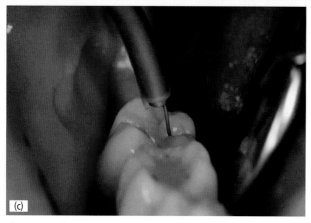

Figure 6.12 (a) Electrical conductance measurements (ECM). The electrical caries monitor with its tip. (b) Air flows through the tube to dry the tooth surface. (c) The measurement of a spot. To prevent the current from 'leaking' through a superficial layer of moisture to the gingiva, an airflow is applied to dry the occlusal tooth surface around the probe.

a much lower electrical impedance (or conduct electricity much better) than sound tooth tissues.

Electrical conductance measurements

The value of site-specific electrical conductance measurements (ECM) in caries diagnosis has been the subject of many *in vitro* (White *et al.*, 1978; Wenzel *et al.*, 1992; Verdonschot *et al.*, 1993; Ricketts *et al.*, 1996; Ashley *et al.*, 1998) and *in vivo* studies (Rock & Kidd, 1988; Verdonschot *et al.*, 1992b; Lussi *et al.*, 1995; Ricketts *et al.*, 1997a, b). The reported sensitivities of ECM in diagnosing dentinal carious lesions of permanent premolar and molar teeth ranged

from 0.67 to 0.96, whereas the specificities ranged from 0.71 to 0.98, reflecting an acceptable performance. When analyzing ECM data obtained by different researchers at different institutions, Huysmans *et al.* (2005) concluded that there was a consistant, systematic, non-random measurement variation. This was assumed to be related to factors such as insufficient and unpredictable probe contact.

The use of ECM in children was investigated in a longitudinal study (Ie *et al.*, 1995). It was found that ECM values obtained from sites that developed caries were significantly higher than those from sites that remained caries free. ECM values obtained from sites that exhibited dentinal caries upon validation were also significantly higher than those obtained from sites that showed no caries or caries limited to enamel. It was concluded from this study that the ECM could aid the detection of fissure caries in recently erupted molar teeth and that the ECM could be used to predict the probability that a sealant or a sealant restoration would be required within 18–24 months after eruption. In another study (Lussi *et al.*, 1995), the electrical resistance was measured *in vivo* on human third molars without existing restorations and without any macroscopic carious cavitation. After measurement, the teeth were extracted, histologically prepared, serially sectioned perpendicular to the occlusal surface and examined for the presence of caries. The electrical resistance monitor was well suited to detect *in vivo* occlusal caries under clinically intact fissures. The rather high value (0.23) of false-positive ratings, however, might lead to a substantial number of sound teeth being restored unnecessarily. Figure 6.12 shows the device and its use on an occlusal surface.

Electrical impedance measurements

The principle of electrical impedance has been applied by researchers to detect caries lesions at approximal sites of teeth (Huysmans *et al.*, 1996; Longbottom *et al.*, 1996). Although the results from these *in vitro* studies were very promising, no follow-up research findings have been reported since.

Are the methods suitable for use in clinical practice or only useful for research?

Digital radiography is a well-established method that is used in many clinical practices. With the price of computer memory becoming cheaper and cheaper, and the high-resolution quality of the screen, it will spread further in the future. As with conventional radiography, digital radiography will not pick up occlusal lesions confined to enamel or very early approximal lesions.

The *DIAGNOdent* (KaVo, Biberach, Germany) is easy to use and able to detect caries in the inner half of enamel as well as dentinal lesions. However, the DIAGNOdent devices also detect deposits such as plaque or fluorescing dental materials, staining and calculus, all of which give false-positive readings. Thorough tooth cleaning must precede the use of laser fluorescence. However, removing spots of calculus and stains on approximal surfaces is difficult and it is not easy to see whether it has been achieved. Moreover, fluorescent polishing paste must be removed with a three-in-one syringe to avoid false-positive measurements (Lussi & Reich, 2005). Despite these reservations, DIAGNOdent is useful in clinical practice as a second opinion during the diagnostic process on occlusal surfaces.

The *QLF* method is now available as Inspektor Pro™ Research QLF System from Inspektor Dental Care (Amsterdam, The Netherlands). The combination of quantitative data and display of the fluorescent image of the tooth on the monitor makes QLF instructive for demonstrating lesion progression and/or regression to the patient. It is an appropriate research tool for *in vivo* monitoring of mineral changes in white-spot enamel lesions up to 400 μm in depth.

The clinical use of QLF may be complicated by several confounding factors in adolescents at risk of caries, such as the presence of plaque and stain. In addition, QLF is only able to demonstrate very initial enamel lesions. Further, the QLF method is an interactive technique and for dentists who are not familiar with image reconstruction software it may be cumbersome in the conventional dental setting. The current cost of the QLF equipment may prevent its use by the clinician.

Advantages of *DIFOTI* include the absence of ionizing radiation, the possiblities for images to be reviewed over time, and the fact that DIFOTI is a user-friendly instrument which is easy to operate. However, training for interpretation of images with this technique is required. Further, currently there is no objective way to quantify caries with the DIFOTI system. Development and evaluation of this method are required before it could become clinically applicable.

An instrument measuring the electrical resistance, called the *Electric Caries Monitor*, is manufactured by Lode Diagnostics (Groningen, The Netherlands). Few practices use the methodology, perhaps because it is time consuming. Thus, this device is mostly used for research purposes, although monitoring of the carious process is hindered by the insufficient and unpredictable probe contact (Huysmans *et al.*, 2005).

Can the methods stand alone or are they only adjuncts to a clinical–visual examination?

Additional diagnostic methods, generally quantitative, may be used as an adjunct to visual inspection. However, to be used in practice the methods must be better than clinical–visual and radiographic examination. They must be convenient to use, not too expensive and, since their value should be in longitudinal monitoring, they must be reproducible.

Of the methods described in this chapter only laser fluorescence (DIAGNOdent) and digital radiography are currently used in practice and seem to be suitable techniques for detection of caries (see Table 6.1). Monitoring the carious process on occlusal surface may be impossible with radiography, but seems possible with the DIAGNOdent.

The resulting quantitative measurements are used by the practitioners as an adjunct to visual examination to obtain a diagnosis. However, the dentist should always remain responsible for the interpretation of the measurements and never pass this responsibility to a machine. Measurements should be considered and weighted against other relevant observations. Dentists who use additional techniques for assistance in caries diagnosis must remain alert and should always be able to explain the measurements from other observations taken from the patient.

The input of Dr E. Verdonschot to this chapter is highly appreciated.

References

Abreu M, Tyndall DA, Ludlow JB. Detection of caries with conventional digital imaging and tuned aperture computed tomography using CRT monitor and laptop displays. *Oral Surg Oral Med Oral Pathol Oral Radiol Endod* 1999a; **88**: 234–8.

Abreu M, Tyndall DA, Platin E, Ludlow JB, Phillips C. Two- and three-dimensional imaging modalities for the detection of caries. A comparison between film, digital radiography and tuned aperture computed tomography (TACT). *Dentomaxillofac Radiol* 1999b; **28**: 152–7.

Abreu M Jr, Yi-Ching L, Abreu AL. Comparative diagnostic performance of TACT slices and its multiple source images: an *in vitro* study. *Dentomaxillofac Radiol* 2004; **33**: 93–7.

Akdeniz BG, Gröndahl H, Magnusson B. Accuracy of proximal caries depth measurements: comparison between limited cone beam computed tomography storage phosphor and film radiography. *Caries Res* 2006; **40**: 202–7.

Alfano RR, Yao SS. Human teeth with and without dental caries, studied by visible luminescent spectroscopy. *J Dent Res* 1981; **80**: 120–2.

Aljehani A, Tranæus S, Forsberg C-M, Angmar-Månsson B, Shi X-Q. *In vitro* quantification of white spot lesions adjacent to fixed orthodontic appliances using quantitative light-induced fluorescence and DIAGNOdent. *Acta Odontol Scand* 2004; **62**: 313–18.

Aljehani A, Bamzahim M, Yousif MA, Shi X-Q. *In vivo* reliability of an infrared fluorescence method for quantification of carious lesions in orthodontic patients. *Oral Health Prev Dent* 2006; **4**: 145–50.

Al-Khateeb S, Oliveby A, de Josselin de Jong E, Angmar-Månsson B. Laser fluorescence quantification of remineralisation *in situ* of incipient enamel lesions: influence of fluoride supplements. *Caries Res* 1997a; **31**: 132–40.

Al-Khateeb S, ten Cate JM, Angmar-Månsson B, *et al*. Quantification of formation and remineralization of artificial enamel lesions with a new portable fluorescence device. *Adv Dent Res* 1997b; **11**: 502–6.

Al-Khateeb S, Forsberg C-M, de Josselin de Jong E, Angmar-Månsson B. A longitudinal laser fluorescence study of white spot lesions in orthodontic patients. *Am J Orthod Dentofac Orthop* 1998; **113**: 595–602.

Ando M. Performance of digital imaging fiber-optic transillumination (DIFOTI) for detection of non-cavitated primary caries. Preliminary report. In: Stookey GK, Kambara M, eds. *Early detection of dental caries*. Proceedings of the 7th Annual Indiana Conference, Indiana University, Indianapolis, 2006: 41–52.

Ando M, Eggertsson H, Isaacs RL, Analoui M, Stookey GK. Comparative studies of several methods for the early detection of fissure lesions. In: Stookey GK, ed. *Early detection of dental caries II*. Proceedings of the 4th Annual Indiana Conference, Indiana University, Indianapolis, 2000: 279–99.

Ando M, Gonzales-Cabezas C, Isaacs RL, Eckert GJ, Stookey GK. Evaluation of several techniques for the detection of secondary caries adjacent to amalgam restorations. *Caries Res* 2004; **38**: 350–56.

Angmar-Månsson B, ten Bosch JJ. Optical methods for the detection and quantification of caries. *Adv Dent Res* 1987; **1**: 14–20.

Armstrong WG. Fluorescent characteristics of sound and carious human dentine preparations. *Arch Oral Biol* 1963; **8**: 79–80.

Ashley PF, Blinkhorn AS, Davies RM. Occlusal caries diagnosis: an *in vitro* histological validation of the Electronic Caries Monitor (ECM) and other methods. *J Dent* 1998; **26**: 83–8.

Bader JD, Shugars DA. A systematic review of the performance of a laser fluorescence device for detecting caries. *J Am Dent Assoc* 2004; **135**: 1413–26.

Bamzahim M, Shi X-Q, Angmar-Månsson B. Secondary caries detection by DIAGNOdent and radiography: a comparative study. *Acta Odontol Scand* 2004; **62**: 61–4.

Bamzahim M, Aljehani A, Shi X-Q. Clinical performance of DIAGNOdent in the detection of secondary caries lesions. *Acta Odontol Scand* 2005; **63**: 26–30.

Benedict HC. Note on the fluorescence of teeth in ultra-violet rays. *Science* 1928; **67**: 442.

Benedict HC. The fluorescence of teeth as another method of attack on the problem of dental caries. *J Dent Res* 1929; **9**: 274–5.

Bjelkhagen H, Sundström F. A clinically applicable laser luminescence method for the early detection of dental caries. *IEEE J Quant Elect* 1981; **17**: 266–86.

Bjelkhagen H, Sundström F, Angmar-Månsson B, Rydén H. Early detection of enamel caries by the luminescence excited by visible laser light. *Swed Dent J* 1982; **6**: 1–7.

Booij M, ten Bosch JJ. A fluorescent compound in bovine dental enamel matrix compared with synthetic dityrosine. *Arch Oral Biol* 1982; **27**: 417–21.

ten Bosch JJ. Light scattering and related methods. In: Stookey GK, ed. *Early detection of dental caries*. Proceedings of the 1st Annual Indiana Conference, Indiana University, Indianapolis, 1996: 81–90.

Boston DW. Initial *in vivo* evaluation of DIAGNOdent for detecting secondary carious lesions associated with resin composite restorations. *Quintessence Int* 2003; **34**: 109–16.

Deery C, Iloya J, Nugent ZJ, Srinivasan V. Effect of placing a clear sealant on the validity and reproducibility of occlusal caries detection by a laser fluorescence device: an *in vitro* study. *Caries Res* 2006; **40**: 186–93.

Emami Z, Al-Khateeb S, de Josselin de Jong E, Sundström F, Trollsås K, Angmar-Månsson B. Mineral loss in incipient caries lesions quantified with laser fluorescence and longitudinal microradiography. *Acta Odontol Scand* 1996; **54**: 8–13.

Gonzales-Cabezas C, Fontana M, Gomes-Moosbauer D, Stookey GK. Early detection of secondary caries using quantitative light-induced fluorescence. *Oper Dent* 2003; **28**: 415–22.

Hafström-Björkman U, Sundström F, ten Bosch JJ. Fluorescence of dissolved fractions of human enamel. *Acta Odontol Scand* 1991; **49**: 133–8.

Hafström-Björkman U, Sundström F, de Josselin de Jong E, Oliveby A, Angmar-Månsson B. Comparison of laser fluorescence and longitudinal microradiography for quantitative assessment of *in vitro* enamel caries. *Caries Res* 1992; **26**: 241–7.

Halse A, Espelid I, Tveit AB, White SC. Detection of mineral loss in approximal enamel by subtraction radiography. *Oral Surg Oral Med Oral Pathol* 1994; **77**: 177–82.

Harase Y, Araki K, Okano T. Accuracy of extraoral tuned aperture computed tomography (TACT) for proximal caries detection. *Oral Surg Oral Med Oral Pathol Oral Radiol Endod* 2006; **101**: 791–6.

Heinrich-Weltzien R, Kühnisch J, Ifland S, Tranæus S, Angmar-Månsson B, Stösser L. Detection of initial caries lesions on smooth surfaces by quantitative light-induced fluorescence and visual examination: an in vivo comparison. *Eur J Oral Sci* 2005; **113**: 494–8.

Hibst R, Paulus R, Lussi A. Detection of occlusal caries by laser fluorescence. Basic and clinical investigations. *Med Laser Applic* 2001; **16**: 205–13.

Huysmans MC, Longbottom C, Pitts NB, Los P, Bruce PG. Impedance spectroscopy of teeth with and without approximal caries lesions – an *in vitro* study. *J Dent Res* 1996; **75**: 1871–8.

Huysmans MC, Kühnisch J, ten Bosch JJ. Reproducibility of electrical caries measurements: a technical problem? *Caries Res* 2005; **39**: 403–10.

Ie YL, Verdonschot EH, Schaeken MJM, van't Hof MA. Electrical conductance of fissure enamel in recently erupted molar teeth as related to caries status. *Caries Res* 1995; **29**: 94–9.

de Josselin de Jong E, Sundström F, Westerling H, Tranaeus S, ten Bosch JJ, Angmar-Månsson B. A new method for *in vivo*-quantification of mineral loss in enamel with laser fluorescence. *Caries Res* 1995; **29**: 2–7.

Keem S, Elbaum M. Wavelet representations for monitoring changes in teeth imaged with digital imaging fiber-optic transillumination. *IEEE Trans Med Imaging* 1997; **16**: 653–63.

König K, Flemming G, Hibst R. Laser-induced autofluorescence spectroscopy of dental caries. *Cell Mol Biol (Paris)* 1998; **44**: 1293–300.

Krause F, Braun A, Frentzen M. The possibility of detecting subgingival calculus by laser-fluorescence *in vitro*. *Laser Med Sci* 2003; **18**: 32–5.

Lennon AM, Buchalla W, Switalski L, Stookey GK. Residual caries detection using visible fluorescence. *Caries Res* 2002; **36**: 315–19.

Longbottom C, Huysmans MC, Pitts NB, Los P, Bruce PG. Detection of dental decay and its extent using a.c. impedance spectroscopy. *Nat Med* 1996; **2**: 235–7.

Lussi A, Hellwig E. Performance of a new laser fluorescence device for the detection of occlusal caries *in vitro*. *J Dent* 2006; **34**: 467–71.

Lussi A, Reich E. The influence of toothpastes and prophylaxis pastes on fluorescence measurements for caries detection *in vitro*. *Eur J Oral Sci* 2005; **113**: 141–4.

Lussi A, Firestone A, Schoenberg V, Hotz P, Stich H. *In vivo* diagnosis of fissure caries using a new electrical resistance monitor. *Caries Res* 1995; **29**: 81–7.

Lussi A, Imwinkelried S, Pitts NB, Longbottom C, Reich E. Performance and reproducibility of a laser fluorescence system for detection of occlusal caries *in vitro*. *Caries Res* 1999; **33**: 261–6.

Lussi A, Megert B, Longbottom C, Reich E, Francescut P. Clinical performance of a laser fluorescence device for detection of occlusal caries lesions. *Eur J Oral Sci* 2001; **109**: 14–19.

Lussi A, Hibst R, Paulus R. DIAGNOdent: an optical method for caries detection. *J Dent Res* 2004; **83**: C80–3.

Lussi A, Longbottom C, Gygax M, Braig F. Influence of professional cleaning and drying of occlusal surfaces on laser fluorescence *in vivo*. *Caries Res* 2005; **39**: 284–6.

Lussi A, Hack A, Hug I, Megert B, Stich H. Detection of approximal caries with a new laser fluorescence device. *Caries Res* 2006; **40**: 90–6.

Minah GE, Vandre RH, Talaksi R. Subtraction radiography of dentinal caries-like lesions induced *in vitro* by cariogenic bacteria. *Pediatr Dent* 1998; **20**: 345–9.

Nair MK, Tyndall DA, Ludlow JB, May K. Tuned aperture computed tomography and detection of recurrent caries. *Caries Res* 1998a; **32**: 23–30.

Nair MK, Tyndall DA, Ludlow JB, May K, Ye F. The effects of restorative material and location on the detection of simulated recurrent caries. A comparison of dental film, direct digital radiography and tuned aperture computer tomography. *Dentomaxillofac Radiol* 1998b; **27**: 80–4.

Nummikoski PV, Martinez TS, Matteson SR, McDavid WD, Dove SB. Digital subtraction radiography in artificial recurrent caries detection. *Dentomaxillofac Radiol* 1992; **21**: 59–64.

Pretty IA, Hall AF, Smith PW, Edgar WM, Higham SM. The intra- and inter-examiner reliability of quantitative light-induced fluorescence (QLF) analyses. *Br Dent J* 2002; **193**: 105–9.

Pretty IA, Edgar WM, Higham SM. A review of the effectiveness of quantitative light-induced fluorescence (QLF) to detect early caries. In: Stookey GK, ed. *Early detection of dental caries III*. Proceedings of the 6th Annual Indiana Conference, Indiana University, Indianapolis, 2003a: 253–89.

Pretty IA, Smith PW, Edgar WM, Higham SM. Detection of *in vitro* demineralization adjacent to restorations using quantitative light induced fluorescence (QLF). *Dent Mater* 2003b; **19**: 368–74.

Ricketts DN. The eyes have it. How good is DIAGNOdent at detecting caries? *Evid Based Dent* 2005; **6**: 64–5.

Ricketts DN, Kidd EA, Liepins PJ, Wilson RF. Histological validation of electrical resistance measurements in the diagnosis of occlusal caries. *Caries Res* 1996; **30**: 148–55.

Ricketts DN, Kidd EA, Wilson RF. The effect of airflow on site-specific electrical conductance measurements used in the diagnosis of pit and fissure caries *in vitro*. *Caries Res* 1997a; **31**: 111–18.

Ricketts DN, Kidd EA, Wilson RF. Electronic diagnosis of occlusal caries *in vitro*: adaptation of the technique for epidemiological purposes. *Community Dent Oral Epidemiol* 1997b; **25**: 238–41.

Rock WP, Kidd EAM. The electronic detection of demineralisation in occlusal fissures. *Br Dent J* 1988; **164**: 243–7.

Scharf F. Über die natürliche Lumineszenz der Zahnhartgewebe 'Schmelz und Dentin'. *Stoma* 1971; **24**: 11–25.

Shi X-Q, Welander U, Angmar-Månsson B. Occlusal caries detection with KaVo Diagnodent and radiography: an *in vitro* comparison. *Caries Res* 2000; **34**: 151–8.

Shi X-Q, Han P, Welander U, Angmar-Månsson B. Tuned-aperture computed tomography for detection of occlusal caries. *Dentomaxillofac Radiol* 2001a; **30**: 45–9.

Shi X-Q, Tranæus S, Angmar-Månsson B. Comparison of QLF and DIAGNOdent for quantification of smooth surface caries. *Caries Res* 2001b; **35**: 21–6.

Spitzer D, ten Bosch JJ. The total luminescence of bovine and human dental enamel. *Calcif Tiss Res* 1976; **20**: 201–8.

Staudt CB, Lussi A, Jacquet J, Kiliaridis S. White spot lesions around brackets: *in vitro* detection by laser fluorescence. *Eur J Oral Sci* 2004; **112**: 237–43.

Takamori K, Hokari N, Okomura Y, Watanabe S. Detection of occlusal caries under sealants by use of a laser fluorescence system. *J Clin Laser Med Surg* 2001; **19**: 267–71.

Tranæus S, Lussi A, de Josselin de Jong E, Angmar-Månsson B. Quantification of occlusal caries – an *in vitro* study with laser fluorescence, electrical resistance measurement and histologic examination. *J Dent Res* 1997a; **76**: 101.

Tranæus S, Lussi A, de Josselin de Jong E, Angmar-Månsson B. Quantitative light induced fluorescence for assessment of enamel caries around fillings – a pilot study. *Caries Res* 1997b; **4**: 324.

Tranæus S, Al-Khateeb S, Björkman S, Twetman S, Angmar-Månsson B. Application of quantitative light-induced fluorescence to monitor incipient lesions in caries-active children. A comparative study of remineralisation by fluoride varnish and professional cleaning. *Eur J Oral Sci* 2001; **109**: 71–5.

Tranæus S, Shi X-Q, Lindgren L-E, Trollsås K, Angmar-Månsson B. *In vivo* repeatability and reproducibility of the quantitative light-induced fluorescence method. *Caries Res* 2002; **36**: 3–9.

Tranæus S, Lindgren L-E, Karlsson L, Angmar-Månsson B. *In vivo* validity and reliability of IR fluorescence measurements for caries detection and quantification. *Swed Dent J* 2004; **28**: 173–82.

Tyndall DA, Clifton TL, Webber RL, Ludlow JB, Horton RA. TACT® imaging of primary caries. *Oral Surg Oral Med Oral Pathol Oral Radiol Endod* 1997; **84**: 214–25.

Vaarkamp J, ten Bosch JJ, Verdonschot EH, Bronkhorst EM. The real performance of bitewing radiography and fiber-optic transillumination in approximal caries diagnosis. *J Dent Res* 2000; **79**: 1747–51.

Verdonschot EH, Bronkhorst EM, Wenzel A. Approximal caries diagnosis using fiber-optic transillumination: a mathematical adjustment to improve validity. *Community Dent Oral Epidemiol* 1991; **19**: 329–32.

Verdonschot EH, Kuijpers JMC, Polder BJ, De Leng-Worm MH, Bronkhorst EM. The effects of digital grey-scale modification on the diagnosis of small approximal carious lesions. *J Dent* 1992a; **20**: 44–9.

Verdonschot EH, Bronkhorst EM, Burgersdijk RCW, König KG, Schaeken MJM, Truin GJ. Performance of some diagnostic systems in examinations for small occlusal carious lesions. *Caries Res* 1992b; **26**: 59–64.

Verdonschot EH, Wenzel A, Truin GJ, König KG. Performance of electrical resistance measurements adjunct to visual inspection in the early diagnosis of occlusal caries. *J Dent* 1993; **21**: 332–7.

Webber RL, Horton RA, Tyndall DA, Ludlow JB. Tuned-aperture computed tomography (TACT). Theory and application for three-dimensional dento-alveolar imaging. *Dentomaxillofac Radiol* 1997; **26**: 53–62.

Wenzel A. Digital imaging for dental caries. *Dent Clin North Am* 2000; **44**: 319–38.

Wenzel A. Bitewing and digital bitewing radiography for detection of caries lesion. *J Dent Res* 2004; **83** (Spec. Iss.) C72–5.

Wenzel A, Halse A. Digital subtraction radiography after stannous fluoride treatment for occlusal caries diagnosis. *Oral Surg Oral Med Oral Pathol* 1992; **74**: 824–8.

Wenzel A, Verdonschot EH, Truin GJ, König KG. Accuracy of visual inspection, fiber-optic transillumination, and various radiographic image modalities for the detection of occlusal caries in extracted non-cavitated teeth. *J Dent Res* 1992; **71**: 1934–7.

White GE, Tsamtsouris A, Williams DL. Early detection of occlusal caries by measuring the electrical resistance of the tooth. *J Dent Res* 1978; **57**: 195–200.

Wicht MJ, Haak R, Stutzer H, Strohe D, Noack MJ. Intra- and interexaminer variability and validity of laser fluorescence and electrical resistance readings on root surface lesions. *Caries Res* 2002; **36**: 241–8.

Wicht MJ, Haak R, Lummert D, Noack MJ. Treatment of root caries lesions with chlorhexidine-containing varnishes and dentin sealants. *Am J Dent* 2003; **16** (Spec. No.): 25–30A.

7

The foundations of good diagnostic practice

V. Baelum, B. Nyvad, H.-G. Gröndahl and O. Fejerskov

Introduction

It is a common claim that dentistry is an artistic craft, as in the expression 'the art of dentistry', whose means and methods can only be learned and optimized by accumulating clinical experience. This is not true. There are also concepts and principles, rules and guidelines, and dental professionals must evaluate the evidence and acquire scientific knowledge to gain a platform, a knowledge base, upon which to build their clinical experience.

This chapter reviews the scientific and conceptual underpinnings of caries diagnosis. Dental students and professionals alike may then gain a deeper understanding of the building blocks necessary for creating a good diagnostic strategy for use in their daily clinical practice. The dental professional, who wants to be able to adapt his or her core diagnostic skills to different settings, and be able to choose the best treatment alternatives, must have a thorough understanding of the building blocks that provide the fundament of clinical decision making. The activities and the decision processes involved in caries diagnosis are not identical for all patients or for different populations with different caries profiles. Nor can it be assumed that caries diagnosis will remain unchanged for all future to come. It is therefore vital that the dental professionals have a clear understanding of the factors influencing their diagnostic practices.

The foundations for diagnostic practices are laid during undergraduate training. This chapter will therefore begin by exploring how dentistry is commonly taught to the bright, but innocent student. It will then proceed to explore why dentists are concerned with caries diagnosis, and it is shown that two rather different lines of thinking operate in the approach to caries diagnosis. Finally, it is emphasized that caries diagnosis, irrespective of the method(s) used, is an error-prone enterprise, and that diagnostic decisions are made under uncertainty. The addition of different caries diagnostic methods, or the repetition of caries diagnostic methods, inevitably results in more diagnostic errors. This fundamental diagnostic uncertainty demands that the dentist exercises a considerable degree of restraint when making caries diagnoses that may have irretrievable negative consequences if the diagnosis is incorrect. In most contemporary populations, there is a continued decline in the caries prevalence, the caries incidence, and carious lesion severity. Thus, the risk of causing adverse health outcomes stems from overzealous operative intervention rather than from overlooking caries lesions.

The making of a dentist

Clinical dentistry is taught under the auspices of the master clinician (Ismail & Bader, 2004), the clinical 'expert'. The 'art and craft' of diagnostic and therapeutic decision-making is learned mainly through a chairside apprenticeship. Unfortunately, the scientific and conceptual underpinnings of the practices taught during these clinical sessions may not receive adequate attention. Certainly, master clinicians and general dentists alike tend to be very reluctant to formalize the clinical decision-making processes they use, and prefer to view these decisions as embedded in the 'art of dentistry' (Bader & Shugars, 1995a). The 'art of dentistry' concept implies that the clinical decision-making process is informal and intuitive, and can only be optimized through accumulated clinical experience. The dental students learn to reproduce what they have been told and shown by the clinical master, whose opinions, perceptions, biases and value judgments therefore determine the practices adopted. The lack of a strategy for training the master clinicians results in inconsistent, and even contradictory, teachers.

The 'art of dentistry' and caries scripts

When inconsistencies or contradictions become obvious, dental students are typically told that they result from 'the natural variation in the best clinical judgment of individual dentists concerning individual patients' (Bader & Shugars, 1995a), i.e. they reflect 'the art of dentistry' to be learned by the student. The students are not supposed to explore the differences, nor are they expected to challenge the argument. Instead, they are encouraged to try to understand and memorize as much as possible the particulars of each single patient ('no two patients are the same!') and each clinical situation to incorporate these details into a mental inventory of clinical scripts (Bader & Shugars, 1997). These clinical scripts incorporate differential diagnostic considerations, i.e. the distinction between carious lesions on the one hand and fluorotic lesions, enamel opacities and hypoplasias on the other. Thus, the caries scripts serve as manuals for the entire clinical decision-making process to use whenever the dentist next encounters a similar clinical presentation.

Thereby, the clinical decision making in dentistry cannot be compartmentalized into distinct diagnostic and therapeutic entities. Caries diagnosis is not an activity undertaken completely independently of the options for intervention, and clinical decision making is more characterized by the execution of 'this-clinical-picture-needs-this-intervention'-like scripts (Bader & Shugars, 1997).

Variation in clinical decisions

In view of the learning process described, it is no wonder that many dentists focus on the minutiae of each single clinical representation, and value expert opinions and clinical experience much higher than scientific evidence and evidence-based practice guidelines. It is likewise not surprising that a huge variation exists in the way dentistry is practiced (Kay *et al.*, 1992; Kay & Nuttall, 1994, 1995a; Bader & Shugars, 1995b) (see Chapter 31). This variation is characteristic for both diagnostic and therapeutic decision making, and implies that some dentists provide better or more efficient dental care than other dentists when faced with similar patients.

Is this variation a problem? Can't we just leave things the way they are and continue to let dentists develop their own particular catalogue of clinical scripts? Our answer is a clear no! While the considerable variation does not seem to be an area of major concern among dental professionals, it will be a tangible problem for the patients if they realize that they receive different standards of care with different practitioners. In times of growing patient expectations and increasing patient-initiated litigations, it may therefore be a wise move for the dental profession to face the variation in order not to fall prey to accusations of deliberate unethical practice (Kay & Nuttall, 1995b), whereby credibility may be irretrievably lost among the populations it serves (Ecenbarger, 1997; Renshaw, 2005).

Can caries scripts be changed?

Dentists' caries scripts are influenced by a large number of factors (Bader & Shugars, 1997), including personal dentist characteristics, such as age and experience, skill and diligence, and knowledge and tolerance for uncertainty; dentist biases concerning the perceived utility of restorations, treatment preferences, diagnostic techniques used and experience with outliers (such as the innocuous looking lesion that turns out to cover a soft carious lesion extending all the way to the pulp); and, finally, practice characteristics such as business size, delivery system, equipment, guidelines and personnel.

If the variation in the clinical decisions made by dentists is to be reduced, some dentists must change their clinical caries scripts. This can be achieved in one of two ways (Bader & Shugars, 1997): either by means of the introduction to the caries scripts of a new salient factor or, more likely, by a reinterpretation of existing salient factors. Examples of such reinterpretations are many: it is known that older dentists tend to be less aggressive in their decisions to intervene (Bader & Shugars, 1992), probably owing to accumulated clinical experience allowing them gradually to reinterpret some of the factors determining their caries scripts. Hence, older dentists may have had the experience that caries does not progress at the rate they once thought, or that restorations do not last for as long as they were once led to believe. Other examples comprise the observation that Australian dentists practicing in a water-fluoridated area have been found to be more inclined to adopt a wait-and-see attitude when presented with a given radiographic lesion than dentists practicing in Norway (Espelid et al., 1994). This was ascribed to Australian dentists having different experiences of carious lesion progression. Others have noted that teeth with decay or 'unsatisfactory' fillings are less likely to be restored when located in patients resid-ing in a fluoridated area than when found in patients from a non-fluoridated area (Grembowski & Milgrom, 1988; Grembowski et al., 1997).

In this context, it is important to realize that the patients seen in the dental schools are typically not representative of the general population. Dental school patients tend to be admitted based on a need for the specific mechanical and technical procedures taught during undergraduate dental training. This means that the oral disease spectrum presented to the dental student may be heavily biased towards more prevalent and severe oral disease than is actually characteristic for the general population. Thereby, the dental student may be left with the impression that good dental practice hinges more on mechanical/technical intervention than is appropriate.

The above examples all concern the propensity to intervene, i.e. whether and how to intervene therapeutically for a given clinical or radiographic presentation. However, numerous steps have been taken before reaching the stage of deciding upon interventions. Decisions have been made regarding the clinical recording methods used and the addition of bitewing radiography or other sense-enhancing diagnostic methods. These decisions are not made consciously and de novo for each single tooth in each single patient, but are dictated by the routines and practices of the dentist, as first learned at dental school and subsequently modified through experience. Thereby, these diagnostic decisions also contribute as a source of variation in the clinical decisions made among dentists.

Fortunately, evidence suggests that variation from this source can be reduced. Hence, a study of the diagnostic performance of dentists before and after attending a 1.5 h seminar explaining the key elements in clinical diagnosis showed that diagnostic decisions improved and became more consistent as a result of a short education in probabilistic reasoning (Choi et al., 1998). While it may seem quite paradoxical that learning about uncertainty will enhance diagnostic consistency, there are analogous examples from other branches of dentistry illustrating that clinical experience and expertise do not guarantee the most consistent diagnoses (Fleiss et al., 1991).

The dental examination: in the best interest of patients

Patients go to the dentist for one of two different reasons: they either have a concrete and tangible dental problem, such as toothache or tooth mobility, for which they seek help; or they go for a routine check-up. In many high-income countries, the routine screening examinations dominate dentist–patient contacts, whereas in low-income countries, symptom-driven contacts are much more frequent, as indeed they were decades ago in the high-income countries.

The symptom-driven dental visit

These two scenarios, the symptom-driven dental visit and the routine (screening) check-up visit, have fundamentally different implications for the patients. The symptom-driven dental visit is strictly patient initiated and prompted by actual symptoms, i.e. the patient has concrete and tangible complaints, which make them seek help to obtain symptom relief. The success or failure of the dentist is obvious in such circumstances. If the diagnostic activities undertaken result in the identification of the sources and causes of the problem, and if the ensuing intervention results in symptom relief, gratification is immediate for both the dentist and the patient: the diagnosis was correct, the dentist solved the problem, and the patient got rid of his or her symptoms.

The routine (screening) check-up visit

The routine check-up visit involves an asymptomatic patient, and thereby amounts to a screening examination. In fact, the routine dental visit is most likely to have been prompted by some recall scheme devised by the dentist, rather than being strictly patient initiated. During this routine visit, the dentist looks for signs of oral diseases, which includes an examination of all tooth surfaces for the presence of signs of caries, and if such signs are found, some form of intervention is carried out to prevent disease progress. Thereby, the gratification of both the dentist and the patient is based on a set of assumptions that can be summarized as follows: if the screening examination had not been carried out and the interventions had therefore not been made, the patient would have fared worse in the future.

The two situations have one thing in common, however: the dental professionals will say that they undertake their activities in the best interest of the patient. In other words, the dentist looks for caries to find the causes of tangible symptoms presented by the patient, or to prevent asymptomatic carious lesions from developing into tangible symptoms with all the unfortunate sequels that this may have.

What are we looking for – what is caries?

The shrewd reader of this textbook will undoubtedly already have spotted that the notion of caries varies. Many of the terms aired in preceding and ensuing chapters all pertain to dental caries, but from rather different perspectives, such as chemistry, bioimaging, microbiology, pathology and epidemiology. This illustrates a lack of a common understanding of what is meant by the term 'caries' (Baelum *et al.*, 2006). This ambiguity stems, in turn, from a more fundamental lack of clarity about what constitutes a 'disease' (Scadding, 1967, 1996; Wulff, 1979). A popular understanding of the disease 'dental caries' (Fig. 7.1) holds that the disease caries is a process – a sort of engine usually termed the 'caries process' – that converts the direct causes of caries (the microbial biofilm on the tooth surfaces and the fermentable carbohydrates from the diet) into the signs and symptoms of caries, i.e. the carious lesions. This understanding, which is termed essentialistic (Wulff, 1979; Scadding, 1996), may be shown to be logically erroneous (Baelum *et al.*, 2006). Nonetheless, this essentialistic thinking has led to the unfortunate belief in the existence of a fixed caries 'truth', placed somewhere in the limbo between the causes of caries and the signs and symptoms of caries. The meaning of this is perhaps best understood if we apply a timeline. Hence, the causes of caries must, by virtue of the definition of a cause, precede the caries process which, if the caries process causes signs and symptoms, must precede the signs and symptoms of caries that it generates (Fig. 7.1). This mistaken belief is the basis for statements such as 'diagnosis is the act or art of identifying a disease from its signs and symptoms' (Kidd *et al.*, 2003) and 'diagnosis is defined as the determination of disease, but not as the determination of the signs and symptoms thereof' (ten Bosch & Angmar-Mansson, 2000).

However, there is no disease, called caries, which differs from its signs and symptoms. This is illustrated by the notable absence of the term 'dental caries' in Fig. 1.1, which also shows that the 'caries process' is no more than a convenient descriptor for the entire complex of causal factors (see Chapters 10–12 for details) that produces certain signs and symptoms labeled 'carious lesions'. The result of the causal processes is the formation of carious lesions. Dental caries is therefore no more than a label attached to tooth surfaces that share certain defining characteristics. In other words, 'dental caries' is a name that describes the signs and symptoms resulting from the completion of the caries causal complex (Fig. 1.1). This caries view is termed nomi-

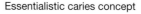

Essentialistic caries concept

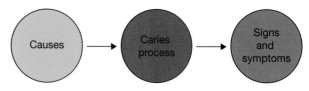

Nominalistic caries concept

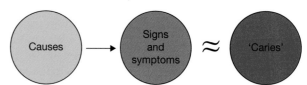

Figure 7.1 Essentialistic versus nominalistic caries concepts. The essentialistic concept holds that a caries truth exists interposed between the causes and the signs and symptoms. The nominalistic concept holds that dental caries is no more than a label attached to tooth surfaces sharing certain defining characteristics, i.e. a convenient and succinct way of describing the signs and symptoms.

nalistic (Fig. 7.1). Nominalism is the underpinning of the old dictum 'there are no diseases, just sick people'. This dictum merely states the fact that the clinical management of sick people is greatly facilitated by the use of disease classifications, because a disease name can, in a very short form, be used to communicate all the knowledge about etiology, pathogenesis, treatment and prognosis that is relevant to a patient with a particular set of signs and symptoms.

Essentialistic versus nominalistic caries concepts

Understanding the distinction between the essentialistic and the nominalistic caries concept is important for understanding the logical underpinnings of caries diagnosis. The essentialistic view leads to the belief in the existence of a caries truth, a key, which is termed the caries 'gold standard', against which caries diagnostic methods and criteria can be evaluated. Caries diagnosis thereby becomes a matter of searching for the caries truth, and this view assumes that a universal and fixed distinction exists between 'caries' and 'sound'. However, as will be shown, the truth about caries is hard to pin down, and the distinction between caries and sound is indefinable.

The nominalistic view of caries leads to a more patient-centered approach, because dental professionals label dental caries and caries lesions to suit their particular needs, i.e. in a way that makes it possible to achieve the best long-term health outcome for the tooth or patient in question. In the nominalistic view, dentists are not particularly concerned with the caries 'truth', because they know it is indefinable. The focus is on the health benefits of undertaking our diagnostic activities. Dentists seek to optimize the health outcome by selecting diagnostic methods and categories that lead to the best interventions and thereby to the best long-term health outcome for the patient. The close link between the management options and the relevant caries diagnostic categories is a centerpiece of the nominalistic caries concept.

The elusive truth about caries

The truth is necessarily elusive about a causal process (Fig. 1.1) that cannot be observed (Wulff, 1979). Some of the essential components, such as the biofilm on the tooth surfaces, can be observed. Related scientific fields (see Chapters 10–12) show that something (the caries causal processes) is happening in the interface between the tooth and the biofilm, and this something we might choose to call 'caries' (this is what essentialists will do). However, this would lead to the conclusion that carious lesion formation is ubiquitous wherever a biofilm is attached to a tooth surface (Fejerskov & Manji, 1990), which is not true. Moreover, if one were to follow this logic through, the dentist should simply use the presence of a biofilm to diagnose caries, and would not really need to inspect the tooth surface for anything else. This has not happened, because it is

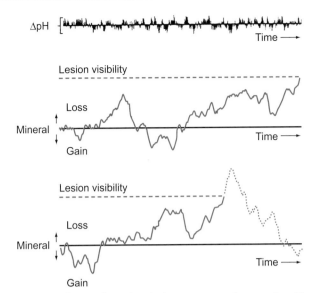

Figure 7.2 Schematic illustration of microevents at a surface over time. The upper fluctuating line indicates pH fluctuations in a biofilm over time (minutes, hours, days). The curves show different examples of fluctuating mineral loss (up) or gain (down) in enamel as a result of innumerable fluctuations in pH. The horizontal dotted lines indicate where loss of mineral may be seen clinically as a white spot.

known that the processes taking place in the interface between the biofilm and tooth are not one-way processes that only lead to demineralization and carious lesion formation. For example, these processes may sometimes drift in the opposite direction, towards calculus formation in the plaque, which is not compatible with the understanding of caries (Fig. 7.2).

Attempts have been made to define caries as a net mineral loss (Hintze, 2004), but problems have immediately arisen. Hence, a logical next question is: how much loss of mineral should be present to deserve the diagnosis of dental caries? Any net mineral loss, no matter how infinitesimally small, is nonetheless a net mineral loss. Thereby, the assessment of the caries truth becomes dependent on the resolution of the measuring instruments and techniques available. In principle, it is possible to conceive of measuring devices with infinitely high resolution, as high-resolution transmission electron microscopy can record loss of mineral at crystal level. It is, therefore, not possible to state a fixed caries truth that is independent of the scale of measurement. Decades ago, Mandelbrot (1967) showed that the length of geographical curves, such as coastlines, has no true value and that any given estimate obtained always refers to a particular scale of measurement. The same holds for caries: the diagnosis 'sound' or 'caries free' always refers to a particular scale of measurement, reflected in the diagnostic instrument resolution.

Even if it were indeed possible to measure the very first mineral loss from the enamel surface, this would make little sense from a clinical perspective. As shown in Fig. 7.2, the metabolic activities taking place in the biofilm on the tooth surface result in pH fluctuations. These fluctuations may be small and erratic (Scheie *et al.*, 1992; Fejerskov *et al.*, 1992a, b) and may even occur in the absence of obvious external stimuli such as sucrose intake (Scheie *et al.*, 1992). When the effects of such pH fluctuations are accumulated over time, they describe a series of mineral losses (demineralization) or gains (remineralization) of the dental hard tissues (Manji *et al.*, 1991), depending on the chemical composition of the plaque fluid. Most episodes of mineral losses will be balanced by episodes of gains, and the whole series of events will not cause discernible signs and symptoms of caries (i.e. caries lesions), let alone jeopardize the integrity of the tooth structure. As long as the results of the processes stay within these limits no one needs to be concerned with the exact state of affairs (the 'truth') with respect to mineral losses or gains, because these are transient and self-limiting in nature. The biological processes described are physiological processes occurring in any biofilm on a tooth surface and should not be confused with caries.

The key messages are two-fold:

- It is meaningless for dentists to continue to pester themselves with attempts to refine the search for the 'truth' about caries. Rather, they need to consider what is sensible and meaningful from a clinical patient-oriented health outcome perspective. The essentialistic gold-standard caries paradigm is unhelpful, because it leads into a blind alley in search of an intangible caries 'truth'.
- For the future, dental professionals should base themselves in the nominalistic, patient-centered paradigm, according to which those caries diagnostic criteria are chosen that correspond to the interventions resulting in the best long-term health outcomes for the tooth and the patient.

The wealth of caries diagnostic methods

As indicated in Chapters 4–6, the caries diagnostic options available to the dentist are abundant and wide ranging. Broadly speaking, they fall into one of three groups, which may be designated the 'classics', the 'newcomers' and the 'prospects'. The 'classics' comprise visual–tactile inspection, which may include fiber-optic transillumination (FOTI), and bitewing radiography, including digital radiography [Chapters 4 and 5; Ismail, 1997, 2004; Ismail & Sohn, 1999; Nyvad *et al.*, 1999; Analoui & Stookey, 2000; Ekstrand, 2004; Wenzel, 2004; Hintze, 2004; International Caries Detection and Assessment System (ICDAS) Coordinating Committee, 2005a, b)]. The 'newcomers' encompass laser fluorescence (DIAGNOdent®), quantitative laser fluorescence (QLF) and the electrical caries monitor (Chapter 6; van der Veen & de Josselin de Jong, 2000; Stookey, 2004; Longbottom & Huysmans, 2004; Lussi *et al.*, 2004; Kühnish & Heinrich-Weltzien, 2004; Haak & Wicht, 2004; Bader &

Shugars, 2004; Pretty & Maupomé, 2004; Tranæus *et al.*, 2005; Stookey, 2005); and the 'prospects' are based on techniques such as multiphoton imaging, thermography, infrared fluorescence, optical coherence tomography, ultrasound and terahertz imaging (Chapter 6; Colston *et al.*, 2000; Hall & Girkin, 2004) not yet developed for clinical use.

... and the wealth of caries diagnostic criteria

Within each diagnostic method, several different sets of criteria exist. The classic methods illustrate this, as Ismail (2004) identified 29 different sets of visual–tactile caries diagnostic criteria reported in the literature between 1966 and 2000. Within these criteria the actual maneuvers undertaken during the visual–tactile clinical examination may vary a lot, e.g. with respect to the use of explorers (Hamilton & Stookey, 2005), or in the perceived necessity to clean and dry the teeth before the examination (Ismail, 2004). Similarly, bitewing radiography covers a host of options (Wenzel, 1995, 2004; Hintze, 2004), including conventional versus digital radiography, number of exposures, different film and storage phosphor plate types, as well as different criteria used to describe the radiographic observations.

The evolution in caries diagnostic methods

There is little doubt that most of the caries diagnostic activities undertaken in modern clinical practice have evolved from tradition. They are therefore deeply rooted in the history of dentistry. Until the beginning of the twentieth century the only caries diagnostic option available to the dental professional was the visual–tactile clinical inspection or ocular-instrumental examination (Raper, 1925) as it was then called. The early twentieth century was the prime time for proponents of the focal infection theory (Burt, 1978; Weintraub & Burt, 1985; Baelum, 1998) (Chapter 32), and a main concern among dental professionals was not so much caries per se, but rather the danger that caries could lead to 'pulpless teeth'. The pulpless tooth was considered a serious risk for grave systemic diseases in other parts of the body, and for decades, periapical radiographs had been used to diagnose such teeth. However, in 1925, a different form of radiography was proposed (Raper, 1925) – the bitewing radiographic examination – to be used annually or biannually to detect cavities of decay before they caused pain, as pain is indicative of pulp involvement. Raper noted that dentists overlook many carious cavities when using only ocular-instrumental examination, and demonstrated this by letting a young woman with a 'pretty good set of teeth' undergo a radiographic bitewing examination, which revealed five cavities and two insufficient fillings (Raper, 1925). The woman subsequently went to each of 10 independent dentists for an 'ordinary ocular, instrumental examination' focussed on observations 'in between the teeth'. This resulted in 'ten out of ten … not find[ing] what the roentgen ray had revealed' (Raper, 1925). This reasoning marked the birth of the concept of the additional caries diagnostic yield, which is discussed in more detail later.

Evaluating caries diagnostic methods

Although the clinical and the bitewing radiographic examination have remained the centerpieces of caries diagnosis ever since the early twentieth century, a more formal approach to the evaluation of the clinical and radiographic caries diagnostic methods had to await the middle and latter half of the twentieth century. As World War II approached, focus moved away from focal infection being the main concern in relation to caries. Increasing attention was paid to issues concerning the best ways to treat and prevent the disease. In the late 1930s the beneficial effects of fluoride on caries incidence began to crystallize, and the correctness (validity) of clinical and radiographic caries diagnosis gradually became an area of concern (Burket, 1941; Arnold et al., 1944). Beginning with formal statistical evaluations of the reproducibility (reliability) of the radiographic diagnostic methods (Backer Dirks et al., 1951), such formal statistical evaluations were also instigated of the correctness (validity) of the caries diagnoses made (Downer, 1975), using a gold-standard methodology. The issues of the correctness and reproducibility of caries diagnostic methods were further expanded when caries epidemiology gained interest and called for standardization of diagnostic methods and criteria and calibrated examiners. The diagnostic test evaluation methods then outlined have increasingly gained ground in response to the host of new diagnostic options that have been developed and offered for use in dental practice over the past few decades.

Diagnostic test assessment in the essentialistic gold-standard paradigm

Despite the obvious flaws of the essentialistic gold-standard paradigm, the dental profession has almost exclusively based approaches to the evaluation of caries diagnostic methods on a mistaken faith in the existence of a caries 'truth', a caries gold standard. In view of the popularity of the reasoning that follows from this belief, it is important to understand in some detail the methods used and their limitations.

In the gold-standard paradigm, the focus of attention is the degree of correctness of the diagnosis. This correctness is estimated by comparing the actual findings using the diagnostic test method with the 'truth' as expressed by the gold-standard reference method.

The observations made in caries diagnosis belong to one of four measurement scales (Table 7.1): the dichotomous, the nominal, the ordinal or the numerical scale, which may be continuous or discrete. A dichotomous (or binary) measurement scale is one where observations occur in one of two possible categories, such as cavity present/cavity absent. A nominal scale of measurement is one where observations belong to one of several categories, such as sound/enamel caries/dentin caries/filled. For observations belonging to an ordinal scale, it is possible to rank order the categories, such as none/mild/moderate/severe, but the distance between categories is not known. For measurements belonging to a numerical scale, one can both rank order the observations and tell exactly how far apart they are. In the discrete numerical scale the observations are restricted to integer values (e.g. number of teeth with caries), whereas the continuous scale does not restrict the observations to particular values. An example of the latter is age, which, if we had the right measurement instruments, could be expressed in nanoseconds rather than in years or months, if such served any reasonable purpose.

Clinical and radiographic caries diagnostic recordings typically belong to the dichotomous, the nominal or the ordinal scale (Table 7.1), whereas the more advanced methods, such as laser fluorescence (DIAGNOdent) and electrical resistance measurement in principle produce recordings on a continuous numerical scale.

Diagnostic accuracy: sensitivity and specificity

If caries diagnostic observations originate in a dichotomous scale, it is very easy to compare the findings with the

Table 7.1 Examples of measurement scales used in caries diagnosis

	Measurement scale			
	Dichotomous	Nominal	Ordinal	Numerical
Diagnostic method	Visual–tactile	Visual–tactile or radiographic	Radiographic	Laser fluorescence
Possible outcomes	Cavity present Cavity absent	Sound Decayed Filled Filled with decay Missing	Sound Lesion < ½ into enamel Lesion > ½ into enamel, but not in dentin Lesion into dentin, but < ½ through Lesion > ½ through dentin	Readings in the range from 0 to 99

caries 'truth' as expressed by a gold-standard reference method. This is done in a simple 2 × 2 table (Table 7.2). From this table the diagnostic test sensitivity can be calculated as TP/(TP + FN) and the test specificity as TN/(FP + TN). The test sensitivity expresses the probability that the diagnostic method (the test) indicates 'caries', when caries is truly present; and the test specificity expresses the probability that the test indicates 'no caries', when caries is truly not present. The ideal caries diagnostic test method has sensitivity = specificity = 1, indicating that the test always reflects the true state of affairs.

From a clinical perspective, sensitivity and specificity values are not overly interesting, because they are based on a priori knowledge of the true state of affairs: caries presence or absence. In the real-life clinical diagnostic situation, the caries 'truth' is unknown, and the probabilities of interest to the dental clinician would instead be the predictive value positive and negative of the caries diagnostic test in question. Referring to Table 7.2, it is more interesting for the clinician to know whether a positive diagnostic test result can be trusted as evidence of caries (predictive value positive), and whether a negative test result is indeed indicative of a sound surface (predictive value negative).

Predictive values, positive and negative

In caries diagnostic research, predictive values have been calculated from the very same data sets that gave rise to the accuracy parameters (i.e. based on the data corresponding to Table 7.2), or by application of Bayes' theorem. Bayes' theorem may be used to convert prior disease probabilities (by means of sensitivity and specificity values) to posterior disease probabilities (expressed in the predictive values positive and negative). The concepts of prior and posterior probabilities are perhaps best understood by considering an example. Suppose a man phones you at your dental clinic, asking whether you think he might have caries. In the absence of any other information, your best estimate of the probability of caries is 0.50, corresponding to the 50–50 chance of being correct when guessing. Thinking that the older the man is, the more probable is caries, you would probably attempt to come up with a more informed estimate, for example by asking the man about his age. Such is a part of taking the patient history, and this can be considered a (very simple) diagnostic test. If, moreover, you happen to know that the prevalence of caries among

50–59-year-old men (which happens to be the age group of the man on the phone) in your area is 90%, you can revise your prior caries probability estimate of 0.50 to a posterior probability estimate of 0.90. This is precisely what Bayes' theorem is about: the revision of prior (not so informed) disease probabilities into posterior (more informed) disease probabilities using new evidence (diagnostic test information).

Bayes' theorem dictates that the caries predictive values positive (PV+) and negative (PV−) can be calculated using these formulae:

$$PV+ = Prev \cdot Sens/[Prev \cdot Sens + (1-Prev) \cdot (1-Spec)]$$

and

$$PV- = (1-Prev) \cdot Spec/[(1-Prev) \cdot Spec + Prev \cdot (1-Sens)]$$

where Sens and Spec denote the sensitivity and specificity, respectively, and Prev denotes the prevalence (probability) of caries.

A closely related method involves the use of likelihood ratios (Fletcher *et al.*, 1996) to convert prior disease odds to posterior disease odds. The likelihood ratio for a positive test result is defined as sensitivity/[1 − specificity], and the likelihood ratio for a negative test result is [1 − sensitivity]/specificity. Odds are mathematically related to disease probabilities by the formula Odds = p/[1 − p], and the relevant predictive values are therefore easily calculated.

Receiver operating characteristic curves

When the caries diagnostic observations belong to an ordinal scale, or a numerical scale (Table 7.1), it is possible to calculate pairs of sensitivity and specificity estimates for each possible threshold value that can be used to turn the measurement scales into a dichotomous scale. The pairs of accuracy estimates defined by (1−specificity, sensitivity) are defining points for a curve, termed the receiver operating characteristic (ROC) curve (Fig. 7.3). The ideal diagnostic test in the gold-standard paradigm has sensitivity = 1, indicating that all caries lesions are found; and 1−specificity = 0, indicating that no sound surface is erroneously deemed carious. This corresponds to the point defined by the left-hand upper corner in the diagram in Fig. 7.3.

ROC curves are commonly summarized by calculating the area under the curve (AUC), as a fraction ranging between 0 and 1. The numerical value of the AUC for a given caries diagnostic test can be interpreted as the probability that a randomly chosen carious lesion will elicit a higher diagnostic test value than a randomly chosen sound surface (Hanley & McNeil, 1982; Lee, 1999). An AUC value of 0.50, which corresponds to the area under the diagonal in Fig. 7.3, thus indicates a 50–50 chance that a carious surface will elicit a higher test value than a sound surface. In other words, an AUC value of 0.50 indicates a useless caries diagnostic test.

Table 7.2 Diagnostic test matrix for a dichotomous test result (T) in the diagnosis of caries

		True caries status = gold standard	
		Caries present	Caries absent
Test result	T+	True positive (TP)	False positive (FP)
	T−	False negative (FN)	True negative (TN)

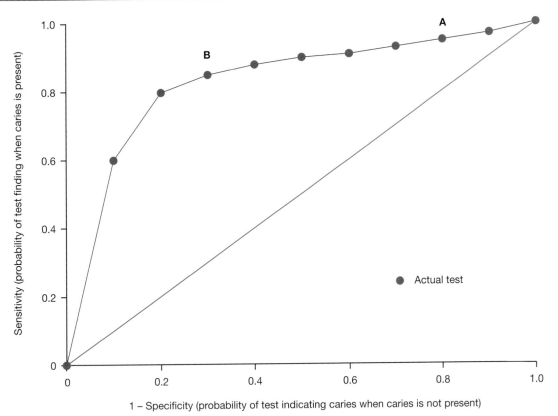

Figure 7.3 The receiver operating characteristic (ROC) curve connecting points determined by (1 – specificity, sensitivity). The test is a hypothetical caries test with nine threshold values [the endpoints (0,0) and (1,1) do not count as threshold values because they correspond to never declaring caries present or always declaring caries present, respectively]. See text for explanation of points A and B (p. 113).

Leaps in the essentialistic gold-standard reasoning

Which is the caries gold standard?

The preceding text has shown that the truth about caries is elusive. It is therefore not surprising that a wealth of different methods has been proposed and used for establishing the caries gold-standard (Wenzel & Hintze, 1999; Huysmans & Longbottom, 2004; Hintze, 2004). The variation is so great in the gold-standard reference methods that the test method investigated in one study may be serving as the reference gold-standard method in other studies (Hintze & Wenzel, 2003; Hintze, 2004). Not only may so many gold standards lead to circular reasoning, but there is also a considerable danger that new reference methods are adopted merely on the grounds of showing no statistically significant difference from older ones. Since a new test method can never be observed to perform better than the reference method (Wenzel & Hintze, 1999) there is a real danger that this confused use of the gold-standard methodology may make new tests seem worse even when they are actually better (Fletcher *et al.*, 1996).

Spectrum bias and transferability

The gold-standard reference for caries is often established using *in vitro* methods involving extracted teeth that are assessed for the presence or depth of demineralization (Huysmans & Longbottom, 2004; Hintze, 2004) using radiographic, visual or histological methods. The tooth materials available for such assessment are often limited and selective, and the use of these *in vitro* methods usually results in a distorted disease spectrum compared to the disease spectrum that would be observed *in vivo* in the free-living populations, for which the caries diagnostic methods are intended. Comprehensive reviews by Bader *et al.* (2001, 2002) have shown that the caries 'prevalence' in the tooth 'populations' used for 'gold-standard' evaluation of caries diagnostic methods is often exceedingly high (50–90%) compared to the situation encountered in free-living natural populations, where estimates of less than 20% are more probable. This means that caries lesions are grossly overrepresented in the tooth populations studied, while sound surfaces are severely underrepresented. It is increasingly recognized that the diagnostic accuracy parameters, sensitivity and specificity, are not diagnostic test constants, but vary according to the disease spectrum (Ransohoff & Feinstein, 1978; Begg & Greenes, 1983; Knottnerus & Leffers, 1992; Fletcher *et al.*, 1996; Guggenmoos-Holzmann & van Houwelingen, 2000). The disease spectrum is, in turn, influenced by a host of sociodemographic factors, including age, gender, place of residence and access to dental health care. This means that there is a considerable risk that most of the accuracy estimates provided in the literature may have limited relevance and transferability for caries diagnosis in free-living populations. This problem also affects the predictive values, whether calculated by means of Bayes' theorem, the likelihood ratio method, or the biased tables that gave rise to the sensitivity and specificity parameters. Either way, the predictive values obtained will attain a similarly limited transferability to free-living populations and are therefore likely to be of limited relevance for clinical caries diagnostic decision making.

Problems in interpreting sensitivity and specificity

As indicated above, the ideal caries diagnostic test has sensitivity and specificity values of 1, predictive values of 1 and an area under the ROC curve of 1. However, in real life these parameters never reach 1, and some trade-offs must be made. One rule devised for the evaluation of the appropriateness of a diagnostic test from sensitivity and specificity estimates is based on Youden's index (Youden, 1950). The index value is the maximal value of the sum of the accuracy parameters minus 1 (i.e. max[sensitivity + specificity − 1]), over all possible cut-points (threshold values; see section on ROC curves) if applicable. Youden's index ranges between 0, indicating a limited correctness of the test, and 1, indicating a high degree of correctness of the test (Schisterman *et al.*, 2005). The Youden index values required for a test to be considered useful are typically above 0.6, and no caries diagnostic test has consistently been shown to fulfill this requirement, as evidenced by the extensive reviews of caries diagnostic methods by Bader *et al.* (2001, 2002).

In Youden's index the same weight is attached to the sensitivity and specificity of the test, meaning that the consequences of making a false-positive diagnosis are considered equivalent to the consequences of a false-negative diagnosis. That, however, is not a valid assumption. There is a world of difference between the long-term consequences of erroneously inserting a restoration and those of overlooking a carious lesion. This difference becomes even greater in regular dental attendees in low-caries populations, in whom an overlooked lesion is likely to be found on the next appointment, before having progressed to an extent that would alter the treatment needed.

Carious lesion: ruled in or ruled out?

Diagnostic tests are expected to help clinicians to achieve the dual aim of ruling in and ruling out disease. However,

diagnostic tests are usually good in only one or the other, rarely in both (Verdonschot *et al.*, 1992). When the sensitivity approaches 1, the test is good at detecting disease when it is present, whereas when specificity approaches 1 the test is good at detecting health. However, great care must be exercised when interpreting the absolute values of sensitivity and specificity, as the example provided in Table 7.3 shows. The data shown originate in an *in vivo* study (Hintze *et al.*, 1998) of three commonly used diagnostic methods for cavity detection in approximal surfaces: the conventional visual–tactile clinical examination, bitewing radiography and FOTI. Neither FOTI nor bitewing radiography allows for immediate detection of cavities; with FOTI a shadow extending into dentin was interpreted as evidence of cavitation, and with bitewing radiography a radiolucency extending into dentin was assumed to indicate cavitation. The true cavitation status of the surfaces was subsequently established by a direct visual inspection of the surfaces following a 3-day tooth separation using orthodontic rubber rings or separation springs.

The visual–clinical method was observed to produce the lowest total number of diagnostic errors (5.3% of all diagnoses), closely followed by FOTI (5.9%), whereas bitewing radiography nearly doubled the total number of errors (9.2%).

The direction of the errors differed: whereas the errors made in the visual–tactile clinical examination and with FOTI were biased towards overlooking carious cavities (74–98% of the cavities were overlooked), bitewing radiography produced an overweight of false-positive cavity diagnoses (76% of the positive diagnoses were false). This occurred despite the fact that bitewing radiography had the highest Youden index value (0.556 for bitewing radiography versus 0.327 for the visual–tactile clinical examination and 0.040 for FOTI), the highest sensitivity (0.631 versus 0.342 and 0.041) and a slightly lower specificity (0.925) compared to the values for the visual–tactile clinical examination (0.985) and FOTI (0.999). However, it is

Table 7.3 Number of errors resulting from the application of three caries diagnostic methods used to detect cavitated lesions

| The 'truth' | n | Visual–tactile | | FOTI | | Radiographic | |
		C	NC	C	NC	C	NC
C	60	21	39	2	58	38	22
NC	940	14	926	1	939	70	870
Total n	1000	35	965	3	997	108	892
Predictive values		0.60	0.96	0.67	0.94	0.35	0.98

The methods include visual-tactile clinical examination (sensitivity 0.342, specificity 0.985), fiber-optic transillumination (FOTI) (sensitivity 0.041, specificity 0.999) and bitewing radiography (sensitivity 0.631, specificity 0.925). A true cavity prevalence of 6% is assumed.
C: cavitation; NC: no cavitation.

precisely the combination of the slightly lower specificity and the high occurrence of non-cavitated surfaces (i.e. the low caries prevalence) that results in bitewing radiography producing substantially more false-positive diagnoses than the visual–tactile clinical examination (see also Chapter 25, Tables 25.3 and 25.4).

The predictive values given in Table 7.3 indicate that cavitation is best ruled out by bitewing radiography (PV– = 0.98), whereas cavitation is best ruled in by the visual–tactile clinical examination (PV+ = 0.60). (FOTI appeared to have a slightly higher predictive value positive than the clinical examination, but a calculation based on only three positive diagnoses may be quite unreliable.) In other words, if these results were universally applicable, they would indicate that the positive visual–tactile clinical findings and the negative bitewing findings should be trusted.

Problems interpreting receiver operating characteristic curves

AUC values have often been used to compare caries diagnostic test methods (Hintze *et al.*, 2002; Mileman & van den Hout, 2002; Ellwood & Côrtes, 2004; Haak & Wicht, 2005), typically by testing the null hypothesis that the AUC values for two alternative methods do not differ statistically significantly. Rarely do these studies discuss the fundamentally important distinction between clinical and statistical significance, just as the observation of no statistically significant difference between two methods often (mis-)leads researchers to conclude equality of the methods. This is very problematic owing to the lack of agreement among caries researchers about the most appropriate caries gold standard, leading to the aforementioned confusion of diagnostic test methods with gold-standard reference methods.

ROC curves are interpreted as global measures of diagnostic test performance because they produce a single summary, the curve or the AUC, which condenses several alternative options for the diagnostic threshold (cut-point) used to declare caries presence or absence into a single number. This means that the ROC curves and their areas do not have immediate applicability for the clinical diagnostic situation. In the clinical situation, the dentist cannot act on an ROC curve or an AUC value; he or she needs to select the diagnostic threshold level by selecting only one point among the many alternative points that have defined the ROC curve. This is perhaps best understood considering Fig. 7.3, which shows the ROC curve for a hypothetical caries diagnostic test with nine possible threshold values. Let us assume that these are: lesion <0.25 into enamel, ⩾0.25 into enamel, ⩾0.5 into enamel, ⩾0.75 into enamel, into dentin but <0.25, ⩾0.25 into dentin, ⩾0.5 into dentin, ⩾0.75 into dentin, or reaching pulp. A dentist choosing the diagnostic threshold level at point A = ⩾0.25 into enamel will find more carious lesions than one choosing a more

restrictive threshold level for a positive diagnosis, say at point B = ⩾0.5 into dentin. If threshold A is chosen, caries will be diagnosed with a high sensitivity (0.95), but a low specificity (0.20); whereas if threshold B is chosen, caries will be diagnosed with a somewhat lower sensitivity (0.85), but a higher specificity (0.70). This leads back to the situation described above on the interpretation of sensitivity and specificity estimates. For the purpose of selecting the diagnostic threshold, a trade-off must be made between sensitivity and specificity. This is a decision as to whether we are happier with false-positive diagnoses (i.e. overaggressive lesion diagnosis) or with false-negative diagnoses (i.e. overlooking lesions), and this decision cannot be made merely on the basis of the ROC curve or the AUC estimate.

Caries diagnostic correctness: a blind alley

Dentistry is a craft that has grown from its cottage industry roots to attempt to embrace a professional and scientific evidence-based approach to the activities undertaken (Chapter 32). Seen in this light, the evaluations carried out of the correctness of caries diagnostic methods based on the essentialistic 'gold-standard' reasoning must be complimented. However, as shown above, the essentialistic thinking leads to failure when the 'truth'-defining characteristics are found in naturally occurring physiological processes, such as those determined by microbial activity in biofilms located on tooth surfaces. Biological systems and processes tend to involve a multitude of self-regulating mechanisms. This influences diagnosis because a potentially deleterious sequence of events in a biological system is often naturally countered by a subsequent beneficial sequence of events, and therefore requires neither diagnosis nor intervention. Just think of the countless 'errors' occurring during the innumerable daily cell divisions necessary for maintaining human organ function, which are taken care of by naturally occurring clean-up mechanisms. This self-regulation means that diagnostic research will increasingly come to recognize that trying to identify the first step in a potentially deleterious sequence of events may amount to entering a blind alley. Researchers and clinicians alike should rather be concerned with the identification of clinically relevant points of no return. These may be defined as points that, if they are surpassed, tangibly alter the prognosis for the patient towards the worse, or substantially alter the treatment options.

Diagnostic test evaluation in the nominalistic caries paradigm

So far, this chapter has shown that there is no easy or objective way to decide whether a caries diagnosis is correct or not. The key to appropriate caries diagnosis is not found in a gold-standard reference method, but in the outcomes of caries diagnostic activities. The best caries diagnostic method is the one that results in the best long-term dental health outcome for the tooth and the patient. It follows that the more relevant approach to caries diagnostic test evaluation uses the randomized, controlled clinical trial (RCCT) to determine whether a new caries diagnostic method results in better long-term health outcomes than does the traditional method. The use of the RCCT design allows evaluation of the professionally determined dental health outcome and may also include evaluation of patient preferences and cost aspects. However, no such RCCTs exist yet, and therefore a different approach must be used.

The approach taken is a clarification and elucidation of the key salient factors involved in the making of caries scripts (Bader & Shugars, 1997). As pointed out earlier in this chapter, several factors determine the nature and content of the 'this-clinical-picture-needs-this-intervention'-like caries scripts used by dentists for caries management purposes.

Long-term health outcomes: the management options?

As previously pointed out, the caries management options are crucial in determining what should be diagnosed. Cavitated carious lesions usually need restorations because it is very difficult to keep such lesions under sufficient plaque control to prevent further progress of the lesion. Cavities located in easily accessible buccal surfaces, and occasionally occlusal surfaces, could be exempted from this general rule, as it is possible to keep such cavities fairly plaque free and thus arrest further progression (Nyvad & Fejerskov, 1986). However, aesthetic considerations may prevent the patient from accepting this management option, as arrested carious lesions tend to be dark and aesthetically displeasing. Non-cavitated lesions may be classified as either arrested, inactive lesions, or active, ongoing lesions (Chapter 4). An arrested non-cavitated carious lesion needs no intervention unless the patient expresses aesthetic concerns. The management options for the active, non-cavitated caries lesion are found in the non-operative package, and include plaque control, use of topical fluorides and dietary intervention.

It follows that the information sought when performing clinical caries diagnostic examinations concerns lesion cavitation and lesion activity, as these features are decisive for the best management options and therefore the best long-term health outcome. We now know not only what we are looking for, but also why this is so!

Interexaminer and intraexaminer errors in caries diagnosis

Any caries diagnostic test method is prone to errors owing to less than perfect intraexaminer and interexaminer reliability (Hintze *et al.*, 1998; Machiulskiene *et al.*, 1999; Nyvad

et al., 1999). Dentists cannot reproduce completely either their own caries recordings or those of a fellow dentist. A real-life example of this is shown in Table 7.4 (Nyvad *et al.*, 1999). A dentist was asked to repeat on different days the clinical caries examinations made in 50 children. During the first examination, the dentist observed 90 cavities in the 5510 tooth surfaces examined. During the second examination, a similar number (87) of cavities was observed, indicating a difference of 'only' three cavities between the two examinations. In the dental diagnostic research literature, it is commonplace to describe the agreement between examinations, or between examiners, by means of the percentage agreement. Table 7.4 shows that this was high, amounting to 95% of all diagnoses made. However, owing to the fact that some of the agreement may have been obtained by chance, it is also customary to account for this by means of calculating the chance-corrected agreement in the form of Cohen's kappa (Cohen, 1960). In the example provided in Table 7.4, kappa was 0.82, indicating an agreement that was 82% of the maximum obtainable chance-corrected one.

Is this good or bad agreement? The dental research literature commonly answers this question by referring the kappa value to one of the normative scales published for the interpretation of kappa values (Landis & Koch, 1977; Byrt, 1996). Depending on the choice of reference scale, a kappa value of 0.82 would justify descriptors such as 'very good', 'excellent' or 'almost perfect'. Unfortunately, such descriptors often lead dental researchers to ignore completely the existence of measurement errors, and this is a fundamental flaw in much dental diagnostic reasoning. Table 7.4 shows that a total of 104 teeth received a cavity diagnosis at one or the other examination. Only 73 (70%) of these were from the same teeth, and from a clinician's point one may indeed wonder whether confirmation of only 70% of the cavities is suggestive of the near-perfect reliability of the caries diagnostic method. In real-life, the dentist would probably restore all 90 cavities observed at the first examination, even though 17 of these could not be confirmed, had a second examination taken place. Examination of the children again, e.g. after a recall period of 6 months, might therefore result in an additional 14

Table 7.4 Example of a data table arising when assessing the intraexaminer reliability of caries diagnoses made at the cavity level

		Second examination		
		No cavity	Cavity	
First examination	No cavity	5406	14	5420
	Cavity	17	73	90
		5423	87	5510

Percentage agreement = (5406 + 73) × 100/5510 = 99.4%.
Kappa = $(p_{obs} - p_{exp})/(1 - p_{exp})$ = 0.82.

cavities being detected and restored. Undoubtedly, most dentists would perceive the additional cavities observed at the second visit as resulting from caries progression, just as they would never realize the probable overtreatment of the 17 unconfirmed cavities that they restored following the first examination (Table 7.4).

The example highlights the facts that diagnostic decisions are made under uncertainty, and that repeating less-than-perfect diagnostic methods leads to an accumulation of diagnostic errors. As the error-free diagnostic method does not exist, dentists must acknowledge this uncertainty and integrate it into their clinical script inventory. Routine dental screening examinations involve the regular repetition of less-than-perfect diagnostic methods in asymptomatic patients, and call for a consideration of the intraexaminer agreement for diagnostic methods. The interexaminer agreement in dental diagnosis is typically lower than the intraexaminer agreement (Hintze *et al.*, 1998; Machiulskiene *et al.*, 1999; Nyvad *et al.*, 1999), and these findings imply that it can indeed be risky to undergo routine dental examinations too often, just as they illustrate the additional risk of diagnostic errors from changing dentist too often. As many dentists continue to consider restorative treatment *the* treatment of caries (Elderton, 2003), these diagnostic errors only add to the risk of entering the patient into the cycle of re-restorations (Elderton, 1985a, b, 1990, 1992, 1993), termed 'iatrogenesis' (Elderton, 1992).

A famous tonsillectomy example published more than 70 years ago (American Child Health Association, 1934; Bakwin, 1945), and later confirmed for other treatments (Ayanian & Berwick, 1991), may be used to illustrate the potential problem involved. The tonsillectomy study was based on a screening of 1000 11-year-old children for the need for tonsillectomy. Children who were deemed negative on the first physical examination were reexamined by another physician and this scheme continued for three rounds. The study clearly demonstrated that undergoing more screening examinations will cause more 'disease' to be found, and the absurd end result was that only 65 of 1000 children would still remain untreated after three routine screening examinations. Although this example is extreme, it is nevertheless worth keeping in mind, considering that the dental professions encourage the populations served to adopt dental attendance patterns involving routine screening examinations, typically every 6–12 months (NHS National Institute for Clinical Excellence, 2004; Mettes *et al.*, 2005).

How do we deal with the unavoidable diagnostic uncertainty?

The first necessary realization is that it is only human to err. Perfection is simply not compatible with human observation. The dental profession should clearly strive to reduce diagnostic errors as much as possible, and can undoubtedly achieve much in this respect. Regular calibration exercises might reduce differences between dental clinicians, and make them see more eye to eye on different clinical presentations. However, no one has ever been able to demonstrate that diagnostic errors can be eradicated by means of intense calibration. The data presented on intraexaminer reproducibility in caries diagnosis testify to this, as no examiner has been reported consistently to be able to avoid diagnostic errors in caries diagnosis. The bottom line is that dental professionals should accommodate the fact that they cannot completely eradicate diagnostic errors in caries diagnosis, whereby the diagnostic errors become inevitable facts that need to be taken into account in clinical decisions.

The key question to answer is this: What will happen if I make a diagnostic mistake? The false-positive diagnosis of a cavity where no cavity exists may needlessly enter the tooth into the vicious cycle of re-restoration (Brantley *et al.*, 1995; Elderton, 2003). Restorations have a limited survival in relation to the human lifespan (Brantley *et al.*, 1995; Qvist *et al.*, 1997; Wendt *et al.*, 1998; Qvist, 2002; Roeleveld *et al.*, 2006), and tend to grow bigger for each replacement (Brantley *et al.*, 1995; Elderton, 2003) (Chapter 20). Each replacement carries a risk of adverse effects on the pulp (Chapter 21), a considerable risk of iatrogenic damage to neighboring teeth (Qvist *et al.*, 1992; Lussi & Gygax, 1998; Medeiros & Seddon, 2000; Lenters *et al.*, 2006), as well as economic costs to the patient.

The consequences of a false-negative diagnosis of a cavity, i.e. overlooking a carious cavity, depend on a number of factors. If the patient in question is at a high risk of rapid caries progression, and only attends the dentist in case of symptoms, there is a real risk that an overlooked carious cavity may progress to pulp involvement and serious dental hard tissue breakdown, causing pain and endangering tooth survival, before a dentist has had a chance to detect it. However, evidence suggests that this risk may often be exaggerated. Studies show that the risk of a primary tooth being extracted (Tickle *et al.*, 1999; Milsom *et al.*, 2002b), developing pain (Milsom *et al.*, 2002a), or becoming extracted owing to pain (Tickle *et al.*, 2002; Milsom *et al.*, 2002a) is not influenced by whether the tooth is restored or not. While these results may in part be explained by difficulties in making adequate restorations in children (Roeleveld *et al.*, 2006), they also serve to challenge a widely held treatment philosophy.

If, however, the patient in whom we have overlooked a carious cavity is characterized by slow caries progression, and attends the dentist fairly regularly, it is likely that the overlooked cavity will be detected at a later dental visit before any serious additional tissue destruction has occurred. If such is the case, the health outcome consequences of having overlooked the lesion may be considered negligible.

The false-positive diagnosis of an active non-cavitated caries lesion will result not in operative treatment but in non-operative intervention, including plaque control, topical fluorides and dietary intervention. While this represents a cost for the patient, it does not result in a deleterious health outcome.

The consequences of overlooking an active non-cavitated caries lesion (a false-negative diagnosis) depend on several factors. If the patient is caries active and an irregular dental attendee, there is a risk that the lesion may progress to the cavitation stage before it is detected. Thereby, the consequence could be unnecessary entry into the cycle of re-restoration as detailed above. If, however, the patient shows low risk/slow caries progression and/or is a regular attendee, it is probable that the carious lesion will be detected at a later visit before having progressed to the cavitation stage.

The major sections of the populations living in high-income countries are characterized by continued declines in the prevalence and severity of carious lesions, indicating a continued lowering of the caries progression rates (Chapters 8 and 32). The answers to the key questions discussed above indicate that in such circumstances dentists should adopt very stringent caries diagnostic criteria, and allow all diagnostic doubts to benefit the tooth by choosing the non-operative options over the irreversible operative options. In populations living in high-caries countries characterized by increasing caries incidence, dental clinicians should exercise diligence and meticulousness in the detection of signs of non-cavitated stages of caries lesion formation, to postpone the entry to the vicious cycle of re-restorations for as long as possible. In such high-caries populations, the benefit of the doubt concerning the presence or absence of non-cavitated lesions should be biased towards providing non-operative caries treatment. In other words, the possible cost of unnecessarily carrying out such non-operative treatments should not preclude their routine use if non-cavitated lesions are suspected. Having said so, it is also clear (Chapter 28) that classical chairside dentistry stands little chance of exerting influence over the caries situation in populations where caries is increasing, and that population strategies must be implemented to bring about effective control of the caries situation.

The additional diagnostic yield argument

As mentioned previously, bitewing radiography was introduced as an adjunct to the clinical–visual caries examination based on the argument that bitewing radiography leads to detection of lesions that would otherwise be overlooked. This additional diagnostic yield argument is effectively a sensitivity enhancement argument, although this does not imply adherence to the 'gold-standard' tradition. The additional yield argument is still frequently invoked in the caries diagnostic literature, although the focus has moved away from the detection of cavities towards the detection of earlier stages of carious lesion formation (Kidd & Pitts, 1990; Hintze, 1993; Hintze & Wenzel, 1994) and 'hidden' caries in occlusal surfaces (Weerheijm et al., 1992b, 1997).

Indeed, most studies comparing the diagnostic yield of a clinical and a radiographic caries examination conclude that substantially more lesions are detected in approximal surfaces (de Vries et al., 1990; Kidd & Pitts, 1990; Poorterman et al., 1999; Hopcraft & Morgan, 2005; Llena-Puy & Forner, 2005) and occlusal surfaces (Creanor et al., 1990; Weerheijm et al., 1992a; Poorterman et al., 2000; Fracaro et al., 2001) using bitewing radiographs than by clinical examination alone, hence the common recommendation to use bitewing radiography as an adjunct to the clinical examination. It is implicit in the additional diagnostic yield argument that a positive diagnosis has been reached when at least one of the diagnostic test methods used is positive. However, while this decision rule increases the sensitivity of the combined diagnostic test, it also diminishes the specificity, and this is likely to have the unintentional consequence of actually increasing the total number of diagnostic errors. Using the data in Table 7.3, it can be shown that the addition of bitewing radiography to the visual–tactile examination, and considering a positive diagnosis reached when at least one of the diagnostic tests is positive, results in an increase in the total number of errors from 53 (visual–tactile examination alone) to 97 (both methods combined). More cavities are correctly detected, but this occurs at the expense of an increase in the number of false-positive diagnoses from 14 to 83. Therefore, adding diagnostic test methods also means adding diagnostic errors.

The potential magnitude and seriousness of this problem have been highlighted in a study of the variation among dentists in radiographic caries diagnoses (Espelid & Tveit, 2001). The study indicated that dentists generally produce many false-positive diagnoses of dentin caries when examining approximal or occlusal surfaces that are either sound or with caries confined to the enamel, as are indeed most surfaces. Overall, 21% of the diagnoses made were false-positive diagnoses and more than 70% of the dentists had at least three false-positive diagnoses out of a possible 16.

In the land of the blind the one-eyed is king

It is a serious limitation of the additional diagnostic yield argument that the actual yield observed depends on the diagnostic criteria used with the diagnostic methods being added. The additional yield of bitewing radiography is really only apparent when the clinical criteria have been restricted to recording cavitated lesions only. When the clinical caries examination also comprises recording of the non-cavitated stages of lesion formation, the added value of bitewing radiography is no longer obvious (Machiulskiene *et al.*, 1999, 2004). In fact, these studies indicate that in such circumstances the clinical caries examination will result in the detection of many more lesions than will the bitewing radiographic examination, indicating that the clinical examination is superior in detecting the early carious lesions (Machiulskiene *et al.*, 1999, 2004) that can be controlled by non-operative means (see Figs 4.29, 25.3).

Different diagnostic methods tell different stories

When considering whether to add another caries diagnostic method to the basic clinical examination, one must account for the fact that the different diagnostic methods portray rather different aspects of carious lesions. Depending on the specifics of the diagnostic criteria used, the visual–tactile clinical examination focusses primarily on surface characteristics (Chapter 4) and to a lesser extent on lesion size/depth. Conversely, the bitewing radiographic observations primarily reflect the depth of penetration of demineralization into the dental hard tissues (Chapter 5). The more advanced methods reflect yet other physico-chemical aspects of caries lesions (Chapter 6).

Adding observations is therefore no simple matter, and involves a number of assumptions about the criteria to use which best portray the same underlying dimension or the feature sought. Returning to the example given in Table 7.3, the bitewing radiographic diagnostic criterion used to indicate cavitation was a radiolucency extending at least into the outer third of the dentin (Hintze *et al.*, 1998). Thereby, the assumption has been made that all radiolucencies extending into the outer third of the dentin represent cavitated caries lesions. But is this a tenable assumption? Figure 7.4 shows that it is not. The scientific literature also leans towards a negative answer, as only two small studies (Rugg-Gunn, 1972; Mejàre *et al.*, 1985) have been able to demonstrate clinical cavitation in all (100%) of the approximal radiographic lesions extending into dentin. Most other studies indicate a high frequency of cavitation (75–90%) (Mejàre & Malmgren, 1986; de Araujo *et al.*, 1992, 1996; Akpata *et al.*, 1996) or a substantially lower cavitation frequency (28–65%) (Bille & Thylstrup, 1982; Thylstrup *et al.*, 1986; Pitts & Rimmer, 1992; Lunder & von der Fehr, 1996; Ratledge *et al.*, 2001) of radiographic dentin lesions (see also Table 20.1). Therefore, if a dentist uncritically uses the observation of a radiographic dentin lesion to overrule the clinical observation, the risk may be substantial that an unnecessary restoration is inserted. There are many adverse effects associated with the insertion of a restoration, including iatrogenic damage to neighboring teeth (Qvist *et al.*, 1992; Lussi & Gygax, 1998; Medeiros & Seddon, 2000; Lenters *et al.*, 2006) and limited restoration longevity (Brantley *et al.*, 1995; Qvist *et al.*, 1997; Wendt *et*

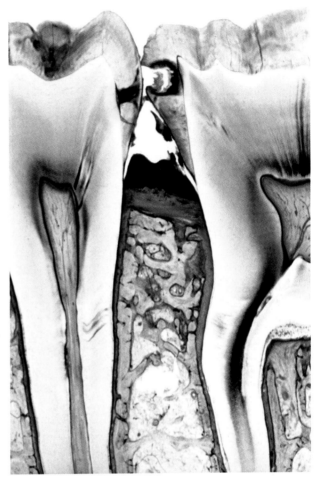

Figure 7.4 Undemineralized section of lower first molar and second premolar both showing caries lesions with complications in the pulpo-dentinal complex. Only the first molar shows a cavity and the premolar might be recorded as sound. (Hanagawa Collection, Ciba University, Japan. Courtesy of Professor Yanigazawa.)

al., 1998; Qvist, 2002; Roeleveld *et al.*, 2006) (Chapter 24). While these adverse effects have to be accepted when the restoration is necessary, they are intolerable wherever they could have been avoided.

Concluding remarks

This chapter has shown that two different lines of thinking exist in caries diagnostic reasoning. The essentialistic view pursues a search for the caries 'truth', while the nominalistic view is more concerned with making diagnoses that reflect the best caries management options. Until now, the former has dominated caries diagnostic research and caries diagnostic test evaluation, although the changing caries concepts have rendered this 'gold-standard' paradigm increasingly inadequate. According to the nominalistic view, the crux of caries diagnosis is to categorize carious lesions to reflect the best management options, which in turn necessitates a profound understanding of the caries causal processes and how they may be interfered with.

The central role of the clinical inspection and the bitewing radiographic examination for caries diagnosis does not originate in formal diagnostic test evaluations, but is deeply rooted in the history of dentistry. Bitewing radiography was introduced in the 1920s as an adjunct to the clinical caries examination, using the additional diagnostic yield argument. However, an additional diagnostic yield of bitewing radiography is discernible only when the clinical examination is limited to cavity diagnosis. The additional benefit of bitewing radiography may indeed be questioned when the clinical examination encompasses the non-cavitated stages of carious lesion formation. The visual–tactile clinical examination and the bitewing radiographic examination capture different features of carious lesions, and the features most relevant for the selection of the best management options are those reflected in the visual–tactile caries examination.

Based on these considerations, good caries diagnostic practice may involve the following elements:

- selection of a visual–tactile diagnostic method that links directly to the management options for caries: cavitated versus non-cavitated, and active versus arrested are the features that determine the management options, and hence should be recorded
- full exhaustion of the visual–tactile diagnostic method, i.e. recording of non-cavitated lesions is a must
- careful consideration of the pros and cons of adding other diagnostic test methods, such as bitewing radiography, to the visual–tactile method
- continued attention to the possibility of diagnostic errors, such that doubt should always bias towards less invasive decisions.

References

Akpata ES, Farid MR, Al-Saif K, Roberts EAU. Cavitation at radiolucent areas on proximal surfaces of posterior teeth. *Caries Res* 1996; **30**: 313–16.

American Child Health Association. *Physical defects: the pathway to correction*. New York: American Child Health Association, 1934: 80–96.

Analoui M, Stookey GK. Direct digital radiography for caries detection and analysis. *Monogr Oral Sci* 2000; **17**: 1–19.

de Araujo FB, Rosito DB, Toigo E, dos Santos CK. Diagnosis of approximal caries: radiographic versus clinical examination using tooth separation. *Am J Dent* 1992; **5**: 245–8.

de Araujo FB, de Araujo DR, dos Santos CK, de Souza MA. Diagnosis of approximal caries in primary teeth: radiographic versus clinical examination using tooth separation. *Am J Dent* 1996; **9**: 54–6.

Arnold FA, Dean HT, Singleton DE. The effect on caries incidence of a single topical application of a fluoride solution to the teeth of young adult males of a military population. *J Dent Res* 1944; **23**: 155–62.

Ayanian JZ, Berwick DM. Do physicians have a bias toward action? A classic study revisited. *Med Decis Making* 1991; **11**: 154–8.

Backer Dirks O, van Amerongen J, Winkler KC. A reproducible method for caries evaluation. *J Dent Res* 1951; **30**: 346–59.

Bader JD, Shugars DA. Understanding dentists' restorative treatment decisions. *J Publ Health Dent* 1992; **52**: 102–10.

Bader JD, Shugars DA. Variation in dentists' clinical decisions. *J Publ Health Dent* 1995a; **55**: 181–8.

Bader JD, Shugars DA. Variation, treatment outcomes, and practice guidelines in dental practice. *J Dent Educ* 1995b; **59**: 61–95.

Bader JD, Shugars DA. What do we know about how dentists make caries-related treatment decisions? *Community Dent Oral Epidemiol* 1997; **25**: 97–103.

Bader JD, Shugars DA. A systematic review of the performance of a laser fluorescence device for detecting caries. *J Am Dent Assoc* 2004; **135**: 1413–26.

Bader JD, Shugars DA, Bonito AJ. Systematic reviews of selected caries diagnostic and management methods. *J Dent Educ* 2001; **65**: 960–8.

Bader JD, Shugars DA, Bonito AJ. A systematic review of the performance of methods for identifying carious lesions. *Publ Health Dent* 2002; **62**: 201–13.

Baelum V. *The epidemiology of destructive periodontal disease. Causes, paradigms, problems, methods and empirical evidence.* Dissertation. Aarhus: University of Aarhus, 1998.

Baelum V, Heidmann J, Nyvad B. Dental caries paradigms in diagnosis and diagnostic research. *Eur J Oral Sci* 2006; **114**: 263–77.

Bakwin H. Pseudodoxia pediatrica. *N Engl J Med* 1945; **232**: 691–7.

Begg CB, Greenes RA. Assessment of diagnostic tests when disease verification is subject to selection bias. *Biometrics* 1983; **39**: 207–15.

Bille J, Thylstrup A. Radiographic diagnosis and clinical tissue changes in relation to treatment of approximal carious lesions. *Caries Res* 1982; **16**: 1–6.

ten Bosch JJ, Angmar-Mansson B. Characterization and validation of diagnostic methods. *Monogr Oral Sci* 2000; **17**: 174–89.

Brantley CF, Bader JD, Shugars DA, Nesbit SP. Does the cycle of restorations lead to larger restorations? *J Am Dent Assoc* 1995; **126**: 1407–13.

Burket LW. The accuracy of clinical and roentgenologic diagnosis of dental caries as determined by microscopic studies. *J Dent Res* 1941; **20**: 70–6.

Burt BA. Influences for change in the dental health status of populations: an historical perspective. *J Publ Health Dent* 1978; **38**: 272–88.

Byrt T. How good is that agreement? *Epidemiology* 1996; **7**: 561.

Choi BCK, Jokovic A, Kay EJ, Main PA, Leake JL. Reducing variability in treatment decision-making: effectiveness of educating clinicians about uncertainty. *Med Educ* 1998; **32**: 105–11.

Cohen J. A coefficient of agreement for nominal scales. *Educ Psychol Meas* 1960; **20**: 37–46.

Colston BW Jr, Everett MJ, Sathyam US, DaSilva LB, Otis LL. Imaging of the oral cavity using optical coherence tomography. *Monogr Oral Sci* 2000; **17**: 32–55.

Creanor SL, Russell JI, Strang DM, Stephen KW, Burchell CK. The prevalence of clinically undetected occlusal dentine caries in Scottish adolescents. *Br Dent J* 1990; **169**: 126–9.

Downer MC. Concurrent validity of an epidemiological diagnostic system for caries with the histological appearance of extracted teeth as validating criterion. *Caries Res* 1975; **9**: 231–46.

Ecenbarger W. How honest are dentists? *Readers Digest* 1997; (February); 50–6.

Ekstrand KR. Improving clinical visual detection – potentials for caries clinical trials. *J Dent Res* 2004; **83**(Special Issue C): C67–71.

Elderton RJ. Implications of recent dental health services research on the future of operative dentistry. *J Publ Health Dent* 1985a; **45**: 101–5.

Elderton RJ. Scope for change in clinical practice. *J R Soc Med* 1985b; **78**(Suppl): 27–32.

Elderton RJ. Clinical studies concerning re-restoration of teeth. *Adv Dent Res* 1990; **4**: 4–9.

Elderton RJ. Iatrogenesis in the treatment of dental caries. *Proc Finn Dent Soc* 1992; **88**: 25–32.

Elderton RJ. Overtreatment with restorative dentistry: when to intervene? *Int Dent J* 1993; **43**: 17–24.

Elderton RJ. Preventive (evidence-based) approach to quality general dental care. *Med Princ Pract* 2003; **12**(Suppl 1): 12–21.

Ellwood RP, Côrtes DF. *In vitro* assessment of methods of applying the Electrical Caries Monitor for the detection of occlusal caries. *Caries Res* 2004; **38**: 45–53.

Espelid I, Tveit AB. A comparison of radiographic occlusal and approximal caries diagnoses made by 240 dentists. *Acta Odontol Scand* 2001; **59**: 285–9.

Espelid I, Tveit AB, Riordan PJ. Radiographic caries diagnosis by clinicians in Norway and Western Australia. *Community Dent Oral Epidemiol* 1994; **22**: 214–19.

Fejerskov O, Manji F. Reactor paper: Risk assessment in dental caries. In: Bader JD, ed. *Risk assessment in dentistry*. Chapel Hill, NC: University of North Carolina Dental Ecology, 1990. 215–7.

Fejerskov O, Scheie AA, Birkhed D, Manji F. Effect of sugarcane chewing on plaque pH in rural Kenyan children. *Caries Res* 1992a; **26**: 286–9.

Fejerskov O, Scheie AA, Manji F. The effect of sucrose on plaque pH in the primary and permanent dentition of caries-inactive and -active Kenyan children. *J Dent Res* 1992b; **71**: 25–31.

Fleiss JL, Mann J, Paik M, Goultchin J, Chilton NW. A study of inter- and intra-examiner reliability of pocket depth and attachment level. *J Periodont Res* 1991; **26**: 122–8.

Fletcher RH, Fletcher SW, Wagner EH. *Clinical epidemiology. The essentials*, 3rd Baltimore, MD: Lippincott Williams & Wilkins, 1996: 1–276.

Fracaro MS, Seow WK, McAllan LH, Purdie DM. The sensitivity and specificity of clinical assessment compared with bitewing radiography for detection of occlusal dentin caries. *Pediatr Dent* 2001; **23**: 204–10.

Grembowski D, Milgrom P. The influence of dentist supply on the relationship between fluoridation and restorative care among children. *Med Care* 1988; **26**: 907–17.

Grembowski D, Fiset L, Milgrom P, Conrad D, Spadafora A. Does fluoridation reduce the use of dental services among adults? *Med Care* 1997; **35**: 454–71.

Guggenmoos-Holzmann I, van Houwelingen HC. The (in)validity of sensitivity and specificity. *Stat Med* 2000; **19**: 1783–92.

Haak R, Wicht MJ. Caries detection and quantification with DIAGNOdent: prospects for occlusal and root caries? *Int J Comput Dent* 2004; **7**: 347–58.

Haak R, Wicht MJ. Grey-scale reversed radiographic display in the detection of approximal caries. *J Dent* 2005; **33**: 65–71.

Hall A, Girkin JM. A review of potential new diagnostic modalities for caries lesions. *J Dent Res* 2004; **83**(Special Issue C): C89–94.

Hamilton JC, Stookey G. Should a dental explorer be used to probe suspected carious lesions? *J Am Dent Assoc* 2005; **136**: 1526–32.

Hanley JA, McNeil BJ. The meaning and use of the area under a receiver operating characteristic (ROC) curve. *Radiology* 1982; **143**: 29–36.

Hintze H. Screening with conventional and digital bite-wing radiography compared to clinical examination alone for caries detection in low-risk children. *Caries Res* 1993; **27**: 499–504.

Hintze H. *Radiography for the detection of dental caries lesions*. Dissertation. Aarhus: University of Aarhus, 2004.

Hintze H, Wenzel A. Clinically undetected dental caries assessed by bite-wing screening in children with little caries experience. *Dentomaxillofac Radiol* 1994; **23**: 19–23.

Hintze H, Wenzel A. Diagnostic outcome of methods frequently used for caries validation. *Caries Res* 2003; **37**: 115–24.

Hintze H, Wenzel A, Danielsen B, Nyvad B. Reliability of visual examination, fibre-optic transillumination, and bite-wing radiography, and reproducibility of direct visual examination following tooth separation for the identification of cavitated carious lesions in contacting approximal surfaces. *Caries Res* 1998; **32**: 204–9.

Hintze H, Wenzel A, Frydenberg M. Accuracy of caries detection with four storage phosphor systems and E-speed radiographs. *Dentomaxillofac Radiol* 2002; **31**: 170–5.

Hopcraft MS, Morgan MV. Comparison of radiographic and clinical diagnosis of approximal and occlusal dental caries in a young adult population. *Community Dent Oral Epidemiol* 2005; **33**: 212–18.

Huysmans M-CDNJM, Longbottom C. The challenges of validating diagnostic methods and selecting appropriate gold standards. *J Dent Res* 2004; **83**(Special Issue C): C48–52.

International Caries Detection and Assessment System (ICDAS) Coordinating Committee. *Criteria manual (draft). International Caries Detection and Assessment System (ICDAS II)*. Indianapolis: Indiana Conference, 2005a: 1–31.

International Caries Detection and Assessment System (ICDAS) Coordinating Committee. *Rationale and evidence for the International Caries Detection and Assessment System (ICDAS II) (draft)*. Indianapolis: Indiana Conference, 2005b: 1–43.

Ismail AI. Clinical diagnosis of precavitated carious lesions. *Community Dent Oral Epidemiol* 1997; **25**: 13–23.

Ismail AI. Visual and visuo-tactile detection of dental caries. *J Dent Res* 2004; **83**(Special Issue C): C56–66.

Ismail AI, Bader JD. Evidence-based dentistry in clinical practice. *J Am Dent Assoc* 2004; **135**: 78–83.

Ismail AI, Sohn W. A systematic review of clinical diagnostic criteria of early childhood caries. *J Publ Health Dent* 1999; **59**: 171–91.

Kay EJ, Nuttall NM. Relationship between dentists' treatment attitudes and restorative decisions made on the basis of simulated bitewing radiographs. *Community Dent Oral Epidemiol* 1994; **22**: 71–4.

Kay E, Nuttall N. Clinical decision making – an art or a science? Part I: An introduction. *Br Dent J* 1995a; **178**: 76–8.

Kay E, Nuttall N. Clinical decision making – an art or a science? Part II: Making sense of treatment decisions. *Br Dent J* 1995b; **178**: 113–16.

Kay EJ, Nuttall NM, Knill-Jones R. Restorative treatment thresholds and agreement in treatment decision-making. *Community Dent Oral Epidemiol* 1992; **20**: 265–8.

Kidd EAM, Pitts NB. A reappraisal of the value of the bitewing radiograph in the diagnosis of posterior approximal caries. *Br Dent J* 1990; **169**: 195–200.

Kidd EAM, Mejáre I, Nyvad B. Clinical and radiographic diagnosis. In: Fejerskov O, Kidd E, eds. *Dental caries: the disease and its clinical management*. Oxford: Blackwell Munksgaard, 2003: 111–28.

Knottnerus JA, Leffers P. The influence of referral patterns on the characteristics of diagnostic tests. *J Clin Epidemiol* 1992; **45**: 1143–54.

Kühnish J, Heinrich-Weltzien R. Quantitative light-induced fluorescence (QLF) – a literature review. *Int J Comput Dent* 2004; **7**: 325–38.

Landis JR, Koch GG. The measurement of observer agreement for categorical data. *Biometrics* 1977; **33**: 159–74.

Lee WC. Probabilistic analysis of global performances of diagnostic tests: interpreting the Lorenz curve-based summary measures. *Stat Med* 1999; **18**: 455–71.

Lenters M, van Amerongen WE, Mandari GJ. Iatrogenic damage to the adjacent surfaces of primary molars, in three different ways of cavity preparation. *Eur Arch Paediatr Dent* 2006; **7**: 6–10.

Llena-Puy C, Forner L. A clinical and radiographic comparison of caries diagnosed in approximal surfaces of posterior teeth in a low-risk population of 14-year-old children. *Oral Health Prev Dent* 2005; **3**: 47–52.

Longbottom C, Huysmans M-CDNJM. Electrical measurements for use in caries clinical trials. *J Dent Res* 2004; **83**(Special Issue C): C76–9.

Lunder N, von der Fehr FR. Approximal cavitation related to bite-wing image and caries activity in adolescents. *Caries Res* 1996; **30**: 143–7.

Lussi A, Gygax M. Iatrogenic damage to adjacent teeth during classical approximal box preparation. *J Dent* 1998; **26**: 435–41.

Lussi A, Hibst R, Paulus R. DIAGNOdent: an optical method for caries detection. *J Dent Res* 2004; **83**(Special Issue C): C80–3.

Machiulskiene V, Nyvad B, Baelum V. A comparison of clinical and radiographic caries diagnoses in posterior teeth of 12-year-old Lithuanian children. *Caries Res* 1999; **33**: 340–8.

Machiulskiene V, Nyvad B, Baelum V. Comparison of diagnostic yields of clinical and radiographic caries examinations in children of different age. *Eur J Paediatr Dent* 2004; **5**: 157–62.

Mandelbrot B. How long is the coast of Britain? Statistical self-similarity and fractional dimension. *Science* 1967; **156**: 636–8.

Manji F, Fejerskov O, Nagelkerke NJD, Baelum V. A random effects model for some epidemiological features of dental caries. *Community Dent Oral Epidemiol* 1991; **19**: 324–8.

Medeiros VAF, Seddon RP. Iatrogenic damage to approximal surfaces in contact with class II restorations. *J Dent* 2000; **28**: 103–10.

Mejáre I, Malmgren B. Clinical and radiographic appearance of proximal carious lesions at the time of operative treatment in young permanent teeth. *Scand J Dent Res* 1986; **94**: 19–26.

Mejáre I, Grondahl HG, Carlstedt K, Grever AC, Ottoson E. Accuracy at radiography and probing for the diagnosis of proximal caries. *Scand J Dent Res* 1985; **93**: 178–84.

Mettes TG, Bruers JJM, van der Sanden WJM, *et al*. Routine oral examinations: differences in characteristics of Dutch general dental practitioners related to type of recall interval. *Community Dent Oral Epidemiol* 2005; **23**: 219–26.

Mileman PA, van den Hout WB. Comparing the accuracy of Dutch dentists and dental students in the radiographic diagnosis of dentinal caries. *Dentomaxillofac Radiol* 2002; **31**: 7–14.

Milsom KM, Tickle M, Blinkhorn AS. Dental pain and dental treatment of young children attending the general dental service. *Br Dent J* 2002a; **192**: 280–4.

Milsom KM, Tickle M, King D, Kearney-Mitchell P, Blinkhorn AS. Outcomes associated with restored and unrestored deciduous molar teeth. *Prim Dent Care* 2002b; **9**: 16–19.

NHS National Institute for Clinical Excellence. *Dental recall. Recall interval between routine dental examinations.* London: National Institute for Clinical Excellence, 2004. 1–38.

Nyvad B, Fejerskov O. Active root surface caries converted into inactive caries as a response to oral hygiene. *Scand J Dent Res* 1986; **94**: 281–4.

Nyvad B, Machiulskiene V, Baelum V. Reliability of a new caries diagnostic system differentiating between active and inactive caries lesions. *Caries Res* 1999; **33**: 252–60.

Pitts NB, Rimmer PA. An *in vivo* comparison of radiographic and directly assessed clinical caries status of posterior approximal surfaces in primary and permanent teeth. *Caries Res* 1992; **26**: 146–52.

Poorterman JHG, Aartman IH, Kalsbeek H. Underestimation of the prevalence of approximal caries and inadequate restorations in a clinical epidemiological study. *Community Dent Oral Epidemiol* 1999; **27**: 331–7.

Poorterman JHG, Weerheijm KL, Groen HJ, Kalsbeek H. Clinical and radiographic judgement of occlusal caries in adolescents. *Eur J Oral Sci* 2000; **108**: 93–8.

Pretty IA, Maupomé G. A closer look at diagnosis in clinical dental practice: Part 5. Emerging technologies for caries detection and diagnosis. *J Can Dent Assoc* 2004; **70**: 540–540i.

Qvist V. Longevity of restorations in primary teeth. In: Hugoson A, Falk M, Johansson S, eds. *Consensus Conference on Caries in the Primary Dentition and its Clinical Management.* Jönköping, Sweden: Institute for Postgraduate Dental Education, 2002: 69–83.

Qvist V, Johannessen L, Bruun M. Progression of approximal caries in relation to iatrogenic preparation damage. *J Dent Res* 1992; **71**: 1370–3.

Qvist V, Laurberg L, Poulsen A, Teglers PT. Longevity and cariostatic effects of everyday conventional glass-ionomer and amalgam restorations in primary teeth: three-year results. *J Dent Res* 1997; **76**: 1387–96.

Ransohoff DF, Feinstein AR. Problems of spectrum and bias in evaluating the efficacy of diagnostic tests. *N Engl J Med* 1978; **299**: 926–30.

Raper HR. Practical clinical preventive dentistry based upon periodic roentgen-ray examinations. *J Am Dent Assoc* 1925 (September); 1084–100.

Ratledge DK, Kidd EAM, Beighton D. A clinical and microbiological study of approximal carious lesions. Part 1: The relationship between cavitation, radiographic lesion depth, the site-specific gingival index and the level of infection of the dentine. *Caries Res* 2001; **35**: 3–7.

Renshaw J. After the first 125 years of the BDJ where might clinical dentistry be heading? *Br Dent J* 2005; **199**: 331–7.

Roeleveld AC, van Amerongen WE, Mandari GJ. Influence of residual caries and cervical gaps on the survival rate of class II glass ionomer restorations. *Eur Arch Paediatr Dent* 2006; **7**: 85–90.

Rugg-Gunn AJ. Approximal carious lesions. A comparison of the radiological and clinical appearances. *Br Dent J* 1972; **133**: 481–4.

Scadding JG. Diagnosis: The clinician and the computer. *Lancet* 1967; **ii**: 877–82.

Scadding JG. Essentialism and nominalism in medicine: logic of diagnosis in disease terminology. *Lancet* 1996; **348**: 594–6.

Scheie AA, Fejerskov O, Lingström P, Birkhed D, Manji F. Use of palladium touch microelectrodes under field conditions for *in vivo* assessment of dental plaque pH in children. *Caries Res* 1992; **26**: 44–51.

Schisterman EF, Perkins NJ, Liu A, Bondell H. Optimal cut-point and its corresponding Youden index to discriminate individuals using pooled blood samples. *Epidemiol* 2005; **16**: 73–81.

Stookey GK. Optical methods – quantitative light fluorescence. *J Dent Res* 2004; **83**(Special Issue C): C84–8.

Stookey GK. Quantitative light fluorescence: a technology for early monitoring of the caries process. *Dent Clin North Am* 2005; **49**: 753–70.

Thylstrup A, Bille J, Qvist V. Radiographic and observed tissue changes in approximal carious lesions at the time of operative treatment. *Caries Res* 1986; **20**: 75–84.

Tickle M, Milsom K, Kennedy A. Is it better to leave or restore carious deciduous molar teeth? A preliminary study. *Prim Dent Care* 1999; **6**: 127–31.

Tickle M, Milsom K, King D, Kearney-Mitchell P, Blinkhorn A. The fate of the carious primary teeth of children who regularly attend the general dental service. *Br Dent J* 2002; **192**: 219–23.

Tranæus S, Shi X-Q, Angmar-Månsson B. Caries risk assessment: methods available to clinicians for caries detection. *Community Dent Oral Epidemiol* 2005; **33**: 265–73.

van der Veen MH, de Josselin de Jong E. Application of quantitative light-induced fluorescence for assessing early caries lesions. *Monogr Oral Sci* 2000; **17**: 144–62.

Verdonschot EH, Bronkhorst EM, Burgersdijk RCW, König KG, Schaeken MJM, Truin GJ. Performance of some diagnostic systems in examinations for small occlusal carious lesions. *Caries Res* 1992; **26**: 59–64.

de Vries HCB, Ruiken HMHM, König KG, Van't Hof MA. Radiographic versus clinical diagnosis of approximal carious lesions. *Caries Res* 1990; **24**: 364–70.

Weerheijm KL, Groen HJ, Bast AJJ, Kieft JA, Eijkman MAJ, van Amerongen WE. Clinically undetected occlusal dentine caries: a radiographic comparison. *Caries Res* 1992a; **26**: 305–9.

Weerheijm KL, Gruythuysen RJM, van Amerongen WE. Prevalence of hidden caries. *J Dent Child* 1992b; **59**: 408–12.

Weerheijm KL, Kidd EAM, Groen HJ. The effect of fluoridation on the occurrence of hidden caries in clinically sound occlusal surfaces. *Caries Res* 1997; **31**: 30–4.

Weintraub JA, Burt BA. Oral health status in the United States: tooth loss and edentulism. *J Dent Educ* 1985; **49**: 368–76.

Wendt LK, Koch G, Birkhed D. Replacements of restorations in the primary and young permanent dentition. *Swed Dent J* 1998; **22**: 149–55.

Wenzel A. Current trends in radiographic caries imaging. *Oral Surg Oral Med Oral Pathol* 1995; **80**: 527–39.

Wenzel A. Bitewing and digital bitewing radiography for detection of caries lesions. *J Dent Res* 2004; **83**(Special Issue C): C72–5.

Wenzel A, Hintze H. The choice of gold standard for evaluating tests for caries diagnosis. *Dentomaxillofac Radiol* 1999; **28**: 132–6.

Wulff HR. What is understood by a disease entity? *J R Coll Physicians Lond* 1979; **13**: 219–20.

Youden WJ. An index for rating diagnostic tests. *Cancer* 1950; **3**: 32–5.

Part II
Clinical caries epidemiology

8

The epidemiology of dental caries

B.A. Burt, V. Baelum and O. Fejerskov

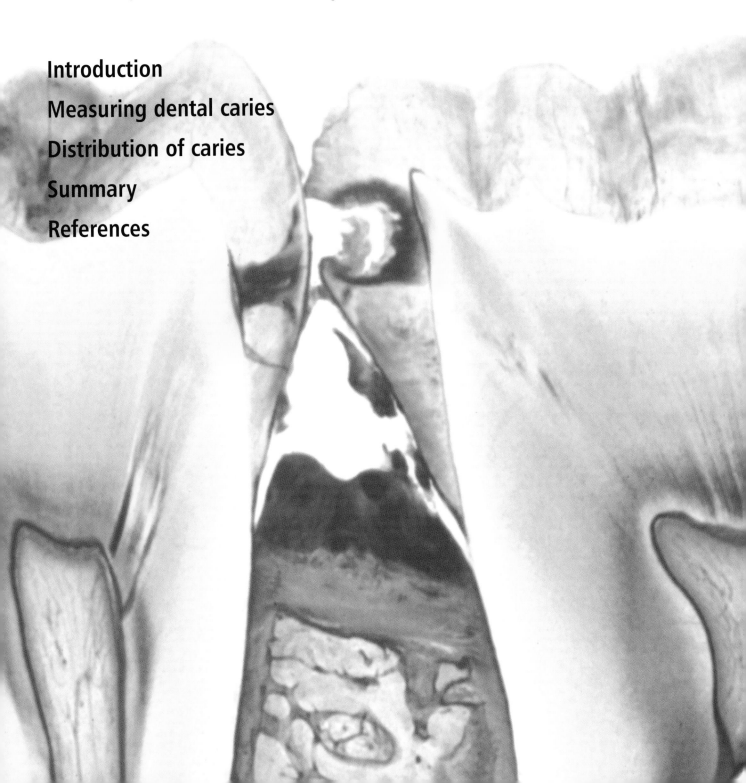

Introduction

Epidemiology is the study of health and disease in populations, and of how these states are influenced by heredity, biology, physical environment, social environment and human behavior. It differs from clinical studies in that epidemiology's focus is on groups of people, often whole populations, rather than on individuals or patients. The goal of epidemiological study is to identify the risk of disease that follows certain exposures, so that appropriate preventive interventions may be carried out at the public health and individual levels. To achieve this goal, epidemiological study uses a number of different research designs. All of them, however, include people with and without the disease in question, and with and without exposure to the correlates of interest. While research designs can become quite involved, Figure 8.1 shows the simple matrix that is the core of all epidemiological investigations.

Many factors are considered to be part of the causal chain in dental caries: bacteria, diet, plaque deposits, saliva quantity and quality, enamel quality, genetic history and tooth morphology have all been studied as possible risk factors for caries (Chapter 29). A risk factor is defined as:

An environmental, behavioral, or biologic factor confirmed by temporal sequence, usually in longitudinal studies, which if present directly increases the probability of a disease occurring, and if absent or removed reduces the probability. Risk factors are part of the causal chain, or expose the host to the causal chain. Once disease occurs, removal of the risk factor may not result in a cure (Beck, 1998).

Epidemiology's role is to identify the risk factors for disease. As stated in the definition above, determining whether exposure to a potential risk factor leads to a particular disease requires longitudinal study. Where there is evidence to suggest that a particular exposure is a risk factor, but the relationship cannot be confirmed through prospective study, the exposure is referred to as a risk indicator.

Major intraoral entities that are part of the causal chain (e.g. oral microflora, specific dental plaques, and saliva

quality and quantity) are dealt with in detail elsewhere in this book and so will not be part of this chapter. Instead, the distribution of dental caries in populations, and the factors that influence that distribution, are examined here. A major theme is that severe caries today is increasingly being recognized as a disease that closely follows a social gradient, so this chapter is broadened to emphasize the important role of the social environment in caries distribution. After a brief look at some of the issues in caries measurement, the relationships between caries experience and national income levels (as a broad measure of social resources) are examined. Then, following a brief consideration of how caries distribution is related to those individual attributes that cannot be changed, e.g. age, race, gender and genetic predisposition, the relationship between caries and socioeconomic status (an individual measure) and social determinants (a community measure) is explored. These community-based factors, sometimes called neighborhood characteristics, are now recognized as having a strong influence on caries extent and severity.

Caries is an ancient disease

Dental caries has been making people miserable since at least the time when humans began to develop agriculture. From palentological remains from the Iron Age, it appears that carious lesions in young people sometimes began in occlusal fissures, but developed no further because attrition progressed faster than caries. This pattern of development can still be seen today, e.g. in some African populations, where the rate of progression on approximal surfaces may also be so low that these lesions are ground away. Most lesions found in human remains from the Iron Age were cervical or root caries; coronal caries was relatively uncommon at this time, although it became more common during the time of the Roman Empire. Roman remains give evidence that some teeth with large coronal cavities had obviously been treated. The moderate caries experience found in Britain during the Anglo-Saxon period (sixth to seventh centuries) had changed little by the end of the Middle Ages (Moore & Corbett, 1971, 1973).

Increased consumption of processed food and greater availability of sugar were probably chiefly responsible for the development of the modern pattern of caries. Import duties on sugar in Britain were relaxed in 1845 and completely removed by 1875, a period during which the severity of caries increased greatly (Corbett & Moore, 1976; Lennon *et al.*, 1974). By the end of the nineteenth century, dental caries was well established as an epidemic disease of massive proportions in most of the economically developed countries (Burt, 1978). The severity of the caries epidemic in the late nineteenth century led directly to the establishment of public dental services, which first appeared in the Scandinavian countries.

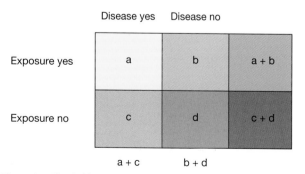

Figure 8.1 The simple matrix that is the core of all epidemiological investigations.

Measuring dental caries

To study caries and its distribution in populations, it must be possible to measure it validly and reliably, and then put those measurements together in some systematic fashion so that caries distribution in one group can be compared with that in another. Since the disease of dental caries occurs on a continuum, from the earliest demineralization to cavitation, it is clearly important to have clear rules, or criteria, for the conditions under which caries is judged to be present. (Chapter 9 shows the impact of using differing measurement criteria on prevalence and severity data). Valid and reliable measurement is the basis of any science, including epidemiology, where an index (a numerical scale with upper and lower limits, with scores on the scale that correspond to specific criteria) is usually required to obtain a precise expression of disease distribution in a group. The properties of an ideal index are listed in Box 8.1. Index scores usually give no picture of clinical conditions (e.g. what does a plaque index score of 1.2 look like?), and in the past were often statistically mistreated when averages were computed from ordinal scales, but they have value when compared with the index scores from other groups measured in a similar way.

While various indexes for measuring caries were suggested during the 1920s to the early 1930s, it was only with Dean's studies of naturally occurring fluoridated water in the 1930s that a practical method was developed and used. Dean and his colleagues (Dean *et al.*, 1942) counted the numbers of teeth in the mouth with obvious caries (i.e. cavities). Filled teeth and teeth missing due to caries were added in, so that the index score included all teeth that had been attacked by caries. The first description of what is now known as the DMF index came from extensive studies of dental caries among children in Hagerstown, Maryland,

USA, in the 1930s (Klein *et al.*, 1938). After that, the DMF index became the most used of all dental indexes.

The DMF index

As originally described, D was for decayed teeth, M for teeth missing due to caries and F for teeth that had been previously filled. Filled teeth were assumed to have been unequivocally decayed before restoration. The index could be applied to teeth as a whole (designated as DMFT), or applied to all surfaces of the teeth (DMFS). The DMFT score for any one individual can range from 0 to 32, in whole numbers, while the mean DMFT score for a group can have decimal values. The index can be modified to deal with such factors as filled teeth that have redecayed, crowns, bridge pontics and any other particular attribute required for study. It can also be applied with varying criteria for what constitutes caries. The original intention to score D only when there was cavitation has largely given way to scoring systems which record caries at all stages from the earliest enamel caries through to cavitation. An example of the latter is the International Caries Detection and Assessment System (ICDAS), which records caries on a six-point ordinal scale (Pitts, 2004). Another example is a scale that distinguishes between caries progress in active and inactive lesions (Nyvad *et al.*, 1999). As a result, DMF scores where caries is measured over its full range of development are higher than those where only cavitation, i.e. a later stage of caries progression, is used as the criterion for decayed teeth.

The DMF index has been used widely since its introduction in 1938 because it meets a number of the criteria for an ideal index (Box 8.1). For example, it is simple, versatile, statistically manageable and reliable when examiners have been trained. However, the DMF does have its limitations, and the main ones are listed in Box 8.2.

The limitations of the DMF index today frequently relate to modern preventive and restorative technology. For example, there were no sealants or adhesive resins when the DMF index was first developed. There are two reasonable approaches for adapting the DMF to deal with sealants. One says that the sealed tooth is not restored in the usual sense and should therefore be considered sound. The other says that it has required hands-on, one-to-one dental attention, and so should be considered a filled tooth. Probably the best way to deal with sealed teeth is to put them in a category by themselves, S for sealed. The DMFS index would then become DMFSS. Depending on the study's purpose, the S teeth can be left separate, included with F or regarded as sound.

The DMF index today is really outdated as a measure of caries incidence and severity, and may actually be more valid as a measure of treatment received. It is philosophically questionable to use an index for a disease that is so dependent upon the treatment judgments of many practitioners,

---

- *Validity.* The index must measure what it is intended to measure, so it should correspond with clinical stages of the disease under study at each point.
- *Reliability.* The index should be able to measure consistently at different times and under a variety of conditions. The term *reliability* is virtually synonymous with *reproducibility, repeatability* and *consistency*, meaning the ability of the same or different examiners to interpret and use the index in the same way.
- *Clarity, simplicity and objectivity.* The criteria should be clear and unambiguous, with mutually exclusive categories. Ideally, it should be readily memorized by an examiner after some practice.
- *Quantifiability.* The index must be amenable to statistical analysis, so that the status of a group can be expressed by a distribution, mean, median or other statistical measures.
- *Sensitivity.* The index should be able to detect reasonably small shifts, in either direction, in the condition.
- *Acceptability.* The use of the index should not be painful or demeaning to the subject.

Box 8.1 Properties of an ideal index

The DMF index has received remarkably little challenge over some 70 years of life, probably because it is conceptually simple and versatile in practice. But it was developed for use in children a long time ago, and accordingly it shows its age in a few areas. The principal limitations of the DMF index are:

- DMF values are not related to the number of teeth at risk. A DMF score for an individual is a simple count of those teeth that in the examiner's judgment have been affected by caries; it has no denominator. A DMF score thus does not directly give an indication of the intensity of the attack in any one individual. A 7-year-old child with a DMF score of 3.0 may have only nine permanent teeth in the mouth; thus, one-third of these teeth have already been attacked by caries in a short space of time. An adult may have a DMF score of 8.0 from a full complement of 32 teeth; thus, over a longer period only one-quarter of the teeth have been affected. DMF scores therefore have little meaning unless age is also stated.
- The DMF index gives equal weight to missing, untreated decayed or well-restored teeth. Common sense suggests that this philosophical basis is faulty for many purposes.
- The DMF index is invalid when teeth have been lost for reasons other than caries. Teeth can be lost for periodontal reasons in older adults, and for orthodontic reasons in teenagers. Decision rules, which go along with criteria, are required to determine how to deal with these instances.
- The DMF index can overestimate caries experience in teeth with 'preventive restorations'. In an epidemiological survey, such teeth must be included in the F component of DMF, although had they not been filled in the first place they might have been diagnosed as sound teeth. DMF scores will thus be inflated (Bader et al., 1993). Composite restorations judged to have been placed only for cosmetic reasons likewise should not be included in DMF counts.
- Composite and resin restorations not only may have been placed on non-carious teeth, but are often hard for an examiner to detect, thus leading to underestimation.
- DMF scores cannot be compared from one group to another without considering the criteria by which caries was considered present or absent. There is no universal criterion for what is a decayed tooth. Comparing one group where caries was recorded across the full disease continuum to one which only recorded caries at cavitation is clearly invalid.
- DMF data are of little use for estimating treatment needs.
- DMF cannot account for sealed teeth. Sealants did not exist in 1938, so are obviously not included in the description of the index. Sealants and other composite restorations for cosmetic purposes have to be dealt with separately.

Box 8.2 Limitations of the DMF index

and the combination of previous treatment (i.e. the M and F components) with current treatment need (the D component) is not used elsewhere in public health surveillance. An objective measure of caries activity (e.g. a marker of active disease) would be preferable to clinical judgment for many purposes, but because valid markers for caries are elusive, scoring caries activity is still based on clinical acumen (Nyvad et al., 1999). On the credit side, DMF has been used for generations and still has some use in monitoring trends over time. Its mix of treated and untreated caries measures also gives it some value in health services research. Until a more objective measure is developed and accepted then some modification of DMF will continue

to be the principal index used to express the caries status of a population.

Other measures of caries

Other methods of measuring dental caries, using different philosophical bases, have been suggested from time to time. One is Grainger's hierarchy, an ordinal scale designed to simplify the recording of the caries status of a population, which uses five zones of severity of the carious attack (Grainger, 1967). This method was based on a landmark paper of Klein and Palmer (1941), which presented a caries-susceptibility order for the teeth, an ordering which has changed little down the years (Macek et al., 2003). Several studies confirmed the validity of the hierarchy (Katz & Meskin, 1976; Kingman, 1979; Poulsen & Horowitz, 1974). The Grainger hierarchy could be useful in public health surveillance, but it has received little further use.

'Composite' indicators have been suggested that attempt to measure health rather than disease by statistically weighting healthy restored teeth differently from missing or decayed teeth (Sheiham et al., 1987). The first of these is the FS-T, which sums the sound and well-restored teeth. The second is T-Health, which seeks to measure the amount of healthy dental tissue and ascribes descending numerical weights for a sound healthy tooth, a well-restored tooth and a decayed tooth. These are conceptually sound approaches to measuring dental health and function (rather than disease), and they probably deserve more attention than they have received.

An offshoot of the present-day skewed distribution of caries is the significant caries index (SiC) (Bratthall, 2000; WHO, 2005). The SiC is not a new index, but rather is a form of data presentation to help give a better picture of caries distribution in the population. It is the mean DMF score for the third of the population that is most affected by caries, intended to be used alongside the mean DMF of the whole population to give a more complete summary of its caries distribution. The more skewed the distribution, the greater the gap between the mean DMF and the SiC.

Criteria for diagnosing coronal caries

There is no global consensus on the criteria for diagnosing dental caries, despite a vast quantity of words on the subject. Apart from the inherent problem of diagnosing a borderline lesion, the major philosophical issue comes with scoring the early carious lesion which has not yet become cavitated. These lesions appear as discolored fissures without loss of substance, as a 'white spot' on visible smooth surfaces, or radiographically as an early interproximal shadow. The issue is that not all non-cavitated lesions progress to dentinal lesions requiring restorative treatment, and active non-cavitated lesions should receive non-operative treatment to prevent any further caries progression. With non-operative treatment (or sometimes even without it), a good proportion of them will remain static or even remineralize (Pitts, 1993). These lesions are thus reversible, as opposed to dentinal lesions, which are usually considered irreversible. Because there are usually more non-cavitated than cavitated lesions at any one time in both high-caries and low-caries populations (Pitts & Fyffe, 1988; Bjarnason *et al.*, 1992; Ismail *et al.*, 1992; Machiulskiene *et al.*, 1998), the decision of whether to include or exclude them, and how to express them if included, can make a substantial difference in the oral health profiles obtained (Chapter 9). This is illustrated in Fig. 8.2, where in surveys in Kenya the carious lesions were recorded as both cavitated and enamel-only (i.e. non-cavitated). There is a marked difference in any caries profile depending on whether non-cavitated lesions are included or not.

Examples of these two broad approaches to diagnostic criteria for dental caries are shown in Box 8.3. European investigators have long recorded caries on a scale that extends through the full range of disease from the earliest detectable non-cavitated lesion through to pulpal involvement (Backer Dirks *et al.*, 1961). The criteria in Box 8.3 were first published by the World Health Organization (WHO) in 1979 (WHO, 1979), and will be referred to as the $D_1–D_3$ scale. (There is a D4 for pulpal involvement, but that recording is seldom contentious.) More recently, clinical researchers in Europe have expanded on this concept to produce a scale with up to 10 points, combining increasing depths of lesion development with clinical signs of activity or inactivity (Machiulskiene *et al.*, 1999; Nyvad *et al.*, 1999; Pitts, 2004). However, investigators in North America, Britain and other English-speaking countries have until

recently used visual–tactile means to record caries as a dichotomous condition, meaning that caries was recorded only as present or absent. (This is referred to here as the dichotomous scale.) In the dichotomous recording, caries was only noted when it reached the level of dentinal involvement (Horowitz, 1972), i.e. the D_3 level. The $D_1–D_3$ scale requires the teeth to be dried and receive a longer, more meticulous examination, although with well-trained examiners this can be done even under fairly primitive field conditions.

A scoring system based on the $D_1–D_3$ scale is a necessity in cariology research studies, for it permits identification of lesion initiation, progression and regression. Research questions on the conditions under which early lesions progress, regress or remain static can only be answered with a measurement scale of this nature. Its use demands meticulous examiner training, since because D_1 lesions are capable of remineralizing back to sound enamel it becomes difficult to differentiate examiner error from natural phenomena. This may influence the assessment of absolute changes, although in the absence of bias it should not affect the contrast between groups. There is less consensus on whether the $D_1–D_3$ scale should be used in large-scale surveillance surveys, for arguments can be made both ways. Surveillance surveys are conducted at multiyear intervals to address the broad questions of whether disease levels are increasing or decreasing so that appropriate public policy can be formulated. For comparisons over time, it is clear that disease-measurement criteria need to be similar, and generally the simpler the system the better the examiner reliability. However, measuring caries only when cavitation can be

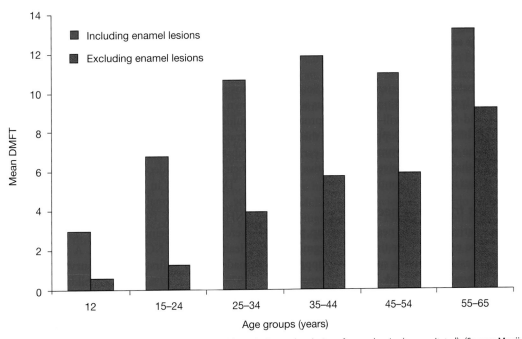

Figure 8.2 Mean DMFT scores by age in a Kenyan population, recorded for inclusion and exclusion of enamel caries (non-cavitated). (Source: Manji *et al.*, 1989.)

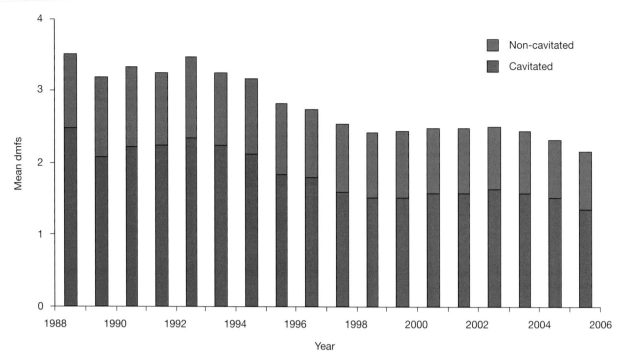

Figure 8.9 Trends in caries experience in the primary dentition in Danish 5-year-old children between 1988 and 2005. (Source: Danish National Board of Health, Copenhagen, 2006.)

uses of fluoride as the main reason (Bratthall *et al.*, 1996). However, fluoride alone does not explain more than about 50% of the reduction (Marthaler *et al.*, 1996), and we still do not have a clear understanding of the relative strength of caries risk factors. Sugar consumption, in the USA at least, has increased rather than diminished, and there is no good evidence concerning the roles of better oral hygiene, changes in the bacterial ecology of the oral cavity and the widespread use of pediatric antibiotics on oral bacteria. Many see a likely impact, though as yet unquantified, from raised living standards that come with indoor plumbing, and elevated social norms concerning laundry, personal hygiene and grooming. Better oral hygiene can easily be seen as part of more meticulous personal hygiene and grooming rather than a conscious act to improve oral health. As with the cyclical nature of other diseases over time, however, it is quite likely that there are factors operating that have not been identified (see discussion later in this chapter on the effect of the social environment).

The uneven distribution of caries

For many years, the results of national surveys were presented only as mean DMF values, usually with only a standard deviation to indicate the distribution. While means are valid and useful, they 'compress' extreme values, meaning those with no caries and those with a lot, into an average figure which sometimes can be misleading. A break from this convention in the USA came with the results of a major preventive study in the mid-1980s, which drew attention to the fact that while average caries experience in children was lower than the researchers had originally expected, there was still a significant minority with severe caries (Graves *et al.*, 1986). This type of distribution is illustrated in Fig. 8.10, which shows data from the US national surveys of schoolchildren in 1979–1980 and 1988–1994. Rather than mean DMF scores, this graph illustrates the distributional changes and shows a classic skewed distribution. It is evident that in the more recent survey the proportion of children with low DMF scores had increased, while the proportion with high scores (i.e. severe caries) had decreased. Even so, the shape of the distribution remained much the same: highly skewed toward zero or few DMFS teeth, but with a persistent 'tail', meaning children at the severe end of the scale. It is these children in the tails who are considered to be at high risk, and who thus absorb a lot of attention from public health services. It is generally accepted today that in any population some 60–70% of all carious lesions are found in 15–25% of the children. Whether these children should be targeted for special preventive treatment or not remains a subject for active debate (see Chapters 28 and 29).

Age and gender

Mean DMF scores increase with age. Caries used to be considered just a childhood disease, a perception from those days of high caries severity when most susceptible surfaces were usually affected by adolescence. With younger people now reaching adulthood with many surfaces free of caries,

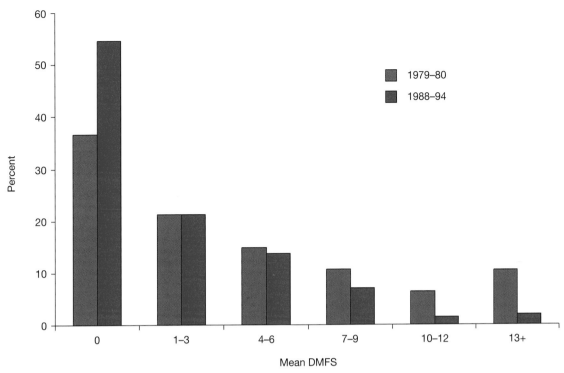

Figure 8.10 Distribution of mean DMFS values in US schoolchildren, aged 5–17 years, in a national survey in 1979–1980 and in another national survey in 1988–1994. (Source: US Public Health Service, National Institute of Dental Research, 1981; US Department of Health and Human Services, National Center for Health Statistics, 1997.)

the carious attack is spread out more throughout life. Adults of all ages can, and do, develop new coronal lesions (Hand *et al.*, 1988; Drake *et al.*, 1994; Luan *et al.*, 2000), and caries has to be viewed as a lifetime disease. Even the skewed disease distribution seen in youth can be seen among the elderly (McGuire *et al.*, 1993). In populations where caries experience is severe the disease starts early in life and is common in the young. A more even occurrence of new lesions throughout life is characteristic of a lower community attack rate.

Root caries

One important offshoot of the age–caries relationship is root caries, defined as caries that begins on cemental root surfaces exposed to the oral environment, and hence when bacterial plaque can accumulate around these exposed roots. As mentioned above, root caries has been with humankind since our earliest days. Even so, awareness of root caries in the high-income countries only grew around the early 1980s with the realization that older adults were keeping more teeth than they used to. Root caries is highly prevalent among older people in high-income countries (Salonen *et al.*, 1989; Beck, 1993; Lo & Schwarz, 1994; Hawkins *et al.*, 1998; Gilbert *et al.*, 2001; Chalmers *et al.*, 2002; Morse *et al.*, 2002), although it too has declined in recent years, just as coronal caries has. Figure 8.11 shows the decline in root lesions in the USA, despite greater tooth

retention, between the two most recent national surveillance surveys.

Root caries, by definition, is strongly associated with the loss of periodontal attachment (Locker & Leake, 1993; Slade *et al.*, 1993; Whelton *et al.*, 1993; Lawrence *et al.*, 1995; Ringelberg *et al.*, 1996). Other correlates associated with root caries are primarily socioeconomic: years of education, number of remaining teeth, use of dental services, oral hygiene levels and preventive behavior (Vehkalahti & Paunio, 1988; DePaola *et al.*, 1989; Beck, 1993;). Another important risk factor is the use of multiple medications among the elderly (Kitamura *et al.*, 1986), a common practice in institutions, and one that can promote xerostomia. Xerostomia has long been known as a major risk factor for caries among people of any age, and is particularly prevalent among those who have received radiation treatment for cancer. Other risk factors identified in a representative British sample of people aged 65 or more were poor oral hygiene, wearing partial dentures, sucking candies in a dry mouth and living in an institution (Steele *et al.*, 2001). Root caries is less prevalent in high-fluoride areas than in low-fluoride communities (Burt *et al.*, 1986; Stamm *et al.*, 1990), smokers exhibit more root caries than non-smokers, and prevalence tends to be inversely related to the number of teeth remaining (Beck, 1993; Locker & Leake, 1993).

Root caries seems to be a particular problem among older people of lower socioeconomic status, those who have

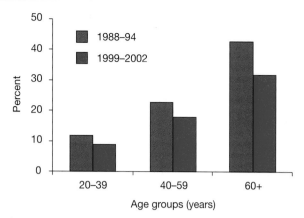

Figure 8.11 Prevalence of carious or restored root lesions in US adults in two national surveys, one in 1988–1994 and the other in 1999–2002. (Source: Beltrán-Aguilar *et al.*, 2005.)

lost some teeth, who do not maintain good oral hygiene and do not visit the dentist regularly. Because of our aging populations and increasing retention of teeth, it could be that the dimensions of the root caries problem will continue growing in the years ahead. However, the decline shown in Fig. 8.11 adds strength to the argument that root caries, while not exactly going away, will continue to diminish in the population.

Regarding gender, women usually have higher DMF scores than do men of the same age, although this finding is not universal. When observed in children, the difference has been attributed to the earlier eruption of teeth in girls, but this explanation is hard to support when the differences are seen in older age groups. In those instances a treatment factor is more likely because in national survey data men usually have more untreated decayed surfaces than women, while women have more restored teeth. Women visit the dentist more frequently, so this observation is perhaps to be expected. In a national survey in the USA, girls aged 12–17 years had the same mean number of decayed and missing surfaces as their male counterparts, but 25% more filled surfaces (Kaste *et al.*, 1996). One cannot conclude from these figures that women are more susceptible to caries than are men; a combination of earlier tooth eruption plus a treatment factor is a more likely explanation for the observed differences.

Race and ethnicity

Global variations in caries experience result from environmental rather than from inherent racial attributes. To illustrate that point, there is evidence that some racial groups, once thought to be resistant to caries, quickly developed the disease when they migrated to areas with different cultural and dietary patterns (Beal, 1973; Russell, 1966). In the United States, to choose one example of a multiracial and multiethnic society, most surveys before the 1970s found that whites had higher DMF scores than African–Americans,

although the latter usually had more decayed teeth. One of the early national surveys in 1960–1962 showed that whites had higher DMF scores than did African–American adults of the same age group, a difference that remained even when the groups were standardized for income and education (US Public Health Service, NCHS, 1967). This difference was still evident in a national survey from the 1970s (US Public Health Service, NCHS, 1981). By the time of the 1988–1994 national survey, however, there was little difference in total DMF scores between whites and African–Americans, although whites still had a higher filled component and lower scores for decayed and missing surfaces. DMF values for Mexican–Americans were in between. This turnaround probably reflects improving access to care for African–Americans, although it still reflects socio-economic and cultural contrasts between the groups.

Even though overall caries experience in the permanent dentition continues to decline in the USA, disparities between racial and ethnic groups in the prevalence and severity of dental caries still remain in the twenty-first century (Beltrán-Aguilar *et al.*, 2005). However, the overall pattern is that there is no evidence to support inherent differences in caries susceptibility between racial and ethnic groups. Far more important are socioeconomic differences and contrasting social environments, meaning differences in education, available income and access to health care. More difficult to measure are long-held cultural beliefs that affect values and behavior related to dental health. However, no one doubts that these factors are present and influencing caries incidence.

Familial and genetic patterns

Familial tendencies ('bad teeth run in families') are seen by many dentists and have been recorded (Klein & Palmer, 1938; Klein & Shimizu, 1945; Ringelberg *et al.*, 1974). However, these studies have not identified whether such tendencies have a true genetic basis, or whether they stem from bacterial transmission or continuing familial dietary or behavioral traits. Husband–wife similarities clearly have no genetic origin, and intrafamilial transmission of cariogenic flora, especially from mother to infant, is considered by some to be a primary way for cariogenic bacteria to become established in children (Kohler *et al.*, 1983; Caufield *et al.*, 2000). The lack of a demonstrable genetic influence by race, discussed above, weakens the case for genetic inheritance of susceptibility or resistance to caries, although it is interesting that Klein, years ago, concluded that the similarities within families involved 'strong familial vectors which very likely have a genetic basis, perhaps sex-linked' (Klein, 1946).

With the explosion of research discoveries of genetic influences in many diseases, dental caries is being looked at in a different light. It is plausible that host attributes that could affect an individual's caries experience, such as salivary flow and composition, tooth morphology and arch width, are genetically determined, and the genetics of the cariogenic bacteria themselves may have an effect. However, the ready preventability of caries, indicated by the caries decline, strongly counters (if not refutes) the idea of any genetic component worth mentioning. At present, no genetic role in caries experience has been demonstrated.

Socioeconomic status

Socioeconomic status (SES), or social class, is intended to be a broad summary of an individual's attitudes, values and behavior as determined by such factors as education, income, occupation or place of residence. Attitudes toward health are often part of the set of values that follow from an individual's social standing in the community, and can help to explain some of the observed variance in health measures. Obtaining a valid measure of SES, however, is always a problem because of the construct's complexity. The most commonly used measures are income and years of formal education, despite acknowledged shortcomings with the latter measure (Hadden, 1996).

SES is used in research as an attribute specific to the individual, rather than to the community. It is usually inversely related to the occurrence of many diseases, and to characteristics thought to affect health (Marmot & Wilkinson, 1999). The reasons for disparities in health status between various SES strata can often seem obvious, but that is not always the case (Link & Phelan, 1996). For example, higher infant mortality in lower SES strata can be partly explained by the facts that higher SES women have easier access to prenatal care, can better afford such care, and have more time to obtain it, a deeper educational base to permit better understanding of the condition and probably less fatalistic attitudes, and perhaps some other factors. However, even after all these likely variables have been factored into explaining the differences, there is still a considerable gap which defies explanation (Fuchs, 1974). Measurements used in science cannot always pick up all the subtleties embedded in SES.

These subtleties have also been seen in dental health. In one Finnish study, for instance, differences in caries experience between children in the higher and lower social classes still remained after accounting for the reported frequency of tooth brushing, consumption of sugars and ingestion of fluoride tablets (Milen, 1987). These are all individual behaviors that would be more common in higher SES strata. Another instance comes from Sweden, where even with the extensive Swedish welfare system a social gradient in oral health is still evident (Flinck et al., 1999; Kallestal & Wall, 2002).

As part of his landmark research in caries epidemiology during the 1930s and 1940s, Klein observed that overall DMF values did not vary much between SES groups, but aspects of treatment certainly did (Klein & Palmer, 1940). Lower SES groups had higher values for D and M, lower for

F. In the first national survey of US children in 1963–1965, white children in the higher SES strata actually had higher DMF scores than did white children in the lower strata, but African–American children showed the opposite profile (US Public Health Service, NCHS, 1971). In the white children, the F component ballooned so much with increasing SES that it lifted the whole DMF index. By contrast, the F component in the African–American children did not change with SES, with the net result that their DMF scores diminished with increasing SES. As mentioned earlier, these results from 1963–1965 showed that a 'treatment effect' was artificially inflating the DMF data in the white children.

In today's lower overall caries experience, however, the position has been reversed. During the period when the caries decline was first recognized, it was soon found that the higher SES groups enjoyed the sharpest decline in caries experience (Graves et al., 1986), so that the DMF values of children in higher SES strata are now generally well below those of children in lower SES strata. This is illustrated in Fig. 8.12, which shows the components of the DMFS index for 15-year-old children in low, medium and high SES groups from a national survey in the USA during 1988–1994. Figure 8.13 illustrates two features of the caries decline. The first, the secular decline in caries, has already been illustrated (Figs 8.6–8.10) and is seen again with the reductions over time in each poverty-status group in Fig. 8.13, showing that, even over this fairly short period of 8–11 years, caries levels across all age and socioeconomic groups have continued to decline. The second aspect illustrated here is how caries levels are related to SES. The children are grouped by poverty status as defined by the US federal government (a socioeconomic measure used to determine eligibility for government programs), and it can be seen that children in the higher SES groups (i.e. those at ⩾200% of

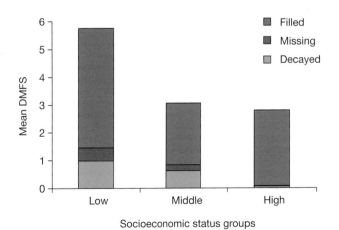

Figure 8.12 Mean DMFS scores for 15-year-old children at three socioeconomic levels in the United States, 1988–1994. (Source: US Department of Health and Human Services, 1997. Reprinted with permission of Elsevier from Burt & Eklünd, *The dentist, dental practice and the community*. Elsevier, Philadelphia, PA; p. 244.)

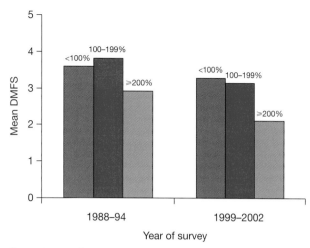

Figure 8.13 Decline in mean DMFS scores in children aged 6–19 years between 1988–1994 and 1999–2002, as seen in three levels of poverty status as defined by the US federal government. (US government's poverty guidelines: http://aspe.cos.dhhs.gov/poverty/06poverty.shtml; accessed 14 March 2006.) The green bars indicate the highest SES groups.

the poverty level) have lower caries scores than do children below the poverty level or only just above it.

As noted above, it is difficult for any one measure to capture all the nuances of SES. British studies have explored the issue by introducing broader measures of SES determinants, such as private housing and car ownership, that go beyond just education and income (Palmer & Pitter, 1988; Carmichael *et al.*, 1989; Gratrix & Holloway, 1994). These measures were all related to caries levels in the population. A better sense of coherence among poor parents of adolescent children, i.e. people who have a more structured life than do others in the same social circumstances, is related to lower caries levels among their children (Freire *et al.*, 2002). This is an intriguing area for further research. Caries levels are also related to the degree of neighborhood deprivation, where several area summary measures have been used (Jones *et al.*, 1997a; Jones & Worthington, 1999; Gray *et al.*, 2000). These broad measures of area deprivation lead directly into the role of social determinants.

Caries and the social environment

A useful definition of public health is '… assuring conditions in which people can be healthy' (IOM, 1988) (with emphasis on the word *can*). That covers everything from maintaining the stratospheric ozone layer to picking up the garbage, to providing recreational facilities, decent housing or dental care where needed. While it stresses the public responsibility for a healthy physical and social environment, it still leaves room for individuals to exercise personal choice in their health-related behavior and how they use health-care services. The term social determinants is related to this definition in that it refers to factors that affect health outcomes for everyone in the community, and whose pres-

ence or absence influences the environment 'in which people can be healthy'. Social determinants can include such factors as the quality of housing, extent of community services, availability of transport, prospects for employment, crime levels, and access to parks, open space and suitable recreational facilities.

There are substantial and well-documented differences in health status between people who reside in upscale areas and those who reside in more deprived areas. These contrasts have been documented in a number of countries and in a variety of cultures, although they have been best studied in the high-income countries (Kaplan, 1996). The data show with remarkable consistency that people who live in the more affluent areas are invariably in better health than those from poorer areas, and this observation has endured well over time (Syme & Berkman, 1976; Kaplan *et al.*, 1987; Marmot *et al.*, 1987; Haan *et al.*, 1989). This finding is not dependent on how health status is measured, for it has been documented in terms of overall mortality, heart disease, diabetes or even subjective perceptions of ill-health (Pappas, 1994; Blane, 1995; Kaplan *et al.*, 1996; Link & Phelan, 1996; Goodman, 1999).

While there are numerous individual behavioral determinants involved in this profile (e.g. smoking, use of alcohol, quality of diet, regular exercise), there is also evidence that social determinants, i.e. those risk factors that apply to the whole community rather than to specific individuals, play a key role in determining health outcomes. When any of these basic community necessities are deficient or absent, the quality of life is diminished. When they are mostly deficient, as is not uncommon in rundown parts of major cities, quality of life is diminished to the degree that a high level of emotional stress ensues from the demands of day-to-day coping with the cumulative burden of living in deprived circumstances. Poor social circumstances are linked to disease by way of material, psychosocial and behavioral pathways. Social and environmental disadvantages can lead directly to poor health behavior and the subsequent biological disturbances that lead directly to ill-health. This argument therefore holds that social stresses in themselves can negatively affect health (Brunner & Marmot, 1999). As one example, the gap in both mortality rates and cardiovascular disease levels between Western European countries and those that were formerly part of the Soviet bloc were accentuated sharply around the time of the break-up of the Soviet Union. This phenomenon has been attributed to the high degree of social stress that accompanied the political break-up (Bobak & Marmot, 1996).

Dental research in this area has not developed to the extent it has in medical research, but there is some indication that the same relations between social determinants and oral health are generally evident. Parents' employment status and attitudes have been identified as determinants of the dental health of young children in Belfast (Freeman *et al.*, 1997) and work stress was related to oral health among workers in Brazil (Marcenes & Sheiham, 1992). British studies, using a variety of measures to characterize the nature and extent of social deprivation in contrasting neighborhoods, have shown how the severity of dental caries is related both to the presence/absence of fluoridated drinking water (Chapter 18) and to the social deprivation level of the residential areas (Jones *et al.*, 1997b, c; Jones & Worthington, 1999; Riley *et al.*, 1999). The effects of social inequalities in youth can be enduring; both low birth weight and social deprivation in youth are related to caries levels at age 13 years (Nicolau *et al.*, 2003, 2005). Contrasts between social inequalities in youth are similarly related to caries severity in adolescence (Pattussi *et al.*, 2001).

These studies collectively demonstrate that dental caries today should be looked upon as a disease of poverty or deprivation as much as being a disease of diet, oral hygiene and other aspects of individual behavior. The great reductions in caries experience among more affluent people in the high-income countries stand in contrast to the much lower reductions in the more socially deprived groups. Further advances in closing these disparities will require sweeping changes in social circumstances as much as changes in individual behavior. Since diet is a prime example of a personal behavior affected by neighborhood characteristics, its relationship to caries deserves some special attention.

Diet and dental caries

Dietary practices are a complex mix of food availability, community and personal affluence, history, culture, marketing practices, and personal affluence, behavior and tastes. Dietary quality is a major determinant of caries levels in a community, and is a major factor in the social environment.

The word diet refers to the food and drink that passes through the mouth, whereas nutrition is concerned with the absorption and metabolism of nutrients from dietary sources. Although a link between malnutrition and caries would be intuitively expected, there is actually little evidence to support it. Studies of children in Peru have concluded that chronic and severe malnutrition during the first year of life is associated with increased caries years later, although this association is difficult to demonstrate because malnutrition delays eruption and exfoliation of the primary teeth (Alvarez, 1995). Chronic malnutrition among children in India has been shown to reduce salivary flow, which could be one reason for a causative link (Johansson *et al.*, 1992).

By contrast, diet has a clear influence on caries development. The relation between the intake of refined carbohydrates, especially sugars, and the prevalence and severity of caries is so strong that sugars are clearly a major etiological factor in the causation of caries. Added sugars are the primary culprit, although a limited degree of caries occurs in populations for whom the only sugars they consume are naturally occurring (Schamshula *et al.*, 1978).

While the evidence is strong that consumption of sugars is a major risk factor for caries, sugars are not the only food sources involved in the carious process. Cooked or milled starches can be broken down to low molecular weight carbohydrates by the salivary enzyme amylase and thus act as a substrate for cariogenic bacteria. It has long been asserted that sugar–starch mixtures are more cariogenic than sugars alone (Bibby, 1975), and there is some animal evidence to support that view (Firestone *et al.*, 1984). The issue may never be totally clarified in humans, but it is reasonable and prudent to view all sugar-containing food and drinks, as well as cooked or milled starches, as potentially cariogenic. By contrast, the large molecular weight carbohydrates in lightly cooked vegetables are considered non-cariogenic because so little breakdown of these foods occurs in the mouth (Lingstrom *et al.*, 2000).

The evolving understanding of diet and caries

The great exploratory voyages of the seventeenth and eighteenth centuries led to the discovery of peoples previously unknown to Europeans, such as the islanders of the South Pacific, who appeared to live an idyllic life free of the diseases that afflicted Europe at the time. The concept of the 'noble savage' (Dubos, 1959) thus developed during the latter part of the eighteenth century. An offshoot from this ideal was the belief that the apparent freedom from caries enjoyed by so-called 'primitive' races could be attributed to the 'natural' diet on which they existed. Eating hard, fibrous and unprocessed food, so the theory went, led to better development of the jaws and teeth and helped to clear food debris from the teeth. By contrast, Europeans were even then eating a lot of processed food, high in fermentable carbohydrates, which was thought to exercise the masticatory apparatus insufficiently and lead eventually to tooth decay. Against the background of these beliefs, Miller, in the late nineteenth century, put forward his chemoparasitic theory of the development of dental caries. Miller's theory, developed during the 'golden age of bacteriology', was based on the action of microorganisms upon fermentable carbohydrates that adhered to the tooth's surface (Miller, 1883). Modern research shows that Miller got the overall picture pretty right.

Theories about the preventive value of hard and fibrous foods became more widespread in the early twentieth century and became established dogma in many places. One such article of faith stated that accumulations of fermentable carbohydrates could be removed by eating hard and fibrous foods (Wallace, 1902), the so-called 'cleansing' or 'detersive' foods. Another view was that if a meal was finished with a salivary stimulant such as an apple, the mouth would be kept free of fermentation both by the physical cleansing effect of the fibrous food and also because of the salivary flow induced by it (Pickerill, 1923). However, 'protective' factors in a diet based on unprocessed foods have proven hard to identify. High-fiber diets with a good proportion of vegetables and fruit are today recommended by all health authorities, and these dietary guidelines are seen as promoting good oral health as well as general health. Their value, however, is attributable less to the presence of hard and fibrous foods than to the relative absence of fermentable carbohydrates.

In this historical context, the best known attempt to conduct an experimental study on the effect of diet on dental decay in humans was the Vipeholm study, conducted in Sweden between 1945 and 1952 (Gustafsson *et al.*, 1954). The study was conducted in a mental institution (and by today's standards it would be considered unethical because the participants were unable to give their informed consent to potentially harmful exposures). Vipeholm's conclusions profoundly influenced the way in which the role of sugars in dental decay was viewed, despite its complicated and flawed study design. In brief, inmates of the institution were divided into groups with controlled consumption of refined sugars which varied in amount, frequency, physical form, and whether they were taken with or between meals. The extremes of intake were (a) no added sugars at all, to (b) daily between-meal consumption of 24 sticky toffees, each of which was too large to be swallowed and so had to be sucked and chewed. The differences in caries incidence between the groups were pronounced, although some of the Vipeholm conclusions can be challenged in the light of more recent research.

Sugars–caries relationships in today's low-caries environment

Many of the views on diet and caries are carry-overs from the pre-fluoride era, when caries was widespread and severe in high-income countries. In light of modern research protocols, design and analysis can be criticized in virtually all of them: all studies except for Vipeholm were cross-sectional, measurement of dietary intakes was often sloppy, and data analysis usually did not take likely confounders into account. In the period of caries decline, however, researchers have to think that the 'Vipeholm rules' have changed. Are all the children with no detectable caries seen today not consuming sugar, or are other factors having a major influence? Studies such as those concluding that oral hygiene is an important covariable in the sugar–caries relationship (Hausen *et al.*, 1981; Kleemola-Kujala & Rasanen, 1982; Sundin *et al.*, 1992) have served to question the validity of the Vipeholm findings.

Two prospective studies reported in the 1980s, one in Britain and one in the USA, measured diet and caries incidence concurrently and included more analytical detail than did any previous research. The British study followed 405 children with an average initial age of 11.5 years for 2 years (Rugg-Gunn *et al.*, 1984). The children, all from a low-fluoride area near Newcastle, completed five food diaries, each for a 3-day period, for a total of 15 days of recorded diet over the 2 years. Interviews with a dietitian followed each 3-day period to clarify uncertainties and to quantify amounts. The mean DMFS incidence of the group was 3.63 over the 2 years, with 57% of new lesions in pits and fissures, a lower caries increment than the authors had expected. Average consumption of all sugars was 118 g per day, providing 21% of energy intake. The results showed that caries increment was weakly but significantly correlated with total intake of sugars, but poorly correlated with frequency of intake. The authors stated that because of the lower-than-expected caries increment, more clear-cut results would have been likely if the study had been extended for another year.

The second study was based in the low-fluoride area of Coldwater, Michigan, USA. It followed 499 children, initially aged 11–15 years, for 3 years (Burt *et al.*, 1988). The majority completed four 24 h dietary recall interviews with a dietitian, although 27% completed more interviews. The boys in the study averaged 156 g of sugar intake per day from all sources, the girls 127 g, and sugars accounted for 26% of total energy intake. Both of these measures are higher than was found in the British group. Caries incidence, however, was lower than in the British group, averaging 2.9 DMF surfaces over the 3 years, of which 81% were pit-and-fissure lesions (buccal pits and lingual extensions as well as occlusal lesions). Nearly 30% of the group developed no caries at all over the 3 years, and only 51 children (10.2%) developed two or more proximal lesions during the study. Only among the latter 'high-risk' group was caries experience related to total intake of sugars, and that relationship was weak. No relationships between caries experience and frequency of consumption were found. The relative risk of caries from high sugar consumption relative to low sugar consumption was low (Burt & Szpunar, 1994); each additional 5 g of sugars ingested daily was associated with a 1% increase in the probability of developing caries (Szpunar *et al.*, 1995).

Despite some differences in study protocols, findings across these two independent studies were generally similar. Between them, the studies indicated that consumption of sugars is not a major risk factor for many children (i.e. those with no incident caries despite eating a lot of sugar), but it is for those who are still clearly susceptible to caries (broadly defined here as the minority who developed two or more proximal-surface lesions during the study). A systematic review of the present-day caries–sugars relationship (Burt & Pai, 2001) also concluded that the sugar–caries relationship was not as strong as generally supposed. This report identified 36 studies since 1980, all conducted in countries where there is widescale exposure to fluoride, which met the quality criteria for inclusion in the review. Eighteen of these studies found only a weak relationship between sugar consumption and incident caries, 16 found a moderate relationship and only two identified a strong relationship. The evidence from these more recent studies suggests that sugars still play a modest role as a risk factor for caries, especially among more high-risk children, but that this relationship is by no means linear.

The much stressed role of frequency of consumption of sugars ('it's not how much you eat, it's how often you eat it') is clearly questioned by the results of the Newcastle and Michigan studies, as it has been by other studies in Sweden (Sundin *et al.*, 1983; Bergendal & Hamp, 1985; Stecksen-Blicks *et al.*, 1985). The importance of frequency of consumption was a major finding of the Vipeholm study, and it has been prominent in dental health education ever since. However, the importance of frequency in Vipeholm was principally based on the caries experience of the group which consumed 24 large toffees between meals each day, a frequency of consumption that was not even approached in either the British or the Michigan study. The results from the highly artificial circumstances and non-representative sample of the Vipeholm study thus may be misleading when generalized to the population at large. Even so, frequency and amount of fermentable carbohydrate are related, and this issue has come to light again with recent evidence on the role of soft drinks in caries development.

Caries and soft drinks

Sugar in liquid form is cariogenic; it served well to demonstrate demineralization in landmark experimental caries studies (Von der Fehr *et al.*, 1970). There is more recent evidence to show that soft drink consumption is related to caries: the more often soft drinks are consumed, the greater the extent and severity of caries (Ismail *et al.*, 1984; Jones *et al.*, 1999; Watt *et al.*, 2000; Marshall *et al.*, 2003). Soft drinks have also been implicated as part of the cause of the global epidemic of obesity in children (Mann, 2003), for it is now common to find soft drinks and juices replacing formula and milk in children up to 2 years of age (Marshall *et al.*, 2003). A study among low-income adults found that 54% of their total energy intake came from several types of soft drinks and juices, and that high consumption of soft drinks when linked to poor oral hygiene was associated with higher caries levels (Burt *et al.*, 2006). Soft drinks seem to have replaced confectionery as the prime source of sugar in several populations.

The subject therefore has serious health implications that go beyond dentistry, and is yet another example of a general public health problem having clear dental overtones. Soft drinks thus can be viewed as a 'common risk factor' in public health (Sheiham & Watt, 2000).

Summary

The epidemiology of caries has traditionally been expressed in terms of bad diet, poor oral hygiene, cariogenic bacteria in plaque, 'acid attacks' and demineralization, salivary flow and exposure to fluoride. Those factors and others are all part of how and why caries develops, but this is too narrow a view for full understanding of the disease. In recent years there has been a growing awareness that there is a wider social dimension to caries, just as there is with other diseases. The growth of social and lifecourse epidemiology has shown the importance of the social environment in caries, and how youthful influences can years later affect adult disease. A comprehensive view of caries epidemiology includes all environments, from those at the plaque–enamel interface to the social environment in which a person lives. Caries is a disease of social deprivation, just as it is a disease of bad diet (indeed, those two factors are frequently found together). The key to eventual control of caries thus lies in improving the broad social environment for affected populations just as much as it does in intervening to improve the intraoral environment.

References

Alvarez JO. Nutrition, tooth development, and dental caries. *Am J Clin Nutr* 1995; **61**: 410–16S.

Anderson RJ, Bradnock G, James PMC. The changes in the dental health of 12-year-old school children in Shropshire. *Br Dent J* 1981; **150**: 278–81.

Athanassouli I, Mamai-Homata E, Panagopoulos H, Koletsi-Kounari H, Apostolopoulos A. Dental caries changes between 1982 and 1991 in children aged 6–12 in Athens, Greece. *Caries Res* 1994; **28**: 378–82.

Backer-Dirks O, Houwink B, Kwant GW. The results of 6½ years of artificial drinking water in the Netherlands; the Tiel-Culemborg experiment. *Arch Oral Biol* 1961; **5**: 284–300.

Bader JD, Shugars DA. What do we know about how dentists make caries-related treatment decisions? *Community Dent Oral Epidemiol* 1997; **25**: 97–103.

Bader JD, Shugars DA, Rozier RG. Relationship between epidemiologic coronal caries assessments and practitioners' treatment recommendations in adults. *Community Dent Oral Epidemiol* 1993; **21**: 96–101.

Baelum V, Fejerskov O, Manji F. The 'natural history' of dental caries and periodontal diseases in developing countries: some consequences for health care planning. *Tandlaegebladet* 1991; **95**: 139–48.

Barnard PD. Tamworth dental survey, summary report 1963–1988. Westmead, Australia: Westmead Centre for Oral Health, 2005.

Beal JF. The dental health of five-year-old children of different ethnic origins resident in an inner Birmingham area and a nearby borough. *Arch Oral Biol* 1973; **18**: 305–12.

Beck JD. The epidemiology of root surface caries: North American studies. *Adv Dent Res* 1993; **7**: 42–51.

Beck JD. Risk revisited. *Community Dent Oral Epidemiol* 1998; **26**: 220–5.

Beltrán-Aguilar ED, Barker LK, Canto MT, *et al.* Surveillance for dental caries, dental sealants, tooth retention, edentulism, and enamel fluorosis – United States, 1988–1994 and 1999–2002. *MMWR* 2005; **54**(SS-3): 1–44.

Bergendal B, Hamp SE. Dietary pattern and dental caries in 19-year-old adolescents subjected to preventive measures focused on oral hygiene and/or fluorides. *Swed Dent J* 1985; **9**: 1–7.

Bibby BG. The cariogenicity of snack foods and confections. *J Am Dent Assoc* 1975; **90**: 121–32.

Bjarnason S, Kohler B, Ranggard L. Dental caries in a group of 15 to 16-year-olds from Göteborg. Part I. *Swed Dent J* 1992; **16**: 143–9.

Bjarnason S, Finnbogason SY, Holbrook P, Kohler B. Caries experience in Icelandic 12-year-old urban children between 1984 and 1991. *Community Dent Oral Epidemiol* 1993; **21**: 195–7.

Blane D. Social determinants of health – socioeconomic status, social class, and ethnicity. *Am J Public Health* 1995; **85**: 903–5.

Bobak M, Marmot MG. East-West mortality divide and its potential explanations: proposed research agenda. *BMJ* 1996; **312**: 421–5.

Bohannan HM. Caries distribution and the case for sealants. *J Public Health Dent* 1983; **43**: 200–4.

Bratthall D. Introducing the Significant Caries Index together with a proposal for a new oral health goal for 12-year-olds, *Int Dent J* 2000; **50**: 378–84.

Bratthall D, Hänsel Petersson G, Sundberg H. Reasons for the caries decline: what do the experts believe? *Eur J Oral Sci* 1996; **104**: 416–22.

Brown LJ, Kingman A, Brunelle JA, Selwitz RH. Most US schoolchildren are caries free in their permanent teeth: this is no myth. *Public Health Rep* 1995; **110**: 531–3.

Brunner E, Marmot MG. Social organization, stress, and health. In: Marmot M, Wilkinson RG, eds. *Social determinants of health*. New York: Oxford University Press, 1999: 17–43.

Bryan ET, Collier DR, Vancleave ML. Dental health status of children in Tennessee; a 25-year comparison. *J Tenn Dent Assoc* 1982; **62**: 31–3.

Burt BA. Influences for change in the dental health status of populations: an historical perspective. *J Public Health Dent* 1978; **38**: 272–88.

Burt BA. The future of the caries decline. *J Public Health Dent* 1985; **49**: 368–76.

Burt BA, Pai S. Sugar consumption and caries risk: a systematic review. *J Dent Educ* 2001; **65**: 1017–23.

Burt BA, Szpunar SM. The Michigan Study: the relationship between sugars intake and dental caries over three years. *Int Dent J* 1994; **44**: 230–40.

Burt BA, Ismail AI, Eklund SA. Root caries in an optimally-fluoridated and a high-fluoride community. *J Dent Res* 1986; **65**: 1154–8.

Burt BA, Eklund SA, Morgan KJ, *et al.* The effects of sugars intake and frequency of ingestion on dental caries increment in a three-year longitudinal study. *J Dent Res* 1988; **67**: 1422–9.

Burt BA, Kolker JL, Sandretto AM, Yuan Y, Sohn W, Ismail AI. Dietary patterns related to caries in a low-income adult population. *Caries Res* 2006; **40**: 473–80.

Carmichael CL, Rugg-Gunn AJ, Ferrell RS. The relationship between fluoridation, social class and caries experience in 5-year-old children in Newcastle and Northumberland in 1987. *Br Dent J* 1989; **167**: 57–61.

Carvalho JC, Van Nieuwenhuysen JP, D'Hoore W. The decline in dental caries among Belgian children between 1983 and 1998. *Community Dent Oral Epidemiol* 2001; **29**: 55–61.

Caufield PW, Dasanayake AP, Li Y, Pan Y, Hsu J, Hardin JM. Natural history of *Streptococcus sanguinis* in the oral cavity of infants: evidence for a discrete window of infectivity. *Infect Immun* 2000; **68**: 4018–23.

Chalmers JM, Carter KD, Fuss JM, *et al.* Caries experience in exissting and new nursing home residents in Adelaide, Australia. *Gerodontology* 2002; **19**: 30–40.

Chen M, Andersen RM, Barmes DE, Leclerq M-H, Lyttle SC. *Comparing oral health systems. A second international collaborative study*. Geneva: World Health Organization, 1997.

Chironga L, Manji F. Dental caries in 12-year-old urban and rural children in Zimbabwe. *Community Dent Oral Epidemiol* 1989; **17**: 31–3.

Corbett ME, Moore WJ. Distribution of dental caries in ancient British populations. IV: The 19th century. *Caries Res* 1976; **10**: 401–14.

Dean HT, Arnold FA Jr, Elvove E. Domestic water and dental caries. V. Additional studies of the relation of fluoride domestic waters to dental caries experience in 4,425 white children aged 12–14 years of age in 13 cities in 4 states. *Public Health Rep* 1942; **57**: 1155–79.

DePaola PF, Soparkar PM, Tavares M, Kent RL Jr. The clinical profiles of individuals with and without root caries. *Gerodontology* 1989; **8**: 9–16.

Downer MC. Caries prevalence in the United Kingdom. *Int Dent J* 1994; **44**(Suppl 1): 365–70.

Drake CW, Hunt RJ, Beck JD, Koch GG. Eighteen-month coronal caries incidence in North Carolina older adults. *J Public Health Dent* 1994; **54**: 24–30.

Dubos R. *The mirage of health*. New York: Doubleday, 1959.

Espelid I, Tveit AB, Haugejorden O, Riordan PJ. Variation in radiographic interpretation and restorative treatment decisions on approximal caries among dentists in Norway. *Community Dent Oral Epidemiol* 1985; **13**: 26–9.

Fejerskov O, Antoft P, Gadegaard E. Decrease in caries experience in Danish children and young adults in the 1970s. *J Dent Res* 1982; **61** (Special Issue): 1305–10.

Firestone AR, Schmid R, Mühlemann HR. Effect on the length and number of intervals between meals on caries in rats. *Caries Res* 1984; **18**: 128–33.

Flinck A, Kallestal C, Holm AK, Allebeck P, Wall S. Distribution of caries in 12-year-old children in Sweden. Social and oral health-related behavioural patterns. *Community Dent Health* 1999; **16**: 160–5.

Freeman R, Breistein B, McQueen A, Stewart M. The dental health status of five-year-old children in north and west Belfast. *Community Dent Health* 1997; **14**: 253–7.

Freire M, Hardy R, Sheiham A. Mothers' sense of coherence and their adolescent children's oral health status and behaviours. *Community Dent Health* 2002; **19**: 24–31.

Fuchs V. *Who shall live?* Health, economics, and social choice. New York: Basic Books, 1974.

Gilbert GH, Duncan RP, Dolan TA, Foerster U. Twenty-four month incidence of root caries among a diverse group of adults. *Caries Res* 2001; **35**: 366–75.

Glass RL. Secular changes in caries prevalence in two Massachusetts towns. *Caries Res* 1981; **15**: 445–50.

Goodman E. The role of socioeconomic status gradients in explaining differences in US adolescents' health. *Am J Public Health* 1999; **89**: 1522–8.

Grainger RM. Epidemiological data. In: Chilton NW, ed. *Design and analysis in dental and oral research*, 1st edn. Philadelphia, PA: Lippincott, 1967: 311–53.

Gratrix D, Holloway PJ. Factors of deprivation associated with dental caries in young children. *Community Dent Health* 1994; **11**: 66–70.

Graves RC, Bohannan HM, Disney JA, Stamm JW, Bader JD, Abernathy JR. Recent dental caries and treatment patterns in US children. *J Public Health Dent* 1986; **46**: 23–9.

Gray M, Morris AJ, Davies, J. The oral health of South Asian five-year-old children in deprived areas of Dudley compared with white children of equal deprivation and fluoridation status. *Community Dent Health* 2000; **17**: 243–5.

Gustafsson BE, Quensel C-E, Swenander Lanke L, *et al.* The Vipeholm dental caries study. The effect of different levels of carbohydrate intake on caries activity in 436 individuals observed for five years. *Acta Odont Scand* 1954; **11**: 232–364.

Haan MN, Kaplan GA, Syme SL. Socioeconomic status and health: old observations and new thoughts. In: Bunker JP, Gomby DS, Kehrer BH, eds. *Pathways to health: the role of social factors*. Menlo Park, CA: Henry J Kaiser Family Foundation, 1989: 76–135.

Hadden WC. The use of educational attainment as an indicator of socioeconomic position. *Am J Public Health* 1996; **86**: 1525–6.

Hand JS, Hunt RJ, Beck JD. Incidence of coronal and root caries in an older adult population. *J Public Health Dent* 1988; **48**: 14–19.

Hargreaves JA, Wagg BJ, Thompson GW. Changes in caries prevalence of Isle of Lewis children, a historical comparison from 1937 to 1984. *Caries Res* 1987; **21**: 277–84.

Hausen H, Heinonen OP, Paunio I. Modification of occurrence of caries in children by toothbrushing and sugar exposure in fluoridated and non-fluoridated areas. *Community Dent Oral Epidemiol* 1981; **9**: 103–7.

Hawkins RJ, Main PA, Locker D. Oral health status and treatment needs of Canadian adults aged 85 years and over. *Special Care Dent* 1998; **18**: 164–9.

Horowitz HS. Clinical trials of preventives for dental caries. *J Public Health Dent* 1972; **32**: 229–33.

Hughes JT, Rozier RG. The survey of dental health in the North Carolina population; selected findings. In: Bawden JW, De Friese GH, eds. *Planning for dental care on a statewide basis; the North Carolina dental manpower project*. Chapel Hill, NC: Dental Foundation of North Carolina, 1981: 21–37.

Hugoson A, Koch G, Hallonsten A-L, Ludvigsson N, Lundgren D, Rylander H. Dental health 1973 and 1978 in individuals aged 3–20 years in the community of Jonkopping, Sweden. *Swed Dent J* 1980; **150**: 217–29.

Hunter PBV. The prevalence of dental caries in 5-year-old New Zealand children. *N Z Dent J* 1979; **75**: 154–7.

Institute of Medicine. *The future of public health*. Washington DC: National Academy Press, 1988.

Ismail AI, Burt BA, Eklund SA. The cariogenicity of soft drinks in the United States. *J Am Dent Assoc* 1984; **109**: 241–45.

Ismail AI, Brodeur JM, Gagnon P, *et al.* Prevalence of non-cavitated and cavitated carious lesions in a random sample of 7–9-year-old schoolchildren in Montreal, Quebec. *Community Dent Oral Epidemiol* 1992; **20**: 250–5.

Johansson I, Saellstrom AK, Rajan BP, Parameswaran A. Salivary flow and dental caries in Indian children suffering from chronic malnutrition. *Caries Res* 1992; **26**: 38–43.

Jones CM, Worthington H. The relationship between water fluoridation and socioeconomic deprivation on tooth decay in 5-year-old children. *Br Dent J* 1999; **186**: 397–400.

Jones C, Taylor G, Woods K, Whittle G, Evans D, Young P. Jarman underprivileged area scores, tooth decay and the effect of water fluoridation. *Community Dent Health* 1997a; **14**: 156–60.

Jones CM, Taylor GO, Whittle JG, Evans D, Trotter DP. Water fluoridation, tooth decay in 5 year olds, and social deprivation measured by the Jarman score: analysis of data from British dental surveys. *BMJ* 1997b; **315**: 514–17.

Jones CM, Woods K, Taylor GO. Social deprivation and tooth decay in Scottish schoolchildren. *Health Bull* 1997c; **55**: 11–15.

Jones C, Woods K, Whittle G, Worthington H, Taylor G. Sugar, drinks, deprivation and dental caries in 14-year-old children in the north west of England in 1995. *Community Dent Health* 1999; **16**: 68–71.

Kallestal C, Wall S. Socioeconomic effect on caries. Incidence data among Swedish 12–14-year-olds. *Community Dent Oral Epidemiol* 2002; **30**: 108–14.

Kaplan GA. People and places: contrasting perspectives on the association between social class and health. *Int J Health Serv* 1996; **26**: 507–19.

Kaplan GA, Haan MN, Syme SL, Minkler M, Winkelby M. Socioeconomic status and health. In: Amler RW, Dull HB, eds. *Closing the gap: the burden of unnecessary illness.* New York: Oxford University Press, 1987: 125–9.

Kaplan GA, Pamuk E, Lynch JW, Cohen RD, Balfour JL. Inequality in income and mortality in the United States: analysis of mortality and potential pathways. *BMJ* 1996; **312**: 999–1003.

Kaste LM, Selwitz RH, Oldakowski RJ, Brunelle JA, Winn DM, Brown LJ. Coronal caries in the primary and permanent dentition of children and adolescents 1–17 years of age: United States, 1988–1991. *J Dent Res* 1996; **75**(Special Issue): 631–41.

Katz RV, Meskin LH. Testing the internal and external validity of a simplified dental caries index on an adult population. *Community Dent Oral Epidemiol* 1976; **4**: 227–31.

Kingman A. A method of utilizing the subject's initial caries experience to increase efficiency in caries clinical trials. *Community Dent Oral Epidemiol* 1979; **7**: 87–90.

Kitamura M, Kiyak HA, Mulligan K. Predictors of root caries in the elderly. *Community Dent Oral Epidemiol* 1986; **14**: 34–8.

Kleemola-Kujala E, Rasanen L. Relationship of oral hygiene and sugar consumption to risk of caries in children. *Community Dent Oral Epidemiol* 1982; **10**: 224–33.

Klein H. The family and dental disease. IV. Dental disease (DMF) experience in parents and offspring. *J Am Dent Assoc* 1946; **33**: 735–43.

Klein H, Palmer CE. Studies on dental caries. V. Familial resemblance in the caries experience of siblings. *Public Health Rep* 1938; **53**: 1353–64.

Klein H, Palmer CE. Community economic status and the dental problem of school children. *Public Health Rep* 1940; **55**: 187–205.

Klein H, Palmer CE. Studies on dental caries. XII. Comparison of the caries susceptibility of the various morphological types of permanent teeth. *J Dent Res* 1941; **20**: 203–16.

Klein H, Shimizu T. The family and dental disease. I. DMF experience among husbands and wives. *J Am Dent Assoc* 1945; **32**: 945–55.

Klein H, Palmer CE, Knutson JW. Studies on dental caries: I. Dental status and dental needs of elementary school children. *Public Health Rep* 1938; **53**: 751–65.

Kohler B, Bratthall D, Krasse B. Preventive measures in mothers influence the establishment of the bacterium *Streptococcus mutans* in their infants. *Arch Oral Biol* 1983; **28**: 225–31.

Kumar J, Green E, Wallace W, Bustard R. Changes in dental caries prevalence in upstate New York schoolchildren. *J Public Health Dent* 1991; **51**: 158–63.

Lawrence HP, Hunt RJ, Beck JD. Three-year root caries incidence and risk modeling in older adults in North Carolina. *J Public Health Dent* 1995; **55**: 69–78.

Lennon MA, Davies RM, Downer MC, Hull PS. Tooth loss in a 19th century British population. *Arch Oral Biol* 1974; **19**: 511–16.

Lingstrom P, van Houte J, Kashket S. Food starches and dental caries. *Crit Rev Oral Biol Med* 2000; **11**: 366–80.

Link BG, Phelan JC. Understanding sociodemographic differnces in health; the role of fundamental social causes [editorial]. *Am J Public Health* 1996; **86**: 471–3.

Lo EC, Schwarz EC. Tooth and root conditions in the middle-aged and the elderly in Hong Kong. *Community Dent Oral Epidemiol* 1994; **22**: 381–5.

Locker D, Leake JL. Coronal and root decay experience in older adults in Ontario, Canada. *J Public Health Dent* 1993; **53**: 158–64.

Luan W, Baelum V, Fejerskov O, Chen X. Ten-year incidence of dental caries in adult and elderly Chinese. *Caries Res* 2000; **34**: 205–13.

McDonald SP, Sheiham A. The distribution of caries on different tooth surfaces at varying levels of caries – a compilation of data from 18 previous studies. *Community Dent Health* 1992; **9**: 39–48.

Macek MD, Beltran-Aguilar ED, Lockwood SA, Malvitz DM. Updated comparison of the caries susceptibility of various morphological types of permanent teeth. *J Public Health Dent* 2003; **63**: 174–82.

McEniery TM, Davies GN. Brisbane dental survey 1977. A comparative study of caries experience of children in Brisbane, Australia, over a 20-year period. *Community Dent Oral Epidemiol* 1979; **7**: 42–50.

McGuire SM, Fox CH, Douglass CW, Tennstedt SL, Feldman HA. Beneath the surface of coronal caries: primary decay, recurrent decay, and failed restorations in a population-based survey of New England elders. *J Public Health Dent* 1993; **53**: 76–82.

Machiulskiene V, Nyvad B, Baelum V. Prevalence and severity of dental caries in 12-year-old children in Kaunas, Lithuania, 1995. *Caries Res* 1998; **32**: 175–80.

Machiulskiene V, Nyvad B, Baelum V. A comparison of clinical and radiographic caries diagnoses in posterior teeth of 12-year-old Lithuanian children. *Caries Res* 1999; **33**: 340–8.

Manji F, Fejerskov O. Dental caries in developing countries in relation to the appropriate use of fluoride. *J Dent Res* 1990; **69**(Special Issue): 733–41.

Manji F, Fejerskov O, Baelum V, Luan W-M, Chen X. The epidemiological features of dental caries in African and Chinese populations: implications for risk assessment. In: Johnson NW, ed. *Risk markers for oral diseases*, Vol. 1, *Dental caries markers of high and low risk groups and individuals.* Cambridge: Cambridge University Press, 1991: 62–100.

Mann J. Sugar revisited – again [editorial]. *Bull WHO* 2003; **81**: 552.

Marcenes WS, Sheiham A. The relationship between work stress and oral health status. *Soc Sci Med* 1992; **35**: 1511–20.

Marmot M, Wilkinson RG, eds. *Social determinants of health.* New York: Oxford University Press, 1999.

Marmot MG, Kogenivas M, Elston MA. Social/economic status and disease. *Ann Rev Public Health* 1987; **8**: 111–35.

Marshall TA, Levy SM, Broffitt B, Eichenberger-Gilmore JM, Stumbo PJ. Patterns of beverage consumption during the transition stage of infant nutrition. *J Am Diet Assoc* 2003; **103**: 1350–3.

Marthaler TM, O'Mullane DM, Vrbic V. The prevalence of dental caries in Europe 1990–1995. *Caries Res* 1996; **30**: 237–75.

Milen A. Role of social class in caries occurrence in primary teeth. *Int J Epidemiol* 1987; **16**: 252–6.

Miller WD. Agency of micro-organisms in decay of human teeth. *Dent Cosmos* 1883; **25**: 1–12.

Møller IJ. Impact of oral diseases across cultures. *Int Dent J* 1978; **28**: 376–80.

Moore WJ, Corbett ME. The distribution of dental caries in ancient British populations. I. Anglo-Saxon period. *Caries Res* 1971; **5**: 151–68.

Moore WJ, Corbett ME. The distribution of dental caries in ancient British populations. II. Iron Age, Romano-British and Mediaeval periods. *Caries Res* 1973; **7**: 139–53.

Morse DP, Holm-Pedersen P, Holm-Pedersen J, *et al.* Dental caries in persons over the age of 80 living in Kungsholmen, Sweden: findings from the KEOHS project. *Community Dent Health* 2002; **19**: 262–7.

Mosha HJ, Robison VA. Caries experience of the primary dentition among groups of Tanzanian urban preschoolchildren. *Community Dent Oral Epidemiol* 1989; **17**: 34–7.

Mosha HJ, Scheutz F. Dental caries in the permanent dentition of schoolchildren in Dar es Salaam in 1979, 1983 and 1989. *Community Dent Oral Epidemiol* 1992; **20**: 381–2.

9

The impact of diagnostic criteria on estimates of prevalence, extent and severity of dental caries

N. Pitts

Introduction

This chapter seeks to help students of all ages to understand a range of important, but frequently subtle, caries measurement issues. The chapter covers the types of diagnostic criteria used in epidemiology, in contrast to those used in clinical practice and research (so that by learning from the past we can synthesize evidence to inform future choices), and then considers in turn the impact of diagnostic criteria on estimates of the prevalence of the disease, its extent and its severity. Finally, a framework is outlined to help in the choice and understanding of diagnostic criteria that are appropriate for particular types of epidemiological study.

Diagnostic criteria for dental caries: an epidemiological perspective

In the control of dental caries, a common risk factor approach (see Chapter 28) provides the public health foundation; this should be built upon and complemented by appropriate non-operative and operative care in dental practice. This challenge to control the caries process is a lifelong one (Fejerskov, 1997, 2004; Selwitz *et al.*, 2007), extending from very early childhood to death.

The terminology, case definitions and conventions used to define and subdivide the signs of caries have to be carefully and consistently framed. Unfortunately, there is very considerable variation in this area (Ismail, 2004). There is also wide variation in both clinical research and clinical practice about the terms associated with caries diagnosis. Throughout this chapter the terminology and conventions developed at an international workshop (Pitts & Stamm, 2004) will be used. It was decided to define three key terms relevant to diagnostic criteria and their use:

- '*lesion detection* (which implies an objective method of determining whether or not disease is present)
- *lesion assessment* (which aims to characterise or monitor a lesion, once it has been detected)
- *caries diagnosis* (which should imply a human professional summation of all available data)'.

These terms will be used throughout this chapter.

Impact of caries diagnostic thresholds on reported caries estimates

To appreciate the epidemiological caries data currently available on a global basis, together with its strengths, limitations and degree of generalizability, it is very important to understand the concepts underlying the D_1, D_2, D_3 and D_4 (see Chapters 4 and 8) diagnostic thresholds and their impact on the estimates of caries prevalence, extent or severity. This is an area where clinicians and dental public health dentists often use similar terminology very differently. Figure 9.1 shows an iceberg metaphor for caries (Pitts & Longbottom, 1995) which, in Fig. 9.1a, provides a graphical representation or summary of the range of caries diagnostic levels and thresholds typically used in epidemiology, research and clinical practice. In Fig. 9.1b a similar presentation is linked to patient advice and treatment need, as information about both operative and non-operative care will increasingly be needed from epidemiological studies.

As has been emphasized in Chapters 2 and 4, the caries lesion, irrespective of its size and extent, is the manifestation of long-lasting metabolic activity in biofilms on tooth surfaces. The iceberg conceptualizes the potential sum of the metabolic processes by stacking lesions of increasingly severe stages of disease on top of each other, starting from the smallest carious demineralizations at the base, through to established open dentin lesions penetrating into the pulp at the tip. At a certain point in time, a lesion can only exist at one particular level of the iceberg, although it has previously passed through the more modest (or lower) levels. Clinically detectable lesions can be graded from D_1 to D_4 lesions, using terms that were in widespread use with the World Health Organization (WHO) in the 1970s (WHO, 1979). This gradation of the extent of individual lesions should not be confused with the commonly used diagnostic thresholds (or cut-offs) which share similar names (e.g. D_1 and D_3).

The horizontal lines (or water levels) of Fig. 9.1a illustrate the impact of changing the diagnostic threshold (or cut-off) on what is considered to constitute 'diseased' or 'sound' tooth tissue. At this stage the sole concern is with the detection stage of the diagnostic process. The arrows to the left of the figure illustrate just how much of the caries process is often misclassified as 'caries free' if only the D_3 threshold is used when collecting and reporting epidemiological data.

The D_3 (caries into dentin) diagnostic threshold includes only D_3 and D_4 grades of lesion and has been used (in several ways, with and without the use of sharp explorers) for many years in classical caries epidemiological studies to provide comparative data on the more severe manifestations of the caries disease process. When using results of epidemiological studies where data are collected and/or reported only at the D_3 (caries into dentin only) threshold, the proportion of the population classified as 'caries free' conveys a mistaken impression that there is no disease at all present in these groups (or in the individuals within them). This paradox means that many clinicians, educators, planners and politicians are often not clear about the limitations of data reported solely at the D_3 threshold.

The situation is further complicated by the decision around what constitutes dentin caries when using clinical–visual methods. For many years in North America and elsewhere, the convention was (and in many places still is) that D_3 'caries' was only recognized epidemiologically when macroscopic cavitation was seen ('open' cavities).

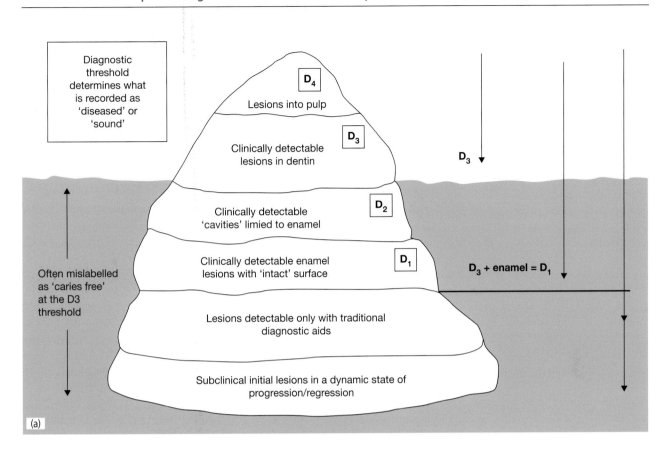

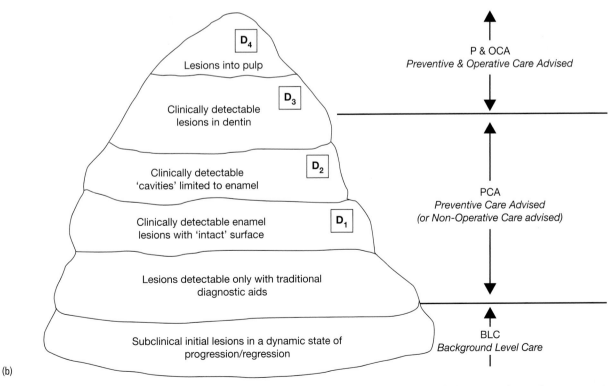

Figure 9.1 The iceberg metaphor for dental caries: (a) diagnostic thresholds for lesion extent; (b) caries extent linked to patient advice and treatment need.

There has been a long-running debate over whether or not the sharp probe (explorer) actually contributes any diagnostic benefit and also whether it may result in clinically significant iatrogenic damage, particularly to white-spot lesions with macroscopically intact surface zones (Ekstrand *et al.*, 1987). Diagnostic criteria from the USA have typically used a sharp explorer (Radike, 1968), while European systems have favoured a more visual approach where the probe is only used to assess surface texture and roughness. However, today, North American authors tend to apply classifications that rely upon the visual appearance of both enamel and dentin caries (Ismail, 2004; Pitts & Stamm, 2004).

It should, however, be appreciated that visually discernible non-cavitated dentin lesions are an important subset of the total number of dentin lesions (Ismail, 1997). They should be included in caries counts and can have a significant impact on results, particularly for children and young adults (Pitts & Harker, 2004). These dentinal lesions are often of equivalent size to frank cavities, and may be seen clinically owing to the changed colour of the dentin caries visible through the apparently 'intact' or whitened enamel. In fact, the enamel is not intact; there is often a small hole (or very small discontinuity) which may, or may not, be associated with stain (Fig. 9.2a), but such a lesion will not admit the 0.5 mm diameter ball end of the probe, previously used to help define a 'cavity' in these studies (Fig. 9.2b).

Moving further down the icebergs in Fig. 9.1, one can visualize the D_1 diagnostic threshold level. In addition to the detection of lesions at the caries into dentin level, this threshold includes the detection of 'white-spot' and 'brown-spot' caries in enamel. It has been accepted and in use for many years in a wide range of countries for clinical practice, research examinations and, in some cases, caries epidemiological studies. The D_1 threshold systems are not new, they have evolved from studies of Backer-Dirks in the 1950s (Backer-Dirks *et al.*, 1951), Marthaler and Moller in the 1960s (Marthaler, 1965; Moller, 1966) and the WHO in the 1970s (WHO, 1979), while examples of data collection at this threshold come from places as diverse as Hong Kong (Pitts & Fyffe, 1988), Africa (Manji *et al.*, 1991) and China (Luan *et al.*, 2000), for example. During the 1990s, it was gradually accepted that the use of the D_1 threshold is important in order to be able to adopt the concept of caries control.

Caries diagnostic thresholds and epidemiological estimates of treatment need

The impetus to record at the D_1 diagnostic threshold comes from a desire to link epidemiological estimates of caries prevalence with needs for non-operative and operative dental care in populations and groups. In using epidemiological data to make estimates of treatment need, one should first establish which diagnostic threshold(s) have been used in data collection and in reporting and then see how the information obtained may be used to assess needs. The concepts of non-operative treatment (NOT) and operative treatment (OT) (Nyvad & Fejerskov, 1997) outlined for the treatment of individual patients in Chapters 14 and 20 are pertinent here. In some countries the established terms used are preventive and operative care advised (P&OCA) and operative care advised (OCA) (Pitts & Longbottom, 1995) (see Fig. 9.1b).

Once again there are considerable variations between and within countries in assessing treatment need. The non-operative treatment approach has been in use in Scandinavian countries for decades and represents the trend in many other areas (Pitts, 2004a). However, in some parts of the world the more traditional, restorative-only philosophy from the 1960s has persisted and the pace of change is slower.

Epidemiological data will need to identify and quantify the proportion of lesions in need of non-operative care alone as well as those requiring both non-operative and operative care. In all of these considerations, the need for clinicians

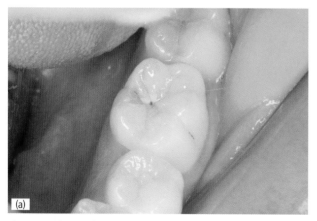 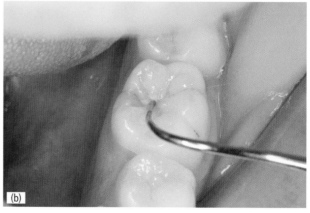

Figure 9.2 (a) Clinical appearance of an occlusal surface of molar tooth with equivocal signs of dentin caries; (b) the same tooth surface being explored with a 0.5 mm blunt probe, which is not admitted to the fissure.

to tailor treatment decisions to individual patients with their own needs, wants and circumstances should also be recognized, along with the inherent and long-recognized difficulty of estimating precisely operative treatment need at the individual level from surveys (Nuttall, 1983; Burt, 1997).

Caries diagnostic thresholds and specific epidemiological considerations

Diagnostic criteria for epidemiology are different from those in the world of clinical care. Epidemiology studies the distribution and determinants of health-related states or events in specified populations and applies this study to control health problems. Not only are the epidemiological questions different, but the clinical resources, the types of staff, the time and the financial constraints available at the community level may also be different.

Diagnostic criteria and conventions for the epidemiological recording of caries

Recording dental caries
Worldwide, dental caries has been recorded for years using variations of the decayed, missing and filled (DMF) index developed in the 1930s by Klein, Palmer and Knutson (Klein *et al.*, 1938). The index is still in use 70 years after its first description, indicating how successful it has been and how difficult it is to develop and gain acceptance for any alternative. The DMF score, whether calculated by teeth (DMFT) or surfaces (DMFS) affected, can be collected for both permanent (DMF) and primary (dmf) teeth. The index has come to have a particular meaning to dental epidemiologists and researchers.

The method is understood internationally and facilitates the ready comparison of data sets. However, it has disadvantages. The terminology is not understood by other health professionals. A further challenge is that the index is also poorly understood by patients, lay audiences and policy makers. In addition, the index is not sensitive to non-operative interventions or sealants and becomes saturated for older age groups.

Recording visual caries at the dentin-only level
Figure 9.3 comprises a series of schematic caries icebergs recording the sequential stages of dental caries. Figure 9.3a shows that when epidemiologists record caries with clinical–visual criteria that only recognize as caries either pulpal decay (severe decay) or visible dentin decay (established decay), they are underrecording the disease manifestations. This is both in terms of unseen dentin lesions (beyond the resolution of a clinical-only visual examination) and in terms of the less severe lesions lower down in the iceberg which are, at this threshold, classed as 'sound'. This becomes a real issue if those conducting the survey and those receiving the results are unaware of the intrinsic limitations of this diagnostic threshold. For this reason it is becoming increasingly common in Europe to refer to the proportion of subjects examined with dentin lesions as those 'with obvious decay experience', as this term seems to convey a more accurate impression of the data collected to both lay and professional groups.

Although properly conducted and reported studies at this d_3/D_3 threshold continue to be valuable, there is a significant gap between traditional practice and contemporary needs for planning, delivering and monitoring non-operative oral health-care services.

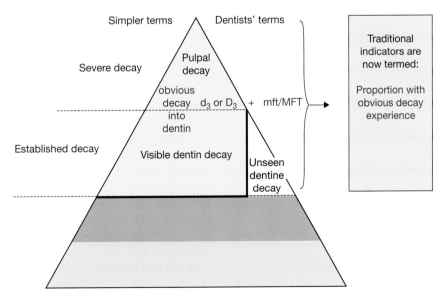

(a)

Figure 9.3 (a–e) Series of graphics depicting the extent of the total caries experience present in a tooth (or person, or population) which is recorded at different levels. (a) Visual caries at the dentin-only level.

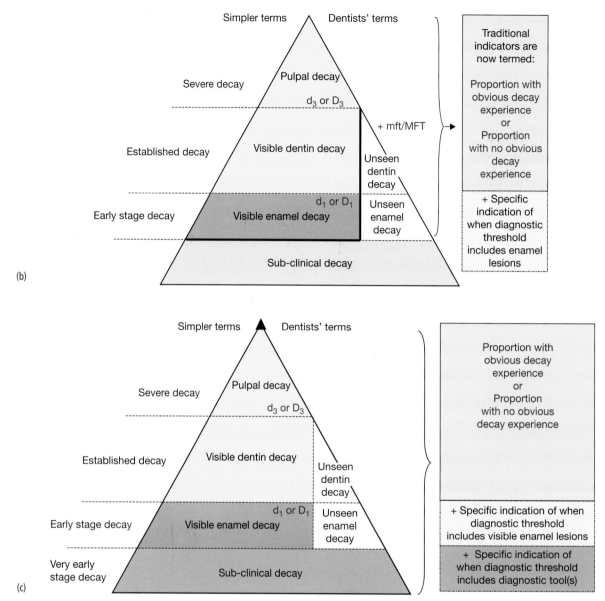

Figure 9.3 (b) Visual caries at the enamel plus dentin level. (c) 'Ideal' recording of total caries experience.

Recording clinical visual caries at the enamel plus the dentin level

Figure 9.3b illustrates the impact of adding in the next level of the iceberg, 'visual enamel' lesions (early-stage decay), to supplement all the information available, as before, about caries into dentin. Studies at this d_1/D_1 threshold capture more of the caries present in the population being examined, and the criteria include the spectrum of clinical lesions in enamel that clinicians increasingly recognize, chart and try to manage non-operatively as a routine. Note that the graphic indicates that there is a proportion of unseen enamel decay to add to the unseen dentin decay from the higher level. There is a continuing need for clarity over exactly what diagnostic thresholds are used in different surveys,

studies and projects, and these must be reported explicitly to inform the report users and readers as well as to help those who have later to conduct systematic reviews of the literature.

As the ability to look at trends over time is often important, any change in diagnostic threshold may be seen as a threat to comparisons with data collected earlier. However, if clinical epidemiological data are collected with suitable codes, the results can be reported at either the D_1 or D_3 diagnostic threshold, or at both thresholds.

In the past it has been argued that enamel lesions could not be included in epidemiological assessments of caries because they could not be reproducibly assessed. However, it now appears that this is not the case, as excellent repro-

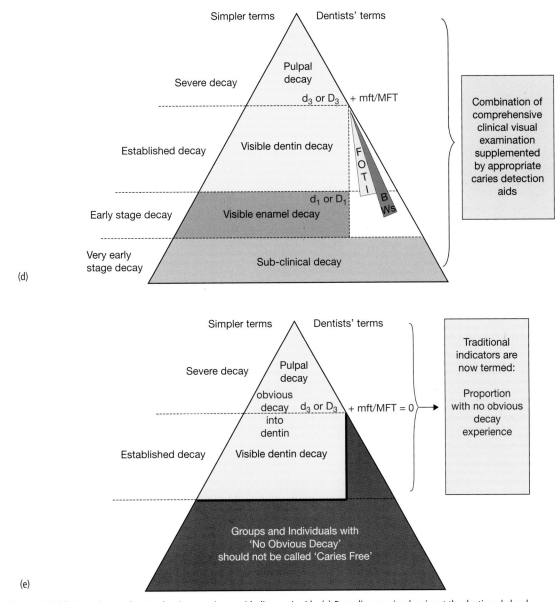

Figure 9.3 (d) Towards recording total caries experience with diagnostic aids. (e) Recording no visual caries at the dentin-only level.

ducibility has been achieved by a range of examiners from different countries when using the D_1 threshold in clinical trials (Deery, 1997; Nyvad *et al.*, 1998; Deery *et al.*, 2000; Forgie *et al.*, 2000; Chesters *et al.*, 2002) and survey-type settings (Glass *et al.*, 1987; Ismail *et al.*, 1992; Forgie, 1999; Luan *et al.*, 2000).

Moves towards recording total caries

Figure 9.3c illustrates ongoing moves towards being able to record more of the total caries picture where information on very early-stage decay is also captured. At present, this theoretical ideal is not achievable, but when the survey or study question requires this type of data, comprehensive clinical–visual examinations can be supplemented by tradi-

tional diagnostic aids (Fig. 9.3d), such as bitewing radiographs and fiber-optic transillumination (FOTI), which may show additional information (see Chapters 5 and 6). It may even be possible in the future to pick up very early-stage decay that is beyond the resolution of the naked eye.

Importance of correct terminology when recording no visual dentin caries

It must be remembered that in epidemiological surveys, the combination of the limitations imposed by the diagnostic criteria chosen, the challenging environment of field conditions and the lack of diagnostic aids available to the clinician will inevitably mean that epidemiological results systematically underscore caries prevalence, extent and severity (Pitts, 1997). It is unfortunate and misleading, for politicians and decision makers, to continue to use the term 'caries free'. Figure 9.3e demonstrates the magnitude of uncertainty when working at the d_3/D_3 threshold with clinical–visual examination alone and outlines the more descriptive term for groups or individuals who have 'no obvious decay'.

Impact of diagnostic criteria on estimates of caries prevalence

It is important to understand the clinically and statistically significant impact that apparently subtle changes in the wording and use of diagnostic criteria and conventions can have on the results of epidemiological investigations. For the purposes of providing a brief example relating to the impact of criteria and conventions upon prevalence, the data from the most recent (2003) United Kingdom Child Dental Health Survey are illustrative (Pitts & Harker, 2004).

This survey is part of a series that has been repeated at 10 yearly intervals, collecting data at the D_3 (dentin-only) level. In planning the survey there was an awareness that, even when working at the D_3 diagnostic threshold, variation in epidemiological practice was occurring, with many centers becoming unhappy about excluding from the caries count dentinal lesions which, although they did not have macroscopic cavitation in dentin sufficient to admit the tip of a blunted or ball-ended dental probe (explorer) of specified dimensions (the criteria used in earlier studies in the series), did have a clear visible change in color arising from dark carious dentin shining through the translucent enamel as a darkened gray shadow. Therefore, in 1992 a change was made in the specification of the criteria for the relevant clinical code (Code 2) used in the UK British Association for the Study of Community Dentistry co-ordinated program of epidemiological surveys (Pitts, 1992) to include visual dentin caries. These criteria have been in successful use ever since. The organizers of the UK Child Dental Health Survey were keen to update the diagnostic criteria to be used in 2003, but were also very aware of the need to ensure 'backwards compatibility' of the results with those of the 1993 and earlier surveys.

The solution adopted was to score caries using criteria that allowed the results to be calculated as a best current estimate (including dentin cavitation and visual dentin caries) or as a separate estimate to permit the evaluation of trends in caries prevalence over decades (including dentin cavitation, but excluding visual dentin caries). These two measures were reported in the results as 2003a estimates ($D_{3CV}MFT$) and 2003b estimates ($D_{3C}MFT$), respectively (Pitts & Harker, 2004; Pitts et al., 2006a).

Let us look first at the impact of diagnostic criteria for caries into dentin upon estimates of prevalence at the subject level. Figure 9.4 shows the Child Dental Health 2003

results for the proportion of children at the ages of 8, 12 and 15 years with obvious decay in permanent teeth, both including (2003a) and excluding (2003b) visual dentin caries. The inclusion of the visual element of the criteria for dentin caries resulted in a doubling of the prevalence of decayed permanent teeth (D_3T) at the age of 8 years and a 2.5-fold increase at the age of 15 years. The change in the result of a national survey estimating the proportion of 15-year-old children affected by dentinal caries from 32% to 13% would be deemed as of public health significance and newsworthy if it were measured over a specific period. The fact that changes of this magnitude can be seen purely as a result of changing the diagnostic threshold of the criteria being used by trained and calibrated examiners underlines the importance of the criteria and their framing.

The impact of the criteria on the prevalence of overall dentinal caries experience (D_3MFT) across the three age groups was more modest, but still marked. This impact on measuring the prevalence of dentin caries was, however, age and dentition related. In primary teeth at the age of 5 years there was little difference in the values of $d_{3CV}t$ and $d_{3C}t$. These findings demonstrate the need to be very clear and consistent with the definition and wording of diagnostic criteria and in the training of examiners in their use.

Epidemiological criteria for estimating the prevalence of root caries also vary widely (Nyvad & Fejerskov, 1986; Manji et al., 1988; Fejerskov et al., 1991, 1993; Kelly et al., 2000) and again this diversity adds to the uncertainty when making comparisons between surveys and when relating findings to clinical data (Fejerskov et al., 1993). Criteria for recurrent or secondary caries (primary caries associated with a restoration or sealant) are a further area where there is a dearth of validated, practical, reliable epidemiological measures.

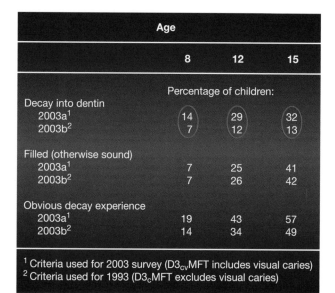

	Age		
	8	**12**	**15**
	Percentage of children:		
Decay into dentin			
2003a[1]	14	29	32
2003b[2]	7	12	13
Filled (otherwise sound)			
2003a[1]	7	25	41
2003b[2]	7	26	42
Obvious decay experience			
2003a[1]	19	43	57
2003b[2]	14	34	49

[1] Criteria used for 2003 survey ($D3_{cv}MFT$ includes visual caries)
[2] Criteria used for 1993 ($D3_cMFT$ excludes visual caries)

Figure 9.4 Impact of using alternative diagnostic criteria relating to dentin caries illustrated with results from the UK Child Dental Health Survey, 2003.

Impact of diagnostic criteria on estimates of caries extent

The impact of criteria on measures of the extent of the caries can be seen by reference to changes in the estimates of mean values for the number of teeth or surfaces affected in typical individuals within entire populations or subgroups. For instance, this impact could be seen in changes in mean values between D_3MFS and D_1MFS, or between d_3mft and d_1mft. Examples in this section are taken from (i) the 1998 UK Adult Dental Health Survey, (ii) a comparison of international methods made on the same subjects on the same day, and (iii) sequential assessments of caries extent in primary teeth made of over 1200 preschool children.

1998 UK Adult Dental Health Survey

For the 1998 UK Adult Dental Health Survey, it was decided (in a similar way to that described above for the 2003 Child Dental Health Survey above) to ensure comparability between the contemporary data for dentin caries experience collected with modern caries criteria, while at the same time allowing trend information to be collected with criteria compatible with those used decades earlier. The diagnostic criteria ultimately used in the 1998 Adult Dental Health Survey (Kelly *et al.*, 2000) were set at the D_3 (caries into dentin) threshold, as before in this series of surveys. However, this time they included an additional code allowing the inclusion of lesions scored as 'visual (dentin) caries' without any gross cavitation, in addition to the previously used code for cavitated dentin caries scored in surveys (which had previously attracted some critical comment; Kidd, 1991).

A comparison of excluding and then including the clinical–visual dentin lesions in the adult survey showed that, overall for the UK, the proportion of the population with one or more decayed or unsound teeth changed from 42% to 55% when the visual dentin caries scores were included. Similarly, when the extent of the disease recorded as the overall mean number of teeth affected was examined, this estimate rose by 50%, a mean of 1.0 to 1.5 teeth. The impact of this criteria change was greatest for the younger adult age groups, when the mean number of decayed and unsound teeth in the 16–24-year-old group doubled, from 0.8 without the visual dentin caries lesions to a mean of 1.6 when the new code was used (Kelly *et al.*, 2000).

Eurocaries: a comparison of international epidemiological methods made on the same subjects on the same day

The impacts described above were demonstrated within the same tightly organized surveys with examiners using exactly the same criteria and receiving the same training. The impact of subtle, as well as major, differences in caries diagnostic criteria is most marked when making comparisons across studies conducted by different teams with different training, even when they aim to follow a common diagnostic standard. This type of unintended variation can have dramatic and unintended impacts when data are used to make comparisons between countries, when politicians and policy makers attempt to look at regional variations within a country or region, or when researchers attempt a systematic review of published data.

The need for caution when comparing data collected with differing diagnostic criteria is illustrated by a study comparing the findings of nine trained and calibrated examiners (seven from Europe and two from the USA) using established methods from several European countries (all said to be equivalent to the WHO's 'Basic Methods') and two new clinical systems, one from the USA (Pitts, 2001). Each examiner was selected as a benchmark examiner responsible for training and/or calibrating examiners in their country or region. They clinically examined the same groups of 10 6-year-old and 10 12-year-old children in a school setting in rotation using their own methods and criteria. Even when standardizing all results for the D_3 diagnostic threshold, the range for mean D_3MFT estimates for the 12-year-old group was from 2.9 to 5.1. For the 6-year-old group the mean d_3mft ranged from 2.0 to 3.2.

Figure 9.5 shows the findings for the 12-year-old group expressed as 'total DMFT count' for the group of 12-year-old children seen by all examiners on the same day in the same school. Despite their best diligent and professional efforts, the nine 'gold-standard' examiners achieved poor agreement among themselves in estimating caries experience when using supposedly comparable criteria. The degree of variation in the caries into dentin values was unexpectedly high; all systems were expected by the examiners and proponents of the systems to give broadly similar estimates at the caries into dentin level. Those systems recording D_2 and D_1 caries also produced a wide range of estimates. The examiners could not even agree on the number of teeth that were filled. This study demonstrates that

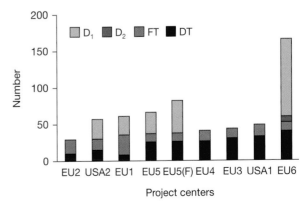

Figure 9.5 Illustration from the Eurocaries project of variation seen between experienced examiners using supposedly similar diagnostic criteria.

there is a need for improved harmonization in the details of diagnostic criteria, conventions and coding if comparability of results across regions and countries is to be achieved.

Caries extent in cohorts of Scottish preschool children

Figure 9.6 provides a graphic demonstration of the pattern of caries development in preschool children with and without information on carious lesions that are clinically confined to enamel. These data are derived from sequential assessments of caries extent made by a single examiner assessing a cohort of children born in Dundee, Scotland, at the ages of 1, 2, 3 and 4 years (Ballantyne, 2000). The children, 1419 at 1 year old, 1394 at 2 years old, 1219 at 3 years old and 1365 at 4 years old, were dentally examined in either nurseries or their homes using criteria that captured caries at both the enamel and dentin thresholds. The mean data for

the primary dentition for each year have been assembled into a tooth chart format in the figure.

The results highlight the different outputs that are possible according to the purpose required. If all that is needed is an indication at the age of 3 or 4 years about the restorative treatment need of the children, or an idea about which teeth will become involved, then recording at the caries into dentin level will be sufficient. However, consideration at the level of requiring a filling seems a totally outdated management concept. Caries is controllable before a filling is required. Thus, if the purpose of the study is to examine the pattern of caries attack in these children and to be able to plan or evaluate strategies to control the lesions in order to minimize subsequent restorative or extractive therapy, then including lesions at the enamel threshold is essential. With a trained examiner, collecting this information from preschool children proved to be entirely feasible. Using these criteria

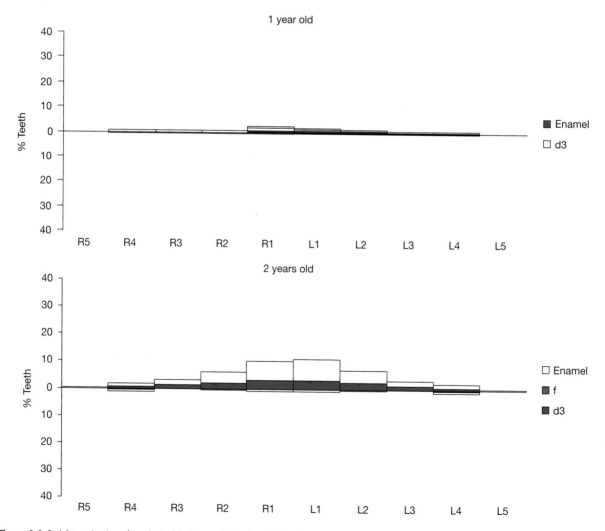

Figure 9.6 Serial examination of a cohort of 1–4-year-old Dundee children demonstrating how the pattern of caries development is seen very differently when including or excluding enamel lesions.

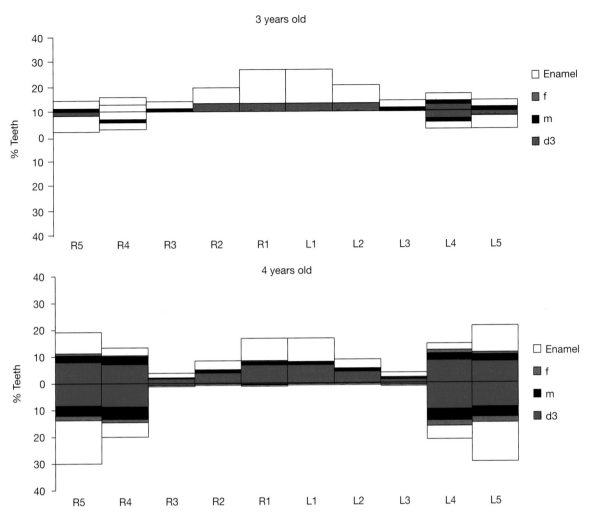

Figure 9.6 Continued.

also allows a much more valid assessment of the total burden of disease suffered by a typical child at a particular age, even though the data are derived by clinical examination alone and will be an underestimate (see Fig. 9.3b).

In looking at the impact of diagnostic criteria on caries extent it should be borne in mind that including diagnostic aids such as bitewing radiography or FOTI may affect the results. They would also be altered if it were decided to give means for only the individuals affected by caries, rather than the whole population. Even modest changes in the inclusion criteria and definitions of age may also have an impact. An example is seen when a change in schools available for access results in generating data for 11-year-old children, as opposed to 12-year-olds examined for many years previously (Pitts et al., 2006b).

Impact of diagnostic criteria on estimates of the severity of dental caries

Although severity may be assessed in terms of how many surfaces are typically involved and with what degree of

caries, there is an increasing emphasis now on the severity of caries attack, whether through an attack rate or assessment of caries activity status. This is a reflection of the importance of the severity of the caries challenge in determining outcomes for individuals, groups and populations.

One way in which diagnostic criteria can have an impact on estimates of severity is in the ability to distinguish more rapidly between groups with different caries rates. An illustration is in the ability of visual caries criteria to differentiate between groups using fluoride toothpastes. Differences between groups could be found in 12 months when enamel and dentin lesions were included, but a 24-month period was required with the more traditional caries into dentin criteria (Chesters et al., 2002).

Another way to judge the severity of caries is through measurement of caries activity. Nyvad and co-workers have, over recent years, described a visual system that uses the subjective judgment of the trained examiner to differentiate active white-spot lesions from inactive ones on the basis of surface roughness perceived by the examiner drawing a sharp probe (explorer) over the lesion surface (Nyvad et al.,

1998). Lesion status has been compared according to differences in subsequent lesion behavior in groups with different fluoride exposure (Nyvad *et al.*, 2003). This is a significant step forward in methodological development, although it has yet to be established whether the performance achieved by these workers with this system can be transferred readily to other examiners. However, this group has shown the method to be highly reproducible.

Ismail *et al.* (1992) also reported data on the validity of detecting non-cavitated caries lesions using broadly similar criteria in the early 1990s. More recently, the challenges in defining robust criteria for lesion activity that can be readily transferred to different examiners have been illustrated (Ekstrand *et al.*, 2005). This important area of caries activity assessment is a focus for further research and development to complement the more established criteria for visual lesion detection.

A framework for considering the choice of appropriate diagnostic criteria for epidemiological studies

This chapter has focussed on the diagnostic criteria used in epidemiology, rather than those used in clinical practice and research. The size of the (frequently unintended) impacts on estimates of caries prevalence, extent and severity associated with using even slightly different diagnostic criteria has prompted an international collaborative group to provide a framework for individuals and groups to choose diagnostic criteria appropriate to the task at hand from a range of standardized 'tools' that are supported by the best evidence available to date. The system, which has been developed since 2002, is known as ICDAS (the International Caries Detection and Assessment System). The system has been designed to meet the needs of epidemiology, clinical research and clinical practice (Pitts *et al.*, 2004b). The focus here is on epidemiology.

International Caries Detection and Assessment System framework

The concept of ICDAS is that its widespread adoption should lead to better quality information to inform decisions about appropriate diagnosis, prognosis and clinical management at both the individual and public health levels. Figure 9.7 shows, in the form of a graphic, the design objective within ICDAS to overcome the traditional barriers and to seek to achieve explicit linkages between the diagnostic criteria used in clinical practice, epidemiology, clinical research and dental education. The epidemiological objectives have been set out in some detail (Pitts, 2004b).

ICDAS is not a new system per se, but rather is an integrated system for caries detection and assessment building on the already demonstrated ability to achieve reliable (if not very sensitive) clinical–visual examination of lesions in both

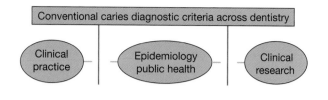

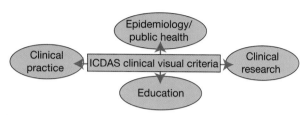

Figure 9.7 Overview of how the International Caries Detection and Assessment System (ICDAS) has been designed to allow intrinsic comparability of data derived from epidemiology, clinical practice, clinical research and educational settings.

enamel and dentin. The detection component of ICDAS is based on reviews of the evidence from previous research (Ismail, 2004) carried out since the publication of such criteria as those of Backer-Dirks from the 1950s (Backer-Dirks *et al.*, 1951). The format of the ICDAS criteria is based on a series of systems developed since the late 1980s (Pitts & Fyffe, 1988; Ismail *et al.*, 1992; Ekstrand *et al.*, 1997; Fyffe *et al.*, 2000).

The rationale, validity and reliability of the ICDAS system for detecting coronal lesions have been outlined with reference to the Detroit Cohort Study (Ismail *et al.*, 2007) and the full system has been used in a recent paper investigating diet related to caries in a low-income adult population (Burt *et al.*, 2006).

Summary

This chapter has discussed diagnostic criteria used in epidemiology, with particular reference to diagnostic thresholds and just how little or how much of the total caries experience of an individual or a population is captured by using different types of criteria. The impacts of using even slightly different diagnostic criteria on estimates of caries prevalence, extent and severity have been demonstrated with a series of examples.

References

Backer-Dirks O, van Amerongen J, Winkler KE. A reproducible method for caries evaluation. *J Dent Res* 1951; **30**: 346–59.

Ballantyne H. *Identification of infants at high risk to developing dental caries using microbiological and social factors.* PhD Thesis, University of Dundee, 2000.

Burt BA. How useful are cross-sectional data from surveys on dental caries? *Community Dent Oral Epidemiol* 1997; **25**: 36–41.

Burt BA, Kolker JL, Sandretto AM, Yuan Y, Sohn W, Ismail AI. Dietary patterns related to caries in a low-income adult population. *Caries Res* 2006; **40**: 473–80.

Chesters RK, Pitts NB, Matuliene G, *et al*. An abbreviated caries clinical trial design validated over 24 months. *J Dent Res* 2002; **81**: 637–40.

Deery CH. *An evaluation of the use of pit and fissure sealants in the General Dental Service in Scotland*. PhD Thesis, University of Dundee, 1997.

Deery CH, Care R, Chesters R, Huntington E, Stelmachonoka S, Gudkina Y. Prevalence of dental caries in Latvian 1- to 15-year-old children and the enhanced diagnostic yield of temporary tooth separation, FOTI and electronic caries measurement. *Caries Res* 2000; **34**: 2–7.

Ekstrand K, Qvist V, Thylstrup A. Light microscope study of the effect of probing in occlusal surfaces. *Caries Res* 1987; **21**: 368–74.

Ekstrand KR, Ricketts DN, Kidd EA. Reproducibility and accuracy of three methods for assessment of demineralization depth of the occlusal surface: an *in vitro* examination. *Caries Res* 1997; **31**: 224–31.

Ekstrand KE, Ricketts DN, Longbottom C, Pitts NB. Visual and tactile assessment of arrested initial enamel caries lesions: an *in vivo* examination. *Caries Res* 2005; **39**: 173–7.

Fejerskov O. Concepts of dental caries and their consequences for understanding the disease. *Community Dent Oral Epidemiol* 1997; **25**: 5–12.

Fejerskov O. Changing paradigms in concepts on dental caries: consequences for oral health care. *Caries Res* 2004; **38**: 182–91.

Fejerskov O, Luan WM, Nyvad B, Budtz Jorgensen E, Holm Pedersen P. Active and inactive root surface caries lesions in a selected group of 60- to 80-year-old Danes. *Caries Res* 1991; **25**: 385–91.

Fejerskov O, Baelum V, Ostergaard ES. Root caries in Scandinavia in the 1980s and future trends to be expected in dental caries experience in adults. *Adv Dent Res* 1993; **7**: 4–14.

Forgie A. *Eyesight and magnification in dentistry*. PhD Thesis, University of Dundee, 1999.

Forgie AH, Paterson M, Pine CM, Pitts NB, Nugent ZJ. A randomised controlled trial of the caries preventive efficacy of a chlorhexidine containing varnish in high caries risk adolescents. *Caries Res* 2000; **34**: 432–9.

Fyffe HE, Deery CH, Nugent, ZJ, Nuttall NM, Pitts NB. *In vitro* validity of the Dundee Selectable Threshold Method for caries diagnosis (DSTM). *Community Dent Oral Epidemiol* 2000; **28**: 52–8.

Glass RL, Alman JE, Chauncey HH. A 10-year longitudinal study of caries incidence rates in a sample of male adults in the USA. *Caries Res* 1987; **21**: 360–7.

Ismail AI. Clinical diagnosis of precavitated carious lesions. *Community Dent Oral Epidemiol* 1997; **25**: 13–23.

Ismail A. Visual and visuo-tactile methods of caries detection. *J Dent Res* 2004; **83** (Special Issue C): 56–66.

Ismail AI, Brodeur J-M, Gagnon P, *et al*. Prevalence of non-cavitated and cavitated carious lesions in a random sample of 7–9-year-old schoolchildren in Montreal, Quebec. *Community Dent Oral Epidemiol* 1992; **20**: 250–5.

Ismail AI, Sohn W, Tellez M, *et al*. Rationale, validity and reliability of the coronal caries detection criteria of the International Caries Detection and Assessment System (ICDAS). Development and Experiences from the Detroit Cohort Study. *Community Dent Oral Epidemiol* 2007; **35**: 170–8.

Kelly M, Steele J, Nuttall NM, *et al*. In: Walker A, Cooper I, eds. *Adult Dental Health Survey – oral health in the United Kingdom 1998*. London: Stationery Office, 2000.

Kidd EAM. A critical evaluation of caries diagnostic methods and epidemiological methods. Can we trust the available data? In: Johnson NW, ed. *Risk markers for oral diseases*, Vol. 1, *Dental caries markers of high and low risk groups and individuals*. Cambridge: Cambridge University Press, 1991: 15–32.

Klein H, Palmer CE, Knutson JW. Studies on dental caries. I. Dental status and dental needs of elementary school children. *Public Health Rep* 1938; **53**: 751–65.

Luan W-M, Baelum V, Fejerskov O, Chen X. Ten-year incidence of dental caries in adult and elderly Chinese. *Caries Res* 2000; **34**: 205–13.

Manji F, Baelum V, Fejerskov O. Tooth mortality in an adult rural population in Kenya. *J Dent Res* 1988; **67**: 496–500.

Manji F, Fejerskov O, Baelum V, Luan W-M, Chen X. The epidemiological features of dental caries in African and Chinese populations: implications for risk assessment. In: Johnson NW, ed. *Risk markers for oral diseases*, Vol. 1, *Dental caries markers of high and low risk groups and individuals*. Cambridge: Cambridge University Press, 1991: 62–100.

Marthaler TM. The caries-inhibiting effect of amine fluoride dentifrices in children during three years of unsupervised use. *Br Dent J* 1965; **119**: 153–63.

Moller IJ. Clinical criteria for the diagnosis of the incipient carious lesion. *Adv Fluor Res Dent Caries Prevent* 1966; **4**: 67–72.

Nuttall NM. Capability of a national epidemiological survey to predict general dental service treatment. *Community Dent Oral Epidemiol* 1983; **11**: 296–301.

Nyvad B, Fejerskov O. Active root surface caries converted into inactive caries as a response to oral hygiene. *Scand J Dent Res* 1986; **94**: 281–4.

Nyvad B, Fejerskov O. Assessing the stage of caries lesion activity on the basis of clinical and microbiological examination. *Community Dent Oral Epidemiol* 1997; **25**: 69–75.

Nyvad B, Machiulskiene V, Baelum V. Reliability of a new caries diagnostic system differentiating between active and inactive caries lesions. *Caries Res* 1998; **33**: 252–60.

Nyvad B, Machiulskiene V, Baelum V. Construct and predictive validity of clinical caries diagnostic criteria assessing lesion activity. *J Dent Res* 2003; **82**: 117–22.

Pitts NB. Safeguarding the quality of epidemiological caries data at a time of changing disease patterns and evolving dental services. *Community Dent Health* 1992; **10**: 1–9.

Pitts NB. Diagnostic tools and measurements – impact on appropriate care. *Community Dent Oral Epidemiol* 1997; **25**: 24–35.

Pitts NB. Clinical diagnosis of dental caries: a European perspective. *J Dent Educ* 2001; **65**: 973–80.

Pitts NB. Are we ready to move from operative to non-operative/preventive treatment of dental caries in clinical practice? *Caries Res* 2004a; **38**: 294–304.

Pitts NB. 'ICDAS' – an international system for caries detection and assessment being developed to facilitate caries epidemiology, research and appropriate clinical management. *Community Dent Health* 2004b; **21**: 193–8.

Pitts NB, Fyffe HE. The effect of varying diagnostic thresholds upon clinical caries data for a low prevalence group. *J Dent Res* 1988; **67**: 592–6.

Pitts NB, Harker R. Obvious decay experience. Children's dental health in the United Kingdom 2003. Office for National Statistics, October 2004. http://www.statistics.gov.uk/children/dental/health.

Pitts NB, Longbottom C. Preventive care advised (PCA)/operative care advised (OCA) – categorising caries by the management option. *Community Dent Oral Epidemiol* 1995; **23**: 55–9.

Pitts NB, Stamm J. International Consensus Workshop on Caries Clinical Trials (ICW-CCT) – final consensus statements: agreeing where the evidence leads. *J Dent Res* 2004; **83** (Special Issue C): 125–8.

Pitts NB, Chestnutt IG, Evans D, White D, Chadwick B, Steele JG. The dentinal caries experience of children in the United Kingdom, 2003. *Br Dent J* 2006a; **200**: 313–20.

Pitts NB, Boyles J, Nugent ZJ, Thomas N, Pine CM. BASCD survey report: the dental caries experience of 11 year old children in Great Britain 2004/2005. Surveys co-ordinated by the British Association for the Study of Community Dentistry. *Community Dent Health* 2006b; **23**: 44–57.

Radike AW. Criteria for diagnosing dental caries. In: American Dental Association. *Proceedings of the Conference on the Clinical Testings of Cariostatic Agents*. Chicago, IL: American Dental Association, 1968: 87–8.

Selwitz RH, Ismail AI, Pitts NB. Dental caries. *Lancet* 2007; **369**: 51–9.

World Health Organization. *A Guide to Oral Health Epidemiological Investigations*. Geneva: WHO, 1979.

Part III
Dental caries in a biological context

10

The oral microflora and biofilms on teeth

P.D. Marsh and B. Nyvad

these organisms (often 20–30 distinct types) being able to predominate at an individual site (Aas *et al.*, 2005).

Ecological factors affecting the growth and metabolism of oral bacteria

The mouth provides both a friendly and a hostile environment for microbial growth. Resident oral microorganisms are adapted to use endogenous (host-derived) nutrients for growth (e.g. salivary proteins and glycoproteins), but superimposed on this can be sudden and irregular intakes of dietary carbohydrates in excess (e.g. readily fermentable sugars such as glucose, fructose and sucrose). The mouth is overtly aerobic, and yet obligate anaerobes and facultatively anaerobic bacteria are able to persist within biofilms on oral surfaces (tongue, teeth) and comprise the most numerous group of bacteria at these sites. Organisms have to attach firmly to a surface to avoid being washed away by the flow of saliva and swallowed. Thus, the majority of organisms (and the most disease) are found at protected and stagnant sites around the dentition (Figs 10.1, 10.2).

Saliva plays other roles in regulating the growth and metabolic activity of the oral microflora. Saliva helps to maintain the pH in the oral cavity at values around 6.75–7.25 and the temperature at around 35–36°C, which is optimal for the growth of many organisms. Saliva contains glycoproteins and proteins that act as the primary source of carbohydrates, peptides and amino acids for microbial growth. Bacteria co-operate to degrade the oligosaccharide side-chains of glycoproteins such as mucins. Acid is produced relatively slowly from the metabolism of these compounds, and so there is little risk of enamel demineralization. Importantly, saliva is a sufficient source of nutrients to sustain the growth of a natural and diverse oral microflora in the absence of other nutrients. Lastly, saliva delivers a spectrum of innate and specific immune host defense factors which are essential to the maintenance of a healthy mouth (Marsh, 2000b; see Chapter 11).

A carbohydrate-rich diet increases the acid production (Fig. 10.3) and growth rate of many oral bacteria. Thus, it has been shown that the accumulation of dental plaque after 4 days, as regards extension, weight and actual numbers of bacteria, is higher when individuals consume a diet supplemented with sucrose candies compared with a control diet

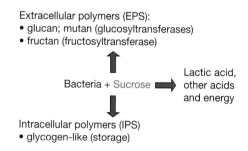

Figure 10.3 The metabolism of sucrose by oral bacteria.

without added sucrose (Rateitschak-Plüss & Guggenheim, 1982). What may be clinically more important, however, is that a sucrose-rich diet could change the composition of the microflora by generating a low pH capable of inhibiting the growth of many of the bacteria found naturally in dental plaque, thereby selecting for the more aciduric (acid-loving) species (see later for details). In addition, sucrose can be converted by bacterial enzymes, glucosyltransferases (GTF) and fructosyltransferases (FTF), into glucans and fructans. Glucans can consolidate bacterial attachment and contribute to the biofilm matrix, while fructans are highly labile (i.e. easily metabolized) and can act as extracellular nutrient storage compounds (Fig. 10.3). Excess dietary carbohydrate is stored by some species as intracellular glycogen-like storage compounds, which can be metabolized to acid at a later time in the absence of fermentable exogenous substrates. All of these factors can contribute towards increasing the likelihood of developing caries.

Dental biofilms: development, structure, composition and properties

In order to persist, oral micro-organisms have to attach to a surface and grow; otherwise they will be lost from the habitat. An important relatively recent discovery is that the properties of microbial cells forming a biofilm (a community of microorganisms growing on a surface) are distinct from those expressed when microorganisms are growing as individual cells in a liquid culture (Costerton *et al.*, 1995; Marsh, 2004, 2005). This has led to a novel interest in trying to understand the dental biofilm mode of growth. This chapter describes how such biofilms develop on teeth, what are their composition and properties, and what is the significance of the biofilm lifestyle to oral microorganisms. Throughout the chapter the term 'biofilm' has been used to signify the common features among biofilms forming on teeth and biofilms forming in other natural environments. However, in the dental literature the terms dental plaque and dental biofilm are often used interchangeably. Note that dental plaque is a biofilm, but not all biofilms are dental plaque.

Development of dental biofilms

The development of dental biofilms can be divided into several arbitrary stages, as revealed by experimental studies *in situ* (Nyvad, 1993):

1. pellicle formation
2. attachment of single bacterial cells (0–24 h)
3. growth of attached bacteria leading to the formation of distinct microcolonies (4–24 h)
4. microbial succession (and coadhesion) leading to increased species diversity concomitant with continued growth of microcolonies (1–7 days)
5. climax community/mature biofilm (1 week or older).

It should be appreciated that biofilm formation is a highly dynamic process, and that attachment, growth, removal and reattachment of bacteria may occur at the same time (Marsh, 2004).

Pellicle formation

Microorganisms do not colonize directly on the mineralized tooth surface. The teeth are always covered by an acellular proteinaceous film; this is the pellicle that forms on the 'naked' tooth surface within minutes to hours. In uncolonized areas the pellicle reaches a thickness of 0.01–1 μm within 24 h. The major constituents of the pellicle are salivary glycoproteins, phosphoproteins, lipids and, to a lesser extent, components from the GCF (Levine et al., 1985) (see Chapter 11). Remnants of cell walls from dead bacteria, and other microbial products (e.g. glucosyltransferases and glucans), have also been identified in the pellicle. Some salivary molecules undergo conformational changes when they bind to the tooth surface; this can lead to exposure of new receptors for bacterial attachment (cryptitopes; see later).

The pellicle plays an important modifying role in caries and erosion because of its permeable-selective nature restricting transport of ions in and out of the dental hard tissues. The presence of a pellicle inhibits subsurface demineralization of enamel *in vitro* (Zahradnik et al., 1976). Frequent mouth rinses with milk or cream increase the thickness and electron density of the pellicle (Nyvad & Fejerskov, 1984), but it is not clear whether such modification of the pellicle provides additional protection against demineralization of the enamel.

The composition of the pellicle has received considerable interest because of its potential role in determining the composition of the initial microflora. It has been speculated that the surface characteristics of different dental hard tissues and dental materials may influence the profile of amino acids in the pellicle and thereby modify the number of potential adsorption sites for different bacterial species (Sönju & Glantz, 1975; Öste et al., 1981). However, so far there is little evidence that variations in the amino acids in the pellicle between different supporting materials can markedly influence the pattern of microbial colonization *in vivo*.

Microbial colonization

Microbial colonization of teeth requires that bacteria adhere to the surface. The mechanisms involved in adherence are complex and are still being investigated. As the microbial cell approaches the pellicle-coated surface, long-range but relatively weak physicochemical forces between the two surfaces are generated. Initially, bacteria are non-specifically associated with the tooth surface under the net influence of van der Waal's attractive forces as well as repulsive electrostatic forces. Within a short time, these weak physicochemical interactions may become stronger owing to adhesins on the microbial cell surface becoming involved in specific, short-range interactions with complementary receptors in the acquired pellicle. A high degree of surface hydrophobicity may facilitate attachment.

Initial microbial colonization

Irrespective of the type of tooth surface (enamel or root), the initial colonizers constitute a highly selected part of the oral microflora, mainly *S. sanguinis*, *S. oralis* and *S. mitis* biovar 1 (Fig. 10.4) (Nyvad & Kilian, 1990a). Together, these three streptococcal species account for 95% of the streptococci and 56% of the total initial microflora. In addition, the initial microflora comprises *Actinomyces* spp. and Gram-negative bacteria, e.g. *Haemophilus* spp. and *Neisseria* spp.

The selective manner by which bacteria attach to the tooth surface supports the fact that bacteria contain a recognition system on their surfaces that enables bacterial surface adhesins to bind to complementary molecules (receptors) in the pellicle (Gibbons, 1989) (Fig. 10.5). Some receptors have been identified as oligosaccharides on the protein backbone of the pellicle glycoproteins. For example, *S. sanguinis* and *S. oralis* bind specifically to terminal sialic acid residues in human salivary glycoproteins. In addition, *S. oralis* has a galactose-binding adhesin. *Actinomyces naeslundii* possesses surface appendages termed fimbriae; type 1 fimbriae mediate adherence to proteins such as proline-rich protein and statherin in the pellicle (i.e. protein–protein interactions), whereas type 2 fimbriae are involved in cell adherence to

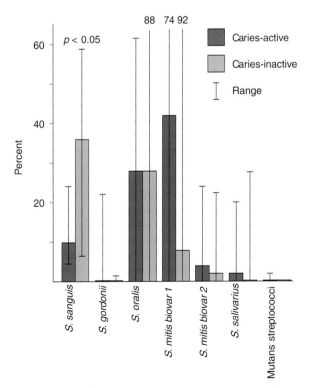

Figure 10.4 Proportions of various streptococci (%) from 4 h dental plaque in caries-active and caries-inactive individuals (Nyvad & Kilian, 1990a).

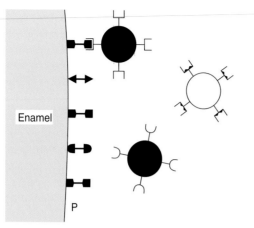

Figure 10.5 Simplified explanation of the principle of selective adherence of bacteria to enamel. Successful attachment is achieved when the surface characteristics of a bacterium fit with a receptor in the pellicle (P).

already attached bacteria (a process termed coaggregation or coadhesion; see later) by lectin-like interactions (i.e. carbohydrate–protein interactions). However, *Actinomyces* species can also bind to galactosyl residues in glycoproteins exposed as a result of enzymic action of bacterial neuraminidases. The modification of pellicle constituents, either enzymically (e.g. by neuraminidase) to expose new receptors, or by conformation changes following adsorption to a surface to reveal previously hidden receptors (termed cryptitopes; Gibbons *et al.*, 1990), is probably an important factor in the regulation of colonization. Knowledge of the biochemical mechanisms involved in attachment could potentially be exploited to develop biofilms with reduced acidogenic properties, for example, by using molecules to saturate receptors used by aciduric bacteria, thereby blocking their adhesion. However, this preventive approach has not yet been tested clinically.

For many years it was believed that mutans streptococci constituted a significant part of the initial microflora because of their ability to elaborate sticky extracellular polysaccharides from sucrose *in vitro*. However, clinical studies have shown that mutans streptococci comprise only 2% or less of the initial streptococcal microflora, irrespective of an individual's exposure to sucrose (Nyvad & Kilian, 1987) and irrespective of *Streptococcus sobrinus* possessing an adhesin that binds to glucan (Gibbons *et al.*, 1986). Apparently, glucan production from sucrose does not promote *de novo* colonization of tooth surfaces by mutans streptococci. Rather, the low recovery of mutans streptococci in initial dental biofilm *in vivo* is likely to reflect the relatively low concentration of these species in saliva. A positive correlation has been demonstrated between the concentration of specific microorganisms available in saliva for adsorption and the actual number of adsorbed microbial cells. *Streptococcus mutans* is much less efficient than *S. sanguinis* in adhering to the tooth surface. Approximately 10^4–10^5 cells of *S. mutans*

per milliliter of saliva must be present before one cell can be recovered from a cleaned tooth surface, while the equivalent concentration for *S. sanguinis* is about 10^3 cells/ml (van Houte & Green, 1974).

Microbial succession

As the microbiota ages the most striking change is a shift from a *Streptococcus*-dominated plaque to a plaque dominated by *Actinomyces* (Syed & Loesche, 1978). Thus, the initial establishment of a streptococcal flora appears to be a necessary antecedent for the subsequent proliferation of other organisms. Such population shifts are known as microbial succession.

The principle of microbial succession is, briefly, that pioneer bacteria create an environment that is either more attractive to secondary invaders or increasingly unfavorable to themselves because of a lack of nutrients, accumulation of inhibitory metabolic products, and/or increase in anaerobiosis, etc. In this way the resident microbial community is gradually replaced by other species more suited to the modified habitat. The secondary colonizers also attach to the established pioneer species via adhesin–receptor interactions (termed coaggregation or coadhesion) (Kolenbrander *et al.*, 2000). As dental biofilms develop, some of the bacteria produce polysaccharides, especially from the metabolism of sucrose (Fig. 10.3), and these contribute to the biofilm matrix. The biofilm matrix is not just a physical scaffold that helps to support the structure of the biofilm; the matrix is also biologically active and is involved in retaining nutrients, water (thereby preventing desiccation) and key enzymes within the biofilm (Branda *et al.*, 2005). As the composition of the developing biofilm becomes more diverse, the bacteria can interact both in a conventional biochemical manner and via specific signaling molecules. These will be described in more detail in a later section.

As the bacterial deposits become thicker, a lowering of the oxygen concentration (increased anaerobiosis) is one of the factors that help to drive microbial succession. Thus, in developing coronal plaque, a progressive shift is observed from mainly aerobic and facultatively anaerobic species in the early stages to a situation in which facultatively and obligately anaerobic organisms predominate after 9 days (Fig. 10.6) (Ritz, 1967).

Microbial composition of the climax community (mature biofilm)

Environmental conditions on a tooth are not uniform. Differences exist in the degree of protection from oral removal forces and in the gradients of many biological and chemical factors that influence the growth of the resident oral microflora on particular surfaces. These differences will be reflected in the composition of dental biofilms, particularly at sites so obviously distinct as approximal surfaces, occlusal fissures and gingival crevices. The predominant organisms are spatially organized into a three-dimensional structure enclosed in a matrix of extracellular material derived from both the cells and the environment. The following section describes the structural features of initial and mature biofilms that have developed on natural tooth surfaces in the oral cavity.

Pattern of initial colonization

Four hours after a tooth surface has been exposed to the oral environment following professional tooth cleaning surprisingly few bacteria are found. The enamel is covered by a granular deposit reflecting the pellicle, which is unevenly distributed over the surface (Figs 10.9, 10.10). The pellicle is

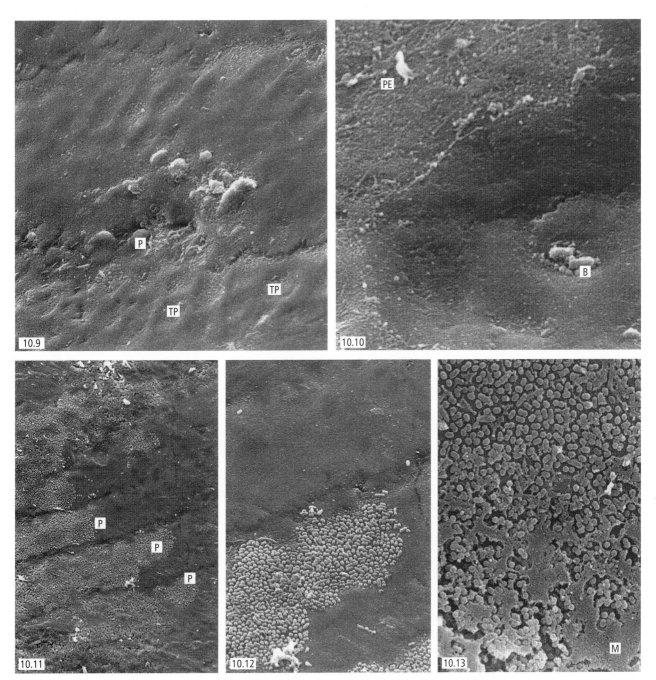

Figures 10.9–10.13 Scanning electron micrographs demonstrating sequential stages in microbial colonization of human enamel during the initial 12 h after cleaning (Nyvad & Fejerskov, 1987). Figure 10.9: After 4 h exposure, the enamel is covered by pellicle which is a granular deposit, primarily located in Tomes' processes pits (TP) and in perikymatal grooves (P). Figure 10.10: The first bacteria to colonize the tooth surface are of the coccobacillary type (B). Note that the granular deposit does not cover the tooth surface in a uniform layer (PE). Figures 10.11, 10.12: In 12-h-old bacterial deposits (biofilms) the microorganisms spread in a monolayer along the perikymata (P). Figure 10.13: The monolayer of bacteria (upper part), is gradually replaced by a multilayer of cells (lower part), which is embedded in an intermicrobial matrix (M).

primarily located corresponding to depressions in the enamel (pits and perikymatal grooves), but it does not completely mask the anatomical characteristics of the enamel surface. Whenever bacteria are encountered at this early stage they are of the coccoid or coccobacillary type, and always reside in shallow depressions on the surface (Fig. 10.10).

A certain lag-phase exists before colonization by bacteria proceeds. After 8 h only a few small groups of microorganisms are found on the surface, sheltered by the perikymata. Numerous bacteria, many of which occur in a stage of division, spread across the surface as a monolayer (Figs 10.11, 10.12). A rapid increase in the number of bacteria is only observed after 8–12 h. In some areas multiplying microorganisms form multilayers (Fig. 10.13) in which the individual organisms are embedded in an intermicrobial matrix. Within 1 day the tooth surface is almost completely covered by a blanket of microorganisms. However, the microbial deposits are not uniform in thickness. Areas of monolayers are intermingled with multilayers, and some uncolonized areas are still covered by a thick, bacteria-free pellicle. At this early stage of colonization, Gram-positive and Gram-negative bacteria are not organized according to any particular pattern.

After 1 day the surface of the microbiota is mainly made up of coccoid bacteria with scattered filaments (Fig. 10.14). However, during the course of the second day the biofilm becomes colonized by multiple filamentous organisms with a perpendicular orientation to the surface (Fig. 10.15).

Colonization of root surfaces occurs in principle as outlined for enamel surfaces, but growth of the microbiota proceeds more rapidly on root surfaces because of the irregular surface topography. After 2 days the thickness of the microbial deposits varies distinctly across enamel surfaces, probably reflecting the undulating pattern of the perichymata, whereas on root surfaces the biofilm exhibits a more homogeneous thickness (Figs 10.16, 10.17).

Mature biofilms

Detailed information about morphological changes of the microbiota over the first few weeks of plaque formation is not available. It is believed that during the initial days, biofilm growth occurs predominantly as a result of cell division, as evidenced by the development of columnar microcolonies perpendicular to the tooth surface. However, continuous adsorption of single microorganisms from saliva also contributes to the expansion of the bacterial deposit. In the surface layer some microorganisms coaggregate with other species to form 'corn-cob' structures (Fig. 10.18). The 'corn cobs' are composed of a central filament coated with spherical organisms, and appear to have a direct interspecies relationship mediated by surface fibrils (Fig. 10.19).

As the biofilm becomes older (2 weeks or older), characteristic structural changes are noted deep to the surface. The most striking change is the formation of an inner layer of densely packed Gram-positive pleomorphic bacteria next to the tooth surface (Fig. 10.20). These bacteria,

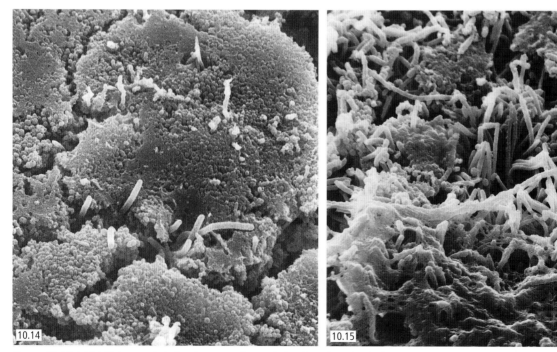

Figures 10.14, 10.15 Distinct morphological changes may be recorded on the surface of the biofilms when comparing the microflora on teeth after 24 h (Fig. 10.14) and 48 h (Fig. 10.15). Whereas the 24-h-old biofilm comprises a mass of coccoid bacteria from which a few filaments extend, the 48-h-old microflora is almost entirely dominated by filamentous organisms (Nyvad & Fejerskov, 1987).

which show ultrastructural characteristics in common with *Actinomyces* species, are found in association with both enamel and root surfaces. The outer part of mature biofilms is usually more loosely structured and varies in composition (Figs 10.21–10.23) (Nyvad & Fejerskov, 1989). In some individuals the outer microbiota may be organized in spheres of one particular type of organism (Fig. 10.21), whereas in others, layers of different bacterial species are

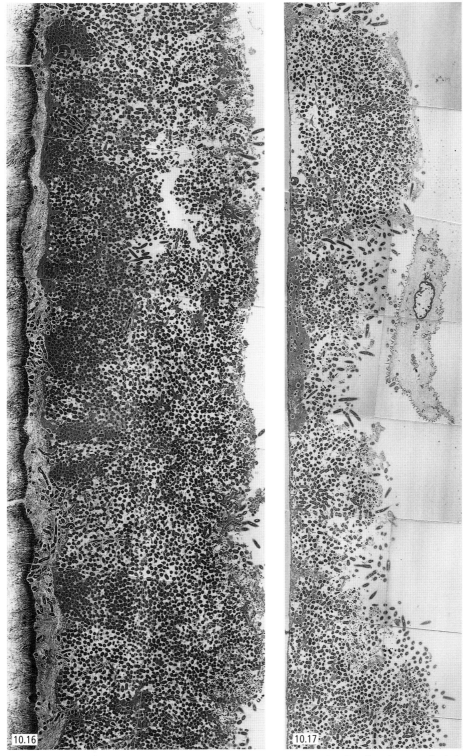

Figures 10.16, 10.17 Forty-eight-hour-old biofilms on root cementum (Fig. 10.16) and enamel (Fig. 10.17) surfaces from the same individual. Note that the microbial biofilms are thicker and more densely packed on root cementum (Nyvad, 1983).

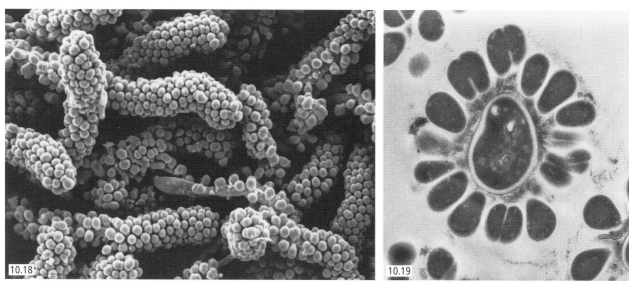

Figures 10.18, 10.19 Some bacteria in the surface of plaque biofilms coaggregate to form 'corn-cob' structures (Fig. 10.18). Individual 'corn cobs' are composed of a central filament covered by spherical microorganisms (Fig. 10.19, cross-section) (Nyvad & Fejerskov, 1994).

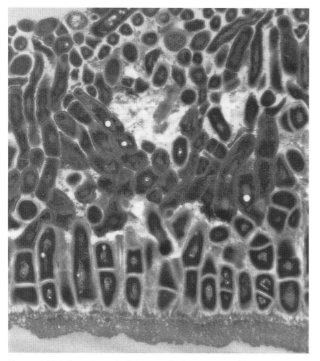

Figure 10.20 Densely packed pleomorphic bacteria resembling *Actinomyces* form palisades along the tooth surface in 3-week-old dental biofilms (Nyvad & Fejerskov, 1989).

organized roughly parallel to the tooth surface (Fig. 10.23). In some cases the outer microbiota is loosely structured and does not show any characteristic pattern (Fig. 10.22). Irrespective of the dominating pattern of colonization, the bacteria are embedded in an intermicrobial matrix of highly varying amount and electron density. This heterogeneous composition, combined with the observation that young dental biofilms contain fluid-filled channels and

voids (Wood *et al.*, 2000), is believed to create concentration gradients and influence the diffusion properties of biofilms. For example, it has been shown that short-term exposures to fluoride solutions (1000 ppm F⁻) for 30 or 120 s (equivalent to tooth brushing) result in restricted penetration of fluoride into 7-day-old dental biofilms (Watson *et al.*, 2005). Thus, the caries-controlling effect of fluoride delivery from tooth brushing may be reduced where oral hygiene is poor.

Along with these observations, it is interesting that dental biofilms must be up to 2 days old before the acid formation in response to a sucrose challenge is sufficient to cause demineralization of the enamel (Fig. 10.24) (Imfeld & Lutz, 1980). This does not mean, however, that people should refrain from cleaning their teeth every day. Most individuals are not able to clean their teeth perfectly every time they brush, and bacteria left on the teeth at inaccessible sites may contribute to continued plaque growth and acid production when tooth brushing is insufficient to remove dental plaque.

Properties of dental biofilms

As stated earlier, the microbial deposits on teeth are an example of a biofilm the physiological and genetic properties of which will differ substantially from those of planktonic cells (i.e. the same organisms growing in liquid culture). Novel imaging and molecular techniques have confirmed that dental biofilms display properties that are consistent with those of biofilms present in other natural habitats (Table 10.2). Thus, the free movement of molecules can be reduced in oral biofilms which, coupled with bacterial metabolism, leads to gradients in key factors (oxygen, nutrients, pH, etc.) over short distances throughout the depth of the biofilm. The use of live/dead stains has shown

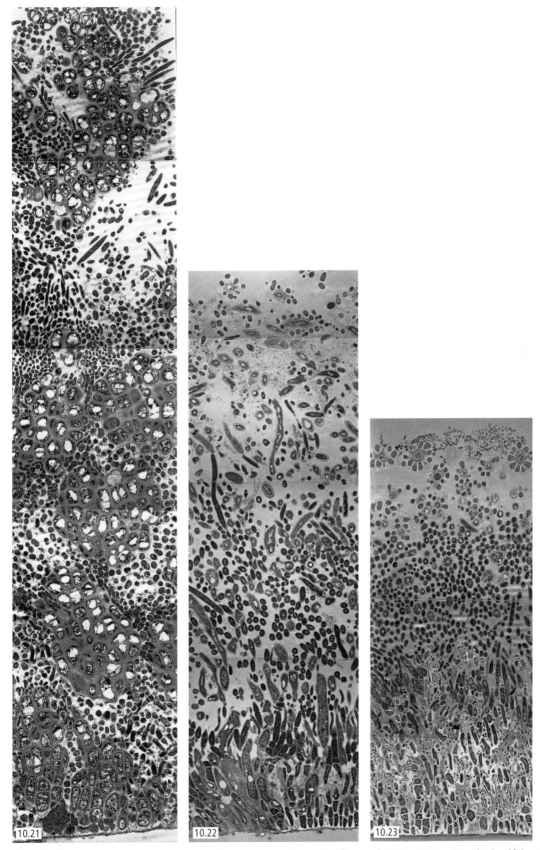

Figures 10.21–10.23 Ultrastructure of 2-week-old dental biofilms from three individuals with different colonization patterns. Note that in addition to differences in thickness, the outer part of the biofilms varies in composition and structure (Nyvad & Fejerskov, 1989).

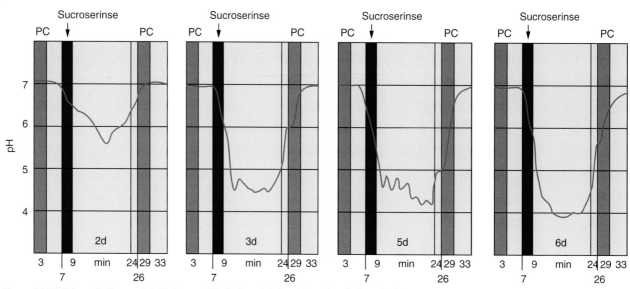

Figure 10.24 Telemetrically recorded pH changes of 2-, 3-, 5- and 6-day-old interdental plaque biofilms in a 62-year-old male volunteer during and after 2 min rinses with 10% sucrose rinse. PC: paraffin chewing. Note that the rate and amount of acid formation increase with the age of the biofilm. (Adapted from Imfeld & Lutz, 1980.)

that bacterial vitality varies, with the greatest concentration of viable microorganisms present in the central parts of the biofilm, and lining any voids or channels. Culture-independent approaches (e.g. 16S rRNA gene amplification, fluorescent *in situ* hybridization) have also demonstrated an increased richness in bacterial diversity in dental biofilms, with many novel and currently unculturable bacteria being described for the first time (for examples, see Paster *et al.*, 2001; Brinig *et al.*, 2003).

There are direct- and indirect-mediated changes in bacterial gene expression during biofilm development. For example, the binding of oral bacteria to salivary proteins can induce genes encoding adhesins. During the initial stages of *in vitro* biofilm formation by *S. mutans* (first 2 h after attachment), 33 proteins were differentially expressed (25 proteins up-regulated; eight proteins down-regulated; i.e. this is a direct effect following attachment to a surface), and there was an increase in the relative synthesis of enzymes involved in carbohydrate catabolism (Welin *et al.*, 2004). In contrast, some glycolytic enzymes were down-regulated in older (3 day) *S. mutans* biofilms, while proteins associated with other biochemical functions were up-regulated

Table 10.2 Properties of biofilms and microbial communities.

General property	Dental biofilm example
Open architecture	Presence of channels in dental plaque
Protection from host defenses, desiccation, etc.	Production of extracellular polymers to form a functional matrix; physical protection from phagocytosis
Enhanced tolerance to antimicrobials	Reduced sensitivity to chlorhexidine and antibiotics; transfer of resistance genes; microbial community effects provide mutual protection (see below)
Neutralization of inhibitors	Catalase production by neighboring cells to protect sensitive organisms from hydrogen peroxide
Novel gene expression[a]	Synthesis of novel proteins upon attachment; up-regulation of glucosyltransferases in mature plaque
Cell–cell signaling	Production of bacterial cell–cell signaling molecules (e.g. CSP) to co-ordinate gene expression
Spatial and environmental heterogeneity	pH and O_2 gradients; coadhesion between distinct bacterial species
Broader habitat range	Oral obligate anaerobes grow in an overtly aerobic environment; acid-sensitive species survive
More efficient metabolism	Complete catabolism of complex host macromolecules (e.g. mucins) by consortia; development of microbial food webs
Enhanced virulence	Pathogenic synergism in abscesses

[a] A consequence of altered gene expression can also be an increased tolerance to antimicrobial agents.
CSP: competence stimulating peptide.

(Svensater *et al.*, 2001). Expression of glucosyltransferases by *S. mutans* was markedly up-regulated in older biofilms, but this was assumed to be due to indirect effects of biofilm formation (e.g. nutrient limitation, reduced pH) (Li & Burne, 2001). As biofilms develop, there are increasing opportunities for cells to interact both with each other via cell signaling systems, and with other species in a range of conventional synergistic and antagonistic biochemical interactions (some of which will be discussed in more detail in the next section; see Table 10.3).

It is clear from the above statements that the behavior of microorganisms on a surface as part of a biofilm can be very different to that observed in the laboratory in conventional homogeneous liquid culture growth systems (planktonic culture). Of particular clinical relevance is the finding that the sensitivity of oral bacteria to antimicrobials is reduced during growth on a surface, particularly in mature biofilms. Thus, four times the concentration of chlorhexidine was necessary to kill older compared with younger biofilms of *S. sanguinis*. Similarly, biofilms of diverse mixed cultures of oral bacteria were unaffected by concentrations of chlorhexidine that were equivalent to the minimum inhibitory concentration (MIC) of the component species (as determined in liquid culture). Ten-fold higher concentrations were needed to demonstrate some effectiveness, but even at these elevated levels some species were unaffected (Kinniment *et al.*, 1996). Similar findings have been reported with other antimicrobial agents used in toothpastes and mouthrinses, while up to 500 times the MIC of amoxicillin and doxycycline (as determined for liquid cultures) was required to eliminate *S. sanguinis* biofilms (Larsen & Fiehn, 1996). Studies of natural plaque biofilms showed that chlorhexidine only affected the outer layers of cells in 24 and 48 h biofilms, suggesting either quenching of the agent at the biofilm surface or a lack of penetration (Zaura-Arite *et al.*, 2001). Such observations may partly explain why antimicrobial treatment has so far not been a totally successful approach to the control of dental caries (Chapter 16).

Significance of the biofilm lifestyle

Dental plaque is an example of a biofilm which functions as a microbial community, i.e. as a consortium of interacting microorganisms (Marsh & Bradshaw, 1999; Marsh, 2005). The significance of this is that the properties of a microbial community are more than the sum of those of the constituent species (Table 10.2). In a complex biofilm such as dental plaque, populations of bacteria are in close proximity to one another and interact as a consequence. These interactions can be beneficial to one or more of the interacting species, while others can be antagonistic (Table 10.3). As stated earlier, the production of antagonistic compounds is a mechanism by which exogenous microbial species can be excluded from the mouth (colonization resistance). In addition, the production of inhibitors can provide an organism with a competitive advantage when interacting with other community members. Although competition for nutrients will be a highly significant factor in determining the prevalence of a species within a habitat such as the mouth, it has been proven that bacteria also have to collaborate to catabolize completely host-derived, biochemically complex nutrients such as salivary mucins. The concerted and sequential actions of individual species with complementary patterns of glycosidase and protease activity are required to metabolize fully such glycoproteins. Likewise, a primary feeder (an organism that initially metabolizes a substrate) generates products that can be metabolized to even simpler products by secondary feeders (organisms that utilize the products generated by the metabolism of primary feeders), thereby generating food chains (Carlsson, 2000). A classic example is the utilization by *Veillonella* spp. of lactate produced from the metabolism of sugars by saccharolytic bacteria. Such metabolic interdependencies make a major contribution to the maintenance of microbial homeostasis in dental plaque.

Some dental biofilm bacteria can secrete small, diffusible signaling molecules that enable them to co-ordinate their activities. Gram-positive bacteria use small peptides, and *S. mutans* synthesizes a competence stimulating peptide (CSP). This peptide is believed to enhance acid tolerance and induce genetic competence in neighboring cells of *S. mutans*, so that the ability to take up DNA (transformation) was greater for biofilm-grown cells. Thus, bacteria may be able to transfer genetic material more readily in biofilms, including virulence or antibiotic resistance traits. Different communication systems operate among Gram-negative bacteria (e.g. auto-inducer-2, AI-2), and these may operate among many genera of bacteria to co-ordinate gene expression, emphasizing the need to view plaque as a consortium of microorganisms working in a partnership. Biofilms also facilitate communication via horizontal gene transfer (Marsh, 2005). Evidence of horizontal gene transfer between resident oral bacteria (*S. mitis*, *S. oralis*) and opportunistic pathogens (*S. pneumoniae*) has come from the identification of penicillin resistance genes with a common mosaic structure, emphasizing the need for care when prescribing antibiotics.

Microbial metabolism within plaque produces localized gradients in factors affecting the growth of other species

Table 10.3 Microbial interactions in dental plaque.

Beneficial	Antagonistic
Enzyme complementation	Nutrient competition
Food chains/food webs	Production of:
Coaggregation	• bacteriocins
Inactivation of inhibitors	• hydrogen peroxide
Subversion of host defenses	• organic acids
	Low pH generation

(e.g. pH, dissolved oxygen, essential nutrients, and the accumulation of products of metabolism and inhibitors) (Marsh, 2000b). In this way, bacteria are able to modify their local environment. These gradients lead to the development of environmental heterogeneity, and ensure the coexistence of species that would be incompatible with one another in a homogeneous habitat, enabling a more diverse microbial community to establish. A consequence of a 'community lifestyle' is that microorganisms experience a wider habitat range and demonstrate an increased metabolic efficiency than might be predicted from laboratory data generated from pure culture studies (Marsh & Bowden, 2000). Microbial communities are also better able to cope with minor environmental perturbations and stresses and, in some instances, the component bacteria demonstrate an enhanced pathogenic potential, which is often seen in dental abscesses, which generally have a polymicrobial etiology.

Caries microbiology: a brief historical perspective

Over a century ago, Dr W. D. Miller (Miller, 1890) recognized the role of the resident oral microflora in caries. Miller introduced the 'chemico-parasitic' theory of caries by suggesting that in order for caries to develop, 'two factors always have to be in operation; the action of acids and the action of germs'. However, unlike his contemporary colleagues (G. V. Black and J. L. Williams), Miller was not aware of the crucial etiological role of dental biofilm and believed that the bacteria producing organic acids were mainly living in saliva. It was not until after the end of the 1940s, with the development of antibiotics, that experimental studies using germ-free animals provided a further insight into the microbiology of caries. Experiments showed that rodents developed caries when infected with specific bacteria, and that caries could be transmitted from animal to animal, while other studies proved the essential role of fermentable sugars in the diet (Keyes, 1960; Fitzgerald & Keyes, 1960). Bacteria could be ranked in terms of their cariogenicity, and the most cariogenic group were the mutans streptococci, especially *S. mutans* and *S. sobrinus*. The role of bacteria was also confirmed in treatment studies. Antibiotics and immunization against the inoculated strain caused a decrease in the numbers of both bacteria in plaque and caries lesions compared with control animals. It is important to understand, however, that the experimental conditions applied in the above studies were highly artificial as in most studies the animals were inoculated with only a single bacterial strain. This experimental set-up is very different from the human oral cavity, which contains a pool of bacteria interacting with each other. Nevertheless, in spite of these limitations, such observations were taken by leading scientists to indicate that dental caries is a specific infection, with mutans streptococci as the main 'pathogens' (Loesche, 1986;

Tanzer, 1989), a view that is still prevalent in many countries today.

However, dental caries does not fulfill the classical principles of a specific infectious disease (Fejerskov & Nyvad, 2003). Historically, for a microorganism to be considered responsible as an etiological agent for a disease, it would need to satisfy Koch's postulates. Thus:

- the microorganism should be found in all cases of the disease, with a distribution corresponding to the observed lesions
- the organism should be grown on artificial media for several subcultures
- a pure subculture should produce the disease in a susceptible animal.

As stated previously, the relationship between mutans streptococci and caries is not absolute. Relatively high proportions of mutans streptococci may survive on tooth surfaces without caries developing, while the opposite is also true, i.e. caries may arise in the apparent absence of these organisms (Nyvad, 1993; Marsh & Martin, 1999). Therefore, rather than necessarily initiating the caries process, an outgrowth of mutans streptococci may reflect a disturbance in the homeostasis of the dental biofilm. If the homeostatic balance is broken down, changes in the relative proportions of the microorganisms making up the microbial community can occur, and this could predispose a site to disease (an opportunistic infection). Hence, it may be more appropriate to think about dental caries as an endogenous infection (see later).

Methodological problems in microbiological studies of dental caries

The high species diversity of dental biofilms makes it rather laborious to perform microbiological studies of caries. Therefore, for many years, with easy access to selective culture media, many researchers were tempted to study only the primary suspects of caries: mutans streptococci and lactobacilli. In view of the discussion above it should be clear, however, that such a simplified microbiological approach could be very misleading when trying to understand the etiology of caries.

Traditionally, the composition of dental plaque has been determined by growing the constituent organisms on a range of selective and non-selective agar plates, incubated under appropriate conditions, for various lengths of time. The identity of the resultant microbial colonies is achieved by the application of physiological, biochemical and serological tests. However, recent comparisons of total viable versus total microscopic counts have demonstrated that only about 40–50% of the oral microflora can be cultivated, and that many groups of microorganism are being underestimated. Some contemporary studies are now using culture-independent (molecular) approaches in which DNA (mainly 16S rRNA gene sequences) is amplified from a specimen of dental plaque using universal primers, partially sequenced, and compared with known sequences in international databases. Novel organisms, and organisms previously found only in low numbers using culture, have been identified, particularly from advanced lesions. Findings from these studies will be presented in a later section.

Attention should also be given to the study design when evaluating the results of microbiological investigations of caries. Evidence for the role of plaque bacteria in dental caries in humans has come from both cross-sectional and longitudinal studies in which the microbial composition of plaque was related to the integrity of the underlying tooth surface (Fig. 10.25). In cross-sectional studies, predetermined caries-prone surfaces are sampled at a single timepoint, and the microbial composition of plaque is related to the caries status of the tooth surface at that time. A limitation of this type of study is that it cannot be established whether the species that are isolated at the time of lesion diagnosis caused the decay or are present as a result of the lesion; thus, these studies only demonstrate associations. In contrast, longitudinal studies regularly sample, over a set period, surfaces that are initially clinically sound. The microflora can then be compared (i) at the same site before and after the diagnosis of a lesion, and (ii) between those surfaces that decayed and those that remained caries free

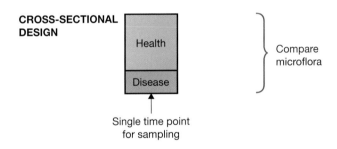

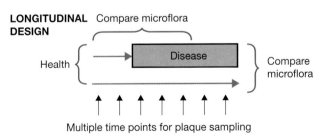

Figure 10.25 Distinction between cross-sectional and longitudinal study designs to investigate the role of dental biofilm bacteria in caries. Cross-sectional studies are relatively quick and easy to perform on different population groups, but they only show associations between the microflora and caries because each site is sampled only at a single time point. Longitudinal studies provide more insights into the microbial etiology of dental caries because the microflora can be compared (a) before and after the diagnosis of a lesion and (b) between sites that developed caries and those that remained caries free. All sites to be investigated are caries free at the start of sampling.

throughout the study. This type of study design is more expensive and difficult to conduct, but can establish true cause-and-effect relationships. Nonetheless, both the cross-sectional design and the longitudinal study design suffer from the fact that it is often difficult to say exactly when a non-cavitated lesion may be detected clinically, as this is essentially a question about the refinement of the diagnostic method (Chapter 7). Likewise, in longitudinal studies of lesion development, the clinical caries diagnostic criteria applied should be sensitive enough to reflect changes in lesion activity (Chapter 4). Alternatively, the latter problem may be solved by using an experimental *in situ* model in which the mineral content of natural tooth surfaces, worn in intraoral appliances in human volunteers, is monitored in parallel with changes in the composition of the biofilm (Nyvad & Kilian, 1990b).

Microbiology of caries

The following paragraphs provide an outline of selected microbiological studies that have attempted to describe the microflora associated with or implied in the causation of caries. A full description of the caries microflora is beyond the scope of this chapter. However, considering the diversity of clinical designs and differences in sampling techniques and microbiological methods, it seems safe to conclude that no single microorganism or group of microorganisms may be held solely responsible for the initiation and progression of caries. It may be comforting for the dental student to know that it is less important to remember the specific names of the bacteria than to understand their potential role in the biofilm community in health and disease.

Enamel caries

Fissures are the most caries-prone sites of the dentition, and the strongest correlations between the plaque levels of mutans streptococci and caries have been found at these sites. For example, in a classical cross-sectional study, 71% of carious fissures had viable counts of mutans streptococci >10% of the total cultivable plaque microflora, whereas 70% of fissures that were caries free had no detectable mutans streptococci (Loesche *et al.*, 1975). In a longitudinal study of fissures, the proportions of mutans streptococci increased significantly at the time of lesion diagnosis (Loesche & Straffon, 1979). However, mutans streptococci were only minor components of plaque from five fissures that became carious, but these sites had relatively high levels of lactobacilli, and these bacteria may have been responsible for the observed demineralization. A subsequent longitudinal study confirmed these findings, and demonstrated an even stronger relationship between mutans streptococci and caries initiation (Table 10.4), while lactobacilli, when present, were strongly associated with sites requiring restoration (Loesche *et al.*, 1984).

Table 10.4 Mean proportions of mutans streptococci (MS) and lactobacilli (L) on teeth in schoolchildren (7–8 years old) who remained caries free or who developed a caries lesion during a longitudinal study[a]

Time (months) before caries diagnosis	Mean proportions in fissure plaque					
	Caries sites		Filled sites		Caries-free sites	
	MS	L	MS	L	MS	L
0	29	8	–	–	9	2
6	25	8	15	3	17	1
12	16	1	20	2	9	3
18	9	<1	16	1	11	1

[a] Loesche *et al.* (1984).

A major prospective study of young Swiss children (aged 7–8 years) found that both fissures and smooth surfaces of first permanent premolars that suffered demineralization without cavitation were heavily colonized with mutans streptococci (10^4–10^5 cfu/ml sample) around 12–18 months before the clinical diagnosis of the lesion (Lang *et al.*, 1987). The proportions of mutans streptococci markedly increased 6–9 months before lesion detection, to reach 11–18% and 10–12% of the total streptococcal microflora of fissures and smooth surfaces, respectively. Some lesions 'remineralized', and the levels of mutans streptococci fell dramatically from around 20% to 2–5% of the total streptococcal count in the period 6–9 months before the diagnosis of the reversal. As with most studies on the microflora of caries, this study found some fissures with high levels of mutans streptococci but no discernible lesions, while other sites that were carious had no detectable mutans streptococci at any time.

Microbiological studies based on examination of the total fissure content may not be suitable to reveal changes in the composition of the microflora in relation to the initiation and progression of caries. It is well known that the early signs of fissure caries develop along the fissure entrance rather than within the fissure proper (see Chapter 3). Microbiological studies of fissure caries should therefore allow for sampling at discrete sites. One study that adopted this approach showed that the relative proportion of various groups of bacteria differs between different parts of the fissure (Meiers & Schachtele, 1984). In particular, the percentage of streptococci was higher at the fissure entrance than within the fissure proper.

Similarly, a problem with studies of approximal surfaces lies with the difficulty in accurately diagnosing early lesions, and with the fact that the biofilm is inevitably removed from the whole interproximal area, including that overlying sound as well as carious enamel. Early cross-sectional studies reported a positive correlation between elevated mutans streptococci levels and lesion development. A less clear-cut association was found in a large longitudinal study of 11–15-year-old UK children. At some sites, mutans streptococci could be found in high numbers before the radiographic detection of demineralization, while some lesions also developed in the apparent absence of these bacteria (Hardie *et al.*, 1977). Mutans streptococci could also be present at some sites for prolonged periods in high numbers without any evidence of caries. The isolation frequency and proportions of mutans streptococci tended to increase after the first diagnosis of a lesion, especially in those that progressed deeper into the enamel, suggesting that the composition of the microflora may shift as the lesion progresses through the tooth. Similar findings were found in a study of Dutch Army recruits, aged 18–20 years (Huis in't Veld *et al.*, 1979). Mutans streptococci were isolated from 40% and 86% of sites from caries-free and caries-active recruits, respectively. In this study, distinct differences in association were found when the mutans streptococci were subdivided: *S. mutans* (serotype *c*) was isolated from caries-free and caries-active individuals, whereas *S. sobrinus* (originally *S. mutans* serotype *d*) was recovered almost exclusively from caries-active recruits.

Rampant caries can occur in people who experience an exceptional change in the oral environment, such as those with markedly reduced salivary flow rates due to, for example, radiation therapy or medication. Longitudinal studies of patients undergoing radiation treatment showed large increases in the proportions of mutans streptococci and lactobacilli in plaque and saliva. These organisms also reach high levels in 'nursing-bottle' caries, which occurs in young infants fed from bottles containing formulae with a high concentration of fermentable carbohydrate (Loesche, 1986).

Collectively, the data from numerous surveys of various tooth surfaces, of different patient age groups from numerous countries, and populations with different dietary habits, etc., have shown a strong positive association between increased levels of mutans streptococci and the initiation of demineralization. However, not all of the studies relating biofilm composition to the initiation of dental caries attempted to identify all of the bacteria present in the clinical samples, and many studies inevitably focussed only on groups of organisms already implicated in disease, e.g. mutans streptococci and lactobacilli. Other bacteria may also contribute to demineralization, while others may reduce the impact of acid production by either utilizing the lactate produced from sugar metabolism (e.g. *Veillonella* spp.) or producing alkali from saliva components (*S. salivarius*, *S. sanguinis*, *A. naeslundii*). It should also be appreciated that mutans streptococci is a general term for several closely related species of streptococcus originally described as different serotypes of *S. mutans*. The specific name, *S. mutans*, is now limited to human isolates previously belonging to serotypes *c*, *e* and *f*. This is the most common species isolated from human dental biofilms. The next most prevalent species is *S. sobrinus* (previously *S. mutans* serotypes *d* and *g*). Some of these strains produce more acid from sucrose than *S. mutans* (de Soet *et al.*, 2000), and it is preferable, therefore, that mutans streptococci be identified at the species or serotype level in future studies of the microbiology of caries.

Root-surface caries and infected dentin

Early studies using animal models, and epidemiological surveys in humans, suggested a key role for Gram-positive filamentous bacteria, especially *Actinomyces* spp., in root-surface caries. Recent studies have failed to confirm such an association, possibly because the early studies focussed exclusively on infected root dentin. In cross-sectional studies of plaque overlying carious root surfaces, mutans streptococci, alone or in combination with lactobacilli, have been isolated more frequently or in higher proportions than on sound root surfaces (Billings *et al.*, 1985; Brown *et al.*, 1986; Fure *et al.*, 1987; Keltjens *et al.*, 1987; Bowden *et al.*, 1990; van Houte *et al.*, 1990). However, as with enamel caries, this relationship is not absolute. Mutans streptococci can be isolated from sound surfaces (Brown *et al.*, 1986; Keltjens *et al.*, 1987), and in some studies it has not been possible to detect any differences in the proportion of mutans streptococci between sound and carious surfaces (Ellen *et al.*, 1985; Emilson *et al.*, 1988).

For reasons of simplicity many microbiological studies have applied selective media for identification of target species. However, selective media may detect only a limited fraction of the total cultivable microflora. Recent studies using non-selective media and anaerobic sampling techniques clearly show that the microflora of root caries is much more diverse than previously thought and, in addition to mutans streptococci and lactobacilli, commonly includes species belonging to *Actinomyces*, non-mutans streptococci, *Bifidobacterium*, *Rothia*, *Veillonella*, *Candida*, enterococci and anaerobic Gram-negative species (Bowden, 1990; Nyvad & Kilian, 1990b; Schüpbach *et al.*, 1995) (Table 10.5). In one study it was not possible to detect clear differences in the microbial composition of dental plaque on sound and carious root surfaces (Scheie *et al.*, 1996).

As pointed out before, a crucial problem with most microbiological studies of caries is the lack of an accurate definition of the onset of lesion formation and/or the demineralization activity of the lesions studied. Because of the dynamic nature of caries, the mineral loss varies over time, not only between different lesions, but also within the individual lesion depending on the metabolic activity of the microflora. Studies of associations between the microflora and caries should therefore preferably be performed on lesions with known age and history in the oral cavity. One study that applied this approach suggested that lesions presenting the highest mineral loss (as assessed by microradiography of root caries lesions developed during 3 months *in situ*) were dominated by a few acidogenic species, such as *Actinomyces* spp., or a combination of mutans streptococci and lactobacilli (Nyvad & Kilian, 1990b). Lesions that lost only a small amount of mineral were associated with a much more diverse microflora, including various acidogenic (mutans streptococci, *Actinomyces* spp., *Lactobacillus* spp. and *S. mitis* biovar 1) and lactate-metabolizing species (*Veillonella* spp.). Such differences in the pattern and acidogenic potential of the microflora are likely to reflect differences in the ecology of the lesions and imply that in order to understand the ecology of caries it may be necessary to recover the total microflora of a site.

A diverse microflora was recovered from plaque overlying sound or carious root surfaces when a more specialized sampling technique was used. The microflora on sound root surfaces included both Gram-positive (predominantly *Actinomyces* spp., but also *Streptococcus*, *Bifidobacterium*, *Corynebacterium*, *Lactobacillus*, 'Peptostreptococcus' and *Propionibacterium* spp.) and Gram-negative bacteria (predominantly *Prevotella* spp., but including *Campylobacter*, *Capnocytophaga*, *Fusobacterium*, *Leptotrichia*, *Selonomonas* and *Veillonella* spp.), in approximately equal proportions (Schüpbach *et al.*, 1995). This diversity was also observed in active non-cavitated root surface lesions, although there were substantial increases in the proportions of *A. naeslundii*, together with increases in some Gram-negative species such as *Prevotella intermedia* and *Capnocytophaga* spp. The presence of these latter organisms may be significant since root caries involves both demineralization of the tissues due to acid production and proteolysis of the dentin collagen matrix. Perhaps some of the above Gram-negative bacteria are able to degrade protein under acidic conditions, whereas other proteolytic species associated with advanced periodontal diseases require a neutral or alkaline pH. Lower numbers of Gram-negative bacteria were found in arrested root lesions (Schüpbach *et al.*, 1995).

In advanced cavitated lesions, notably higher levels of *S. mutans* were reported, possibly at the expense of *Actinomyces* spp., while lactobacilli were more common from sites with soft and necrotic dentin (Schüpbach *et al.*, 1996). Other studies have also reported high proportions of

Table 10.5 Mean proportions of selected bacteria from biofilms developing on root surfaces with and without caries (Bowden, 1990)

| Bacterium | Sound | Root-surface caries | |
		Initial (soft)	Advanced (hard)
Mutans streptococci	2	34	8
Streptococcus sanguinis	19	11	48
Actinomyces naeslundii	12	13	13
Lactobacillus	ND	1	1
Veillonella	ND	4	2

A range of other *Actinomyces* species has been isolated from infected dentin of active root caries lesions, including *A. gerencseriae*, *A. israelii*, *A. odontolyticus* and *A. georgiae* (Brailsford *et al.*, 1999).
ND: not determined.

lactobacilli and other Gram-positive rods from infected dentin (Beighton *et al.*, 1993), including several species of *Actinomyces* such as *A. israelii* and *A. gerencseriae* (Brailsford *et al.*, 1999). Obligately anaerobic Gram-negative bacteria are also present, but in lower levels than in the plaque overlying the lesion. Their role would still be important in contributing to the proteolytic and collagenolytic activities associated with breakdown of the tissue. The anaerobe *Eubacterium saburreum* also formed a considerable proportion of the bacteria in advanced cavitated dentinal lesions. Indeed, the majority of the bacteria from cavitated root lesions were isolated from the outermost segments of the lesion.

Recently, molecular analyses have been performed on carious dentin to describe more fully the microbial diversity of lesions. A range of lactobacilli, comprising 50% of the species detected, were identified, with novel *Prevotella* spp. also being abundant. Other taxa present included those more commonly seen in subgingival plaque, including *Selenomonas* spp., *Dialister* spp., *Eubacterium* spp. and *Fusobacterium* spp. (Nadkarni *et al.*, 2004; Chhour *et al.*, 2005); a novel *Propionibacterium* species has also been reported (Munson *et al.*, 2004). Thus, it is plausible that the diversity and proportions of the organisms within the microflora change as the lesion progresses through the dental tissues, probably in direct response to alterations in critical environmental conditions. These include shifts in pH, the degree of anaerobiosis and changes to the primary sources of nutrients.

In summary, many studies have shown that mutans streptococci can be isolated more often and in higher numbers from a range of caries lesions, although some advanced lesions generally yield a more diverse microflora including acidogenic and proteolytic species working in concert. A consistent feature of clinical studies has been the finding that the association of mutans streptococci with caries is not absolute. Thus, mutans streptococci can persist at some sites without evidence of demineralization, while they cannot be recovered from a proportion of lesions, implying a role for other bacteria. The involvement of other species should not be unexpected when the features that are associated with the cariogenic potential of an organism are considered; these will be described in the next section.

Cariogenic features of dental biofilm bacteria

In order that bacteria can be claimed to play a role in caries they must possess certain caries-promoting characteristics. Such distinctive characteristics (Loesche, 1986) include:

- the ability rapidly to transport fermentable sugars when in competition with other plaque bacteria, and the conversion of such sugars to acid. Mutans streptococci possess several sugar transport systems, including high-affinity phosphoenolpyruvate–phosphotransferase (PEP-PTS) systems, which are able to scavenge sugars even when they are present in the oral environment only in low concentrations

- the ability to maintain sugar metabolism under extreme environmental conditions, such as at a low pH. Few oral bacteria are able to tolerate acidic conditions for prolonged periods; however, mutans streptococci and lactobacilli not only remain viable at a low pH, but preferentially grow and metabolize, i.e. they are both acidogenic and aciduric (acid loving). This ability relies on (i) the ability to maintain a favorable intracellular environment, and pump out protons even under acidic conditions, (ii) the possession of enzymes with a more acidic pH optimum, and (iii) the production of specific acid-stress response proteins.

- the production of extracellular (EPS) and intracellular polysaccharides (IPS). EPS include glucans and fructans, both of which contribute to the biofilm matrix. In addition to supporting the structure of the biofilm, this may help to concentrate acids in distinct regions of the biofilm. Furthermore, fructans are labile and can be metabolized by biofilm bacteria under carbohydrate-restricted conditions. IPS are glycogen-like storage compounds that can be used for energy production and converted to acid when free sugars are not available in the mouth. Thus, the metabolism of IPS can prolong periods over which biofilms can generate acids (and, therefore, a low pH).

It should be noted, however, that these properties are not specific to mutans streptococci in the same way that the possession of some virulence factors (e.g. cholera toxin for *Vibrio cholerae*, pertussis toxin for *Bordetella pertussis*) help to define certain classical medical pathogens. Indeed, the acidogenic and aciduric profile of particular species lie along a continuum, with increasing evidence of considerable overlap. Recent studies have recovered strains of non-mutans streptococcal species (van Houte, 1994; van Ruyven *et al.*, 2000), e.g. *S. mitis*, *S. gordonii*, *S. anginosus* and *S. oralis* (de Soet *et al.*, 2000) that can be as acidogenic and acid tolerating as some mutans streptococci (Fig. 10.26). As these species are prevalent among the early colonizers of teeth (Nyvad & Kilian, 1990a) they could play an important role in preparing the environment to make it suitable for the outgrowth of more aciduric species such as mutans streptococci and lactobacilli. Hence, the importance of the three caries-promoting properties described above may vary depending on the stage and activity of lesion formation. Therefore, it is not surprising that mutans streptococci and bacteria with similar caries-promoting traits are found in elevated proportions at caries sites. However, it should be appreciated that other bacteria may also contribute to the cariogenic potential of the biofilm. Some of these issues are developed further in the following section.

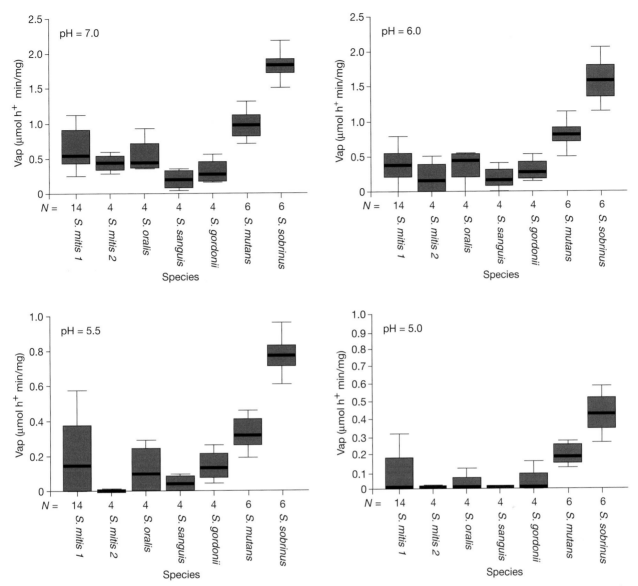

Figure 10.26 Velocity of acid production by six oral streptococcal species at different pH values. The bold line represents the median, and the box and error bars the 95% and 75% confidence intervals, respectively (de Soet *et al.*, 2000).

The ecological plaque hypothesis to explain the role of dental biofilm bacteria in the etiology of dental caries

For many years, there were two main schools of thought on the role of plaque bacteria in the etiology of caries. The specific plaque hypothesis proposed that, out of the diverse collection of organisms comprising the resident plaque microflora, only a single or very small number of species were actively involved in disease. This proposal has been easy to promote because it focussed efforts on controlling disease by targeting preventive measures and treatment against a limited number of organisms, such as by vaccination or gene therapy (Chapter 17), or by antimicrobial treatment (Chapter 16). In contrast, the non-specific plaque hypothesis considered that disease is the outcome of the overall activity of the total plaque microflora, so not just those that make acid, but also species that produce alkali or consume lactate need to be considered. Thus, a heterogeneous mixture of microorganisms could play a role in disease. In some respects, the arguments about the relative merits of these hypotheses may be about semantics, since biofilm-mediated diseases are essentially mixed culture (polymicrobial) infections, but in which only certain (perhaps a limited number of) species are able to predominate. The arguments then centre around the definitions of the terms specific and non-specific. More recently, an alternative hypothesis has been proposed (the ecological plaque hypothesis), which reconciles key elements of the earlier two hypotheses (Marsh, 1994, 2003). In brief, the ecological plaque hypothesis proposes that the organisms associated with disease may also be present at sound sites, but at levels too low to be clinically relevant. Disease is a result of a shift in the balance of the resident microflora driven by a change in local environmental conditions. In the case of dental caries, repeated conditions of low pH in plaque following frequent sugar intake (or decreased sugar clearance following low salivary secretion) will favor the growth of acidogenic and aciduric species, and thereby predispose a site to caries (Fig. 10.27).

A consistent feature of most of the clinical studies described earlier has been the occasional but regular finding of carious sites from which no mutans streptococci can be isolated. As discussed previously, this suggests that acidogenic bacteria other than mutans streptococci can make a biologically significant contribution to the strength of the cariogenic challenge at a site (van Houte, 1994; van Ruyven *et al.*, 2000). The converse situation is also not uncommon, where mutans streptococci are found in high numbers in plaque but in the apparent absence of any demineralization of the underlying enamel. This may be due to:

- the structure of the biofilm and the localization of mutans streptococci in plaque
- the presence of lactate-consuming species (e.g. *Veillonella*)
- the production of alkali to raise the local pH (e.g. by ammonia production from urea or arginine by *S. salivarius* and *S. sanguinis*, respectively).

Other factors will also be significant, and these include the influence of the diet and enamel chemistry. These observations serve to emphasize the multifactorial nature

of caries (Chapter 3), which involves the interaction of an acidogenic/aciduric microflora on a tooth surface, fueled by a diet consisting of frequent intakes of rapidly fermentable carbohydrates.

Collectively, these findings allow a dynamic model to be constructed to explain the changes in the ecology of dental plaque that lead to the development of a caries lesion (Fig. 10.27). Potentially acidogenic/aciduric bacteria may be found naturally in dental biofilm, but at neutral pH, these organisms are weakly competitive and may be present only as a small proportion of the total plaque community. In this situation the acid production by such bacteria is clinically insignificant or may be counteracted by other bacteria, and the processes of demineralization and remineralization are in equilibrium. If the frequency of fermentable carbohydrate intake increases and/or salivary flow is impaired, then the biofilm spends more time below the critical pH for enamel demineralization (approximately pH 5.5). The effect of this on the microbial ecology would be two-fold. Conditions of low pH favor the proliferation of aciduric (and acidogenic) bacteria (especially mutans streptococci and lactobacilli, but not exclusively so) (van Houte, 1994), while tipping the balance towards demineralization. Greater numbers of aciduric bacteria such as mutans streptococci and lactobacilli in plaque would result in more acid being produced at even faster rates, thereby enhancing demineralization still further. Other bacteria could also make acid under similar conditions, but at a slower rate, or could initiate lesions in the absence of other (more overt) aciduric species in a more susceptible host. If

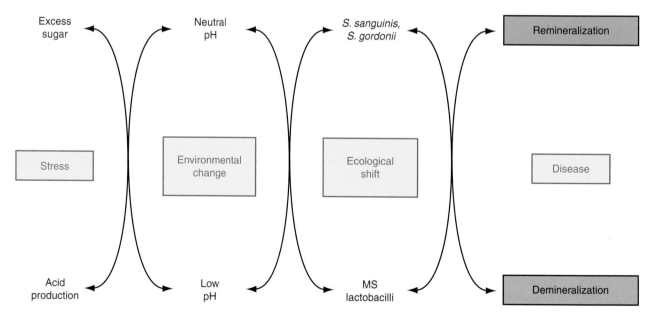

Figure 10.27 The ecological plaque hypothesis and the etiology of dental caries. The diagram shows a dynamic relationship whereby an environmental change in the biofilm (e.g. low pH) drives a shift in the balance of the resident microflora, thereby shifting the balance towards enamel demineralization. Caries could be controlled by inhibiting the putative pathogens, e.g. mutans streptococci (MS) or other acid producers, by interfering with the environmental changes driving the ecological shift, e.g. by reducing the acid challenge by the use of sugar control, saliva stimulation and/or biofilm removal. (Adapted from Marsh, 1994.)

highly aciduric species were not present initially, then the repeated conditions of low pH coupled with the inhibition of competing organisms might increase the likelihood of colonization by mutans streptococci or lactobacilli. This sequence of events would account for the lack of specificity in the microbial etiology of caries and explain the pattern of bacterial succession observed in many clinical studies. This model forms the basis of the ecological plaque hypothesis (Fig. 10.27) (Marsh, 1994, 2003). In this hypothesis, caries is a consequence of changes in the natural balance of the resident plaque microflora brought about by an alteration in local environmental conditions (e.g. repeated conditions of high sugar and low plaque pH). The hypothesis also acknowledges the dynamic relationship that exists between the microflora and the host, so that the impact of alterations in key host factors (such as diet and saliva flow) on plaque composition is also taken into account. This has a great significance for caries prevention, since implicit in the hypothesis is the concept that disease can be controlled by targeting the putative pathogens (mutans streptococci and other acidogenic/aciduric species) through interference with the factors that are driving the deleterious shifts in the balance of the microflora. Identification of such critical control points (e.g. mechanical biofilm removal, saliva stimulation and/or dietary control) can lead to the selection of appropriate caries-preventive strategies that are tailored to the needs of individual patients (see Chapter 27). In this way, the clinician not only treats the end result of the disease process, but also attempts to identify and interfere with the factors that, if left unaltered, will inevitably lead to more disease.

Concluding remarks

This chapter has presented evidence for a hypothesis by which it may be possible to explain the etiology of dental caries: the ecological plaque hypothesis of caries. According to this hypothesis it is postulated that dental caries is a naturally occurring biological phenomenon that takes place in the dental biofilm as a result of ecological disturbances in the biofilm community. Such imbalances in the biofilm community may originate in the host's own microflora in response to various external factors. For example, increased sugar exposure or impaired salivary clearance may lead to an outgrowth of mutans streptococci and other aciduric bacterial species. This hypothesis is compatible with previous clinical observations of increased proportions of aciduric species in caries lesions, while at the same time acknowledging the lack of absolute specificity of the microflora involved. The ecological hypothesis may also help to explain why tooth surfaces that are constantly covered by biofilm do not always develop caries lesions. Hence, because of the many interactions among different types of bacteria in the biofilm, the outcome may not necessarily be a net mineral loss over time (Chapter 3).

Knowledge about the role of bacteria in caries is not merely a theoretical issue. The way in which dental professionals interpret the microbiological features in caries has strong implications for the choice of strategy for caries control. If dentists believe that dental caries results from an ecological disturbance in the biofilm, they should focus their preventive strategies on such methods that restore the ecological balance of the microbial community, such as mechanical plaque removal (Chapter 15), salivary stimulation (Chapter 11) and/or sugar control (Chapter 19).

Background literature

Beighton D, Brailsford, SR. Plaque microbiology of root caries. In: Newman HN, Wilson M, eds. *Dental plaque revisited: oral biofilms in health and disease.* Cardiff: BioLine, 1999: 295–312.

Hamilton IR. Ecological basis for dental caries. In: Kuramitsu HK, Ellen RP, eds. *Oral bacterial ecology: the molecular basis.* Wymondham: Horizon Scientific Press, 2000: 219–74.

References

Aas JA, Paster BJ, Stokes LN, Olsen I, Dewhirst FE. Defining the normal bacterial flora of the oral cavity. *J Clin Microbiol* 2005; **43**: 5721–32.

Beighton D, Lynch E, Heath MR. A microbiological study of primary root caries lesions with different treatment needs. *J Dent Res* 1993; **72**: 623–9.

Billings RJ, Brown LR, Kaster AG. Contemporary treatment strategies for root surface dental caries. *Gerodontics* 1985; **1**: 20–7.

Bowden GHW. Microbiology of root surface caries in humans. *J Dent Res* 1990; **69**: 1205–10.

Bowden GH, Hardie JM, Slack GL. Microbial variations in approximal dental plaque. *Caries Res* 1975; **9**: 253–77.

Bowden GHW, Ekstrand J, McNaughton B, Challacombe SJ. The association of selected bacteria with the lesions of root surface caries. *Oral Microbiol Immunol* 1990; **5**: 345–51.

Brailsford SR, Tregaskis RB, Leftwich HS, Beighton D. The predominant *Actinomyces* spp. isolated from infected dentin of active root caries lesions. *J Dent Res* 1999; **78**: 1525–34.

Branda SS, Vik S, Friedman L, Kolter R. Biofilms: the matrix revisited. *Trends Microbiol* 2005; **13**: 20–6.

Brinig MM, Lepp PW, Ouverney CC, Armitage GC, Relman DA. Prevalence of bacteria of division TM7 in human subgingival plaque and their association with disease. *Appl Environ Microbiol* 2003; **69**: 1687–94.

Brown RL, Billings RJ, Kaster AG. Quantitative comparisons of potentially cariogenic microorganisms cultured from noncarious and carious root and coronal tooth surfaces. *Infect Immun* 1986; **11**: 765–70.

Carlsson J. Growth and nutrition as ecological factors. In: Kuramitsu HK, Ellen RP, eds. *Oral bacterial ecology: the molecular basis.* Wymondham: Horizon Scientific Press, 2000: 67–130.

Caufield PW, Cutter GR, Dasanayake AP. Initial acquisition of mutans streptococci by infants: evidence for a discrete window of infectivity. *J Dent Res* 1993; **72**: 37–45.

Chhour K-L, Nadkarni MA, Byun R, Martin FE, Jacques NA, Hunter N. Molecular analysis of microbial diversity in advanced caries. *J Clin Microbiol* 2005; **43**: 843–9.

Costerton JW, Lewandowski Z, Caldwell DE, Korber DR, Lappin-Scott HM. Microbial biofilms. *Annu Rev Microbiol* 1995; **49**: 711–45.

Ellen RP, Banting DW, Fillery ED. *Streptococcus mutans* and *Lactobacillus* detection in the assessment of dental root surface caries risk. *J Dent Res* 1985; **64**: 1245–9.

Emilson CG, Klock B, Sanford CB. Microbial flora associated with presence of root surface caries in periodontally treated patients. *Scand J Dent Res* 1988; **96**: 40–9.

Fejerskov O, Nyvad B. *Is dental caries an infectious disease? Diagnostic and treatment consequences for the practitioner. Nordic Dentistry 2003.* Copenhagen: Quintessence, 2003: 141–52.

Fejerskov O, Silness J, Karring T, Löe H. The occlusal fissure of unerupted third molars as an experimental caries model in man. *Scand J Dent Res* 1976; **84**: 142–9.

Fitzgerald RJ, Keyes PH. Demonstration of the etiological role of streptococci in experimental caries in the hamster. *J Am Dent Assoc* 1960; **61**: 9–19.

Fure S, Romaniec M, Emilson CG, Krasse B. Proportions of *Streptococcus mutans*, lactobacilli, and *Actinomyces* spp. in root surface plaque. *Scand J Dent Res* 1987; **95**: 119–23.

Gibbons RJ. Bacterial adhesion to oral tissue: a model for infectious diseases. *J Dent Res* 1989; **68**: 750–60.

Gibbons RJ, Cohen L, Hay DI. Strains of *Streptococcus mutans* and *Streptococcus sobrinus* attach to different pellicle receptors. *Infect Immun* 1986; **52**: 555–61.

Gibbons RJ, Hay DI, Childs WC III, Davis G. Role of cryptic receptors (cryptitopes) in bacterial adhesion to oral surfaces. *Arch Oral Biol* 1990; **35**: 107–14S.

Hardie JM, Thomson PL, South RJ, *et al*. A longitudinal epidemiological study on dental plaque and the development of dental caries – interim results after two years. *J Dent Res* 1977; **56** (Special Issue C): C90–8.

van der Hoeven JS, Rogers AH. Factors affecting the stability of the dental plaque microflora of specific pathogen-free rats in relation to the ability to resist colonization by *S. mutans*. *Arch Oral Biol* 1979; **24**: 787–90.

van Houte J. Role of micro-organisms in caries etiology. *J Dent Res* 1994; **73**: 672–81.

van Houte J, Green DB. Relationship between the concentration of bacteria in saliva and the colonization of teeth in humans. *Infect Immun* 1974; **9**: 624–30.

van Houte J, Jordan HV, Laraway R, Kent R, Soparkar PM, DePaola PF. Association of the microbial flora of dental plaque and saliva with human root surface caries. *J Dent Res* 1990; **69**: 1463–8.

Huis in't Veld JHJ, van Palenstein Heldeman WH, Backer Dirks O. *Streptococcus mutans* and dental caries in humans: a bacteriological and immunological study. *Antonie van Leeuwenhoek* 1979; **45**: 25–33.

Imfeld TN, Lutz F. Intraplaque acid formation assessed *in vivo* in children and young adults. *Pediatr Dent* 1980; **2**: 87–93.

Keltjens HMAM, Schaeken MJM, van der Hoeven JS, Hendriks JCM. Microflora of plaque from sound and carious root surfaces. *Caries Res* 1987; **21**: 193–9.

Keyes PH. The infectious and transmissible nature of experimental dental caries. Findings and implications. *Arch Oral Biol* 1960; **1**: 304–20.

Kinniment SL, Wimpenny JWT, Adams D, Marsh PD. The effect of chlorhexidine on defined, mixed culture oral biofilms grown in a novel model system. *J Appl Bacteriol* 1996; **81**: 120–5.

Köhler B, Andréen I, Jonsson B. The effect of caries-preventive measures in mothers on dental caries and the oral presence of the bacteria *Streptococcus mutans* and lactobacilli in their children. *Arch Oral Biol* 1984; **29**: 879–83.

Kolenbrander PE, Andersen RN, Kazmerak KM, Palmer RJ. Coaggregation and coadhesion in oral biofilms. In: Allison DG, Gilbert P, Lappin-Scott HM, Wilson M, eds. *Community structure and co-operation in biofilms* (Society for Microbiology Symposium Vol. 59). Cambridge: Cambridge University Press, 2000: 65–85.

Lang NP, Hotz PR, Gusberti FA, Joss A. Longitudinal clinical and microbiological study on the relationship between infection with *Streptococcus mutans* and the development of caries in humans. *Oral Microbiol Immunol* 1987; **2**: 39–47.

Larsen T, Fiehn N-E. Resistance of *Streptococcus sanguis* biofilms to antimicrobial agents. *APMIS* 1996; **104**: 280–4.

Levine MJ, Tabak LA, Reddy M, Mandel ID. Nature of salivary pellicles in microbial adherence: role of salivary mucins. In: Mergenhagen SE, Rosan B, eds. *Molecular basis of oral microbial adhesion*. Washington, DC: American Society of Microbiology, 1985: 125–30.

Li Y, Burne RA. Regulation of the *gtfBC* and *ftf* genes of *Streptococcus mutans* in biofilms in response to pH and carbohydrate. *Microbiology* 2001; **147**: 2841–8.

Li Y, Caufield PW. The fidelity of initial acquisition of mutans streptococci by infants from their mothers. *J Dent Res* 1995; **74**: 681–5.

Loesche WJ. Role of *Streptococcus mutans* in human dental decay. *Microbiol Rev* 1986; **50**: 353–80.

Loesche WJ, Straffon LH. Longitudinal investigation of the role of *Streptococcus mutans* in human fissure decay. *Infect Immun* 1979; **26**: 498–507.

Loesche WJ, Rowan J, Straffon LH, Loos PJ. Association of *Streptococcus mutans* with human dental decay. *Infect Immun* 1975; **11**: 1252–60.

Loesche WJ, Eklund S, Earnest R, Burt B. Longitudinal investigation of bacteriology of human fissure decay: epidemiological studies in molars shortly after eruption. *Infect Immun* 1984; **46**: 765–72.

Marsh PD. Microbial ecology of dental plaque and its significance in health and disease. *Adv Dent Res* 1994; **8**: 263–71.

Marsh PD. Role of the oral microflora in health. *Microb Ecol Health Dis* 2000a; **12**: 130–7.

Marsh, PD. Oral ecology and its impact on oral microbial diversity. In: Kuramitsu HK, Ellen RP, eds. *Oral bacterial ecology: the molecular basis*. Wymondham: Horizon Scientific Press, 2000b: 11–65.

Marsh PD. Are dental diseases examples of ecological catastrophes? *Microbiology* 2003; **149**: 279–94.

Marsh PD. Dental plaque as a microbial biofilm. *Caries Res* 2004; **38**: 204–11.

Marsh PD. Dental plaque – biological significance of a biofilm and community life-style. *J Clin Periodontol* 2005; **32** (Suppl 6) 7–15.

Marsh PD, Bowden GHW. Microbial community interactions in biofilms. In: Allison DG, Gilbert P, Lappin-Scott HM, Wilson M, eds. *Community structure and co-operation in biofilms* (Society for Microbiology Symposium Vol. 59). Cambridge: Cambridge University Press, 2000: 167–98.

Marsh PD, Bradshaw DJ. Microbial community aspects of dental plaque. In: Newman HN, Wilson M, eds. Dental plaque revisited. *Oral biofilms in health and disease*. Cardiff: BioLine, 1999: 237–53.

Marsh PD, Martin MV. *Oral microbiology*, 4th edn. Oxford: Wright, 1999.

Meiers JC, Schachtele CF. Fissure removal and needle scraping for evaluation of the bacteria in occlusal fissures of human teeth. *J Dent Res* 1984; **63**: 1051–5.

Miller WD. *The micro-organism of the human mouth*. Unaltered reprint of the original work by Willoughby D. Miller (1853–1907) published in 1890 in Philadelphia. Basel: Karger, 1973.

Munson MA, Banerjee A, Watson TF, Wade WG. Molecular analysis of the microflora associated with dental caries. *J Clin Microbiol* 2004; **42**: 3023–9.

Nadkarni MA, Caldon CE, Chhour KL, *et al*. Carious dentine provides a habitat for a complex array of novel *Prevotella*-like bacteria. *J Clin Microbiol* 2004; **42**: 5238–44.

Nyvad B. Tidlig bakterieakkumiulation på emelje-og rodoverflader *in vivo*. PhD Thesis, Royal Dental College, Aarhus, Denmark, 1983. (In Danish.)

Nyvad B. Microbial colonization of human tooth surfaces. *APMIS* 1993; **101** (Suppl 32): 1–45.

Nyvad B, Fejerskov O. Experimentally induced changes in ultrastructure of pellicle on enamel *in vivo*. In: ten Cate JM, Leach SA, Arends J, eds. *Bacterial adhesion and preventive dentistry*. Oxford: IRL Press, 1984: 143–51.

Nyvad B, Fejerskov O. Scanning electron microscopy of early microbial colonization of human enamel and root surfaces *in vivo*. *Scand J Dent Res* 1987; **95**: 287–96.

Nyvad B, Fejerskov O. Structure of dental plaque and the plaque–enamel interface in human experimental caries. *Caries Res* 1989; **23**: 151–8.

Nyvad B, Fejerskov O. Development, structure and pH of dental plaque. In: Thylstrup A, Fejerskov O, eds. *Textbook of clinical cariology*. Copenhagen: Munksgaard, 1994: 89–110.

Nyvad B, Kilian M. Microbiology of the early microbial colonization of human enamel and root surfaces *in vivo*. *Scand J Dent Res* 1987; **95**: 369–80.

Nyvad B, Kilian M. Comparison of the initial streptococcal microflora on dental enamel in caries-active and in caries-inactive individuals. *Caries Res* 1990a; **24**: 267–72.

Nyvad B, Kilian M. Microflora associated with experimental root surface caries in humans. *Infect Immun* 1990b; **58**: 1628–33.

Öste R, Rönström A, Birkhed D, Edwardsson S, Stenberg M. Gas–liquid chromatographic analysis of amino acids in pellicle formed on tooth surfaces and plastic film *in vivo*. *Arch Oral Biol* 1981; **26**: 335–41.

Paster BJ, Bosches SK, Galvin JL, *et al*. Bacterial diversity in human subgingival plaque. *J Bacteriol* 2001; **183**: 3770–83.

Percival RS. Changes in oral microflora and host defences with advanced age. In: Percival S, Hart A, eds. *Microbiology and ageing: clinical manifestations*. Totowa: Human Press, 2007: in press.

Rateitschak-Plüss EM, Guggenheim B. Effects of a carbohydrate-free diet and sugar substitutes on dental plaque accumulation. *J Clin Periodontol* 1982; **9**: 239–51.

Ritz HL. Microbial population shifts in developing human dental plaques. *Arch Oral Biol* 1967; **12**: 1561–8.

van Ruyven FOJ, Lingström P, van Houte J, Kent R. Relationship among mutans streptococci, 'low-pH' bacteria, and iodophilic polysaccharide-producing bacteria in dental plaque and early enamel caries in humans. *J Dent Res* 2000; **79**: 778–84.

Scheie AA, Luan W-M, Dahlen G, Fejerskov O. Plaque pH and microflora of dental plaque on sound and carious root surfaces. *J Dent Res* 1996; **75**: 1901–8.

Schüpbach P, Ostervalder V, Guggenheim B. Human root caries: microbiota in plaque covering sound, carious and arrested carious root surfaces. *Caries Res* 1995; **29**: 382–95.

Schüpbach P, Ostervalder V, Guggenheim B. Human root caries: microbiota of a limited number of root caries lesions. *Caries Res* 1996; **30**: 52–64.

de Soet JJ, Nyvad B, Kilian M. Strain-related acid production by oral streptococci. *Caries Res* 2000; **34**: 486–90.

Sönju T, Glantz PO. Chemical composition of salivary integuments formed *in vivo* on solids with some established surface characteristics. *Arch Oral Biol* 1975; **20**: 687–91.

Svanberg M, Loesche WJ. The salivary concentration of *Streptococci mutans* and *Streptococci sanguis* and their colonization of artificial tooth fissures in man. *Arch Oral Biol* 1977; **22**: 441–7.

Svensater G, Welin J, Wilkins JC, Beighton D, Hamilton IR. Protein expression by planktonic and biofilm cells of *Streptococcus mutans*. *FEMS Microbiol Lett* 2001; **205**: 139–46.

Syed SA, Loesche WJ. Bacteriology of human experimental gingivitis: effect of plaque age. *Infect Immun* 1978; **21**: 821–9.

Tanzer JM. On changing the the cariogenic chemistry of coronal plaque. *J Dent Res* 1989; **68** (Special Issue): 1576–87.

Theilade E, Fejerskov O, Karring T, Theilade J. A microbiological study of old plaque in occlusal fissures of human teeth. *Caries Res* 1978; **12**: 313–19.

Theilade E, Fejerskov O, Karring T, Theilade J. Predominant cultivable microflora of human dental fissure plaque. *Infect Immun* 1982; **36**: 977–82.

Watson PS, Pontefract AH, Devine DA, *et al*. Penetration of fluoride into natural biofilms. *J Dent Res* 2005; **84**: 451–5.

Welin J, Wilkins JC, Beighton D, Svensater G. Protein expression by *Streptococcus mutans* during initial stage of biofilm formation. *Appl Environ Microbiol* 2004; **70**: 3736–41.

van Winkelhoff AJ, Boutaga K. Transmission of periodontal bacteria and models of infection. *J Clin Periodontol* 2005; **32**: 16–27.

Wood SR, Kirkham J, Marsh PD, Shore RC, Nattress B, Robinson C. Architecture of intact natural human plaque biofilms studied by confocal laser scanning microscopy. *J Dent Res* 2000; **79**: 21–7.

Zahradnik RT, Moreno EC, Burke EJ. Effect of salivary pellicle on enamel subsurface demineralization *in vitro*. *J Dent Res* 1976; **55**: 664–70.

Zaura-Arite E, van Marle J, ten Cate JM. Confocal microscopy study of undistorbed and chlorhecidine-treated dental plaque. *J Dent Res* 2001; **80**: 1436–40.

11

The role of saliva

A. Bardow, F. Lagerlöf, B. Nauntofte and J. Tenovuo

Introduction

Who made the first observation of the influence of saliva on the caries process is hidden in the mists of time, but around 1900 there were several case reports on the deleterious effects of absence of saliva. The father of cariology, Willoughby D. Miller, described as early as 1903 a woman suffering from excessive dryness of the mouth as follows: 'the teeth began decaying in a frightful manner, especially at the necks and along the free margins of fillings'. This is something that most experienced clinicians have seen in patients with severe impairment of saliva secretion. Since the time of Miller many reports on the relationship between caries and saliva have been published, and it is apparent that caries cannot be attributed to a single factor in saliva, but more to interplay among several salivary factors.

As shown in Fig. 11.1, saliva protects the teeth through a number of mechanisms that relate to both its fluid characteristics and specific components. Functions such as the rinsing effect, food and bacterial clearance, dilution of detritus, lubrication of dental surfaces, protection of the teeth by neutralization of acid by buffering actions, maintenance of supersaturation with respect to hydroxyapatite, and participation in enamel pellicle formation and antimicrobial defense are all examples of the many roles that saliva plays in determining oral health and disease. This chapter focusses on the multiple functions of saliva with relevance to caries.

Formation of saliva

To understand the complex interplay between the teeth and their surrounding fluid bath, it is of importance to understand how saliva is secreted and how its flow and composition are dynamic parameters that are controlled by the physiological and pathological conditions of the host. Factors such as the type of stimulus behind saliva formation, the host's medical history including systemic diseases and daily intake of medicines are examples of conditions that have great impact on saliva flow and composition and thereby are likely to affect the integrity of the teeth, perhaps leading to an increased number of caries lesions.

What is saliva?

Saliva is composed of more than 99% water and less than 1% solids, mostly electrolytes and proteins, the latter giving saliva its characteristic viscosity. The term 'saliva' refers to the mixed fluid in the mouth in contact with the teeth and oral mucosa, which is often called 'whole saliva'. Normally, the daily production of whole saliva ranges from 0.5 to 1.0 liters. Ninety per cent of whole saliva is produced by three paired major salivary glands, the parotid, submandibular and sublingual glands (Fig. 11.2). Secretions from the many minor salivary glands in the oral mucosa also contribute, although only somewhat less than 10%. In addition, whole saliva contains contributions from non-glandular sources such as gingival crevicular fluid in an amount that depends

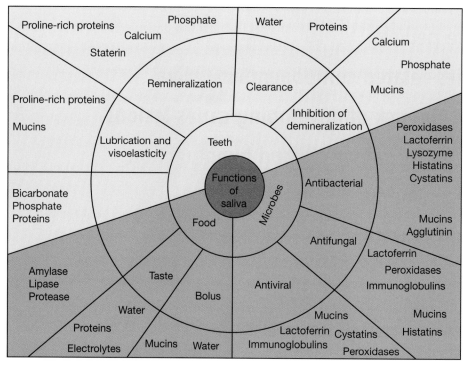

Figure 11.1 Multiple functions of saliva in relation to teeth, food intake and oral microbiology. As shown, both the quantity of saliva and its inorganic and organic composition have wide arrays of functions. (Modified from Amerongen & Veerman, 2002, and Van Nieuw Amerongen et al., 2004.)

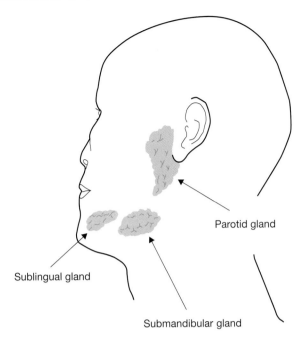

Figure 11.2 Location of the major salivary glands, the parotid, the submandibular and the sublingual in humans.

on the periodontal status of the patient. Whole saliva, in contrast to glandular saliva, also contains vast amounts of epithelial cells from the oral mucosa and millions of bacteria. These components give whole saliva its cloudy appearance, which is different from glandular saliva, which is transparent like water.

Salivary gland anatomy

The largest of the salivary glands are the parotid glands, which are purely serous glands that produce thin, watery, amylase-rich saliva. Upon saliva stimulation the parotids, just like the submandibular glands, contribute a little less than half of the volume of whole saliva. In the unstimulated state (i.e. the basal saliva secretion that occurs without stimulus in the mouth), however, the parotids contribute much less to the total volume of whole saliva, because the submandibular glands produce around two-thirds. The latter are mixed glands comprising both mucous and serous acinar cells, although they are mainly serous glands. In contrast to the parotids, they secrete more viscous, slimy, mucin-rich saliva. The sublingual glands, the smallest of the major glands, consisting mainly of mucous acinar cells, also produce such viscous secretion, although they only contribute a few per cent of the volume of whole saliva in both the unstimulated and stimulated state. In spite of their relatively low contribution to the volume of whole saliva, the minor glands secrete a large fraction of the total secretion of saliva protein with great importance for oral tissue lubrication. They are found in many parts of the oral mucosa and named according to their location, e.g. labial, buccal,

palatine, lingual or glossopalatine glands. The minor glands are mixed glands largely composed of mucous acinar cells, except for the palatine glands, which are strictly mucous, and the lingual von Ebner's glands, which are strictly serous.

The salivary glands, both the acinar and ductal segments, have a rich blood supply. In general, the secretory endpiece consisting of acinar cells represents about 80% of the gland mass. The duct system of the human parotid and submandibular glands is well developed and branched, containing intercalated, striated and excretory ducts, where the striated ducts make up the bulk of the duct tissue (Fig. 11.3). In sublingual glands and in a number of minor glands, the intercalated and striated ducts are sparsely distributed or even absent. In contrast to the duct of the major glands, the minor glands have short, small-diameter ducts. Around the secretory endpieces and intercalated ducts are contractile myoepithelial cells that aid in promoting the flow of saliva into the duct system by stimulus-activated constriction. The parotid duct opens into the mouth in the buccal mucosa (the parotid papilla) opposite the second maxillary molar. The saliva secreted from the submandibular and sublingual glands enters the mouth mostly through the submandibular duct, which ends on the sublingual caruncula just lateral to the frenulum of the tongue behind the mandibular front teeth, but the sublingual gland also secretes through several small ducts along the sublingual fold in the floor of the mouth lateral to the side of the tongue.

Control of saliva secretion

Saliva secretion is initiated by afferent signals from sensory receptors in the mouth transmitted by the trigiminal, facial and glossopharyngeal nerves (Fig. 11.3). These carry nerve impulses from chewing-activated mechanoreceptors in the periodontal ligament (masticatory–salivary reflex) and from taste-activated chemoreceptors in the taste buds within the lingual papillae (gustatory–salivary reflex) to the salivary nuclei in the medulla oblongata of the brain. The salivary nuclei then convey information to the efferent part of the reflex arch consisting of two branches, the parasympathetic and the sympathetic autonomic nerve bundles traveling separately to the glands. The sympathetic fibers follow the blood vessels supplying the glands and then separately innervate the glands, and the parasymathetic fibers follow the efferent facial or glossopharyngeal nerves.

The masticatory–salivary and the gustatory–salivary reflexes are referred to as unconditioned reflexes. However, the saliva secretion is also controlled by conditioned reflexes. Besides receiving impulses from the afferents, the salivary nuclei also receive impulses from higher centers of the brain. This gives rise to the release of a variety of neurotransmitters and neuropeptides resulting in facilatory or inhibitory effects on the preganglionic efferents. Accordingly, the integration of nervous output to the salivary glands is a result of a complicated central modulation of the incoming signals

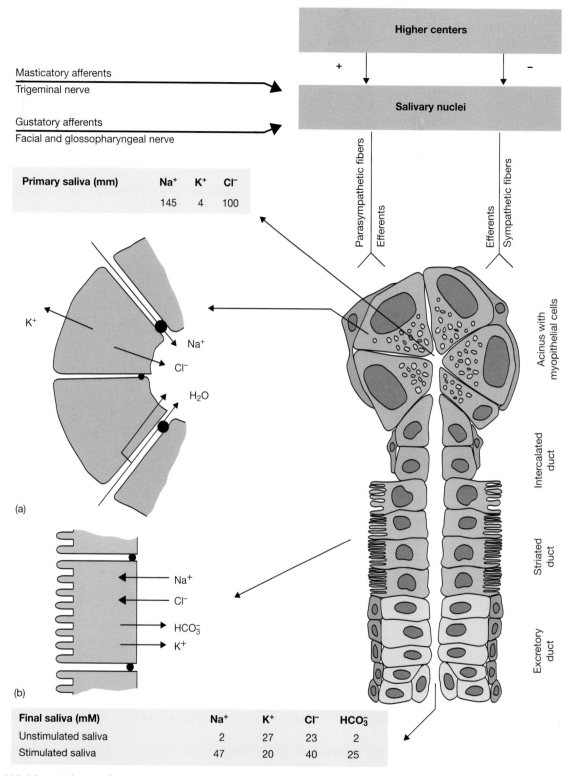

Higher centers

Salivary nuclei

Masticatory afferents
Trigeminal nerve

Gustatory afferents
Facial and glossopharyngeal nerve

Primary saliva (mm)	Na$^+$	K$^+$	Cl$^-$
	145	4	100

K$^+$

Na$^+$

Cl$^-$

H$_2$O

(a)

Na$^+$

Cl$^-$

HCO$_3^-$

K$^+$

(b)

Parasympathetic fibers

Efferents

Efferents

Sympathetic fibers

Acinus with myoepithelial cells

Intercalated duct

Striated duct

Excretory duct

Final saliva (mM)	Na$^+$	K$^+$	Cl$^-$	HCO$_3^-$
Unstimulated saliva	2	27	23	2
Stimulated saliva	47	20	40	25

Figure 11.3 Schematic drawing of a parotid secretory unit with nerve supply and with saliva composition before and after modification in the duct system. Usually, the ducts are branched, thereby serving several acini. Many of the ion transport mechanisms (pumps, ion channels, co-transporters and exchangers) and the cell signal transduction pathways of the acinar and ductal tissue are functionally similar. However, the ductal tissue has a low water permeability as opposed to the highly water-permeable acinar tissue. Upon stimulation, neurotransmitters bind to specific receptors that via coupling to different G-proteins activate cell signaling pathways, which result in the activation of a number of ion transporters in the cell membrane. Acinar cells [insert (a)] show some of the key events leading to the formation of primary saliva. Ductal cells [insert (b)] show some of the key events involved in the modification of primary saliva as it passes through the ducts to yield the final saliva, which is secreted to the oral cavity.

to the salivary nuclei. As a result of such central control, unstimulated salivation is normally inhibited during sleep, fear and mental depression. Stress may increase saliva flow when it produces a will to fight, but may also decrease saliva flow when it produces a feeling of anxiety or defeat.

Formation of saliva is a result of a unilateral, central reflex. Thus, stimulation of one side of the mouth induces ipsilateral salivation where the flow rate is dependent on the stimulus intensity applied, be it the intensity of taste or chewing. In general, the parasympathetic pathway provides the predominant control path of the salivary glands. The outcome of such stimulation is saliva with a high flow rate. Sympathetic stimulation leads to a lower flow rate and more protein-rich saliva. There are many other factors that influence the flow rate of saliva, including the water balance of the body, the nature and duration of the stimulus, previous stimulation and gland size.

At the peripheral salivary gland level, the control of salivation depends on neurotransmitter release from the parasympathetic and sympathetic nerve endings in the vicinity of salivary glands. The classical transmitters that activate secretion of saliva are acetylcholine and norepinephrine, but other substances released from the peripheral nerve endings also have important modulator effects on formation of saliva by the glands. Binding of neurotransmitters and neuropeptides to specific cell-surface membrane receptors on the richly innervated secretory endpieces and ductal systems activates a large number of biochemical events within the gland tissue. One of the most important is the rise in the intracellular free calcium concentration. This activates a number of transporters, and eventually leads to the formation of saliva.

Salivary secretion: the two-step model

Formation of saliva is not dependent on pressure filtration. It is due to active transport of solutes by the gland tissue and a dramatic increase in the metabolic turnover on stimulation. Basically, the formation of saliva occurs in two steps (Thaysen *et al.*, 1954) and includes activation of a number of plasma membrane transporters such as ion channels, pumps, co-transporters and exchange systems (Fig. 11.3).

The first step in the two-step model is the formation of the primary saliva. The secretion rate of saliva to the mouth is determined by the formation rate of primary saliva by the acinar cells. This formation is initiated by binding of neurotransmitters (e.g. acetylcholine or norepinephrine) to specific cell-surface receptors at the level of acinar cell membranes in the secretory endpieces. Thereby, a number of biochemical cascade reactions within the cell membranes and cytoplasm occurs which leads to secretion of primary saliva from the secretory endpiece. The general principle is that the acinar cell loses potassium to the interstitium and chloride to the lumen. These events occur in response to a receptor-activated intracellular increase in the free calcium concentration, which activates calcium-regulated potassium and chloride channels localized in the basolateral and luminal parts of the plasma membrane, respectively. In the lumen the gain of chloride creates a negative potential compared with the surroundings that drives interstitial sodium, via a paracellular transport route through cation-selective tight junctions, into the lumen, thereby restoring electroneutrality. A water flux, probably occurring by paracellular and transcellular pathways owing to the high water permeability of the acinar tissue, follows the net movement of salt into the lumen for osmotic reasons, resulting in acinar cell shrinkage. The outcome is the formation of isotonic primary saliva with concentrations of sodium and chloride resembling that of plasma (Nauntofte, 1992). The release of proteins from the acinar cells to the primary saliva also stands under nervous control and includes release of synthesized proteins by exocytosis.

The second step in the two-step model is the modification of the primary saliva in the ducts. Like in the acinar cells, binding of neurotransmitters to specific cell-surface receptors in the ductal tissues initiates a number of biochemical cascade reactions within the cell membranes and cytoplasm that leads to modification of the electrolyte composition of this fluid in the ductal system. As saliva passes along through the duct system it becomes modified, mostly by the selective reabsorption of sodium and chloride (without water) that occurs in the striated duct. In parallel to the reabsorption of sodium and chloride, a certain release of potassium and bicarbonate takes place. Owing to the low ductal water permeability the final saliva secreted into the mouth becomes hypotonic, with concentrations of sodium and chloride much below those of primary saliva. Some release of proteins to the saliva also occurs in the duct system.

Composition of saliva: a dynamic process

As shown in Fig. 11.4, the final composition of saliva secreted to the mouth depends strongly on the saliva flow rate (Dawes, 1969, 1974). Because the mechanisms involved in the reabsorption process have a maximal transport capacity and the ducts have limited time to modify the electrolyte composition at high stimulated flow rates, the reabsorption of salt falls behind and the stimulated saliva becomes less hypotonic, with higher concentrations of sodium and chloride than that of unstimulated saliva. The concentration of bicarbonate, an important buffer in saliva, is not constant but varies with the flow rate in such a way that unstimulated saliva contains only a few millimoles per liter, whereas stimulated saliva contains much higher levels depending on the stimulus intensity (Fig. 11.4). Owing to the flow-dependent variations in the saliva bicarbonate concentration, saliva pH is strongly dependent on the secretion rate. In healthy individuals it normally varies between about 6.0 and 7.5, with the most alkaline values obtained under stimulated flow rates. The latter is a result of the salivary gland tissue's

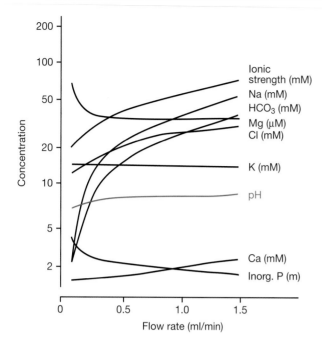

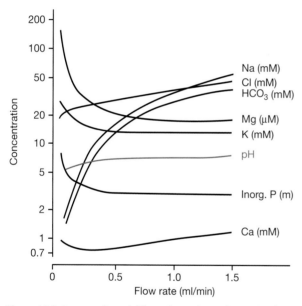

Figure 11.4 Concentrations of different inorganic constituents in saliva as a function of flow rate. Upper curves: submandibular/sublingual saliva; lower curves: parotid saliva. Note that the ordinates have logarithmic scales. The red line represents the saliva pH ($-\log [H^+]$).

high metabolic turnover during stimulation. The secreted bicarbonate is derived from carbon dioxide (CO_2) owing to the presence of carbonic anhydrase in the acinar and ductal cells as well as in saliva.

Hypofunction of salivary glands

Salivary gland hypofunction may be used as a term to cover both subjective symptoms and objective signs of dry mouth

(Nederfors, 2000). Xerostomia is defined as a subjective feeling of daily oral dryness, which often impairs oral functions such as swallowing and speech, and thus the overall health-related quality of life. Hyposalivation is a term based on objective measures of the saliva production, describing a condition where the flow rates of saliva are abnormally low. The cut-off value for unstimulated whole saliva flow rate is ≤0.1 ml/min and that of paraffin-chewing stimulated whole saliva is ≤0.5–0.7 ml/min (for women and men, respectively). These flow rates are significantly lower than the generally accepted 'normal values' in healthy individuals of around 0.3 ml/min for the unstimulated whole saliva flow rate and 1.5 ml/min for the chewing stimulated one. It should be noted that taste stimulation, especially sour taste, results in much higher flow rates. Xerostomia may exist without the patient fulfilling the criteria for the diagnosis of hyposalivation and hyposalivation may be symptomless, although xerostomia most often is associated with low saliva flow rates (Bergdahl, 2000).

In general, individuals may complain of oral dryness when the unstimulated (resting) whole saliva flow rate falls to about 50% of normal (Dawes, 1987). Such a large decrease in flow implies that more than one major salivary gland must be affected. The most common symptoms and signs in relation to xerostomia and hyposalivation are summarized in Table 11.1.

During childhood, the salivary secretion rate increases gradually with age, and adult levels are reached as late as at 14–16 years. In children hyposalivation is an unusual condition, whereas in elderly populations it is much more common owing to the increased prevalence of systemic

Table 11.1 Oral symptoms and signs related to oral dryness (xerostomia and hyposalivation)

Patient's complaints
Oral dryness and soreness
Burning sensation of oral mucosa and tongue
Difficulties in speech
Difficulties in chewing dry food
Taste impairment and disturbances
Difficulties in wearing removable dentures
Dry lips
Acid reflux, nausea, heartburn
Sensation of thirst
The oral symptoms are often associated with other symptoms such as dry skin, dry nose, dry eyes, dry vaginal mucosa, dry throat, dry cough and constipation

Signs
Mucosal dryness: dry glazed and red oral mucosa
Lobulation or fissuring of the dorsal part of the tongue
Atrophy of filiform papillae
Dry lips, angular cheilitis
Increased caries experience and activity with atypical pattern (in particular cervically)
Oral candidiasis

diseases and medication intake. However, old age per se does not reduce the whole saliva flow rates in healthy, non-medicated adults, despite the histological appearance of the salivary glands in elderly people suggesting decreased function.

Iatrogenic causes and diseases

Many medications induce complaints of oral dryness and influence saliva flow rate and/or composition (Table 11.2). Among these are antidepressants, antihypertensives (including diuretics) and antihistamines (Sreebny & Schwartz, 1997). Some of these medications may have peripheral interactions with the salivary gland muscarinic cholinergic receptor systems (antidepressants and antihistamines), thereby inducing impaired saliva volume. Others, such as diuretics, may induce compositional changes via their action on the body's salt and water balance and inhibitory effects on the electrolyte transporters in the salivary glands. The risk of salivary gland hypofunction also increases with the number of drugs taken and becomes especially high when more than three different drugs are taken per day. Another iatrogenic cause is radiotherapy against cancer in the head and neck region, where the radiation field has included one of the major salivary glands. This treatment leads to significantly impaired saliva secretion and irreversible damage to the salivary gland tissue (Jensen et al., 2003).

The presence of systemic disease is a common cause of impaired saliva secretion and compositional changes in the saliva (Table 11.2). The autoimmune disease Sjögren's syndrome, which has a prevalence as high as 3% and in particular affects women in the age range of 40–60 years, is the most prominent example (Pedersen & Nauntofte, 2001). Impaired saliva secretion is often observed in elderly patients because of the higher frequency of systemic diseases and high intake of medication in this population.

Oral clearance

The oral cavity is frequently exposed to substances with potentially harmful properties. Some of these substances have a direct influence on the caries process, for example different kinds of fermentable carbohydrates, most notably sucrose. An important function of saliva is therefore to dilute and eliminate substances. This is a physiological process usually referred to as salivary clearance or, more commonly, oral clearance.

The total volume of saliva spread out in a thin film on teeth and mucosa varies depending on several factors, but is usually small, 0.8–1.2 ml (Lagerlöf & Dawes, 1984). Since the mucosal surface area of the oral cavity is approximately 200 cm^2, the saliva film is only about 100 μm thick and varies between sites in the oral cavity. For example, the film is only about 10 μm in the palate and it has been shown that individuals experiencing xerostomia often have a saliva film less than that. The saliva film is moving slowly towards the throat with a speed varying from about 1 to 8 mm/min (Dawes, 1989); the slowest movement is in the front of the upper jaw and the fastest in the lower jaw. The main stream of saliva goes over the floor of the mouth at each side of the tongue with little exchange between the two streams. For example, a fluoride tablet placed in one side of the mouth will mainly raise the salivary fluoride concentration on that side only and very little fluoride is distributed to the other side (Weatherell et al., 1984).

Sucrose dissolved in the small volume of saliva may give rise to very high concentrations that will vary locally and with time after the exposure. Just a few sugar granules can cause high concentrations locally in the mouth. This means that patients with active caries who have frequent intake of sugar need to give up the sugar, not just reduce it. This is especially important for patients with low salivary flow rates. After an intake of sugar the salivary glands will be stimulated by taste or chewing to increase the flow rate, resulting in a swallow, which eliminates some of the sugar

Table 11.2 Some causes of salivary gland hypofunction comprising low saliva flow rates and/or changes in saliva composition

Diseases	
Autoimmune diseases	Sjögren's syndrome, rheumatoid arthritis, systemic lupus erythematosus, autoimmune thyroiditis
Hormonal disorders	Diabetes mellitus (labile)
Hereditary disorders	Cystic fibrosis, ectodermal dysplasia, familial amyloidotic polyneuropathy, sphingolipid storage disease (Gaucher disease), hereditary amyloidosis, Papillon–Lefèvre syndrome, thalassemia major
Infections	Human immunodeficiency virus, cytomegalovirus, hepatitis C, epidemic parotitis
Metabolic disturbances	Eating disturbances (anorexia nervosa, bulimia), malnutrition
Neurological disorders	Depression, cerebral palsy, Bell's palsy (idiopathic disruption of the facial nerve), Holmes–Adie syndrome
Local salivary diseases	Sialolithiasis, sialadenitis, carcinoma
Iatrogenic causes	
Medication	Antidepressants, antipsychotics, antianxiety agents, diuretics, antihypertensives, antihistamines, opiates, polypharmacy
Cancer treatment	Radiotherapy to head and neck, chemotherapy
Surgical trauma	

For review see von Bültzingslöwen et al. (2007).

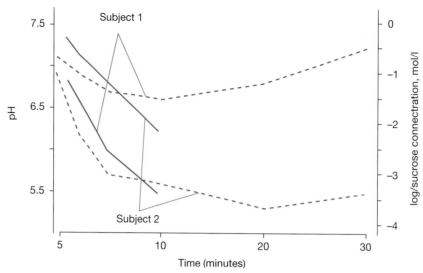

Figure 11.5 Two subjects have rinsed with a sucrose solution. They differ considerably in clearance rate (solid lines), causing a large difference in pH decrease (dashed lines) in the dental plaque. Subject 1 had a higher salivary flow rate than subject 2.

from the oral cavity. For each swallow the concentration of sugar will gradually decrease in a manner similar to a serial dilution in the laboratory. If the sugar concentration is plotted against time a fast initial decrease is found, after which the concentration gradually reaches zero (Fig. 11.5). To compare the clearance rate between different individuals a suitable measure of salivary clearance is needed. The time it takes to reach a certain detectable low level has been used in a measure called clearance time. The clearance half-time is a measure of the time it takes for the salivary sugar concentration to reach half of its initial concentration.

The clearance rate for a certain individual is fairly constant over time, but it varies to a great extent between individuals. Thus, the clearance rate depends on several factors, the most important being the salivary flow rate. A striking example is shown in Fig. 11.5, where the sugar concentration after 10 min differs by about 10 times between two individuals with different salivary flow rates (Lindfors & Lagerlöf, 1988). Figure 11.5 also shows that the clearance rate is fastest during the first minutes after sugar exposure owing to the effect of stimulated salivary flow.

The sucrose in the thin salivary film will rapidly diffuse into the plaque layer, which is usually many times thicker. The amount of sugar passing the saliva–plaque interface is dependent on the concentration gradient of sucrose between saliva and plaque fluid. Since this gradient is very steep during the first minutes, the sugar concentration in the plaque will increase rapidly. After only a few minutes it will be higher than in the saliva, where the concentration will diminish owing to the clearance process. It is important for both the therapist and the patient to know that sugar is available for bacteria in the plaque long after the sugar concentration in saliva has reached levels below the taste threshold for sugar.

Inorganic saliva composition

The ability of saliva to keep the oral environment supersaturated with respect to hydroxyapatite offers a protective and reparative environment for the teeth. The salivary components involved in maintaining supersaturation are salivary calcium and phosphate ions. Under physiological conditions the salivary buffer capacity will work in concert with these ions to maintain supersaturation by keeping a pH near neutral in the oral environment.

Saliva calcium

The concentration of calcium in saliva increases slightly from unstimulated to stimulated states of secretion, but remains mostly within the range from 1 to 2 mmol/l (Fig. 11.4). In whole saliva some calcium (around 20%) is bound to proteins such as statherin and proline-rich proteins. The salivary calcium that is not firmly bound to proteins can be divided into ionized and non-ionized calcium. Half of the non-protein-bound calcium is normally ionized and half is non-ionized. How much is in either form depends on saliva pH and ionic strength. The ionized and free form of calcium, at a given pH and ionic strength, is equal to the saliva calcium activity, and combined, all three forms (protein bound, ionized and non-ionized) make up the total calcium concentration.

Non-ionized calcium that is not bound to proteins is more or less firmly bound to inorganic ions, such as phosphate and bicarbonate as well as small organic ions (Lagerlöf & Lindqvist, 1982). When saliva pH and ionic strength increase at high flow rates (Fig. 11.4) more calcium will be in the non-ionized form. These relations are due to an increased likelihood of ions to meet and form pairs with many ions in solution (i.e. high ionic strength) and formation of various ion complexes with calcium at high pH. Calcium, which carries two positive charges, can also be strongly bound to ion species with two negative charges and a suitable steric configuration forming a chelate ring. Such compounds could be citrate originating from citric acid rich foodstuffs such as soft drinks and fruits. After exposure to such foodstuffs, the concentration of citrate in saliva becomes much higher than the concentration of calcium. Thereby, the ionized free calcium concentration in saliva can be reduced to very low values, which affect the saturation level with respect to hydroxyapatite (Bashir & Lagerlöf, 1996) and further accelerate demineralization of the teeth.

Saliva phosphate

Phosphates are phosphorus-containing compounds. As shown in Fig. 11.6, inorganic phosphate consists of phosphoric acid (H_3PO_4), dihydrogen phosphate ($H_2PO_4^-$), hydrogen phosphate (HPO_4^{2-}) and phosphate (PO_4^{3-}). As for calcium, some saliva phosphate is ionized, making up the phosphate activity (different for each form), and some is non-ionized (bound phosphate). The lower the pH, the lower the concentration of phosphate and the higher the concentration of phosphoric acid, and vice versa. Thus, the concentration of the individual ion relative to the other is determined by the saliva pH and by the dissociation constants (pK) for each of the three equilibriums involved in the phosphate buffer system. The sum of all four ions equals the total phosphate concentration. In contrast to calcium, the concentration of total phosphate decreases dramatically with increasing saliva flow rates. From a state of resting to a state of very high saliva stimulation the saliva total phosphate concentration may drop from nearly 10 mmol/l to 2–4 mmol/l (Fig. 11.4). Therefore, the total phosphate concentration is determined by the saliva flow rate. In contrast,

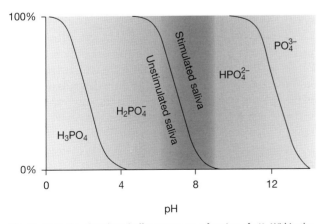

Figure 11.6 The phosphate buffer system as a function of pH. Within the physiological pH range (6.0–7.5) most phosphate is in the dihydrogen and hydrogen phosphate forms. In unstimulated saliva most is in the dihydrogen form and in stimulated saliva most is in the hydrogen form owing to higher pH in stimulated saliva compared with unstimulated. The gray area represents the normal pH range of human saliva

the saliva phosphate (PO_4^{3-}) concentration is determined by the saliva pH because it will be reduced to very low values by a low saliva pH (Fig. 11.6). This is why low saliva pH values are more harmful for the teeth than low total phosphate concentration in saliva.

Degree of saturation

It is important that saliva has a composition that protects the teeth against demineralization (see Chapter 12). Here, the salivary activities of calcium and phosphate (ionized forms) become important because both ions are part of the hydroxyapatite unit cell ($Ca_{10}(PO_4)_6(OH)_2$). In a repeated form the unit cells make up the large hydroxyapatite crystals that are the main inorganic component of human teeth. When the calcium, phosphate and hydroxyl ion activities are known, the ion activity product for hydroxyapatite (IAP_{HAp}) in saliva can be calculated by the formula:

$$IAP_{HAp} = (Ca^{2+})^{10} (PO_4^{3-})^6 (OH^-)^2$$

From this expression it can be seen that the ion activity product increases with increasing activities of these ions in saliva and vice versa. Although both the total calcium and total phosphate concentrations of saliva influence the ion activity product, the most important factor is the saliva pH. Thus, a drop in pH of one unit from pH 6 to pH 5 will reduce the hydroxyl ion activity 10-fold and the phosphate ion activity nearly 100-fold (Fig. 11.6), thereby reducing the overall ion activity product for hydroxyapatite many times (Lagerlöf, 1983). In a pure aqueous solution where complete equilibration between tooth substance and water has taken place, the ion activity product will be equal to the solubility product of tooth substance. Thus, the solubility product is a constant that needs to be determined. At mouth temperature the solubility product for human tooth substance is on average 10^{-117} mol^{18} l^{-18} (McDowell *et al.*, 1977). If the ion activity product is larger than the solubility product the saliva is supersaturated and remineralization may occur. If the ion activity product is smaller than the solubility product the saliva is undersaturated and demineralization may occur. However, saliva supersaturation or undersaturation does not imply that something will happen with the tooth substance, only that it can happen. This is because saliva contains specific proteins with inhibitory effects on these processes (see later).

Critical pH

When the ion activity product is equal to the solubility product of hydroxyapatite the solution is saturated and no demineralization or remineralization will occur. In dental literature, the pH value that corresponds to this level of saturation is often denoted as the critical pH value. The critical pH value is frequently referred to as a fixed value of pH 5.5 and used as a threshold value for determining when demineralization of human teeth can occur in the oral cavity. The value was determined in human saliva (Schmidt-Nielsen, 1946) and therefore it only refers to this fluid and not to other fluids such as soft drinks or water with different chemical compositions. The main determinants of critical pH are the total calcium and phosphate concentrations in saliva. As flow-dependent variations in total calcium and total phosphate concentrations occur constantly in human saliva, the saliva critical pH may vary by up to one pH unit from the mean critical pH with different flow rates (Dawes, 2003). Unstimulated saliva will generally have a lower critical pH than stimulated saliva owing to a higher total phosphate concentration in unstimulated saliva. Different individuals may also have different critical pH values owing to interindividual variations in saliva total calcium and phosphate concentrations. Thus, the critical pH in saliva is not constant, but more a dynamic variable, which varies around a mean pH value of 5.5.

Saliva buffer capacity and pH regulation

After intake of sugar-containing foodstuffs the pH in plaque will drop and remain lowered until the sugar is cleared from the mouth and the bacterial produced acid is buffered (Fig. 11.7). The magnitude of the pH drop is determined by the amount of acid that is produced by bacteria and by the saliva buffer capacity, the latter working at counteracting the pH drop. As tooth demineralization can occur when the actual pH drops below the critical pH, it is crucial to reduce the time that the actual pH stays below this value.

Various terms have been used for evaluation of saliva buffering capacity (Ericsson, 1959). One is the amount of acid that is needed to lower the pH from the original saliva pH value to a predetermined lower value. This term could be denoted the 'titratable base'. As shown in the upper part of Fig. 11.7, the titratable base for stimulated whole saliva down to pH 4 normally ranges between 20 and 30 mmol/l hydrogen ions. A more simple measure for the buffering capacity of human saliva is the 'buffer effect'. The buffer effect is determined by adding a fixed amount of acid to a fixed amount of saliva and then reading off a final pH value. The higher the final pH value the better the buffering capacity and vice versa. Test systems that use this method are available in various chairside versions for the dental clinic (see later for comments on the usefulness of these tests). The common chemical definition of buffer capacity, which is called β, has been used to determine the buffering capacity of human saliva in the laboratory. From titration curves the saliva buffer capacity can be determined in millimoles of hydrogen ions/(litre saliva · pH unit) in a certain pH interval:

$$\beta = \Delta C_A / \Delta pH$$

where ΔC_A is the increase in saliva acid concentration and ΔpH is the change in saliva pH (in pH units) caused by the addition of acid. If the addition of large amounts of acid

results in only a minor pH change the buffer capacity is high and vice versa. Because the buffer capacity can be determined for a limited pH range, this method has allowed for a detailed description of the buffer systems in human saliva, namely the phosphate, bicarbonate and protein buffer systems.

The phosphate buffer system

The dominant forms of phosphate within the physiological pH range are the hydrogen and dihydrogen phosphate forms. Unstimulated saliva has mainly dihydrogen phosphate and stimulated saliva mainly hydrogen phosphate (Fig. 11.6). The pK value for this equilibrium is around 7 in human saliva, where the pK value is the dissociation constant indicating when half of the buffer system is in the base form and half in the acid form. In general, buffers such as the phosphate and bicarbonate have their best effects in the range of ±1 pH unit around their pK values and with the highest capacity at the pK value (area 1 in Fig. 11.7). At this value a buffer system will buffer hydrogen ions equal to a little more than half its total concentration in moles or millimoles. As the saliva total phosphate concentration decreases with increasing flow rate, the contribution from phosphate to the overall buffer capacity decreases from around half in resting saliva to as little as 10% in highly stimulated saliva.

The bicarbonate buffer system

The saliva bicarbonate concentrations vary from about 3–5 mmol/l in resting saliva to a venous plasma level of 25–28 mmol/l in highly stimulated saliva. Owing to these variations, the contribution from the bicarbonate buffer system to the overall buffer capacity varies from a little less than half in resting saliva to more than 90% in stimulated saliva produced at high flow rates. The equilibrium for the bicarbonate buffer system is:

$$CO_2 + H_2O \leftrightarrow H_2CO_3 \leftrightarrow HCO_3^- + H^+$$

where CO_2 is carbon dioxide, H_2CO_3 is carbonic acid and HCO_3^- is bicarbonate. The hydration of CO_2 to carbonic acid and vice versa is catalyzed by the enzyme carbonic anhydrase, which is present in the salivary glands as well as in saliva. In saliva, CO_2 is present primarily as dissolved gas with a partial pressure (P_{CO_2}) in parotid saliva of around 6 kPa, which is equal to the P_{CO_2} in blood. A small drop in saliva P_{CO_2} occurs when it enters the mouth owing to nearly instantaneous CO_2 equilibration between saliva and exhaled air. The magnitude of the drop in P_{CO_2} varies with the flow of air passing over the thin salivary film and may be somewhat dependent on the breathing pattern. When CO_2 is lost from saliva the P_{CO_2} will drop and the pH increase, the latter because hydrogen ions are removed.

Upon buffering in a closed system the bicarbonate buffer system basically works in the same way as the phosphate buffer system by buffering hydrogen ions equal to around half its concentration at the pK value for carbonic acid,

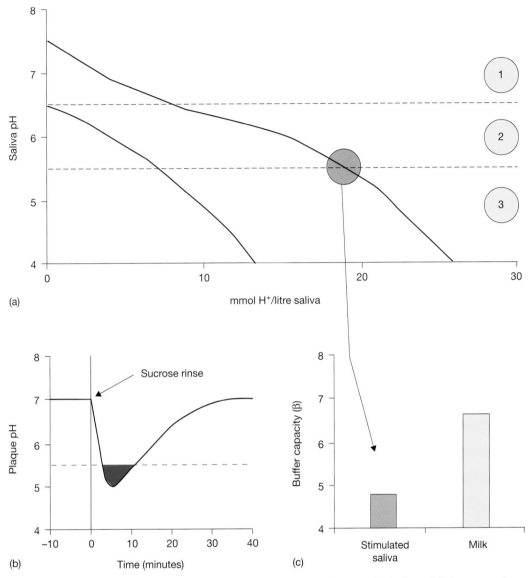

Figure 11.7 (a) Titration of whole saliva with strong acid in a closed system. The upper curve shows stimulated saliva and the lower curve shows unstimulated saliva. Above pH 5.5 the buffering capacity is high owing to the buffering ability of the phosphate (1) and bicarbonate buffer system (2). At low pH values the slope of the curve becomes steeper, indicating a lower buffer capacity mainly from salivary proteins (3). (b) Typical Stephan curve of plaque pH in response to an oral sucrose rinse. In spite of the saliva buffer capacity the plaque pH will drop immediately after the rinse to values below the critical pH of human saliva (red area), whereafter it slowly returns to baseline. The reason for this drop is that plaque may form a diffusion barrier that prevents diffusion of salivary buffer systems into the plaque. Moreover, the saliva buffer capacity is only moderate compared to, for example, many common foodstuffs when determined at pH 5.5 and in the range from pH 4 to 7, which is indicated by the circle and the arrow from (a). Thus as shown in (c), the buffer capacity of whole saliva is much less than that of, for example, milk.

which is near 6 in human saliva (area 2 in Fig. 11.7). The bicarbonate buffer system also has the ability to change form during buffering. Thus, as a result of the buffering action, CO_2 may be lost from the buffer system. This type of buffering is called phase buffering and adds an actual pH-rising capacity to the buffer system. In the mouth, which should not be considered a closed system, extensive phase buffering may occur, allowing for further buffering of remaining bicarbonate (Jensdottir *et al.*, 2005). As a result, the buffer capacity of the bicarbonate buffer system may be boosted more than four-fold compared with its own buffer capacity in a closed system (Izutsu, 1981). However, in spite of these effects the buffer capacity of human saliva is still only moderate compared with, for example, the buffer capacity of milk (Fig. 11.7). In the mouth the saliva buffer capacity therefore works in concert with the clearing effect of saliva. After some dilution has taken place the buffer systems in saliva can overcome the remaining acidic challenge in acid producing dental plaque and thereby increase plaque pH, as shown on the Stephan curve in Fig. 11.7.

The protein buffer system

Saliva contains many different proteins, which can act as buffers when the pH is above or below their isoelectric point. Below their isoelectric point proteins can accept protons and above it they can release protons. Many salivary proteins have their isoelectric point between pH 5 and 9 and therefore they become good buffers at alkaline and especially at acidic pH values (area 3 in Fig. 11.7). Although the buffering effect of the proteins is far less than bicarbonate and phosphate in human saliva, there are loci where saliva macromolecules are found in high concentrations, e.g. in integuments on both mucosa and teeth, and in these microenvironments the proteins become the dominant buffering substances. In addition to their chemical buffering, some of the saliva proteins increase the viscosity of the saliva when the pH becomes acidic and thereby physically protect the teeth against acid load by forming a diffusion barrier.

Saliva proteins

One milliliter of whole saliva contains between 1 and 2 mg of proteins and it is these proteins that give saliva its characteristic viscosity. There are distinct differences between the proteins from different glands depending on whether they are serous, mucous or a mixture of both. In its pure form parotid saliva has a viscosity close to that of water. In contrast, submandibular and sublingual salivas have a distinct ropy viscosity owing to their content of mucins, and this is given on to whole saliva. Almost all salivary proteins are glycoproteins, i.e. they contain variable amounts of carbohydrates linked to the protein core. Glycoproteins are often classified according to their cell origin and are further subclassified based on their biological properties. A characteristic feature is that glycoproteins may occur in multiple forms (polymorphism) having several functions and functional differences (Levine, 1993). Thus, most salivary properties are supported by a concerted action of several proteins.

Mucous glycoproteins

Mucous glycoproteins, mucins, are of acinar cell origin, have a high molecular weight and contain more than 60% carbohydrates (Tabak, 1995). The major mucins constitute a family with two members, MUC5B and MUC7 (Amerongen & Veerman, 2002). These are often also designated as high and low molecular weight mucins, respectively. Mucins are asymmetrical molecules with an open, randomly organized structure in which the carbohydrate side-chains often end in negatively charged groups, such as sialic acid. Mucins are hydrophilic, hold water and are therefore effective in lubricating and maintaining a moist mucosal surface, which is a prerequisite for the subjective feeling of a healthy mouth. Mucins also aggregate oral bacteria, thereby accelerating the clearance of bacteria from the mouth. Some oligosaccharides in mucins mimic those in mucosal cell surfaces and thus competitively inhibit the adhesion of bacterial cells to soft tissues by blocking reactive groups, adhesins, on bacterial cell surfaces. Thus, mucins help to protect the mucosa from infections. Mucins also interact with dental hard tissues and may mediate specific bacterial adhesion to the tooth surface (Slomiany et al., 1996). All of these functions will be compromised when the secretion of these proteins is reduced, as would be the case in dry-mouth patients with low saliva flow rates. Thus, several studies have reported an inverse relationship between the agglutinating activity of saliva and colonization by *Streptococcus mutans*.

Serous glycoproteins

Serous glycoproteins have a much lower molecular weight than mucins and contain less than 50% carbohydrate. Many of them belong to a group called proline-rich glycoproteins. These proteins are secreted from human parotid and submandibular glands. The variability of the side-chains contributes to the polymorphism of glycoproteins and adds different functional properties to them. The collective name glycoprotein for all carbohydrate-linked proteins makes this group heterogeneous and large. Most salivary proteins, such as secretory immunoglobulin A (IgA), lactoferrin, peroxidases and agglutinins, belong to this group.

Calcium binding proteins

Because human saliva is supersaturated with respect to most calcium phosphate salts, some proteins are needed to inhibit spontaneous precipitation of these salts in the salivary glands and their secretions. Such calcium-binding proteins are statherin and proline-rich proteins (PRPs). These proteins are never absent from saliva. The resulting stable, but individually to a varying degree, supersaturated state of saliva with respect to calcium salts constitutes a protective and reparative environment, which is important for the integrity of the teeth (see Chapter 12).

Statherin is present in both parotid and submandibular saliva. Although proteases of oral microflora are able to degrade statherin, it seems that concentrations of statherin remain high enough to exert its action as long as saliva remains in the mouth before swallowing. As an example of multifunctionality, statherin is also known to promote the adhesion of *Actinomyces viscosus* to tooth surfaces.

Acidic PRPs, which constitute as much as 25–30% of all proteins in saliva, form a complex group with a large number of genetic variants. Some of these can inhibit the spontaneous precipitation of calcium phosphate salts. PRPs are readily adsorbed from saliva to hydroxyapatite surfaces and they are present in initially formed acquired enamel pellicle. The multifunctional properties of PRPs, like statherins, are shown by their ability to promote selectively the attachment of bacteria, e.g. *A. viscosus* and *Streptococcus gordonii*, to apatitic surfaces. The modulation of bacterial adhesion is mediated by the carboxy-terminal region of the molecule, which is not able to bind to tooth surfaces.

Digestive enzymes

α-Amylase is the most abundant salivary enzyme, accounting for as much as 40–50% of the total salivary gland-produced protein. About 80% of amylase is synthesized in the parotid glands and the rest in the submandibular glands. The biological role of amylase is to split starch into maltose, maltotriose and dextrins. Maltose can be further fermented by oral bacteria, and also hydrolysis of maltotriose produces glucose as an endproduct. Amylase in saliva clears food debris, containing starch, from the mouth, but in this process bacteria-produced acids may be formed. Thus, starch has some cariogenic potential, as shown in pH measurements after the intake of processed starch *in situ*. It is recommended to avoid foods with processed starch, particularly among people with dry mouth owing to their slow oral clearance and the retention of such foodstuffs, which gives more time for the amylase to work.

Antimicrobial proteins and peptides

The major antimicrobial proteins of saliva are listed in Table 11.3. Most of these proteins can inhibit the metabolism, adherence or even the viability of cariogenic microorganisms *in vitro*, but their clinical role in the human mouth is largely unknown (Tenovuo, 1998). Nevertheless, oral hygiene products containing such proteins may alleviate

Table 11.3 Major antimicrobial proteins of human whole saliva

Protein	Major target/function
Non-immunoglobulin (innate) proteins	
Lysozyme	Gram-positive bacteria, *Candida*
Lactoferrin	Bacteria, yeasts, viruses
Salivary peroxidase and myeloperoxidase	Antimicrobial, decomposition of H_2O_2
Histatins	Antifungal, antibacterial
Cystatins	Antiviral, protease inhibitors
Agglutinins	
Parotid saliva glycoproteins	Agglutination/aggregation of a number of microorganisms
Mucins	Same
$β_2$-Microglobulin	Same
Immunoglobulins	
Secretory IgA	Inhibition of adhesion
IgG	Enhancement of phagocytosis
IgM	Enhancement of phagocytosis (?)

Adapted from Tenovuo (1998).
H_2O_2: hydrogen peroxide; IgA: immunoglobulin A; IgG: immunoglobulin G; IgM: immunoglobulin M.

symptoms among patients with dry mouth (Pedersen *et al.*, 2002) and reduce inflammatory conditions (Van Nieuw Amerongen *et al.*, 2004). Among healthy individuals with normal saliva flow, an increase in antimicrobial protein concentration in saliva by some oral hygiene products does not usually give better protection against dental caries. In healthy individuals these proteins seem mainly to be important for the control of microbial overgrowth in the mouth, but how selective they are against pathogens is not yet fully understood. Lysozyme in whole saliva comes from major and minor salivary glands, gingival crevicular fluid and salivary leukocytes. Salivary lysozyme is present in newborn babies at levels equal to those of adults and thus exerts antimicrobial functions before tooth emergence. The classical concept of the antimicrobial action of lysozyme is based on its muramidase activity, i.e. the ability to hydrolyze the β(1–4) bond between *N*-acetylmuramic acid and *N*-acetylglucosamine in the peptidoglycan layer of the bacterial cell wall. In addition to its muramidase activity, lysozyme, as a strongly cationic protein, can activate bacterial autolysins, which can also destroy the cell walls.

Lactoferrin is an iron-binding glycoprotein secreted by the serous cells of major and minor salivary glands. Leukocytes are also rich in lactoferrin and release this protein into gingival fluid and whole saliva. The biological function of lactoferrin is attributed to its high affinity for iron and its consequent expropriation of this essential metal from pathogenic microorganisms. Lactoferrin has bacteriostatic, bactericidal, fungicidal, antiviral and anti-inflammatory activity (Amerongen & Veerman, 2002).

Peroxidase systems in human saliva comprise two enzymes, salivary gland-derived peroxidase (SP) and leukocyte-derived myeloperoxidase (MP), together with thiocyanate (SCN⁻) ions and hydrogen peroxide (H_2O_2). Thiocyanate is a filtrate from serum and most H_2O_2 originates from aerobic oral bacteria. Peroxidases catalyze the oxidation of SCN⁻ by H_2O_2 to the antimicrobial component, hypothiocyanite (OSCN⁻):

$$\text{SP and/or MP}$$
$$H_2O_2 + SCN^- \rightarrow OSCN^- + H_2O$$

Salivary peroxidase systems have two major biological functions: antimicrobial activity, and protection of host proteins and cells from the toxicity of H_2O_2. Peroxidase systems are effective against a variety of microorganisms, such as mutans streptococci, lactobacilli, yeasts, many anaerobes (periodontal pathogens) and also some viruses (herpes simplex type 1, human immunodeficiency virus). *In vivo* the antimetabolic activity may be of importance, since the more hypothiocyanite in saliva, the less dental plaque produces acids after stimulation with glucose (Fig. 11.8). In Fig. 11.8 red circles indicate subjects with variable OSCN⁻ concentrations, and white circles those whose saliva has been supplemented with peroxidase-generated OSCN⁻. Thus, hypothiocyanite

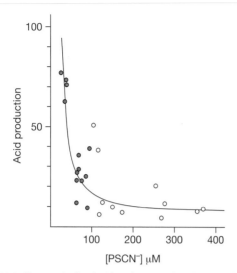

Figure 11.8 Glucose-stimulated acid production in dental plaque of subjects with different concentrations of hypothiocyanite [OSCN⁻] in whole saliva. Red circles indicate subjects with variable OSCN⁻ concentrations, and white circles subjects whose saliva has been supplemented with peroxidase-generated OSCN⁻.

concentration in saliva seems to have an important effect on plaque acidogenicity.

Cystatins (cystein-containing phosphoproteins) are considered to be protective by inhibiting unwanted proteolysis. Cystatins in saliva and acquired pellicle inhibit selected bacterial proteases, and proteases originating from lyzed leukocytes. Cystatins also affect calcium phosphate precipitation and may have some antiviral activity, suggesting multifunctionality of these molecules.

Of the salivary antimicrobial peptides, histatins have attracted most attention during the past few decades (Helmerhorst *et al.*, 1999). They have a broad antimicrobial spectrum against bacteria as well as oral yeasts. The histatins are synthesized in the parotid and submandibular glands, which means that they are practically always present in whole saliva. The possible association of histatins (and cystatins) with dental caries is unknown, although some cariogenic bacteria and *Candida albicans* are also sensitive to histatins *in vitro*.

Agglutinins

Agglutinins are glycoproteins, which have the capacity to interact with unattached bacteria, resulting in clumping of bacteria into large aggregates, which are more easily flushed away by saliva and swallowed. Therefore, the term aggregation is often used synonymously with agglutination. Some of the agglutinating proteins are listed in Table 11.3. The most potent one is a high molecular weight glycoprotein gp340, which has been found in human parotid saliva. The concentration of this agglutinin in parotid saliva is less than 0.1%, but as little as 0.1 µg of it can agglutinate 10^8–10^9 bacteria, including mutans streptococci.

Role of the pellicle

Saliva is seldom in direct contact with the tooth surface. The saliva compartment is separated from the surface of the tooth by a thin, bacteria-free biofilm called the acquired pellicle (Lendenmann *et al.*, 2000), which is an acellular layer of adsorbed salivary proteins and other macromolecules. The thickness of the pellicle varies between oral sites and may amount to 1–10 µm, becoming thicker with time. This thin layer forms the base for subsequent adhesion of microorganisms. The pellicle layer, even if thin, plays an important role in protecting the tooth against mechanical and chemical damage, but it also serves as a diffusion barrier (e.g. to acids). In the pellicle molecule movements due to forces other than diffusion are slower than in most other parts of the salivary film. The relatively undisturbed layer of liquid in the pellicle will therefore reduce the solubility of the enamel surface compared with whole saliva because of its high concentrations of calcium and phosphate. The pellicle is not removed mechanically by regular tooth brushing, but detergents from dentifrice and polishing with rubber cups and powders as well as acid etching and bleaching remove the pellicle. It is re-formed, however, within minutes except in a dry mouth, where it takes much longer. The lack of a pellicle will make tooth surfaces more susceptible to acids and thus demineralization.

The adsorption of macromolecules, usually originating from the saliva, to the tooth surfaces is selective, i.e. certain macromolecules show a higher affinity for the mineral surface than others. The surface of enamel is charged negatively in the normal oral pH range. This negative net charge is caused by the structure of hydroxyapatite, in which phosphate groups are arranged close to the surface. Counterions of opposite charge, e.g. calcium, are attracted to the surface, forming a hydration layer in which charges are unevenly distributed. The exact composition of this layer will be determined by several factors, e.g. pH, ionic strength and type of ions present in the saliva. Normally, this hydration layer contains mainly calcium and phosphate ions in the proportion 10:1, but other ions such as sodium, potassium and chloride are also present. Because of the domination of calcium, the resulting net charge of the enamel surface with its hydration layer is positive, implying that the hydration layer will attract negatively charged macromolecules. Negative charges on macromolecules are found in acidic side-chains of salivary macromolecules, such as MUC5B, which is a characteristic constituent of acquired pellicle.

The adsorption of the first molecule layer on a clean surface is instantaneous. The rate of formation of the pellicle is fast during the first hour, after which it decreases. The rate varies between individuals, owing to differences in salivary flow and composition. Because of the variation in salivary composition and influx at different areas inside the mouth, pellicle formation and composition are site specific (Hannig *et al.*, 2005). Many of the proteins that contribute to the pellicle are quite well defined, e.g. most glycoproteins identified in saliva are also found in the pellicle. Macromolecules, such as α-amylase, lysozyme, peroxidase, sIgA, IgG, carbonic anhydrases and glycosyltransferases, participate selectively in pellicle matrix formation, together with mucins and breakdown products from macromolecules of salivary, bacterial and even dietary background. Salivary enzymes exist in the pellicle as immobilized proteins and their enzymic activity *in situ* is affected by possible conformational changes during absorption. Many salivary constituents in the pellicle seem to be in a dynamic state of adsorption and desorption, but owing to their intimate closeness to both tooth surface and bacterial biofilm, these protein components are likely to exert their main biological activities on surfaces rather than in the liquid phase. Some proteins and peptides of the pellicle act as receptors for oral bacteria such as *Streptococcus* and *Actinomyces* species. These receptor proteins display genetic polymorphism, which may be linked to the adhesion of pathogenic/non-pathogenic microorganisms.

Other caries-related components in saliva

Saliva contains numerous substances other than those of pure salivary origin, and these substances may also have an effect on dental caries. Some of these substances are present in high concentrations in only a few individuals and very low concentrations in most other individuals. One example is the saliva level of urea, which can become very high in patients with chronic renal failure. In the mouth, an elevation of the saliva urea level will lead to binding of hydrogen ions and a more alkaline saliva pH. Therefore, it is not unusual to experience that such patients may have little caries in spite of having high plaque scores (Al-Nowaiser *et al.*, 2003). Another example of a caries-related substance in saliva is glucose, which may be high in diabetic patients with poor metabolic control. Such patients have been shown to develop more caries than diabetes patients with good metabolic control (Twetman *et al.*, 2002). Other substances may be ions coming from foodstuffs and geochemically via drinking water. One such ion, namely fluoride, has an important role against caries for all individuals.

Fluoride

The fluoride concentration in the secreted saliva is low and similar to that in blood and extracellular fluids. The concentrations of most saliva constituents are influenced by the salivary flow rate, but this is not the case for fluoride, although the concentration is slightly higher in unstimulated saliva (Shannon *et al.*, 1976). The fluoride concentration in the secreted saliva and the oral fluid depends strongly on the fluoride present in the environment, above all in the drinking water. In areas with low concentrations of fluoride in the drinking water the basal concentration of fluoride in whole saliva may be lower than 1 μmol/l. In areas with higher levels of fluoride in the drinking water the basal salivary concentration may be much higher. With increasing fluoride concentration in the drinking water the risk of systemic fluorosis of the enamel increases, while the prevalence of caries decreases (see Chapter 18). Other important sources of fluoride are foodstuffs and drinks, with fish and tea, in particular, being rich in fluoride. Products used for caries control, e.g. dentifrices and rinse solutions, are partly or fully swallowed and a minute amount of the ingested fluoride is excreted via the saliva. After ingestion the level of fluoride in the blood increases, reaching a peak after 30 min to 1 h. The concentration of fluoride in the duct saliva follows the plasma values, although at a 20–40% lower level. Crevicular fluid with fluoride concentrations roughly similar to plasma will contribute to the whole saliva concentration of fluoride, especially in the microenvironment close to the gingiva. As previously stated, the volume of saliva present in the mouth is small, perhaps only a milliliter spread out in a thin film. Even a very small amount of fluoride dissolved in this small volume of saliva will result in a high fluoride concentration that may be more than 10 000 times the basal levels. Close to the fluoride source, e.g. remnants of toothpaste after brushing, even higher fluoride concentrations could be expected. This fact stresses the importance of locally applied fluoride preparations for caries control. After the initial fluoride exposure of the oral cavity, the salivary concentration of fluoride decreases rapidly owing to oral clearance. The most important factor for the fluoride clearance rate is, as for sugar, the salivary flow rate, which is mainly dependent on the degree of stimulation. Fluoride preparations vary greatly as salivary stimuli depending on their taste properties. A strong-tasting topical fluoride, e.g. toothpaste, may counteract its own aim as a fluoride source, in that the stimulated saliva flow inevitably will increase the rate of clearance of the applied fluoride. Tooth brushing before bedtime will increase the fluoride concentration during sleep when the clearance is very slow, and thus give a long period with high fluoride concentrations in the oral cavity.

The current approach to caries control stresses the importance of fluoride present in the oral fluids close to sites of action, i.e. where the dissolution of the hard tissues takes place. Therefore, most strategies to control caries involve measures to increase the fluoride concentration locally in the oral fluids. Fluoride will diffuse from the thin saliva film into the plaque, elevating the fluoride concentration in the plaque fluid considerably in a short time. Both in saliva and, more importantly, in plaque, mineral calcium fluoride will form. The calcium fluoride functions as a slow releaser of fluoride (Chapter 18). Fluoride also forms a complex ion with magnesium, the concentration of which in both saliva and plaque is only about 10% of the calcium concentration. In that way, fluoride diffusing into the microorganisms prevents the enzyme enolase from taking part in the glycolytic pathway by binding magnesium, which is needed for the optimum function of the enzyme.

Saliva and the risk of developing caries lesions

In general, caries can develop in all individuals regardless of their saliva flow and saliva composition. Thus, from a physiological point of view no one has saliva that would make them resistant to caries. However, there are notable differences in caries between individuals, some of which can be explained by saliva (Rudney, 1995). Patients suffering from salivary gland hypofunction often have increased caries activity and progression compared with individuals with normal saliva function. In such patients caries is often observed in relation to retention sites for dental plaque, especially along the gingival margin on root surfaces and adjacent to dental fillings. In patients who have received radiation therapy to the head and neck region, but also in patients with autoimmune diseases of the salivary glands such as primary Sjögren's syndrome, the lack of saliva can lead to rapidly developing caries even in atypical places such as lingual, incisal and cuspal tooth surfaces (Figs 11.9,

11.10). Thus, knowledge about the salivary status of a given patient is a valuable tool in identifying patients at risk, and may give the clinician the possibility of evaluating prognosis and planning treatments on an individual level (Chapter 27). Whenever saliva is part of an evaluation one should distinguish between the effects of the quantity of saliva and the effects of the quality of saliva.

Quantity of saliva

In patients with reduced quantity of saliva the mechanistic and cleaning properties of saliva in the mouth are impaired. A slow oral sugar clearance rate inevitably increases the risk of caries. Thus, numerous clinical studies have shown that a reduced ability to produce saliva is associated with an increased caries experience (Leone & Oppenheim, 2001). Concerning this relation, the unstimulated flow rate has been found to be diagnostically more important than the stimulated one (Bardow et al., 2003). Although many clinicians have observed that patients suffering from chronically impaired saliva secretion are prone to dental decay, no cut-off value has been defined for the increased risk of developing dental caries with regard to unstimulated or stimulated flow rates (Tenovuo, 1997). It seems that individuals with subnormal unstimulated saliva flow rates (<0.2 ml/min) as a group have an elevated demineralization rate and a higher risk of developing caries. Unstimulated saliva flow rates below this level will also markedly increase the clearance time compared with flow rates above this level (Dawes, 1983). This will prolong periods with low pH values in the plaque. A low saliva flow rate, and especially a low unstimulated saliva flow rate, also seems to favor an acidic and more cariogenic dental microflora rich in acidogenic and aciduric bacteria, such as lactobacilli and mutans streptococci. Thus, a low saliva flow rate not only will prolong clearance time and periods with low plaque pH, but also may change the ecology of the mouth. The long-term effects of a low saliva flow rate may become much more complex

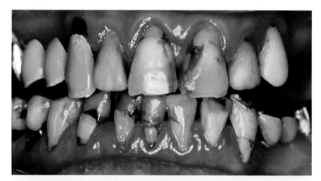

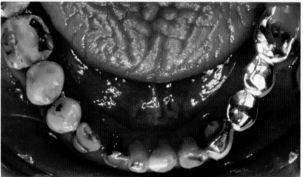

Figure 11.9 Clinical manifestations of dry mouth in a woman with Sjögren's syndrome. The upper picture shows multiple caries lesions and the lower picture shows dry mucosal surfaces and tongue in the same patient.

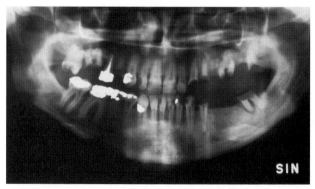

Figure 11.10 A patient with hyposalivation due to a unilateral radiation dose of >40 Gy to an area including the left parotid and submandibular glands. Note the extensive dental caries and loss of teeth on the left side of the maxilla and mandible, which has occurred over time following irradiation.

than the purely mechanistic considerations relating to long clearance times. Patients with low saliva flow rates generally experience a faster caries lesion progression rate than individuals with normal saliva flow rates. Where it may take years for caries to progress through the enamel in individuals with normal saliva flow rates it may take only months in patients with low saliva flow rates. Therefore, regular dental examinations at short time intervals are important in these patients (Fig. 11.9 and Chapter 27).

Measurements of whole saliva flow rates

Ideally, evaluation of salivary function should be a routine part of any oral examination. The first step in identifying an individual with potential salivary gland hypofunction includes a thorough questioning of the patient. This must include questions about medication intake, chronic diseases and previous radiation therapy in the head and neck region (Table 11.2). It should also include questions about symptoms of oral dryness and compromised oral functions related to saliva secretion (Table 11.1). As an absolute minimum, measurements of whole saliva output should be performed in patients with symptoms of xerostomia (Narhi *et al.*, 1999), and in patients where the routine clinical inspection of the oral cavity shows that the patient's caries activity is increased or if mucosal integrity is affected (dryness or yeast infection). It is certainly not sufficient to draw any conclusion regarding the salivary status solely on interview and clinical inspection of the saliva pool in the floor of the mouth. It is also important to follow regularly saliva flow rates among caries-prone individuals, since single-point measurement has limited diagnostic value of the individual's salivary function. The following is a description of a relatively simple method for the measurement of secretion rates of whole saliva that easily can be conducted in the dental clinic.

The tools required are a watch, an electronic weight with two digits, a plastic cup and 1 g of paraffin (inert chewing material) for saliva stimulation. For comparisons of salivary gland function over time, collections in a certain patient should be carried out at the same time of day. In general, patients must have nothing by mouth, including smoking, for at least 90 min before the measurement of unstimulated secretions and stimulation must be done in a reproducible manner. Measurement of the production of unstimulated whole saliva is usually performed for 15 min and for chewing-stimulated saliva for 5 min.

Before the saliva collection procedure starts, the subject must be seated in a chair to relax for a few minutes. The collection of unstimulated saliva occurs without any masticatory or gustatory stimulus, and is just based on passive drooling (or gentle drips every minute) of the saliva into a cup (Fig. 11.11). The patient should be seated in a relaxed position with elbows resting on knees and with the head tilted forward between the arms to allow the saliva to drain

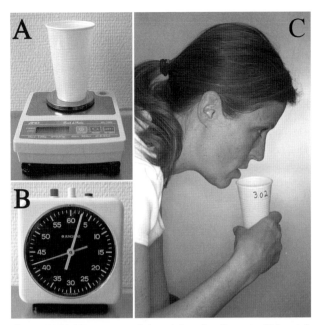

Figure 11.11 Measurement of the whole saliva flow rate (sialometry). Materials required are a plastic cup for collection and weight with two digits (A) and a stopwatch (B). During saliva collection the patient is placed in a relaxed, hunched-over position, with the face tilted slightly downwards (C).

passively from the lower lip into a preweighed plastic cup. Even slight movements of the tongue, cheeks, jaws or lips should be avoided during the collection period. After an initial swallowing action the collection starts at time zero. At the end of the collection period, the patient must empty all residual saliva from the mouth into the cup. After weighing the saliva-containing plastic cup and subtracting the weight of the cup, the flow rate can be calculated in g/min, which is almost equivalent to ml/min (Navazesh & Christensen, 1982). Collection of stimulated whole saliva should be performed after the collection of unstimulated saliva and the procedure includes almost the same steps described above, except for a much shorter collection time and the application of a chewing stimulus at the natural chewing frequency of the patient. Every 30 s during the collection, the patient should let the saliva drip into the preweighed plastic cup for a few seconds, after which the saliva collection continues.

With these simple methods it is possible for clinicians to test whether a patient has a subnormal saliva flow rate, and thus whether, for salivary reasons, the patient should be expected to have an increased risk of developing caries.

The quality of saliva

The teeth that are most bathed in saliva, the lower canines and lower incisors, are less susceptible to caries than the teeth in other oral locations. Such intraoral differences in caries susceptibility are in part due to intraoral differences in clearance, and also to the numerous substances in saliva that protect against caries. Early studies on caries and saliva composition mainly related the inorganic composition of saliva to caries. In those times, with high caries incidence and before fluoride dentifrice, relationships were often obtained between saliva composition and caries. Thus, by comparing large groups of individuals with caries to groups without caries it was often shown that high saliva buffer capacity and high saliva concentrations of calcium and phosphate were caries protective (Tenovuo, 1997). Therefore, several simple tests of the saliva buffer capacity have been developed over the years and used as 'caries tests'. The usefulness of these tests for predicting caries risk is, however, questionable, because what can be shown for a group may still have little predictive value on an individual level. In addition, the introduction of powerful caries-control measures such as fluoride dentifrice may to some extent have reduced the importance of weaker biological factors such as saliva buffer capacity and saturation levels with respect to hydroxyapatite.

Apart from determining the inorganic chemistry of the mouth, a steady supply of saliva will also guarantee a continuous presence of both non-immune and immune proteins in the mouth (Tenovuo, 2002). The immunological factors, such as secretory IgA and serum IgG antibodies, are present in saliva at an early age, but their capacity to inactivate pathogens is highest among adults. Most non-immunoglobulin factors, however, work at almost full capacity during early childhood, thus providing protection while the humoral immune system is still immature. In relatively infrequent cases of immunodeficiency, it has been observed that the non-immunoglobulin factors of saliva form a back-up system, which compensates for the lack of antibodies. Therefore, for example, IgA-deficient patients or patients with common variable immunodeficiency do not seem to have an increased risk of dental caries. Furthermore, there is no evidence, despite extensive study, that any single salivary antimicrobial protein is more important than the others (Tenovuo, 1998). Instead, they seem to form a network (Rudney, 1995) with concerted effects because additive or synergistic interactions have been found between many salivary antimicrobial proteins. Quantification of these factors does not provide diagnostic help in the assessment of individual caries risk. Enhancement of individual antimicrobial systems, or an increase in individual antimicrobial protein concentration in saliva (e.g. by some oral hygiene products), does not usually give better protection against dental caries in individuals with normal saliva flow. In another view, however, several studies have reported an inverse relationship between the agglutinating activity of saliva and colonization by *Streptococcus mutans*, and also a positive correlation between the adhesion-promoting activity for pathogenic microorganisms of saliva and dental caries. As the individual profile of salivary proteins that mediate agglutination and inhibition of bacterial adhesion

seems to be genetically determined (Rudney, 1995), new aspects of saliva composition for dental caries may arise in the future.

Management of salivary gland hypofunction

Patients with salivary gland hypofunction are predisposed for caries and oral mucosal infections. Thus, intensive caries preventive care including an individually tailored prophylactic dental program is often necessary. The key concepts of preventive dental management include careful oral hygiene instruction to improve the patient's oral hygiene and regular (at least every 3 months) follow-up at a dental clinic, including dental plaque control, dietary instruction and advice, as well as regular application of topical fluoride to reduce caries activity and help preserve dentition. Sugar-free chewing gum containing fluoride may be a useful tool. In patients with low saliva flow rates, the beneficial effect of fluoride on tooth substance is prolonged owing to reduced oral clearance. During meals, hyposalivating patients should be advised to sip water and after the meal the mouth should be rinsed thoroughly with water. Gustatory and/or masticatory stimulation with regular use of sugar-free sweets or sugarless chewing gum are stimulants to increase the secretion of saliva. Pharmacological sialogogues (e.g. pilocarpine and cevimeline), via activation of muscarinic cholinergic receptors in the salivary gland tissue, may lead to increased salivary secretion in patients with remaining functional gland tissue. They should be prescribed only in collaboration with the patient's physician, to avoid unexpected side-effects such as the aggravation of heart disease or interactions with other drugs. The patient's medication should be checked for 'saliva-inhibiting xerostomic' effects (Sreebny & Schwartz, 1997) and, if possible, changed to drugs with fewer adverse effects. The systemic disease has a higher treatment priority and the necessary medication should not be changed for dental reasons alone. Symptoms of oral dryness may be alleviated by the use of mouth gels, oral sprays or artificial saliva. Some of the latter products contain carbomethylcellulose, mucins or electrolytes.

Concluding remarks

Saliva has numerous effects working towards protection against caries, some by inhibition of bacteria, some by dilution and elimination of bacteria and their substrates, some by buffering bacterial acids, and some by offering a reparative environment after bacterial-induced demineralization of teeth. Patients suffering from salivary gland hypofunction are therefore at risk of developing caries and should receive an individually tailored prophylactic dental program including intensive caries preventive care. This includes instructions to improve the patient's oral hygiene, appropriate dietary advice, and targeted use of antimicrobials and regular topical fluoride treatments to help preserve dentition when the natural protection from saliva is reduced.

Background literature

Bardow A, Pedersen AM, Nauntofte B. Saliva. In: Miles T, Nauntofte B, Svensson P, eds. *Clinical oral physiology*. Copenhagen: Quintessence, 2004: 17–51.

Edgar WM, Dawes C, O'Mullane DM. *Saliva and oral health*, 3rd edn. London: British Dental Association, 2004.

Ferguson DB. The salivary glands and their secretions. In: Ferguson DB, ed. *Oral bioscience*. Edinburgh: Churchill Livingstone, 1999: 117–50.

Garrett JR, Proctor GB. Control of salivation. In: Linden RWA, ed. *The scientific basis of eating*. Basel: Front Oral Biol, Karger, 1998: 135–55.

Nauntofte B, Jensen JL. Salivary secretion. In: Yamada T, Alpers DH, Laine L, Owyang C, Powell DW, eds. Textbook of gastroenterology, 3rd edn. Philadelphia, PA: Williams & Wilkins, 1999: 263–78.

Tenovuo J. *Human saliva: clinical chemistry and microbiology*, Vols I and II. Boca Raton, FL: CRC Press, 1989.

References

Al-Nowaiser A, Roberts GJ, Trompeter RS, Wilson M, Lucas VS. Oral health in children with chronic renal failure. *Pediatr Nephrol* 2003; **18**: 39–45.

Amerongen AV, Veerman E. Saliva – the defender of the oral cavity. *Oral Dis* 2002; **8**: 12–22.

Bardow A, ten Cate JM, Nauntofte B, Nyvad B. Effect of unstimulated saliva flow rate on experimental root caries. *Caries Res* 2003; **37**: 232–6.

Bashir E, Lagerlöf F. Effect of citric acid clearance on the saturation with respect to hydroxyapatite in saliva. *Caries Res* 1996; **30**: 213–17.

Bergdahl M. Salivary flow and oral complaints in adult dental patients. *Community Dent Oral Epidemiol* 2000; **28**: 59–66.

Dawes C. The effects of flow rate and duration of stimulation on the concentrations of protein and the main electrolytes in human parotid saliva. *Arch Oral Biol* 1969; **14**: 277–94.

Dawes C. The effects of flow rate and duration of stimulation on the concentrations of protein and the main electrolytes in human submandibular saliva. *Arch Oral Biol* 1974; **19**: 887–95.

Dawes C. A mathematical model of salivary clearance of sugar from the oral cavity. *Caries Res* 1983; **17**: 321–34.

Dawes C. Physiological factors affecting salivary flow rate, oral sugar clearance, and the sensation of dry mouth in man. *J Dent Res* 1987; **66**: 648–53.

Dawes C. An analysis of factors influencing diffusion from dental plaque into a moving film of saliva and the implications for caries. *J Dent Res* 1989; **68**: 1483–8.

Dawes C. What is the critical pH and why does a tooth dissolve in acid? *J Can Dent Assoc* 2003; **69**: 722–4.

Ericsson Y. Clinical investigations of the salivary buffering action. *Acta Odontol Scand* 1959; **97**: 131–65.

Hannig C, Hannig M, Attin T. Enzymes in the acquired enamel pellicle. *Eur J Oral Sci* 2005; **113**: 2–13.

Helmerhorst EJ, Hodgson R, van't Hof W, Veerman EC, Allison C, Nieuw Amerongen AV. The effects of histatin-derived basic antimicrobial peptides on oral biofilms. *J Dent Res* 1999; **78**: 1245–50.

Izutsu KT. Theory and measurement of the buffer value of bicarbonate in saliva. *J Theor Biol* 1981; **90**: 397–403.

Jensdottir T, Nauntofte B, Buchwald C, Bardow A. Effects of sucking acidic candy on whole-mouth saliva composition. *Caries Res* 2005; **39**: 468–74.

Jensen SB, Pedersen AM, Reibel J, Nauntofte B. Xerostomia and hypofunction of the salivary glands in cancer therapy. *Support Care Cancer* 2003; **11**: 207–25.

Lagerlöf F. Effects of flow rate and pH on calcium phosphate saturation in human parotid saliva. *Caries Res* 1983; **17**: 403–11.

Lagerlöf F, Dawes C. The volume of saliva in the mouth before and after swallowing. *J Dent Res* 1984; **63**: 618–21.

Lagerlöf F, Lindqvist L. A method for determining concentrations of calcium complexes in human parotid saliva by gel filtration. *Arch Oral Biol* 1982; **27**: 735–8.

Lendenmann U, Grogan J, Oppenheim FG. Saliva and dental pellicle – a review. *Adv Dent Res* 2000; **14**: 22–8.

Leone CW, Oppenheim FG. Physical and chemical aspects of saliva as indicators of risk for dental caries in humans. *J Dent Educ* 2001; **65**: 1054–62.

Levine MJ. Development of artificial salivas. *Crit Rev Oral Biol Med* 1993; **4**: 279–86.

Lindfors B, Lagerlöf F. Effect of sucrose concentration in saliva after a sucrose rinse on the hydronium ion concentration in dental plaque. *Caries Res* 1988; **22**: 7–10.

McDowell H, Gregory TM, Brown WE. Solubility of $Ca_5(PO_4)_3OH$ in the system $Ca(OH)_2$–H_3PO_4–H_2O at 5, 15, 25, and 35.5°C. *J Res Natl Bur Stand* 1977; **72**: 773–82.

Narhi TO, Meurman JH, Ainamo A. Xerostomia and hyposalivation. Causes, consequenses and treatment in the elderly. *Drugs Aging* 1999; **15**: 103–16.

Nauntofte B. Regulation of electrolyte and fluid secretion in salivary acinar cells. *Am J Physiol* 1992; **263**: G823–37.

Navazesh M, Christensen CM. A comparison of whole mouth resting and stimulated salivary measurement procedures. *J Dent Res* 1982; **61**: 1158–62.

Nederfors T. Xerostomia and hyposalivation. *Adv Dent Res* 2000; **14**: 48–56.

Pedersen AM, Nauntofte B. Primary Sjögren's syndrome: oral aspects on pathogenesis, diagnostic criteria, clinical features and approaches for therapy. *Expert Opin Pharmacother* 2001; **2**: 1415–36.

Pedersen AM, Andersen TL, Reibel J, Holmstrup P, Nauntofte B. Oral findings in patients with primary Sjogren's syndrome and oral lichen planus – a preliminary study on the effects of bovine colostrum-containing oral hygiene products. *Clin Oral Investig* 2002; **6**: 11–20.

Rudney J. Does variability in salivary protein concentrations influence oral microbial ecology and oral health? *Crit Rev Oral Biol Med* 1995; **6**: 343–67.

Schmidt-Nielsen B. The solubility of tooth substance in relation to the composition of saliva. *Acta Odontol Scand* 1946; **7**(Suppl 2): 1–88.

Shannon IL, Feller RP, Chauncey HH. Fluoride in human parotid saliva. *J Dent Res* 1976; **55**: 506–9.

Slomiany BL, Murty VLN, Piotrowski J, Slomiany A. Salivary mucins in oral mucosal defence. *Gen Pharmacol* 1996; **27**: 761–71.

Sreebny LM, Schwartz SS. A reference guide to drugs and dry mouth – 2nd edition. *Gerodontology* 1997; **14**: 33–47.

Tabak LA. In defence of the oral cavity: structure, biosynthesis, and function of salivary mucins. *Annu Rev Physiol* 1995; **57**: 547–64.

Tenovuo J. Salivary parameters of relevance for assessing caries activity in individuals and populations. *Community Dent Oral Epidemiol* 1997; **25**: 82–6.

Tenovuo J. Antimicrobial function of human saliva – how important is it for oral health? *Acta Odontol Scand* 1998; **56**: 250–6.

Tenovuo J. Antimicrobial agents in saliva – protection for the whole body. *J Dent Res* 2002; **81**: 807–9.

Thaysen JH, Thorn NA, Schwartz IL. Excretion of sodium, potassium, chloride and carbon dioxide in human parotid saliva. *Am J Physiol* 1954; **178**: 155–9.

Twetman S, Johansson I, Birkhed D, Nederfors T. Caries incidence in young type 1 diabetes mellitus patients in relation to metabolic control and caries-associated risk factors. *Caries Res* 2002; **36**: 31–5.

Van Nieuw Amerongen A, Bolscher JG, Veerman EC. Salivary proteins: protective and diagnostic value in cariology? *Caries Res* 2004; **38**: 247–53.

von Bültzingslöwen I, Sollecito TP, Fox PC, Daniels T, Jonsson R, Lockhart PB, et al. Salivary dysfunction associated with systemic diseases: systematic review and clinical management recommendations. *Oral Surg Oral Med Oral Pathol Oral Radiol Endod* 2007; **103**(Suppl 1): S57.e1–S57.e15.

Weatherell JA, Robinson C, Ralph JP, Best JS. Migration of fluoride in the mouth. *Caries Res* 1984; **18**: 348–53.

12

Chemical interactions between the tooth and oral fluids

J.M. ten Cate, M.J. Larsen, E.I.F. Pearce and O. Fejerskov

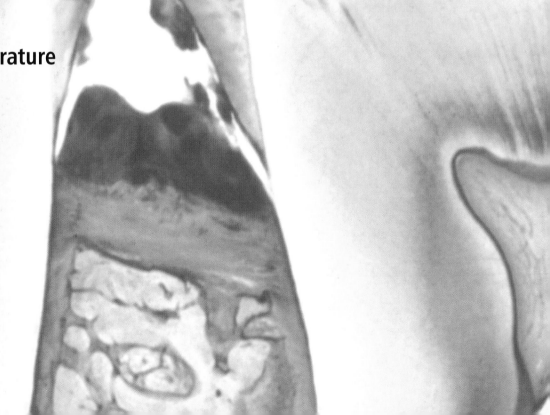

Introduction

It is commonly said that the teeth are 'bathed in saliva'. This gives the erroneous impression of the oral cavity as a closed sink filled with saliva. However, as is evident from Chapter 11, saliva only covers the teeth with a film of about 10 μm thickness. This thin fluid film is constantly moved along the tooth surfaces as swallowing, chewing, talking, etc., take place. The composition of saliva, as well as the velocity of the salivary film, play a significant role in maintaining the integrity of tooth tissues because saliva is in 'direct contact' with them.

In children and young adults only dental enamel is exposed to the oral environment, but with increasing age and accompanying recession of the gingivae the root surfaces may become exposed. Often, as a result of tooth brushing and dental scaling, the cementum of the root surface is removed and the tooth surface comprises exposed dentin. This mineralized tissue consists of minute apatite crystals embedded in a collagenous matrix but, as a result of the numerous dentinal tubules, exposure of the root surfaces results in direct communication between the oral environment and the pulpo-dentinal complex. Exposed root surfaces may therefore give rise to painful reactions, especially when sudden shifts in temperature (drinking hot tea and coffee or ice-cold drinks) or pH (eating sugar-containing products, drinking soft drinks) occur.

Although enamel does not contain cells, this does not mean that there is no transport through the fully mature enamel tissue. The crystals in dental enamel are much larger than those of cementum and dentin, and therefore the crystals have a less reactive surface area. However, from a purely inorganic chemical point of view the biological apatite reacts to chemical challenges similarly in enamel, cementum and dentin. From a structural point of view the enamel can be considered as a microporous solid (see Chapter 3), but this microporosity, represented by the intercrystalline spaces, does not mean that the enamel simply reacts as a sponge for the oral fluids. In fact, in vital teeth, there is a slight pressure of tissue fluid from the pulpo-dentinal organ through the enamel towards the enamel surface. Thus, in these vital teeth any chemical interaction with the dental enamel will have to operate against such a gradient.

When chemical reactions of the biological apatites in the dental hard tissues are discussed, it should be appreciated that the situation is not as simple as having a pure hydroxyapatite exposed to a surrounding liquid phase of known composition. As mentioned above, the small crystals in the mesenchymally derived tissues (cementum and dentin) are embedded in a collagen matrix, whereas the enamel crystals are surrounded by proteins of developmental origin left behind in the tissue as the long-lasting process of enamel maturation occurs. Although these proteins only constitute about 1% by weight, they cover the crystals in a fine meshwork and as such they influence the chemical behavior of the enamel.

Moreover, proteins of salivary origin will cover any exposed tooth tissue. The very thin organic film on tooth surfaces is called the pellicle and is formed as a result of selective adsorption of salivary proteins to tooth surfaces (Bernardi & Kawasaki, 1968; Sønju & Rølla, 1973). The surface of hydroxyapatite is amphoteric, which means that it binds acidic and basic proteins equally well. However, acidic proteins can be desorbed by phosphate or other anions, whereas basic proteins can be desorbed by calcium. The hydroxyapatite surface has a net negative charge because the phosphate groups close to the surface of the crystals more or less shield the positively charged calcium groups.

This chapter will consider how the oral fluids interact with the complex chemical situation on and within tooth surfaces. The chapter not only deals with the effect and interaction of saliva on tooth surfaces, but also describes in detail what is known about the fluid phase at the interface between the biofilms and the tooth surfaces, i.e. the interface that plays a key role when disturbances occur in the chemical equilibrium between the tooth surface and dental plaque. Plaque fluid is likely to be influenced by the saliva on most surfaces. However, the biofilms along the cervical rim of gingiva will also be modified by the crevicular fluid, which is a constant outflux of inflammatory exudate from the gingival crevice.

So, the subsequent sections investigate the composition of these oral fluids and how they are able to maintain the integrity of the tooth tissues. Particular emphasis will be placed on what happens when disturbances in equilibrium between mineral and the fluids result in a net loss of minerals from the tooth, giving rise to a carious lesion. As dental caries is not the only chemical damage to the dental hard tissue that may occur in the oral cavity, the chemical events leading to dental erosions will also be mentioned and further discussed in Chapter 13.

The importance of the mineral phase in enamel

Dental enamel is a highly mineralized acellular tissue in which microscopic calcium phosphate crystals comprise some 99% of the dry weight (Table 12.1). The crystals resemble the mineral hydroxyapatite, $Ca_{10}(PO_4)_6(OH)_2$, in the way that the calcium, phosphate and hydroxyl ions are arranged in a repeating pattern in the crystal lattice structure. Inclusions of carbonate, sodium, fluoride and other ions make it an impure form of the mineral. While apatite is commonly found in biological hard tissues such as enamel, calcium phosphates can exist in various other mineral forms, each having its own unique properties, e.g. brushite, $CaHPO_4.2H_2O$, β-tricalcium phosphate, $Ca_3(PO_4)_2$, and octacalcium phosphate, $Ca_8(PO_4)_4(HPO_4)_2.5H_2O$. Enamel

Table 12.1 Composition of dental hard tissues (% dry weight)

	Enamel	Dentin	Cementum
Calcium	34–39	29	26
Phosphorus	16–18	14	13
Carbonate	2.0–3.6	5.6	5.5
Sodium	0.3–0.9	0.7	?
Magnesium	0.3–0.6	0.9	?
Chloride	0.2–0.3	0.4	?
Mineral	99	80	77
Organic	1	20	23

apatite crystals are long and thin, approximately 50 nm wide in cross-section and more than 100 μm long in the C-axis, and are tightly packed in a repeating arrangement which forms the enamel prisms. Some individual crystals may run the full thickness of enamel and fuse with adjacent crystals at places along their length (Daculsi *et al.*, 1984). The space between the crystals is occupied by water (11% by volume) and organic material (2% by volume). Because of its very high mineral content and minimal acellular matrix, the color, hardness and other physical properties of enamel are similar to those of hydroxyapatite. For example, the density of hydroxyapatite is 3.16 g/cm^3 and that of enamel is 2.95 g/cm^3. Hydroxyapatite is a colorless mineral and enamel is also colorless; the slight yellowish color of tooth crowns is due to the color of dentin showing through. Although hydroxyapatite crystals are transparent, the fact that they have a refractive index (RI) of 1.62 while surrounded by water with an RI of 1.33 renders enamel translucent. If water is replaced by air then enamel appears opaque chalky white. Hydroxyapatite has a hardness of about 430 KHN (Knoop hardness number) and enamel 370 KHN; however, this not only reflects hydroxyapatite hardness but is also related to how strongly the individual crystals adhere to one another. Most importantly, the solubility of enamel apatite corresponds to the solubility of enamel as a tissue. Since dental caries and erosion of enamel are intimately concerned with mineral stability issues, i.e. what makes crystals dissolve, precipitate or grow in aqueous solutions, it is important to look at this closely.

Crystal dissolution

All minerals have an inherent and fixed solubility in water at any given temperature. Dissolution in pure water is relatively fast at first, but then slows as ions making up the crystal accumulate in solution. Eventually net dissolution ceases and the solution is then said to be saturated with respect to that mineral, although there remains a slow exchange of ions between crystal and solution. Water is almost unique in its ability to dissolve inorganic crystals. Water molecules work their way into the crystal surface and dislodge ions from the lattice by virtue of their ability to reduce the attractive forces between oppositely charged ions, a func-

tion of water's high dielectric constant. In addition, water molecules surround the newly released ions, and this energy of hydration overcomes the lattice energy holding the crystal together.

Whether or not a solution is saturated with respect to hydroxyapatite can be determined from the solubility product principle. This theory is derived from the law of mass action, which states that the velocity of a reaction is proportional to the product of the masses of the reacting substances, each raised to a power equal to the number of molecules taking part. By convention, when one unit mass of solid hydroxyapatite dissolves, five calcium ions, three trivalent phosphate ions and one hydroxyl ion are released into solution:

$$Ca_5(PO_4)_3OH \leftrightarrow 5Ca^{2+} + 3PO_4^{3-} + OH^-$$

Thus, the ion activity product of hydroxyapatite (IAP$_{HA}$) is determined by multiplying the calcium ion concentration (or rather the chemical activity) raised to the fifth power by the trivalent phosphate concentration raised to the third power by the hydroxyl concentration, all in mol/l:

$$IAP_{HA} = (Ca^{2+})^5 \times (PO_4^{3-})^3 \times (OH^-)$$

In very dilute solution the activity of an ion is similar to its concentration, but as the soluble salt concentration increases, the activity becomes significantly less than the concentration because of ion interactions. Activity is related to concentration by the activity coefficient, which can be calculated with knowledge of the ionic strength, the saltiness of a solution. The concentration in turn is affected by the extent of formation of complex ions, e.g. $CaH_2PO_4^+$.

When a solution containing hydroxyapatite is saturated and the mineral is in equilibrium with the ions in solution, the IAP$_{HA}$ equals the solubility product of hydroxyapatite (KSP$_{HA}$), a constant which has a value of 7.41×10^{-60} mol^9/l^9 at 37°C.

Thus, at equilibrium:

$$KSP_{HA} = (Ca^{2+})^5 \times (PO_4^{3-})^3 \times (OH^-) = 7.41 \times 10^{-60} \text{ mol}^9/l^9$$

This value could also result, for example, from solution calcium and phosphate concentrations of 0.2925 mmol/l at pH 6 and 37°C (Table 12.2, case 2).

Many salts, e.g. NaCl, are much more soluble in hot water than in cold, but hydroxyapatite and most other calcium phosphates are slightly more soluble in cold water, e.g. KSP$_{HA}$ = 3.72×10^{-58} at 25°C. Therefore, when a person drinks a hot fluid, their teeth are not liable to dissolve any more than when they drink the same fluid cold.

Why is apatite solubility increased by acid?

The solubility of hydroxyapatite and other calcium phosphates is greatly affected by the pH of the water in which it is dissolving, unlike many salts such as table salt, NaCl, the solubility of which is relatively unaffected by pH. As explained

Table 12.2 Calcium and phosphate concentrations, activities and activity product with respect to hydroxyapatite for the same solution at pH 5, 6 and 7, and 37°C

	Case 1	Case 2	Case
pH	5.0	6.0	7.0
Basic strength (mol/l)	8.887×10^{-4}	8.926×10^{-4}	9.653×10^{-4}
Total calcium concentration (mol/l)	2.925×10^{-4}	2.925×10^{-4}	2.925×10^{-4}
Ca^{2+} activity (mol/l)	2.553×10^{-4}	2.539×10^{-4}	2.452×10^{-4}
Total phosphate concentration (mol/l)	2.925×10^{-4}	2.925×10^{-4}	2.925×10^{-4}
Total PO_4^{3-} concentration (mol/l)	1.652×10^{-13}	1.546×10^{-11}	9.395×10^{-10}
PO_4^{3-} activity (mol/l)	1.215×10^{-13}	1.136×10^{-11}	6.822×10^{-10}
OH^- activity (mol/l)	4.787×10^{-10}	4.787×10^{-9}	4.787×10^{-8}
Total activity product (mol^9/l^9) $(Ca^{2+})^5 \times (PO_4^{3-}) \times OH^-$	9.31×10^{-67}	7.41×10^{-60}	1.35×10^{-53}

In each case the total calcium and phosphate concentrations are the same, 0.2925 mmol/l. In case 2, $IAP_{HA} = KSP_{HA}$ (7.41×10^{-60}), thus this solution is saturated with respect to hydroxyapatite.

above, when PO_4^{3-} and and OH^- accumulate in solution, together with calcium ions, dissolution of hydroxyapatite slows and stops as the solution becomes saturated. If acid is added, PO_4^{3-} ions and OH^- ions combine with H^+ to form HPO_4^{2-} ions and H_2O, respectively, thereby removing a proportion of PO_4^{3-} ions and OH^- ions from solution:

$$Ca_5(PO_4)_3OH \leftrightarrow 5Ca^{2+} + 3PO_4^{3-} + OH^-$$
$$\downarrow H^+ \quad \downarrow H^+$$
$$HPO_4^{2-} \quad H_2O$$
$$\downarrow H^+$$
$$H_2PO_4^{2-}$$

In this case the IAP decreases, the solution is then said to be unsaturated and more hydroxyapatite dissolves until saturation is re-established. For example, in Table 12.2, case 1, where the pH of the solution containing 0.2925 mmol/l calcium and phosphate is changed to pH 5, the IAP_{HA} is now much less than the KSP_{HA} and the solution is unsaturated. Conversely, when the pH is 7, the IAP_{HA} is greater than the KSP_{HA} and the solution is then said to be supersaturated with respect to hydroxyapatite (Table 12.2, case 3). When the pH of a supersaturated solution is gradually lowered, the point at which the solution becomes just saturated with respect to the mineral in question is called the 'critical pH'. In the example in Table 12.2, the critical pH is 6. Physically, dissolution of a hydroxyapatite crystal is not isotropic but proceeds more rapidly along the C-axis. This may result in a central cavity in partly dissolved crystals, a phenomenon sometimes seen in electron-microscopic images of carious enamel (Tohda et al., 1987).

One can see from the solubility product equation that if there is an excess of one ion in solution, then less of the others is required to attain the KSP_{HA}. This is sometimes called the 'common ion' effect and explains why addition of either calcium or phosphate to a solution in which hydroxyapatite is dissolving reduces the amount that will dissolve. The solubility product principle also explains why removal

of calcium from a solution in equilibrium, e.g. with a calcium-binding agent such as ethylenediaminetetra-acetic acid (EDTA), will cause more hydroxyapatite to dissolve.

Since the activity product of hydroxyapatite is a function of the calcium ion concentration raised to the fifth power, one might predict that a change in solution calcium concentration would have the most profound effect on IAPHA. However, change in pH affects both OH^- and the proportion of the total phosphate present as PO_4^{3-}, as well as complex ion formation, and with typical concentrations found in oral fluids, doubling the OH^- concentration has a greater effect on the activity product than doubling the calcium concentration (Pearce, 1991).

In summary, hydroxyapatite crystals dissolve in acid because the surrounding solution becomes unsaturated owing to the removal of one or more component ions from solution. The driving force for dissolution is the degree of undersaturation.

Crystal growth

It is well known that under suitable conditions new crystals can precipitate from solution and small crystals can grow in size. Hydroxyapatite is no different to other minerals in this regard. For growth to occur the solution must be supersaturated with respect to hydroxyapatite, i.e. the IAP_{HA} must exceed the KSP_{HA}. With many salts a supersaturated solution can be made by cooling an already saturated solution, but with hydroxyapatite it is necessary to add the constituent ions to a solution until these conditions are met, either by adding calcium and/or phosphate separately as soluble salts, or by raising the pH (which increases PO_4^{3-} and OH^- concentrations) or both. Supersaturated solutions are unstable, and adding a single crystal will seed the precipitation of new crystals if the level of supersaturation is high enough. The concentration of ions in solution will then drop until the solution is just saturated. Crystal growth is, however, quite susceptible to poisoning by foreign substances, and pyrophosphate and certain salivary proteins are important hydroxyapatite growth inhibitors.

Crystals do not grow to an indefinite size, but each mineral has crystals of an inherent shape and maximum size (at fixed temperature and pressure). Hydroxyapatite crystals formed under biological conditions are usually very small in size, but apatite formed geologically may be found with macroscopic hexagonal crystals. The apatite crystals of enamel are extremely elongated considering their formation conditions, and no one has yet been able to reproduce them in the laboratory. In contrast, the apatite crystals of dentin and cementum are small, like those formed *in vitro* in the laboratory. Crystal formation and growth are of great interest in the repair of dental hard tissues. While the presence of a supersaturated solution and the effect of inhibitors have already been noted, there may also be physical restraints on crystal growth. For example, enamel crystals are so tightly packed in the tissue that there is very little space for them to grow larger.

Crystals constantly bathed in a large volume of solution saturated with respect to the mineral will tend to perfect themselves. Newly precipitated crystals are usually small and contain many defects, e.g. missing ions in the lattice, which make the crystal more soluble. Over time, these more soluble parts tend to re-form and the crystals grow to reach their maximum natural size, a process called Ostwald ripening.

Stability of calcium phosphates

At the pH of tissue fluids, 7.4, hydroxyapatite is the most stable calcium phosphate mineral, and it is understandable why it is the form laid down during tissue development. However, after eruption of the tooth the apatite of outer enamel and dentin may be exposed to a wide variation in pH through dietary and plaque effects. A phase diagram such as that shown in Fig. 12.1 can be used to predict that below pH 4.3 brushite is more stable than hydroxyapatite and that brushite may precipitate as separate crystals or cover existing enamel crystals. However, above pH 4.3 hydroxyapatite is more stable than any of the other three calcium phosphates shown. Moreover, the presence of additional ions, fluoride or magnesium, can result in other stable calcium phosphate minerals such as whitlockite and fluorapatite precipitating in preference to hydroxyapatite.

Enamel mineral and oral fluids

Enamel crystals differ from pure hydroxyapatite in that they contain several foreign inorganic ions. The apatite lattice is particularly 'flexible' and will allow the inclusion of extraneous ions in sites normally reserved for calcium, phosphate or hydroxyl ions. In enamel crystals some phosphate ions, for example, are replaced by carbonate ions, often with the simultaneous replacement of calcium by sodium. There is, however, a limit to how much carbonate

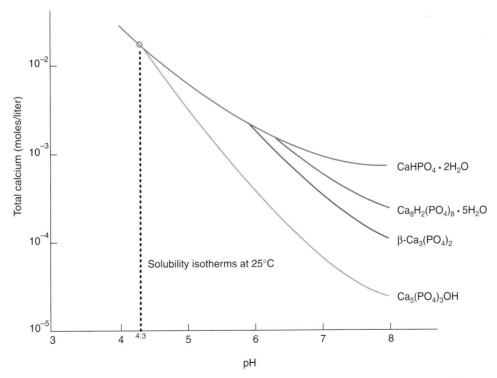

Figure 12.1 Phase solubility diagram at 25°C for calcium and phosphate, which may form under physiological conditions. (Adapted from Brown, 1971.)

can be accommodated in this way without disrupting the lattice. In addition, some hydroxyl ions are replaced by fluoride ions, but there is no limit to the possible extent of this substitution; 100% replacement results in fluorapatite, but this mineral is rarely found in biological tissues (an exception is shark enameloid). One can tell that carbonate and fluoride are embedded within the crystal because they change the lattice dimensions. Enamel apatite and most other biological apatite is, therefore, a carbonated fluorhydroxyapatite. Other ions that are normally incorporated in biological apatite, but to a smaller extent, are chloride and magnesium. Yet other substitutions are possible, e.g. strontium for calcium, but are not quantitatively important.

Effect of carbonate and fluoride on apatite dissolution and growth

Ionic substitutions influence the physical and chemical properties of the mineral and, most importantly with respect to enamel, change its solubility. Carbonate inclusion makes hydroxyapatite more soluble (Nelson, 1981), but fluoride inclusion has the opposite effect, decreasing the effective KSP. Fluorapatite, which has a KSP_{FA} of 3.2×10^{-61}, is less soluble than hydroxyapatite, but approximately 50% replacement produces the least soluble mineral: $KSP_{FHA0.5} = 6.6 \times 10^{-63}$ (Moreno et al., 1974). Because of the relatively small amount of fluoride in native enamel, carbonate has

an overriding effect on enamel solubility, decreasing the KSP_{enamel} to 5.5×10^{-55} (Moreno & Zahradnik, 1974), although there is evidence that only prism junction material is quite as soluble (Shellis, 1996), the bulk of the enamel mineral having a KSP closer to 10^{-58}. When determining the saturation status of oral fluids with respect to enamel, a KSP of this order should be used, rather than KSP_{HA}. However, because of the changeable nature of enamel mineral the exact KSP_{enamel} is difficult to determine.

Traces of fluoride in solution when hydroxyapatite dissolves render the solution highly supersaturated with respect to fluorapatite and especially fluorhydroxyapatite, which then tends to precipitate or overgrow on the existing hydroxyapatite. Small amounts of fluoride are therefore removed from solution during apatite crystal regrowth. However, since carbonate-free or low-carbonate apatite is less soluble, this will tend to form in preference to the original apatite. Thus, when a carbonated fluorhydroxyapatite crystal dissolves and reprecipitation occurs, fluoride tends to be reincorporated, whereas carbonate is discarded. The overall effect of this solution fluoride is to reduce dramatically the amount of calcium that may be liberated from enamel in acid solution. This is the scientific basis for the current view that low concentrations of fluoride in solution in the environment of the tooth are more beneficial in reducing caries than high concentrations of fluoride incorporated into enamel (Fig. 12.2).

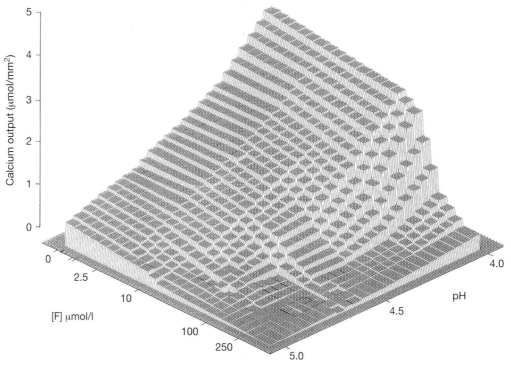

Figure 12.2 Calcium output for enamel during demineralization in solutions initially containing 2.2 mmol/l calcium chloride and 2.2 mmol/l potassium phosphate, adjusted to the pH and fluoride [F] levels indicated. (For original figure refer to ten Cate & Duijsters, 1983a.)

Trace elements in enamel

Because enamel crystals are so small they have a very large surface area, allowing great opportunity for the adsorption of foreign ions. It is likely that all the previously mentioned ions are to some extent also adsorbed at the surface, or near it in a bound water layer, the 'hydration shell', including HPO_4^{2-} and Ca^{2+} ions. These ions are readily exchangeable, unlike ions in the lattice. Also adsorbed on the crystal surface are enamel trace elements such as potassium, zinc, lead and copper (Curzon & Cutress, 1983).

Homogeneity of enamel and enamel crystals

In addition to variations on the crystal surface due to adsorption, the bulk of the enamel crystal is probably not homogeneous. There is reason to believe that enamel crystals are covered with an indistinct layer of apatitic mineral which has a greater stability, e.g. less carbonate and/or more fluoride. Thus, the extent of the substitutions is not constant throughout the crystal.

If powdered enamel is repeatedly exposed to acid its dissolution is incongruous, meaning that the initial products are not those expected from enamel mineral. Carbonate, sodium and magnesium are released preferentially during the first exposure (Larsen et al., 1993), and this may reflect either the release of adsorbed ions or the dissolution of enamel mineral and simultaneous reprecipitation of a more perfect fluorhydroxyapatite with a lower solubility. During such a reprecipitation process crystals may become coated with a different calcium phosphate phase, e.g. brushite, which then becomes the 'solubility-controlling' phase (Pearce et al., 1995). Moreover, separate whitlockite crystals may precipitate (Shellis et al., 1997), which may lead to the formation of 'caries crystals', the relatively large rhomboidal crystals sometimes seen at the prism periphery in carious enamel.

Enamel as a tissue is also not homogeneous, in that crystals near the outer surface have more fluoride and less carbonate than crystals in the enamel interior. This renders the outer enamel less soluble than most of the tissue. Another interesting phenomenon is the irregular dissolution of crystals in relation to enamel prisms, which accentuates the cross-striations of the prisms and the striae of Retzius (Fig. 12.3). Why crystals or parts of crystals at certain points in the prism should be more soluble than crystals elsewhere is not well understood, but may be related to variations in carbonate content.

State of saturation of oral fluids

Saliva contains considerable amounts of calcium and phosphate and is nearly always supersaturated with respect to enamel mineral and other biological apatites (Table 12.3). In the most studied secretion, parotid fluid, both pH and calcium concentration increase with increasing flow rate, so that the ion activity product increases with increasing flow rate. Parotid saliva is supersaturated with respect to hydroxyapatite at all flow rates and slightly undersaturated or just saturated with respect to brushite (Lagerlöf, 1983). Most importantly, unstimulated whole saliva is supersaturated with respect to hydroxyapatite and the level increases when the flow rate is stimulated (Dawes & Dong, 1995). By implication, if saliva is supersaturated with respect to hydroxyapatite, then it will also be supersaturated with respect to native enamel crystals since they are more soluble. Thus, it is clear that enamel mineral will not dissolve in saliva under normal conditions, i.e. provided it is not acidified with dietary, gastric or medicinal acids. Research indicates that parotid saliva must be acidified to below about pH 5.5 before the secretion becomes unsaturated with respect to hydroxyapatite and enamel is at risk of dissolution, i.e. its critical pH is about 5.5.

It might be expected that because of this high supersaturation, enamel crystals would continue to grow or that saliva would seed new crystals at the tooth surface. The principal reason why this does not happen on plaque-free surfaces is that saliva contains protein inhibitors of hydroxyapatite crystal growth. These include a tyrosine-rich peptide, statherin, and various proline-rich proteins that coat the enamel surface and prevent seeding by exposed crystals (Moreno et al.,

Table 12.3 Minerals in oral fluids and their saturation status

	Mixed saliva Flow unstimulated	Parotid saliva Flow stimulated	Fluid from resting plaque[a]	Fluid from fermenting plaque[b]
Calcium (mmol/l)	1.32	1.17	3.5	8.2
Prosphate (mmol/l)	5.40	3.60	13.2	13.5
Potassium (mmol/)	19.4	16.0	51.5	52.6
Fluoride (mmol/l)	1–2.6	1.0	6.0	5.0
pH	7.06	7.70	6.89	5.29
$IAP_{HA}(mol^9/l^9)$	6.13×10^{-48}	2.69×10^{-47}	1.42×10^{-47}	1.02×10^{-55}

Data recalculated from Shannon et al. (1974), Bruun et al. (1982), Lagerlöf (1983), Margolis et al. (1993), Dawes & Dong (1995) and Tanaka & Margolis (1999).
[a] Overnight starved plaque from caries-free individuals.
[b] Plaque collected 3 min after a 5% sucrose rinse in caries-positive individuals.
$KSP_{enamel} = 5.5 \times 10^{-55}$.

1979). These inhibitors also prevent spontaneous precipitation in the salivary ducts.

Dental plaque, the bacterial biofilm that covers enamel at protected sites, generally prevents access of saliva to enamel, so the interbacterial fluid of plaque is of greater importance here. Plaque fluid, normally isolated by centrifugation, has a composition markedly different to that of saliva (Table 12.3). For example, calcium and phosphate levels are higher by a factor of 2–3. Fluid in non-fermenting, 'resting' plaque is highly supersaturated with respect to enamel mineral and all other biological calcium phosphates. This can be expected to be beneficial for the remineralization of underlying carious enamel, but it also provides necessary preconditions for the calcification of plaque and may lead to supragingival calculus formation. Fluid in plaque made metabolically active by exposure to sucrose has, however, a much reduced degree of supersaturation, and in caries-positive subjects is frequently unsaturated with respect to enamel mineral (Margolis et al., 1993) (Table 12.3). Plaque fluid tends to become more unsaturated the higher the concentration of sucrose applied to plaque, even in caries-free individuals.

This change in saturation status of plaque fluid is largely due to reduction in pH as a consequence of lactic acid production by bacteria. However, a simultaneous increase in calcium in plaque fluid tends to counteract the pH change (Table 12.3). In one study, the calcium ion concentration in plaque fluid rose from 2.8 to 9.6 mmol/l after a sugar rinse (Margolis & Moreno, 1992). This calcium comes from reservoirs in plaque, either amorphous granules of calcium phosphate or ionic calcium bound to bacterial cell walls (Rose et al., 1993). The latter is largely released into plaque fluid as the pH drops from 7 to 5. It has been postulated that metabolic activity of plaque may remove inorganic phosphate from plaque fluid for phosphorylation purposes, and thereby contribute to the decrease in degree of saturation, but recent studies show only small changes in phosphate on sugar exposure, possibly because of the concomitant release of phosphate from mineral stores. However, it seems that frequent sugar exposures, cycling the pH down and up repeatedly, may deplete calcium and phosphate reservoirs in plaque and thereby promote the pH-induced reduction in degree of saturation, and the cariogenic potential of plaque fluid. This is one reason why frequency of sugar intake is regarded as more harmful than the total sugar ingested in caries-active individuals.

Diffusion pathways

Enamel crystals are in intimate contact with the small amount of water in enamel. It may be assumed, therefore, that a state of equilibrium exists between the crystals and enamel fluid, i.e. that the fluid is nearly always just saturated with respect to enamel mineral. If an overlying plaque is exposed to sugar an increase in acid in the plaque fluid will decrease the concentration of OH^- and PO_4^{3-} ions in

the fluid. This will allow these ions, together with appropriate counter-ions in enamel fluid, to diffuse from the enamel fluid to the exterior. Initially, acid penetrates enamel with little regard for anatomical detail, but as the lesion becomes established acid penetrates into the underlying sound enamel via widened prism junctions. Equilibrium is quickly re-established by the dissolution of a small amount of native enamel mineral and the re-formation of a low-carbonate, less soluble apatite as supersaturation conditions allow. Studies show that diffusion of H^+ into carious lesions is very slow, often taking days (Larsen & Pearce, 1992), and that a thick, well-mineralized surface layer retards diffusion even more. Thus, there is not a close temporal correspondence between cariogenic events in plaque and net dissolution events in enamel. The rate of enamel dissolution and carious lesion development is a function of both the degree of understaturation of plaque fluid and rates of diffusion of ions into and out of enamel.

Mineral transformations

When a relatively soluble calcium phosphate mineral dissolves and equilibrium is attained with that mineral, the solution is often then supersaturated with respect to a less soluble calcium phosphate, which will tend to precipitate if a suitable seeding site is present. Transformations within the apatite series are, perhaps, the most important. If under the influence of plaque cariogenic activity a small amount of native high-carbonate, low-fluoride mineral of enamel dissolves, then the enamel fluid at that site will be supersaturated with respect to low-carbonate and/or high-fluoride hydroxyapatite. It is likely that the native crystals in the developing lesion will only be partly dissolved, and will attempt to regrow using the remains of the original crystal as a template. The repaired section will contain less carbonate and will be less soluble and therefore more resistant to future dissolution events. As mentioned previously, fluoride ions in solution are likely to be incorporated, so that the repaired section will be not only lower in carbonate but also higher in fluoride, provided that fluoride is available in solution. After repeated dissolution episodes enamel crystals may become entirely transformed from their original state. This is seen most clearly in outer enamel overlying a white-spot caries lesion, and is the explanation for the high fluoride concentration in this enamel. In the body of the lesion it is thought that H^+ ions diffuse from the prism junction inwards towards the prism center, dissolving the more soluble mineral. The prism periphery then becomes re-formed by re-deposition of mineral from the prism interior (see Fig. 12.3B). Thus, what happens in the individual prisms appears to reflect what happens in enamel as a whole.

While apatite is the only calcium phosphate that can incorporate fluoride into its lattice, fluoride has some important effects on the relative stability of other calcium phosphates. For example, fluoride promotes the conversion

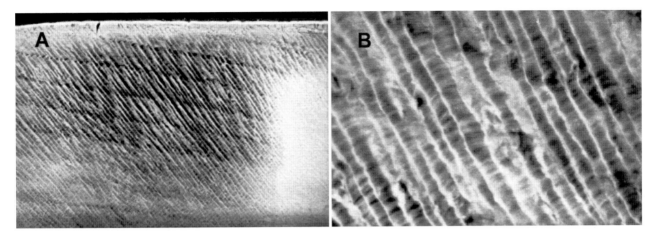

Figure 12.3 Back-scattered scanning electron micrograph images of a natural caries lesion in permanent human enamel. (B) High-magnification view of the body of the lesion in (A). White areas are highly mineralized, while in gray and black areas the mineral has been partly dissolved. The enamel prisms are decalcified irregularly along their length, and areas of strong decalcification line up in adjacent prisms, corresponding to the striae of Retzius. A highly mineralized layer covers the whole lesion (A) consisting of re-formed low-carbonate, high-fluoride mineral. Prism peripheries are highly mineralized and probably also consist of re-formed mineral.

of brushite and octacalcium phosphate to apatite, and allows the formation of fluorhydroxyapatite in acidic conditions when brushite might form or when magnesium is present and β-tricalcium phosphate might form. In both these instances the explanation is that fluorhydroxyapatite is more stable than either brushite or β-tricalcium phosphate.

Demineralization and remineralization of the dental hard tissues

Under physiological conditions saliva and the oral fluids are supersaturated with respect to hydroxyapatite and fluorapatite (Fig. 12.4). That is the necessary precondition for the existence of dental apatite in the mouth. If the oral fluids were unsaturated with respect to apatite the dental hard tissues would dissolve without any other reason. In general, the higher the supersaturation with respect to the actual salt the greater is the tendency for its formation. Thus, the bars in Fig. 12.4 indicate a considerable tendency to form fluorhydroxyapatite and hydroxyapatite, and this explains why most supragingival calculus consists of mixed fluorhydroxyapatite and hydroxyapatite. Occasionally, octacalcium phosphate or brushite has been observed as a component of calculus. Further, the supersaturation with respect to apatites may lead to mineral deposition in porous areas in the teeth, such as observed during developmental maturation of enamel or remineralization of carious lesions. Figure 12.4 shows that saliva is unsaturated with respect to calcium fluoride, which explains why this salt only exists in the oral cavity for a limited period and invariably will dissolve.

When the pH in the surrounding medium decreases, the solubility of the tooth mineral apatite increases considerably (Fig. 12.5). (In Fig. 12.4 a pH drop would result in a

decrease in the height of the bars.) In general, the solubility of apatite increases by a factor of 10 with a drop of each single pH unit, which is what makes the mineral vulnerable to an acidic environment. Exposure to acids may lead to two types of lesion, the carious lesion (Fig. 12.6) and erosion (Fig. 12.7). In short, the initial stages of the carious lesion are characterized by a partial dissolution of the tissue, leaving a 20–50-μm-thick, rather well-mineralized surface layer and a subsurface body of the lesion with a mineral loss of up to 30–50% extending deep into the enamel and dentin. In contrast, the erosion lesion shows features of complete demineralization and dissolution layer by layer. Thus, the dental hard tissues remaining after even extensive erosion do not show signs of demineralization except that some of the enamel is gone. The mineral content of the remaining enamel is unchanged.

The histological features are reflected in the clinical appearance: the carious lesion is chalky white and softened (Fig. 2.11), while the appearance of eroded enamel is usually unaltered; it is hard and shiny (Fig. 13.2).

A third type of enamel dissolution by acids is seen when enamel is conditioned for the retention of resin fillings. The etch pattern is similar to the erosion (see Chapter 13) in the sense that it is a surface etching without formation of a surface layer covering a subsurface demineralization. However, the etching acid penetrates considerably deeper into the enamel and exposes the prism pattern to a much larger extent than is seen in eroded enamel. When the water in these surface etchings is removed by drying the etched area appears white and chalky (Fig. 12.8).

Caries is defined as chemical dissolution of the dental hard tissues by acidic bacterial products from degradation of low molecular weight sugars. In contrast, erosion is defined as dissolution of apatite mineral caused by acids of

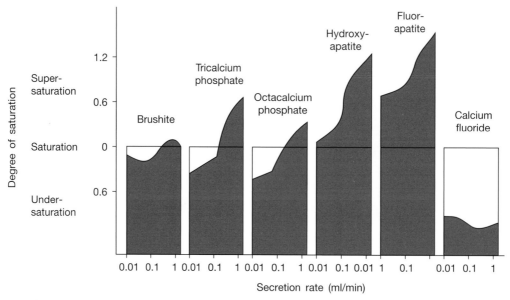

Figure 12.4 Degrees of saturation with respect to various calcium phosphates and to calcium fluoride in parotid saliva (after McCann, 1968). The degrees of saturation are given by $\log \sqrt[n]{}$ (ion product in saliva)/(solubility product), in which n is the number of ions in the actual salt. The salts may all at least occasionally occur in the oral cavity as part of teeth or calculus, or as a precipitate after topical fluoride application. Saliva is highly supersaturated with respect to the apatites, which is the basis of the integrity of the teeth in the mouth. The saturation with respect to the other calcium phosphates explains their occurrence in calculus, while the undersaturation with respect to calcium fluoride shows that saliva invariably dissolves that salt.

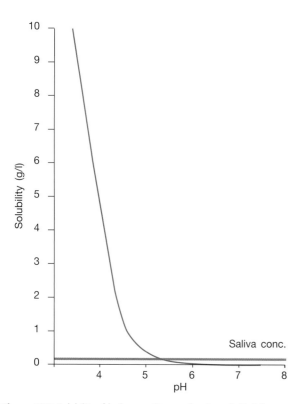

Figure 12.5 Solubility of hydroxyapatite as a function of pH. Salivary concentrations of calcium and phosphate are indicated by the horizontal line. The solubility of apatite increases considerably as pH decreases. It should be noted that caries develops in the pH range around 4.0–5.5, while teeth are eroded in the pH range 2.5–4.0.

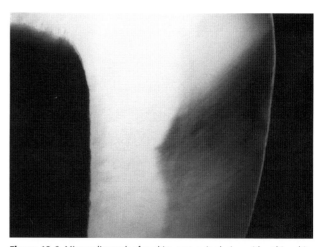

Figure 12.6 Microradiograph of a white-spot caries lesion with a thin white surface layer covering the demineralized lesion body that extends halfway through the enamel. When the subsurface lesion becomes further demineralized the support of the surface layer becomes insufficient to prevent the layer from collapsing and breaking apart.

any other origin, except for acids used for conditioning of enamel and dentin for retentive purposes.

Caries demineralization

Under normal conditions the oral fluids are supersaturated with respect to both hydroxyapatite and fluorapatite (see above), indicative of a tendency for the formation of these two minerals, i.e. formation of apatite in calculus and remineralization of demineralized areas in carious lesions.

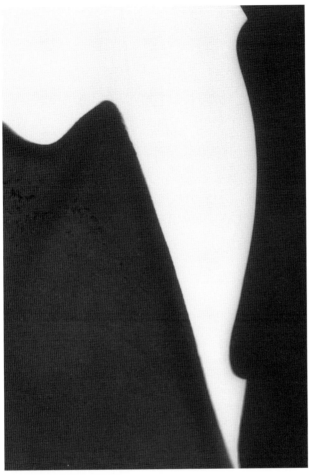

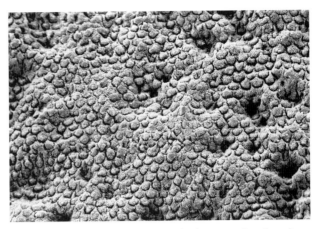

Figure 12.8 Scanning electron micrograph of an enamel surface after a conditioning etching with phosphoric acid. The prism pattern is clearly seen, with accentuated arcade-shaped prism boundaries.

As pH is lowered in the oral fluids, saliva and plaque fluid, the supersaturation with respect to hydroxyapatite is reduced and replaced by saturation at critical pH. Below this critical pH the fluids are undersaturated with respect to hydroxyapatite. Because fluorapatite is less soluble than is hydroxyapatite, plaque fluid remains supersaturated with respect to fluorapatite when it is undersaturated with respect to hydroxyapatite (Fig. 12.9). Under these conditions a carious lesion forms. Subsurface hydroxyapatite is dissolved, while fluorhydroxyapatite is formed in the surface layers of enamel. In general, the more undersaturated the plaque fluid, with respect to hydroxyapatite, i.e. the lower the pH, the greater the tendency for dissolution of the enamel apatite.

Figure 12.7 Eroded human tooth. No subsurface demineralization is seen as teeth are eroded layer by layer.

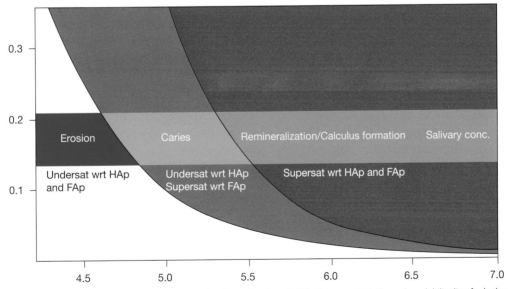

Figure 12.9 Solubility of hydroxyapatite (HAp) and fluorapatite (FAp) as a function of pH in the range 4–6. Above the solubility line for hydroxyapatite, solutions will be supersaturated with respect to (wrt) both HAp and FAp. In saliva, formation of calculus and remineralization of caries lesions may occur. Between the two solubility lines solutions will be undersaturated with respect to HAp and saturated with respect to FAp. In saliva, HAp tends to dissolve and FAp may form, i.e. a caries lesion may develop. Below the solubility line for FAp, both apatites may dissolve and erosions develop.

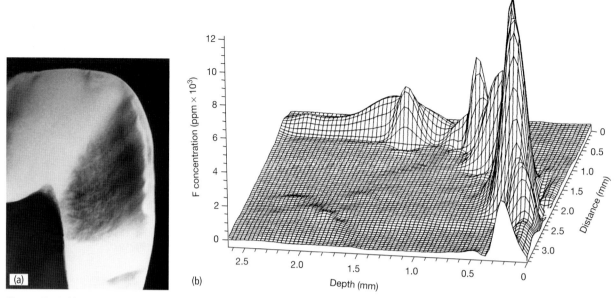

(a)   (b)

Figure 12.10 (a) Microradiogram of a caries lesion with a well-mineralized surface layer, under which the subsurface demineralization extends to and further into the dentin. (b) The graph demonstrates a high fluoride content in the surface layer and very little fluoride in the subsurface lesion body, despite a high exposure to fluoride. A slight increase at the border between the enamel and dentin can be distinguished.

The concurrent supersaturation with respect to fluorapatite is responsible for the maintenance and integrity of the surface layer. Experimentally, the more supersaturated the solution, with respect to fluorapatite, the thicker and less demineralized the surface layer remains. This formation of fluorapatite at the expense of hydroxyapatite in surface enamel leads in time to a high content of fluorhydroxyapatite in the surface layer of the carious lesion (Fig. 12.10).

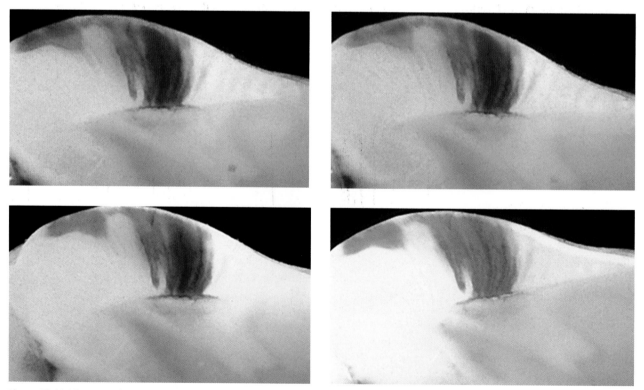

Figure 12.11 Microgram of a caries lesion in which the pores have been filled with blue litmus. Diffusion of acid (0.1 mol/l HCl) through the surface layer can be monitored by the color change from before (top left), after 24 h (top right), to after 13 days (bottom left). A control micrograph with purple red litmus is shown in the bottom right. Note that the pH of the smaller and narrow lesions shifts more quickly than that of the larger lesion.

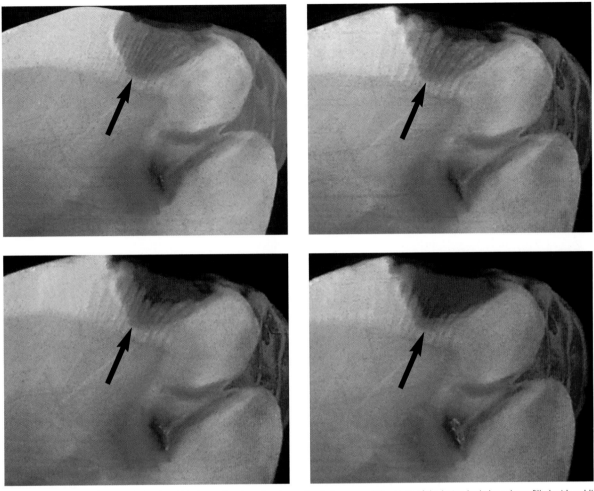

Figure 12.12 Microgram of a caries lesion in which the surface layer has been abraded away and the pores of the lesion body have been filled with red litmus (arrow). The 0.1 mol/l NaOH changes the pH of the lesion as it diffuses into the lesion during the first hour of exposure. Top left: before; top right: after 17 min; bottom left: after 40 min; bottom right: after 60 min.

In Fig. 12.10, it should be noted that the fluoride concentration in subsurface enamel is not increased. As long as the surface layer remains intact and has a reasonable mineral content, fluoride does not seem to diffuse into the body of the lesion. Rather, it reacts as it diffuses inwards, causing fluorhydroxyapatite formation in the outer layers. In a number of respects the surface layer exerts a protective effect to prevent further dissolution of the lesion body.

Diffusion in the caries lesion

In an experiment, natural caries lesions were slit in half, the pores of the lesions were filled with a litmus (pH indicator) solution and the cut faces of the lesions were painted with a transparent varnish that allowed monitoring of the pH as acids or alkali diffused through the surface layer of the lesion. It was observed that a pH shift took days or even weeks. The rate of change of color indicated that the diffusion through the surface layer is slow compared with the diffusion through the larger pores of the lesion body (Fig. 12.11). In general, the larger the lesion and the thicker the surface layer, the more time required for the shift. In particular, when the lesion included demineralized dentin below the enamel lesion the color shift was delayed. The appearance of the color shift was completely different when the surface layer was removed: the color shift appeared as a wave of one color moving quickly (within 1 h) inwards, with a rather distinct border between the red and the blue parts of the lesion (Fig. 12.12).

This experiment illustrates that the diffusion of demineralizing agents, and in general ions, into a lesion with an intact surface layer is slow. A single pH drop fall-and-rise cycle in plaque is unlikely to affect the pH in lesion fluid, but the effect of a pH drop is much larger when the surface layer is broken down and lost. From these observations it is evident that filling up the pores with a topical fluoride solution is not possible and that remineralization of a subsurface lesion body is, at best, a very slow process.

Remineralization

Remineralization of dental lesions requires the presence of partially demineralized apatite crystals that can grow to their original size as a result of exposure to solutions supersaturated with respect to apatite. The formation of entirely new crystals in a lesion is not common. The two conditions set limits to what can be expected from remineralization. First, as the erosion is characterized as a lesion in which enamel is etched away layer by layer and the crystals are lost layer by layer, very little, if any, remineralization of eroded enamel can be expected, despite the lesion being exposed to supersaturated saliva for long periods.

In contrast, the carious lesion contains partially demineralized crystals and considerable remineralization of surface enamel in lesions free of plaque has been observed. Thus, surface remineralization of carious lesions developed during orthodontic treatment is not uncommon, leaving the body of the lesion as a white scar under a shiny hard surface. Owing to slow diffusion, however, it does not seem possible to maintain the necessary supersaturation in the lesion fluid and therefore remineralization of the lesion body is not obtained. The surface layer of the lesion protects the underlying lesion body not only from demineralization, but also from remineralization.

On rare occasions the lesion body may be remineralized when the surface layer has been lost and plaque in the rough area is controlled. Under such conditions there is free access for salivary calcium, phosphate and fluoride ions (Fig. 12.13). However, it must be noted that the loss of the surface layer also means free access of cariogenic acids and thus an increase in the demineralization rate. Therefore, with the possible exception of orthodontic lesions, therapeutic removal of the surface layer to increase remineralization is not recommended.

Dentin caries

In the oral cavity dentin is covered by either enamel (in the tooth crown) or cementum (in the root). The role of the enamel is to provide the teeth with a mechanically strong and chemically resistant surface layer. Nevertheless, during life the dentin may become exposed to the oral cavity. In former times, the dentition was generally used for grinding food, and the enamel was easily worn away, as can be seen on skulls from ancient times. Today the dentition suffers more from the chemical insults imposed by the dental plaque. Dental caries occurs first in enamel (see previous section) and then as the lesion develops on a smooth surface, it is seen as a cone-shaped defect, wide at the tooth surface and becoming narrow towards the dentino-enamel junction. At that point the defect becomes wider again, and may extend all the way to the pulp. Various studies have shown that the broadening of the carious defect at the dentino-enamel junction is not the effect of a lateral spread of acids, but rather the result of the early stages of decalcification not being seen in enamel, when they are already visible in dentin. This shows that dental caries affects enamel and dentin to significant depth while the outer surface may remain intact.

The roots of the teeth are covered by periodontal ligaments and fibers. However, after gingival retraction or surgery, the root is exposed. Owing to its low wear resistance, the cementum is removed rapidly during brushing.

Composition of dentin

Dentin is comprised of 70% by weight (50% by volume) mineral and 20% by weight (50% by volume) organic matrix. The mineral phase is hydroxyapatite, similar to enamel, but the crystallites have much smaller dimensions than in enamel. The hexagonal or plate-like dentinal crystallites are 3–30 nm in cross-section and about 50 nm in length. This results in a much larger surface area to crystallite volume ratio and therefore a more reactive mineral phase. Consequently, the percentage of foreign ions, ions other than calcium, phosphate and hydroxyl ions, is higher in dentin than in enamel.

The organic matrix (unlike enamel) is composed of collagen. It is present as a very structured triple helix of three, intertwined, polypeptide chains. Typically, such a helix is about 300 nm long and has a diameter of about 1.5 nm. In addition, there are many non-collagenous components that determine the properties of the matrix, e.g. phosphoproteins, phospholipids and proteoglycans. These compounds play a role in the nucleation and regulation of mineral formation during dentinogenesis. By a similar mode of action they may interfere with the demineralization and remineralization process. Collagen is the structural backbone of dentin, which holds together the apatite crystallites, some of which are precipitated within the fine structure of the collagen helix. With this structure there is a synergism between matrix and apatite; the mineral phase can only be partly dissolved during acid attack, while the matrix cannot be digested by enzymatic action as its surface is protected by apatite crystallites.

Structural aspects

As will be apparent from Chapter 3, the natural root-surface carious lesion is characterized by a subsurface loss of mineral very similar to that seen in enamel caries. This is true irrespective of whether it develops while the root surface is still covered by cementum or has dentin exposed. From a chemical point of view it is therefore tempting to suggest that the basic physicochemical events leading to an established natural root-surface lesion are very similar to those occurring during enamel caries development. Having

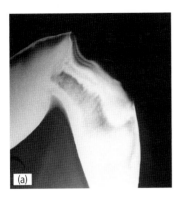

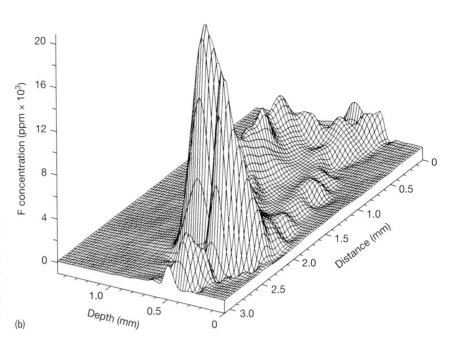

Figure 12.13 (a) Microradiograph of caries lesion remineralized for years *in vivo*. The surface layer of this third molar has been abraded away, giving the saliva access to the lesion body and resulting in a considerable uptake of mineral. (b) The graph of the fluoride scan shows uptake of extraordinary amounts of fluoride in the remineralized zones of the lesion.

said this, it is important to realize that the overall structural composition of cementum and dentin results in substantial differences in the way in which microorganisms interact with dentin and root surfaces during carious lesion development (see Chapter 3). Thus, in addition to the inorganic chemical events, there will be substantial proteolytic activity in order to remove the collagenous matrix. To understand the chemical events occurring during carious lesion development in dentin and cementum, different *in situ* models have been used for experimentation. An *in situ* model is a specimen of tooth tissues inserted into the human oral environment to study lesion formation. However, the outcome of *in situ* caries models may differ substantially depending on their design (Fejerskov *et al.*, 1994) and, therefore, the choice of model may influence the conclusions drawn from these studies. For example, root specimens have been mounted in a sheltered position underneath orthodontic bands in palatal appliances and exposed to the oral environment for 1–4 weeks (Ögaard *et al.*, 1988). The type of root-surface lesion created under these conditions is characterized by a shallow surface etching. In contrast, this section will consider chemical events occurring when root-surface lesions are developed over 3–6 months under conditions where the surfaces are freely exposed to the oral fluids (Nyvad *et al.*, 1997). Figure 12.14 shows microradiographs of experimental root carious lesions developed *in situ* after 3 and 6 months. The microbial deposits on the tooth surface were not removed during the first 3 months

of the study. During the second 3-month period two topical treatments with a 2% solution of sodium fluoride were given for 2 min, one at the beginning of the treatment period when plaque removal was started and the second after 1.5 months of regular plaque removal. The illustration shows that the treatment resulted in an overall mineral gain in the surface layer or within the body of the lesion. In a separate experiment during the second 3-month period no additional oral hygiene measures were taken, resulting in additional mineral loss (Fig. 12.15). It is not possible on the basis of such experiments to draw conclusions about the relative importance of fluoride toothpaste, topical fluoride treatment and plaque removal on the outcome of lesion development. It is remarkable that no studies have attempted to distinguish the effect of plaque removal from that of fluoride alone on lesion development. However, topical fluorides inhibit caries, especially when dental cleaning is insufficient (Ögaard *et al.*, 1990).

Notice that actively progressing root carious lesions can arrest with an increase in mineral content of the surface layer. Perhaps this increased mineral results from daily fluoride exposure from toothpaste combined with a reduced cariogenic challenge due to regular plaque removal. In many ways the basic chemical events occurring during carious lesion development in enamel, dentin and cementum appear similar. As stressed earlier in this chapter, it is thus to be expected that fluoride will gradually accumulate in the surface of the tissues as a result of ongoing demineralizing and remineralizing processes. Hence, a subsurface enamel carious lesion is covered by a surface layer with a high fluoride content – higher than that of surrounding normal enamel – and likewise the well-mineralized surface layer covering a subsurface dentin or cementum lesion contains a much higher fluoride content than that of normal tissues (Tohda *et al.*, 1996).

Root surfaces (exposed cementum/dentin) appear to be more susceptible to carious attack than enamel surfaces. A clinical manifestation of this is the occurrence of dentin caries in some patients with dry mouths, where the enamel is caries free (Figs 27.6 and 27.7). In the above-mentioned *in situ* study it was striking that even with daily plaque control, root surfaces, sound but previously unexposed to the oral environment, undergo changes in mineral distribution. This may lead to a subsurface mineral loss, which is only detectable at the microscopic level. Unerupted root surfaces that become exposed to the oral environment as a result of gingival recession or periodontal surgery are very prone to lesion development (Selvig & Zander, 1962; Furseth, 1970). The very small apatite crystals in dentin and cementum, compared with those of enamel, have a much more highly reactive surface. Thus, unerupted root surfaces

exposed to the oral environment may undergo substantial modification of the mineral as a result of metabolic activity in the biofilms. This may explain the differences in crystal packing and size in the root surfaces of unexposed and exposed carious root surfaces Fig. 12.16). These processes reflect a substantial uptake and redeposition of minerals into crystals that are partly dissolved. The permeability and reactivity of the root surfaces may change so that they become less susceptible to future cariogenic challenges (ten Cate *et al.*, 1987).

The complex events leading to mineral loss and deposition in dental hard tissues exposed to the oral environment are not fully understood. Although the *in situ* models may mimic the physicochemical events occurring during lesion formation *in vivo*, it should be remembered, for example, that teeth with a vital pulpo-dentinal organ will respond to most exogenous stimuli through the apposition of minerals along and within the dentinal tubules (Frank & Vogel, 1980). This phenomenon, together with the outward flow of dentinal fluid from the pulp, may be expected to reduce the rate of lesion progression *in vivo* significantly in dentin (Shellis, 1994). This may explain why caries seems to progress more rapidly in non-vital teeth.

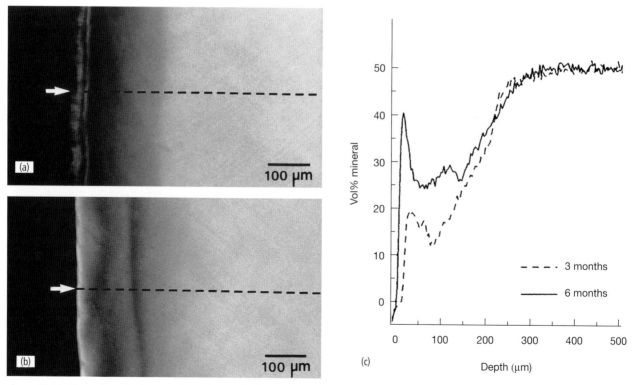

Figure 12.14 Microradiograph of an experimental root caries lesion *in situ* after (a) 3 months without plaque removal, followed by (b) 3 months with daily plaque removal and topical fluoride treatment. (c) The mineral content as a function of depth corresponding to the dotted lines in (a) and (b). The treatment resulted in an overall mineral gain because of an increase of the mineral content in the surface layer and formation of a mineral zone in the body of the lesion 125 μm deep to the surface. Scale bar = 100 μm. (For original figure refer to Nyvad *et al.*, 1997.)

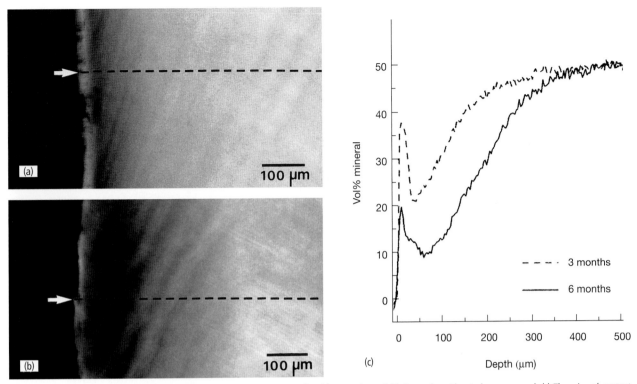

Figure 12.15 Microradiographs of experimental root caries lesion *in situ* after (a) 3 months and (b) 6 months without plaque removal. (c) The mineral content as a function of depth corresponding to the dotted lines in (a) and (b). Note that the lesion depth increased and that the mineral content in the surface layer decreased over time. Scale bar = 100 μm. (For original figure refer to Nyvad *et al.*, 1997.)

Fluoride reactions in the oral environment

Formation of fluorhydroxyapatite

When enamel is exposed to ionic fluoride it may be taken up with the formation of either fluorhydroxyapatite or calcium fluoride. Fluorhydroxyapatite is formed when the fluoride concentration in solution is low, less than around 50 ppm, and in an acidic environment:

$$Ca_{10}(PO_4)_6(OH)_2 + F^- + H^+ \rightarrow Ca_{10}(PO_4)_6(OH)F + H_2O$$

The fluorhydroxyapatite formed will be situated in the outermost layers of enamel and form an integral part of the tissue that is only lost if the entire mineral is worn away or dissolved entirely. In particular, under neutral conditions, the formation of the fluorhydroxyapatite is slow and unable to keep pace with normal wear of the tooth surface. Therefore, despite the use of fluoride toothpaste, thorough daily tooth brushing reduces the fluoride content of buccal enamel surfaces over the years. In contrast, under plaque, e.g. in approximal areas, the conditions are more favorable and the fluoride content of surface enamel generally increases over a lifetime.

The above explains why the fluoride content of buccal surface enamel to some extent depends on the prevalence of dental caries (Fig. 12.17). When the prevalence of caries is low the fluoride content of enamel is not affected by the carious challenge and varies considerably according to the intake of fluoride during the mineralization of the tooth and to wear after eruption. However, in subjects with a high prevalence of caries the fluoride content of the enamel is higher owing to the frequent pH drops.

The necessary condition in the mouth for fluorapatite formation is that the oral fluids, saliva and plaque fluid are supersaturated with respect to fluorapatite. This is usually the case when the pH is above 4.5. Below pH 4.5 the oral fluids become increasingly unsaturated with respect to fluorapatite as well, and fluorhydroxyapatite dissolves increasingly with lower pH.

Formation of calcium fluoride

When the fluoride concentration in the solution bathing the enamel is above 100 ppm calcium fluoride is formed thus:

$$Ca_{10}(PO_4)_6(OH)_2 + 20\ F^- + 8\ H^+ \rightarrow 10\ CaF_2 + 6\ HPO_4^{2-} + 2\ H_2O$$

The above reaction indicates what happens when the teeth are given a topical treatment or exposed to fluoride toothpaste containing NaF. The higher the fluoride concentra-

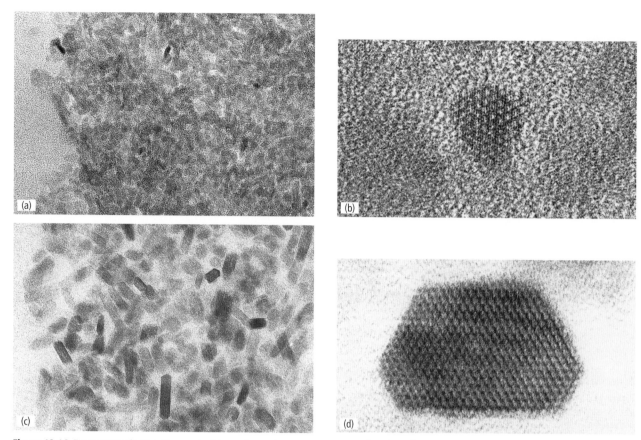

Figure 12.16 Transmission electron microscopic pictures of normal cementum not exposed to the oral environment (a, b) and exposed root surface (c, d). Note the difference in crystal size showing evidence of crystal growth when apatite crystals in cementum had been exposed to the oral cavity. (For original figure refer to Tohda *et al.*, 1996.)

tion the more calcium fluoride is formed. Further, a low pH in the solution has a very strong effect on the calcium fluoride formation. What happens is that in a low pH solution the solubility of enamel increases considerably. The enamel dissolution provides amounts of calcium for a substantial calcium fluoride formation. In a topical treatment for 2 min with a neutral 2% NaF solution containing 9000 ppm fluoride the formation of calcium fluoride is limited because the necessary dissolution of the enamel apatite is slow and leads to low concentrations of ionic calcium. In contrast, fluoride solutions acidulated with phosphoric acid dissolve enamel slightly and deposit substantial amounts of calcium fluoride on the tooth surface.

It should be realized that calcium fluoride is not only formed on sound enamel surfaces. Presumably the most important calcium fluoride is that which precipitates in plaque, in pellicle, in enamel porosities and in other inaccessible, stagnation areas. In such areas the concentration of free ionic calcium is high and a considerable formation can be assumed.

The calcium fluoride is formed in the shape of spherical globules scattered over the surface. Recent studies have shown a structure radiating from the center outwards (Fig. 12.18), indicating that the globules are formed from a central nidus from where their mineralization radiates. The globules consist of calcium fluoride of a rather poor crystalline nature mixed with phosphate.

Dissolution of calcium fluoride

The precipitated calcium fluoride acts as a temporary storage of fluoride from where the active ion gradually is released. This preventive effect is presumed to last as long as the released fluoride is able to maintain an increased concentration level in the near surroundings.

Thus, calcium fluoride does not survive in the oral fluids because the fluids are unsaturated with respect to that salt. To saturate saliva with respect to calcium fluoride, the fluoride concentration must be increased 100-fold, from the physiological 0.02–0.05 ppm to 3–7 ppm. Therefore, in the mouth calcium fluoride will invariably dissolve (Figs 12.19, 12.20). However, this will occur at varying rates. Calcium fluoride situated on open, exposed surfaces disappears within a day, while in protected sites, in plaque and in rough surfaces of active carious lesions, the salt survives for days and

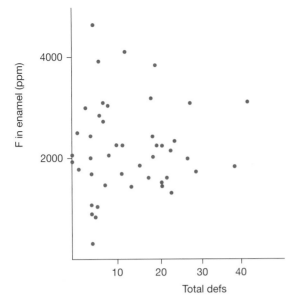

Figure 12.17 Scatter plot of fluoride concentration in surface enamel depending on the prevalence of caries in the deciduous teeth. It may be expected that a low fluoride concentration would be related to a high caries prevalence and vice versa. However, it is seen that when the prevalence is low the fluoride concentration varies from low to high values, and when the caries prevalence in the mouth is high the fluoride concentration in the surface enamel is also high. (Data from Poulsen & Larsen, 1975.)

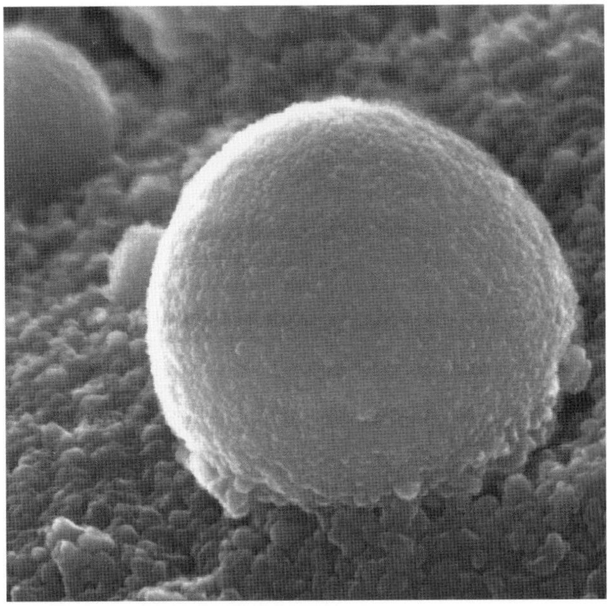

Figure 12.18 Scanning electron micrograph of a calcium fluoride globule (about 0.6 μm in diameter) sitting on the enamel surface. The globule is round with a nodular surface. In transmission electron microscopy the structure of the globule radiates from the center outwards, indicating its growth from a central nidus. (For original figure refer to Petzold, 2001.)

weeks. In particular, considerable survival of calcium fluoride has been observed after topical treatment with acidified fluoride solutions on surfaces that after the treatment were covered with pellicle and plaque. Presumably the acid had created deep irregularities in which the salt was well protected.

A special situation arises when an attempt is made to prevent further development of erosions by frequent application of topical fluoride solutions. The drinks that induce erosion of the teeth are acidic, with pH usually below 3.2. As the p*Ka* value of hydrofluoric acid is 3.2, a considerable part of the fluoride in the drink is present in the form of this acid, which greatly increases the dissolution of calcium fluoride. In theory, a single liter of Coca Cola (pH 2.5) could dissolve calcium fluoride that has been deposited on the surface of more than 5000 teeth. Therefore, it is not expected that calcium fluoride would survive for long in a mouth through which a notable amount of soft drinks passes, in particular where the drink washes over the tooth surface. In conclusion, there is no theoretical background to support the idea that topical fluoride has a notable effect either on remineralization of erosive lesions, or on prevention of further development of these lesions (see also Chapter 13).

Under normal conditions the dissolution of calcium fluoride gives rise to increased concentrations of fluoride in saliva in the period after the topical application (Fig. 12.20).

After a few days, however, the concentrations are back to normal, physiological levels.

It should be noted that the formation and dissolution of calcium fluoride are the only events after a topical treatment that are measurable by chemical means. After the dissolution of the calcium fluoride all chemical traces of the topical treatment have disappeared. Only one other result has been observed: a reduced caries incidence in the months after the topical treatment.

Commercial fluoride varnish

Varnishes with up to 5% sodium fluoride are marketed for caries prevention. Calcium fluoride may also be incorporated in the product. After the setting of the varnish on the tooth or over plaque, fluoride is released partly to the saliva and partly towards the underlying enamel surface with a caries lesion or into the underlying plaque. Locally, high fluoride concentrations can be obtained and calcium fluoride formed. Eventually, the varnish is worn away, the calcium fluoride dissolves and the preventive effect tapers off.

Fluoride toothpaste and calcium fluoride

Fluoride toothpastes contain 500–1500 ppm fluoride either in the form of sodium fluoride (NaF), in the complexed form monofluorophosphate (MFP, Na_2PO_3F), in which oxygen in the phosphate molecule has been replaced by fluoride, or in mixtures of the two salts, NaF and MFP. In NaF

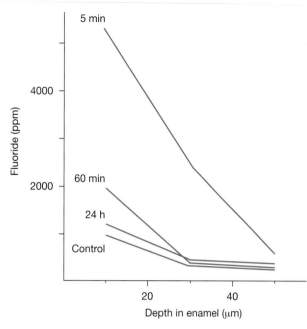

Figure 12.19 Fluoride concentration in enamel after a topical treatment with 2% NaF solution. In the first few hours after treatment most of the deposited CaF$_2$ is dissolved. (From Brudevold, 1974.)

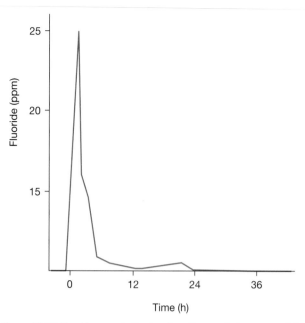

Figure 12.20 Fluoride concentration in saliva after a topical treatment of the dentition with 2% NaF. The fluoride concentration decreases quickly. Overnight a slight increase can be observed. (Data from Lambrou et al., 1981.)

toothpaste the sodium fluoride is dissociated and the fluoride is present in free ionic form. The MFP molecule is hydrolyzed by non-specific bacterial phosphatases when it meets the oral fluids and tissues and when it diffuses into plaque (Pearce & Dibdin, 1995):

$$PO_3F^{2-} + H_2O \rightarrow H_2PO_4^- + F^-$$

It is generally believed that the MFP molecule is unable to diffuse through plaque to the enamel surface without being hydrolyzed. Therefore, basically the fluoride concentration in the mouth, and the preventive effects of the two types of toothpaste are similar. Fluoride toothpastes are also formulated by including various amine fluorides. These are amphipathic compounds where amines substituted with long hydrocarbon chains are the cations for ionic fluoride. The amine parts are intended to improve delivery of fluoride to the tooth surface and possess antimicrobial properties.

Fluoride toothpaste, especially MFP toothpaste, is unlikely to induce any notable calcium fluoride formation on free, well-brushed enamel surfaces, but the extent to which toothpaste causes deposition of calcium fluoride in the plaque remains unknown. Little evidence is available to show its deposition under clinical conditions. If it is present in plaque after tooth brushing it dissolves again with release of fluoride.

Recently, toothpastes with fluoride contents of 2500 and 5000 ppm have been marketed for high-caries individuals. To minimize the risk of inducing fluorosis the opening of the tube is narrow, allowing only a slim line of toothpaste

on the brush. A few studies have shown a beneficial effect of the high concentration of fluoride, but for the time being it remains an open question whether an extra brushing of the teeth a day would not give the same result.

Dentin

The physicochemical rationale to explain the demineralization and remineralization processes described for enamel also applies to dentin, as do the fluoride interactions.

Fluoride treatments on dentin reduce its solubility. Microscopic analysis shows that a thick layer is formed in the surface layer of the dentinal lesion. When dentin specimens are placed in solutions to form caries-like lesions, the presence of fluoride inhibits the demineralization of dentin, as it does with enamel (ten Cate & Duijsters, 1983a, b; ten Cate et al., 1998). However, the fluoride levels required to inhibit demineralization are 10 times higher for dentin than for enamel (Fig. 12.21). Another difference is that when demineralization occurs in the presence of fluoride the surface layer of the specimens is preserved, while the mineral loss of the lesion occurs at greater depth, that is beyond the surface layer. Without fluoride, demineralization creates an erosion-like defect, but with fluoride a subsurface lesion is formed (Fig. 12.22). Histological analysis shows that when dentinal lesions are subjected to pH cycling (a simulation of the pH changes occurring in the mouth) the remineralization occurs primarily in the former lesion area, while mineral is removed from deeper layers in the dentin.

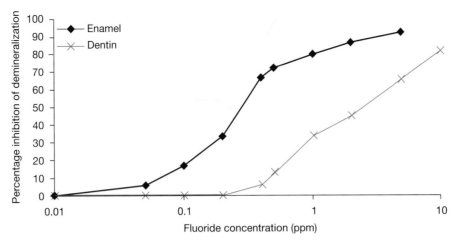

Figure 12.21 Inhibition of demineralization of enamel and dentin at various levels of fluoride in the ambient solutions, expressed as a percentage of the demineralization at 0 ppm fluoride. The data show that dentin requires higher levels of fluoride to reach an inhibition similar to that of enamel. (Adapted from ten Cate & Duijsters, 1983a; ten Cate *et al.*, 1998.)

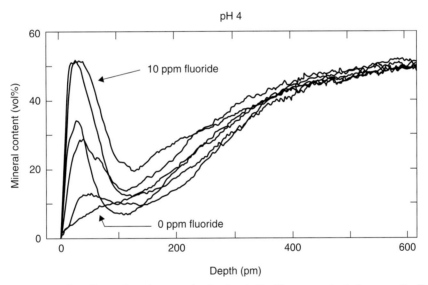

Figure 12.22 Mineral content depth profiles of lesions formed at pH 4, showing that the fluoride concentration in the surrounding fluid determines the mineral content in the surface layer. (For original figure refer to ten Cate *et al.*, 1998.)

Recently it has been shown that very deep lesions, extending through the enamel into the dentin, can still be remineralized when brought into contact with a mineralizing solution. This is a very slow process, but it opens up possibilities for a non-operative approach to very deep lesions.

Dental calculus

The supersaturation of oral fluids with respect to calcium phosphates is the reason (more specifically the thermodynamic driving force) for the maturation and remineralization of enamel and dentinal lesions. However, by the same mechanism it may cause the calcification of dental plaque, resulting in calculus formation. Calculus is also called calcified or petrified dental plaque, and the bacteria play a role in this calcification process. Calculus may occur either subgingivally or supragingivally, and these two types of calculus have a different etiology and different relationships with periodontal inflammation. Supragingival calculus is formed at sites of the dentition close to the ducts of salivary glands and where little caries occurs. This points towards the etiological factors of pH and higher calcium and phosphate concentrations in determining the formation of calculus. The mineral ions are not only are supplied by saliva but may also come from crevicular fluid. Likewise, exudate from

Table 12.4 Prevalence (%) of mineral phases occurring in human dental calculus according to X-ray diffraction

Apatite	Whitlockite	OCP	Brushite
100	80	–	14
100	65	–	–
99.5	80.7	94.8	43.6
98	71	95	44
93	86	99	18
100	–	–	40

Data from Driessens (1982).

periodontally inflamed tissue may contain alkaline substances that could increase the precipitation of mineral salts. Subgingival calculus may form around any tooth. Its position is not related to the ducts of the salivary glands. Calculus is primarily composed of an impure hydroxyapatite, but brushite, whitlockite and octacalcium phosphate are also found in substantial amounts (Table 12.4). In most mineral deposits the more soluble calcium phosphates (such as brushite) slowly convert into hydroxyapatite. For calculus this is apparently a very slow process. Perhaps it is inhibited by other components, because a diversity of minerals was found in calculus obtained from individuals living in the Neolithic times.

Besides calcium and phosphate, magnesium and carbonate are chemical elements found in calculus. The composition of calculus differs significantly between animals, with dogs and cats showing much higher amounts of calcium carbonate than humans. Bacteria are directly or indirectly involved in calculus formation. Specific bacteria have been associated with calculus formation, e.g. *Corynebacterium matruchotii* (Boyan *et al.*, 1989). This bacterium produces membrane-associated proteolipids that are capable of inducing hydroxyapatite formation *in vitro*. Bacteria are constantly subject to invasion by ions present in high concentrations in the surrounding plaque fluid, e.g. calcium and fluoride. They are only able to keep such intruders out by effective metabolism and ion pumps. A dying or less vital microorganism is therefore likely to be killed by high concentrations of mineral ions and intracellular precipitation of minerals. On histological assessment, older calculus shows many bacterial ghost cells, associated with mineral deposits. In addition, enzymes are produced by bacteria that cause the pH in plaque to rise to values where mineral deposition also occurs spontaneously, that is, without the need for a mineral phase on which to precipitate.

While bacteria may facilitate calculus formation, saliva contains many inhibitors of precipitation. The simplest explanation for this is that, in general, they inhibit the formation of mineral deposits in the salivary glands and ducts. Research on calculus formation has shown that calculus is also inhibited by mineralization inhibitors administered as ingredients of a toothpaste. To this end, pyrophosphate and zinc citrate have been investigated and shown to be clinically effective (White, 1997).

Background literature

Elliot JC. *Structure and chemistry of the apatites and other calcium orthophosphates.* Amsterdam: Elsevier, 1994.

Holden A, Morrison P. *Crystals and crystal growing.* Cambridge, MA: MIT Press, 1982.

LeGeros RZ. *Calcium phosphates in oral biology and medicine.* Basel: Karger, 1991.

Schroeder HE. *Formation and inhibition of dental calculus.* Berne: Hans Huber, 1969.

References

Bernardi G, Kawasaki T. Chromatography of polypeptides and proteins on hydroxyapatite columns. *Biochim Biophys Acta* 1968; **13**: 160: 301–10.

Boyan BDE, Swain LD, Boskey AL. Mechanisms of microbial calcification. In: Cate JM ten, ed. *Recent advances in the study of dental calculus.* Oxford: IRL Press, 1989: 29–35.

Brown WE. *Solubilities of phosphates and other sparingly soluble compounds.* National Bureau of Standards Report 10 599. Washington, DC: US Department of Commerce, 1971.

Brudevold F. Fluoride therapy. In: Bernier JL, Muhler JC, eds. *Improving dental practice through preventive measures.* St Louis, MO: Mosby, 1974: 77–103.

Bruun C, Lambrou D, Larsen MJ, Fejerskov O, Thylstrup A. Fluoride in mixed human saliva after different topical fluoride treatments and possible relation to caries inhibition. *Community Dent Oral Epidemiol* 1982; **10**: 124–9.

ten Cate JM, Duijsters PP. Influence of fluoride in solution on tooth demineralization. I. Chemical data. *Caries Res* 1983a; **17**: 193–9.

ten Cate JM, Duijsters PP. Influence of fluoride in solution on tooth demineralization. II. Microradiographic data. *Caries Res* 1983b; **17**: 513–19.

ten Cate JM, Jongebloed WL, Simons YM, Exterkate RAM. Adaptation of dentin to the oral environment. In: Thylstrup A, Leach SA, Qvist V, eds. *Dentine and dentine reactions in the oral cavity.* Oxford: IRL Press, 1987: 67–76.

ten Cate JM, Damen JJM, Buijs MJ. Inhibition of dentin demineralisation by fluoride *in vitro. Caries Res* 1998; **32**: 141–7.

Curzon MEJ, Cutress TW. *Trace elements and dental disease.* Bristol: John Wright, 1983.

Daculsi G, Menanteau J, Kerebel LM, Mitre D. Length and shape of enamel crystals. *Calcif Tiss Int* 1984; **36**: 550–5.

Dawes C, Dong C. The flow rate and electrolyte composition of whole saliva elicited by the use of sucrose-containing and sugar-free chewing-gums. *Arch Oral Biol* 1995; **40**: 699–705.

Driessens FCM. Calculus. In: Myers HM, ed. *Mineral aspects of dentistry.* Basel: Karger, 1982: 154–8.

Fejerskov O, Nyvad B, Larsen MJ. Human experimental caries models: intra-oral environmental variability. *Adv Dent Res* 1994; **8**: 134–43.

Frank RM, Vogel JC. Ultrastructure of the human odontoblast process and its mineralisation during dental caries. *Caries Res* 1980; **14**: 367–80.

Furseth R. A study of experimentally exposed and fluoride treated dental cementum in pigs. *Acta Odontol Scand* 1970; **28**: 833–50.

Lagerlöf F. Effects of flow rate and pH on calcium phosphate saturation in human parotid saliva. *Caries Res* 1983; **17**: 403–11.

Lambrou D, Larsen MJ, Fejerskov O, Tachos B. The effect of fluoride in saliva on remineralization of dental enamel in humans. *Caries Res* 1981; **15**: 341–5.

Larsen MJ, Pearce EIF. Some notes on the diffusion of acidic and alkaline agents into natural human caries lesions *in vitro. Arch Oral Biol* 1992; **37**: 411–16.

Larsen MJ, Pearce EIF, Jensen SJ. Notes on the dissolution of human dental enamel in dilute acid solutions at high solid/solution ratio. *Caries Res* 1993; **27**: 87–95.

McCann HG. The solubility of fluorapatite and its relationship to that of calcium fluoride. *Arch Oral Biol* 1968; **13**: 987–1001.

Margolis HC, Moreno EC. Composition of pooled plaque fluid from caries-free and caries positive individuals following sucrose exposure. *J Dent Res* 1992; **71**: 1776–84.

Margolis HC, Zhang YP, van Houte J, Moreno EC. Effect of sucrose concentration on the cariogenic potential of pooled plaque fluid from caries-free and caries-positive individuals. *Caries Res* 1993; **27**: 467–73.

Moreno EC, Zahradnik RT. Chemistry of enamel subsurface demineralisation *in vitro*. *J Dent Res* 1974; 53: 226–35.

Moreno EC, Kresak M, Zahradnik RT. Fluoridated hydroxyapatite solubility and caries formation. *Nature* 1974; **247**: 64–5.

Moreno EC, Varughese K, Hay DI. Effect of human salivary proteins on the precipitation kinetics of calcium phosphate. *Calcif Tiss Int* 1979; **28**: 7–16.

Nelson DGA. The influence of carbonate on the atomic structure and reactivity of hydroxyapatite. *J Dent Res* 1981; **60**: 1621–9.

Nyvad B, ten Cate JM, Fejerskov O. Arrest of root surface caries *in situ*. *J Dent Res* 1997; **76**: 1845–53.

Ögaard B, Rølla G, Arends J. *In vivo* progress of enamel and root surface lesions under plaque as a function of time. *Caries Res* 1988; **22**: 302–5.

Ögaard B, Arends J, Rølla G. Action of fluoride on initiation of early root surface caries *in vivo*. *Caries Res* 1990; **24**: 142–4.

Pearce EIF. Relationship between demineralisation events in dental enamel and the pH and mineral content of plaque. *Proc Am Dent Soc* 1991; **87**: 527–39.

Pearce EIF, Dibdin GH. The diffusion and enzymic hydrolysis of monofluorophosphate in dental plaque. *J Dent Res* 1995; **74**: 691–7.

Pearce EIF, Larsen MJ, Cutress TW. Studies on the influence of fluoride on the equilibrating calcium phosphate phase at a high enamel/acid ratio. *Caries Res* 1995; **29**: 258–65.

Petzold M. The influence of different fluoride compounds and treatment conditions on dental enamel: a descriptive *in vitro* study of the CaF$_2$ precipitation and microstructure. *Caries Res* 2001; **35** (Suppl 1): 45–51.

Poulsen S, Larsen MJ. Dental caries in relation to fluoride content in the primary dentition. *Caries Res* 1975; **9**: 59–65.

Rose RK, Dibdin GH, Shellis RP. A quantitative study of calcium binding and aggregation in selected oral bacteria. *J Dent Res* 1993; **72**: 78–84.

Selvig KA, Zander HA. Chemical analysis and microradiography of cementum and dentin from periodontally diseased teeth. *J Periodontol* 1962; **33**: 303–10.

Shannon IL, Suddick RP, Dowd FJ Jr. Saliva: composition and secretion (review). *Monogr Oral Sci* 1974; **2**: 1–103.

Shellis RP. Effects of a supersaturated pulpal fluid on the formation of caries-like lesions on the roots of human teeth. *Caries Res* 1994; **28**: 14–20.

Shellis RP. A scanning electron-microscope study of solubility variations in human enamel and dentine. *Arch Oral Biol* 1996; **41**: 473–84.

Shellis RP, Heywood BR, Wahab FK. Formation of brushite, monetite and whitlockite during equilibration of human enamel with acid solutions at 37°C. *Caries Res* 1997; **31**: 71–7.

Sønju T, Rølla G. Chemical analysis of the acquired pellicle formed in two hours on cleaned human teeth *in vivo*. Rate of formation and amino acid analysis. *Caries Res* 1973; **7**: 30–8.

Tanaka M, Margolis HC. Release of mineral ions in dental plaque following acid production. *Arch Oral Biol* 1999; **44**: 253–8.

Tohda H, Takuma S, Tanaka N. Intracrystalline structure of enamel crystals affected by caries. *J Dent Res* 1987; **66**: 1647–53.

Tohda H, Fejerskov O, Yanagisawa T. Transmission electron microscopy of cementum crystals correlated with Ca and F distribution in normal and carious human root surfaces. *J Dent Res* 1996; **75**: 949–54.

White DJ. Dental calculus: recent insights into occurrence, formation, prevention, removal and oral health effects of supragingival and subgingival deposits. *Eur J Oral Sci* 1997; **105**: 508–22.

13

Erosion of the teeth

M.J. Larsen

Introduction

After eruption, three types of acid dissolution may remove tooth mineral: caries, erosion and acid etching to create retention for resin fillings. Each of these lesions has a specific etiology, a specific microscopic and macroscopic appearance and diagnostic challenges and, for the two first lesions, specific treatment solutions. The caries lesion and its related problems are dealt with elsewhere in this book and retentive etching in Chapter 22, while erosion of the teeth is presented below.

Clinical manifestations and diagnosis

Erosion is characterized by dissolution and removal of an ultrathin layer of enamel each time it is exposed to an acidic challenge. This is in contrast to caries, which develops with a subsurface lesion body and the surface layer preserved so long as it remains supported by subsurface structures. The color of active eroded enamel remains unaltered, the surface becomes smooth and usually shiny, and surface details such as perichymata and lobi disappear. It is characteristic that the tooth becomes rounded and often lacks attrition facets because enamel often is eroded away more rapidly than it is worn by attrition.

Only surfaces directly exposed to the acidic matter are affected. Enamel under plaque, approximal surfaces, and areas in the vicinity of and under gingiva are not exposed and remain unaffected. Primary caries develops under plaque close to gingiva, approximally under contact points and deep in fissures. Thus, the location of erosion is different from that of caries.

Lingual surfaces of maxillary incisors are often more affected than are labial surfaces, with early removal of the lingual tuberculum of the tooth (Figs 13.1–13.5). Further, initial exposure of dentin often occurs lingually at the edge, the incisal enamel prisms become unsupported with some transparency when viewed *en face* and, as the prisms are torn away, the incisal edge often becomes serrated (Fig. 13.2). Occlusally in premolars and molars and in lower incisors where the incisal enamel is worn or eroded away, the dentin can be hollowed out (Fig. 13.17).

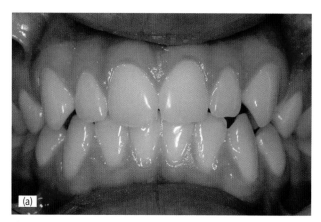 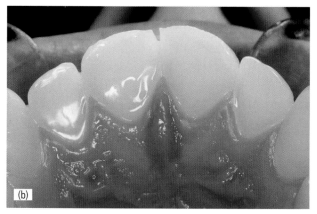

Figure 13.1 Early stage of eroded anterior teeth. Viewed *en face*, the contours are rounded (a). The lingual surfaces have been flattened and the tubercula eroded away (b). The enamel is smooth and shiny.

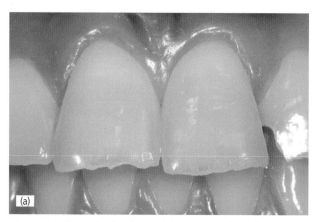 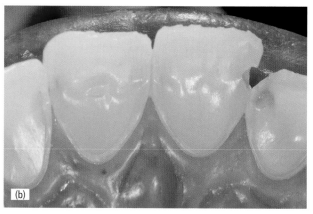

Figure 13.2 The erosion has flattened the anterior surface (a) and removed most of the enamel of the lingual surface (b), leaving a narrow shelf of enamel protected by gingiva. The incisal edge appears bluish and serrated as incisal enamel prisms become unsupported by dentin.

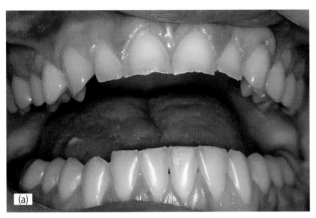

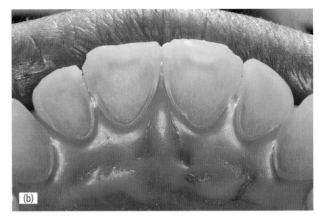

Figure 13.3 The erosion has shortened the anterior maxillary teeth (a), removed all enamel of lingual surfaces (b) and is close to the pulp, still leaving a narrow shelf of enamel protected by gingiva. The enamel has a silk-like surface, indicating an aggressive stage of erosion.

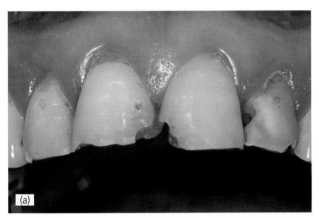

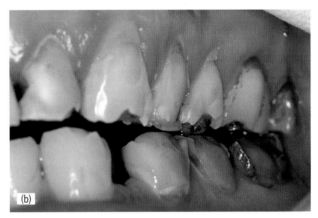

Figure 13.4 Subject with serious erosion and caries after long-lasting consumption of still red fruit lemonade. The surface enamel of anterior teeth is silk-like (a); elsewhere, the buccal enamel has been almost entirely eroded away leaving dentinal surfaces (b) that are too sore for careful brushing. Such surfaces often turn yellow–brownish. The fillings can be seen to be raised over the tooth substance.

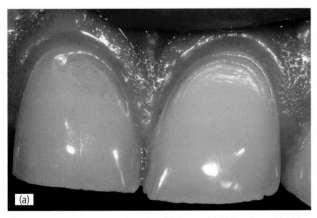

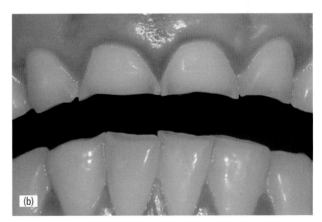

Figure 13.5 Two outcomes of erosion: (a) flattened labial surface with kidney-shaped exposure of yellowish dentin and (b) considerable shortening of the clinical crown.

Occasionally, when dentin is exposed the surface becomes sensitive to cold and warm foods and to tactile stimuli. The subject may then abstain from careful tooth brushing of such areas and the exposed dentin becomes yellowish or brownish.

Erosion and wear

Clinical features of erosion are characterized by a smoothening of the surface, a removal of lobi and a rounding of the enamel contours. In contrast, attrition leaves wear facets, matching the cusps and incisal edges of the antagonists.

Occasionally, lower incisors may develop a groove in the lingual surface of maxillary incisors without signs of facets (Fig. 13.6). Wear facets are rarely observed in eroded teeth.

Occlusal surfaces of molars and premolars rarely show wear facets, but are rounded with time (Fig. 13.7). When the combination of wear and erosion has removed the enamel

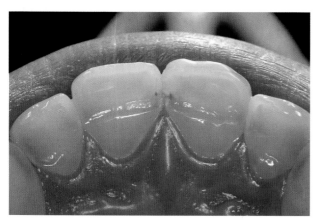

Figure 13.6 Lingual surface of incisors showing a shelf-like furrow fretted by the mandibular teeth. Note that no wear facets are seen.

and penetrated to the dentin, the dentin is eroded more rapidly than the surrounding enamel and if fillings are present the tooth substance around it is removed, leaving a protruding filling that looks as if it is being extruded from the tooth.

Whether daily tooth brushing with abrasive toothpaste removes significant and observable amounts of enamel from eroded surfaces remains to be shown *in vivo*. It has conclusively been shown that *in vitro* etched and 'presoftened' enamel is more vulnerable to tooth brushing than normal enamel. It is likely that tooth brushing with an acidic drink in the mouth also removes more dental material than does tooth brushing after neutralization with a neutral saliva/toothpaste mixture in the mouth. However, it has never been demonstrated whether the presoftened enamel is a caries-like lesion with partially demineralized enamel vulnerable to wear or an erosion-like lesion with a glass-like, wear-resistant surface.

Histological and chemical features

The caries lesion is characterized by a subsurface partial demineralization in which the subsurface lesion body is

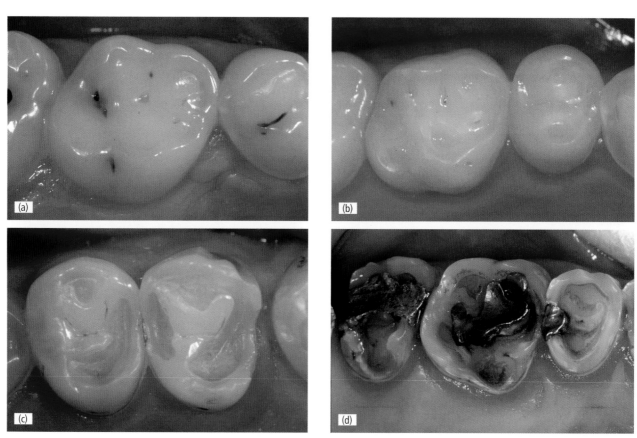

Figure 13.7 Eroded occlusal surfaces from a rounding of the contours over partial exposure of dentin with deepened hollowed out areas to complete enamel removal, leaving fillings and an enamel rim elevated over the dentin. Note that no sign of wear facets can be seen.

covered by a surface layer with a fluoride content higher than the surrounding sound enamel (Chapter 12, Fig. 12.6). The partial demineralization of both surface and subsurface renders the enamel softer by further demineralization. The lesion is at least to some extent theoretically subject to remineralization of partially dissolved apatite crystals. In contrast, erosion of the teeth is characterized by a complete dissolution of the apatite mineral of enamel and dentin and the lesion appears hard (Larsen, 1973; Meurman & ten Cate, 1995). As remineralization in the oral cavity is a regrowth of partially destroyed apatite crystals, remineralization of eroded enamel is hardly possible (Chapter 12, Fig. 12.7).

When the dental hard tissues are exposed to a solution that is unsaturated with respect to hydroxyapatite and supersaturated with respect to fluorapatite, subsurface hydroxyapatite dissolves and fluorapatite is formed in the surface layer (Chapter 12). The more fluoride present in the oral environment, the more fluorapatite is formed in the surface and the thicker and more well mineralized the surface layer remains. When the dental hard tissues are exposed to a solution that is unsaturated with respect to both hydroxyapatite and fluorapatite, both apatites dissolve and the tooth is eroded (Larsen, 1975). Thus, in development of the caries lesion, fluoride plays an important role by being taken up in surface enamel under the formation of fluorapatite, and thereby forms the basis for formation and maintenance of the surface layer (Larsen, 1973). Without fluoride uptake the surface layer is not formed and the lesion becomes an erosion (Chapter 12, Figs 12.6; 12.7).

As fluoride is part of the caries process, by creating and maintaining the surface layer, fluoride interaction and caries control are explainable. In erosion of the teeth, fluoride plays no role and fluoride is not found to prevent erosion.

Classification by depth of the lesion

Erosion is classified after two principles: the depth of the lesion and the pathogenesis of the erosion. Classification of erosion according to the depth of the lesion is based on observation of exposure of the dentin (Larsen *et al.*, 2000):

0: Intact, sound, no sign of erosion.
1: Erosion exclusively of enamel; no sign of exposure of dentin. The surface appears smooth with no sign of perichymata, lobi and other signs of minor anatomical details that have been eroded away. In the single surface, dentin is not exposed.
2: Erosion through enamel with exposure of dentin, the area of dentin exposure is less than 50% of the area of the single surface.
3: Erosion through enamel with exposure of dentin being more than 50% of the surface area.

Other classification systems have been suggested and used with success (Imfeld, 1995; Lussi, 1995). The above

system has the advantage that the limits between classes are reasonably well defined, i.e. dentinal exposure can usually be identified. The system has two main weaknesses. First, it is extremely difficult to identify the first erosion of a surface, partly because the signs are so weak and uncharacteristic, and the surface appears similar to normal intact enamel, and partly because everybody has some slight erosion of the teeth that may be considered normal. This weakness is shared with any classification index of erosion. Secondly, class 1 is very wide and roomy, extending from slight signs of erosion that may be ignored, to a state where almost all the enamel is eroded away. It has been suggested that class 1 may be divided into two classes by a limit halfway through enamel, but the identification of such a limit presents severe problems. The width of class 1 makes it impossible to monitor development of erosion from an early lesion to maturity by simple written records. Photographs, casts or other measures are needed.

Classification by etiology

Erosion is also classified according to the pathogenesis of the lesion. Various classification systems have been used. A simple classification is:

- erosion caused by foods and drinks
- erosion caused by stomach acid (regurgitation, vomit, eating disorders)
- occupational erosion by airborne acids
- idiopathic erosion (the cause is unknown).

Erosion caused by foods and drinks is widespread in younger age groups, whereas regurgitation seems to be a frequent cause in adults and elderly. Presumably every grown individual living in a modern society has at least some erosion from consumption of fresh fruit and soft drinks. Erosion caused by regurgitated or vomited stomach contents and occupational airborne acids shows a distribution within the dentition that usually differs from that of erosion caused by fruits and drinks. The group idiopathic erosion is often suggested to accommodate erosion with no apparent pathogenesis. Most often, idiopathic erosion has been caused by food and drinks that have been long forgotten.

The distribution in the mouth usually reflects the pathogenesis, as shown below.

Erosion and dry mouth

A reduced rate of saliva secretion is an aggravating factor, just as it increases the risk of caries, presumably owing to delayed removal of acid and sugar from the mouth and because many patients suffering from dry mouth wet their mouth with a fresh acidic drink that may contain sugar. Treatment with cytotoxic drugs often causes nausea and vomiting combined with dry mouth. Slaking the mouth with a fresh acidic soft drink may be assumed to be particularly erosive.

Erosion caused by food and drinks

Distribution in the mouth

The teeth are eroded where the fresh and acidic food and drinks hit the enamel surfaces before they are diluted and neutralized by saliva. Primarily, the labial and lingual surfaces of maxillary anterior teeth are affected, presumably as a result of drinking habits. Both prevalence and distribution within the mouth depend on food habits, selection of foods and drinks preferred locally, the age, prehistory and habits of the individual, etc.

A special subgroup is formed by consumers of acidic medicine.

Events in the mouth

When a soft drink enters the mouth it flows over the tongue, and seeps down between its papillae on its way towards the throat. There is, by and large, a seal between the tongue and the mandibular teeth and their supporting gums. During swallowing, the tongue is pressed up against the palate and the maxillary teeth. As the drink flows over the lingual surfaces of the maxillary incisors and premolars it may erode these surfaces. The erosive effect of the drink is assumed to be enhanced by remains of the drink between the papillae of the tongue. Often, lips and cheeks may cover and protect the labial and buccal surfaces of maxillary and mandibular teeth, but occasionally an individual may enjoy letting the drink swish around in vestibulum oris, eroding labial and buccal tooth surfaces as well as occlusal surfaces.

The erosive effect of most drinks is short lived and limited to the seconds during which it washes over the tooth surface. The drink that is harbored between the papillae of the tongue may protract the effect up to a few minutes, in particular when the drink has a high content of fruit acids and the buffering capacity is high (Figs 13.8–13.11). Within minutes the drink in the tongue surface and elsewhere in the mouth is neutralized by saliva stimulated by the acidity of the drink. Stimulated saliva has a high content of bicarbonate and thus a high buffer capacity. Overall, the drink and what is left in the mouth is neutralized within minutes, in contrast to the pH drop in plaque after consumption of fermentable carbohydrates. Those pH drops may last for half an hour.

In the next few minutes the surface of the tongue harbors the drink and the tongue is able to lick away an ultrathin layer of enamel, in particular when the drink has a high buffer capacity that keeps the pH of the tongue surface low for a minute or two more than a drink with a small content of acids (Fig. 13.9). Measurement of pH of the dorsum of the tongue has demonstrated that pH initially drops to a value not much higher than that of the drink itself. Within 1 min the pH has risen to above 5.5, unless the buffer capacity is high, as it is in orange juice. The pH drop after orange juice remains low for up to around 2 min. If the drink contains fermentable carbohydrates a secondary pH drop is induced after about 5 min, presumably due to the bacterial flora of the back of the tongue (Figs 13.8–13.10). In most patients the secondary drop is just a small lowering of the pH curve, whereas in other subjects the pH drops to 5 even if the acid of the drink was neutralized before it was

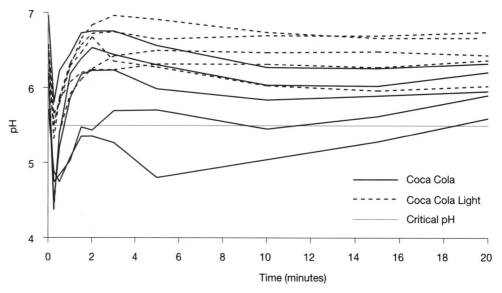

Figure 13.8 pH of tongue saliva among five subjects after consumption of 2 × 20 ml of Coca Cola and Coca Cola Light. Standard Coca Cola causes a deeper immediate pH and a secondary pH drop after a few minutes. Coca Cola Light does not seem to induce a secondary pH drop.

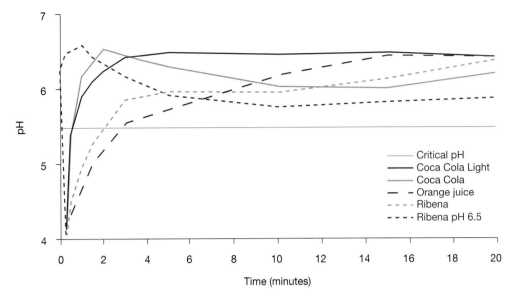

Figure 13.9 Tongue saliva pH of a single individual after drinking 2 × 20 ml of Coca Cola, Coca Cola Light, orange juice, Ribena fruit drink (diluted for drinking) and Ribena pH 6.5 (diluted for drinking and neutralized with HCl). Critical pH is given for reference. The Coca Cola drinks have been neutralized by saliva within 1 min, whereas the drinks with more buffering fruit acids maintain a low pH for up to 3 min. Note that drinks with sugars tend to establish a secondary pH drop after 5 min, presumably due to tongue flora bacterial metabolism. The strongest secondary pH drop seems to be caused by neutralized Ribena fruit drink.

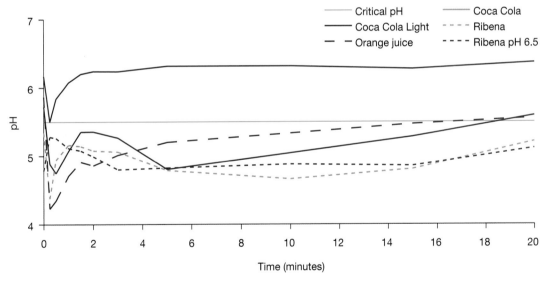

Figure 13.10 Tongue saliva pH of a single individual after drinking 2 × 20 ml of Coca Cola, Coca Cola Light, orange juice, Ribena fruit drink (diluted for drinking) and Ribena pH 6.5 (diluted for drinking and neutralized with HCl). Critical pH is given for reference. In comparison with the subject in Fig. 13.9, this subject harbored an acidogenic tongue flora that was able to extend the low pH in the tongue saliva for 15 min or more. The absence of fermentable carbohydrates in diet Coca Cola Light caused pH not to establish a secondary pH drop.

consumed. Whether this secondary pH drop has clinical importance, and may make some subjects more susceptible to erosion, is unknown.

In conclusion, the primary pH drop after drinking an acidic drink is short-lived. It may be assumed that enamel is eroded when the drink flushes over the teeth and this is terminated within this short period. Therefore, to have any chance at all of preventing erosion, the mouth and the tongue must be rinsed within the first 30 s after drinking some fresh drink. However, such preventive action seems impractical because people do not usually consume a drink in one go. Indeed, they are more likely to sip.

Another consequence of the short-lived pH drop is that sipping a drink extends the time of exposure considerably and therefore the way in which a drink is consumed may be an erosive risk factor of significance.

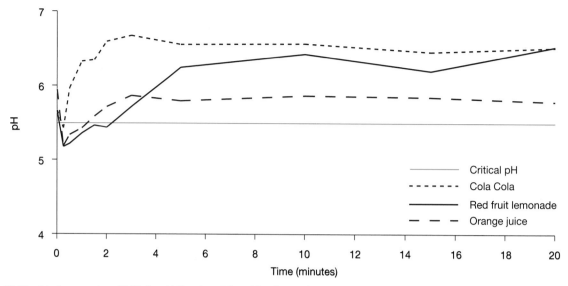

Figure 13.11 pH in the upper buccal fold after drinking Coca Cola, red fruit lemonade and orange juice. Drinking habits vary and other people may habitually let a drink swish around in the buccal folds, which will give another curve.

Epidemiology

The epidemiology of erosion presents a number of problems that make the description less reliable than the epidemiology of other lesions and disorders of humans. First, erosion is widespread. Presumably, every individual who has consumed some fresh fruit, juice and/or soft drinks has at least some, and initially insignificant erosion of the teeth that may develop with time. Therefore, only readily observable and distinct erosion should appear in an epidemiological description. Whatever the level of inclusion may be, the limit between a sound surface and an eroded surface is difficult to identify. No international concept has been established.

Further, both prevalence and distribution within the mouth depend on age, the lifestyle of the person and the way in which he or she consumes acidic drinks and fresh fruit. It should be noted that in a large number of articles a distinction between wear and erosion is not made because the two lesions appear visually similar. In such articles the term erosive wear is used. It should, however, not be so extraordinarily difficult to distinguish between the two lesions, as wear creates and is associated with wear facets that can be checked with the antagonist, whereas erosion smooths off the surface and is not confined to sites in contact with antagonists.

In caries, prevalence data are usually given by the average number of decayed, missing and filled teeth or surfaces, DMFT or DMFS. No such concept has been developed for studies of erosion. In erosion studies, a single occurrence, occurrence in the anterior teeth, and occurrence in four or more sites have been used as criteria for inclusion of an individual in the group of subjects affected by erosion.

The most serious obstacle for a reliable epidemiological description is diagnostic difficulties. Because the surface of the tooth does not change in either color or texture, the identification and diagnosis of erosion are difficult and much more inconsistent than those of caries. After an in-depth discussion of diagnostic criteria and having stressed the rule 'if in doubt, don't score', nine examiners recorded erosion among 10 15–17-year-old subjects (Table 13.1) (Larsen *et al.*, 2005). The interexaminer reliability was low, indicating that any comparison of erosion studies should be made with the utmost caution. The results indicate further that clinicians often may fail to see erosion in general everyday practice, even if they make an effort to identify eroded surfaces or teeth. These features make any epidemiological description of dental erosion and comparison of studies difficult.

Table 13.1 Number of eroded surfaces among 10 subjects identified by nine independent blinded examiners: erosion confined exclusively to enamel, erosion also involving dentin and total number of eroded surfaces

Examiner	Erosion of enamel	Erosion exposing dentin	Erosion, total
A	3.9	0.2	4.1
B	6.4	2.5	8.9
C	10.3	0.1	10.4
D	10.1	0.5	10.6
E	11.6	0	11.6
F	11.6	1.3	12.9
G	13.2	1.2	14.4
H	17.6	0.8	18.4
I	21.3	0	21.3

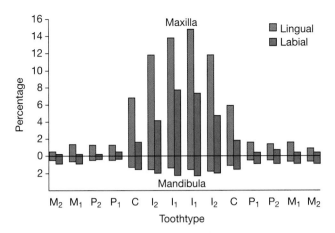

Figure 13.12 Percentual prevalence of eroded surfaces within the mouth among 14–16-year-old adolescents. The lingual surfaces of maxillary anteriors in particular, and to a lesser extent their labial surfaces are eroded. Premolars and molars are rarely affected. This indicates that the place to look for erosion is the lingual surfaces of the maxillary incisors.

The prevalence and distribution of erosion among 14–16-year-olds was examined in a Danish population (Fig. 13.12). In this group the maxillary incisors in particular had been eroded, and mostly their lingual surfaces. Molars, premolars and lower incisors were only slightly affected. The distribution of erosion is derived from local drinking habits. Different drinking and eating habits will be likely to create different erosive patterns.

Acidity of drinks, juice and fruit

Two factors in erosive food items are of importance in relation to tooth erosion: pH and the content of fruit acids. The relation between the pH of the drink and the content of acids appears in Fig. 13.13. The content of acids is equivalent to the amount of alkali sufficient to neutralize the drink, as given in the abscissa, while pH is the pH value given where the curves intersect the ordinate. Although the pH of Coca Cola is low, at 2.5, the content of acid is moderate. In contrast, the pH in orange juice and ready-made fruit drinks ranges between 3 and 4, although they contain considerable amounts of fruit acids. Grape tonic combines a low pH with significant amounts of acids. A list of the pH of various fruits and drinks is provided in Table 13.2.

The term erosive potential is not well defined. The term expresses how much enamel apatite a drink or a food item may dissolve in the period it is supposed to be in the mouth before it is neutralized. It is generally believed that the erosive potential is closely related to the pH of the drink because drinks only briefly in contact with enamel as they wash over it are quickly neutralized by saliva in the mouth (Fig. 13.14) (Jensdottir *et al.*, 2006). The effect of drinks harbored between the papillae of the tongue can be assumed to be somewhat prolonged, in particular if the content of organic fruit acids is high.

Organic acids and carbohydrates in soft drinks

In principle, a non-carbohydrate, diet soft drink erodes enamel to the same extent as does the corresponding soft

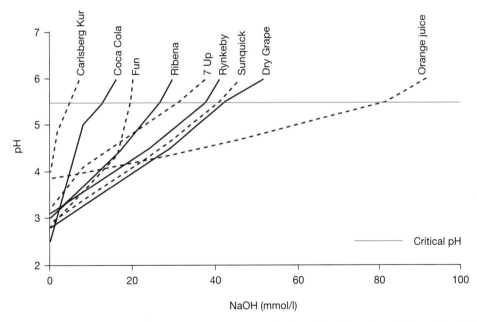

Figure 13.13 pH in various drinks and orange juice as a function of added sodium hydroxide. At the ordinate, the original pH of the drink is given. In general, the more NaOH necessary to neutralize the drink, the more fruit acid the drink contains, the higher the buffer capacity and the longer the drink is able to maintain a low pH in the mouth, at least in the tongue saliva. Coca Cola has the lowest pH and thus a high erosive potential when flushing over the tooth surface. In contrast, orange juice is able to maintain a pH in the range below pH 5 owing to its high buffer capacity.

Table 13.2 Some soft drinks and fruits, with their pH

	pH		pH
Soft drinks		*Fresh fruits*	
Schweppes Indian Tonic	2.5	Jonagold apple	3.2
Coca Cola	2.5	Belle de Boskop apple	3.2
Schweppes Dry Grape	2.8	Granny Smith apple	3.2
Fanta Orange	2.9	Orange	3.4–3.5
Sprite Light	3.0	Grapefruit	3.0
7up	3.0	Apricot	3.9–4.8
		Green grapes	3.2
Juice		Blue grapes	3.7
Orange juice	3.5–4.0	Kiwi fruit	3.5
Apple juice	3.5		
Tomato juice	4.2	*Mineral water*	
		Carlsberg mineral water	4.6
Fruit drinks, non-carbonated		Carlsberg mineral water with lemon and lime	4.0
Fun Light	2.8		
Fruiss, Sirop de Fruits	2.8	Aqua Minerale	5.1
Sunquick Trope	3.0	Aqua Minerale with lemon and lime	5.0
Ribena	3.1		
Rynkeby Black Currant	3.1	Tuborg mineral water	5.4

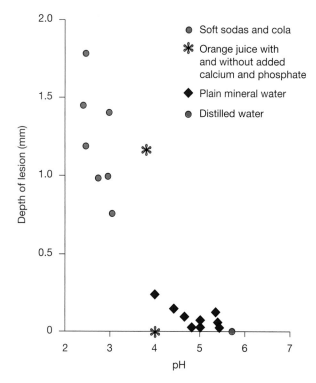

Figure 13.14 Depth of enamel lesion after exposure to gently agitated drinks for a week as a function of pH of the drink. The depth of the lesion is a function of pH, and a curve through the points has a shape similar to that of enamel solubility (cf. Fig. 12.5). The orange juice containing 40 mmol/l calcium and 30 mmol/l phosphate is non-erosive, in contrast to that without calcium and phosphate.

drink with low molecular carbohydrates in it. However, a sugar-containing drink provides fermentable carbohydrates for the plaque that induces acid production and a pH drop there, which may contribute to carious demineralization. Diet soft drinks have not been shown to affect either plaque pH or pH in the caries lesion.

Consumption of soft drinks and fruit

The consumption of soft drinks in the USA has been on the increase since the late 1970s, but seems to have stabilized in the twenty-first century (http://www.statpub.com, 2006). In the USA annual soda production ranges around 600 12-oz cans per person per year or 200 liters per person per year, which is twice as much as it was in 1977. In particular, the age groups below 40 years accounted for a high consumption (Nielsen & Popkin, 2004). In Denmark the annual consumption of soda, fruit drinks and juice increased from 126 liters per person in 1993 to 157 liters per person in 1998. There is nothing to indicate that the trends differ elsewhere in the Western world.

The consumption of fruit in the USA ranges around 115–135 kg per capita per year, including fresh fruit, canned and dried fruit, fruit juice, etc. Of the fresh fruit, bananas with a moderate pH, around 5, account for one-third. The amount of fruit thus has a volume comparable to that of soft drinks.

It may be assumed that the prevalence of erosion is linked to the consumption of fresh fruit and soft drinks and, in particular, to the cumulated consumption over the years, as erosion is cumulated over such periods. Therefore, it can be expected that a steady high consumption of these foods will lead to increasing erosion in the future.

Apatite solubility and pH

The solubility of a mineral is the amount of mineral dissolved at equilibrium between a solid phase and a solution. The solubility is given in grams of dissolved mineral per liter or in moles of dissolved apatite per liter. The solubility of tooth mineral, apatite, depends on the pH of the medium that surrounds it. In the pH range of particular interest, between pH 2 and 6, the solubility increases by a factor of 10 for each pH drop of one pH unit. Thus, the solubility of apatite increases 10-fold when the pH drops from 5 to 4, for example (Chapter 12, Fig. 12.5). The solubility curve describes the amount of dissolved material, i.e. dissolved calcium and phosphate, as a function of pH.

When an acidic drink washes over a tooth surface, equilibrium is not attained. However, the rate of apatite dissolution is a function of the solubility, so that the higher the solubility, the faster the apatite dissolves. This means that low pH products such as Coca Cola, and tonic water at pH 2.5, are more aggressive than orange juice at pH 4 (Table 13.2, Fig. 13.14). However, the high content of fruit acids in orange juice gives it its ability to keep pH low, allowing it more time for dissolution (Figs 13.9, 13.10).

Erosion caused by medicine

Frequently consumed acidic medicine may erode the teeth where it hits directly and where medicine dissolved in tongue saliva comes into contact with maxillary teeth.

Erosion caused by stomach contents

Stomach acid may enter the mouth as a consequence of an eating disorder, rumination or gastroesophageal reflux, often in connection with indigestion, chronic alcoholism, pregnancy, etc. (Holst & Lange, 1939; Scheutzel, 1995). Vomiting may be a feature of eating disorders, which may be classified as:

- anorexia nervosa
- bulimia nervosa
- other eating disorders.

The latter may have characteristics of both anorexia and bulimia.

Anorexia is Greek and means absence of appetite. The patient slims excessively by abstaining from eating and despite a low body mass index still considers that further weight loss is attractive. It is estimated that around 1% of the population in the Western countries is affected. In particular, younger women, from 14 to 40 years, are affected. The condition is also found in men, but is less common. Anorexia may be serious, with a death rate of 25% among seriously affected patients. As the patients rarely vomit, the teeth usually are not eroded by gastric contents.

In contrast, bulimia (Greek: ox hunger) is characterized by normal to inordinate eating, followed by self-induced vomiting. The vomiting is induced after excessive eating to reduce the intake of nutritious matter as part of a slimming program.

The pathophysiology and psychology of these disorders are poorly understood and the treatment is complicated and multifactorial. The role of the dentist is limited to early identification of the disorder and preventing serious damage to the dentition.

Some people are human ruminants. They voluntarily regurgitate food, chew on it, and then swallow again. The resulting tooth erosion can be quite excessive. A sympathetic manner is required in history taking to extract this information. Those to whom it applies may be reluctant to admit the habit, while those who do not do it can be both revolted and insulted by the questioning. The prevalence of rumination is unknown.

Gastroesophageal reflux disease is characterized by a reflux of stomach contents from the stomach through the esophagus, past its sphincters and into the oropharynx (Bartlett *et al.*, 1996). The symptoms include heartburn,

difficulty in swallowing and chest pain combined with regurgitation. The prevalence of gastric reflux is difficult to assess. Its erosive significance varies, as some subjects with reflux are free of erosion whereas others present with severely eroded teeth. Presumably, if the individual manages to keep the stomach content from entering the mouth the erosion can be held at a low level.

In general, acidic gastric content entering the mouth may, in time, erode the teeth. The pH of gastric juice ranges around 1.5–3.0 with a concentration of acid around 40 mmol/l. Although it will be somewhat buffered and diluted by the foods, gastric juice is considered to be strongly erosive.

Distribution in the mouth

When the regurgitated or vomited stomach content enters the oral cavity from the oropharynx, it spreads over the dorsum of the tongue. Where the dorsum is in contact with the teeth they are eroded, so that primarily the lingual cusps and lingual surfaces of maxillary premolars and molars are at risk (Fig. 13.15). Even the palatal surfaces of maxillary incisors and canines are often affected. Occlusal surfaces of the teeth are also affected by erosion around fillings, which may leave them protruding, elevated over the enamel. Lingual cusps of maxillary molars and premolars are flattened. When lingual enamel is eroded away, the surface becomes sensitive and less well brushed, which may lead to a brownish discoloration. Rarely, buccal and labial surfaces are affected.

Erosion caused by airborne acids

In certain industries, e.g. the steel industry, galvanizing of tanks and the accumulator industry, the air may contain acidic fumes. Years ago, under poor factory hygiene standards and with poor protection of workers, the fumes

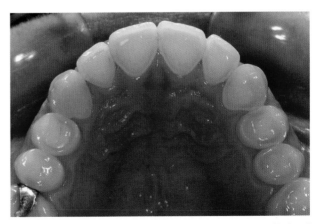

Figure 13.15 Maxillary dentition of a young woman complaining of habitual vomiting after eating (bulimia). The lingual surfaces of incisors, occlusal and lingual surfaces of premolars (and of molars) are eroded. The enamel surface is smooth and without wear facets.

caused rapid erosion of the teeth. This is now a rare phenomenon in the Western world.

Distribution in the mouth

When the air contains evaporated acids it tends to burn the nasal mucosa. To ease the discomfort in the nose, the exposed individual starts to breathe through the mouth. The evaporated acids are then dissolved in saliva, covering the teeth, the tongue and elsewhere in contact with the airstream. The enamel and dentin exposed below the upper lip are eroded away (Figs 13.16, 13.17) to the extent that the patient may look almost edentulous. Once the acidic saliva on the tongue erodes the lingual enamel surfaces in the maxilla the erosive pattern is similar to erosions caused by fresh drinks and foods.

Idiopathic erosion

Distribution in the mouth

The label idiopathic erosion covers those cases where no pathogenesis can be identified by anamnestic questioning. Although a pathogenetic cause cannot be identified and the erosion appears unexplained, this does not mean that there is no cause. Some acidic agent must have passed the mouth and dissolved the tooth substance. No case of erosion has been shown to be caused by unsaturated saliva; unsaturated saliva has never been reported. Therefore, enamel is not eroded unless acids are brought into the mouth by foods, regurgitated stomach contents, vomit or air. Thus, the distribution of 'idiopathically eroded' teeth and surfaces is as described above.

Prophylaxis and treatment of erosion

Fluoride and erosion

Topical fluoride has been suggested as a control strategy without scientific evidence shown by double-blind trials. It must be admitted that such studies are difficult to run and may bring the researcher close to unethical behavior, which

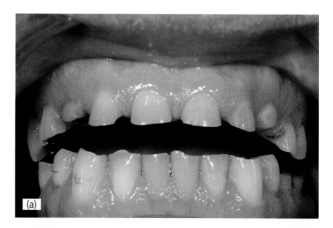

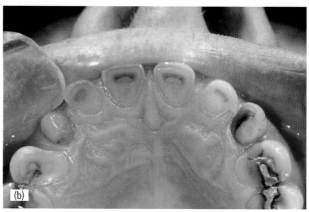

Figure 13.17 Typical dentition of a subject who for many years has worked in the galvanizing industry. The teeth are shortened and the lingual surfaces of most teeth are severely eroded. (Although the statement 'worked in the galvanizing industry' strongly suggests airborne erosion, it does not exclude the possibility that part of the clinical outcome may be caused by food and drinks, or by any other cause.)

presumably is the reason why no such studies have been undertaken.

A topical fluoride treatment leaves calcium fluoride (CaF_2) on the tooth surface, in plaque, etc. To obtain information on how long this deposited material stays in the mouth, dissolution of CaF_2 in saliva has been examined (Chapter 12, Figs 12.19, 12.20). CaF_2 on smooth enamel surfaces is short-lived in the mouth and hardly survives for the day on exposed smooth surfaces. Similarly, to examine the resistance of CaF_2 in erosive foods, its solubility in various soft drinks has been examined (Fig. 13.18). The solubility of CaF_2 in acidic drinks is quite high, owing to conversion of the fluoride ion to hydrogen fluoride (Larsen, 2001). Generally, the more acidic and aggressive the drink, the more CaF_2 can be dissolved in it. Thus, 1 liter of Coca Cola is able to dissolve all of the CaF_2 left by topical fluoride treatments of 5000 teeth. The conclusion is that CaF_2 does not survive for long in a mouth through which considerable amounts of acidic drinks pass, in particular on surfaces over which the drink washes.

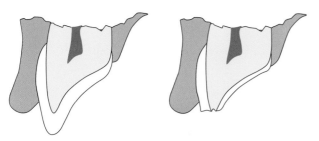

Figure 13.16 Schematic drawing to illustrate the most eroded areas of subjects exposed to occupational airborne acids. The airborne acid will irritate the mucosa of the nose and force the subject to breathe through the mouth. It will concentrate in the saliva film of exposed tooth surfaces and erode away tooth substance visible *en face*. Further, the acid will dissolve in the saliva on the tongue, which will lick away enamel where tongue and teeth meet.

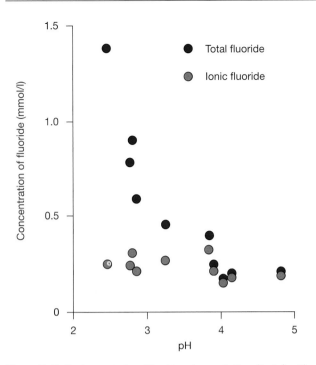

Figure 13.18 Total concentration of fluoride and concentration of ionic fluoride in soft drinks with various pH in which calcium fluoride has been suspended under gentle agitation for 72 h. The more acidic the drink the higher the total fluoride concentration and the more calcium fluoride is dissolved owing to formation of hydrogen fluoride.

In vitro solubility studies have shown that fluoride, even in high concentrations in excess of 20 ppm in the aqueous solution below pH 3, has absolutely no effect on enamel dissolution (Larsen & Richards, 2002). At higher pH a weak effect has been observed of 6–11 ppm fluoride, however, at a concentration that does not occur in soft drinks.

In vitro and *in vivo* studies have shown a dissolution-reducing effect of topical stannous fluoride. The effect is presumably due to the stannous ion and its ability to co-ordinate hydroxyl, i.e. various stannohydroxide ions are formed that adhere to solid surfaces and form a somewhat acid-resistant layer. Stannous hydroxide ion layers have been observed to cause tooth discoloration that can be removed by tissue-removing polishing.

In a similar way, a 1000 ppm fluoride varnish based on polyurethane has been demonstrated to prevent enamel dissolution. It is an open question whether 1000 ppm fluoride, at a concentration similar to that of toothpaste, prevents erosion or it is the adhering polyurethane varnish covering the tooth that prevents the erosion.

Calcium phosphates and erosion

Dissolution of the dental hard tissues occurs only when the apatite is bathed in a solution unsaturated with respect to apatites. If the solution is saturated with respect to apatites,

enamel does not dissolve. Functional foods based on orange juice with a pH around 4 and with calcium and phosphate concentrations similar to those in dairy milk products (40 mmol/l calcium and 30 mmol/l phosphate or 4.5 g apatite/l) are exactly saturated with respect to apatites and unable to erode enamel, just as milk products such as yogurt and junket, with pH around 4, are non-erosive (Fig. 13.19). However, at pH significantly below 4 an adjustment of the concentration of calcium and phosphate to prevent enamel dissolution becomes futile without altering the drink considerably, because the solubility of apatite increases so much. Thus, at pH 3 the amount of apatite required to saturate a drink is around 80 g/l.

In conclusion, chemical prevention by means of fluoride has not been supported by experimental evidence and double-blind trials that warrant clinical use. Addition of calcium and phosphate to acidic foods has been shown to prevent enamel dissolution at moderate pH (Grenby, 1996; Jensdottir *et al.*, 2007). However, producers for the vast soda and fruit markets have not implemented their use. Only very few products contain sufficient calcium phosphates and so far they play a limited role.

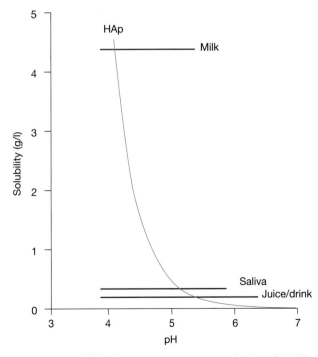

Figure 13.19 Solubility of enamel hydroxyapatite as a function of pH. The horizontal bars indicate the amount of calcium and phosphate in orange juice and many soft drinks, in saliva, and in milk and most dairy milk products. Juice low in calcium and phosphate starts the dissolution of enamel early at a rather high pH, whereas saliva requires a pH drop to around 5.2. Milk has a high content of the two ions and pH must be below 4 for dissolution of enamel apatite. As milk products such as yogurt have a pH above 4 they are no threat to the teeth. Saturation of drinks at pH below 4 becomes futile.

Early diagnosis

Early identification of patients with erosion is important so that the dentist can help the patient to establish the cause. Sometimes the patients' complaint of sensitive tooth surfaces draws attention to the problem because dentin is exposed. However, the dentist may have seen the problem much earlier than this. In particular, lingual surfaces of maxillary incisors should be examined as they are the surfaces most often eroded. Careful history taking is essential to try to determine the likely cause, and counseling is mandatory. However, quite often the anamnestic questioning does not reveal any cause because the history taking is sensitive (Kidd & Smith, 1993). Even if no cause is established, counseling should be provided.

Monitoring of erosion development

Treatment of eroded teeth is often not necessary in the early stages. However, it is important to monitor whether an eroded surface is stabilized or is still being eroded. As noted, the range of class 1 erosion, from slight dissolution of surface enamel that can be ignored to removal of most of the enamel, makes written records unsuitable for monitoring. Casts and photographs are preferable, although there needs to be a considerable further removal of enamel to identify erosive activity. A more sensitive method is insertion of a small amalgam or gold filling in an area not too exposed to attrition. After polishing, an impression is taken and a cast made for later comparison with future casts. If the surface is still eroded the filling will be found to be elevated above the surface. If so, the development should be discussed, the cause should be further elucidated and counseling repeated.

Prevention

Where the cause is deemed to be mainly diet, prophylaxis focusses primarily on reducing the exposure by changing drinking and eating habits. The amount of erosive foods and drinks consumed should be reduced and sipping avoided. Occasionally, when a patient is warned not to drink an erosive soda, he or she may shift to a still fruit drink that contains twice as much acid and is just as erosive as the original soda. The patient should be advised not to brush the teeth immediately after consuming acidic food and drink. After a few minutes the saliva will have neutralized the drink and the teeth may be brushed with no harm.

If erosion continues to progress there will come a time when operative intervention may be justified because of tooth sensitivity or disfiguration of teeth, because the erosion is approaching the pulp or because the tooth has become practically unrestorable without root canal retention. In the early stages etch-retained two-component resin may prove helpful, in particular if sufficient retentive enamel remains. When all the enamel has gone, retention of the resin is compromised and often insufficient to withstand occlusion and daily wear. In the later stages, veneering, full coverage and porcelain crowns may be the treatments of choice. As such restoration is difficult, expensive, laborious and requires lifelong maintenance, it is the goal of early diagnosis and preventive reduction of exposure not to let the situation go that far.

Conclusion

Erosion of the teeth is quite common, most often caused by acidic foods and soft drinks, regurgitated acid, vomit and occasionally acid fumes. Teeth are eroded where the agent hits the enamel directly. The erosive exposure is short-lived, usually less than 1 min, but acidic remnants around the papillae of the tongue may lengthen the exposure time, in particular if the content of fruit acids and the buffer capacity are high. In general, the more acidic the drink, the more aggressive is it. Identification of erosion is difficult and most eroded teeth are not identified as eroded. The most important part of management is to establish the diagnosis, find the cause and control progression by reducing the causative factors. Restorative treatments are a final port of call when all else has failed.

Background literature

Lussi A, ed. *Dental erosion. From diagnosis to therapy*. Basel: Karger, 2006.

Pindborg JJ. *Pathology of the dental hard tissues.* Copenhagen: Munksgaard, 1970.

Zero DT. Etiology of dental erosion – extrinsic factors. *Eur J Oral Sci* 1995; **104**: 162–77.

References

http://www.statpub.com/stat. US fruit consumption declines for second year. Canada: Stat Communications, 2006.

Bartlett DW, Evans DF, Smith BGN. The relationship between gastro-oesophageal reflux disease and dental erosion [review]. *J Oral Rehabil* 1996; **23**: 289–97.

Grenby TH. Lessening erosive potential by product modification. *Eur J Oral Sci* 1996; **104**: 221–8.

Holst JJ, Lange F. Perimylolysis. A contribution towards the genesis of tooth wasting from non-mechanical causes. *Acta Odont Scand* 1939; **1**: 36–48.

Imfeld T. Dental erosion, definition, classification and links. *Eur J Oral Sci* 1995; **104**: 151–5.

Jensdottir T, Holbrook P, Nauntofte B, Buchwald C, Bardow A. Immediate erosive potential of cola drinks and orange juices. *J Dent Res* 2006; **85**: 226–30.

Jensdottir T, Nauntofte B, Buchwald C, Bardow A. Effects of calcium on the erosive potential of acidic candies in saliva. *Caries Res* 2007; **41**: 68–73.

Kidd EAM, Smith BGN. Toothwear histories: a sensitive issue. *Dent Update* 1993; **20**: 174–8.

Larsen MJ. Dissolution of enamel. *Scand J Dent Res* 1973; **81**: 518–22.

Larsen MJ. Degrees of saturation with respect to apatites in fruit juices and acidic drinks. *Scand J Dent Res* 1975; **83**: 7–12.

Larsen MJ. Prevention by means of fluoride of enamel erosion as caused by soft drinks and orange juice. *Caries Res* 2001; **35**: 229–34.

Larsen MJ, Richards A. Fluoride is unable to reduce dental erosion from soft drinks. *Caries Res* 2002; **36**: 75–80.

Larsen IB, Westergård J, Larsen AI, Gyntelberg F, Holmstrup P. A clinical index for evaluating and monitoring dental erosion. *Community Dent Oral Epidemiol* 2000; **28**: 211–17.

Larsen MJ, Poulsen S, Hansen I. Erosion of the teeth: prevalence and distribution in a group of Danish school children. *Eur J Paediatr Dent* 2005; **7**: 44–7.

Lussi A. Dental erosion. Clinical diagnosis and case history taking. *Eur J Oral Sci* 1995; **104**: 191–8.

Meurman JH, ten Cate JM. Pathogenesis and modifying factors of dental erosion. *Eur J Oral Sci* 1995; **104**: 1199–206.

Nielsen JS, Popkin BM. Changes in beverage intake between 1977 and 2001. *Am J Prev Med* 2004; **27**: 205–10.

Scheutzel P. Etiology of dental erosion – intrinsic factors. *Eur J Oral Sci* 1995; **104**: 178–90.

Part IV
Non-operative therapy

14

The control of disease progression: non-operative treatment

E.A.M. Kidd and O. Fejerskov

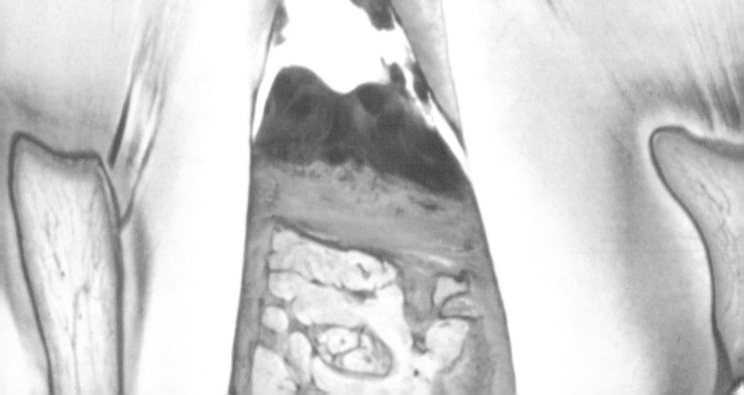

Introduction

From the previous chapters it will be apparent that although dental caries is considered an infectious dental disease, it should not be considered a result of an infection with one specific type of microorganism (once thought to be *Lactobacillus acidophilus* and later, and still by some, thought to be *Streptococcus mutans*). As presented in Chapter 10, the infectious agents are the indigenous flora of the oral cavity. Although there are some 500 different species present in the oral environment, they only present a possible insult to the dental hard tissues if they are allowed to form a biofilm on the tooth surfaces, i.e. dental plaque.

The bacterial metabolism in the microbial deposits that constitute the plaque biomass results in fluctuations in pH. These fluctuations influence the dynamic equilibrium between the mineral in the tooth and the degree of saturation in the plaque fluid with respect to the apatites. This causes dissolution and redistribution of mineral in the underlying dental hard tissues (see Chapter 12). A range of factors determines the extent to which and the rate at which the metabolic events may result in a net loss of mineral (development or progression of a lesion). These include the composition of the bacterial biofilm, the composition and flow rate of saliva, the presence of fermentable carbohydrates, and the concentrations of fluoride, calcium and phosphate in the oral fluids (Fejerskov & Manji, 1990) (see schematic illustration in Chapter 1, Fig. 1.1).

The interplay of these factors affects what happens in the interface between the biomass and the tooth surface, and therefore mineral dissolution and reprecipitation are dynamic processes, as described in Chapters 2, 3 and 12. If the caries challenge is high (the rate of dissolution exceeds the rate of redeposition) the clinical appearances will be different from those observed where the local environment favors redeposition of minerals. The rate of progression of the lesion reflects the activity of the biofilm. This means that a clinician can gauge the net activity of the biofilm by looking at the surface features of the caries lesion that is beneath it. Lesions may appear 'active' or 'arrested', as described in Chapter 2.

Can the caries process be prevented?

The formation of a biofilm on a tooth surface cannot be prevented in surface irregularities such as occlusal fissures, or in the gingival or approximal niches. In these areas occlusal function or attrition (friction) from cheeks, lips and tongue does not occur. All bacterial deposits, irrespective of their stage of maturation, are metabolically active. These metabolic activities will affect the tooth surface beneath and a plaque that is only a few days old will produce a classical Stephan response to sugar. If, over time, such regular pH fluctuations are able to result in a net loss

of mineral, then the caries process results in a detectable lesion. The formation of cavities can be prevented by controlling the caries process, but metabolic fluctuations in the biofilm cannot be prevented. Thus, caries is a ubiquitous, natural process (Manji *et al.*, 1991a; Fejerskov, 1997).

A tooth surface covered over long periods by a metabolically active biofilm will gradually be chemically modified. For instance, the biological apatite in newly erupted enamel contains a variety of impurities such as carbonate and magnesium which make the apatite more soluble (see Chapter 12). If chemical conditions with fluctuations in pH prevail, a gradual loss of magnesium and carbonate in surface enamel should be expected. This chemical change in surface enamel is therefore to be considered the earliest sign of the caries process. If, however, fluoride is available during this process, the fluoride will become incorporated in the biological apatite over time, to such an extent that the fluoride content in the clinically 'normal' cervical enamel surface (where plaque accumulates) increases significantly over a period of 6–7 years (Richards *et al.*, 1977; Fig. 18.10). All this can happen without any clinically recordable changes in porosity or, for that matter, changes assessed by different microscopic methods. Thus, the metabolically active biofilm results in a permanent chemical modification of the tooth surface. As explained in Chapter 3, the process known as posteruptive enamel maturation may be considered a part of the caries process at a subclinical level.

Thus, accepting that biofilms constantly form and grow on any tooth surface, these regular demineralizations and remineralizations, which occur at random (Manji *et al.*, 1991b), cannot be prevented, because they are a ubiquitous and natural process. Their effect on tooth surfaces over time can, however, be influenced and the metabolic processes can be modified. Thus, caries lesion development and progression can be controlled. Therefore, by controlling the metabolism in the microbial biomass, it is possible to prevent cavities from occurring. An already formed subsurface lesion, presenting itself as a thin, white opaque line or the extensive white-spot lesion, does not have to progress. Any lesion, at any stage of tissue destruction, noncavitated or cavitated, can become arrested. This statement is true irrespective of the age of the patient.

Controlling disease progression

Disease control concerns influencing biofilm formation and growth, or modifying the dissolution kinetics of the apatites, or both. The following may have a role to play:

- mechanical/chemical removal of plaque (oral hygiene)
- chemical (antimicrobial) modification of plaque
- use of fluorides
- dietary composition
- salivary composition and stimulation.

Each of these topics is discussed in this text, but it is salutary to realize that most of these measures depend on a degree of patient co-operation, and behavioral considerations are a very important part of this. Potentially, any non-medicated and physically normal individual can learn to control lesion development and progression. As such, dental caries, progressing to the stage of frank cavities in teeth, can be prevented in the majority of any population, and in most patients white-spot lesions may also be prevented or their appearance modified.

It is important to realize that on an individual patient basis there is great variation in the complex interplay between all known and unknown determinants involved in caries lesion development. Therefore, an assessment of the individual patient's relative risk is an important prerequisite to planning appropriate treatment.

Should disease control be considered as 'treatment' of the caries lesion?

Disease control measures, such as showing a patient how to remove plaque, applying topical fluoride and discussing their diet and whether it needs modification, have classically been described as 'prevention'. As already discussed, this may not be an accurate term because the caries process as such is not prevented; rather, the likely outcome (a lesion with a cavity) can be prevented or most often postponed (Haugejorden et al., 1990). Unfortunately, 'preventive' on the one hand has been contrasted with 'treatment' on the other, with 'treatment' implying operative intervention. Sadly, operative intervention is seen by many patients, dentists and politicians as the way to manage the process. This is despite the fact that once a tooth has been subject to an operative treatment procedure, the likelihood of losing the tooth with age is higher than for a sound tooth and, in certain populations, may be as high as having a non-treated caries lesion (Luan et al., 2000).

Many patients do not understand, or do not believe, that they will not necessarily need fillings. Some expect this management when they visit the dentist and may not question what can be done to prevent fillings being needed in the future. Moreover, fillings were considered by the profession as 'secondary prevention', adding to the belief that inserting a filling would not only restore form and function, but also prevent further damage. However, even the best performed restorative procedure does not result in a lifelong restoration (see Chapter 24). The dental profession is by tradition focussed on pain relief by the extraction or restoration of severely damaged teeth. For years dentists have been paid for filling teeth but sometimes not paid, or very poorly remunerated, for taking measures to prevent disease progression. Even in public dental services the efficiency of the dental staff has been measured in numbers of fillings inserted (or fissure sealants placed in recent years).

There are several examples of attitudes that may have to be reconsidered to render dentists more cost-effective. For instance, patient education in measures that prevent disease progression is often delegated to another member of the dental team, perhaps a dental hygienist. This individual has received a shorter training and has a lower salary than the dentist. Does this mean that this treatment is easier to perform or less important than operative treatment? What about turning the present situation on its head and training ancillary personnel to place fillings, leaving the dentist with diagnosis, treatment planning, decisions on whether to perform non-operative treatments and conventional filling, and patient education?

As another example, for years dental epidemiologists have recorded decayed teeth, in the DMFT/S recording, as being a reflection of 'the disease' (Pitts, 1997). Thus, decayed is considered synonymous with an 'untreated' cavity (i.e. a cavity in need of a filling). Moreover, some public health dentists have been content to tell their political masters that a certain percentage of their child population is 'caries free'. These figures are produced on the basis of the most peremptory clinical examination at the level of cavitation or caries into dentin. The politicians seize on the good news that caries prevalence and incidence are falling in young people and they erroneously believe that the disease has been eradicated. The fact that this is delayed disease progression (Haugejorden et al., 1990) and that the disease may present at the cavitation level in older populations unless controlled, has not been made sufficiently clear.

In all fairness, the dental schools should also bear some responsibility for the current attitude to restorative dentistry. The school may fuel the 'treatment equals fillings' philosophy by giving points for restorative procedures but not rewarding non-operative treatments. A school has a responsibility to train competent operators and the amount of experience each student has must be recorded; however, a points system that only rewards operative procedures may engender the attitude that it is 'filling holes in teeth' that counts in monetary terms. Efficient cutting automatons may be hatched from the dental school egg confident of their own ability to treat caries lesions by restorations. This is an important message: restorations have a role to play in managing some caries lesions, and this role will be discussed in Chapter 20, but operative dentistry must go hand in hand with non-operative treatment to control further disease progression, otherwise restorations may not survive. To ignore non-operative treatment would be biologically illogical and ethically unacceptable. Disease control should be seen as 'treatment' of ongoing caries processes and hence of the lesions at different stages of development.

Why use the term 'non-operative treatment'?

The perceptive reader will have noticed the term 'non-operative treatment' creep into this chapter. It is used to encompass all those measures that attempt to control disease progression. The aim of this is to set non-operative treatment alongside operative treatment, implying that both 'treat' the disease process and both are time-consuming, skillful and worthy of payment.

Does the approach work? Is it cost-effective?

At this point it would be reassuring to direct the reader to a series of practice-based, randomized control trials showing the value of non-operative treatment in terms of reduced caries incidence. Unfortunately, this work is not particularly positive. These studies have targeted preventive efforts at individuals judged to be a high risk. Work focussing on advising preschool mothers in tooth brushing with fluoride toothpaste and sugar control achieved an 18% difference in the mean DMFT between the test and control groups. However, this was not a statistically significant difference, despite the test group having 4-monthly counselling over 2 years compared with a single session for the control group (Blinkhorn et al., 2003).

Two Finnish studies (Seppä et al., 1991; Hausen et al., 2000) targeted 'high-risk' adolescents with intensified non-operative treatments, with modest results. Recent work from Sweden (Kallestal, 2005) also concentrated on 'high-risk' adolescents over 5 years and could find no significant differences in mean 5-year increment among four different programs. These were:

- information on tooth-brushing techniques
- prescription of fluoride lozenges
- semi-annual application of fluoride varnish
- quarterly appointments for oral hygiene and diet instruction and fluoride varnish application.

The results showed all programs to have a rather low efficacy.

Perhaps it is relevant that none of these studies had a true control group that received no advice on oral care. Inclusion of such a group would be unethical, but it would also probably be impossible in countries where all dentists are giving basic preventive advice. The studies are important because they appear to show that preventive interventions targeted only at 'high-risk' individuals may not be cost-effective, and this topic will be raised again in Chapters 28 and 29. Perhaps it is patient compliance that is the all-important factor, or maybe there is a ceiling through which further preventive effort cannot break. It must be remembered that there are no tests with sufficient predictive power to identify individuals at 'high risk' (Chapter 29). However, recent work from a child population with an overall low caries experience (Hausen et al., 2007), targeting caries control at all children in an area with an active lesion, recorded a significantly reduced increment in dental decay. Indeed the prevented fraction was similar to studies on non-operative caries management conducted in areas of high or moderate levels of dental caries (Ekstrand et al., 2000; Curnow et al., 2002).

An attempt has been made to carry out an economic evaluation of preventive programs (Kallestal et al., 2003). Five studies were considered worthy of inclusion, but the authors were frustrated in their attempt to draw a conclusion because the studies gave contradictory results, some negative, some positive.

It has also been pointed out (Seppä, 2001) that there will be relevant intercountry differences. In countries with a high caries rate, a low level of basic prevention and an unorganized dental care system, any preventive program seems effective, whereas in other countries, often described as economically developed, the effectiveness of preventive programs seems to have diminished. One aspect of prevention that seems indisputable is the importance of fluoride toothpaste as a cost-effective and feasible method of fluoride delivery and this will hold good in all countries, irrespective of the caries level and dental care systems.

The other side of the coin is concentrating on reparative treatment, and experiences from New Zealand are a cautionary tale indicating how wrong it may be to take this course (Hunter, 1998). Despite a comprehensive child and adolescent restorative program in New Zealand, there was a high rate of tooth extraction in adults. Teenagers had little untreated dental decay but many fillings. It is even tempting to think, with today's knowledge, that the high extraction rate was a direct result of the restorative program! When a policy change discouraging early operative intervention was made in the late 1970s, the rapid decline in DMFT was the result of the F component (and hence the M component) being dramatically reduced. In other words, the 'disease pattern' was partly a reflection of the treatment orientated concept. Sheiham (1997) discussed this concept and also pointed out that the literature indicates that dental care has a small impact on the incidence of dental caries in children, with social factors being more important.

References

Blinkhorn AS, Gratix D, Holloway PJ, Wainwright-Stringer YM, Ward SJ, Worthington HV. A cluster randomised, controlled trial of the value of dental health educators in general dental practice. *Br Dent J* 2003; **195**: 395–400.

Curnow MM, Pine CM, Burnside G, Nicholson JA, Chesters RK, Huntington E. A randomised controlled trial of the efficacy of supervised tooth brushing in high-caries risk children. *Caries Res* 2002; **36**: 294–300.

Ekstrand KR, Kuzmina IN, Kuzmina E, Christiansen ME. Two and a half-year outcome of caries-preventive programs offered to groups of children in the Solntsevsky district of Moscow. *Caries Res* 2000; **34**: 8–19.

Fejerskov O. Concepts of dental caries and their consequences for understanding the disease. *Community Dent Oral Epidemiol* 1997; **25**: 5–12.

Fejerskov O, Manji F. *Risk assessment in dental caries*. In: Bader JD, ed. Risk assessment in dentistry. Chapel Hill, NC: University of North Carolina Dental Ecology, 1990: 215–17.

Haugejorden O, Lervik T, Birkeland JM, Jorlgend L. An 11-year follow-up study of dental caries after discontinuation of school-based fluoride programs. *Acta Odontol Scand* 1990; **48**: 257–63.

Hausen H, Kärkkäinen S, Seppä L. Application of the high risk strategy to control dental caries. *Community Dent Oral Epidemiol* 2000; **28**: 26–34.

Hausen H, Seppa L, Poutanen R, Niinimaa A, Lahti S, Karkkainen S, *et al.* Non-invasive control of dental caries in children with active initial lesions. *Caries Res* 2007; **41**: 384–91.

Hunter PB. Documenting the changing face of New Zealand. *N Z Dent J* 1998; **94**: 106–9.

Kallestal C. The effect of five years' implementation of caries-preventive methods in Swedish high-risk adolescents. *Caries Re*s 2005; **39**: 20–6.

Kallestal C, Norlund A, Soder B, *et al.* Economic evaluation of dental caries prevention: a systematic review. *Acta Odontol Scand* 2003; **61**: 341–6.

Luan W-M, Baelum B, Fejerskov O, Chen X. Ten-year incidence of dental caries in adult and elderly Chinese. *Caries Res* 2000; **34**: 205–13.

Manji F, Fejerskov O, Baelum V, Luan W-M, Chen X. The epidemiological features of dental caries in African and Chinese populations: implications for risk assessment. In: Johnson NW, ed. *Risk markers for oral diseases*, Vol. 1, *Dental caries. Markers of high and low risk groups and individuals.* Cambridge: Cambridge University Press, 1991a: 62–99.

Manji F, Fejerskov O, Nagelkerke NJD, Baelum V. A random effects model for some epidemiological features of dental caries. *Community Dent Oral Epidemiol* 1991b; **19**: 324–8.

Pitts NB. Diagnostic tools and measurements – impact on appropriate care. *Community Dent Oral Epidemiol* 1997; **25**: 24–35.

Richards A, Joost Larsen M, Fejerskov O, Thylstrup A. Fluoride content of buccal surface enamel and its relation to caries in children. *Arch Oral Biol* 1977; **22**: 425–8.

Seppä L. The future of preventive programs in countries with different systems for dental care. *Caries Res* 2001; **35**:(Suppl 1): 26–9.

Seppä L, Hausen H, Pollänën L, Kärkkäinen S, Helasharju K. Effect of intensified caries prevention on approximal caries in adolescents with high caries risk. *Caries Res* 1991; **25**: 392–5.

Sheiham A. Impact of dental treatment on the incidence of dental caries in children and adolescents. *Community Dent Oral Epidemiol* 1997; **25**: 104–12.

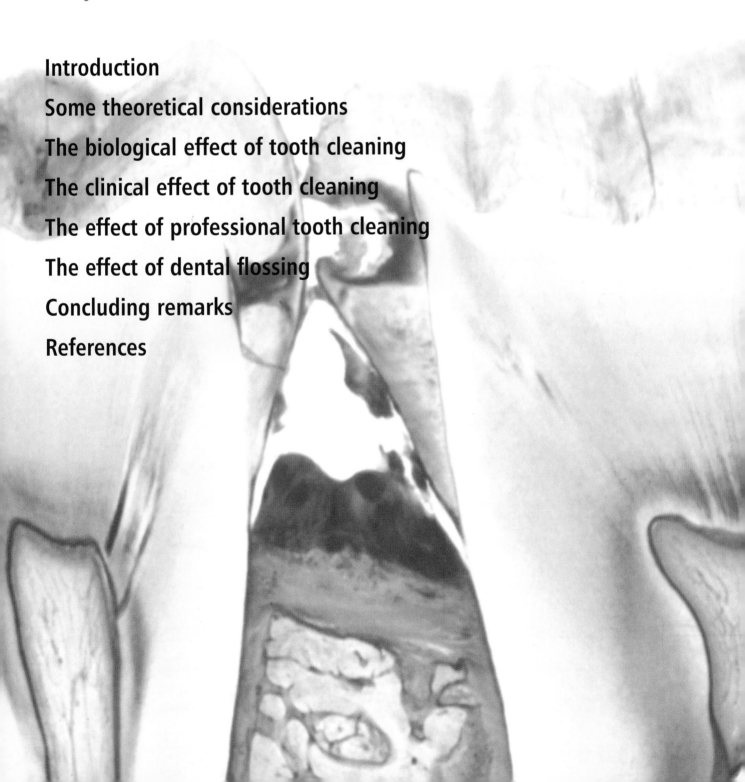

15

Role of oral hygiene

B. Nyvad

Introduction

Motivation and instruction in oral hygiene form the basis of school-based caries-preventive programs for children in many populations. Today, 80% of 11-year-old schoolchildren in Scandinavia report that they brush their teeth at least twice a day (Kuusela *et al.*, 1997). Daily tooth brushing with fluoride toothpaste is believed to be the primary reason for the caries decline observed in many populations since the 1970s (Marthaler, 1990). However, the role of oral hygiene in caries control has been questioned. Dental practitioners have seen that many patients do not develop cavities, in spite of the fact that they perform rather poor oral hygiene and consume candy and soft drinks on a regular basis. Furthermore, it has been claimed that the effect of tooth cleaning is primarily an effect of fluoride in the paste rather than an effect of biofilm removal per se (Lewis & Ismail, 1995). Other researchers have placed more emphasis on the fact that dental caries is a biofilm-mediated disease by promoting the old saying that 'a clean tooth never decays'. In a systematic review, Sutcliffe (1996) proposed a more balanced view by concluding that 'there is no unequivocal evidence that good oral cleanliness reduces caries experience, nor is there sufficient evidence to condemn the value of good oral cleanliness as a caries preventive measure'.

The aim of this chapter is to present and discuss some of the literature that has evaluated the caries-preventive effect of oral hygiene in an attempt to explain why there are such diverging opinions on the usefulness of this important method in preventive dentistry.

Some theoretical considerations

It is not surprising that it is not always possible to find a strong positive association between the presence of dental biofilm and caries. According to the caries concept proposed by Fejerskov and Manji (1990) (see Chapter 1), biofilms on teeth are the one and only prerequisite for caries; they are a necessary but not a sufficient cause. Because of the multi-factorial nature of the disease there are numerous determinants that may influence the outcome by either increasing or decreasing the rate of demineralization. Increased sugar consumption and decreased salivary secretion are typical examples of determinants that speed up the carious process because of acidification of the dental plaque (see Chapter 10). Fluoride, in contrast, owing to its stabilizing effect on the mineral balance, tends to decrease the rate of mineral loss (see Chapter 12). It is the combined effect of all the determinants, positive and negative, rather than the amount of biofilm itself, that determines whether a carious lesion develops and progresses. Therefore, there is no standard level of oral hygiene to be recommended (Nyvad & Fejerskov, 1997). In fact, it might be expected that given a perfectly balanced combination of determinants, no lesion progres-

sion will occur if individuals suspend their regular tooth-cleaning habits!

To evaluate the importance of dental cleanliness per se it is necessary to take into account all the determinants that may potentially influence the association between plaque and caries. Unfortunately, studies describing the caries-preventive effect of tooth brushing often fail to use such an analytical approach. For example, most studies published after the introduction of fluoride toothpaste have not made an attempt to separate the effect of cleaning from the effect of the toothpaste itself.

The biological effect of tooth cleaning

Before describing the clinical effect of tooth cleaning it may be helpful to illustrate the extent to which tooth cleaning can influence the metabolism of the biofilm. Most people believe that every time they brush their teeth, the dentition becomes perfectly free from debris. The truth is that this goal is seldom achieved in the hands of the patient. This is clearly shown in Fig. 15.1. Cleaning of an approximal surface with dental floss significantly reduces the production of organic acids after a carbohydrate challenge, but residual biofilm maintains the ability to elicit a moderate pH drop (Firestone & Mühlemann, 1985). Thus, even after carefully performed plaque removal, teeth are never 'clean' from a microbiological point of view. Bacteria will often be retained in surface irregularities and in areas that are diffi-

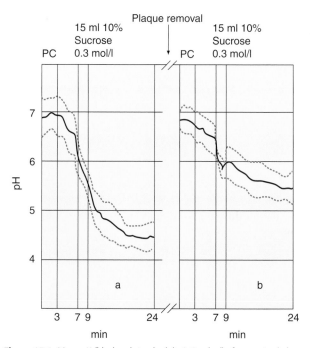

Figure 15.1 Mean pH (blue) and standard deviation (red) of approximal plaque following a 2 min rinse with 10% sucrose solution (a) before and (b) after plaque removal with dental floss ($n = 8$). PC: paraffin chewing. (From Firestone & Mühleman, 1985.)

cult to reach, such as approximal surfaces and fissures. Therefore, it is not surprising that dental cleanliness plays a crucial role in the effect of tooth brushing.

The clinical effect of tooth cleaning

When evaluating the results from clinical studies assessing the caries-preventive effect of tooth brushing, it is important to appreciate that the design of the study, as well as the method of analysis, will affect the conclusions. Depending on the design of the study, the outcome may reflect either the efficacy or the effectiveness of the preventive measure (Abramson, 1990). Efficacy is used to refer to the benefits observed when a procedure is applied as it 'should' be, and with full compliance by all concerned. The term efficacy is usually reserved for benefits at the individual level (or the tooth/site level), e.g. as measured by a controlled clinical trial, and answers the question: 'Can the procedure work?' Effectiveness refers to the degree of realization of desirable effects observed at the population level, or among people to whom a procedure is offered. Hence, the term effectiveness answers the question: 'Does the procedure work?' As shall be demonstrated in the following sections, these distinctions are very useful when discussing the effects of oral hygiene. For the purpose of clarity the discussion will therefore be dealt with at the following levels: the tooth/site level, the level of the individual and the population level.

The tooth/site level

The strongest evidence supporting an effect of oral hygiene on caries stems from experimental *in vivo* studies. In a study conducted in dental students by von der Fehr *et al.* (1970), it was shown that withdrawal of oral hygiene procedures for 23 days led to the emergence of whitish, opaque, non-cavitated enamel lesions along the gingival margin of the teeth. Not surprisingly, students who performed nine daily mouthrinses with 50% sucrose solution during the test period developed more lesions than students who did not rinse. Equally important, however, was the observation that irrespective of whether sucrose had been applied or not, the early manifestations of caries were reversible. Thus, after 30 days of careful oral hygiene (possibly using non-fluoride toothpaste) and daily mouthrinses with 0.2% sodium fluoride (NaF) the clinical appearance of the enamel had almost returned to pre-experimental levels. These observations have been confirmed by other studies showing that improved oral hygiene, including daily use of fluoride toothpaste, favors the arrest of active enamel and dentin caries lesions (Årtun & Thylstrup, 1986; Nyvad & Fejerskov, 1986; Lo *et al.*, 1998).

More recently, modified orthodontic bands have been applied as an experimental model to study the effect of prolonged protection from mechanical forces on the buccal surfaces of premolars. When using this technique it has been demonstrated both clinically and histologically that undisturbed biofilm formation under the band leads to the development of progressive stages of white-spot carious lesions within a period 4 weeks (Holmen *et al.*, 1985a, b). After such lesions were re-exposed to the natural oral environment, including normal oral hygiene with a non-fluoride toothpaste, they showed evidence of regression and microwear of the surface (Holmen *et al.*, 1987a, b) (for further details, see Chapter 3). Increased microwear with time supported the concept that mechanical biofilm removal was the main factor responsible for the arrest of the initial lesions.

The role of biofilm removal as an essential mode of caries control has also been addressed in *in situ* studies. *In situ* studies are experimental studies carried out under conditions that closely mimic the natural conditions in the oral cavity, e.g. by inserting tooth specimens into lower partial dentures and exposing them to the oral environment for varying periods, while subjecting them to a well-defined experimental procedure. Before the start of the experiment the volunteers are told to comply carefully with the instructions, and often compliance is monitored and reinforced at regular intervals during the study. After the experimental period, changes in the mineral content of the tooth specimens can be measured by quantitative microradiography and compared with specimens obtained from a control group. Provided that full compliance is achieved, such studies provide information about the efficacy of a procedure.

In one *in situ* study Dijkmann *et al.* (1990) assessed the effect of two oral hygiene regimens – twice-daily brushing with a fluoride toothpaste (1250 ppm F) and twice-daily brushing with a non-fluoride toothpaste – relative to no brushing, on the mineral content of shallow enamel lesions that were developed under artificial conditions in the laboratory. After 10 weeks *in situ* the authors observed a distinct mineral uptake in the lesions after brushing with the fluoride toothpaste. The mineral content of the lesions that were cleaned with a non-fluoride toothpaste did not change, while the control lesions that were not subjected to any treatment at all became deeper and lost considerable mineral (Fig. 15.2). The authors calculated that twice-daily brushing with fluoride toothpaste resulted in a 90% reduction in mineral loss compared with the control group that did not brush. The effect was ascribed to a combination of two factors, a cleaning effect and a fluoride effect, both of which were of the same order of magnitude. These findings suggest that there may be an additive effect of brushing the teeth with fluoride toothpaste. Therefore, individuals who either do not use a paste containing fluoride or neglect the importance of mechanical biofilm removal are unlikely to achieve maximum protection against caries.

Another *in situ* study was designed to test whether a caries-preventive program consisting of careful daily brushing with a 1100 ppm fluoride toothpaste, supplemented with two

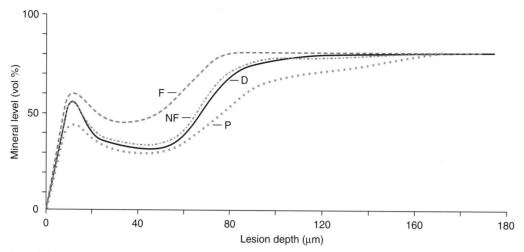

Figure 15.2 Mineral distribution curves of enamel specimens after different experimental tooth-brushing regimens *in situ*. The mineral content is plotted versus the distance from the outer surface. P: no tooth brushing for 3 months, NF: brushing with a non-fluoride toothpaste for 3 months; F: brushing with a fluoride toothpaste for 3 months; D: artificially demineralized control specimen. (From Dijkman *et al*. 1990.)

topical 2% NaF applications, had a controlling effect on natural actively progressing root-caries lesions over a 3-month period (Nyvad *et al*., 1997). The preventive non-operative treatment program applied in this study had previously been shown to arrest root-caries lesions in clinical studies (see Chapter 3). Assessment of the mineral content of the root lesions after 3 months of treatment revealed that most lesions did not experience further mineral loss, whereas in control specimens (no brushing with fluoride toothpaste and no topical fluoride application) the mineral loss continued (Fig. 15.3). Importantly, the non-operative treatment also had a pronounced inhibitory effect on lesion progression in newly exposed root surfaces. Unfortunately, the study did not include a test group that brushed with a non-fluoride toothpaste. Hence, it was not possible in this study to determine the impact of the oral hygiene procedures relative to the impact of the fluoride component.

Collectively, studies at the tooth/site level have shown that when meticulous oral hygiene and fluoride toothpaste are applied together and targeted specifically at sites with a high rate of lesion progression it is possible to control the development and progression of caries. Thus, tooth cleaning with fluoride toothpaste can be highly efficacious.

The level of the individual

Conclusions from studies analyzing the effect of tooth cleaning at the individual level are less consistent. While some clinical trials have shown that children brushing their teeth more than once a day may develop fewer new carious lesions than children who brush their teeth less frequently (Tucker *et al*., 1976; Chestnutt *et al*., 1998), other studies have not been able to confirm such a relationship (Horowitz & Thompson, 1967). This is probably because reported tooth brushing in itself does not say anything about the quality of the oral hygiene procedures (Bellini *et al*., 1981). When

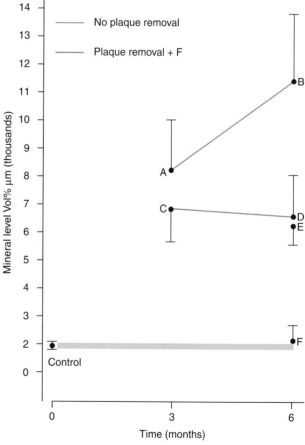

Figure 15.3 Mineral loss of root-caries specimens after different treatments *in situ*. The red and green lines indicate periods with an without plaque removal, respectively. The solid data points (A–D) and error bars give the mean values and SEM for the amount of mineral removed in each group (*n* = 9). E and F indicate the mean amount of mineral removed from sound root surfaces after a 3-month period without and with tooth cleaning, respectively. The mean mineral content value for sound control surfaces (blue horizontal line) is included for comparison (*n* = 5). (From Nyvad *et al*., 1997.)

examining the effect of tooth brushing expressed in terms of oral cleanliness, a clearer picture has been obtained. Thus, children whose dental cleanliness is consistently good may experience lower caries increments than those whose cleanliness is consistently bad (Sutcliffe, 1973; Tucker et al., 1976; Beal et al., 1979; Naylor & Glass, 1979).

Only one clinical trial has so far allowed evaluation of the effect of tooth cleaning as an isolated variable relative to the effect of fluoride (Koch & Lindhe, 1970). The overall aim of this study was to assess the effect of daily supervised tooth brushing in groups of 9–11-year-old children over a 3-year period. Brushing at school was supervised as a means to control compliance. The design of the study was very elaborate (Table 15.1). There were two supervised brushing regimens, one with and one without a fluoride toothpaste. Three experimental groups served as controls, one group not performing supervised brushing at school, and two groups rinsing fortnightly with either distilled water or a 0.5% NaF solution. The results demonstrated that fortnightly fluoride rinses reduced dental caries increments significantly. However, daily brushing with fluoride toothpaste was more efficacious than fortnightly fluoride rinses. The effect of tooth brushing with fluoride toothpaste was most pronounced on smooth surfaces that are easy to clean and easily accessible to fluoride. Another observation from the study was that supervised tooth brushing with a non-fluoride toothpaste did not appear to have a detectable effect.

The findings of the study suggest that in most people tooth-brushing performance (even under supervision) may be insufficient to obtain a caries-preventive effect when using a fluoride-free toothpaste. However, when tooth brushing is performed with a fluoride-containing toothpaste it can have a very significant caries-preventive effect. Moreover, the fact that supervised brushing with fluoride toothpaste had a better clinical effect than did plain rinsing with a fluoride solution supports the contention that dental cleanliness plays an important role in the outcome. This assumption is further supported by the results from clinical trials in which it was demonstrated that children performing unsupervised tooth brushing with toothpaste, with or without fluoride,

developed significantly less caries with better oral hygiene (Beal et al., 1979; Naylor & Glass, 1979). A closer look at the data in the latter studies revealed that the caries-preventive effect was higher in the groups using the fluoride paste, again suggesting that biofilm removal and fluoride, when acting together, have an additive effect. It should also be appreciated, however, that poor oral hygiene cannot be compensated for by the intensive use of fluorides. Thus, the effect of professional administration of fluorides in the form of gels, rinses or tablets has been shown to be limited in individuals who do not practice good oral hygiene (Wellock et al., 1965; Mathiesen et al., 1996).

To summarize, the above findings indicate that the most simple and efficacious way to control the development and progression of caries at the level of the individual is to suppress the presence of dental biofilm in conjunction with the regular use of fluoride, preferably in the form of a fluoride toothpaste. Tooth brushing can be efficacious without the additional help of fluoride, provided that brushing is supervised and the degree of cleanliness is high (Fogels et al., 1982). However, most individuals will find it difficult to achieve and maintain such a high proficiency of cleaning.

The population level

Self-performed tooth brushing is not particularly effective in controlling dental caries at the population level. Of the investigations quoted in the review by Sutcliffe (1996), only about half of the cross-sectional studies showed a positive association between plaque removal and caries. However, multivariate analyses have shown that oral hygiene status is a strong risk indicator of caries when controlling for various other factors such as sugar consumption and fluoride exposure (Stecksen Blicks & Gustafsson, 1986; Bjertness, 1991; Vehkalathi et al., 1997; Mascarenhas, 1998).

It is hardly surprising that there is no clear-cut association between oral hygiene and caries in population studies. Because of the multifactorial nature of caries, the presence of dental biofilm does not by itself imply a high rate of lesion progression. Furthermore, cross-sectional studies have often measured the level of dental cleanliness by indices developed for periodontal purposes. However, gingival

Table 15.1 Caries increment (DS) during the final year of a 3-year experiment of different preventive measures

Prophylactic measure		New carious surfaces				
	n	Total	Proximal	Occlusal	Buccal	Lingual
Daily supervised tooth brushing with a sodium fluoride dentifrice	57	4.4	2.3	1.6	0.2	0.4
Daily supervised tooth brushing with a non-fluoride dentifrice	56	8.3	4.7	2.5	0.5	0.6
Fortnightly rinsing with a 0.5% sodium fluoride solution	69	6.3	3.3	2.2	0–5	0–3
Fortnightly rinsing with distilled water	71	8.4	4.8	2.3	0.8	0.5
Control	46	9.0	5.2	2.0	0.9	0.8

Adopted from Koch & Lindhe (1970).

plaque is probably a poor predictor of caries on occlusal surfaces and on root surfaces. Thus, in a study of periodontal patients followed over an 8-year maintenance period, Ravald *et al.* (1986) reported that only about 7% of the new lesions occurred along the gingival margin. The majority of new carious lesions developed along the cemento-enamel junction (25%) or in relation to margins of restorations (51%).

Because of the low clinical effectiveness of tooth brushing, as revealed by cross-sectional studies, some researchers believe that the primary purpose of tooth brushing is to serve as a vehicle for the application of fluoride (Lewis & Ismail, 1995). As discussed in the previous sections, this belief is hardly justified. It is true that at the population level the effect of brushing with a fluoride toothpaste often does not exceed that obtained by water fluoridation (Ainamo & Parvinen, 1989) or by fortnightly fluoride rinses (Heidmann *et al.*, 1992). However, this does not mean that careful tooth brushing should not be advocated. Tooth brushing is cheap and easy to implement and, when performed properly, has the potential to control both caries and gingivitis.

Furthermore, it should be appreciated that biofilm removal could play a significant role in caries control by an interaction with the diet. Kleemola-Kujala and Räsänen (1982) suggested that there may be a synergistic interaction between dental biofilm and sugar consumption, i.e. the effect of the two factors in combination is higher than the sum of the separate effects. The authors calculated the relative risks of caries in three groups of children with increasing levels of biofilm and sugar consumption, respectively, relative to a group of children with low biofilm levels and low sugar consumption (Fig. 15.4). The data showed that at low levels of biofilm an increase in the total sugar consumption did not increase the risk of caries notably. However, the risk of caries increased significantly (up to three-fold) with increasing levels of biofilm at all levels of sugar consumption. The increase was greatest at the highest levels of sugar consumption. These findings may be taken to indicate that when sugar consumption is high biofilm removal can be a powerful method to control the development and progression of caries.

The effect of professional tooth cleaning

In an attempt to overcome the difficulties encountered in obtaining improved biofilm control for individuals, alternative strategies for non-operative caries control have been suggested. One such strategy, commonly referred to as the Karlstad program, was developed by Axelsson and Lindhe (1974). In addition to the traditional components of a caries-preventive program (repeated oral hygiene instruction, dietary counseling and topical fluorides), this program included a new treatment component, namely professional cleaning of the teeth at regular intervals by specially trained personnel. The idea was based on the results of the experimental *in vivo* studies described previously in this chapter, showing that when dental biofilm was allowed to accumulate on a clean tooth surface, white-spot lesions developed in the enamel within a period of 2–3 weeks (von der Fehr *et al.*, 1970). In the classical Karlstad program, biofilm was therefore removed professionally from all tooth surfaces of the dentition every fortnight to control the progression of caries (for details of the clinical procedure, see Chapter 27).

When the Karlstad program was carried out in children every fortnight during the school term, the number of carious lesions per year went down from about three per child to a single lesion in every 10 children (Table 15.2). Later studies by the Karlstad group (Axelsson *et al.*, 1991) summarizing experiences with the method for more than 15 years, showed that the caries-controlling effect was largely retained with longer intervals between the appointments (up to 3 months) in well-motivated children and adults (Table 15.2).

Researchers who have applied the Karlstad method in other populations have not been able to obtain quite as impressive results (Badersten *et al.*, 1975; Poulsen *et al.*, 1976; Hamp *et al.*, 1978; Kjaerheim *et al.*, 1980). However, it should be emphasized that professional tooth cleaning is

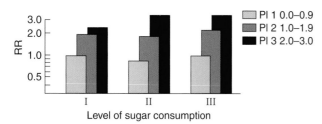

Figure 15.4 Risk of caries (RR) at different levels of plaque accumulation and sugar consumption in terms of unit risk for teeth with PII = 0–0.9 and low (= I) sugar exposure. Primary teeth; 5-year-olds. (From Kleemola-Kujala & Räsänen, 1982.)

Table 15.2 The Karlstad studies (1973–1978): annual caries increments at different professional tooth-cleaning frequencies

Frequency of cleaning	Annual caries increment		Caries reduction (%)	Age group (years)	Period
	Test	Control			
Fortnightly	0.06	3.06	98	7–14	1st year
Fortnightly	0.12	3.25	94	8–15	2nd year
Monthly	0.24	3.56	93	9–13	3rd year
Every 2 months	0.37	4.68	92	15–16	3rd year
Every 2 months	0.28	3.20	91	10–17	4th year
	0.03	1.53	98	<35	
Every 2–3 months	0.00	0.90	100	36–50	3 years
	0.00	0.13	100	>50	

Adopted from Bellini *et al.* (1981).

particularly efficient on tooth surfaces that are difficult to clean, such as approximal surfaces (Badersten *et al.*, 1975; Hamp *et al.*, 1978; Kjaerheim *et al.*, 1980) and erupting occlusal surfaces (Carvalho *et al.*, 1992; Ekstrand *et al.*, 2000). Therefore, this rather costly treatment program may be justified in the management of some highly caries-active patients (see Chapter 27).

The effect of dental flossing

It may come as a surprise to some dental professionals that the widely recommended use of dental floss has not been shown to have a caries-controlling effect on approximal surfaces when used as a supervised preventive measure by children at school (Granath *et al.*, 1979, Horowitz *et al.*, 1980). Only when flossing is performed professionally on a daily basis by trained personnel may a caries reduction be obtained (Wright *et al.*, 1980). This, of course, does not mean that flossing is a poor method to control the amount of biofilm between teeth. Indeed, dental flossing, when performed properly, can be an effective means of reducing the amount of approximal bacterial deposits (Germo & Flötra, 1970; Hill *et al.*, 1973, Bergenholtz *et al.*, 1974). However, when self-performed flossing does not lead to the expected effect this is probably because flossing is difficult to perform. The success of interdental cleaning is greatly dependent on the ease of use and patient motivation (Bergenholtz & Brjthon, 1980). Therefore, implementation of a flossing program should be restricted to selected individuals who are in need of such treatment and who can be expected to practice the method in the recommended way (Granath *et al.*, 1979). For patients who do not master the flossing technique it is helpful to remember that as tooth brushing improves there may be no advantage in following it with flossing (Hill *et al.*, 1973).

Concluding remarks

This chapter provides evidence to support the suggestion that tooth cleaning can be a highly efficacious method for controlling the development and progression of caries, in particular when using a fluoride toothpaste. When tooth brushing is often found to be ineffective it is probably not because of deficiency of the method, but because of delinquency on the part of the individual who applies the method. Controlled clinical trials in children testing the effect of supervised tooth brushing at school have clearly shown that the level of oral cleanliness improves significantly during the course of the trial (Koch & Lindhe, 1970; Machiulskiene *et al.*, 2002). This observation, together with the marked caries-controlling effect obtained by regular professional tooth cleaning, suggests that failure to achieve caries control by self-performed oral hygiene is primarily associated with a lack of compliance. Oral health profes-

sionals should be aware of this problem when motivating their patients in the treatment of dental caries.

In summary, the effectiveness of tooth brushing in caries control (i.e. tooth brushing as normally performed) is not very high. However, when the quality of tooth brushing is high (i.e. tooth brushing as it 'should' be) it can be a very efficacious procedure.

Tooth cleaning and fluoride may have an additive effect in caries control. Therefore, tooth cleaning should always be carried out in conjunction with the use of a fluoride toothpaste.

References

Abramson JH. *Survey methods in community medicine: epidemiological studies, programme evaluation, clinical trials*, 4th edn. New York: Churchill Livingstone, 1990: 47–56.

Ainamo J, Parvinen K. Influence of increased toothbrushing frequency on dental health in low, optimal, and high fluoride areas in Finland. *Community Dent Oral Epidemiol* 1989; **17**: 269–9.

Årtun J, Thylstrup A. Clinical and scanning electron microscopic study of surface changes of incipient enamel caries lesions after debonding. *Scand J Dent Res* 1986; **94**: 193–210.

Axelsson P, Lindhe J. The effect of a preventive programme on dental plaque, gingivitis and caries in schoolchildren. Results after one and two years. *J Clin Periodontol* 1974; **1**: 126–38.

Axelsson P, Lindhe J, Nyström B. On the prevention of caries and periodontal disease. Results of a 15-year longitudinal study in adults. *J Clin Periodontol* 1991; **18**: 182–9.

Badersten A, Egelberg J, Koch G. Effect of monthly prophylaxis on caries and gingivitis in school-children. *Community Dent Oral Epidemiol* 1975; **3**: 1–4.

Beal JF, James PMC, Bradnock G, Anderson RJ. The relationship between dental cleanliness, dental caries incidence and gingival health. *Br Dent J* 1979; **146**: 111–14.

Bellini HT, Arneberg P, von der Fehr FR. Oral hygiene and caries. A review. *Acta Odontol Scand* 1981; **39**: 257–65.

Bergenholtz A, Bjorne A, Vickström B. The plaque-removing ability of some common interdental aids: an intraindividual study. *I Clin Perodontol* 1974; **1**: 157–65.

Bergenholtz A, Brjthon J. Plaque removal by dental floss and toothpicks: an intra-individual comparative study. *J Clin Periodontol* 1980; **7**: 515–24.

Bjertness E. The importance of oral hygiene on variation in dental caries in adults. *Acta Odontol Scand* 1991; **49**: 97–102.

Carvalho JC, Thylstrup A, Ekstrand KR. Results after 3 years of non-operative occlusal caries treatment of erupting permanent first molars. *Community Dent Oral Epidemiol* 1992; **20**: 187–92.

Chestnutt IG, Schäfer F, Jacobson APM, Stephen KW. The influence of toothbrushing frequency and post-brushing rinsing on caries experience in a caries clinical trial. *Community Dent Oral Epidemiol* 1998; **26**: 406–11.

Dijkman A, Huizinga E, Ruben J, Arends J. Remineralization of human enamel *in situ* after 3 months: the effect of not brushing versus the effect of an F dentifrice and an F-free dentifrice. *Caries Res* 1990; **24**: 263–6.

Ekstrand KR, Kuzmina IN, Kuzmina E, Christiansen ME. Two and a half-year outcome of caries-preventive programs offered to groups of children in the Solntsevsky district of Moscow. *Caries Res* 2000; **34**: 8–19.

von der Fehr FR, Löe H, Theilade E. Experimental caries in man. *Caries Res* 1970; **4**: 131–48.

Fejerskov O, Manji F. Risk assessment in dental caries. In: Bader JD, ed. *Risk assessment in dentistry*. Chapel Hill, NC: University of North Carolina Dental Ecology, 1990: 215–17.

Firestone AR, Mühlemann HR. *In vivo* pH of plaque-covered and plaque-free interdental surfaces in humans following a sucrose rinse. *Clin Prev Dent* 1985; **7**: 24–6.

Fogels H, Cancro LP, Bianco J, Fischman SL. The anticaries effect of supervised toothbrushing with a nonfluoride dentifrice. *J Dent Child* 1982; **49**: 424–7.

Germo P, Flötra L. The effect of different methods of interdental cleaning. *J Periodontol* 1970; 5: 230–6.

Granath L, Martinsson T, Matsson L, Nilsson G, Schröder U, Söderholm B. Intraindividual effect of daily supervised flossing on caries in schoolchildren. *Community Dent Oral Epidemiol* 1979; **7**: 147–50.

Hamp S-E, Lindhe J, Fornell J, Johansson L-Å, Karlsson R. Effect of a field program based on systematic plaque control on caries and gingivitis in schoolchildren after 3 years. *Community Dent Oral Epidemiol* 1978; **6**: 17–23.

Heidmann J, Poulsen S, Arnbjerg D, Kirkegaard E, Laurberg L. Caries development after termination of a fluoride rinsing program. *Community Dent Oral Epidemiol* 1992; **20**: 118–21.

Hill HC, Levi PA, Glickman I. The effects of waxed and unwaxed dental floss on interdental plaque accumulation and interdental gingival health. *J Periodontol* 1973; **7**: 411–14.

Holmen L, Thylstrup A, Øgaard B, Kragh F. A polarized light microscopic study of progressive stages of enamel caries *in vivo*. *Caries Res* 1985a; **19**: 348–54.

Holmen L, Thylstrup A, Øgaard B, Kragh F. A scanning electron microscopic study of progressive stages of enamel caries *in vivo*. *Caries Res* 1985b; 19: 355–67.

Holmen L, Thylstrup A, Øgaard B, Kragh F. Surface changes during the arrest of active enamel carious lesions *in vivo*. *Acta Odontol Scand* 1987a; **45**: 383–90.

Holmen L, Thylstrup A, Årtun J. Clinical and histologic features observed during arrestment of active enamel carious lesions *in vivo*. *Caries Res* 1987b; **21**: 546–54.

Horowitz AM, Suomi JD, Peterson JK, Mathews BL, Vogelsong RH, Lyman BA. Effects of supervised daily dental plaque removal by children after 3 years. *Community Dent Oral Epidemiol* 1980; **8**: 171–6.

Horowitz HS, Thompson MB. Evaluation of a stannous fluoride dentifrice for use in dental public health programs III. Supplementary findings. *J Am Dent Assoc* 1967; **74**: 979–86.

Kjaerheim V, von der Fehr FR, Poulsen S. Two-year study on the effect of professional toothcleaning on schoolchildren in Oppegaard, Norway. *Community Dent Oral Epidemiol* 1980; **8**: 401–6.

Kleemola-Kujula E, Räsänen L. Relationship of oral hygiene and sugar consumption to risk of caries in children. *Community Dent Oral Epidemiol* 1982; **10**: 224–33.

Koch G, Lindhe J. The state of the gingivae and the caries-increment in schoolchildren during and after withdrawal of various prophylactic measures. In: McHugh WD, ed. *Dental plaque*. Edinburgh: Livingstone, 1970: 271–81.

Kuusela S, Honkala E, Kannas L, Tynjälä J, Wold B. Oral hygiene habits of 11-year-old schoolchildren in 22 European countries and Canada in 1993/94. *J Dent Res* 1997; **76**: 1602–9.

Lewis DW, Ismail AI. Periodic health examination, 1995 update: 2. Prevention of dental caries. *CMAJ* 1995; **152**: 836–46.

Lo EC, Schwarz E, Wong MC. Arresting dentine caries in Chinese preschool children. *Int J Paediatr Dent* 1998; **8**: 253–60.

Machiulskiene V, Richards A, Nyvad B, Baelum V. Prospective study of the effect of post-brushing rinsing behaviour on dental caries. *Caries Res* 2002; **36**: 301–7.

Marthaler TM. Changes in the prevalence of dental caries: how much can be attributed to changes in diet? *Caries Res* 1990; **24** (Suppl 1): 3–15.

Mascarenhas AK. Oral hygiene as a risk indicator of enamel and dentin caries. *Community Dent Oral Epidemiol* 1998; **26**: 331–9.

Mathiesen AT, Øgaard B, Rølla G. Oral hygiene as a variable in dental caries experience in 14-year-olds exposed to fluoride. *Caries Res* 1996; **30**: 29–33.

Naylor MN, Glass RL. A 3-year clinical trial of calcium carbonate dentifrice containing calcium glycerophosphate and sodium monofluorophosphate. *Caries Res* 1979; **13**: 39–46.

Nyvad B, Fejerskov O. Active root surface caries converted into inactive caries as a response to oral hygiene. *Scand J Dent Res* 1986; **94**: 281–4.

Nyvad B, Fejerskov O. Assessing the stage of caries lesion activity on the basis of clinical and microbiological examination. *Community Dent Oral Epidemiol* 1997; **25**: 69–75.

Nyvad B, ten Cate JM, Fejerskov O. Arrest of root surface caries *in situ*. *J Dent Res* 1997; **76**: 1845–53.

Poulsen S, Agerbæk N, Melsen B, Korts DC, Glavind L, Rölla G. The effect of professional toothcleaning on gingivitis and dental caries in children after 1 year. *Community Dent Oral Epidemiol* 1976; **4**: 195–9.

Ravald N, Hamp SE, Birkhed D. Long-term evaluation of root surface caries in periodontally treated patients. *J Clin Periodontol* 1986; **13**: 758–67.

Stecksen Blicks C, Gustafsson L. Impact of oral hygiene and use of fluorides on caries increment in children during one year. *Community Dent Oral Epidemiol* 1986; **14**: 185–9.

Sutcliffe P. A longitudinal clinical study of oral cleanliness and dental caries in school children. *Arch Oral Biol* 1973; **18**: 765–70.

Sutcliffe P. Oral cleanliness and dental caries. In: Murray JJ, ed. *Prevention of oral disease*. New York: Oxford University Press, 1996: 68–77.

Tucker GJ, Andlaw RJ, Burchell CK. The relationship between oral hygiene and dental caries incidence in 11-year-old children. *Br Dent J* 1976; **141**: 75–9.

Vehkalathi MM, Vrbic VL, Peric LM, Matvoz ES. Oral hygiene and root caries occurrence in Slovenian adults. *Int Dent J* 1997; **47**: 26–31.

Wellock WD, Maitland A, Brudevold F. Caries increments, tooth discoloration, and state of oral hygiene in children given single annual applications of acid phosphate-fluoride and stannous fluoride. *Arch Oral Biol* 1965; **10**: 453–60.

Wright GZ, Feasby WH, Banting DB. The effectiveness of interdental flossing with and without fluoride dentifrice. *Pediatr Dent* 1980; **2**: 105–9.

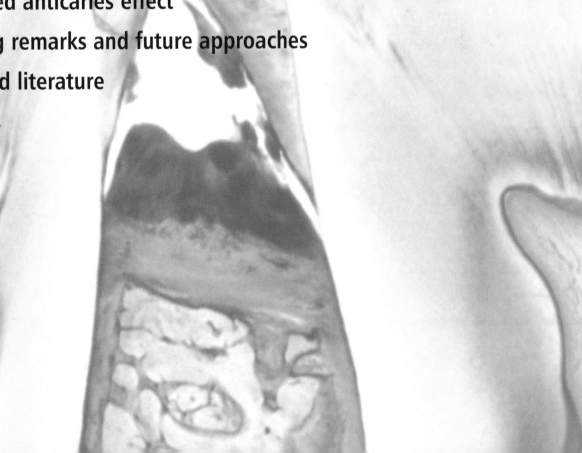

16

Antimicrobials in caries control

A.A. Scheie and F.C. Petersen

Dental plaque: the biofilm lifestyle and the rationale for antimicrobial intervention

Biological activity and mode of action

Modification of dental biofilm biochemistry and ecology

Vehicles for administration of caries-prophylactic agents

Specific agents

Other agents proposed for caries prophylaxis, but without documented anticaries effect

Concluding remarks and future approaches

Background literature

References

Dental plaque: the biofilm lifestyle and the rationale for antimicrobial intervention

The biofilm mode of growth appears to be the preferred lifestyle of microorganisms in nature. Microbial biofilms represent the major cause of diseases of microbial origin, including dental caries and periodontal disease. Dental plaque is a typical biofilm. Ecological imbalance within microbial biofilms on teeth may lead to dental caries (Marsh, 1994). Therefore, control of dental biofilms is fundamental to caries control. Dental biofilms are, however, not easily controlled by mechanical means. Thus, it seems reasonable to control caries by agents that either prevent the formation of, or disrupt biofilms on teeth, or inhibit acid formation or stimulate base formation by dental biofilms. Caries control using chemical agents has been of long-standing interest. Researchers have searched for suitable agents ever since Miller suggested in 1890 that antiseptics that destroy bacteria, or limit their number and activity, could be a way to 'counteract or limit the ravages of dental caries'.

Numerous agents, with varying modes of action, have been tested for their ability to intervene with dental biofilm formation or metabolism, assuming that dental caries development would be reduced by such agents. However, as discussed in this chapter, there are few antimicrobial agents with documented anticaries effect, owing to either a lack of properly controlled clinical studies or the lack of efficacy of the agents. Lack of documentation may be related to use of surrogate endpoints, such as biofilm mass or levels of mutans streptococci to assess the anticaries effect. No direct relationship exists, however, between caries development and biofilm mass or salivary or biofilm levels of mutans streptococci. One, therefore, cannot extrapolate from studies on dental biofilm inhibition or inhibition of mutans streptococci to possible cariostatic properties of an agent. The only way to assess the clinical cariostatic efficacy of an agent is through well-controlled clinical studies with assessment of caries incidence or progression as an endpoint.

Lack of agent efficacy may be related to the fact that the oral microorganisms prefer to organize in complex biofilms. Their properties are then changed markedly from their free-floating (planktonic) condition. Thus, biofilm microorganisms are much less susceptible to antimicrobial agents and to the host immune response than when they are planktonic. An agent that is effective against planktonic cells might require 2–1000 times higher concentrations to kill the same type of microorganisms if they grow in biofilms. *In vitro*, the chlorhexidine concentration needed to kill *Streptococcus mutans* in a biofilm is five times higher than when they grow in suspension (Filoche *et al.*, 2005).

The inherent natural biofilm resistance to antimicrobial agents was not appreciated until recently; therefore, agents generally have been tested against planktonic cells. The biofilm resistance to antimicrobial agents partly explains why many oral prophylactic agents predicted to be efficacious *in vitro*, show only marginal clinical effects. Retarded or incomplete penetration of the agent into the biofilm, and reduced growth rate of the microorganisms due to nutrient limitations, have been considered reasons for lack of efficacy. More importantly, however, is that microorganisms within a biofilm are phenotypically altered by their ability to turn on and off genes. Evidence exists that microorganisms are able to turn on or off genes in response to intermicrobial and environmental signals. Thus, other genes may be expressed by the biofilm microorganisms than those expressed by planktonic cells. The machinery involved in carbohydrate catabolism is, for instance, more active during early stages of *S. mutans* biofilm formation than in planktonic cells (Welin *et al.*, 2004).

Unlike classical infectious diseases, which are caused by microbial pathogens, caries is caused by the resident oral microflora. This flora represents an important line of defense and protects the host against colonization by foreign microorganisms. The goal is therefore not to eliminate the flora, but to prevent a shift from an ecologically favorable to an ecologically unstable biofilm that may lead to disease. Whether this should be achieved by chemical agents or by other means may be discussed. One view is that any reduction in dental biofilms is beneficial if accomplished safely. Since adequate self-performed mechanical control of dental biofilms is difficult and often inadequate, antimicrobials may offer an adjunct. The opposing view is that such agents may disturb the ecological balance within the oral cavity, and that resistant microbial strains may emerge. It is a well-established fact that widespread and sometimes indiscriminate use of antimicrobials may cause treatment failure owing to resistant or multiresistant microorganisms. The oral flora, including the early tooth colonizers *Streptococcus oralis* and *Streptococcus mitis*, may function as a reservoir of antibiotic resistance genes (Hakenbeck *et al.*, 1998; Seppala *et al.*, 2003). Such genes are likely to be transferred to the close relative *Streptococcus pneumoniae*, which may be associated with human infections such as otitis media, sinusitis, meningitis and pneumonia.

Any chemical agent that affects microbial cells may be expected to have some adverse effects against host cells, unless the target structure or metabolic pathway is unique to the microorganism. There is, however, no evidence that the common use of chemical agents against dental biofilms has resulted in demonstrable adverse effects; but there is also a lack of conclusive, controlled studies to demonstrate a health benefit from prolonged use of antimicrobial agents. Thus, possible benefit must be weighed against potential disadvantages on an individual basis.

Biological activity and mode of action

A general requirement for biological activity of an agent is bioavailability, i.e. delivery of the agent to the intended site of action in a biologically active form and at effective doses. Topic application is therefore the choice for agents intended to affect oral biofilms. The clinical efficacy of an orally delivered antimicrobial agent depends both on its potency and on its substantivity. Substantivity refers to the agent's ability to bind to oral surfaces and its subsequent rate of release from its binding sites. After delivery, effective agents are characterized by slow release over time. An agent may be retained in the oral cavity by binding to oral surfaces including mucosal surfaces, tooth surfaces, pellicle and supragingival dental biofilm according to its affinity and binding strength. The equilibrium between bound and free agent molecules determines the subsequent release rate from the binding sites (Fig. 16.1). This binding and release allow for contact of varying duration between the agent and the dental biofilm, depending on agent substantivity. An agent with high substantivity will be retained in the mouth for a prolonged period (Fig. 16.2a), whereas an agent without substantivity will be cleared from the oral cavity with a rate determined by the salivary clearance. This only allows a short-term effect of the agent, and microorganisms may have time to metabolize and multiply between agent applications. A non-substantive agent must therefore be applied frequently to have clinical efficacy similar to a substantive agent (Fig. 16.2a, b).

Most agents used are antimicrobials with a broad spectrum of activity aiming at reducing biofilm accumulation or activity by direct action on the microbial cell. Non-antimicrobial approaches are generally designed to reduce

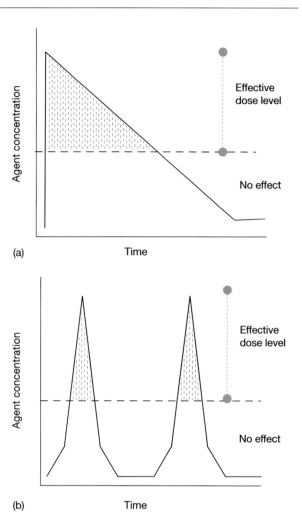

(a)

(b)

Figure 16.2 Dose curves of (a) an agent with high substantivity and (b) an agent with low substantivity. The horizontal dotted lines represent the effective dose levels. The effective dose–time area (circumscribed between the curves and the dotted lines) may be similar if the low substantive agent is applied frequently. (After Pader, 1988.)

biofilm accumulation by interference with microbial adhesion to the tooth surface.

Chemical agents can reduce biofilm mass at various stages of biofilm formation or maturation through one or more of the following mechanisms:

- inhibition of microbial adhesion and colonization
- inhibition of microbial growth and metabolism
- disruption of mature biofilms and detachment of biofilm microorganisms
- modification of biofilm biochemistry and ecology (Table 16.1).

Inhibition of microbial adhesion and colonization

Inhibiting microbial adhesion to tooth surfaces will reduce the accumulation of dental biofilms. *In vitro* studies have shown that agents that reduce the surface free energy will reduce microbial adhesion to that surface. Various

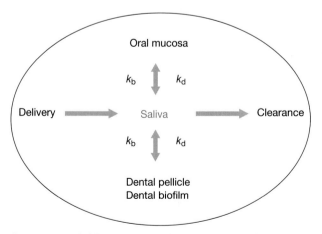

Figure 16.1 Oral delivery, binding, release and clearance of antimicrobial agents in the oral cavity. The agent binds to oral mucosa, tooth surfaces, pellicle and dental biofilm bacteria according to its affinity [K_b], and is released from its binding site depending on its dissociation constant [K_d] and salivary clearance rate. The oral mucosa represents the major reservoir for substantive agents. (After van der Ouderaa & Cummins, 1989.)

Table 16.1 Stages and mechanisms of biofilm formation as targets for interference

Mechanism and stage	Target
Inhibition of microbial adhesion and colonization	Surface physicochemical properties Bacterial cell-surface components Cell communication
Inhibition of microbial growth and metabolism	Transport systems Cell wall Metabolic activity Cell viability Cell communication
Disruption of biofilm maturation Detachment of biofilm microorganisms	Extracellular polymers: *Polysaccharides, DNA* Cell-surface proteins Cell communication Adhesion Coaggregation Release of cell-surface proteins
Modification of biofilm biochemistry and ecology Replacement	Specific microbial niche

approaches have been explored to modify surface characteristics of teeth, pellicle and/or microorganisms. The salivary pellicle, to which the microorganisms adhere through specific and non-specific binding mechanisms, provides a complex array of binding sites. Thus, the composition of the pellicle may modulate bacterial adhesion events. One approach is to change the surface characteristics by manipulating the protein film on the enamel, and thereby reduce bacterial adhesion. Several routes of surface modification have been investigated. Unfortunately, the clinical efficacy has so far been low, but recent progress in material sciences may lead to novel approaches.

Specific surface proteins on the microorganisms are involved in the binding of oral bacteria to pellicle components. Intermicrobial communication may regulate surface protein expression. Targeting surface-associated proteins, directly or through communication interference, may therefore represent a logical strategy to control biofilm formation and activity. Expression of surface adhesins may, for instance, be impaired by subminimal inhibitory concentrations of several antimicrobial agents, thus interfering with microbial adhesion and colonization.

Immunization against dental caries has been a central research topic for many years. The aim is to inhibit adhesion or to reduce virulence, most often by the use of vaccines against epitopes on mutans streptococci. The surface-bound antigen I/II and glucosyltransferases in mutans streptococci are the most studied cell-surface targets for possible immunization against dental caries.

In general, immunization approaches are directed against single microbial species. Knowing the ability of microorganisms to form biofilms and to adapt and transform in such environments, a question is whether immunization will give lasting protection. No clinically applicable immunization scheme directed against dental caries is yet commercially available (see Chapter 17).

Inhibition of microbial growth and/or metabolism

The majority of agents used to limit or inhibit biofilm formation are broad-spectrum antimicrobial agents with bactericidal (killing) or bacteriostatic (growth-inhibiting) effects. They are used according to a non-specific plaque hypothesis and are formulated to be used as supplements to mechanical oral cleaning.

Antimicrobials bind to the microbial membrane and thus interfere with normal membrane functions such as transport. This disturbs the microbial metabolism and in turn may kill the microorganism. Adsorption to microbial membranes may also lead to alterations in the permeability, resulting in leakage of intracellular components, along with denaturation and coagulation of cytoplasmic protein contents. Antimicrobial activity, per se, does not necessarily coincide with clinical effects.

More recent understanding of mechanisms involved in biofilm formation indicates that it may be possible to interfere with microbial activity on surfaces, without affecting cell viability. For several bacteria, communication signals may be necessary to form structured biofilms. Compounds that interfere with signal formation or signal detection are being investigated for several microorganisms, including oral bacteria. Such signals may be involved not only in the formation of structured biofilms, but also in the ability of the cells to adapt to adverse environmental conditions. Different communication systems in *S. mutans* seem to influence, for instance, biofilm formation, antimicrobial resistance and acid tolerance. Studies in this field are, however, in an early stage. A deeper understanding of microbial behaviors regulated by communication will be required before the possibility of interfering with signaling mechanisms can be fully appreciated.

Disruption of mature biofilms and detachment of biofilm microorganisms

It is likely that the mature community dental biofilm is the result of a well-regulated series of processes, each of which may represent a potential target for biofilm control. Adhesive biopolymers such as glucan form important components of the oral biofilms. Approaches to disrupt established biofilms through the hydrolytic action of enzymes therefore seem reasonable. So far, experimental results have, however, been disappointing. For one thing, the dental biofilm matrix contains several types of biopolymers including a variety of polysaccharides and DNA, as well as proteins. Therefore, targeting just one of these may be insufficient. Another barrier is diffusion of the agent into the biofilm.

Disturbance of the structural properties of the dental biofilm during formation could also limit its ultimate mass. For instance, inhibitory effects on glucosyltransferase activity could result in more loosely attached deposits. Glucosyltransferase is an enzyme involved in glucan formation. Studies have shown that, for instance, chlorhexidine may inhibit glucosyltransferase activity. In addition, *in vitro* studies show reduction in the viscosity of glucans synthesized in presence of delmopinol. *In vivo*, frequent applications of chlorhexidine and high concentrations of delmopinol have been shown to possess biofilm-dispersive activity. Any effect on caries has, however, not been documented.

Recent studies indicate that bacteria may have a program leading to detachment from biofilms. Under unfavorable conditions, detachment would allow bacteria to leave the biofilm and find new sites for colonization. For several microorganisms, release of surface proteins used for attachment is a regulated process. Elucidation of such mechanisms may lead to novel strategies to disrupt or prevent the formation of mature dental biofilms.

Modification of dental biofilm biochemistry and ecology

According to the ecological plaque hypothesis, the microbial ecological balance is crucial for the maintenance of dental health. One way to maintain or restore such a balance could be to replace potential pathogens with harmless and beneficial microorganisms through probiotics or replacement therapy. By definition, a probiotic is a live microbial food ingredient that when ingested in a sufficient quantity exerts health benefits on the consumer. Coupled with an understanding of how these microorganisms act, genetic engineering opens the possibility of designing new probiotic strains. Such strains may be enabled to compete against and to replace known pathogens, while being non-virulent themselves. Given the increasing problem of antimicrobial resistance, probiotics may become an attractive future alternative.

With probiotics, naturally occurring harmless microorganisms may exert beneficial action by occupying colonization sites and competing with the pathogen for nutrients. They may also produce harmful metabolites, biosurfactants or antimicrobial agents that inhibit biofilm formation by the pathogen.

Probiotics have been shown to prevent and treat various gastrointestinal disorders (Doron & Gorbach, 2006). They have also been suggested in caries prophylaxis (Meurman, 2005). In a recent project children were given milk containing the probiotic *Lactobacillus rhamnosus* LGG with meals, five days a week for 7 months (Nase *et al.*, 2001). The results indicated that the probiotic milk had a protective effect, since a tendency towards low caries incidence was seen in one of the age groups.

Two main approaches have been pursued to replace mutans streptococci with strains that lack the ability to produce lactate or strains that produce alkaline products. Both approaches would limit the pH drop in dental biofilms. Animal studies have shown promising results, but as with immunization, the approach is directed against a single microbial species, mutans streptococci, disregarding a possible cariogenic role of other microorganisms.

The requirements for prevention through probiotics to be efficacious are:

- They are able to adhere and become part of the biofilm.
- There is a definite pathogen to interact with or to replace.
- The probiotic or replacement organisms must not cause disease themselves.
- They must colonize persistently.
- They must replace or interact with the pathogen effectively.
- They must possess high degrees of genetic stability.

One cannot exclude the possibility that a probiotic strain might acquire new phenotypic traits through DNA exchange with the resident flora or with virulent strains in oral biofilms, later to become an opportunistic pathogen.

As of today, direct approaches to alter the ecology of the biofilm to become less pathogenic are restricted and have not yet led to development of agents appropriate for general clinical use.

Vehicles for administration of caries-prophylactic agents

Caries-prophylactic agents may be delivered to the oral cavity by various delivery formulations (vehicles):

- mouthrinses
- sprays
- dentifrices
- gels
- chewing gum/lozenges
- various sustained-release formulations or devices.

The choice of vehicle depends on compatibility between the active agent and the constituents of the vehicle. For instance, the first fluoride dentifrices were ineffective owing to incompatibility between fluoride and the abrasive system of the dentifrice.

The vehicles should provide optimal bioavailability of the agent at its site of action. Delivery by dentifrices and mouthwashes, which are the most common vehicles, results in immediate high concentrations of the agent. Patient compliance is of vital importance, and is probably reduced with increasing dosing frequency and with increasing length and complexity of the treatment. Therefore, the prophylaxis is most likely to succeed if the delivery vehicle does not require patients to adopt new habits.

Recent developments in material sciences have provided novel systems for drug delivery. Active agents may be packed into microparticles or nanoparticles or incorporated into functional films. In the future, such new approaches may also be used in oral prophylaxis.

Mouthrinses

Mouthrinses represent the simplest vehicle formulation. They are usually a mixture of the active component in water and alcohol, with addition of a surfactant and flavor. Most antimicrobial agents are compatible with this vehicle.

Sprays

Sprays have been evaluated for the delivery of, for instance, chlorhexidine in mouthrinse formulations. An advantage attributed to the spray is that relatively small doses are required to achieve efficacy. Good compliance may be expected with sprays because they are easy for a patient or carer to use. Further investigations into the use of sprays for the delivery of prophylactic agents are warranted, however.

Dentifrices

Dentifrices fill three main functions:

- to debride teeth of stain
- to give the cavity a feeling of freshness and cleanliness
- to serve as a vehicle for prophylactic agents.

Dentifrices contain the following essential ingredients:

- an abrasive system to help remove stain
- a component to carry the abrasive and the active agent
- a surfactant to provide foam and detersive action
- a binder for desirable rheological properties
- flavor to make tooth brushing pleasant.

The complex formulation of dentifrices involves possibilities for component interactions. Care must therefore be taken to secure bioavailability of the active components. Tooth brushing with a dentifrice is a well-adopted habit. Therefore dentifrices should be a suitable vehicle for the delivery of prophylactic agents.

Gels

A gel is a thickened aqueous system, but with neither abrasive material nor foaming agents. Gels are generally compatible with relevant antimicrobial agents. Gels are usually applied in premade or individually made appliances to provide close contact between the agent and the tooth surface.

Chewing gums and lozenges

The effect of chewing gums and lozenges depends on release of the agent during chewing or dissolution. The contact time is longer than, for instance, with mouthrinses, but increased salivation will inevitably increase the oral clearance rate of an agent. Administration of antimicrobials via such vehicles may represent effective and acceptable routes, particularly in patients with low tooth-brushing compliance. For individuals with reduced salivation, stimulated salivary secretion due to chewing may also be beneficial and relieve some discomfort. Increased salivation in itself may be beneficial. Further work on chewing gums and lozenges as vehicles is justified.

Sustained-release vehicles

Sustained-release vehicles such as varnishes may provide a long-term effect of the prophylactic agent. The agent's efficacy depends on its degree and rate of release from the carrying material. Fluoride varnishes and chlorhexidine varnishes are in use and found to be effective. The efficacy of sustained-release agents is independent of patient compliance.

Specific agents

Three agents have received particular interest as caries-prophylactic agents. These are chlorhexidine, which is a cationic antimicrobial agent, triclosan, which is a non-ionic antimicrobial agent, and xylitol, which is a sugar alcohol claimed to have various effects on the oral microflora. These agents will be described in some detail in the following. Other less frequently used agents such as cetylpyridinium chloride, delmopinol, hexetidine, sanguinaria extracts, metal ions, sodium dodecyl sulfate (SDS) and certain enzymes will be discussed briefly.

Cationic agents readily bind to negatively charged microbial surfaces and therefore generally are more potent than anionic or non-ionic agents. Likely binding sites for cations on Gram-positive microorganisms are free carboxyl groups from peptidoglycans, and phosphate groups from teichoic and lipoteichoic acid within the microbial cell wall. In Gram-negative microorganisms lipopolysaccharides have high affinity for cations. Cationic agents thus can interact with both Gram-positive and Gram-negative microorganisms. Cationic agents that have been used as antibiofilm agents include:

- chlorhexidine
- cetylpyridinium chloride
- delmopinol
- hexetidine
- sanguinaria extracts
- metal ions.

Chlorhexidine digluconate is the most thoroughly studied and the most efficacious antibiofilm and antigingivitis agent, and represents a gold standard against which the potency of other antibiofilm agents is compared.

The antimicrobial non-ionic agent triclosan has been used as a preservative in consumer products such as deodorants, soaps and body powder for more than 30 years. More recently, triclosan has been added to dentifrices and mouthrinses as a prophylactic agent with the objective of reducing dental biofilm formation and the development of gingivitis.

Xylitol is a pentitol, which is used as a sugar substitute, for instance, in chewing gums. Like other polyols, which cannot be fermented by oral microorganisms, xylitol does not lead to acid formation.

As will be discussed, evidence for any cariostatic effects of these agents either does not exist or is inconclusive.

Chlorhexidine

Mode of action and clinical use
Chlorhexidine is a bisbiguanide with both hydrophilic and hydrophobic properties (Fig. 16.3).

The positively charged molecule may bind to negatively charged groups, i.e. to phosphate, carboxyl or sulfate groups on the oral mucosa, on microorganisms and in the pellicle. The microbial membrane integrity may be disrupted by interactions with the hydrophobic portion of the molecule, causing disturbance of the membrane function. At high concentrations, chlorhexidine is bactericidal, causing leakage of low molecular weight cell constituents and precipitation of cell contents. This damage is irreversible. At lower concentrations the effect is bacteriostatic, causing interference with normal membrane functions or leakage of cell constituents (Hugo & Longworth, 1964). The *in vitro* antimicrobial effect of chlorhexidine is not outstanding, but the spectrum is broad. Gram-positive microorganisms are generally more sensitive to chlorhexidine than are Gram-negative microorganisms. Mutans streptococci are particularly sensitive, whereas, for instance, *Streptococcus sanguinis* exhibits great variation in susceptibility among strains (Emilson, 1977). Despite the widespread clinical use of chlorhexidine, reports of untoward effects are few. General and systemic effects are rare, and degradation of the chlorhexidine molecule to form potentially dangerous metabolites seems unlikely. Local adverse effects, such as discoloration of teeth, tongue, restorations and dentures, desquamation and soreness of the oral mucosa, taste disturbances and bitter taste, however, are frequently reported. Reducing the concentration of chlorhexidine reduces the local adverse effects. The usually prescribed dosage for chlorhexidine mouthrinses has been 10 ml of a 0.2% solution, with twice-daily mouthrinses. A 0.12% chlorhexidine-mouthrinse is available. By using 15 ml of this rinse a

similar dosage is obtained, and the efficacy is comparable. Similar doses may also be obtained by chlorhexidine-containing chewing gums (20 mg per piece). For long-term term chlorhexidine should be dosed individually.

The clinical antimicrobial and antibiofilm effect of chlorhexidine is better than for other agents with similar or even better *in vitro* antimicrobial efficacy. This superior effect has been ascribed mainly to the substantivity of chlorhexidine and to the fact that chlorhexidine retains its antimicrobial effect even when adsorbed to surfaces. A single mouthrinse with 0.2% chlorhexidine exerts an immediate antimicrobial effect, reducing the oral microbial flora by 80–95% (Schiött, 1973). Twice-daily mouthrinses inhibit dental biofilm accumulation almost completely. As a result of the direct antimicrobial effect, chlorhexidine reduces the metabolic activity of the dental biofilm, thus decreasing acid challenge after sucrose or glucose intake. Chlorhexidine may also inhibit the enzyme glucosyltransferase (Scheie *et al.*, 1987), which is essential for microbial accumulation on tooth surfaces, and the metabolic enzyme phosphoenolpyruvate phosphotransferase, which is involved in the transport and phosphorylation of glucose across the membrane (Marsh *et al.*, 1983).

Caries prophylactic effect
One would expect that these effects on dental biofilm formation and metabolic activity would affect caries development. Intensive prophylaxis with chlorhexidine and fluoride in combination may be indicated in individuals with high caries activity and incidence due, for instance, to hyposalivation after irradiation treatment of the head and neck regions (Katz, 1982). However, the universal use of chlorhexidine as an anticaries agent is controversial. No or very low cariostatic effect has been found in human studies where the chlorhexidine treatment is carried out as part of the individual's home care with either mouthrinses or tooth brushing. In contrast, professional application of chlorhexidine combined with a rigorous prophylactic regimen including oral hygiene instruction, dietary advice, professional dental prophylaxis and topical application of fluoride varnish reduced caries lesion development in children during a 3-year study period (Zickert *et al.*, 1982). The idea was to inhibit caries lesion development by reducing the acidogenic potential of the microflora. The number of new caries lesions in the untreated control group was 9.6, compared with 4.2 for the chlorhexidine-treated group. It is worth noting, however, that a similar prophylactic regimen,

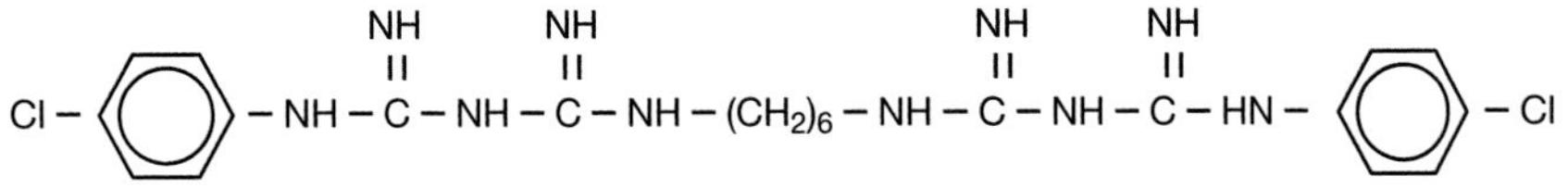

Figure 16.3 Molecular formula of chlorhexidine.

but without chlorhexidine treatment, may give similar caries reduction (Klock & Krasse, 1978).

Professional application of a chlorhexidine gel was shown to perform better than two different fluoride varnishes in a 2-year study in children (Lindquist *et al.*, 1989), and better than a placebo gel when applied to approximal sites (Gisselsson *et al.*, 1988). Quarterly application to approximal sites in 13–14-year-old children of either a 0.1% fluoride varnish or a 1% chlorhexidine varnish had similar caries-prophylactic effects during a 3-year study period (Petersson *et al.*, 1991). In another study, varnishes containing either 40% chlorhexidine or fluoride (Duraphat®) applied every 3 months for 1 year were evaluated for their ability to inhibit the progression of already existing root caries lesions. Both fluoride and chlorhexidine decreased lesion progression compared with the control (Schaeken *et al.*, 1991). In a recent review of chlorhexidine intervention studies performed between 1995 and 2003, chlorhexidine varnish seemed to have an inhibitory effect on fissure caries development in children with low exposure to fluoride. In elderly people and in fluoride-exposed caries-active children and adolescents, evidence for an anticaries effect of chlorhexidine was inconclusive (Twetman, 2004). The inconclusive results from studies on the anticaries effect of chlorhexidine are reflected in two recent publications reporting on the caries-inhibiting effect of 40% chlorhexidine varnish in Chinese children. In one study, the authors conclude that the effect is questionable and only transient (Zhang *et al.*, 2006), whereas 37.3% caries reduction was found in the other study (Du *et al.*, 2006).

Triclosan

Mode of action and clinical use

Triclosan is a non-ionic antimicrobial agent with hydrophilic and hydrophobic properties (Figure 16.4).

Triclosan has a broad antimicrobial spectrum, with activity against both Gram-positive and Gram-negative microorganisms and fungi. Oral microorganisms such as mutans streptococci, *S. sanguinis* and *Streptococcus salivarius* are susceptible to low concentrations of triclosan *in vitro*. At low concentrations, the effect is bacteriostatic. Until recently, triclosan was thought to function as an unspecific biocide, but recent data show that it specifically inhibits lipid synthesis (McMurry *et al.*, 1998). This leads to defective cell-membrane synthesis.

Owing to its poor aqueous solubility, triclosan is solubilized in the flavor/surfactant phase of formulation. In commercial products, triclosan is solubilized in one or more detergents, such as SDS, sodium lauroyl sarcosinate, or in propylene glycol or polyethylene glycol. Thus, when testing the antimicrobial effect of triclosan, one must consider possible additive or synergistic effects with these constituents.

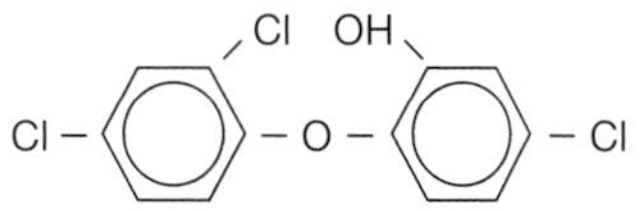

The substantivity of triclosan in the oral cavity is relatively low. For triclosan to be efficacious, a copolymer, polyvinylmethyl–ether maleic acid (PVM/MA, commercially known as Gantrez), or zinc citrate is added to the formulations. Without these retention mediators, triclosan toothpastes have no apparent effect on dental biofilm biomass (Waraaswapati *et al.*, 2005).

Extensive studies have been performed to prove the efficacy of triclosan-containing products. Despite the demonstration in several short- and long-term studies that triclosan prevents dental biofilm formation and gingivitis, its effect must be considered as modest. A metanalysis of 16 clinical studies of the long-term effect of daily unsupervised triclosan use showed reductions in dental biofilm mass by 15% and gingivitis by 12% (Davies *et al.*, 2004). As to the effect on periodontitis development, the effect on the general population is not significant. Triclosan may possibly slow down progression in predisposed individuals, i.e. in individuals who have already increased dental pocket depth (Cullinan *et al.*, 2003b). Notably, this effect appears to be of moderate magnitude (between 10 and 20% compared with placebo) and independent of triclosan's antimicrobial properties (Cullinan *et al.*, 2003a). Data on a possible cariostatic effect of triclosan are scarce. It has been shown that triclosan neither enhances nor interferes with fluoride-enhanced remineralization and that triclosan-containing toothpastes are 'at least as good as' fluoride-containing dentifrices without antimicrobial additives.

Concerns have recently been raised that the widespread use of triclosan-containing products may lead to the development of antimicrobial resistance (Yazdankhah *et al.*, 2006). In high concentrations, triclosan causes disruption of the bacterial cells by targeting multiple non-specific targets. However, triclosan-containing products such as dentifrices leave residues that will dilute to sublethal concentration. At sublethal concentrations triclosan inhibits a specific bacterial target in a similar manner to clinically relevant antibiotics. It has been shown that triclosan use selects triclosan-resistant bacteria. Of particular public health concern is that widespread use of triclosan, in addition to selecting for triclosan resistance, may promote the development of concomitant resistance to other clinically important antimicrobials through cross- or co-resistance mechanisms. It should furthermore be kept in mind that oral streptococci constitute a pool of genetic material and that DNA exchange readily occurs among them. The emergence of resistant pathogenic strains is seen, for instance, in *S. pneumoniae* through gene exchange with *S. mitis* (Hakenbeck *et al.*, 1998; Seppala *et al.*, 2003). The use of

Figure 16.4 Molecular formula of triclosan.

triclosan should therefore be restricted to purposes where there is a well-documented effect. The meager documentation of triclosan's anticaries effect hardly justifies its use in caries prophylaxis for the general population.

Xylitol

Xylitol is a sugar alcohol with five carbon atoms, a pentitol (Fig. 16.5). Xylitol is non-acidogenic and thus does not promote dental caries. Potential effects of xylitol have been extensively studied, particularly in Finland. An interpretation of early results was that xylitol possesses anticaries or even caries-therapeutic properties. It has also been suggested that xylitol exerts effects on microbial growth and metabolism, salivary factors, and demineralization and remineralization processes. Reduced dental biofilm formation has been reported, as well as a decrease in the number of salivary mutans streptococci and less gingivitis. Each factor alone or in combination could theoretically contribute to a cariostatic effect.

A specific xylitol-induced change in salivary factors has been confirmed in neither short- nor long-term studies. Nor has xylitol been shown specifically to interfere with enamel demineralization or to increase remineralization. *In vivo* studies have indicated that remineralization also occurs with other sugar alcohols, e.g. sorbitol. Even sucrose-sweetened gum chewed regularly after meals may enhance remineralization, thus pointing to the effect of increased salivation. Unfortunately, in many clinical studies, caries incidence in subjects chewing xylitol gum has been compared with non-chewing control subjects (Lingstrom *et al.*, 2003). It is therefore difficult to discriminate between a true xylitol effect and the impact of increased salivation through chewing a sweetened gum. Thus, the claim of remineralization being a xylitol-specific effect has not yet been confirmed. On the contrary, it may be concluded that any caries-preventive effect of chewing sugar-free gums sweetened by xylitol or other sweeteners is related to the chewing process, and not to the sweetener itself (Machiulskiene *et al.*, 2002).

Several studies indicate that the levels of mutans streptococci in saliva and in dental biofilm may be reduced after consumption of xylitol, and the view that a specific effect of xylitol on *S. mutans* is a cornerstone of xylitol's anticaries mechanism has been broadly supported.

Xylitol seems to be unique among sugar alcohols in its *in vitro* inhibitory effect on glycolysis, particularly in mutans streptococci. The inhibitory effect has been related to uptake of xylitol via a constitutive transport system specific for fructose and subsequent intracellular accumulation of xylitol-5-phosphate, as part of an energy, phosphoenolpyruvate and adenosine triphosphate-consuming futile xylitol cycle. Concomitant intracellular accumulation of glucose-6-phosphate to confirm an antimetabolic effect of xylitol *in vivo* has, however, not been demonstrated.

Reduced adhesiveness through impaired polysaccharide formation has also been suggested as one of the inhibitory mechanisms of xylitol on mutans streptococci and an explanation for cariostatic effects of xylitol. It is worth noting that long-term xylitol consumption leads to selection of mutans streptococci that are resistant to, or unaffected by xylitol. It has been speculated that xylitol-resistant strains may be less virulent than xylitol-sensitive strains. According to Trahan *et al.* (1996), selection in xylitol consumers of natural mutants with diminished virulence may be one of the mechanisms of the inhibitory action of xylitol. There are, however, no clinical data to support such a contention.

Attempts have been made to incorporate xylitol as an active ingredient in dental hygiene products and, at present, xylitol-containing dentifrices are available on the market. One of three longitudinal xylitol dentifrice studies found a caries-reducing effect of xylitol (Sintes *et al.*, 1995), whereas the two other studies failed to find an additive effect of xylitol when added to fluoride-containing dentifrices (Cutress *et al.*, 1992; Petersson *et al.*, 1991).

Xylitol is an interesting alternative sweetening agent, and could be the sweetening agent of choice when sucrose is to be substituted, e.g. in chewing gums. Chewing in itself increases salivation and therefore is beneficial. However, data to confirm caries-prophylactic effects of xylitol or superiority claims of xylitol over other polyols are lacking. Well-designed randomized clinical studies with proper controls are needed to demonstrate a role of xylitol in caries prophylaxis.

Other agents proposed for caries prophylaxis, but without documented anticaries effect

Cetylpyridinium chloride

Cetylpyridinium chloride (CPC), benzalconium chloride and benzethonium chloride are quaternary ammonium compounds. CPC has been widely used in mouthrinses, mainly because of its antimicrobial property.

The CPC molecule possesses both hydrophilic and hydrophobic groups, thus allowing ionic and hydrophobic interactions. It is assumed that interaction with microorganisms occurs via cationic binding in much the same way as for chlorhexidine.

$$H_2C - OH$$
$$|$$
$$H - C - OH$$
$$|$$
$$HO - C - H$$
$$|$$
$$H - C - OH$$
$$|$$
$$H_2C - OH$$

Figire 16.5 Molecular formula of xylitol.

The antimicrobial activity of CPC is equal to, or better than chlorhexidine, whereas its biofilm-inhibitory property is inferior. This difference in antibiofilm efficacy may be related to the fact that CPC loses part of its antimicrobial activity upon adsorption to surfaces. Notably, the substantive properties are also different. Initial retention of CPC is higher than for chlorhexidine, but CPC is cleared from the oral cavity more rapidly (Bonesvoll & Gjermo, 1978). It has recently been suggested that CPC could be incorporated into dental materials, e.g. in orthodontic adhesives, with the aim of controlling caries lesion formation around orthodontic brackets. Although CPC retains its antimicrobial properties, the clinical effect remains to be assessed. There are no data on CPC's ability to prevent dental caries in humans.

Delmopinol

Delmopinol is a potent surfactant with low molecular weight and is predominantly cationic at pH <7. It has low antimicrobial activity and is believed to act primarily by interfering with the physicochemical properties of oral surfaces. Microbial resistance or major shifts in the microbial composition of dental biofilm have not been observed in clinical experiments with delmopinol. Delmopinol reduces dental biofilm formation, probably by reducing microbial adhesion to the tooth surface. Its inhibitory effect on dental biofilm is less than or comparable to that of chlorhexidine. The effect on dental caries in humans has not yet been assessed.

Hexetidine

Hexetidine is a synthetic hexahydropyridine, which has antimicrobial and antifungal activity *in vitro* and *in vivo*. It is active against Gram-positive and Gram-negative microorganisms, including oral microorganisms such as mutans streptococci, *Streptococcus sobrinus* and *S. sanguinis*. The *in vitro* antimicrobial activity of hexetidine is reported to be inferior to or essentially similar to that of chlorhexidine or CPC. Hexetidine-containing mouthrinses are commercially available, yet at clinically acceptable concentrations hexetidine exerts only a very slight inhibitory effect on dental biofilms. Increasing the concentration of hexetidine from 0.10 to 0.14% increases the antibiofilm efficacy to approach that of 0.2% chlorhexidine. However, the frequency of desquamative lesions increases correspondingly. The exact mechanism for the antibiofilm activity is not clear. Hexetidine has been claimed to inhibit glycolysis, but clinical data do not support this assumption. The antimicrobial effect of hexetidine is reduced in the presence of saliva. Enhanced antibiofilm effects of hexetidine are observed in combination with divalent metal ions, e.g. Zn^{2+} (Saxer & Muhlemann, 1983) or Cu^{2+} (Grytten *et al.*, 1987). This is probably related to increased intracellular uptake of the metal ions. The agent has not been evaluated for its ability to prevent dental caries in humans.

Sanguinaria extracts

Sanguinaria extract (SE) is a herbal preparation, obtained from the bloodroot plant *Sanguinaria canadensis*. SE has been used in homeopathic preparations and folklore medicine for the treatment of topical infections and as an expectorant. It is antimicrobial against Gram-positive and Gram-negative microorganisms, including oral microorganisms. The exact mode of action is not clear, but SE seems to exert a bactericidal effect by interfering with essential steps in the synthesis of the microbial cell wall (Walker *et al.*, 1994). SE, reportedly, suppresses the activity of several enzymes, possibly through oxidation of SH-groups. The antimicrobial activity is thought to be associated with the lipophilic property of the molecules. More important may be, however, that SE is capable of binding metal ions. The marketed preparations of SE contain quite high concentrations of $ZnCl_2$. As will be discussed later, zinc ions have antimicrobial activity. It may be speculated, therefore, that the potential effects of SE are related to the Zn^{2+} content.

SE has substantive properties, but clinical data on the efficacy of mouthrinses with SE are not conclusive. In some studies antibiofilm, as well as antigingivitis and antiglycolytic effects were reported. In others, little or no effect was found. *In vitro* studies have indicated that adherence of oral microorganisms to hydroxyapatite may be inhibited, and SE may increase saliva-mediated aggregation. Both factors may contribute to the inhibition of dental biofilm formation *in vivo*, but clinical effects on caries have not been assessed.

Metal ions

Metal ions have antimicrobial effects depending on the ion concentration, as well as the chemistry of the ion. Their bacteriostatic effects have been recognized for a long time. Miller proposed the use of metal ions to treat rampant caries as early as 1890, and Hanke reported in 1940 that mouthrinses containing certain metal ions have antibiofilm potential. The antimicrobial efficacy is proportional to the concentration of free metal ions, which is the predominant bioactive form (Cummins & Watson, 1989). Hydrolysis of the metal ions and binding of metal ions to other components reduce the metal ion activity. The formulation of the vehicle is therefore crucial.

Metal ions of interest are Cu^{2+}, Sn^{2+} and Zn^{2+}. Cu^{2+} and Sn^{2+} are more potent than Zn^{2+}, but these are only moderately efficacious compared with chlorhexidine. Because of the ability of Zn^{2+} to combine with odoriferous sulfur-containing compounds, zinc salts have a long history in oral hygiene products. Zn^{2+} is also an anticalculus agent. Concerns were raised as to a possible interference of Zn^{2+} with the cariostatic effect of fluoride, but this seems not to be a problem.

Metal ions interact with both Gram-positive and Gram-negative microorganisms. The antimicrobial effect is unspecific. Metal ions form metal–salt bridges with anionic groups of enzymes. This, in turn, may influence substrate interactions owing to altered charge or conformational changes of the enzyme. Metal ions have antiglycolytic effect, as shown both *in vitro* in pure cultures of microorganisms and as reduced acid formation *in vivo*. Divalent metal ions probably inhibit glycolysis in dental biofilm by oxidative inactivation of SH-groups of glycolytic enzymes.

Numerous studies have confirmed the clinical antibiofilm effect of metal ions, both alone and in combination with other agents. The antibiofilm effect relates partly to the antimicrobial activity and partly to displacement of Ca^{2+} from pellicle and microbial surfaces. Binding of metal ions to microorganisms alters their surface charge and adherence ability (Olsson & Odham, 1978).

Cu^{2+}, Sn^{2+} and Zn^{2+} have all shown cariostatic effects in rats. SnF_2 has been used as a prophylactic agent in humans for many years owing to its potential cariostatic effect and antibiofilm properties.

Metal ions are substantive agents. Both salivary and dental biofilm levels of Cu^{2+}, Sn^{2+} and Zn^{2+} are elevated for several hours after a mouthrinse. The ions bind to the same oral receptors as chlorhexidine.

Adverse effects related to metal ions are an unpleasant metallic taste, a tendency to induce a feeling of dryness in the oral cavity, and a yellowish to brownish dental stain. Metal sulfides, which are formed between the metal ions and sulfhydryl groups of pellicle proteins, probably cause these effects. Zn^{2+} ions have the least tendency to stain, because zinc sulfide is yellowish to grayish–white in color. The staining tendency is generally lower for metal ions than for chlorhexidine.

Sodium dodecyl sulfate

SDS is an anionic agent. The molecule has a hydrophilic sulfate group and a hydrophobic carbon chain. It is the most frequently used detergent in commercial dentifrices.

SDS has antimicrobial activity against a range of microorganisms *in vitro*, including mutans streptococci, *S. sobrinus* and *Actinomyces viscosus*. Adsorption of SDS to the microbial surface may interfere with cell-wall integrity, with subsequent leakage of cellular components. At low concentrations SDS is reported to inhibit specific microbial enzymes, such as glucosyltransferase from *S. sobrinus* and *S. mutans*, enzymes of the phosphoenolpyruvate phosphotransferase transport in *S. sobrinus*, and lactate dehydrogenase and glucose-6-phosphate dehydrogenase in *Escherichia coli*. These effects may be related to the strong affinity of SDS for proteins and its denaturing property.

Dental biofilm inhibitory properties of SDS have been shown in humans. These may relate, mainly, to the antimicrobial effect, but competition with negatively charged microorganisms and pellicle proteins for binding sites, with subsequent inhibition of microbial adsorption to the tooth surface, may also contribute to the inhibitory effect. SDS apparently has some degree of substantivity, which may be explained by its high affinity for calcium. SDS in combination with Zn^{2+} shows increased antibiofilm and antimicrobial properties. There are no data to support a cariostatic effect of SDS.

Enzymes

Whole saliva contains two peroxidase enzymes that oxidize thiocyanate (SCN^-) to hypothiocyanite ($OSCN^-$) in the presence of hydrogen peroxide. Hypothiocyanite is antimicrobial and inhibits some streptococci and lactobacilli *in vitro* (Lumikari *et al.*, 1991). The activity of the salivary peroxidase system depends on available hydrogen peroxide. Hydrogen peroxide is produced by various microorganisms as a metabolic endproduct, but in limiting amounts for maximum activity of the salivary peroxidase. The enzyme amyloglucosidase provides glucose, from which glucose oxidase produces hydrogen peroxide. Addition of these enzymes to oral products is suggested to ensure sufficient hydrogen peroxide to control the proliferation of microorganisms through enhanced peroxidase activity.

Mouthrinses containing the enzymes have been tested for their ability to reduce dental biofilm, gingivitis and dental caries, but the effect was not impressive. Dentifrices containing these enzymes show slightly improved antibiofilm and antigingivitis effects compared with non-enzyme dentifrices, but whether this marginal effect is of clinical relevance may be questioned.

Concluding remarks and future approaches

The oral flora, consisting of millions of microorganisms of hundreds of various species, is in balance with its host. The flora responds to various local ecological selective forces and communication signals by adaptive gene regulation, which determines the activity and composition of the flora at various sites within the oral cavity.

Most chemical prophylactic agents are broad-spectrum antimicrobials, which are used according to the non-specific plaque hypothesis. The members of the oral flora show varying degrees of susceptibility to such agents; therefore, the use of broad-spectrum antimicrobial agents may cause an unfavorable ecological imbalance by killing benign and beneficial microorganisms. The eradication of sensitive microorganisms allows the surviving organisms to multiply. Therefore, except for the use of fluoride dentifrices, chemical prophylactic agents should not be instituted routinely. Such agents should be used restrictively and only if the conventional prophylactic methods are likely to be ineffective. This may be the case for individuals with high caries activity and incidence, such as physically or mentally handicapped individuals, or subjects who suffer from hyposalivation due to systemic diseases or medication. They may benefit from intermittent or chronic use of chemical prophylactic agents. Certain conditions such as intraoral fixation or splinting, treatment with orthodontic appliances, insertion of prosthetic restorations or implants, or presurgical and postsurgical treatment where mechanical cleaning is particularly difficult may justify the use of chemical prophylactic agents for periods of varying length. In all cases, expected benefit should be weighed against potential adverse effects, and the choice of agent, treatment length, mode of application and dose should be made on an individual basis.

As discussed in this chapter, the ideal chemical agent for dental biofilm control is not yet available, and documentation for caries-prophylactic effects in humans of available agents, except for fluoride, is sparse. The main reasons lie in the multifaceted nature of the caries disease and the fact that microorganisms causing the disease are organized in complex biofilms. This fact has often been neglected and it is only recently that methods to study gene expression and regulation in biofilm microorganisms have been adopted.

Biofilms are likely to represent a natural scenario for bacterial communication, and the ability to communicate has been shown in both oral streptococci and periodontal pathogens. This communication may regulate pathogenic traits such as biofilm formation and the expression of virulence factors. For most oral biofilm microorganisms, however, the presence and function of communication pathways remain to be clarified.

In the future there may be new developments in caries prevention based on the progress being made in understanding the special features of biofilm microorganisms and their communication systems. Developments in material science may lead to novel vehicles for the delivery of targeted agents. Definite targets, however, remain to be defined.

Background literature

Busscher HJ, Evans LV. *Oral biofilms and plaque control.* Amsterdam: Harwood Academic, 1998.

Gjermo P. Chlorhexidine and related compounds. *J Dent Res* 1989; **68** (Special Issue): s1602–8.

Scheie AAa. Modes of action of currently known chemical antiplaque agents other than chlorhexidine. *J Dent Res* 1989; **68** (Special Issue): 1609–16.

Scheie AAa, Fejerskov OB. Xylitol in caries prevention: what is the evidence for clinical efficacy? *Oral Dis* 1998; **4**: 268–78.

Scheie AAa, Petersen FC. The biofilm concept: consequences for future prophylaxis of oral diseases? *Crit Rev Oral Biol Med* 2004; **15**: 4–12.

References

Bonesvoll P, Gjermo P. A comparision between chlorhexidine and some quaternary ammonium compounds with regard to retention, salivary concentration and plaque-inhibiting effect in the human mouth after mouth rinses. *Arch Oral Biol* 1978; **23**: 289–94.

Cullinan MP, Hamlet SM, Westerman B, Palmer JE, Faddy MJ, Seymour GJ. Acquisition and loss of *Porphyromonas gingivalis*, *Actinobacillus actinomycetemcomitans* and *Prevotella intermedia* over a 5-year period:

effect of a triclosan/copolymer dentifrice. *J Clin Periodontol* 2003a; **30**: 532–41.

Cullinan MP, Westerman B, Hamlet SM, Palmer JE, Faddy MJ, Seymour GJ. The effect of a triclosan-containing dentifrice on the progression of periodontal disease in an adult population. *J Clin Periodontol* 2003b; **30**: 414–19.

Cummins D, Watson GK. Computer model relating chemistry to biologic activity of metal anti-plaque agents. *J Dent Res* 1989; **68**: 1702–5.

Cutress T, Howell PT, Finidori C, Abdullah F. Caries preventive effect of high fluoride and xylitol containing dentifrices. *ASDC J Dent Child* 1992; **59**: 313–8.

Davies RM, Ellwood RP, Davies GM. The effectiveness of a toothpaste containing triclosan and polyvinyl–methyl ether maleic acid copolymer in improving plaque control and gingival health: a systematic review. *J Clin Periodontol* 2004; **31**: 1029–33.

Doron S, Gorbach SL. Probiotics: their role in the treatment and prevention of disease. *Expert Rev Anti Infect Ther* 2006; **4**: 261–75.

Du MQ, Tai BJ, Jiang H, Lo EC, Fan MW, Bian Z. A two-year randomized clinical trial of chlorhexidine varnish on dental caries in Chinese preschool children. *J Dent Res* 2006; **85**: 557–9.

Emilson CG. Susceptibility of various microorganisms to chlorhexidine. *Scand J Dent Res* 1977; **85**: 255–65.

Filoche SK, Soma K, Sissons CH. Antimicrobial effects of essential oils in combination with chlorhexidine digluconate. *Oral Microbiol Immunol* 2005; **20**: 221–5.

Gisselsson H, Birkhed D, Bjorn AL. Effect of professional flossing with chlorhexidine gel on approximal caries in 12- to 15-year-old schoolchildren. *Caries Res* 1988; **22**: 187–92.

Grytten J, Tollefsen T, Afseth J. The effect of a combination of copper and hexetidine on plaque formation and the amount of copper retained by dental plaque bacteria. *Acta Odontol Scand* 1987; **45**: 429–33.

Hakenbeck R, Konig A, Kern I, *et al.* Acquisition of five high-Mr penicillin-binding protein variants during transfer of high-level beta-lactam resistance from *Streptococcus mitis* to *Streptococcus pneumoniae*. *J Bacteriol* 1998; **180**: 1831–40.

Hanke M. Studies on the local factors in dental caries. I. Destruction of plaques and retardation of bacterial growth in the oral cavity. *J Am Dent Assoc* 1940; **27**: 1379–93.

Hugo WB, Longworth AR. Some aspects of the mode of action of chlorhexidine. *J Pharm Pharmacol* 1964; **16**: 655–62.

Katz S. The use of fluoride and chlorhexidine for the prevention of radiation caries. *J Am Dent Assoc* 1982; **104**: 164–70.

Klock B, Krasse B. Effect of caries-preventive measures in children with high numbers of *S. mutans* and lactobacilli. *Scand J Dent Res* 1978; **86**: 221–30.

Lindquist B, Edward S, Torell P, Krasse B. Effect of different caries preventive measures in children highly infected with mutans streptococci. *Scand J Dent Res* 1989; **97**: 330–7.

Lingstrom P, Holm AK, Mejare I, *et al.* Dietary factors in the prevention of dental caries: a systematic review. *Acta Odontol Scand* 2003; **61**: 331–40.

Lumikari M, Soukka T, Nurmio S, Tenovuo J. Inhibition of the growth of *Streptococcus mutans*, *Streptococcus sobrinus* and *Lactobacillus casei* by oral peroxidase systems in human saliva. *Arch Oral Biol* 1991; **36**: 155–60.

Machiulskiene V, Richards A, Nyvad B, Baelum V. Prospective study of the effect of post-brushing rinsing behaviour on dental caries. *Caries Res* 2002; **36**: 301–7.

McMurry LM, Oethinger M, Levy SB. Triclosan targets lipid synthesis. *Nature* 1998; **394**: 531–2.

Marsh PD. Microbial ecology of dental plaque and its significance in health and disease. *Adv Dent Res* 1994; **8**: 263–71.

Marsh PD, Keevil CW, McDermid AS, Williamson MI, Ellwood DC. Inhibition by the antimicrobial agent chlorhexidine of acid production and sugar transport in oral streptococcal bacteria. *Arch Oral Biol* 1983; **28**: 233–40.

Meurman JH. Probiotics: do they have a role in oral medicine and dentistry? *Eur J Oral Sci* 2005; **113**: 188–96.

Miller W. *The microorganisms of the human mouth. The local and general diseases which are caused by them.* Philadaephia; PA, 1890. (Republished Basel: Karger, 1973.)

Nase L, Hatakka K, Savilahti E, *et al.* Effect of long-term consumption of a probiotic bacterium, *Lactobacillus rhamnosus* GG, in milk on dental caries and caries risk in children. *Caries Res* 2001; **35**: 412–20.

Olsson J, Odham G. Effect of inorganic ions and surface active organic compounds on the adherence of oral streptococci. *Scand J Dent Res* 1978; **86**: 108–17.

van der Ouderaa F, Cummins D. Delivery systems for agents in supra- and sub-gingival plaque control. *J Dent Res* 1989; **68**: 1617–24.

Pader M. *Oral hygiene products and practice.* New York: Marcel Dekker, 1988.

Petersson LG, Birkhed D, Gleerup A, Johansson M, Jonsson G. Caries-preventive effect of dentifrices containing various types and concentrations of fluorides and sugar alcohols. *Caries Res* 1991; **25**: 74–9.

Saxer UP, Muhlemann HR. Synergistic antiplaque effects of a zinc fluoride/hexetidine containing mouthwash. A review. *SSO Schweiz Monatsschr Zahnheilkd* 1983; **93**: 689–704.

Schaeken MJ, Keltjens HM, Van Der Hoeven JS. Effects of fluoride and chlorhexidine on the microflora of dental root surfaces and progression of root-surface caries. *J Dent Res* 1991; **70**: 150–3.

Scheie AA, Eggen KH, Rolla G. Glucosyltransferase activity in human in vivo formed enamel pellicle and in whole saliva. *Scand J Dent Res* 1987; **95**: 212–15.

Schiött C. Effect of chlorhexidine on the microflora of the oral cavity. *J Periodontal Res Suppl* 1973; **8**: 7–10.

Seppala H, Haanpera M, Al-Juhaish M, Jarvinen H, Jalava J, Huovinen P. Antimicrobial susceptibility patterns and macrolide resistance genes of viridans group streptococci from normal flora. *J Antimicrob Chemother* 2003; **52**: 636–44.

Sintes JL, Escalante C, Stewart B, *et al*. Enhanced anticaries efficacy of a 0.243% sodium fluoride/10% xylitol/silica dentifrice: 3-year clinical results. *Am J Dent* 1995; **8**: 231–5.

Trahan L, Bourgeau G, Breton R. Emergence of multiple xylitol-resistant (fructose PTS⁻) mutants from human isolates of mutans streptococci during growth on dietary sugars in the presence of xylitol. *J Dent Res* 1996; **75**: 1892–900.

Twetman S. Antimicrobials in future caries control? A review with special reference to chlorhexidine treatment. *Caries Res* 2004; **38**: 223–9.

Walker C, Borden L, Zambon J, Bonta C, DeVizio W, Volpe A. The effects of a 0.3% triclosan-containing dentifrice on the microbial composition of supragingival plaque. *J Clin Periodontol* 1994; **21**: 334–41.

Wara-aswapati N, Krongnawakul D, Jiraviboon D, Adulyanon S, Karimbux N, Pitiphat W. The effect of a new toothpaste containing potassium nitrate and triclosan on gingival health, plaque formation and dentine hypersensitivity. *J Clin Periodontol* 2005; **32**: 53–8.

Welin J, Wilkins JC, Beighton D, Svensater G. Protein expression by *Streptococcus mutans* during initial stage of biofilm formation. *Appl Environ Microbiol* 2004; **70**: 3736–41.

Yazdankhah SP, Scheie AA, Hoiby EA, *et al*. Triclosan and antimicrobial resistance in bacteria: an overview. *Microb Drug Resist* 2006; **12**: 83–90.

Zhang Q, van't Hof MA, Truin GJ, Bronkhorst EM, van Palenstein Helderman WH. Caries-inhibiting effect of chlorhexidine varnish in pits and fissures. *J Dent Res* 2006; **85**: 469–72.

Zickert I, Emilson CG, Krasse B. Effect of caries preventive measures in children highly infected with the bacterium *Streptococcus mutans*. *Arch Oral Biol* 1982; **27**: 861–8.

17

Might caries control involve immunization and gene therapy?

R.R.B. Russell

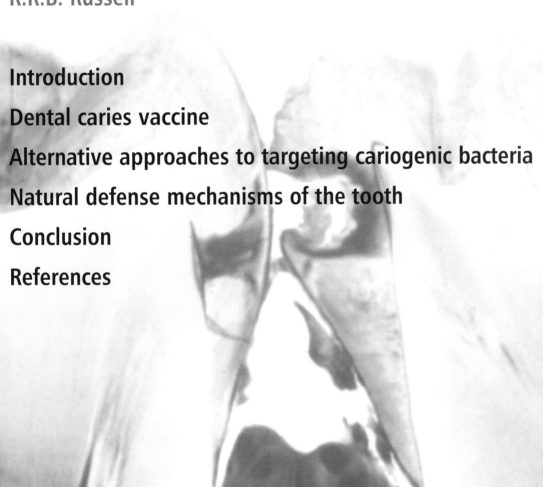

Introduction

Many members of the public, and indeed many old-fashioned dentists, regard caries treatment entirely in mechanical terms rather like road maintenance, whereby an inert hard structure (the tooth enamel) is repaired with another hard substance in the form of amalgam or other restorative material. This view ignores the myriad complex biological processes taking place, and the critical interplay between attack by the bacteria in dental plaque and the defensive response of the living host tissue, particularly the tooth pulp. In recent years there have been rapid developments in our understanding of the mechanisms of the caries process as well as an understanding of how long-established treatments, discovered empirically, actually work. Furthermore, the biological insights have raised the prospect of devising novel approaches to preventing microbial attack or boosting the healing process. The introduction of techniques in molecular biology, in particular, has led to a massive expansion of knowledge, and this chapter will consider how recent discoveries have impacted on the concept of exploiting an immunological approach to caries prevention through a caries vaccine, and exploiting our knowledge of the cellular reactions to insult that might lead to novel therapies that enhance natural rebuilding of damaged tooth substance.

Dental caries vaccine

It is now nearly 40 years since the first reports of successful immunization of experimental animals against dental caries were published (Bowen, 1969) and the feasibility of the approach has been demonstrated many times since, both in rodents and in non-human primates. The subject has been extensively reviewed, with different authors giving different emphasis to the microbiological (Koga *et al.*, 2002), immunological (Russell *et al.*, 1999) or sociomedical aspects (Russell & Johnson, 1987; Smith, 2002). Despite extensive experimental support for a caries vaccine, no clinical trials have yet been undertaken anywhere in the world, although basic research has continued to attract support from funding agencies in a number of countries. There has recently been an upsurge of interest in China, where the rapidly developing economy has the potential to generate an enormous challenge for preventive dentistry.

For any vaccine against an infectious disease, there is a common series of steps that need to be taken in order to make progress (Fig. 17.1).

The caries process and epidemiology

The first two stages, defining the caries process and epidemiology, are the subject of Chapters 1 and 8, but a deep

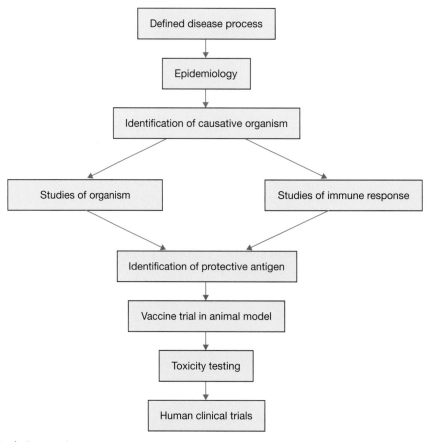

Figure 17.1 Stages in developing a vaccine.

understanding of these facets of the caries process is essential if a rational approach to vaccine development is to be taken. This applies to any infectious disease, but the fact that caries occurs as a consequence of the activities of members of the normal commensal oral microflora adds a new level of complexity. Should we be aiming to prevent initial colonization with cariogenic organisms so that they never become established in plaque, or is it more appropriate to aim at immunological interference with their functioning? Resolution of this issue will determine at which stage a vaccine might be introduced. Hence, an understanding of the transmission and acquisition of oral bacteria is of fundamental importance. A large proportion of infants become colonized by *Streptococcus mutans* during the 'window of infectivity' around the time of eruption of the first molars at the age of 2 years (Caufield *et al.*, 1993). The great increase in sensitivity of detection provided by molecular methods such as polymerase chain reaction (PCR) and various genetic fingerprinting techniques have been major factors in developing knowledge of this area in recent years, and it is now clear that some infants will have *S. mutans* present in their oral cavity from a much earlier age (Milgrom *et al.*, 2000; Tanner *et al.*, 2002; Wan *et al.*, 2003), with the corollary that immunization would need to be started in very young children, with the all the problems associated with vaccine programs in this age group. Although fingerprinting techniques have been invaluable in tracking the transmission of distinctive genotypes of *S. mutans* from mother to child, the fact that distinct genotypes can be observed indicates that not all *S. mutans* are the same. Researchers are only just beginning to understand variability within the species, including the fact that some strains lack some of the target antigens described below, and so would escape the effects of vaccine (Waterhouse & Russell, 2006).

Choosing the target: identification of the causative organism(s)

Numerous publications discuss the evidence that mutans streptococci play a crucial role in dental caries (Tanzer *et al.*, 2001), but authors seeking a paper that points the finger at *S. mutans* frequently cite the major review by Loesche (1986). In fact, Loesche took pains to point out that nearly all the studies on which the conclusions at that time were based did not discriminate between the mutans streptococci, and so indicated that both *S. mutans* and *S. sobrinus* could be of importance. This is principally because no selective growth medium had been devised then (or has been since) that allowed easy counting of the levels of the two species. The fact that *S. mutans* is by far the more prevalent (carried by around 98% of individuals around the world) means that it must be the more important of the two species, but it still remains unclear to what extent *S. sobrinus* may contribute. Certainly, there is evidence that

combined high levels of *S. mutans* and *S. sobrinus* are associated with severe caries (Okada *et al.*, 2005), but there is nothing to suggest that *S. sobrinus* on its own mounts a cariogenic challenge, despite the fact that it is the more acidogenic and more cariogenic of the two species in rats (de Soet *et al.*, 1991). There is a large gap in the knowledge concerning the time of acquisition of *S. sobrinus* or indeed many other aspects of this species. To a large extent, this is because *S. sobrinus* is not naturally transformable (i.e. able to take up foreign DNA) and hence is not amenable to genetic analysis in the same way as *S. mutans*.

Not all readers will be aware of the considerable confusion in the field of taxonomy of the oral streptococci that prevailed during the 1960s and 1970s; it was not until 1974 that the species *S. mutans* was formally described, and *S. sobrinus* a few years later. Before that, they were both included within *S. mutans*, so the choice of organisms for the early vaccine research programs was largely arbitrary. Strain 6715, later clearly identified as *S. sobrinus*, became the model organism of choice for many US laboratories pursuing a vaccine, while in the UK, strain Ingbritt (*S. mutans*) became the object of study. It subsequently became apparent that the macaque monkeys used as experimental animals by the UK research groups were naturally colonized with *S. mutans*, thus providing a suitable model of the human situation. It is thus largely a historical accident, but a central feature of caries vaccine research, that both *S. mutans* and *S. sobrinus* have been investigated in experimental systems. It is, however, questionable whether a vaccine based solely on *S. sobrinus* would be of real value in a human population, although this is not to deny that basic research on *S. sobrinus* can provide valuable lessons. Should other organisms also be considered as potential targets? The group of bacteria long known to be present in large numbers in later stages of caries is the lactobacilli. Here again, there have been major problems in species identification to be overcome and recent results using molecular identification methods have shown the large variety of species that may be detected in carious lesions. However, no individual species correlates with caries and it has been concluded that the lactobacilli are opportunistic late invaders with a dietary or an intestinal origin (Byun *et al.*, 2004; Munson *et al.*, 2004). Of greater interest are those species detected in carious lesions by non-cultural techniques which have revealed the existence of a much greater complexity than deduced from culture-only approaches and potentially implicate species of *Actinomyces* and *Bifidobacterium* (Becker *et al.*, 2002; Chhour *et al.*, 2005) as well as non-mutans streptococci (van Ruyven *et al.*, 2000; Brailsford *et al.*, 2005). All these studies serve to emphasize the differences in the likely contribution of different species of bacteria to caries initiation and progression at different tooth sites and at different stages of the disease.

In summary, developments in recent years have not altered the perception that *S. mutans* is a major etiological agent in dental caries and hence reasonably considered as the prime target for a caries vaccine. There is, however, now a rapidly increasing body of evidence that indicates the importance of other bacteria. Consequently, there must be less confidence in the view that a strategy of specifically targeting *S. mutans* will solve all the problems of caries than there may have been at some times in the past.

The natural immune response to caries

Most of the infectious diseases for which a vaccine can give protection are those against which natural infection also gives protection from subsequent attack, measles for example. Exposure to causative organisms can also result in protective immune responses even in the absence of clinically manifested disease. It is to be expected that exposure to *S. mutans*, once it becomes established in the oral cavity (and also passes through the gut), would induce an immune response, and levels of both secretory immunoglobulin A (IgA) and circulating immunoglobulin G (IgG) antibody do indeed show a correlation with age. Numerous studies have attempted to correlate the level of particular antibody responses with caries experience, but have failed to provide convincing evidence that natural immunity plays any significant part. Whereas earlier studies used immunoassays based on whole bacteria, more recent approaches have examined the level of responses to a range of different proteins and revealed the enormous complexity of the individual immune responses (Bratthall *et al.*, 1997; Nogueira *et al.*, 2005). This may relate to the poorly understood mechanism by which commensal bacteria achieve a stable balance with the host's defense system. It is possible that natural antibody to a particular antigen may be crucial for the development of natural immunity, but the chance of identifying such a relationship remains remote.

Characterization of the target bacteria and identification of protective antigens

The major factors that are believed to contribute to cariogenicity of mutans streptococci are:

- acidogenicity
- aciduricity
- sucrose-independent adhesion
- sucrose-dependent adhesion.

The first two of these are almost entirely determined by functions at the cell membrane or inside the cell, and hence not accessible to antibodies. The search for molecules that may contribute to the efficacy of a caries vaccine, or provide the basis for purified subunit vaccines, has thus been focussed on surface molecules. Although there was some early interest in polysaccharides, by far the most effort has been devoted to a limited number of proteins and enzymes.

It is universally recognized that the optimum vaccines should be as simple as possible, since a clearly defined subunit vaccine allows quality control, exclusion of potentially toxic components that may be present in whole cells and improved monitoring of the immune response.

Interest has focussed on three groups of antigens:

- cell-wall proteins
- glucosyltransferases (GTFs)
- glucan binding proteins.

The first successful experimental vaccines were based on whole cells and it was soon found that cell-wall preparations were also protective, but that the protection was lost following treatment with proteolytic enzymes. This resulted in a search for wall-associated proteins in *S. mutans*, and two have been exploited in vaccines. Most is known about the high molecular weight protein that acts as an adhesin binding to a salivary glycoprotein, and is important in colonization of the tooth (Loimaranta *et al.*, 2005). This is most commonly referred to as antigen I/II, although it has also been referred to as antigen B, SpaP and P1. It is encoded by a gene called *spaP* or *pac*. I/II, or defined fragments generated by genetic engineering, has repeatedly been shown to be capable of inducing protection against caries in both rats and monkeys. The other wall-associated protein is called antigen A, WapA or III (Russell *et al.*, 1995), has also been shown to be protective in rats and monkeys, and is now known to be involved in biofilm formation (Levesque *et al.*, 2005). It is a lucky coincidence that *S. mutans* Ingbritt was the strain originally chosen in the search for wall-associated proteins. This strain is now known to be exceptionally good at releasing such proteins into culture supernatants, since it lacks the sortase enzyme responsible for efficient anchoring (Igarashi, 2004). However, the techniques used to obtain the major antigens failed to detect another wall-anchored protein called WapE, which was only found by analysis of the *S. mutans* genome sequence (Ajdic *et al.*, 2002), but also seems to be required for biofilm formation (Levesque *et al.*, 2005). This has never been tested as a pure vaccine, yet will have been present in the highly protective cell-wall preparations and may be protective on its own.

Glucosyltransferases are the enzymes responsible for synthesizing sticky polymers from sucrose and hence are considered to be important virulence factors owing to their effect on plaque permeability properties and adhesion to the tooth surface. There is extensive evidence that a vaccine based on GTF from *S. mutans* or *S. sobrinus* can protect rats against caries caused by the same species, with most of the protective effect being limited to smooth-surface lesions. GTF-mediated glucan formation is likely to be of major importance for bacterial adhesion to smooth surfaces, which may help to explain the success of GTF vaccines in the experimental rat model, although GTF vaccines failed in monkeys (Russell *et al.*, 1976; Russell & Colman, 1981).

Glucan-binding proteins have also attracted interest as potential vaccine components. This group includes the glucan-binding domain found as a part of GTF (Ferretti *et al.*, 1987) that has been used as a vaccine on its own (Taubman *et al.*, 1995), but also in the GbpA protein and GbpD, which has lipase activity (Shah & Russell, 2004). Since these are all closely related, antibody raised against one molecule is likely to react with other targets. The GbpB protein also binds glucans and is protective (Smith *et al.*, 2003). Its main function may be in maintaining cell-wall integrity (Chia *et al.*, 2001).

Animal models for testing of caries vaccines

One of the stumbling blocks in developing vaccines for some diseases such as AIDS has been the lack of a suitable animal model. Dental caries is also a uniquely human affliction (although a few pampered dogs may suffer from their owners' predilection for sweet things), so it is necessary to examine carefully the relevance to human disease of the animal models available. Rats and mice have tooth morphology and a pattern of decay different from the human and are not naturally colonized by *S. mutans*. Furthermore, many caries vaccine experiments using rats have employed *S. sobrinus* as the challenge organism and it must be remembered that *S. sobrinus* is commonly found in less than one-third of the human population and its contribution to caries in humans is unclear. In monkeys, as in humans, the main points of attack are in occlusal fissures and approximal sites, with *S. mutans* being the principal organism associated with disease progression; protection against smooth-surface attack is therefore of relatively little importance. Monkey experiments may thus offer a more suitable disease model, but present considerable problems in terms of husbandry and cost, with consequentially small experimental groups. Therefore, although it may be desirable to test any proposed vaccine on non-human primates, rats are likely to be more convenient for preliminary experiments so long as caution is exercised in the extrapolation of results to humans.

The big step: clinical trials

In order to carry out any clinical trial, the experimenter would like to have:

- preliminary data indicating prospects of success
- a clear outcome measure of success
- a compliant population with a high incidence of disease
- no confounding external factors likely to come into effect during the trial.

These practical issues can readily be addressed by a competent team of scientists and clinicians. The decision to proceed with a clinical trial, however, will usually rest with a national body charged with assuring the overall health of the population and reaching decisions on the risk–benefit

of any novel preventive strategy or treatment. At this level, proposals to introduce a novel vaccine against a human disease introduce a whole range of ethical and politico-economic issues that extend far beyond laboratory findings and raise questions about the choice of immunogen and validity of animal data. These apply to any novel vaccine, but demand particularly close attention when the proposal is to vaccinate against caries. For a non-life-threatening disease that is regarded as a minor (and avoidable) affliction in medical terms, no adverse reactions can be tolerated.

It should be noted that the introduction of any novel vaccine is fraught with difficulties, not least because of concern that any mishaps (or newspaper scare stories) can have a disastrous effect on public attitudes and participation in immunization schemes, even for unrelated but well-established vaccines such as those for pertussis, polio and diphtheria. The safety requirements for a vaccine against a process that is not life-threatening must be very stringent, not just because of the risk–benefit equation for protection against caries, but because of concerns that public confidence in mass-vaccination campaigns could be damaged. The vulnerability of such campaigns to adverse publicity was vividly illustrated in the UK by the experience with whooping cough vaccine in the 1980s and, more recently, the measles, mumps, rubella (MMR) vaccine. In both cases public concern over one particular vaccine had a knock-on effect on the uptake of other vaccines. As a consequence, many children went unprotected and the result was a resurgence in the incidence of disease in subsequent years.

Serious consideration was given, around 1985, to the initiation of trials in humans of vaccines using *S. mutans* wall-associated proteins in the UK and other countries. Some questions about the extent of the available experimental data remained to be answered, but the overriding concern related to the place of a caries vaccine in national vaccine policies. This was a decisive factor in the decision not to proceed with research leading to trials of an injectable vaccine at that time. A similar conclusion about the prospect of developing a caries vaccine in the foreseeable future was reached in the USA by a NIDCR Expert Panel (http://www.nidcr.nih.gov/Research/LongRangeResearch Opportunities/SummaryOfVaccinePanels.htm).

Where to now? Novel immunogens, DNA vaccines and passive immunization

At the start of the twenty-first century, we are faced with the fact that there is plenty of solid experimental evidence that it is possible to reduce caries in experimental animals, yet a variety of reasons makes it unlikely that a traditional injectable vaccine will be introduced in the foreseeable future, at least in Europe and North America. The vaccine concept has been a powerful driver of research directions in oral microbiology and there is a substantial amount of literature on ingenious research into the identification and characterization of candidate vaccine components. Thanks to knowledge gleaned from gene sequencing, the most important regions of the major antigens that may induce a suitable immune response are now known, and molecular genetic techniques have been applied to construct chimeric (hybrid) molecules consisting of the saliva-binding region of SpaP, catalytic and glucan-binding domains of GTF in various combinations (Zhang et al., 2002; Smith et al., 2005). Novel ways for presenting these immunogens have also been developed, including DNA vaccines where the gene is injected and its product made within the body (Xu et al., 2005). A particularly active area of research has been the induction of a secretory immune response (Russell et al., 1999) or passive immunization. This is the process whereby preformed antibody is introduced to the mouth as a topical application or mouthrinse (Abiko, 2000). The source of this antibody may be the milk of immunized cows, eggs, monoclonal antibodies produced in tissue culture or recombinant antibody generated in transgenic plants or bacteria. The effectiveness of this approach in reducing caries has been repeatedly demonstrated in experimental animals, but studies in humans have been limited to short-term studies of the effect of antibody on levels of S. mutans. Although early reports looked promising (Ma & Lehner, 1990), a recent larger study failed to demonstrate any effect (Weintraub et al., 2005). Part of the problem may be due to the difficulty of achieving and maintaining a sufficient level of inhibitory antibody in plaque, and a recent variation on passive immunization used specific antibody fused to glucose oxidase to target S. mutans (Kruger et al., 2006). However, much work remains to be done to find a cheap, stable source of antibody that can effectively be delivered to gain beneficial effects.

It will be apparent from the discussion above that there is no shortage of bright ideas about how an immune response-based approach might be used to develop a caries-preventive treatment. The need has acted as a stimulus for much innovative research that has indubitably led to much greater insight into the biology of cariogenic bacteria and the disease process. Extensive laboratory and experimental animal research has convincingly demonstrated the potential of a variety of different concepts, although there remain very considerable barriers before the results can be translated into a therapy of practical value in humans.

Alternative approaches to targeting cariogenic bacteria

Replacement therapy

An approach to modifying the oral microflora that has attracted attention in recent years is that of replacement therapy. This is analogous to the use of 'functional foods' or probiotics to modify the gut microflora, and in the case of

S. mutans has been pioneered by Hillman and colleagues (Hillman et al., 2000; Hillman, 2002), who genetically engineered a mutant of S. mutans that lacks lactate dehydrogenase, the enzyme that plays a crucial role in acid production. They had to introduce a number of other changes to ensure metabolic balance and also introduced genes for production of mutacin 1140, a small peptide that inhibits other bacteria and facilitates establishment of the mutant in plaque. The mutant strain was established in rats and found to be non-cariogenic. Approval was granted in 2004 by the US Food and Drug Administration (FDA) to initiate the phase I clinical trial to establish safety in humans, but no reports of progress have yet appeared. As with vaccines, there remain questions about public acceptance for the introduction of a genetically modified organism, and attitudes to this debate are likely to vary from country to country.

Antiadhesin peptides and decoy oligosaccharides

There is now a considerable amount of detailed information available about the nature of the specific interactions between different plaque bacteria and between bacteria and host macromolecules. It is unsurprising that most information has been gathered on the caries-associated bacteria, although it must be realized that the adhesive interactions of a multitude of other bacteria will be even greater contributors to plaque cohesion. Nevertheless, some interesting results have been reported in which either small peptides corresponding to the binding regions of streptococcal adhesins, or carbohydrate receptors, have been used to block adhesion of specific organisms (Kelly et al., 1999; Sharon & Ofek, 2002; Younson & Kelly, 2004; Jakubovics et al., 2005). This approach suffers from the same difficulties as passive immunization, in that it is necessary to achieve an adequate concentration of the competitor in plaque, probably at a crucial moment when the bacteria are first colonizing.

Natural defense mechanisms of the tooth

The response of the dental pulp to carious attack or other injury is considered in Chapter 21. This is an area in which the complex biological processes are beginning to be unraveled, and it may be possible to manipulate the response to hasten repair.

Boosting dentin repair

The ways in which the tooth responds depend on the level of insult. The first line of defense is reactionary dentinogenesis, which involves secretion of a tertiary dentine matrix by primary odontoblasts. The response to more severe caries attack, in which primary odontoblasts are destroyed, involves reparative dentinogenesis by a new generation of odontoblast-like cells. It can thus be seen that recovery of the tooth may be enhanced either by stimulating primary odontoblasts and/or in some way by speeding the supply of new cells differentiated to synthesize reparative dentin. This exciting research area has recently been reviewed (Smith, 2002; Mitsiadis & Rahiotis, 2004). The development of microarray and proteomic techniques, which allow monitoring of the expression of individual genes and proteins in odontoblasts subjected to challenge, helps to identify the crucial molecules involved in the protective response (McLachlan et al., 2005; Paakkonen et al., 2005). Signaling growth factors such as transforming growth factor-β (TGF-β) appear to be of particular importance, and there is now a rational explanation for the effectiveness of calcium hydroxide in inducing dentin bridge formation because of its effect on TGF-β, and gene expression (Graham et al., 2006). Future developments in this field will build on the understanding of the natural cellular response mechanisms, and finding ways to enhance the responses that lead to the formation of reactionary dentin.

In the case of advanced carious attack, primary odontoblasts are destroyed and any repair must be mediated by a new population of cells. There are now many examples of successful tissue engineering being applied in medicine, and three key ingredients have been identified: signals for morphogenesis, undifferentiated stem cells to respond to the morphogens and a scaffold of extracellular matrix (Mitsiadis & Rahiotis, 2004; Nakashima & Akamine, 2005). The major signaling molecules are the bone morphogenetic protein (BMPs), and BMP2 can be applied to exposed pulps to induce dentin formation (Iohara et al., 2004). This approach, however, relies on there being a sufficiently large residual population of viable cells to give an adequate response. Repopulation of the damaged tooth with new cells may be preferable, and the feasibility of this method has been demonstrated by experiments in which growth factor genes were introduced into undifferentiated pulp stem cells before they were transplanted into the lesion (Nakashima et al., 2004). The simple production of unstructured dentin may be adequate in small caries lesions to provide a robust new hard surface. Complete restoration of tooth form and function is the ultimate aim, and there is even the prospect of eventually generating a completely new tooth by bioengineering tooth bud cells or stem cells on appropriate scaffolds. While engineering of a complete new tooth in a human may be some way off, a significant start has been made in experimental animals (Dualibi et al., 2004; Modino & Sharpe, 2005).

Conclusion

The explosion of knowledge of fundamental processes at the molecular level in biological sciences is having a dramatic impact on the understanding of dental caries. Insights into the oral microbial population, mechanisms of biofilm formation and metabolism, and the contribution of different bacterial species to disease have led to a greater realization of the level of complexity involved. In some cases this led to concepts first advanced half a century ago now being regarded as too simplistic. For example, the contribution of bacteria other than S. mutans to caries is now recognized, although there is still irrefutable practical evidence that vaccines based on S. mutans can substantially reduce caries in animals with a complex oral microflora. A host of new opportunities and understanding will allow long-standing problems to be attacked. As with other diseases, there is increasing realization that caries involves interplay between the attack and the host response, and that the disease may be modulated by influencing either of the two. There is no doubt that cariology as a subject area has been, and will continue to be, an exciting and fruitful branch of science. Whether the new biological insights will be translated into practicable approaches of routine clinical value, only time will tell.

References

Abiko Y. Passive immunization against dental caries and periodontal disease: development of recombinant and human monoclonal antibodies. *Crit Rev Oral Biol Med* 2000; **11**: 140–58.

Ajdic D, McShan WM, McLaughlin RE, et al. Genome sequence of *Streptococcus mutans* UA159, a cariogenic dental pathogen. *Proc Natl Acad Sci USA* 2002; **99**: 14434–9.

Becker MR, Paster BJ, Leys EJ, et al. Molecular analysis of bacterial species associated with childhood caries. *J Clin Microbiol* 2002; **40**: 1001–9.

Bowen WH. A vaccine against dental caries: a pilot experiment in monkeys *Macaca irus. Br Dent J* 1969; **126**: 159–60.

Brailsford SR, Sheehy EC, Gilbert SC, Clark DT, et al. The microflora of the erupting first permanent molar. *Caries Res* 2005; **39**: 78–84.

Bratthall D, Serinirach R, Hamberg K, Widerstrom L. Immunoglobulin A reaction to oral streptococci in saliva of subjects with different combinations of caries and levels of mutans streptococci. *Oral Microbiol Immunol* 1997; **12**: 212–18.

Byun R, Nadkarni MA, Chhour K, et al. Quantitative analysis of diverse *Lactobacillus* species present in advanced dental caries. *J Clin Microbiol* 2004; **42**: 3128–36.

Caufield PW, Cutter GR, Dasanayake AP. Initial acquisition of mutans streptococci by infants: evidence for a discrete window of infectivity. *J Dent Res* 1993; **72**: 37–45.

Chhour KL, Nadkarni M, Byun R, et al. Molecular analysis of microbial diversity in advanced caries. *J Clin Microbiol* 2005; **43**: 843–9.

Chia JS, Chang LY, Shun CT, et al. A 60-kilodalton immunodominant glycoprotein is essential for cell wall integrity and the maintenance of cell shape in *Streptococcus mutans. Infect Immun* 2001; **69**: 6987–98.

Dualibi MT, Dualibi SE, Young CS, et al. Bioengineered teeth from cultured rat tooth bud cells. *J Dent Res* 2004; **83**: 523–8.

Ferretti JJ, Gilpin ML, Russell RRB. Nucleotide sequence of a glucosyltransferase gene from *Streptococcus sobrinus* MFe28. *J Bacteriol* 1987; **169**: 4271–8.

Graham L, Cooper PR, Cassidy N, et al. The effect of calcium hydroxide on solubilisation of bio-active dentine matrix components. *Biomaterials* 2006; **27**: 2865–73.

Hillman JD. Genetically modified *Streptococcus mutans* for the prevention of dental caries. *Ant van Leeuwenhoek* 2002; **82**: 361–6.

Hillman JD, Brooks TA, Michalek SM, et al. Construction and characterization of an effector strain of *Streptococcus mutans* for replacement therapy of dental caries. *Infect Immun* 2000; **68**: 543–9.

Igarashi T. Deletion in sortase gene of *Streptococcus mutans* Ingbritt. *Oral Microbiol Immunol* 2004; **19**: 210–13.

Iohara K, Nakashima M, Ito M, et al. Dentin regeneration by dental pulp stem cell therapy with recombinant human bone morphogenetic protein 2. *J Dent Res* 2004; **83**: 590–5.

Jakubovics NS, Stromberg N, van Dolleweerd CJ, et al. Differential binding specificities of oral streptococcal antigen I/II family adhesins for human or bacterial ligands. *Mol Microbiol* 2005; **55**: 1591–605.

Kelly CG, Younson JS, Hikmat BY, et al. A synthetic peptide adhesion epitope as a novel antimicrobial agent. *Nat Biotechnol* 1999; **17**: 42–7.

Koga T, Oho T, Shimazaki Y, Nakano Y. Immunization against dental caries. *Vaccine* 2002; **20**: 2027–44.

Kruger C, Hultberg A, Marcotte H, et al. Therapeutic effect of llama derived VHH fragments against *Streptococcus mutans* on the development of dental caries. *Appl Microbiol Biotechnol* 2006; **72**: 732–7.

Levesque CM, Voronejskaia E, Huang YC, et al. Involvement of sortase anchoring of cell wall proteins in biofilm formation by *Streptococcus mutans*. *Infect Immun* 2005; **73**: 3773–7.

Loesche WJ. Role of *Streptococcus mutans* in human dental decay. *Microbiol Rev* 1986; **50**: 353–80.

Loimaranta V, Jakubovics NS, Hytonen J, et al. Fluid- or surface-phase human salivary scavenger protein gp340 exposes different bacterial recognition properties. *Infect Immun* 2005; **73**: 2245–52.

Ma JK, Lehner T. Prevention of colonization of *Streptococcus mutans* by topical application of monoclonal antibodies in human subjects. *Arch Oral Biol* 1990; **35** (Suppl): 115–22S.

McLachlan JL, Smith AJ, Bujalska IJ, Cooper PR. Gene expression profiling of pulpal tissue reveals the molecular complexity of dental caries. *Biochim Biophys Acta* 2005; **1741**: 271–81.

Milgrom P, Riedy CA, Weinstein P. Dental caries and its relationship to bacterial infection, hypoplasia, diet, and oral hygiene in 6- to 36-month-old children. *Community Dent Oral Epidemiol* 2000; **28**: 295–306.

Mitsiadis TA, Rahiotis C. Parallels between tooth development and repair: conserved molecular mechanisms following carious and dental injury. *J Dent Res* 2004; **83**: 896–902.

Modino SA, Sharpe PT. Tissue engineering of teeth using adult stem cells. *Arch Oral Biol* 2005; **50**: 255–8.

Munson MA, Banerjee A, Watson TF, Wade WG. Molecular analysis of the microflora associated with dental caries. *J Clin Microbiol* 2004; **42**: 3023–9.

Nakashima M, Akamine A. The application of tissue engineering to regeneration of pulp and dentin in endodontics. *J Endodont* 2005; **31**: 711–18.

Nakashima M, Iohara K, Ishikawa M, et al. Stimulation of reparative dentin formation by *ex vivo* gene therapy using dental pulp stem cells electrotransfected with growth/differentiation factor 11 Gdf11. *Hum Gene Ther* 2004; **15**: 1045–53.

Nogueira RD, Alves AC, Napimoga MH, et al. Characterization of salivary immunoglobulin A responses in children heavily exposed to the oral bacterium *Streptococcus mutans*: influence of specific antigen recognition in infection. *Infect Immun* 2005; **73**: 5675–84.

Okada M, Soda Y, Hayashi F, et al. Longitudinal study of dental caries incidence associated with *Streptococcus mutans* and *Streptococcus sobrinus* in pre-school children. *J Med Microbiol* 2005; **54**: 661–5.

Paakkonen V, Ohlmeier S, Bergmann U, et al. Analysis of gene and protein expression in healthy and carious tooth pulp with cDNA microarray and two-dimensional gel electrophoresis. *Eur J Oral Sci* 2005; **113**: 369–79.

Russell MW, Challacombe SJ, Lehner T. Serum glucosyltransferase-inhibiting antibodies and dental caries in rhesus monkeys immunized against *Streptococcus mutans*. *Immunology* 1976; **30**: 619–27.

Russell MW, Harrington DJ, Russell RRB. Identity of *Streptococcus mutans* surface protein antigen III and wall-associated protein antigen A. *Infect Immun* 1995; **63**: 733–5.

Russell MW, Hajishengallis G, Childers NK, Michalek SM. Secretory immunity in defense against cariogenic mutans streptococci. *Caries Res* 1999; **33**: 4–15.

Russell RRB, Colman G. Immunization of monkeys *Macaca fascicularis* with purified *Streptococcus mutans* glucosyltransferase. *Arch Oral Biol* 1981; **26**: 23–8.

Russell RRB, Johnson NW. The prospects for vaccination against dental caries. *Br Dent J* 1987; **162**: 29–34.

van Ruyven FO, Lingstrom P, van Houte J, Kent R. Relationship among mutans streptococci, 'low-pH' bacteria, and lodophilic polysaccharide-producing bacteria in dental plaque and early enamel caries in humans. *J Dent Res* 2000; **79**: 778–84.

Shah DSH, Russell RRB. A novel glucan-binding protein with lipase activity from the oral pathogen *Streptococcus mutans*. *Microbiology* 2004; **150**: 1947–56.

Sharon N, Ofek I. Fighting infectious diseases with inhibitors of microbial adhesion to host tissues. *Crit Rev Food Sci Nutr* 2002; **42**: 267–72.

Smith AJ. Pulpal responses to caries and dental repair. *Caries Res* 2002; **36**: 223–32.

Smith DJ. Dental caries vaccines: prospects and concerns. *Crit Rev Oral Biol Med* 2002; **13**: 335–49.

Smith DJ, King WF, Barnes LA, et al. Immunogenicity and protective immunity induced by synthetic peptides associated with putative immunodominant regions of *Streptococcus mutans* glucan-binding protein B. *Infect Immun* 2003; **71**: 1179–84.

Smith DJ, King WF, Rivero J, Taubman MA. Immunological and protective effects of diepitopic subunit dental caries vaccines. *Infect Immun* 2005; **73**: 2797–804.

de Soet JJ, van Loveren C, Lammens AJ, et al. Differences in cariogenicity between fresh isolates of *Streptococcus sobrinus* and *Streptococcus mutans*. *Caries Res* 1991; **25**: 116–22.

Tanner AC, Milgrom PM, Kent RJ, et al. The microbiota of young children from tooth and tongue samples. *J Dent Res* 2002; **81**: 53–7.

Tanzer JM, Livingston J, Thompson AM. The microbiology of primary dental caries in humans. *J Dent Educ* 2001; **65**: 1028–37.

Taubman MA, Holmberg CJ, Smith DJ. Immunization of rats with synthetic peptide constructs from the glucan-binding or catalytic region of mutans streptococcal glucosyltransferase protects against dental caries. *Infect Immun* 1995; **63**: 3088–93.

Wan AK, Seow WK, Purdie DM, et al. A longitudinal study of *Streptococcus mutans* colonization in infants after tooth eruption. *J Dent Res* 2003; **82**: 504–8.

Waterhouse JC, Russell RRB. Dispensable genes and foreign DNA in *Streptococcus mutans*. *Microbiology* 2006; **152**: 1777–88.

Weintraub JA, Hilton JF, White JM, et al. Clinical trial of a plant-derived antibody on recolonization of mutans streptococci. *Caries Res* 2005; **39**: 241–50.

Xu QA, Yu F, Fan M, et al. Immunogenicity and protective efficacy of a targeted fusion DNA construct against dental caries. *Caries Res* 2005; **39**: 422–31.

Younson J, Kelly CG. The rational design of an anti-caries peptide against *Streptococcus mutans*. *Mol Divers* 2004; **8**: 121–6.

Zhang P, Jespersgaard C, Lamberty-Mallory L, et al. Enhanced immunogenicity of a genetic chimeric protein consisting of two virulence antigens of *Streptococcus mutans* and protection against infection. *Infect Immun* 2002; **70**: 6779–87.

18

Fluorides in caries control

R. Ellwood, O. Fejerskov, J.A. Cury and B. Clarkson

Introduction

The role of fluorides in caries prevention represents one of the most successful stories in general public health. However, as with many successful programs this success is not without cost and it is a story that has resulted in strong emotional debates within the dental profession. These debates have at times split the world into those who advocate the use of fluorides in all populations and those who fight against the use of fluorides in any form.

The views expressed in this chapter are based on what is currently known about the effects of fluorides on developing and erupted teeth to derive a rational way of advocating the use of fluorides in contemporary populations. It is well documented that fluoride can have both beneficial and detrimental effects on the dentition. As a basic principle, the beneficial effects on dental caries are due primarily to the topical effect of fluoride after the teeth have erupted into the oral cavity (for mechanisms of action see Chapter 12). In contrast, the detrimental effects of fluoride are due to its systemic absorption during tooth development, resulting in dental fluorosis. By maximizing topical exposure throughout life and minimizing systemic absorption during the period when the dentition is developing, fluoride can be used to maximize the anticaries benefits while minimizing the risk of fluorosis.

This chapter will discuss:

- how fluoride came into dentistry
- physiological and toxicological aspects of fluoride delivery
- current methods of fluoride delivery
- appropriate use of fluoride in caries control
- recommendations for rational use of fluorides in different populations.

How fluoride came into dentistry

What is remarkable about the fluoride story is that it was the detrimental effects of fluoride on the appearance of tooth enamel (dental fluorosis) that prompted the initial detailed investigations and ultimately the discovery of its anticaries benefits (Fejerskov *et al.*, 1988; Murray *et al.*, 1991).

Throughout history references to dental conditions with similar characteristics to what we now know to be dental fluorosis have been described throughout the world. A good example is the following text from C.I. Gallen (AD131–201):

It is remarkable that above diseases do not attack teeth having a dark yellow colour, although one would have expected the contrary. Thus the teeth receive nourishment and grow, which is clearly seen in teeth which have no opponents, while in other cases their masticating surfaces are worn down from the abrasion of the food.

(Identification of text and translation thanks to the late Professor D. Lambrou, Thessaloniki, Greece.)

In Europe the importance of fluoride to dentistry can be traced back to the late nineteenth century when various preparations containing fluoride, such as powders and pills, were recommended to help combat dental caries. Although many different formulations were available and belief in the benefits was quite widespread, the scientific basis for their use was at best obscure. Denninger must be credited with conducting one of the earliest 'clinical trials' of fluoride in the latter part of the nineteenth century. He prescribed calcium fluoride to children and pregnant women and observed 'great benefits' to their teeth (Cawson & Stocker, 1984).

Although indications of the potential importance of fluoride in preventing and treating dental caries had been highlighted in many parts of the world, the credit for the identification of the scientific basis for fluoride in preventing or treating dental caries can be largely attributed to the work and perseverance of two American dentists, Dr Fredrick McKay and a US Public Health Officer, H. Trendley Dean. Just after graduation in 1901, McKay started work in Colorado Springs, Colorado, USA, and noticed that some of his patients had what was locally known as 'Colorado brown stain'. He later moved out of the area but returned in 1908 and following discussions with other dentists realized that the condition was common but not documented in the dental literature.

His curiosity aroused, McKay turned for help to Dr Greene Vardiman Black, one of America's most eminent experts on tooth enamel. Although Black was at first sceptical that the condition was of any importance, initial epidemiological investigations by McKay and his colleagues convinced him that the condition was endemic in the area, with nearly 90% of children affected. Black's histological investigation of the condition, 'An endemic imperfection of the enamel of the teeth heretofore unknown in the literature of dentistry' (Black, 1916), served to raise the profile of the condition significantly within the dental research community. One thing that puzzled both Black and McKay was that although mottled enamel was clearly hypocalcified and therefore theoretically more susceptible to decay, this did not appear to be the case (McKay, 1928). Coincidentally, Ainsworth in England made a similar observation (Ainsworth, 1933).

Gradually, McKay began to hear reports of mottled enamel similar to the condition he had identified in Colorado, throughout the USA and in other areas of the world such as Italy (Eager, 1902). It became clear that the condition was localized to children born in specific geographical areas and McKay suspected that the water supplies of these districts might be an important etiological factor. This theory was put to the test in Oakley, Idaho, where children's teeth developed brownish discoloration following changes to a water supply in 1908. In 1923 McKay was asked to consider the problem and a pipeline to an alternative water source was laid. McKay returned to the area 10 years later and the problem had disappeared (McKay, 1933).

A similar problem was noticed in Bauxite when changes to a water supply resulted in children having mottled enamel (Kempf & McKay, 1930). The company mining aluminum in Bauxite began to be concerned that aluminum used in cooking utensils might be blamed for the condition. Chemical analysis of the water supply revealed an unexpectedly high level of fluoride in the drinking water (13.7 ppm F) and these high levels were later confirmed in other towns with mottled enamel (Churchill, 1931). This in itself did not establish a cause and effect relationship, but as the condition had been seen in rats fed with drinking water containing fluoride, much of the puzzle was complete (McCollum *et al.*, 1925).

The discovery that fluoride was present in drinking water at high concentrations was of concern, since fluoride at high doses was known to be a poison. The US Public Health Service and particularly Dr H. Trendley Dean took up the investigation and contacted dentists throughout the USA. Dean mapped areas in which mottled enamel appeared to be prevalent and by 1938 had identified 375 areas in 26 states. He also developed a classification system for recording the severity of mottled enamel that is still widely used today (Dean, 1934). Examples of clinical manifestations of dental fluorosis (as 'mottled enamel' is now called) are shown in Figs 18.13–18.19) and will be described later in this chapter.

Travelling throughout the USA in a series of extensive epidemiological investigations. Dean recorded the prevalence and severity of 'mottled enamel' and related this to the fluoride concentration in the drinking water. He identified a clear dose–response relationship and suggested that up to the level of around 1 ppm F the extent and severity of mottled was probably of no public health significance (Dean & Elvove, 1936). Further evidence of the relationship between the prevalence and severity of mottled enamel and the fluoride concentration of the drinking water was identified when the condition disappeared after the drinking water to a number of towns with high levels of fluoride was reduced to less than 1 ppm F (Dean & McKay, 1939).

Dean was also interested in the apparent anomaly that although the enamel appeared to be hypomineralized it did not appear to be any more susceptible to decay. He initially undertook a small study involving 114 children who had used water containing 0.6–1.5 ppm F and found that only 4% were caries free, compared with 22% of 122 children in an area with drinking water containing 1.7–2.5 ppm F (Dean, 1938a). A further larger study suggested that caries experience in two cities with water supplies containing 1.7 and 1.8 ppm was half that of two similar adjacent cities with only 0.2 ppm F in the drinking water (Dean *et al.*, 1939).

The association between the fluoride level in the drinking water and caries levels was then characterized in the '21 city study' (actually a series of studies). Children from cities with fluoride concentrations in their drinking water ranging from around 0 up to 2.6 ppm F were examined, and the results of this classic piece of epidemiological investigation of both fluorosis and caries experience are summarized in Figs 18.1 and 18.2 (Dean, 1942).

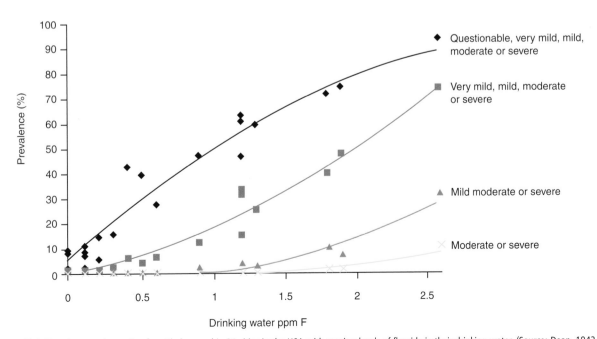

Figure 18.1 Prevalence and severity of mottled enamel in 21 cities in the USA with varying levels of fluoride in their drinking water. (Source: Dean, 1942.)

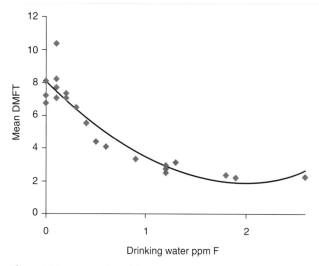

Figure 18.2 Mean number of decayed, missing and filled teeth (DMFT) and fluoride concentration of the drinking water from the 21 city study. (Source: Dean, 1942.)

Dean's index (Dean, 1934, 1938b, 1942) classifies fluorosis as questionable, very mild, mild, moderate and severe. The prevalence of subjects with lesions of any severity is about 50% at the level of 1 ppm F or less in the drinking water (Fig. 18.1). However, it is also interesting to note that the less severe forms of fluorosis (questionable and very mild) account for most cases and there is a very clear dose–response relationship between the fluoride level in the drinking water and the prevalence of fluorosis, even at levels of fluoride in the drinking water below 1 ppm F. Therefore, even at low levels of fluoride in the drinking water there was some risk of fluorosis attached to the use of fluoride.

The use of the term questionable to describe the earliest classification level in Dean's index has been the source of much controversy over the years. It must be remembered that when Dean started his pioneering epidemiological studies he was presented with a spectrum of defects, some of which were due to fluoride and some to other etiologies. Not surprisingly he was unsure of his ability to diagnose fluorosis and a questionable category of defects would seem a reasonable compromise. As Dean's experience in recording enamel defects increased it is likely that his ability to classify defects improved, and there is a suggestion that his recording method evolved so that some defects initially classified as questionable were later recorded in the very mild category. Although it is likely that defects not due to fluoride were recorded in the questionable category, Fig. 18.1 suggests that there is a strong dose–response relationship between this category of defects and the fluoride concentration of the drinking water. In 1983, Myers reviewed the available literature regarding the 'questionable' category of dental fluorosis and demonstrated that it was a distinct entity associated with fluoride.

The association between fluoride levels in the drinking water and dental caries in the 21 cities is shown in Fig. 18.2. There was strong association between caries and the fluoride level in the drinking water up to the level of 1 ppm F, but beyond this, although the trend for the mean DMFT continued to decrease, it did so at a much lower rate. At the level of fluoride of 1 ppm the average number of decayed, missing or filled teeth had reduced by more than 50%. This, in conjunction with the observation that there appeared to be little if any fluorosis of 'cosmetic significance' below this level of fluoride, resulted in the widespread adoption of 1–1.2 ppm F as an 'optimal' level in the drinking water. Although fluoride levels higher than this are not to be recommended, one should consider whether the apparent plateau is an artifact of the recording method or population observed. For example, it is possible that the method of recording dental caries used by Dean and his colleagues at the cavitation level, still widely used today, is insensitive in identifying benefits in arresting enamel lesions at higher levels of fluoride exposure (see Chapters 8 and 9).

The work of Dean and his co-workers used cross-sectional study designs, which were sufficient to identify a strong association between the fluoride level in the drinking water and caries levels, but could not establish a cause and effect relationship. Therefore, intervention studies were required and these began in the Lake Michigan area in 1944. Two towns were selected, Grand Rapids and Muskegon, and baseline caries levels in children aged 4–16 years were recorded. In addition, caries levels were recorded in Aurora, Illinois, an area with naturally occurring fluoride in the drinking water at the level of 1.4 ppm F. At the start of the study caries levels in the two Michigan cities were similar (Dean *et al.*, 1950). Fluoride at the level of 1 ppm was then added to the drinking water of the city of Grand Rapids in January 1945 and caries levels were recorded again after 6½ years of fluoridation. In 'non-fluoride' Muskegon the average number of teeth with decay experience was 5.7, compared with 3.0 in 'fluoridated' Grand Rapids (Arnold *et al.*, 1953). The study was deemed so successful that it was decided to fluoridate the drinking water of Muskegon. After 15 years of fluoridation in Grand Rapids (Fig. 18.3) the number of teeth with decay experience had fallen from 12.5 in 1944 to 6.2 in 1959, a reduction of approximately 50% (Arnold *et al.*, 1962). Caries levels in Grand Rapids were now very similar to those experienced in Aurora, the naturally fluoridated city. This outcome was replicated in a number of studies throughout the USA and other parts of the world, and provided unequivocal evidence of the efficacy of water fluoridation to reduce caries (Murray *et al.*, 1991).

Although it is hard to think how these studies could have been improved, some criticism can be made of the approach taken by Dean and his co-workers. Probably the most important is the possible bias introduced by the fact that

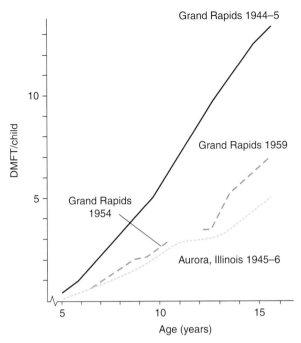

Figure 18.3 Dental caries in Grand Rapids children after 10 and after 15 years of fluoridation (–––––), in Grand Rapids before fluoridation (——) and in the natural fluoride area Aurora (--------).

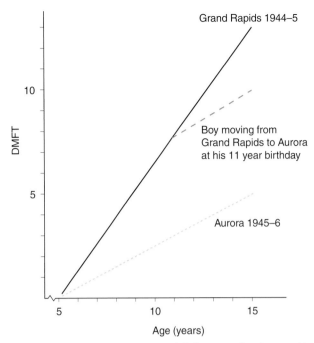

Figure 18.4 Dental caries in Grand Rapids before water fluoridation and in Aurora with fluoride in the water supply. The dashed line indicated caries progression in a boy moving from the non-fluoride to the fluoride area on his 11th birthday. (Source: Luoma *et al.*, 1986.)

the fluoride level of the site investigated was known before the examinations were conducted. This might have resulted in a tendency to underscore fluorosis in the low-fluoride areas and overscore fluorosis in those areas known to have fluoride. A similar bias could also be made in relation to the caries studies and the benefits may have been overestimated. However, the wealth of data now available relating to fluoride use, caries and fluorosis strongly supports the conclusions of Dean and his co-workers, a testament to their skill and ingenuity.

It is clear from our understanding of the mechanisms of action of fluoride (see Chapter 12) and the studies previously discussed that if fluoride is available from the time of eruption and exposure is continued later during the lifetime of the tooth, the maximum benefit is achieved. However, it is also pertinent to consider what might be expected for a child who does not have continuous exposure to fluoride. For example, consider an 11-year-old 'average' boy with a DMFT of 8 from Grand Rapids before fluoridation was introduced, who then moved to Aurora where fluoride in the drinking water was present (Fig. 18.4). On average, one would expect the progression rate of lesions now to parallel that of other children in Aurora, but he would have a higher caries experience than his new contemporaries. Clearly, one would not expect to see a 50% reduction in caries compared with children from Grand Rapids when he was 15 years old. This phenomenon has caused some confusion in the past related to the posterup-

tive and pre-eruptive effects of fluoride, as it was postulated that the difference could largely be attributed to a pre-eruptive fluoride effect. However, from Fig. 18.4 it is clear that what is probably being seen is the influence of the time of initiation and duration of fluoride exposure posteruptively. Likewise, a child born and reared in a fluoride area will on average, if moving to live in a low-fluoride area, experience an increased caries incidence. So, fluoride has to be available in the oral environment and its incorporation in enamel during formation is of much less significance (see Chapter 12).

The concept of an 'optimum' water fluoride level

The studies by Dean and his co-workers in the early 1940s resulted in the wish to add fluoride to numerous water supplies in the USA considered to have too low concentrations. Already at the time it was evident that the water fluoride concentrations had to be determined by balancing the caries-preventive beneficial effect against the risk of development of dental fluorosis. During attempts to decide such water fluoride concentrations, the concept of an 'optimum' water fluoride concentration was developed when Hodge (1950) presented the results of logarithmic transformations of Dean and co-workers' caries data and averaged index values of Dean's original scores of dental fluorosis (Fig. 18.5). It is now appreciated that this way of manipulating data is inappropriate. However, from a public health point of view

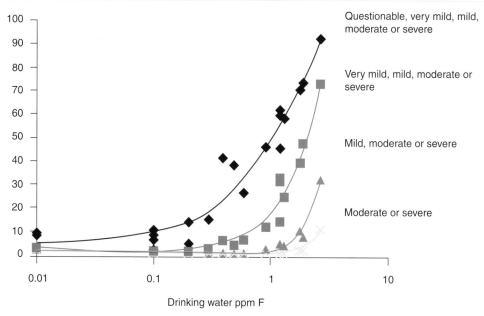

Figure 18.5 Log transformation of the fluoride level in the drinking water and the prevalence and severity of mottled enamel in 21 cities in the USA with varying levels of fluoride in their drinking water. (Source: Dean, 1942.)

it gave rise to a very convincing plot of data which indicated that children born and reared in areas with a fluoride content in water supplies below 1 ppm would only experience a prevalence and severity of fluorosis that was considered of 'negligible biologic (aesthetic) significance'. Moreover, the mean caries experience recorded from the 21 city studies indicated that a maximum caries reduction was obtained around the concentration of about 1–1.2 ppm F in water supplies (Fig. 18.6), so the 'optimum level' was determined as the level of concentration of fluoride in water supplies that gave maximum caries reduction while causing mini-

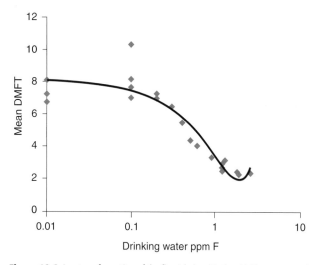

Figure 18.6 Log transformation of the fluoride level in the drinking water and caries prevalence in 21 cities in the USA with varying levels of fluoride in their drinking water. (Source: Dean, 1942.)

mal dental fluorosis of no concern from a public health point of view. This estimate of the optimal water fluoride concentration was subsequently used to determine the amount of fluoride that should be given in other systemic fluoride regimens such as tablets and vitamin drops (see later in this chapter).

The concept of the necessity of ingesting fluoride was based on the belief that fluoride exerted its anticariogenic effect predominantly by becoming incorporated into the crystals in the dental hard tissues. This, it was believed, would make the enamel more resistant to the acid attack on tooth surfaces. With this paradigm it was therefore logical that public health dentists would have to argue that as much fluoride as possible should be ingested during tooth formation to increase the 'resistance of the tooth'. Therefore, early signs of dental fluorosis, considered an undesirable side-effect to the beneficial use of fluoride in water, were looked upon only from the point of view of 'cosmetic disturbances'. In attempts to downplay the significance of a toxicological effect of fluoride, there was much interest in questioning whether it was possible to diagnose the early stages of dental fluorosis. In addition, the position was somewhat distorted by postulating, for example, that 'optimal fluoride concentrations in water supplies result in more perfect mineralized teeth with pearl shine appearance' or 'teeth formed in low fluoride areas are fluoride deficient'.

Dental decay in the middle of the twentieth century was a devastating problem to most child populations in the USA and Europe, and many children had teeth extracted early in life. It was not uncommon in parts of Europe to have all teeth extracted in early adulthood. From this perspective the toxicological effects of fluoride, manifesting as whitish discolorations of teeth, were an acceptable alternative to having deep carious cavities resulting in pain and tooth loss.

It is clear from this chapter and that on the cariostatic mechanisms of fluoride (Chapter 12), that fluoride predominantly exerts its anticaries effect through its topical action on tooth surfaces in the oral cavity (Fejerskov *et al.*, 1981). Fluoride can therefore be used in caries control based on modern scientific evidence of the mechanisms of action and its toxicological effect. Dental caries can be controlled with little risk of dental fluorosis. It is clear that oral health advice recommending the necessity to ingest fluoride is extremely misleading as it is clearly not necessary to ingest fluoride to receive its benefits. Nevertheless, it is striking how many of the recommendations about the use of fluorides are still based on past paradigms and old beliefs from the 1950s and 1960s.

The introduction of fluoride into drinking water was followed by the development of other oral care products, such as toothpaste, tablets, gels and varnishes, and these have had a dramatic impact on the prevalence and severity of dental caries throughout the world. For example, the widespread addition of fluoride to toothpaste in the 1960s and 1970s appears to been mainly responsible for a complete change in the pattern of dental disease in many parts of Europe and in particular Scandinavia and the UK. This is well illustrated by national census data collected for England and Wales in 1973, 1983 and 1993 (Fig. 18.7). Most health professionals agree that although fluoride cannot completely account for these dramatic reductions, an increased availability of fluoride, mainly in toothpaste, has played a major part in the process (Bratthall *et al.*, 1996).

This dramatic decline in caries has had far-reaching implications for the practice of dentistry in the Western world and has had a significant impact on the quality of life of the majority of individuals who avail themselves of this simple preventive and therapeutic intervention.

Physiological and toxicological aspects of fluoride delivery

Introduction

Although fluoride is a trace element it is widely present in the environment. Fluoride reaches the hydrosphere by leaching from soils and minerals into ground waters. Volcanic eruptions and dust storms in areas rich in volcanic rocks add to the fluoride in the atmosphere.

Owing to the small radius of the fluorine atom it is the most electronegative and reactive element and is rarely found in its elemental state. It is most commonly found in combination in the ionic F^- and the electrovalent or covalent form. Most of the ionic fluorides are resoluble in water although some, such as calcium fluorides, are only slightly soluble. Further information is available from the detailed textbook chapters by Smith and Ekstrand (1996) and Glemser (1986).

Water is by far the most common natural source of fluoride, but even in areas with levels of fluoride in the drinking water less than 0.5–0.7 mg/l, importation of commercially prepared beverages and other foods, from areas where water supplies contain higher levels, can add substantially to the amount of fluoride ingested. Some fruit-flavored, carbonated soft drinks and mineral water may also contain significant (0.7–0.9 mg/l) amounts of fluoride (Schulz *et al.*, 1976; Clovis & Hargreaves, 1988). Fish is a particularly good source of fluoride, as are tea leaves. A cup of tea (Duckworth & Duckworth, 1978) or iced tea (Hayacibara *et al.*, 2004) may have a fluoride concentration of 0.5–4 mg/l.

An assessment of the total exposure of a given population to fluoride requires not only a thorough knowledge of the fluoride concentrations of foods and beverages and an understanding of the open markets of a modern society, but also a careful assessment of potential fluoride ingestion from dental products (see later in this chapter).

Fluoride absorption, distribution and elimination in the body

Fluoride ingestion is particularly important in infants as dental fluorosis can only occur when teeth are developing. Fluoride is poorly transported from plasma to milk, even when the mother or animal has a high intake of fluoride, and human and other mammalian milks contain very low concentrations of fluoride (Spak *et al.*, 1983). In contrast, commercially prepared formula milks may have highly

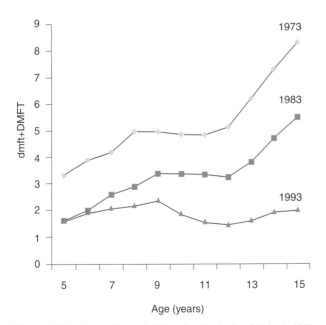

Figure 18.7 Caries experience of children from England and Wales in 1973, 1983 and 1993. (Source: O'Brien, 1994.)

variable fluoride content and if they are furthermore prepared with fluoridated water, children may potentially ingest considerable amounts of fluoride from this source (Levy *et al.*, 1995; Foman & Ekstrand, 1999).

The metabolism and pharmacokinetics of fluoride in humans are dealt with in detail by Ekstrand (1996) and Whitford (1996). Following ingestion, fluoride is rapidly absorbed into the blood plasma, predominantly in the stomach. The stomach content and its composition are important in determining the rate of absorption. Milk, calcium-rich breakfasts and even lunch may reduce the degree of absorption from about 90% to about 60%. The time of fluoride ingestion in relation to meals is critical with respect to how much of the fluoride will become bioavailable (Ekstrand *et al.*, 1990; Cury *et al.*, 2005).

If the absorption of fluoride is high, the major route for the removal of fluoride will be by the kidneys. Fecal fluoride usually accounts for less than 10% of the amount ingested each day (Ekstrand *et al.*, 1984). Fluoride is distributed all over the body by plasma, predominantly as ionic fluoride. Plasma fluoride concentrations vary considerably over the day depending on the intake of fluoride. With increasing age plasma fluoride levels gradually increase because there is a direct relationship between the amount of fluoride accumulating in bone which, as time passes, is gradually released from the bone as part of bone remodeling (Parkins *et al.*, 1974). There is no homeostatic mechanism to maintain the fluoride concentration in any body compartment and fluoride levels are largely dependent on daily intake. This has important implications for the oral environment, which will be described further in this chapter.

Fluoride is distributed from the plasma to all tissues and organs in the body. The degree of blood flow through the different types of tissues determines how rapidly distribution occurs. Of particular interest is that the kidney in general has a higher concentration of fluoride than the corresponding concentration in plasma. In contrast, the central nervous system, like adipose tissue, only contains about 20% of the concentration of that in plasma (Spak *et al.*, 1986).

As previously stressed, fluoride is a highly reactive agent and it reacts rapidly with mineralizing tissues. Over time, the fluoride gradually becomes incorporated into the crystal lattice structure in the form of fluorhydroxyapatite. It is during the growth phase of the skeleton, during active mineralization, that the highest proportion of an ingested fluoride dose will be deposited. Thus, retention of fluoride in infants may be as high as 80%, whereas in adults only about 50% of the fluoride may be retained in the bone.

Fluoride in the bone is not irreversibly bound to the crystals. Bone constantly undergoes remodeling (resorption of bone) and fluoride is thus mobilized slowly from the skeleton. Therefore, when studying cross-sectional samples, fluoride concentrations in plasma and urine will be determined not only by the immediate past intake of fluoride, but also by earlier fluoride exposure and the degree of accumulation of fluoride in bone. Moreover, with age the mobilization rate from bone and how efficient the kidneys are at excreting fluoride will strongly influence such data (Ekstrand *et al.*, 1977). Thus, bone might be considered a fluoride reservoir that maintains the fluoride concentration in the body fluids between the periods that fluoride is not being ingested.

Fluoride concentrations in teeth

Concentrations of fluoride in all mineralized tissues will vary depending on the actual fluoride intake and the length of time during which such an intake has taken place. In general, fluoride levels are greatest at the surface of any tissue since this part of the tissue has the closest proximity to the surrounding tissue fluid from which the fluoride is supplied.

The fluoride concentration of the enamel is highest at the surface, but it falls steeply within the outer 100 μm. After this point it remains fairly constant up to the enamel–dentin junction. The fluoride concentration of dentin is generally higher than that of bulk enamel and usually increases deeper into the tooth (Fig. 18.8). As dentin formation continues slowly throughout life, fluoride steadily accumulates at the dentin–pulp surface.

In Fig. 18.8 the overall shape of the fluoride profile from the surface of the enamel to the enamel–dentin junction is a characteristic 'hockey-stick' shape. The relative concentrations of fluoride in the different layers of enamel reflect the fluoride exposure during tooth development. Hence, the higher the dose of fluoride occurring during development, the higher the concentration of fluoride is to be found in enamel. The effect of different levels of fluoride exposure can be seen in Fig. 18.9. Teeth with more severe forms of fluorosis have significantly higher levels of fluoride in the enamel than those with less severe forms and this difference is maintained even deeper in the enamel. However, the concentration of fluoride at the outermost surface of the enamel is highly dependent on posteruptive changes and therefore it may be a poor indicator of fluoride exposure during the developmental period of the tooth.

Once the enamel is fully formed and mineralized the fluoride content in human enamel can only be permanently altered as a result of chemical traumas to the tooth (dental caries and erosions) or through mechanical abrasion. Unless chemical interactions take place with substantial fluctuations in pH over a prolonged period it is not easy to change significantly the fluoride content in the surface enamel even after several topical fluoride treatments (for details see Chapter 12). However, the fluoride concentration in the surface layers increases whenever demineralization and remineralization processes are ongoing (Weatherell *et al.*, 1977; Cury *et al.*, 2000). This means that in cervical regions, where dental plaque accumulates, fluoride concentrations

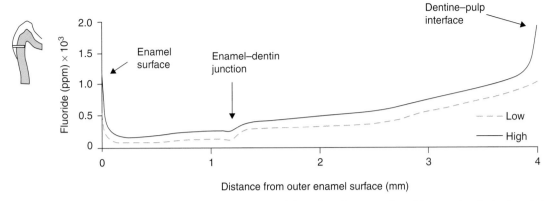

Figure 18.8 Schematic representation of the fluoride concentration in enamel and dentin from the outer surface of the enamel to the dentin–pulp interface for subjects with a low and higher fluoride intake.

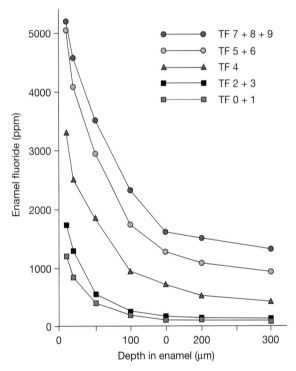

Figure 18.9 Enamel fluoride concentrations in the outer 300 μm of the enamel for erupted teeth with different degrees of fluorosis. See Fig. 18.13 for explanation of the TF index. (Source: Richards *et al.*, 1989.)

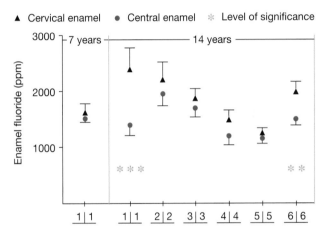

Figure 18.10 Fluoride concentration measured in surface enamel *in vivo* in upper central incisors at the age of about 7 years (shortly after eruption). The concentration is the same in central and cervical enamel. However, after 7 years in the oral environment it is apparent that fluoride in the cervical enamel (where plaque accumulates) increases, whereas it remains unchanged or gradually drops in central parts that have been exposed to attrition/tooth brushing. (Source: Richards *et al.*, 1977.)

What is dental fluorosis?

Clinically, the porosity of the fluorosed enamel is reflected in the opacity of the enamel. Thus, fluoride-induced enamel changes at tooth eruption range from thin, white, opaque lines corresponding to the perikymata running across the tooth surface, to an entirely chalky white surface (Figs 18.13–18.19). Depending on the degree of hypomineralization, this chalky white enamel may then change posteruptively, owing to mechanical damage, resulting in the more severe (aesthetically displeasing) forms of fluorosis.

To appreciate the clinical characteristics of dental fluorosis, it is important to understand the underlying histological features of the pathological changes in the tooth. The earliest manifestation of dental fluorosis is an increase in enamel porosity along the striae of Retzius (Fejerskov *et al.*, 1974). With an increased exposure to fluoride during tooth formation, the enamel exhibits an increased porosity in the tooth surface along the entire tooth surface (Fig. 18.20).

will gradually increase over time (Fig. 18.10). It is also the reason why the surface zone covering a subsurface caries lesion contains significantly higher amounts of fluoride than the surrounding normal enamel (Fig. 18.11).

The differences in fluoride content of enamel formed in low-fluoride areas (<0.2 ppm fluoride in the water supply) and in areas with about 1 ppm of fluoride are so small that they cannot explain differences in caries experience in populations living in low and higher fluoride areas. Moreover, there is little association between the fluoride concentration in the surface zone of teeth and the individual's caries experience for either the primary or permanent teeth (Fig. 18.12).

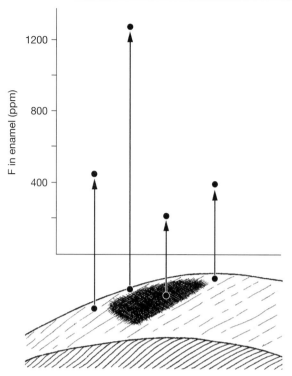

Figure 18.11 Fluoride concentrations in sound and carious enamel. The lowest concentrations are found in body of the lesion and then the sound bulk enamel. The surface enamel layer covering the lesion has picked up considerable amounts of fluoride from the surrounding fluids. (Modified from Weatherell *et al.*, 1977.)

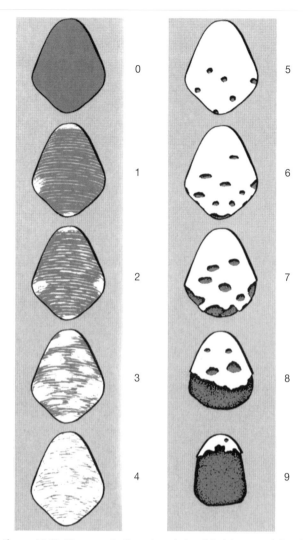

Figure 18.13 Diagrammatic illustration of the clinical features of dental fluorosis from the mildest form (TF 1) to the most severe (TF 9). Compare with Table 18.1.

This porosity, which is a result of a hypomineralization of the enamel, can be seen in microradiographs, mainly in the subsurface enamel (Fig. 18.21). The extent and degree of hypomineralization increase with increasing fluoride exposure during tooth development. In humans the most severe forms of the hypomineralized lesion extend throughout the enamel almost to the enamel–dentin junction in the cervical third of the crowns (Fig. 18.20c), whereas in the occlusal two-thirds of the teeth the band of hypomineralization extends more than half way through the enamel. Such severely hypomineralized enamel will be very fragile and hence when the tooth erupts surface damage may occur due to mastication, attrition and abrasion (Fig. 18.19). It is important to appreciate that in humans fluoride has not been documented to cause true hypoplastic changes; the characteristic pits, bands and loss of extensive areas of enamel occur posteruptively (Fejerskov *et al.*, 1988).

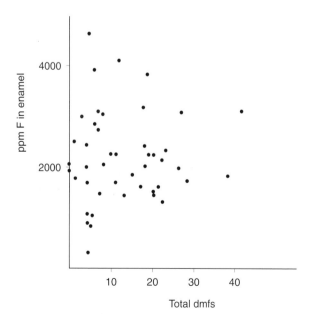

Figure 18.12 Fluoride concentrations in the surface enamel of deciduous canines and dental caries prevalence in the deciduous dentition. No relationship between the two is apparent. (Source: Poulsen & Larsen, 1975.)

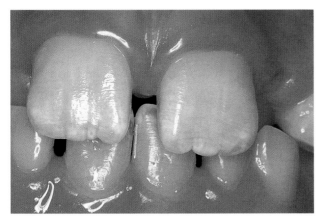

Figure 18.14 TF score 1: the earliest clinical sign of dental fluorosis appears as thin, white, opaque lines running across the tooth surface corresponding to the position of the perikymata.

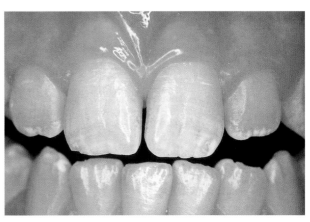

Figure 18.15 In addition to the thin, white, opaque lines, the earliest signs of dental fluorosis may include small, opaque, white areas along cusp tips, incisal edges or marginal ridges.

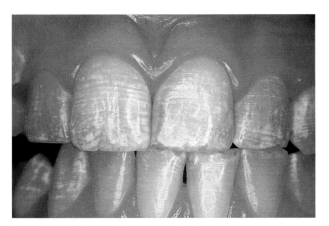

Figure 18.16 In TF score 2 the opaque white lines are more pronounced and frequently merge to form wider bands.

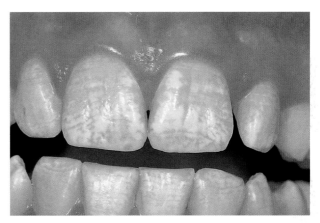

Figure 18.17 In TF score 3 the entire tooth surface exhibits cloudy, white, opaque areas between which accentuated perikymata lines are evident.

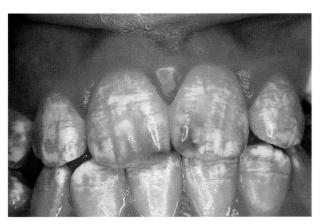

Figure 18.18 Another example of TF score 3 with the addition of posteruptive staining of the porous enamel.

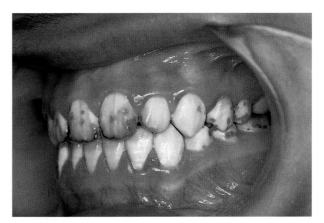

Figure 18.19 TF score 4 represents entirely white opaque enamel (see lower canine). As a reflection of the extension subsurface hypomineralization, part of the surface enamel may break away posteruptively, creating TF scores 5–7. Brown discoloration of the porous enamel, which has occurred posteruptively, is also visible.

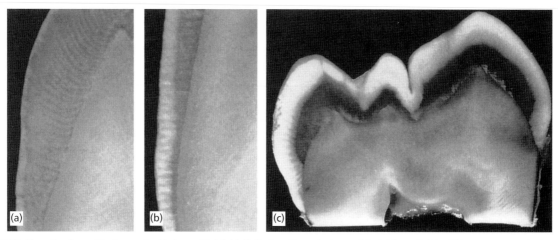

Figure 18.20 Ground sections of teeth examined in transmitted light. Notice how the early stages of dental fluorosis (a) exhibit a porous zone in the outermost enamel. With increasing severity this zone of porosity extends deeper into the enamel (b), and in very severe cases the porosity extends deep into the enamel tissue along the entire tooth crown (c) and in the cervical areas extends to the enamel–dentin junction.

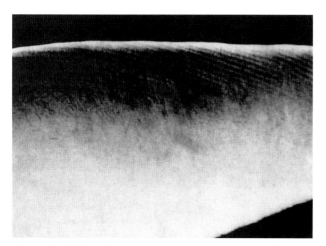

Figure 18.21 Microradiograph showing extensive hypomineralization of fluorosed enamel deep to a well-mineralized surface zone. Note incremental lines of Retzius. This represents a score of 4 according to the TF index.

Dean's way of classifying dental fluorosis was based entirely on his interpretation of clinical appearance. In 1978, Thylstrup and Fejerskov proposed a way of recording dental fluorosis (the TF index) based on the histopathological features of dental fluorosis. It is important to stress that the TF index is a logical extension of the classification principles originally proposed by Dean, but as would be expected with a greater understanding of the underlying pathology, it is a more precise description of how to record early signs of fluorosis as well as the more severe grades. Thylstrup and Fejerskov scored the severity of fluorosis from 0 to 9 (Table 18.1).

A single score in this TF index represents a measurement on an ordinal scale and should therefore be considered only as an arbitrary point along a continuum of changes of the enamel. It is useful to compare the description found in Table 18.1 with the illustrations (Figs 18.13–18.19), but it

Table 18.1 The Thylstrup Fejerskov Index

TF score	
0	The normal translucency of the glossy creamy-white enamel remains after wiping and drying of the surface
1	Thin white lines are seen running across the tooth surface. Such lines are found on all parts of the surface. The lines correspond to the position of the perikymata. In some cases, a slight 'snowcapping' of the cusps/incisal edges may also be seen
2	The opaque white lines are more pronounced and frequently merge to form small cloudy areas scattered over the whole surface. 'Snowcapping' of the incisal edges and cusp tips is common
3	Merging of the white lines occurs, and cloudy areas of opacity occur spread over many parts of the surface. In between the cloudy areas, white lines can also be seen
4	The entire surface exhibits a marked opacity, or appears chalky white. Parts of the surface exposed to attrition or wear appear to be less affected
5	The entire surface is opaque, and there are round pits (focal loss of the outermost enamel) that are less than 2 mm in diameter
6	The small pits may frequently be seen merging in the opaque enamel to form bands that are less than 2 mm in vertical height. In this class are also included surfaces where cuspal and facial enamel has chipped off, and the vertical dimension of the resulting damage is less than 2 mm
7	There is a loss of the outermost enamel in irregular areas, and less than half the surface is so involved. The remaining intact enamel is opaque
8	The loss of the outermost enamel involves more than half the enamel. The remaining intact enamel is opaque
9	The loss of the major part of the outer enamel results in a change of the anatomical shape of the surface/tooth. A cervical rim of opaque enamel is often noted

From Fejerskov *et al.* (1988), as modified from the original work by Thylstrup & Fejerskov (1978).

must be remembered that each score encompasses a spectrum of fluorotic changes. It should also be appreciated that a child who has been exposed to highly varying levels of fluoride during the long-lasting period of tooth development, will have an intraoral distribution of fluorosis severity different from that in a child who has been exposed to more constant fluoride levels throughout the first 10–12 years of life (Thylstrup & Fejerskov, 1979; Larsen *et al.*, 1985b; Fejerskov *et al.*, 1988).

Other suggestions as to how to record fluorosis have been suggested (Horowitz *et al.*, 1984; Pendrys, 1990). The tooth surface fluorosis index (Horowitz *et al.*, 1984) attempts to combine elements from Dean's and Thylstrup and Fejerskov's classifications, but has the aim primarily of recording cosmetic appearance (the teeth are not cleaned and dried). As we are dealing with porosity of enamel, such an approach will not record the early biological effects of fluoride so precisely. The fluorosis risk index (Pendrys, 1990) relates the risk of dental fluorosis to the timing of tooth development and may be used to address the time at which fluoride exposure occurred.

Pathogenesis of dental fluorosis

Until the 1970s it was generally assumed that fluoride caused dental fluorosis by interfering with the process of enamel matrix formation and mineralization and that the secretory ameloblast was highly sensitive to slightly elevated plasma concentrations of fluoride. However, microscopic studies of human enamel (Fejerskov *et al.*, 1974, 1975) showed that enamel fluorosis was a hypomineralization of the enamel in an otherwise normal enamel maturation. Therefore, it was suggested that fluoride predominantly affected enamel by retarding the processes of pre-eruptive enamel maturation (Fejerskov *et al.*, 1977). Moreover, the studies showed that enamel pits resulted from mechanical damage to the enamel after eruption of the tooth (Baelum *et al.*, 1986; Fejerskov *et al.*, 1988).

To test the hypothesis that dental fluorosis might be a result of fluoride delaying otherwise normal enamel maturation, Richards and co-workers (Andersen *et al.*, 1986; Richards *et al.*, 1986) conducted a series of experiments in domestic pigs which clearly showed that fluoride given systemically during enamel maturation only, in dosages comparable to those in humans, would result in subsurface hypomineralized enamel at the time of eruption. How fluoride ingested in just slightly elevated concentrations over several years can influence enamel maturation at the time of pre-eruptive maturation is still unknown.

It should be understood that once the full width of enamel has been laid down the enamel is far from fully mineralized. The transformation of soft, protein-rich enamel into highly mineralized, hard, mature enamel is a result of growth in size of the already seeded crystals. Once a matrix has been laid down the apatite crystals are instan-

taneously seeded and mineral increase occurs as a result of appositional growth of the crystals. In rats it has been calculated that the enamel contains only about 18–20% of mineral after being fully formed (for review see Smith & Ekstrand, 1996). Following this, the enamel matrix proteins have to be broken down and removed from the enamel while calcium and phosphates have to be simultaneously transported into the enamel and allowed to precipitate onto the growing crystal surfaces. The hydroxylapatite crystals grow until the enamel contains about 96% mineral by weight. Enamel crystals grow very slowly and pre-eruptive enamel maturation may last for several years in humans. Despite extensive studies on normal enamel maturation in experimental animals, the processes leading to a fully mineralized enamel are far from understood. Therefore, it is speculative how fluoride in small elevated dosages in plasma may interfere with the processes.

In a review, Aoba and Fejerskov (2002) discussed in depth the various possibilities for how fluoride ions may influence enamel mineralization during tooth development. Enamel mineralization is highly sensitive to free fluoride ions promoting the hydrolysis of acidic precursors to apatite formation such as octacalcium phosphate. This results in precipitation of fluoridated apatite crystals.

Based on the evidence available at present, it seems likely that a slight excess of fluoride ion affects the rates at which enamel matrix proteins break down and/or the rates at which the by-products from this degradation are withdrawn from the maturing enamel. In principle, any interference with enamel matrix removal could retard crystal growth throughout the long-lasting maturation and would result in different magnitudes of enamel hypomineralization at the time of tooth eruption. Fluoride does not, at micromolar levels, affect the proliferation and differentiation of enamel organ cells. Nor does it seem to affect the production and secretion of enamel matrix proteins and proteases within the fluoride dose range that causes dental fluorosis in humans. However, fluoride may modulate the kinetics of enzymic degradation of the matrix proteins in the extracellular environment and may indirectly interfere with protease activities by decreasing the free calcium ion concentration in the mineralizing environment.

Fluoride dose and dental fluorosis

It is remarkable that Dean's original data showed that the toxic effects of fluoride on dental enamel were manifest even in communities exposed to concentrations of fluoride below 1 ppm. Thus, the claim that water fluoride concentrations around 1 ppm are 'of no public health significance' was for Dean not synonymous with saying that no dental fluorosis occurs in such populations.

In general, any pharmaceutical product should be prescribed in relation to the body weight of the individual, but this has not been easy for fluoride-delivery systems. This has

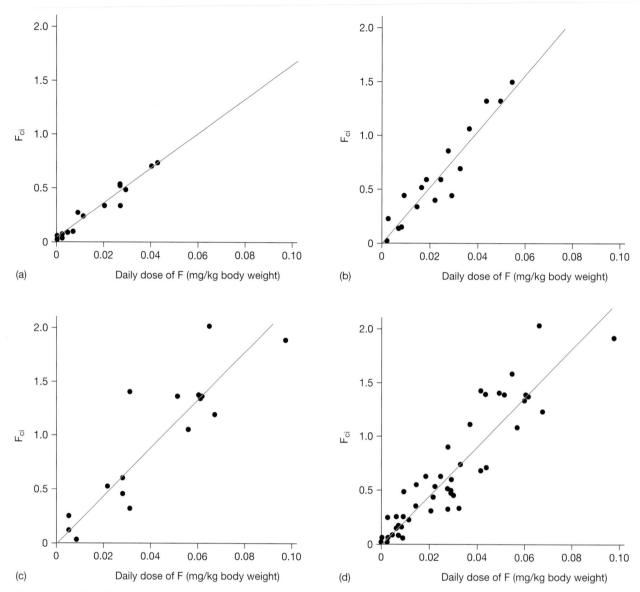

Figure 18.22 Relationship between F_{ci} and daily fluoride dose pooling data. [Sources: (a) Dean *et al.*, 1941, 1942; (b) Butler *et al.*, 1985; (c, d) Richards *et al.*, 1967. All data sets pooled as presented by Fejerskov *et al.*, 1990, 1994.]

made attempts to produce valid estimates of a dose–response relationship between fluoride ingestion and dental fluorosis difficult. An accurate estimate of fluorosis severity can only be made in children when the permanent dentition erupts, hence there is a considerable time lag between the fluoride exposure during tooth formation and the measurement of the effect. In addition, no firm agreement exists as to how much fluoride is actually ingested from foods (Taves, 1983). The bioavailability of fluoride once ingested is relatively uncertain since the fluoride compound in question and the content of the stomach will determine the relative absorption of fluoride by the organism.

However, despite all these difficulties, it is highly relevant to make use of the epidemiological studies throughout the world which have shown a positive relationship between

the water fluoride content and severity of dental fluorosis (Dean, 1942; Richards *et al.*, 1967; Thylstrup & Fejerskov, 1978; Butler *et al.*, 1985; Manji *et al.*, 1986; Larsen *et al.*, 1987). In an attempt to derive an estimate of average water intake, daily consumption of water was related to air temperature and an equation was developed that could describe the average water intake in relation to body weight for children as a function of air temperature (Galagan, 1953; Galagan & Lamson, 1953; Galagan & Vermillion, 1957). For details on how to use these equations and calculate daily dose of fluoride from drinking water, fluoride tablets, etc., the reader is referred to a detailed text by Fejerskov *et al.* (1996). When data from three large American epidemiological surveys conducted in the 1940s, 1960s and 1980s are presented in such a way that the relationship between the average fluorosis score and daily fluoride dose is calculated, a clear dose–response relationship is observed (Fig. 18.22). It can be seen that:

- Regardless of the source of the data, the regression of the amount of fluorosis in a community on the daily dose of fluoride from drinking water clearly demonstrates that even with very low fluoride intake from water a certain level of dental fluorosis will be found.
- The dose–response relationship is clearly linear and the data indicate that for every increase in the dose of 0.01 mg F/kg body weight an increase in dental fluorosis in a population can be anticipated. Thus, there exists no 'critical' value for the fluoride intake below which the effect on dental enamel will not be manifest.
- When the data originating from three distinctly different generations in the USA, and hence very different exposures to diet, commodities and fluoride-containing dental products, are examined, there is no indication that the additional sources of fluoride occurring during the latter half of the twentieth century have led to an upward shift of the dose–response curve.

When these data are kept in mind it is to be expected that whenever more fluoride is ingested during tooth development, in whatever form, both the prevalence and severity of dental fluorosis in a population will increase. Such an increase is not to be blamed, for example, on the fluoride content per se in toothpastes, but is a simple reflection that dental fluorosis is a result of the total intake of fluorides during tooth development, irrespective of the source of the fluoride. The consequence of this is that if the water in any given area contains above 0.5 ppm F it is not acceptable uncritically to add further fluoride for systemic use in such a population (e.g. salt). Furthermore, the estimation of an 'optimal fluoride concentration' based on daily temperature seems not to be valid for tropical regions when additional fluids are consumed and higher daily fluoride intake is estimated (Lima & Cury, 2003).

Calculations of this type are useful, for example, when interpreting the effect of giving fluoride tablets to a population. If such dose–response curves are generated it is possible to predict the subsequent level of fluorosis. Thus, when considering the effect of different fluoride tablet dose regimens in the USA (Aasenden & Peebles, 1974) and Sweden (Granath *et al.*, 1985) it is apparent that had these dose–response curves been generated at the time when the fluoride tablets regimens were developed, it would have been possible to predict the level of fluorosis that would be the outcome of such tablet regimens many years later.

It is also important to understand that, if we assume a constant dose of fluoride, the effects of fluoride are cumulative and hence the longer teeth mineralize the more severe the fluorosis. In Fig. 18.23, which shows data from a very low-fluoride area (Larsen *et al.*, 1985a), the highest prevalence and severity of fluorosis is seen in the second molar teeth, while the prevalence and severity in earlier erupting first molars is much lower.

Figure 18.22 shows the linear relationship between daily fluoride dose and fluorosis prevalence, over the dose range 0–0.1 mg/kg body weight. Therefore, even very low levels of fluoride ingestion (0.02 mg F/kg body weight) constitute a small risk of fluorosis. Ingestion of 0.1 mg F/kg body weight per day would almost certainly result in a significant risk of developing the more aesthetically compromising forms.

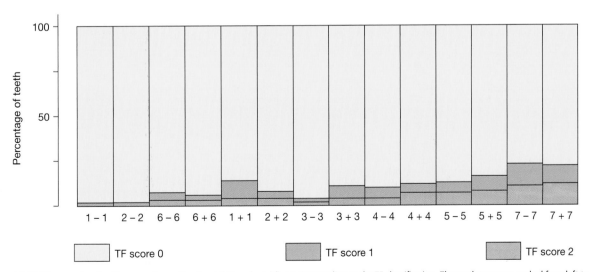

Figure 18.23 Diagram showing the percentage of teeth exhibiting dental fluorosis according to the TF classification. The tooth types are ranked from left to right in the order of mineralization. The data originate from children born and raised in an area of Denmark with less than 0.1 ppm F in the drinking water. (Source: Larsen *et al.*, 1985a.) + Indicates maxillary teeth, − indicates mandibular teeth.

There is only risk of developing dental fluorosis when the dentition is developing, and for upper central incisors the risk is considered to be greatest for children between the ages of 15 and 30 months (Evans & Stamm, 1991). This is in accordance with data from Richards *et al.* (1986) suggesting that dental fluorosis in humans results predominantly from a disturbance of enamel maturation. Although the weight of young children is highly variable, a 2-year-old child might be expected to weigh approximately 12 kg. One can therefore estimate that a fluoride ingestion of 1.2 mg/day would constitute a very high risk of developing aesthetically compromising forms of fluorosis for a 2-year-old. As infants grow older and heavier, the risk of fluorosis moves to the more posterior teeth and because of the greater body weight the dose of fluoride required to be ingested is greater. For example, a 5–6-year-old weighing approximately 20 kg would need to ingest approximately 2.0 mg. It should be remembered that the steady-state level of fluoride in plasma will increase with age, so a child who has been exposed to fluoride since birth is likely to be more at risk than a child of the same weight who has not been exposed for their whole life.

Calculations of fluoride ingestion, although useful, are subject to many errors and must be treated with caution. Figure 18.24 shows the amounts of toothpaste (g) required to be ingested to constitute an intake of 0.1 mg F/kg body weight for 12 and 20 kg children. Covering the head of a child's toothbrush would constitute an application of approximately 0.5–1 g of paste and for a standard-head toothbrush it would be approximately 1–1.5 g of paste. It can be seen therefore that children brushing twice daily may be in contact with sufficient fluoride to constitute a risk of dental fluorosis, particularly when using toothpastes

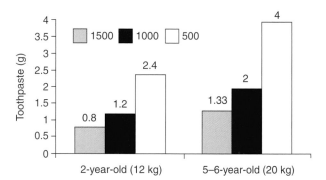

Figure 18.24 Daily amounts of toothpaste (g) required to be ingested to constitute an intake of 0.1 mg F/kg for 12 and 20 kg children for three different fluoride levels in toothpaste (1500, 1000 and 500 ppm F).

containing the higher levels of fluoride. However, children do not generally swallow all the toothpaste applied to the toothbrush. Young children tend to swallow a greater percentage of toothpaste than older ones (Levy, 1993), with 2-year-olds swallowing on average half the toothpaste used and 6-year-olds swallowing one-quarter (Tables 18.2, 18.3). Therefore, on average, the amounts shown in Fig. 18.24 should be multiplied by factors of 2 and 4 for the 2- and 5–6-year-old children, respectively.

In addition, the amount of fluoride absorbed from ingested toothpaste will depend on the gastric content at time of ingestion. Tooth brushing is usually conducted after meals, and this can significantly reduce fluoride bioavailability. Fluoride bioavailability from a 1100 ppm toothpaste ingested after eating can be very similar to that of a 550 ppm toothpaste ingested on fasting (Fig. 18.25).

Tables 18.2 and 18.4 show that the amount of toothpaste children use is fairly consistent between the ages of 2 and

Table 18.2 Amount of dentifrice used per brushing (g) or fluoride per brushing 9(mg)[a] by age

	Age range (years)						
Study	2–3	4	5	6–7	8–10	11–13	16–35
Ericsson & Forsman (1969)[b]		0.45		0.45			
Hargreaves et al. 1972)[c]			0.38			1.10	
Barnhart et al. (1974)[b]	0.86			0.94			1.39
Glass et al. (1975)[b]					1.04[d]		
Dowell (1981)[c]	0.55						
Bruun & Thylstrup (1988)[c]	0.55[d]			0.75[d]	1.10[d]		1.55[d]
Simard et al. (1989)[b]	0.46	0.78	0.65				
Naccache et al. (1990)[b]	0.50		0.47				
Naccache et al. (1992)[b]	0.55	0.45	0.52	0.50			
Mean value	**0.58**	**0.56**	**0.50**	**0.66**	**1.07**	**1.10**	**1.5**
(no. of studies)	(6)	(3)	(4)	(4)	(3)	(1)	(2)

Source: Richards & Banting (1996).

[a] If one assumes that the dentifrice contains 0.1% (1000 ppm), then the ingestion of *x* grams of dentifrice results in the ingestion of *x* mg of fluoride.

[b] Supervised dentifrice use study.

[c] Home use study.

[d] No attempt was made to control for spillage of dentifrice.

Table 18.3 Per cent ingestion of dentifrice fluoride by age

| | Age range (years) | | | | | | |
Study	2–3	4	5	6–7	8–10	11–13	16–35
Ericsson & Forsman (1969)[a]		30		26			
Hargreaves *et al.* (1972)[b]			28				
Barnhart *et al.* (1974)[a]	35			14		6	3
Glass *et al.* (1975)[a]					12[c]		
Simard *et al.* (1989)[a]	59	48	34				
Naccache *et al.* (1990)[a]	41		30				
Naccache *et al.* (1992)[a]	57	49	42	34			
Mean value	**48**	**42**	**34**	**25**	**12**	**6**	**3**
(no. of studies)	(6)	(3)	(4)	(3)	(1)	(1)	(1)

Source: Richards & Banting (1996).
[a] Supervised dentifrice use study.
[b] Home use study.
[c] No attempt was made to control for spillage of dentifrice.

Table 18.4 Estimated median weights of children (source: Documenta Geigy, 1975) and fluoride intake according to age estimated from twice daily use of a 1000 ppm F toothpaste (source: Granath *et al.*, 1985)

Age	Median weight of child (kg)	Toothpaste use per day (g)	Toothpaste ingested (%)	Fluoride intake (mg F/kg for 1000 pm F toothpaste)
2	11.9	1.16	48	0.047
3	14.3	1.16	48	0.039
4	16.3	1.12	42	0.029
5	18.3	1.00	34	0.019
6	20.6	1.32	25	0.013

Source: Fejerskov *et al.* (1996).

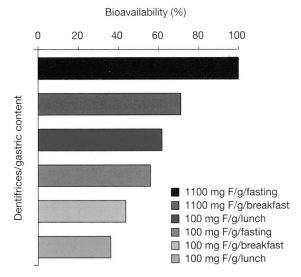

Figure 18.25 Bioavailabity of fluoride ingested from dentifrices, depending on the content of the stomach. (Source: Cury *et al.*, 2005.)

7 years. This has important consequences for fluorosis risk. Young children not only swallow more toothpaste and are often not supervised when brushing, but also are at greater risk of fluorosis as their body weight is lower than the older children. Therefore, particular caution must be exercised when using fluoride toothpaste in the youngest children; small (pea-sized) amounts must be used and children should be encouraged to spit out the waste toothpaste slurry as efficiently as possible (Bentley *et al.*, 1997, 1999).

Although the quantity of fluoride swallowed from toothpaste is not as high as often anticipated, fluoride in toothpaste will add to an increase in overall fluoride consumption and hence increase the risk of developing more fluorosis in populations living in areas with fluoride in the drinking water or using other forms of fluoride such as tablets or salt. Young children should therefore certainly be discouraged from eating toothpaste and care should be taken in using toothpastes containing the higher levels of fluoride (1000–1500 ppm) if multiple fluoride exposures are occurring in a population. Particular care is needed in regions with fluoridated drinking water as there are now a number of studies reporting a relationship between fluoride ingestion from toothpaste and milder forms of dental fluorosis in these areas (Osuji *et al.*, 1988; Pendrys & Katz, 1989; Milsom & Mitropoulos, 1990; Riordan, 1993; Ellwood & O'Mullane, 1995; Pendrys, 1995, 2000; Pendrys *et al.*, 1996; Rock & Sabieha, 1997).

Current methods of fluoride delivery

One of the main reasons for the success of fluoride has been the ease and the variety of ways that it can be administered. The addition of fluoride to water and salt ensures that regular application can be achieved with little or no individual effort. Fluoride can also be readily formulated to produce oral care products providing a range of benefits that become an integral part of the daily hygiene routine. Professionally applied fluoride products can be applied with minimum of patient co-operation and can be timed to coincide with routine dental check-ups or school visits by a community dentist or nurse.

Although the methods of fluoride delivery can be divided into systemic (water, supplements, milk and salt) and topical (toothpaste, gels, varnishes, paint-on applications and mouthrinses), this division is at best arbitrary. There is now strong evidence to suggest that the primary mode of action of fluoride, whether delivered systemically or topically, is the result of its topical activity in the oral cavity (see Chapter 12) and there is little direct benefit from swallowing fluoride. In any of these methods, the primary action of fluoride interfering with the demineralization and re-mineralization process is achieved by the presence of fluoride in the right amount, in the right place and at the right time.

It is also important to understand that there is no homeostatic mechanism to maintain the fluoride concentration in any part of the body and regular exposure of fluoride, either systemical or topical, is required to maintain its concentration in the oral environment and particularly the dental plaque (biofilm). Table 18.5 shows that 2 months after the interruption of water fluoridation, the concentration of fluoride in dental biofilm decreased 16-fold in comparison to when fluoridated water was being regularly ingested. Two months after water fluoridation was restarted the fluoride concentration in dental plaque came back to levels seen before the interruption of fluoridation. The same principle and the need for regular application applies to methods based on topical application, such as dentifrices, solutions or gels (Paes Leme *et al.*, 2004).

Table 18.5 Fluoride concentration in dental plaque from schoolchildren according to the status of water fluoridation (Piracicaba, SP, Brazil, 1986–1987)

Condition of water fluoridation	μg F$^-$/g biofilm wet weight
Fluoridated (0.8 ppm F)	3.2 $\pm$ 1.8
Interrupted (0.06 ppm F)	0.2 $\pm$ 0.09
Refluoridated (0.7 ppm F)*	2.6 $\pm$ 1.9

From Nobre dos Santos & Cury (1988; *unpublished data).

As explained in Chapter 12, dissolution of hydroxyapatite occurs when the pH drops below 5.5. However, if the pH is higher than about 4.5, when fluoride is available at low concentrations, fluorhydroxyapatite may form in the surface layers while hydroxyapatite dissolves in the subsurface enamel, reducing dental demineralization. When the pH rises again above 5.5, fluoride enhances enamel–dentin remineralization. Fluoride therefore provides benefits in terms of reducing demineralization at a lower pH and promoting remineralization at higher pH. In both phenomena, a less soluble mineral is generated and further dissolution may be inhibited.

When fluoride is available in the saliva at higher concentrations (>100 ppm), fluoride reacts with calcium on the tooth surface and in the dental biofilm to form calcium fluoride. The formation of this product is dependent on the fluoride concentration used and it acts as a local reservoir of fluoride, which will later dissolve releasing the ion to interfere with the caries process (see Chapter 12). The rate of calcium fluoride dissolution is increased when the pH falls, coincidentally when the fluoride is most needed. Thus, it can be seen why professional products of high fluoride concentration do not need to be used frequently, whereas those of lower concentration, but used regularly, such as toothpastes, are so important in patients at risk for caries due to frequent acidogenic episodes.

If it is accepted that the primary benefit of fluoride is topical, the distinction between systemic and topical methods of delivering fluoride may not be helpful. An alternative way of classifying the various fluoride delivery systems is to consider community, self-applied and professional methods of application. Community would include those methods introduced on a population basis, such as water, milk and salt fluoridation. Self-applied includes methods used by individuals at home such as toothpaste and mouthrinses. Professional methods of application include those delivered by health-care professionals in the dental office or other settings such as schools. These include methods such as varnishes and gels. However, as with many classification systems there is some overlap, such as the provision of free fluoride toothpastes in community-based schemes or schools.

Before discussing each of these methods in detail it is perhaps important to consider the strengths and weaknesses of the basis of any such recommendations, the human clinical trial.

General considerations when interpreting caries clinical trials

Percentage reductions in caries or caries increment are usually calculated as:

$$\frac{\mathrm{DMF_{control}} - \mathrm{DMF_{test}} \times 100}{\mathrm{DMF_{control}}}$$

In some reports the differences are divided by the increment in the test group, which usually inflates the percentage differences reported. Care must be used when interpreting percentage reductions as the clinical significance of such differences clearly depends on the underlying caries incidence. The estimate of efficacy most widely used in clinical trials of oral care products is the increment. This is the difference in caries scores (DMFS, DFS, DMFT, DFT, etc.) between baseline and the end of the study.

Great care is needed in interpreting the statistical and clinical significance of any data. Large studies may produce statistically significant differences that may be of no clinical importance. Conversely, small or poorly conducted studies may have insufficient statistical power to detect clinically meaningful differences.

Many of the early studies conducted were not double blind, and randomization might have been poor or even based on schools or areas rather than subjects. In some cases group baseline imbalance for risk factors such as caries levels or age may have been present. Studies often did not report the procedures used adequately, particularly in relation to diagnostic methods and calibration of examiners. Poor reporting of drop-outs from a study meant that their potential impact was difficult to interpret. Since the 1990s, the standard of clinical trials conducted in dentistry has improved enormously as the concept of the randomized controlled trial has become better understood.

A particular problem when assessing any intervention is reporting bias. Many clinical studies were conducted to support license applications and marketing claims. It is likely, therefore, that some clinical studies were not reported in the scientific literature, as differences were smaller than expected or not statistically significant. This underreporting would tend to inflate the efficacy of the products when published clinical trials are reviewed as a whole.

Clinical trials can be divided into two broad groups, experimental (proof of concept) and community studies. In experimental studies the design is developed to test the hypothesis that under the conditions specified for the use of the product, one product is better than or equivalent to another. As many variables in the study design as possible are controlled to maximize the ability to detect the differences expected. For example, many studies comparing toothpastes were conducted using supervised brushing regimens in schools using high caries risk populations. In contrast, a community-based study will assess how well a product performs under real-life conditions. For example, if product use is not supervised and for some reason (such as poor taste) is not used regularly, its benefits are unlikely to be demonstrated.

These concepts can be expanded by consideration of the efficacy and effectiveness in relation to an oral care product.

- *Efficacy* is the extent to which a specific intervention, procedure, regimen or service produces a beneficial result under ideal conditions. Ideally, efficacy is determined based on the results of a randomized controlled trial.
- *Effectiveness* is a measure of the extent to which a specific intervention, procedure, regimen or service, when deployed in the field in routine circumstances, does what it is intended to do for a specified population.

When used under ideal conditions a product may be efficacious, but if those conditions cannot be met in real life, the expected benefits are unlikely to be translated into meaningful differences and the product cannot be considered effective. Cost-effectiveness and efficiency must also be considered when assessing the benefits of any product. Efforts should be made to make the best use of resources to obtain the best value for the money.

Community-based fluoride interventions

The main community-based fluoride interventions are based on the addition of small quantities of fluoride to water, milk and salt. As public health measures they can achieve widespread penetration into a population and require little or no individual effort. Their main disadvantage is that fluoride is inevitably ingested and hence mild forms of fluorosis may be prevalent.

Water fluoridation

Fluoride is widely dispersed in the environment and occurs naturally in water supplies, usually at very low concentrations (0.1–1.0 mgF/l) (Smith & Ekstrand, 1996). Following the success of studies that artificially added fluoride to water supplies in the USA, schemes were implemented and evaluated in many parts of the world. Currently, more than 30 countries and over 250 million people participate in water fluoridation programs in countries that include the USA, Canada, the UK, Ireland, Brazil, Australia and New Zealand. In Ireland and Brazil fluoridation is mandatory, but by far the greatest number of individuals receiving fluoridated drinking water live in the USA, that is, more than 50% of the population (Brunelle & Carlos, 1990). In addition to fluoridating the domestic water supply, studies have been conducted to investigate the feasibility and efficacy of fluoridating school water supplies, but these are much less cost-effective (Heifetz et al., 1983). Unfortunately, in many countries with high levels of dental caries and poor access to dental services, such as in Asia, Africa and South America, the infrastructure is often not developed sufficiently to facilitate cost-effective fluoridation programs. Alternatives such as toothpaste may be too costly to provide a realistic alternative.

Although the quality of data is highly variable, there are over 100 reports from more than 23 countries, considering both children and adults, to support the caries-reducing effects of water fluoridation. More than 60 studies present data for the deciduous and over 80 for the permanent dentitions (Murray et al., 1991).

Studies considering the effectiveness of water fluoridation can be divided into two types, self-controlled and controlled. In self-controlled studies, caries prevalence is compared retrospectively to caries levels before fluoridation was introduced. In controlled studies, a fluoridated area is compared to a similar area in which water fluoridation has not been implemented. Ideally, in the latter case, it should be established that before fluoridation was introduced caries levels were similar at the two sites. Self-controlled studies may be difficult to interpret as they do not take account of any changes in caries experience that can be attributed to factors other than water fluoridation, such as increased availability of other forms of fluoride. Hence, caries reductions may be overestimated if there is a concurrent reduction in caries experience in the population as a whole. In *controlled* studies it is possible that changes in populations may occur that are independent of water fluoridation, such as a population migration.

A potential problem with self-controlled studies is illustrated in Fig. 18.26, which shows data from three Danish communities. Vordingborg had fluoride in the drinking water at an average level of 1.2 ppm F and for the 7-year-old children over the period 1973–1980 the mean caries experience remained constant at approximately one surface. In contrast, before the introduction of school-based mouthrinse programs and the increased availability of fluoride toothpastes the mean caries experiences in Hvidovre and Ballerup were much higher in 1973 (1.9 and 3.5 DMFS, respectively). By 1980 both communities had similar caries levels to the fluoride community (Thylstrup *et al.*, 1982). However, it should also be noted that the data are derived from health statistics, and changes in treatment decisions, diagnostic criteria, etc., may also have contributed to the dramatic shift in DMFS from 1972 to 1975.

Most water-fluoridation studies have suffered from a lack of examiner 'blinding', as the residence of the participants was often known and this could introduce bias. To try to overcome this problem some studies have transported participants to a central location for examination (Milsom & Mitropoulos, 1990), but even under these conditions the examiner may be influenced by the presence of fluorosis on the dentition.

Figure 18.27 summarizes the percentage reduction in caries experience from more than 100 studies. In both dentitions the implementation of water fluoridation reduced caries by approximately 50%. For the deciduous dentition the mean percentage reductions were 45% for the controlled studies and 51% for the self-controlled studies. For the permanent dentition they were 50% and 60%, respectively. As might be expected, the self-controlled studies tended to overestimate caries reductions compared with the controlled studies.

It is important to note that the majority of studies were undertaken before 1980. More recent studies suggest that the differences between fluoridated and non-fluoridated communities may be less dramatic, possibly as a result of the widespread use of fluoride toothpaste and other forms of fluoride and an underlying decline in caries experience. For example, in the USA, where less than half the children develop cavities, the difference in caries experience between fluoridated and non-fluoridated areas (Fig. 18.28) was only 18% in 1987 (Brunelle & Carlos, 1990).

If a suitable infrastructure is available in an area with a high incidence and prevalence of disease, water fluoridation is the most cost-effective public health measure to control dental caries. In many parts of the world piped domestic water systems serving large populations are available, so that fluoride can be delivered very cheaply to the majority of a community. Such individuals benefit from the fluoride without any 'active' participation in the intervention and as water is consumed in foods and drinks throughout the day regular applications are made to maximize benefits. Owing to the passive delivery method those individuals who are most difficult to access using other fluoride-delivery methods, usually those with the greatest need, can readily benefit.

Unfortunately, not all water supplies are amenable to cost-effective fluoridation and the strongest reason for its suitability as a public health measure, its 'passive' nature, is also the main reason for its lack of acceptance. Once fluoride is added to the domestic water supply consumers have little choice but to use it, and this has led to strong opposition based on a perception of a lack of freedom of choice. Other problems that have made water fluoridation less appropriate today in many developed parts of the world include the widespread availability of other fluoride-containing products, the possibility of multiple fluoride exposures resulting in an increased risk of fluorosis, the

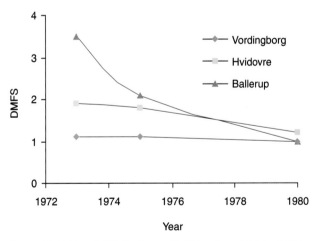

Figure 18.26 Mean DMFS for 7-year-old children from 1973 to 1980 in three Danish communities. Vordingborg is a naturally fluoridated community (1.2 ppm F). (Source: Thylstrup *et al.*, 1982.)

Deciduous dentition

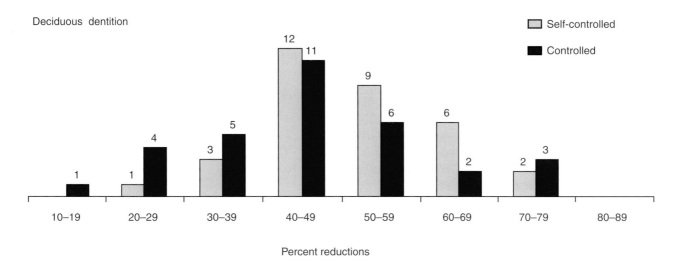

Permanent dentition

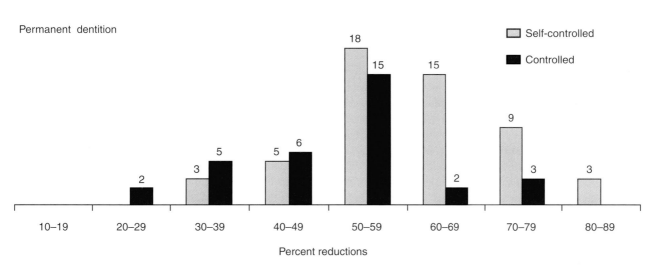

Figure 18.27 Frequency distribution of the percentage reduction in caries experience for self-controlled and controlled studies in the deciduous and permanent dentitions. (Source: Murray *et al.*, 1991.)

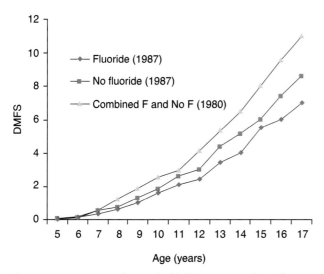

Figure 18.28 Mean DMFS for US schoolchildren in 1980 and 1987 for areas with and without fluoride in the drinking water. (Source: Brunelle & Carlos, 1990.)

variability of domestic water consumption within a community, the operational difficult of each individual water network to keep the fluoride concentration within the 'optimum', a dramatic reduction in caries levels which means that in some cases the risk of fluorosis may outway the benefits, and the knowledge that fluoride need not be ingested to provide substantial benefits.

Unfortunately, many of the pilot schemes initially implemented, such as those in The Netherlands and Finland, although successful in their aim to reduce caries, have been suspended for a variety of political and technical reasons. Although water fluoridation has many problems associated with implementation it still provides the most cost-effective way of solving the caries problem for many communities. However, based on past experience and the current low incidence of disease in many parts of the world, it is unlikely that widespread expansion of water fluoridation programs will occur.

In many parts of the industrialized world it is well documented that the most socially and economically deprived populations have the worst oral health. Water fluoridation is one of the few interventions proven to reduce such oral health inequalities. As fluoridation is a passive fluoride delivery method, individuals in all social strata benefit, but numerically the greatest benefits are seen in those with most disease. Hence, the divide between deprived and non-deprived communities is reduced (Carmichael *et al.*, 1989; Provart & Carmichael, 1995; Riley *et al.*, 1999; Jones & Worthington, 2000). There are several reasons why greater reductions in caries experience may be seen in deprived than in non-deprived communities. First, with similar percentage reductions in caries experience in deprived and non-deprived groups, numerically greater reductions will be seen in those with higher baseline experience. In addition, non-deprived groups tend to have a higher exposure to fluoride from other sources such as fluoride toothpaste and it may be more difficult to see a benefit. However, irrespective of the caries decline in developing countries (Cury *et al.*, 2004; Narvai *et al.*, 2006), water fluoridation alone has not been enough to reduce oral health disparities in countries such as Brazil (Peres *et al.*, 2006).

Salt fluoridation

The idea of adding fluoride to table salt originated in Switzerland following the success of adding iodine to help prevent goiter. This delivery system provides many of the advantages of water fluoridation in that fluoride is delivered in small quantities when food is consumed throughout the day and its use requires little or no modification of the family routine. Unlike water fluoridation, consumers have the choice of buying fluoridated or non-fluoridated salt and hence there is usually relatively little problem with implementation. However, there have been concerns that salt and hence fluoride consumption is quite variable between families, resulting in a risk of fluorosis for those consuming large quantities. In addition, promotion of salt is contrary to other health messages which suggest that its consumption should be reduced to minimize heart disease.

Figure 18.29 shows the caries reductions that occurred in association with the introduction of fluoridated salt in the canton of Glarus. Over approximately 10 years, caries levels reduced by 50%. In comparison, data from the canton of Zurich are presented where a school-based tooth-brushing program with fluoride toothpaste has been carried out since 1963 and a similar, but perhaps less steep, decline can be seen. As with all studies without adequate controls, it is difficult to interpret how much of the decline can be attributed to underlying changes in caries incidence and how much can be attributed to the interventions.

Apart from Switzerland, fluoridated salt has been available in countries such as France, Germany, Costa Rica,

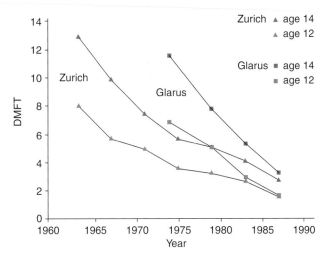

Figure 18.29 Mean DMF teeth per child aged 12 or 14 years in the canton of Zurich, 1963–1987, and in the canton of Glarus, 1974–1987. Glarus uses fluoridated salt in households and bakeries. (Source Marthaler *et al.*, 1988; Steiner *et al.*, 1986, 1989.)

Jamaica, Columbia and Hungary. The fluoride concentration has varied from 90 to 350 mg/kg and the degree of penetration has varied depending on whether it has only been available domestically or has also been used in manufacturing processes such as in bakeries, or in restaurants and schools. The appropriate level of fluoride in salt for a particular community depends on a careful assessment of the expected overall consumption of salt and the expected level of fluoride ingestion from other sources such as toothpaste and drinking water containing natural fluoride.

As with all community-based programs, evaluation of salt fluoridation has been difficult as it is difficult to conduct community randomized controlled double-blind clinical studies with allocation to treatment on an individual level rather than population. Comparing subjects choosing to use salt with those not using it can clearly result in significant bias, and community studies comparing populations in which salt fluoridation is introduced with others without the intervention may also be invalid. Introducing fluoride into one or more communities and comparing this to other populations without salt fluoridation is open to criticism, as it is assumed that all other effects are random between the populations. This is difficult to achieve and validate in this type of study. In addition, effectiveness based on data comparing caries prevalence before and after salt fluoridation was introduced into a population does not take into account the caries decline that has been found, even in developing countries (Cury *et al.*, 2004). Although the weight of evidence suggests that salt fluoridation is effective, with the current emphasis on evidence-based medicine it is mandatory to have better studies conducted so that appropriate data can be provided to document efficacy, efficiency and safety. This is particularly important in this case, given the concerns about potential excessive fluoride ingestion and dental fluorosis and the medical concerns regarding increased salt intake.

Milk fluoridation

Fluoridation of liquid, powdered and long-life milk has been implemented for small groups in some parts of the world, including Eastern Europe, China, the UK and South America (Stephen *et al.*, 1996). It provides both nutritional and anticaries benefits and has the advantage over water fluoridation that it can be targeted directly at segments of a population deemed to be at risk and in which fluoride ingestion can be controlled. Particularly in school-based interventions, the level of fluoride ingestion and the age when it is consumed can be controlled to minimize the risk of fluorosis. The availability of both fluoridated and non-fluoridated milk ensures consumer choice.

Some concerns regarding milk fluoridation have been raised related to both effectiveness of fluoride delivery and the uptake of schemes by different segments of the population. Originally there were concerns that because milk is high in calcium, the fluoride would be inactivated. However, it appears that the majority of fluoride is available in milk up to a concentration of about 5 ppm (Edgar *et al.*, 1992). Fluoride from milk is ultimately absorbed from the alimentary canal, but less quickly than from water (Whitford, 1996).

There are also concerns that some segments of the population choose not to drink milk, and this is particularly true for the lower socioeconomic groups who are most in need (Stamm, 1972). To make milk more widely acceptable, refrigerated milk has been provided in some school-based programs. The cost of providing fluoridated milk has also been raised as a problem, but generally fluoridated milk schemes are implemented where milk schemes already exist. The additional cost of adding fluoride to milk is relatively small, particularly when large quantities are involved. Fluoride fruit juices are an alternative method of fluoride delivery that may be appropriate for warm climates (Gedalia *et al.*, 1981).

Several studies assessing the effectiveness of milk fluoridation schemes have been conducted, but most of these have been poorly designed with flaws including lack of adequate control, high attrition rates and interrupted milk supplies. The educational program that is introduced simultaneously with the distribution of fluoridated milk is a confounding factor that should be taken into account. Well-controlled studies on milk fluoridation are required before this method can be recommended for further implementation.

Self-applied methods of fluoride delivery

Fluoride toothpaste

Preparations for cleaning teeth and protection against oral malodor have been used throughout the ages and are described in early Egyptian, Chinese, Greek and Roman texts. The Romans rubbed their teeth with wool and dentifrices made from burnt stag's horn, animal heads and feet, and they also used pumice mixed with powdered shells of various types. Salt, often mixed with other ingredients, was and still is widely used in many parts of the world as a dentifrice (Fischman, 1992).

It is important to understand that although health-care professionals believe that their patients should use toothpastes for the health benefits they deliver, this is not the reason why most consumers use them. Throughout the ages the most powerful motivation to clean teeth has been the cosmetic benefits related to cleanliness, removal of stains, whiteness and protection against oral malodor (for details see Chapter 15). For most of the population dental caries is important only in so far as it prevents tooth loss and cavities that may affect appearance or result in pain. It is also interesting to note that fluoride up to the level of 1000 or 1500 ppm is considered to be a cosmetic rather than a pharmaceutical product by many governmental regulatory agencies.

Throughout the world fluoride toothpaste is by far the most widely used method of applying fluoride. It is commonly used at home, but has also been used in community and school-based preventive programs. Fluoride toothpastes first became available in 1955 when toothpaste containing 0.4% stannous fluoride was marketed in the USA. Currently, many hundreds of different toothpastes containing fluoride are available.

Over 100 clinical trials of toothpastes of different formulations have been conducted (Clarkson *et al.*, 1993). In the 1960s most of the studies conducted were on toothpastes containing stannous fluoride, but in the 1970s and 1980s interest moved to formulations containing either sodium monofluorophosphate or sodium fluoride (Fig. 18.30).

Most clinical studies comparing fluoride with non-fluoride toothpastes were conducted in the 1960s and 1970s using either sodium monofluorophosphate or stannous fluoride. A wide variety of methods of variable quality was used, and thus any comparisons between studies must be treated with some caution. Figures 18.31 and 18.32 show the results of more than 20 studies lasting for 3 years, all demonstrating significant differences between fluoride test products and non-fluoride controls. Overall, a percentage reduction in caries increment of 25% and a saving of approximately 0.7 carious surfaces per year can be seen. It can also be seen in these figures that there is a wide range in efficacy reported, reflecting differences in study designs, populations and perhaps difficulties in providing clinically effective formulations.

It is often forgotten when comparing the efficacy of various fluoride-delivery systems that the reductions in caries seen with fluoride toothpaste are estimated in relatively short-term trials (2–3 years) and the benefits accrued throughout

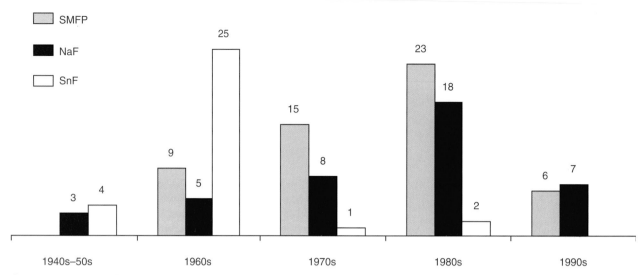

Figure 18.30 Numbers of clinical trials conducted using sodium monofluorophosphate (SMFP), sodium fluoride (NaF) and stannous fluoride (SnF) by decade. (Source: Clarkson *et al.*, 1993.)

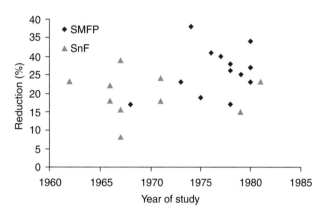

Figure 18.31 Percentage caries reductions per year, for 3-year clinical studies, comparing fluoride (SMFP: sodium monofluorophosphate; SnF: stannous fluoride) and non-fluoride toothpastes. (Source: Clarkson *et al.*, 1993.)

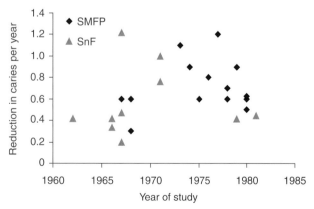

Figure 18.32 Mean caries reductions per year, for 3-year clinical studies, comparing fluoride (SMFP: sodium monofluorophosphate; SnF: stannous fluoride) and non-fluoride toothpastes. (Source: Clarkson *et al.*, 1993.)

a lifetime of exposure may be substantially greater and more likely to mimic water fluoridation (Fejerskov *et al.*, 1981). The efficacy of fluoride toothpastes is now so well documented that it is usually considered unethical to conduct studies using a non-fluoride control toothpaste. Tooth brushing results not only in fluoride delivery, but also in the removal of plaque from the dentition. Modern, well-designed trials are needed to obtain a better understanding of the relative effects of these two benefits, but the efficacy of fluoride alone is well documented from *in situ* studies.

Although fluoride toothpastes have been available for many years, it is only relatively recently that we have gained a clear understanding of the most effective ways they can be used to maximize benefits and minimize risks. As discussed in the following section, the type of toothpaste and the way it is used can have a dramatic effect on anticaries efficacy.

Formulation

The way in which toothpaste is manufactured can have a significant impact on the effectiveness of the product. Some of the earliest fluoride toothpastes were inactive, as they were made with a chalk abrasive that reacted with fluoride to form insoluble calcium fluoride. In some parts of the world toothpastes are still manufactured today using inappropriate combinations of ingredients that result in inactive formulations. It is therefore vital that toothpastes are extensively tested, ideally in human clinical trials, before they are recommended to patients.

A wide variety of fluoride species is used in the manufacture of toothpaste. The two most widely used are sodium fluoride and sodium monofluorophosphate. Stannous fluoride and amine fluoride (Muhlemann *et al.*, 1957) are also available in some parts of the world.

The majority of fluoride toothpastes use sodium mono-fluorophosphate (MFP) as the active ingredient:

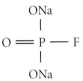

In this form the fluoride is tightly covalently bound and requires enzymic hydrolysis to release fluoride ions (Pearce & Dibdin, 1995):

$$PO_3F^{2-} \cdot + H_2O \rightarrow H_2PO_4^{2-} + F^-$$

However, it is thought that the monofluorophosphate anion may also be incorporated directly into the crystal lattice. The main advantage of this form of fluoride is that it can be combined with chalk-based abrasives to produce cost-effective formulations, widely used in developing countries (Cury *et al.*, 2004).

When sodium fluoride is used as the active ingredient inert abrasives such as silica must be used, as the calcium ions in the chalk-based abrasives react with free fluoride to inactivate the toothpaste. Silica-based formulations tend to be more expensive to produce than the chalk-based alternatives. Recently, silica-based formulations have become more widely used as they enable manufacturers to provide additional benefits such as whitening and gum health by including additional ingredients. Gel toothpastes also enable the formulator to provide a wider range of appearances and color that appeal to consumers.

There is some controversy regarding the comparative anticaries efficacy of sodium fluoride and sodium monofluorophosphate (Bowen, 1995; Volpe *et al.*, 1995). Some authors have claimed superiority for sodium fluoride formulations, whereas others have concluded that they are equivalent. If a difference does exist between these two species it is likely to be of little clinical significance and toothpastes formulated with both fluoride species can be recommended with confidence to patients.

One of the primary determinants of the efficacy of toothpaste is its fluoride concentration. In most of Europe toothpastes are limited to a maximum of 1500 ppm F by the European Cosmetics Directive. In other parts of the world, such as the USA, the fluoride level is restricted to 1000 ppm F in the majority of cases. The amount of fluoride contained within toothpaste can be difficult to ascertain by consumers as the percentage by weight (or volume) of the ingredient is often provided on labeling. The percentages of fluoride by weight are clearly different for sodium fluoride and sodium monofluorophosphate species (Table 18.6).

Labeling of toothpaste for use by children can be a particular problem. Such toothpastes are often flavored and formulated to make them more appealing to children, but

Table 18.6 Percentage by weight of sodium fluoride and sodium monofluorophosphate in toothpastes and the equivalent parts per million fluoride

Fluoride (ppm)	Sodium fluoride (% by weight)	Sodium monofluorophosphate (% by weight)
1500	0.32	1.14
1000	0.22	0.76
500	0.11	0.38

the fluoride concentrations in these pastes can be quite variable. Some manufacturers provide lower levels of fluoride to reduce the risk of excessive fluoride ingestion, whereas others contain the same level of fluoride as in the adult formulations. To help provide more meaningful information to consumers, labeling in parts per million fluoride is now provided by many manufacturers.

As would be expected from our understanding of the cariostatic mechanisms of action (Chapter 12), there is a dose–response relationship between the concentration of fluoride contained in toothpastes and anticaries efficacy. Figure 18.33 shows data from nine clinical studies comparing caries increments over 3–4 years of toothpastes with the same fluoride species at different concentrations. Over the range 1000–2500 ppm F it has been estimated that there is a 6% improvement in efficacy for every 500 ppm increase in fluoride concentration (Stephen *et al.*, 1988). Table 18.7 suggests an average reduction of 8.6% per 500 ppm F for the nine comparisons shown. It is interesting to note in Fig. 18.33 and Table 18.7 that the numerical differences in caries increment are similar even though the baseline prevalences are quite different. Therefore, some of the largest percentage differences are seen at the lower caries incidences, owing to the size of the denominator.

In some parts of the world many children are now using 'low' fluoride toothpaste formulations. For example, in the

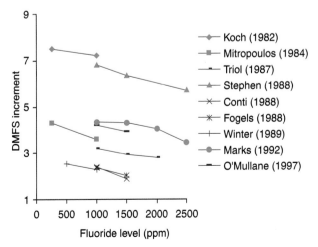

Figure 18.33 Caries increments in 3- and 4-year clinical trials comparing similar toothpastes with different fluoride levels.

Table 18.7 Caries increments and percentage reductions per additional 500 ppm F for studies comparing dentifrices with different fluoride levels

Study	Fluoride (ppm)						Reduction per 500 ppm F	
	250	500	1000	1500	2000	2500	Numeric	%
Koch *et al.* (1982)	7.50		7.20				0.20	3
Mitropolous *et al.* (1984)	4.29		3.61				0.45	10.6
Triol *et al.* (1987)			3.21	2.95			0.26	8.8
				2.95	2.79		0.16	5.4
Stephen *et al.* (1988)			6.80	6.33			0.47	6.9
				6.33		5.71	0.31	4.9
Conti *et al.* (1988)			2.39	1.87			0.52	21.8
Fogels *et al.* (1988)			2.36	2.02			0.34	14.4
Winter *et al.* (1989)		2.52	2.29				0.23	9.1
Marks *et al.* (1992)			4.33	4.27			0.06	1.4
				4.27	4.04		0.23	5.3
					4.04	3.46	0.58	14
O'Mullane *et al.* (1997)			4.19	3.93			0.26	6.2
Mean numeric and percentage reductions per 500 ppm F							0.31	8.6

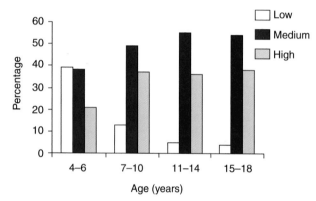

Figure 18.34 Percentages of children using low (<600 ppm), medium (1000 ppm) and high (1450 ppm) fluoride toothpastes by age. (Source: Walker *et al.*, 2000.)

UK, where most drinking water does not contain fluoride, 39% of 4–6-year-old children are reported to be using toothpastes containing less than 600 ppm F (Fig. 18.34). The impact of the increase in availability and use of low-fluoride toothpastes on caries incidence is yet to be seen.

The concept of a clinically significant difference when assessing the results of such studies is clearly subjective. From the above, it can be estimated that lowering or increasing the fluoride level in toothpaste by 500 ppm F would almost certainly result in a small decrease or increase in efficacy over 3 years. However, this difference may be compounded over the lifetime of the individual and this may mean that the difference becomes more important. The community cost of such a change should also be considered; even a 5% decrease or increase in the incidence of caries of a large group could potentially have a massive impact from a public health perspective. It is clear that widespread recommendations to reduce (or increase) fluo-

ride levels in toothpastes should not be conducted without risk and cost-effectiveness analyses of such changes (Ellwood *et al.*, 1998).

For young children, if recommendations are made to reduce the level of fluoride contained within toothpaste to minimize the amount of fluoride ingested and hence fluorosis, the potential benefit will inevitably be reduced. For children at low risk of caries and/or at risk from excessive fluoride intake due to multiple fluoride exposures from water or other products, lower levels of fluoride in toothpaste may be appropriate to help minimize fluoride ingestion. Ultimately, the most appropriate fluoride level to be used in toothpaste for children should be based on a careful risk assessment.

Others would argue that the recommendation of fluoride toothpastes for different age groups and levels of risk is too complicated a message to communicate to the general public and dental health advice should concentrate on ensuring that only small (pea-sized amounts) of conventional toothpaste are used. Dental caries is a multifactorial disease and not just due to insufficient fluoride. Whatever advice is given, it should always be provided with appropriate dietary and oral hygiene advice.

A good example of the provision of toothpaste in a community-based intervention, as an alternative to water, milk or salt fluoridation, is illustrated by a prospective study undertaken in Manchester, UK, in which low- (440 ppm F) and high-fluoride (1450 ppm F) toothpastes were provided by post 'free of charge' to young children from the ages of 12 months to 5–6 years. This study also illustrates the complexity of the problem of providing advice on the use of fluoride toothpastes. The group receiving the 1450 ppm F paste had 16% less caries than a control group who were not provided with toothpaste, but differences between the group receiving the 440 ppm F toothpaste and the controls were not statistically significant (Davies *et al.*, 2002). However, the benefit of the program was also dependent on the deprivation status of the participants. For the most deprived children provision of either a low- or high-fluoride toothpaste provided similar levels of benefit. In the less deprived children only provision of the high-fluoride toothpaste provided a benefit (Ellwood *et al.*, 2004). There was also an association between the use of the high-fluoride toothpaste and fluorosis, with the risk concentrated in the least deprived children. In the most deprived children little fluorosis was seen, whether the children used high- or low-fluoride toothpastes (Tavener *et al.*, 2006).

Although the amount of fluoride ingested by young children must be controlled, there may be a place for toothpastes containing more than 1500 ppm F in high-risk groups such as elderly people, in whom fluorosis is not a problem. Such products are generally only available on prescription or directly from pharmacies as they are classified as medicines in most parts of the world. Toothpastes containing 5000 ppm F or more are available in some parts of the world and if they are used regularly, for limited periods, they will control the rampant forms of caries. In cases when caries is adequately controlled there is no need for universal recommendation of this type of product. During 6 months in a study (Fig. 18.35) conducted in adults, 57% of root-caries lesions became hard in subjects using a 5000 ppm F toothpaste, compared with only 29% for subjects using a 1100 ppm F toothpaste (Baysan *et al.*, 2001), which is again to be expected taking the mechanisms of action of fluoride into account (Chapter 12).

Amount of fluoride applied

The dose of fluoride used is a function of the amount of toothpaste applied and its concentration. There is little evidence to suggest that with normal use the amount (dose) of

fluoride applied is an important determinant of anticaries efficacy. Clinical trials have found little association between the amount of toothpaste used and anticaries efficacy (Ashley *et al.*, 1999), whereas fluoride concentration is an important determinant of plaque fluoride levels and efficacy (Duckworth *et al.*, 1989; Chesters *et al.*, 1992). Fluoride reservoirs in the oral cavity are relatively small compared with the volume of toothpaste applied, and therefore it is the concentration gradient between the toothpaste slurry and the fluoride reservoirs that is responsible for driving in the fluoride.

This has important implications for the way in which dentists should recommend to their patients, particularly children, how they should use fluoride toothpastes. Fluorosis risk is primarily dependent on the overall dose of fluoride ingested, whereas caries benefit appears to be concentration dependent. Therefore, minimizing the amount of paste applied but maximizing its fluoride concentration will maximize anticaries benefit while minimizing the risk of fluorosis. The recommendation for young children to use a pea-sized amount of paste is appropriate.

Brushing frequency and time of application

It is clear from the discussion on the mechanisms of action of fluoride earlier in this chapter that the effectiveness of fluoride is enhanced by maintaining elevated fluoride levels throughout the day through frequent applications of small amounts of fluoride. The association between reported brushing frequency and caries incidence has been considered in a number of clinical studies comparing different toothpaste formulations. Caries increments in 3-year studies were approximately 20–30% greater in subjects brushing once or less a day compared with those brushing twice or more a day (Chesters *et al.*, 1992; O'Mullane *et al.*, 1997; Ashley *et al.*, 1999).

Although such differences are to be expected, they must be treated with some caution. Subjects enrolled in clinical trials comparing different toothpaste formulations or in cross-sectional surveys would not have been randomly assigned to a brushing frequency and data on the reported brushing frequency have been used which may be unreliable. Brushing frequency is strongly linked to other health indicators such as social class and hence to other influences such as dietary intake. The importance of the association of brushing frequency with other oral health behaviors is difficult to quantify, but it is possible that the benefits of more frequent brushing may, to some extent, have been overestimated. The problem is illustrated in Figs 18.36–18.39; for children aged 4–14 years percentage differences in overall caries experience range from 36 to 21% for children brushing twice per day or more and once per day or less. However, there are also percentage differences in caries experience of 15–41% between children of manual and non-manual working parents. As might be expected, the children of

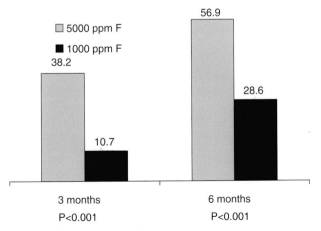

Figure 18.35 Percentage of subjects with one or more root-caries lesions becoming hard after 3 and 6 months for subjects using 5000 and 1000 ppm F toothpastes. (Source: Baysan *et al.*, 2001.)

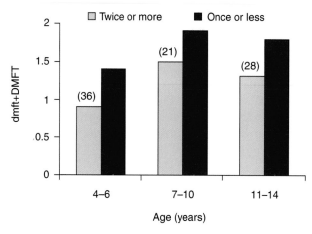

Figure 18.36 Caries experience of children according to brushing frequency per day with percentage difference between groups in parentheses (twice or more and once or less). Sample sizes 350–500 per age group. (Source: Walker *et al.*, 2000.)

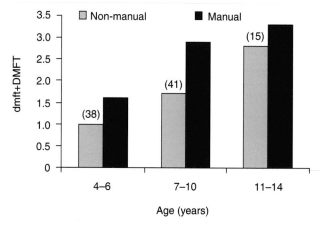

Figure 18.37 Caries experience of children according to social class of head of household with percentage difference between groups in parentheses (manual and non-manual workers). (Source: Walker *et al.*, 2000.)

manual working parents tend to brush less frequently (Fig. 18.38) and also eat more sugary snacks (Fig. 18.39); therefore, disentangling the influence of tooth brushing from the host of other variables influencing caries risk becomes extremely complex. The only way this type of question can be truly resolved is with a randomized controlled clinical trial, but this would mean asking one group of patients to brush less frequently than another which, given the current understanding of fluoride's mechanisms of action, would be unethical. However, given the knowledge of the mechanisms of action of fluoride, the widely accepted guideline that brushing should be conducted at least twice daily would seem appropriate.

The time at which brushing should take place is the subject of some debate (see Chapter 15). It would seem sensible that brushing should take place at mealtimes, when the cariogenic challenge is greatest. Some consider that brushing with fluoride toothpaste should take place before meals, based on the philosophy that the bulk of plaque is reduced by the mechanical action of brushing, so that the cariogenic challenge is minimized and fluoride levels are elevated at the same time as food is taken. However, increased salivation and subsequent eating will clear fluoride quickly; moreover, many people consider that toothpaste interferes with the taste of the food and choose not to brush before meals. Others maintain that fluoride is most beneficial when fluoride is applied directly after eating, so that the concentration is maximized and the fluoride is not flushed so readily from the oral cavity owing to salivary stimulation. It is also well documented that fluoride is less readily absorbed on a full stomach and it is possible that this may help to reduce the risk of fluorosis in young children, as shown in Fig. 18.22.

During sleep, salivary flow levels and buffering capacity are reduced. It is therefore appropriate to brush just before going to bed to reduce the plaque load in the oral cavity and

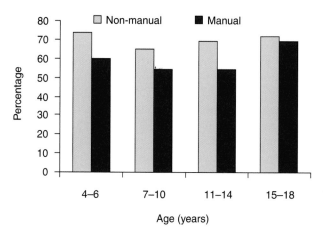

Figure 18.38 Frequency of brushing twice per day or more and social class of head of household. (Source: Walker *et al.*, 2000.)

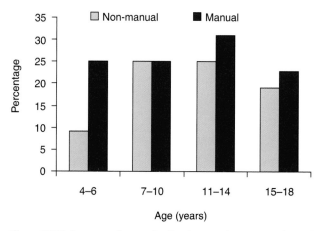

Figure 18.39 Frequency of consuming biscuits more than once per day and social class of head of household. (Source: Walker *et al.*, 2000.)

boost fluoride levels. The reduced flow rate helps to maintain elevated fluoride levels for longer than would be expected during the day. Even these minute elevated levels may significantly impact the ongoing demineralization and remineralization process.

The recommendation to brush just before going to bed and at one other time during the day at a mealtime would seem appropriate in most individuals.

Rinsing behavior

Another important determinant of anticaries efficacy is the method of rinsing used after brushing. Laboratory studies suggest that using larger rather than small volumes of water after brushing results in the removal of significantly more fluoride from the oral reservoirs owing to the concentration gradient effect, and this is probably responsible for the difference in anticaries efficacy (Richards *et al.*, 1988; Duckworth *et al.*, 1991).

The way in which individuals rinse is quite variable: some use a beaker to rinse, some put water on the toothbrush, some use the hand to collect water, while others do not rinse at all. Clinical trials suggest that subjects using a beaker to rinse and hence larger volumes of water have a higher caries risk than those using smaller volumes by using the toothbrush or hand to collect water. Subjects using a beaker to rinse had approximately 20% more caries (Chesters *et al.*, 1992; Sjögren & Birkhed, 1993; O'Mullane *et al.*, 1997) than those using other rinsing methods (Fig. 18.40). However, in another 3-year prospective study of children, representing a high-caries population, rinsing the mouth with a beaker of water after daily supervised toothbrushing at school did not significantly compromise the caries-reducing effect of a fluoride toothpaste (Machiulskiene *et al.*, 2002).

Clinical studies in which some of the participants have been taught to use a small volume of water and the toothpaste slurry left after brushing as a 'mouthrinse' have demonstrated that further reductions in caries are achiev-able. A 26% reduction in the incidence of approximal caries has been claimed for this method (Sjögren *et al.*, 1995).

Overall recommendations for use of fluoride toothpaste

- Use accredited fluoride toothpaste and brush twice daily, before going to bed and at one other time during the day, preferably at a mealtime. Use a small amount of water to remove the waste toothpaste slurry.
- Consider the appropriate fluoride concentration in toothpaste for an individual after assessing potential caries risk and overall fluoride exposure. Consider the use of low-fluoride toothpastes for children with multiple fluoride exposures.
- For young children (6 years or younger), brushing should be supervised and it is important that toothpaste is out of their reach to minimize the risk of children eating toothpaste. When brushing, children should use a very small (pea-sized) amount of paste.

Fluoride tablets

Fluoride tablets were introduced in the late 1940s to try to mimic the 'systemic' fluoride delivery from water fluoridation, and most used sodium fluoride. The dosage was based on an average consumption of 1 liter of water containing 1 ppm F/day, delivering 1 mg of fluoride. However, the toxicity of fluoride, as with other drugs, is related to the dose consumed per kilogram body weight, and the dose prescribed should relate to the weight of the child. Dosing schedules vary throughout the world, but most take into account the weight (age) of the child (Table 18.8).

It was clear more than 20 years ago that fluoride predominantly exerts its cariostatic effect posteruptively (Fejerskov *et al.*, 1981). Hence, ingestion of fluoride provides little if any pre-eruptive effect on caries development, but presents a clear risk of dental fluorosis (Thylstrup *et al.*, 1979). However, many countries still advocate supplements to be taken from birth or shortly afterwards, as recommended by

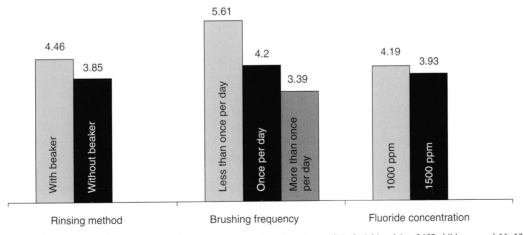

Figure 18.40 Relationship between caries experience and oral hygiene procedures in a 3-year clinical trial involving 3467 children, aged 11–12 years at the start of the study (O'Mullane *et al.*, 1997). All differences were statistically significant ($p < 0.05$).

Table 18.8 Recommended fluoride tablet schedules (mg F/day) for four countries in Europe

	Year of life[a]						
	0–1[a]	1–2	2–3	3–4	4–5	5–6	6+
France	0.25	0.25	0.5	0.5	0.75	0.75	1.0
Switzerland	0.25	0.25	0.5	0.5	0.75	0.75	1.0
Germany	0.25	0.25	0.5	0.75	0.75	0.75	1.0
Austria	0.25	0.25	0.5	0.5	0.75	1.0	1.0

Source: Burt & Marthaler (1996).
[a] In France and Germany it is recommended that intake starts at birth, and in Switzerland and Austria at 6 months.

the American Dental Association in 1958. For example, France and Germany still have dosing schedules starting at birth and Switzerland and Austria start at 6 months (Table 18.8). This clearly demonstrates how slowly some scientific results are transferred into public policy.

Up until quite recently the use of systemic fluoride, particularly in the USA, has not been questioned. Thus, if children were not exposed to fluoride from drinking water having about 1 mg F/l, it was suggested that either the water should be artificially fluoridated or fluoride should be provided in tablets to avoid 'fluoride-deficient teeth', or both. Similarly, in Denmark as in many other countries, as the public would not accept fluoridation of drinking water, fluoride tablets were promoted during the 1970s with the argument that without fluoride the teeth would not develop to be 'pearl-like white and optimally mineralized'. Certainly, in those populations where doctors and dentists followed the recommendations from the National Board of Health children did develop white, opaque teeth as they experienced various degrees of dental fluorosis (Thylstrup et al., 1979; Friis-Hasche et al., 1984). However, a study in which fluoride tablets were originally introduced in a population where artificial water fluoridation had to stop, demonstrated that the only effect of the fluoride tablets was that the children developed obvious signs of dental fluorosis (Kalsbeek et al., 1992).

Moreover, extensive reviews in the 1970s were perhaps uncritical in summarizing the results of efficacy of fluoride supplements (Driscoll, 1974; Binder et al., 1978). Many studies were flawed to an extent that their results were questionable. Selected groups of participants were used, there was often an absence of appropriate controls, many had extensive drop-out of participants during the study period and there were often non-blinded examiners. The weaknesses of these studies are still seen today in those quoted when recommending other types of systemic use of fluoride.

Fluoride supplements are not only produced as tablets (or drops) intended for swallowing, but lozenges intended for chewing and sucking are also available. This is important, as well-designed and well-conducted clinical trials have shown that fluoride supplements provide posteruptive

caries reductions of 20–28% over 3–6 years in school-aged children (DePaola & Lax, 1968; Driscoll et al, 1978). It is likely that slow-dissolution fluoride lozenges can be a method of choice in caries control in certain groups of children, adults and not least elderly people, who may experience a high caries incidence rate. The rationale is that the supplements will help to maintain levels of fluoride in the oral fluids, which will affect caries lesion development and progression (see Chapter 12).

It can therefore be concluded that fluoride supplements used in general public health preventive programs are inappropriate and at present they have limited recommendation even for individual use.

Fluoride rinses

Although mouthrinses containing acidulated phosphate fluoride (APF), stannous fluoride, ammonium fluoride and amine fluoride have been formulated at different concentrations, they are most commonly available as 0.05% NaF (227 ppm F) for daily rinsing and 0.2% NaF (909 ppm F) for weekly rinsing. Typically, 10 ml of the solution is swished around the mouth for 1 min. Clinical trials of both regimens (Figs 18.41, 18.42) demonstrate average caries reductions of approximately 30% (Ripa, 1991). Although the percentage reductions in caries incidence are similar for weekly and daily rinses, the numeric differences in surfaces 'saved' from decay each year are generally higher for the daily rinse regimens, reflecting differences in study populations. In the areas with fluoridated drinking water the number of surfaces 'saved' from decay per year is very much lower, reflecting the lower caries incidence in these populations.

Fluoride mouthrinses have an excellent risk–benefit profile when used correctly. They help to ensure maximal topical exposure while minimizing the risk of fluorosis as little fluoride is ingested. When combining mouthrinsing with other fluoride therapies such as toothpaste it is prudent to use the methods at different times of the day to maximize the overall efficacy (Blinkhorn et al., 1983). Mouthrinsing is not generally recommended for children under the ages of 6 or 7 years because of the possibility that fluoride may be swallowed. As with other fluoride-delivery methods, it is important that the mouthrinse is swished around the mouth to distribute the fluoride effectively. Some care must be taken with many formulations as they may contain high levels of alcohol. Although fairly large quantities of these products must be consumed to risk serious acute toxicity they are packaged and flavored to make them appealing to children and it is important that they are treated with care.

Two studies comparing the daily and weekly regimens reported that both were effective. Although the benefit of daily rinsing was marginally greater than weekly rinsing, the difference was not statistically significant (Driscoll et al., 1982; Heifetz et al., 1982). Weekly rinsing programs

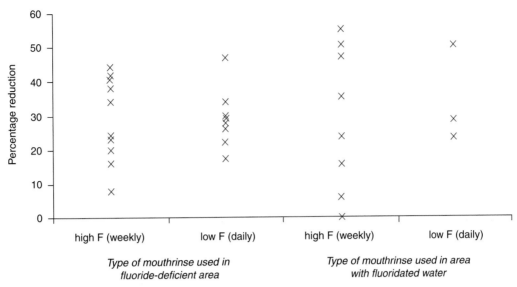

Figure 18.41 Percentage reductions in caries incidence using high-fluoride (900–1000 ppm F) and low-fluoride (200–250 ppm F) mouthrinses in areas with and without fluoride in the drinking water. (Source: Ripa, 1991.)

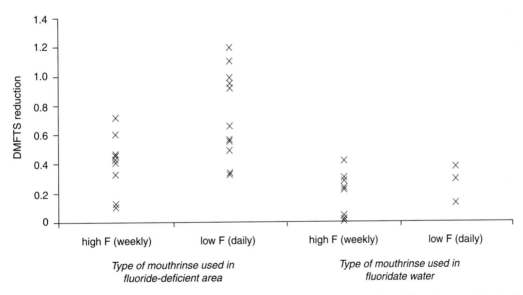

Figure 18.42 DMFS saved per year using high-fluoride (900–1000 ppm F) and low-fluoride (200–250 ppm F) mouthrinses in areas with and without fluoride in the drinking water. (Source: Ripa, 1991.)

have been extensively used in the USA and other parts of the world and are a relatively simple way of targeting fluoride to high-risk groups. They are relatively easy to conduct, well accepted by participants and can be supervised by non-dental personnel. The cost-effectiveness of fluoride mouthrinsing programs clearly depends on the design of the intervention and the caries incidence of the population (Disney *et al.*, 1990). For populations or groups with a high incidence of disease it may be feasible to introduce a cost-effective intervention; however, with a low incidence of disease they are not cost-effective. Hence, in many countries

such as Denmark the regular use of rinsing was stopped during the 1980s.

Fluoride gels and foams

Fluoride gels and foams are available in many parts of the world for self-application. They contain a variety of fluoride levels ranging from similar levels found in mouthrinses to up to 5000 ppm F. Their viscosity makes them easy to apply in trays and excellent fluoride delivery to the dentition is achieved. They are probably equally as effective as their solution counterparts (Horowitz & Doyle, 1971), and the decision to choose one or the other should be made on the basis of cost and ease of use.

Professional fluoride-delivery methods

Fluoride gels

Fluoride gels, foams and solutions containing higher concentrations of fluoride (5000–12 300 ppm F) than those recommended for home use are available for application in the dental office (Ögaard *et al.*, 1994). Some gels are thixotropic so that they flow under pressure and penetrate between the teeth but otherwise remain viscous, aiding retention in trays. To help prevent ingestion it is recommended that the patient sits upright and does not swallow. No more than 2.5 ml of gel per tray should be applied, and custom or properly fitted stock trays with absorptive liners should be used. Suction devices should be used during and after treatment and excess gel removed with gauze. Patients should spit out thoroughly after treatment (LeCompte & Doyle, 1982). The gels are usually recommended to be used twice yearly, but when more severe caries is present they may be used more frequently. Although significant reductions in caries incidence have been achieved using these products (Table 18.9), with the current understanding of cariostatic mechanisms it is hard to justify the use of single infrequent applications of fluoride when the best results for using fluoride are achieved when it is delivered regularly at low doses.

Varnishes

Fluoride varnishes or lacquers have been used in dental office and community programs for over 30 years. They are generally used to provide fluoride delivery to specific at-risk sites or surfaces within the mouth and are usually applied at intervals of 3 or 6 months. They contain high levels of fluoride and are designed to harden on the tooth to aid retention. The most widely used is Duraphat varnish, containing 5% sodium fluoride (22 600 ppm F) in suspension in alcohol with a resin system that sets on contact with saliva. Over 80 studies have been conducted with this product and a meta-analysis (Fig. 18.43) of eight studies

reported a reduction in dental caries of 38% (Helfenstein & Steiner, 1994). It is believed that delivery of high doses of fluoride of this type results in the local formation of calcium fluoride, which can act as a reservoir for the slow release of fluoride (Rolla & Saxegaard, 1990).

Slow-release fluoride

An optimum fluoride-delivery system would be one that supplies small amounts of fluoride throughout the day so that consistent, elevated plaque fluoride levels are maintained with little or no individual effort required. Therefore, not surprisingly there has been considerable interest in methods of releasing fluoride slowly into the oral environment. To be effective the fluoride release has to be constant and sustained and the 'device' must be retained in the mouth without causing damage to soft tissues or becoming loose. Experiments with slow-release glass materials retained on the buccal surface of molar teeth have shown some promise (Toumba & Curzon, 1993), and bioadhesive tablets and other systems have also been evaluated, but there have been significant problems with intraoral retention and maintaining a consistent level of fluoride delivery (ten Cate & van Loveren, 1999).

An alternative approach is to use dental materials to provide fluoride delivery. It is important that addition of fluoride does not compromise the required properties of the restorative material. Materials such as the old silicate restorative materials and glass-ionomer cements contain between 15 and 20% fluoride, and fluoride has also been added to other dental materials such as composite and amalgam (Tveit & Lindh, 1980). These materials could potentially provide a fluoride reservoir to help prevent secondary caries and to prevent or help remineralize caries in adjacent teeth or surfaces (Hatibovic-Kofman *et al.*, 1997). Addition of fluoride to fissure sealants has also been recommended (Vrbic, 1999), but further research is required to demonstrate any additional benefit.

Initially, fluoride release from most methods tends to be high, but it reduces as the available reservoir depletes. Nevertheless, even 1 year after application of a glass-

Table 18.9 Percentage reductions in caries incidence and mean number of carious surfaces saved per year for studies using APF gel topical treatments on the permanent teeth of North American children

Study	No. applications/year	Study duration (years)	DMFS (DFS) saved (n/year)	DMFS (DFS) reduction (%)
Szwejda *et al.* (1967)	1	1	0.04	4
Szwejda (1971)	1	2	0.04	3
Horowitz (1969)	1	2	0.58	22
Horowitz & Doyle (1971)	1	3	0.70	24
Bryan & Williams (1968)	1	1	1.10	28
Ingraham & Williams (1970)	1	2	0.65	41
Cons *et al.* (1970)	1	4	0.23	18
Cobb *et al.* (1980)	2	2	1.44	35
Hagen *et al.* (1985)	2	2	0.66	30

Source: Ripa (1991).

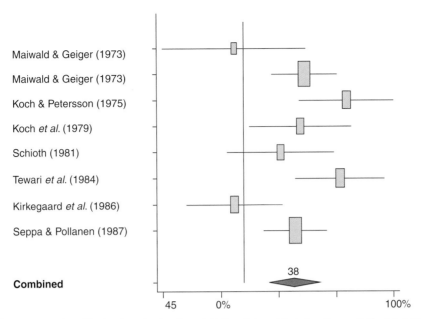

Figure 18.43 Estimates of percentage and combined caries reductions from eight Duraphat varnish studies. (Source: Helfenstein & Steiner, 1994.)

ionomer cement fluoride levels were six times higher than normal in unstimulated saliva (Hatibovic-Kofman & Koch, 1991). It is believed that glass-ionomer cements may act as a reservoir by absorbing fluoride from other sources such as toothpaste and slowly releasing this as fluoride levels diminish in the oral cavity. The extent to which fluoride from different dental materials can provide important therapeutic benefits is open to question and requires further clinical investigation. So far the evidence is lacking.

The future of fluoride delivery?

We are extremely fortunate that many of the methods of fluoride delivery currently available, such as toothpastes, provide a cost-effective method of controlling dental caries. Although dental caries is clearly a multifactorial disease and not due to lack of fluoride, the problems with fluoride generally relate to compliance with appropriate product use, rather than clinical effectiveness. Therefore, there is still a significant research agenda aimed at improving delivery and addressing compliance issues. For example, degradable microspheres are available which adhere to the oral mucosa. These microspheres could be used to release fluoride over time, thus maintaining elevated fluoride concentrations in the oral fluids during periods where pH may be lowered.

One of the unanswered questions in caries and fluoride research is whether the tooth surface has to be free of plaque for the ambient fluoride in the oral cavity to be effective in altering the dynamics of the demineralization and re-mineralization processes. Fluoride does not easily penetrate plaque, but seems to be bound within the matrix of this biofilm (Watson et al., 2005). Therefore, does the mechanical cleaning of the teeth allow plaque-free, caries-active surfaces to be exposed to the relatively high concentrations of fluoride contained in toothpastes, or does the pH drop in the plaque, releasing ionic fluoride from the plaque and/or the tooth surface into the plaque fluid, then enable the fluoride to exert its caries-controlling effect? Perhaps, the future for fluoride and caries research should be focussed on enabling fluoride to penetrate through plaque to the tooth surface. Although plaque is often considered as a well-defined entity, from Chapter 10 it is evident that the age and composition of dental biofilms vary extensively within and between individuals, so there may not be an immediate, easy answer to these apparently simple questions.

Appropriate use of fluoride in caries control

Caries reductions in clinical trials, or clinical studies in general, are usually measured by gross clinical observations of cavitated caries lesions. However, this ignores the fact that before lesions develop to a level where they are cavitated, non-cavitated lesions may have been present for months or even years. It is clear that the conclusion, 'fluoride prevents lesion formation', because a given test group developed fewer cavitated lesions during the test period, does not tell the whole story (Chesters et al., 2002; Nyvad et al., 2003). Fewer lesions have become cavitated, but this is because fluoride interferes with lesion development to the extent that the lesion progression rate has been controlled or even arrested. Elevated levels of fluoride in the oral environment are sufficient to interfere with the demineralization and remineralization processes (see Chapter 12). In this light, fluoride can be seen as an active chemical treatment for caries lesions rather than a preventive measure. Once this is understood, fluoride can be used appropriately as a therapeutic agent that reduces the rate of demineralization and enhances mineral uptake whenever pH drops below a level where plaque fluid is undersaturated with respect to hydroxyapatite. This may happen several times during the day and therefore fluoride has to be present when these events occur. Therefore, when this is appreciated it is understandable why we prefer to talk about 'caries control' rather than prevention, because what fluoride does is to interfere with the dynamics of lesion development and hence control the speed of lesion progression.

Maybe one of the best examples of the importance of this way of interpreting how fluoride controls lesion development can be seen from a re-examination of the data originally developed in the 1950s during a water-fluoridation study (Tiel/Culembourg) in Holland (Backer-Dirks, 1967). It was fortunate that, although at the time the data were not presented, the examiners not only recorded cavitated caries lesions, but also included the earlier, non-cavitated stages. Groeneveld et al. (1990) examined these data, and it can be seen from Figure 18.44 that the above reflections are certainly supported. When lesions are measured as cavities, the well-known 50% reduction in caries experience is seen between the test and control populations. However, when all preceding stages of lesion development, i.e. the non-cavitated lesions, were also recorded there was practically no difference between the two populations. This means that in the water-fluoridated populations the caries challenge was certainly present, but owing to the elevated con-

centrations of fluoride in the environment, only about 50% of the lesions progressed to a stage of cavitation during the test period, whereas the remaining lesions either did not progress at all or progressed very slowly. That this interpretation of data from an observational study may indeed be correct has recently been demonstrated in a very elegantly designed and analyzed controlled clinical trial in Lithuania (Nyvad et al., 2003; Baelum et al., 2003).

These data strongly support fluoride as a therapeutic agent that controls the rate of caries lesion development. Moreover, with this knowledge in mind, it is understandable why children born and raised in an area with about 1.0–1.2 mg F/l in the water supply may have fewer cavitated lesions than contemporary children from low-fluoride areas, but as soon as children in such areas with higher fluoride move to low-fluoride areas later in life they may be seen to develop a caries progression rate similar to those in the low-fluoride area. In other words, fluoride incorporated into the teeth during development does not in and of itself result in 'an increased resistance of the tooth towards caries'.

With the above knowledge in mind, fluoride can be optimized as a therapeutic agent by choosing a regimen that ensures low fluoride concentrations to be present at high frequency in the oral cavity (e.g. fluoride in the water supply and/or regular tooth brushing with fluoride toothpaste). Public health delivery systems will usually have to rely on modes where systemic absorption is inevitable, such as drinking water. These modes of delivery are easily the most cost-effective means of providing fluoride to large

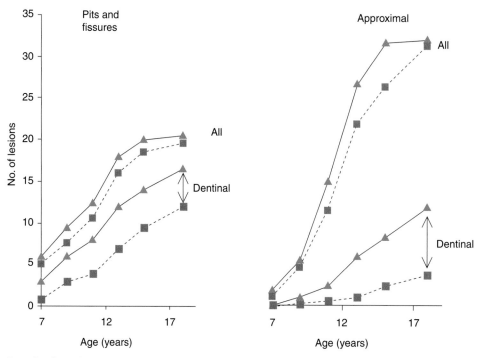

Figure 18.44 Numbers of pit/fissure lesions and approximal lesions at the dentinal level of detection and for all lesions (enamel and dentin) for a fluoridated (------) and non-fluoridated (——) area. (Source: Groeneveld et al., 1990.)

populations and in many instances are the only feasible ways of achieving large-scale fluoride availability. Inevitably, they will result in some prevalence of dental fluorosis in these populations, but so long as the severity of manifestations of fluorosis is within the lower scores (TF scores 1 and 2) of the TF fluorosis index, their public health benefits will be widespread and obvious.

Although fluoride therapy is important for caries control, it must be remembered that fluoride therapy alone will not arrest caries development and progression at every site in every individual. Maximum impact of public health programs can only be achieved concomitant with instructions in proper oral hygiene for the individual patient. As discussed earlier, the public has predominantly considered toothpaste a cosmetic measure. However, the dental team must emphasize to the public, and to the individual patient in the clinic, that the use of toothpaste enhances removal of bacterial deposits on teeth, while introducing to the tooth surface the therapeutic agent (the fluoride ion) during lesion development. When this message is understood it makes sense for the patient that brushing teeth is the best way for each individual to combine plaque removal and provide chemical therapeutic treatment, so that mineral loss may be prevented and even mineral uptake achieved if there are caries lesions under development.

Clinical implications

Once the toxicology and the most likely mechanisms of action of fluoride as a therapeutic agent are understood, it becomes evident that no 'single' fluoride program can be recommended to all populations in all countries throughout the world. It is vital to keep in mind whether the amount of disease 'prevented' justifies the cost of the program in a time of low caries incidence and prevalence for most contemporary populations. As discussed earlier, this was exactly what led to the conclusion that fluoride rinsing programs can no longer be commended in contemporary populations, not because they are not efficacious but because of a very low cost-effectiveness (Heidmann *et al.*, 1992).

Decisions on the most appropriate type of public health program to implement should consider the following factors:

- caries prevalence, incidence and distribution in the population in question
- oral hygiene status
- access to dental services
- living conditions and dietary habits of the population in question
- the socioeconomic character of the community, including information about educational levels in the community
- detailed knowledge about water fluoride concentrations and other fluoride exposures.

The best way to illustrate that there is no 'one and only' appropriate fluoride program is to consider the USA and the different Nordic countries. In general, the caries levels in Scandinavia and the USA are very low, but each country has chosen very different programs to reach this level. It would seem appropriate today to ask the question: how could we develop and maintain the lowest caries experience and incidence with the simplest methods and without building institutions and using expensive personnel to achieve this? There are many different ways to achieve the goal and it is up to each society to determine how much money they would like to spend on this part of the health sector. With the increasing pressure on the health sector in general to become more efficient and to base its activity on scientific evidence, it is time for the dental profession to reconsider how to develop the most appropriate and cost-effective ways of controlling dental caries.

Caries incidence rates have been dramatically reduced in many populations in industrial countries and the relative effectiveness of different fluoride-delivery methods may need to be reassessed. In the USA, the traditional difference (50% reduction) in caries experience between fluoridated and non-fluoridated populations was reduced to about a national 17% difference by 1990 (Brunelle & Carlos, 1990). This has been explained by the 'halo effect', in which products from fluoridated areas spread to non-fluoridated populations, elevating the fluoride exposure to a level that could indirectly influence the caries rate. Such an explanation is speculative and it is also possible that at a lower incidence of caries and in the presence of multiple sources of fluoride, the benefits of water fluoridation are truly less significant.

Data from The Netherlands are particularly interesting. When the decision to stop water fluoridation was taken it was expected that a significant increase in caries would occur. However, in the decades between 1955 and 1975 substantial changes in socioeconomic status, dietary habits and oral health awareness (oral hygiene) took place, resulting in a significant decrease in caries incidence rates. Moreover, attempts to introduce a fluoride tablet regimen, to counteract the anticipated increase in caries incidence, did not in and of itself affect the caries incidence, but only resulted in an increased prevalence of dental fluorosis in the population (Kalsbeek *et al.*, 1992).

In terms of controlling caries by using fluoride, in the 80% of the population with 20% of the disease it will be difficult to find a cost-effective method of improving on the current situation. However, it is still important within this population to ensure individuals will not start to develop active caries lesions if the control of this disease breaks down. This may occur for numerous reasons, including changes in lifestyle, leaving home, medication causing dry mouth, aging and an associated loss of manual dexterity. Targeted individualized caries-control programs, using the standard procedures outlined earlier, should then be used. However, the underlying cause of this breakdown of caries control should be recognized and treated alongside the treatment of dental caries and may require a multidisciplinary approach, involving, for example, the psychologist, the psychiatrist, the physician, the geriatrician and the dentist.

In the 20% of the population who have 80% of the disease, it would seem that fluoride in any form or method of delivery is less effective. This population has been defined as the deprived or low socioeconomic class, where oral health care and perhaps health care in general have a low priority because of other pressures placed upon them, such as housing, jobs and food. Perhaps the way to control the caries in this population is through raising their living standards and health expectations, ensuring the use of fluoride toothpaste and, perhaps, using more passive forms of fluoride delivery such as water, which require little individual participation.

Summary of recommendations for fluoride-delivery methods

For a fluoride-delivery system to be successful it must ensure that:

- fluoride is topically available in the oral cavity at concentrations that can significantly affect the ongoing demineralization and remineralization process
- ingestion of fluoride is minimized
- the method of delivery is cost-effective.

The versatility of fluoride as a preventive and therapeutic agent to control dental caries is outstanding. There can be few other chemical entities that can be delivered in such a flexible manner to provide such important benefits. The versatility of fluoride is also the source of some concern. There is a fine balance between providing fluoride in sufficient quantities to provide anticaries benefits, while ensuring that ingestion is limited so that dental fluorosis is minimized.

Today individuals in many parts of the world are consuming fluoride from multiple sources (Heifetz & Horowitz, 1984), each of which is designed to provide an 'optimal' fluoride delivery to maximize benefit and minimize risk. When combinations of fluoride therapy are used, often unintentionally, there will inevitably be some individuals ingesting too much fluoride and, as might be expected, the prevalence of fluorosis is believed by some to be increasing (Ripa, 1991; Holloway & Ellwood, 1997). Particular problems occur in areas with fluoridated drinking water, such as North America, where excessive quantities of fluoride from the water and toothpaste are ingested and fluoride supplements may be inappropriately prescribed by well-intentioned individuals. The use of fluoride has to be based on a sound scientific understanding, and the outdated maxim 'if a little is good then more is better' has to be avoided at all costs.

The most common combination of methods is the use of fluoride dentifrices in populations with fluoridated drinking water. In this case it is suggested that the benefits of fluoride toothpastes are similar in both populations (Marinho et al., 2003). Any additional benefit of fluoride toothpastes used in combination with other topical methods such as mouthrinses, gels and varnishes is less conclusive and only modest caries reductions might be anticipated (Marinho et al., 2004).

The combination of methods is primarily recommended for patients at high risk for caries, who have insufficient oral hygiene or who are under orthodontic treatment, for example.

The primary mode of action of fluoride is topical and there is little or no benefit to be gained from swallowing it. The methods that should be used to maximize the benefits and minimize the risks are clearly delineated. Methods should be encouraged that ensure that elevated fluoride levels are sustained in the oral cavity and the young swallow as little as possible of the fluoride, so that the risk of fluorosis, particularly the cosmetically important forms, is minimized (Hawley et al., 1996). From a practical point of view, upon eruption of the first permanent molars (6 years) the coronal development of the anterior teeth is near to completion and therefore ingestion of fluoride should have little impact on tooth development after this age. Efforts to minimize fluoride ingestion need therefore to be focussed on the under-sevens.

There is no single method of delivering fluoride that is appropriate for all and consideration of the risks, benefits and cost-effectiveness of any programme must be examined in detail at national, local and individual levels. At a national level one must consider the extent and distribution of caries within the population, existing exposure to fluoride, the infrastructure available, economic development, the availability of personnel, oral hygiene habits and dietary behavior. A fundamental decision to be made by politicians and health-care workers is the distribution of the costs of any program between the individual and the state.

In situations where the caries prevalence and severity is high and evenly distributed throughout the population there can be little argument that water fluoridation provides the most cost-effective and efficient method of fluoride delivery. However, for reasons already discussed, water fluoridation has been difficult to implement as the infrastructure and/or the political will required may not be available. It should be realized, however, that in countries with a high standard of living and where caries prevalence and incidence were among the highest in the world – the Scandinavian countries – reductions in caries of about 90% have occurred without fluoridation. This has been achieved by combining the use of topical fluoride in different ways with good oral hygiene practice, including fluoride toothpastes.

Other community fluoride-delivery schemes such as salt and milk (Burt & Marthaler, 1996) provide alternative methods of delivery that can potentially be targeted to communities at high risk. Importantly, they provide a level of freedom of choice not afforded by fluoridation of drinking water supplies. However, for both these methods well-controlled clinical studies are needed to establish scientific data on which to build health-care recommendations. For salt in particular, the concerns of the medical profession, regarding encouraging ingestion of salt and its potential health implications, need to be very carefully considered. Moreover, fluoridated milk can only be used in child populations controlled by a school health-care system if uncontrolled consumption should be avoided.

Fluoride tablets should no longer be considered an appropriate strategy of fluoride delivery. They are the least efficient way of delivering topical fluoride and inevitably result in a high level of fluoride ingestion when swallowed. They may be appropriate for high-risk adults and elderly people, particularly when used in lozenge form.

Fluoride toothpaste has been by far the most successful fluoride-delivery system to be developed (Cury et al., 2004). The majority of the population use it and methods of application can be tailored to suit the individual. Tooth brushing is the cultural norm in many societies, but it must be remembered that it is probably the cosmetic rather than the therapeutic benefits that have ensured such widespread penetration into the marketplace. It is important that the dental profession realize that fluoride in toothpaste is a highly potent therapeutic agent when used to control ongoing disease. Ensuring a supply of cheap and effective fluoride toothpaste, and ensuring that it is used effectively, should be the key elements in all caries-intervention programs (Davies et al., 1995). Other fluoride-delivery systems such as mouthrinses and gels should be seen as adjuncts to toothpaste use, not an alternative, and predominantly should be used for individuals and groups at high risk of caries.

Background literature

Fejerskov O, Ekstrand J, Burt BA. *Fluoride in dentistry*, 2nd edn. Copenhagen: Munksgaard, 1996.

References

Aasenden R, Peebles TC. Effects of fluoride supplementation from birth on human primary and permanent teeth. *Arch Oral Biol* 1974; **19**: 321–6.

Ainsworth NJ. Mottled teeth. *Br Dent J* 1933; **55**: 233–50.

American Dental Association, Council on Dental Therapeutics. Prescribing supplements of dietary fluorides. *J Am Dent Assoc* 1958; **56**: 589–91.

Andersen L, Richards A, Care AD, Andersen HM, Kragstrup J, Fejerskov O. Parathyroid glands, calcium, and vitamin D in experimental fluorosis in pigs. *Calcif Tissue Int* 1986; **38**: 222–6.

Aoba T, Fejerskov O. Dental fluorosis: chemistry and biology. *Crit Rev Oral Biol Med* 2002; **13**: 155–71.

Arnold FA, Dean HT, Knutson JW. Effect of fluoridated public water supplies on dental caries incidence. Results of the seventh year of study at Grand Rapids and Muskegon, Mich. *Public Health Rep* 1953; **68**: 141–8.

Arnold FA, Likins RC, Russell AL, Scott DB. Fifteenth year of the Grand Rapids fluoridation study. In McClure FJ, ed. *Fluoride drinking waters*. Bethesda, MA: National Institute of Dental Research, 1962: 253–6.

Ashley PF, Attrill DC, Ellwood RP, Worthington HV, Davies RM. Toothbrushing habits and caries experience. *Caries Res* 1999; **33**: 401–2.

Backer-Dirks O. The relationship between the fluoridation of water and dental caries experience. *Int Dent J* 1967; **17**: 582–605.

Baelum V, Manji F, Fejerskov O. Posteruptive tooth age and severity of dental fluorosis in Kenya. *Scand J Dent Res* 1986; **94**: 405–10.

Baelum V, Machiulskiene V, Nyvad B, Richards A, Vaeth M. Survival modelling of caries lesion transitions in community intervention trials of preventive interventions. *Community Dent Oral Epidemiol* 2003; **31**: 252–60.

Barnhart WE, Hiller LK, Leonard GJ, Michaels SE. Dentifrice usage and ingestion among four age groups. *J Dent Res* 1974; **53**: 1317–22.

Baysan A, Lynch E, Ellwood R, Davies R, Petersson L, Borsboom P. Reversal of primary root caries using dentifrices containing 5,000 and 1,100 ppm fluoride. *Caries Res* 2001; **35**: 41–6.

Bentley EM, Ellwood RP, Davies RM. Factors influencing the amount of fluoride toothpaste applied by the mothers of young children. *Br Dent J* 1997; **183**: 412–14.

Bentley EM, Ellwood RP, Davies RM. Fluoride ingestion from toothpaste by young children. *Br Dent J* 1999; **186**: 460–2.

Binder K, Driscoll WS, Schutzmannsky G. Caries-preventive fluoride tablet programs. *Caries Res* 1978; **12**: 22–30.

Black GV, In collaboration with McKay FS. Mottled enamel. An endemic developmental imperfection of the teeth, heretofore unknown in the literature of dentistry. *Dental Cosmos* 1916; **58**: 129–56.

Blinkhorn AS, Holloway PJ, Davies TG. Combined effects of a fluoride dentifrice and mouthrinse on the incidence of dental caries. *Community Dent Oral Epidemiol* 1983; **11**: 7–11.

Bowen WH. The role of fluoride toothpastes in the prevention of dental caries. *J R Soc Med* 1995; **88**: 505–7.

Bratthall D, Hansel-Petersson G, Sundberg H. Reasons for the caries decline: what do the experts believe? *Eur J Oral Sci* 1996; **104**: 416–22.

Brunelle JA, Carlos JP. Recent trends in dental caries in US children and the effect of water fluoridation. *J Dent Res* 1990; **69** (Special No.): 723–7; Discussion 820–3.

Bruun C, Thylstrup A. Dentifrice usage among Danish children. *J Dent Res* 1988; **67**: 1114–17.

Bryan ET, Williams JE. The cariostatic effectiveness of a phosphate-fluoride gel administered annually to school children. I. The results of the first year. *J Public Health Dent* 1968; **28**: 182–5.

Burt BA, Marthaler TM. Fluoride tablets, salt fluoridation, and milk fluoridation In: Fejerskov O, Ekstrand J, Burt BA, eds. *Fluoride in dentistry*, 2nd edn. Copenhagen: Munksgaard, 1996: 291–310.

Butler WJ, Segreto V, Collins E. Prevalence of dental mottling in school-aged lifetime residents of 16 Texas communities. *Am J Public Health* 1985; **75**: 1408–12.

Carmichael CL, Rugg-Gunn AJ, Ferrell RS. The relationship between fluoridation, social class and caries experience in 5-year-old children in Newcastle and Northumberland in 1987. *Br Dent J* 1989; **167**: 57–61.

ten Cate JM, van Loveren C. Fluoride mechanisms [review]. *Dent Clin North Am* 1999; **43**: 713–42, vii.

Cawson RA, Stocker IP. The early history of fluorides as anti-caries agents. *Br Dent J* 1984; **157**: 403–4.

Chesters RK, Huntington E, Burchell CK, Stephen KW. Effect of oral care habits on caries in adolescents. *Caries Res* 1992; **26**: 299–304.

Chesters RK, Pitts NB, Matuliene G, et al. An abbreviated caries clinical trial design validated over 24 months. *J Dent Res* 2002; **81**: 637–40.

Churchill HV. Occurrence of fluorides in some waters of the United States. *Ind Eng Chem* 1931; **23**: 996–8.

Clarkson JE, Ellwood RP, Chandler RE. A comprehensive summary of fluoride dentifrice caries clinical trials. *Am J Dent* 1993; **6** (Special No.): S59–106.

Clovis J, Hargreaves JA. Fluoride intake from beverage consumption. *Community Dent Oral Epidemiol* 1988; **16**: 11–15.

Cobb BH, Rozier GR, Bawden JW. A clinical study of the caries preventive effects of an APF solution and APF thixotropic gel. *Pediatr Dent* 1980; **2**: 263–6.

Cons NC, Janerich DT, Senning RS. Albany topical fluoride study. *J Am Dent Assoc* 1970; **80**: 777–81.

Conti AJ, Lotzkar S, Daley R, Cancro L, Marks RG, McNeal DR. A 3-year clinical trial to compare efficacy of dentifrices containing 1.14% and 0.76% sodium monofluorophosphate. *Community Dent Oral Epidemiol* 1988; **16**: 135–8.

Cury JA, Rebelo MA, Del Bel Cury AA, Derbyshire MT, Tabchoury CP. Biochemical composition and cariogenicity of dental plaque formed in the presence of sucrose or glucose and fructose. *Caries Res* 2000; **34**: 491–7.

Cury JA, Tenuta LMA, Ribeiro CCC, Paes Leme AF, Cury JA The importance of fluoride dentifrices to the current dental caries prevalence in Brazil. *Braz Dent J* 2004; **15**: 167–74.

Cury JA, Del Fiol FS, Tenuta LM, Rosalen PL. Low-fluoride dentifrice and gastrointestinal fluoride absorption after meals. *J Dent Res* 2005; **84**: 1133–7.

Davies GM, Worthington HV, Ellwood RP, *et al.* A randomised controlled trial of the effectiveness of providing free fluoride toothpaste from the age of 12 months on reducing caries in 5–6 year old children. *Community Dent Health* 2002; **19**: 131–6.

Davies RM, Holloway PJ, Ellwood RP. The role of fluoride dentifrices in a national strategy for the oral health of children. *Br Dent J* 1995; **179**: 84–7.

Dean HT. Classification of mottled enamel diagnosis. *J Am Dent Assoc* 1934; **21**: 1421–6.

Dean HT. Endemic fluorosis and its relationship to dental caries. *Public Health Rep* 1938a; **53**: 1443–52.

Dean HT. Chronic endemic dental fluorosis (mottled enamel). In: Gordon SM, ed. *Dental science and dental art.* Philadelphia, PA: Lea and Febinger, 1938b: Chapter 12.

Dean HT. The investigation of physiological effects by the epidemiological method. In: Moulton FR, *Fluorine and dental health.* Publication No. 19. Washington, DC: American Association for the Advancement of Science, 1942: 23–31.

Dean HT, Elvove E. Some epidemiological aspects of chronic endemic fluorosis. *Am J Public Health* 1936; **26**: 567–75.

Dean HT, McKay FS. Production of mottled enamel halted by a change in common water supply. *Am J Public Health* 1939; **29**: 590–6.

Dean HT, Jay P, Arnold FA, Elvove E. Domestic water and dental caries, including certain epidemiological aspects of oral *L. acidophilus. Public Health Rep* 1939; **54**: 862–88.

Dean HT, Jay P, Arnold FA, Elvove E. Domestic water and dental caries II. A study of 2832 white children aged 12–14 years of eight suburban Chicago communities, including *Lactobacillus acidophilus* studies of 1761 children. *Public Health Rep* 1941; **56**: 761–92.

Dean HT, Arnold FA, Elvove E. Domestic water and dental varies. V. Additional studies of the relation of fluoride domestic waters to dental caries experience in 4,425 white children aged 12–14 years of 13 cities in 4 states. *Public Health Rep* 1942; **57**: 1155–79.

Dean HT, Arnold FA, Jay P, Knutson JW. Studies on the mass control of dental caries through fluoridation of the public water supply. *Public Health Rep* 1950; **65**: 1403–8.

DePaola PF, Lax M. The caries-inhibiting effect of acidulated phosphate-fluoride chewable tablets: a two-year double-blind study. *J Am Dent Assoc* 1968; **76**: 554–7.

Disney JA, Bohannan HM, Klein SP, Bell RM. A case study in contesting the conventional wisdom: school-based fluoride mouthrinse programs in the USA. *Community Dent Oral Epidemiol* 1990; **18**: 46–54.

Documeta Geigy. *Scientific tables,* 7th edn. Basel: Ciba-Geigy, 1975: 693–8.

Dowell TB. The use of toothpaste in infancy. *Br Dent J* 1981; **150**: 247–9.

Driscoll WS. The use of fluoride tablets for the prevention of dental caries. In: Forrester DJ, Schulz EM Jr, eds. *International Workshop on Fluorides and Dental Caries Reductions.* Baltimore, MD: University of Maryland School of Dentistry, 1974: 25–93.

Driscoll WS, Heifetz SB, Korts DC. Effect of chewable fluoride tablets on dental caries in schoolchildren: results after six years of use. *J Am Dent Assoc* 1978; **97**: 820–4.

Driscoll WS, Swango PA, Horowitz AM, Kingman A. Caries-preventive effects of daily and weekly fluoride mouthrinsing in a fluoridated community: final results after 30 months. *J Am Dent Assoc* 1982; **105**: 1010–13.

Duckworth SC, Duckworth R. The ingestion of fluoride in tea. *Br Dent J* 1978; **145**: 368–70.

Duckworth RM, Morgan SN, Burchell CK. Fluoride in plaque following use of dentifrices containing sodium monofluorophosphate. *J Dent Res* 1989; **68**: 130–3.

Duckworth RM, Knoop DJM Stephen KW. Effect of mouth-rinsing after brushing with a fluoride dentifrice on human salivary fluoride levels. *Caries Res* 1991; **25**: 287–91.

Eager JM. Denti di Chiaie (Chiaie teeth). *Public Health Rep* 1902; **16**: 2576.

Edgar WM, Lennon MA, Phillips PC. Stability of fluoride milk during storage in glass bottles. *J Dent Res* 1992; **71** (Special Issue): 703 (Abstract 1500).

Ekstrand J. Fluoride metabolism. In: Fejerskov O, Ekstrand J, Burt BA, eds. *Fluoride in dentistry,* 2nd ed. Copenhagen: Munksgaard, 1996: 55–68.

Ekstrand J, Alvan G, Boreus LO, Norlin A. Pharmacokinetics of fluoride in man after single and multiple oral doses. *Eur J Clin Pharmacol* 1977; **12**: 311–17.

Ekstrand J, Hardell LI, Spak CJ. Fluoride balance studies on infants in a 1-ppm-water-fluoride area. *Caries Res* 1984; **18**: 87–92.

Ekstrand J, Spak CJ, Vogel G. Pharmacokinetics of fluoride in man and its clinical relevance [review]. *J Dent Res* 1990; **69** (Special No.): 550–5; Discussion 556–7.

Ellwood RP, O'Mullane DM. Dental enamel opacities in three groups with varying levels of fluoride in their drinking water. *Caries Res* 1995; **29**: 137–42.

Ellwood RP, Blinkhorn AS, Davies RM. Fluoride: how to maximize the benefits and minimize the risks. *Dent Update* 1998; **25**: 365–72.

Ellwood RP, Davies GM, Worthington HV, Blinkhorn AS, Taylor GO, Davies RM. Relationship between area deprivation and the anticaries benefit of an oral health programme providing free fluoride toothpaste to young children. *Community Dent Oral Epidemiol* 2004; **32**: 159–65.

Ericsson Y, Forsman B. Fluoride retained from mouthrinses and dentifrices in preschool children. *Caries Res* 1969; **3**: 290–9.

Evans RW, Stamm JW. An epidemiologic estimate of the critical period during which human maxillary central incisors are most susceptible to fluorosis. *J Public Health Dent* 1991; **51**: 251–9.

Fejerskov O, Johnson NW, Silverstone LM. The ultrastructure of fluorosed human dental enamel. *Scand J Dent Res* 1974; **82**: 357–72.

Fejerskov O, Silverstone LM, Melsen B, Moller IJ. Histological features of fluorosed human dental enamel. *Caries Res* 1975; **9**: 190–210.

Fejerskov O, Thylstrup A, Larsen MJ. Clinical and structural features and possible pathogenic mechanisms of dental fluorosis. *Scand J Dent Res* 1977; **85**: 510–34.

Fejerskov O, Thylstrup A, Larsen MJ. Rational use of fluorides in caries prevention. A concept based on possible cariostatic mechanisms. *Acta Odont Scand* 1981; **39**: 241–9.

Fejerskov O, Manji F, Baelum V, Moller IJ. *Dental fluorosis. A handbook for health care workers.* Copenhagen: Munksgaard, 1988.

Fejerskov O, Manji F, Baelum V. The nature and mechanisms of dental fluorosis in man. *J Dent Res* 1990; **69**: 692–700.

Fejerskov O, Larsen MJ, Richards A, Baelum V. Dental tissue effects of fluoride. *Adv Dent Res* 1994; **8**: 15–31.

Fejerskov O, Baelum V, Richards A. Dose response and dental fluorosis In: Fejerskov O, Ekstrand J, Burt BA, eds. *Fluoride in dentistry.* Copenhagen: Munksgaard, 1996: 153–66.

Fischman SL. Hare's teeth to fluorides, historical aspects of dentifrice use. In: Embery G, Rolla G, eds. *Clinical and biological aspects of dentifrices.* Oxford: Oxford University Press, 1992: 1–8.

Fogels HR, Meade JJ, Griffith J, Miragliuolo R, Cancro LP. A clinical investigation of a high-level fluoride dentifrice. *ASDC J Dent Child* 1988; **55**: 210–15.

Fomon SJ, Ekstrand J. Fluoride intake by infants. *J Public Health Dent* 1999; **59**: 229–34.

Friis-Hasche E, Bergmann J, Wenzel A, Thylstrup A, Pedersen KM, Petersen PE. Dental health status and attitudes to dental cares in families participating in a Danish fluoride tablet program. *Community Dent Oral Epidemiol* 1984; **12**: 303–7.

Galagan DJ. Climate and controlled fluoridation. *J Am Dent Assoc* 1953; **47**: 159–70.

Galagan DJ, Lamson GG. Climate and endemic dental fluorosis. *Public Health Rep* 1953; **68**: 497–508.

Galagan DJ, Vermillion JR. Determining optimum fluoride concentrations. *Public Health Rep* 1957; **72**: 491–3.

Gedalia I, Galon H, Rennert A, Biderco I, Mohr I. Effect of fluoridated citrus beverage on dental caries and on fluoride concentration in the surface enamel of children's teeth. *Caries Res* 1981; **15**: 103–8.

Glass RL, Peterson JK, Zuckerberg DA, Naylor MN. Fluoride ingestion resulting from the use of a monofluorophosphate dentifrice by children. *Br Dent J* 1975; **138**: 423–6.

Glemser O. Inorganic fluorine chemistry, 1900–1945. *J Fluorine Chem* 1986; **33**: 45–69.

Granath L, Widenheim J, Birkhed D. Diagnosis of mild enamel fluorosis in permanent maxillary incisors using two scoring systems. *Community Dent Oral Epidemiol* 1985; **13**: 273–6.

Groeneveld A, Van Eck AAMJ, Backer-Dirks O. Fluoride in caries prevention: is the effect pre- or post-eruptive? *J Dent Res* 1990; **69** (Special Issue): 751–5.

Hagan PP, Rozier RG, Bawden JW. The caries-preventive effects of full- and half-strength topical acidulated phosphate fluoride. *Pediatr Dent* 1985; **7**: 185–91.

Hargreaves JA, Ingram GS, Wagg BJ. A gravimetric study of the ingestion of toothpaste by children. *Caries Res* 1972; **6**: 237–43.

Hatibovic-Kofman S, Koch G. Fluoride release from glass ionomer cement *in vivo* and *in vitro*. *Swed Dent J* 1991; **15**: 253–8.

Hatibovic-Kofman S, Koch G, Ekstrand J. Glass ionomer materials as a rechargeable fluoride-release system. *Int J Paediatr Dent* 1997; **7**: 65–73.

Hawley GM, Ellwood RP, Davies RM. Dental caries, fluorosis and the cosmetic implications of different TF scores in 14-year-old adolescents. *Community Dent Health* 1996; **13**: 189–92.

Hayacibara MF, Queiroz CS, Tabchoury CP, Cury JA. Fluoride and aluminum in teas and tea-based beverages. *Rev Saude Publica* 2004; **38**: 100–5.

Heidmann J, Poulsen S, Arnbjerg D, Kirkegaard E, Laurberg L. Caries development after termination of a fluoride rinsing program. *Community Dent Oral Epidemiol* 1992; **20**: 118–21.

Heifetz SB, Horowitz HS. The amounts of fluoride in current fluoride therapies: safety considerations for children. *ASDC J Dent Child* 1984; **51**: 257–69.

Heifetz SB, Meyers RJ, Kingman A. A comparison of the anticaries effectiveness of daily and weekly rinsing with sodium fluoride solutions: final results after three years. *Pediatr Dent* 1982; **4**: 300–3.

Heifetz SB, Horowitz HS, Brunelle JA. Effect of school water fluoridation on dental caries: results in Seagrove, NC, after 12 years. *J Am Dent Assoc* 1983; **106**: 334–7.

Helfenstein U, Steiner M. Fluoride varnishes (Duraphat): a meta-analysis. *Community Dent Oral Epidemiol* 1994; **22**: 1–5.

Hodge HC. The concentration of fluorides in drinking water to give the point of minimum caries with maximum safety. *J Am Dent Assoc* 1950; **40**: 436–9.

Holloway PJ, Ellwood RP. The prevalence, causes and cosmetic importance of dental fluorosis in the United Kingdom: a review. *Community Dent Health* 1997; **14**: 148–55.

Horowitz HS. Effect on dental caries of topically applied acidulated phosphate-fluoride: results after two years. *J Am Dent Assoc* 1969; **78**: 568–72.

Horowitz HS, Doyle J. The effect on dental caries of topically applied acidulated phosphate-fluoride: results after three years. *J Am Dent Assoc* 1971; **82**: 359–65.

Horowitz HS, Driscoll WS, Meyers RJ, Heifetz SB, Kingman A. A new method for assessing the prevalence of dental fluorosis – the tooth surface index of fluorosis. *J Am Dent Assoc* 1984; **109**: 37–41.

Ingraham RQ, Williams JE. An evaluation of the utility of application and cariostatic effectiveness of phosphate-fluorides in solution and gel states. *J Tenn State Dent Assoc* 1970; **50**: 5–12.

Jones CM, Worthington H. Water fluoridation, poverty and tooth decay in 12-year-old children. *J Dent* 2000; **28**: 389–93.

Kalsbeek H, Verrips E, Dirks OB. Use of fluoride tablets and effect on prevalence of dental caries and dental fluorosis. *Community Dent Oral Epidemiol* 1992; **20**: 241–5.

Kempf GA, McKay FS. Mottled enamel in a segregated population. *Public Health Rep* 1930; **45**: 2923–40.

Kirkegaard E, Petersen G, Poulsen S, Holm SA, Heidmann J. Caries-preventive effect of Duraphat varnish applications versus fluoride mouthrinses: 5-year data. *Caries Res* 1986; **20**: 548–55.

Koch G, Petersson LG. Caries preventive effect of a fluoride-containing varnish (Duraphat) after 1 year's study. *Community Dent Oral Epidemiol* 1975; **3**: 262–6.

Koch G, Petersson LG, Ryden H. Effect of flouride varnish (Duraphat) treatment every six months compared with weekly mouthrinses with 0.2 per cent NaF solution on dental caries. *Swed Dent J* 1979; **3**: 39–44.

Koch G, Petersson LG, Kling E, Kling L. Effect of 250 and 1000 ppm fluoride dentifrice on caries. A three-year clinical study. *Swed Dent J* 1982; **6**: 233–8.

Larsen MJ, Richards A, Fejerskov O. Development of dental fluorosis according to age at start of fluoride administration. *Caries Res* 1985a; **19**: 519–27.

Larsen MJ, Kirkegard E, Fejerskov O, Poulsen S. Prevalence of dental fluorosis after fluoride-gel treatments in a low-fluoride area. *J Dent Res* 1985b; **64**: 1076–9.

Larsen MJ, Kirkegaard E, Poulsen S. Patterns of dental fluorosis in a European country in relation to the fluoride concentration of drinking water. *J Dent Res* 1987; **66**: 10–12.

LeCompte EJ, Doyle TE. Oral fluoride retention following various topical application techniques in children. *J Dent Res* 1982; **61**: 1397–400.

Levy SM. A review of fluoride intake from fluoride dentifrice. *J Dent Child* 1993; **60**: 115–24.

Levy SM, Kiritsy MC, Warren JJ. Sources of fluoride intake in children. *J Public Health Dent* 1995; **55**: 39–52.

Lima YB, Cury JA. Seasonal variation of fluoride intake by children in a subtropical region. *Caries Res* 2003; **37**: 335–8.

Luoma H, Fejerskov O, Thylstrup A. The effect of fluoride on dental plaque, tooth structure and dental caries. In: Thylstrup A, Fejerskov O, eds. *Textbook of cariology*. Copenhagen: Munksgaard, 1986: 299–329.

McCollum EV, Simmonds N, Becker JE, Bunting RW. The effect of additions of fluoride to the diet of rats on the quality of their teeth. *J Biol Chem* 1925; **63**: 553.

Machiulskiene V, Richards A, Nyvad B, Baelum V. Prospective study of the effect of post-brushing rinsing behavior on dental caries. *Caries Res* 2002; **36**: 301–7.

McKay FS. The relation of mottled teeth to caries. *J Am Dent Assoc* 1928; **15**: 1429–37.

McKay FS. Mottled teeth: the prevention of its further production through a change in the water supply at Oakley, Idaho. *J Am Dent Assoc* 1933; **20**: 1137–49.

Maiwald HJ, Geiger L. Local application of fluorine protective varnish for caries prevention in collectivies. *Dtsch Stomatol* 1973; **23**: 56–63.

Manji F, Baelum V, Fejerskov O. Fluoride, altitude and dental fluorosis. *Caries Res* 1986; **20**: 473–80.

Marinho VC, Higgins JP, Sheiham A, Logan S. Fluoride toothpastes for preventing dental caries in children and adolescents. *Cochrane Database Syst Rev* 2003; (1): CD002278.

Marinho VC, Higgins JP, Sheiham A, Logan S. Combinations of topical fluoride (toothpastes, mouthrinses, gels, varnishes) versus single topical fluoride for preventing dental caries in children and adolescents. *Cochrane Database Syst Rev* 2004; (1): CD002781.

Marks RG, D'Agostino R, Moorhead JE, Conti AJ, Cancro L. A fluoride dose–response evaluation in an anticaries clinical trial. *J Dent Res* 1992; **71**: 1286–91.

Marthaler TM, Steiner M, Menghini G, Bandi A. Caries prevalence in schoolchildren in the canton of Zurich. The results in the period of 1963 to 1987. *Schweiz Monatsschr Zahnmed* 1988; **98**: 1309–15.

Milsom K, Mitropoulos CM. Enamel defects in 8 year old children in fluoridated and non fluoridated parts of Cheshire. *Caries Res* 1990; **20**: 286–9.

Mitropoulos CM, Holloway PJ, Davies TG, Worthington HV. Relative efficacy of dentifrices containing 250 or 1000 ppm F⁻ in preventing dental caries – report of a 32-month clinical trial. *Community Dent Health* 1984; **1**: 193–200.

Muhlemann HR, Schmid H, Konig K. Enamel solubility reduction studies with inorganic and organic fluorides. *Helv Odontol Acta* 1957; **1**: 23–33.

Murray JJ, Rugg-Gunn AJ, Jenkins GN. *Fluorides in caries prevention*, 3rd edn. Oxford: Wright, 1991.

Myers HM. Dose–response relationship between water fluoride levels and the category of questionable dental fluorosis. *Community Dent Oral Epidemiol* 1983; **11**: 109–12.

Naccache H, Simard PL, Trahan L, Demers M, Lapointe C, Brodeur JM. Variability in the ingestion of toothpaste by preschool children. *Caries Res* 1990; **24**: 359–63.

Naccache H, Simard PL, Trahan L, *et al.* Factors affecting the ingestion of fluoride dentifrice by children. *J Public Health Dent* 1992; **52**: 222–6.

Narvai PC, Frazão P, Roncalli GA, Antunes JLF. Dental caries in Brazil: decline, polarization, inequality and social exclusion. *Rev Panam Salud Publica* 2006; **19**: 385–93

Nobre dos Santos M, Cury JA. Dental plaque fluoride is lower after discontinuation of water fluoridation. *Caries Res* 1988; **22**: 316–17.

Nyvad B, Machiulskiene V, Baelum V. Construct and predictive validity of clinical caries diagnostic criteria assessing lesion activity. *J Dent Res* 2003; **82**: 117–22.

O'Brien M. *Children's dental health in the United Kingdom 1993.* London: HMSO, 1994.

Ögaard B, Seppa L, Rolla G. Professional topical fluoride applications – clinical efficacy and mechanism of action. *Adv Dent Res* 1994; **8**: 190–201.

O'Mullane DM, Kavanagh D, Ellwood RP, *et al.* A three-year clinical trial of a combination of trimetaphosphate and sodium fluoride in silica toothpastes. *J Dent Res* 1997; **76**: 1776–81.

Osuji OO, Leake JL, Chipman ML, Nikiforuk G, Locker D, Levine N. Risk factors for dental fluorosis in a fluoridated community. *J Dental Res* 1988; **67**: 1488–92.

Paes Leme AF, Dalcico R, Tabchoury CPM, Del Bel Cury AA, Rosalen PL, Cury JA. *In situ* effect of frequent sucrose exposure on enamel demineralization and on plaque composition after APF application and F dentifrice use. *J Dent Res* 2004; **83**: 71–5.

Parkins FM, Tinanoff N, Moutinho M, Anstey MB, Waziri MH. Relationships of human plasma fluoride and bone fluoride to age. *Calcif Tissue Res* 1974; **16**: 335–8.

Pearce EI, Dibdin GH. The diffusion and enzymic hydrolysis of monofluorophosphate in dental plaque. *J Dent Res* 1995; **74**: 691–7.

Pendrys DG. The fluorosis risk index: a method for investigating risk factors. *J Public Health Dent* 1990; **50**: 291–8.

Pendrys DG. Risk of fluorosis in a fluoridated population. Implications for the dentist and hygienist. *J Am Dent Assoc* 1995; **126**: 1617–24.

Pendrys DG. Risk of enamel fluorosis in nonfluoridated and optimally fluoridated populations: considerations for the dental professional. *J Am Dent Assoc* 2000; **131**: 746–55.

Pendrys DG, Katz RV. Risk of enamel fluorosis associated with fluoride supplementation, infant formula, and fluoride dentifrice use. *Am J Epidemiol* 1989; **130**: 1199–208.

Pendrys DG, Katz RV, Morse DE. Risk factors for enamel fluorosis in a nonfluoridated population. *Am J Epidemiol* 1996; **143**: 808–15.

Peres MA, Antunes JLF, Peres KG. Is water fluoridation effective in reducing inequalities in dental caries distribution in developing countries? *Soz Präventiv Med* 2006; **51**: 1–9.

Poulsen S, Larsen MJ. Dental caries in relation to fluoride content of enamel in the primary dentition. *Caries Res* 1975; **9**: 59–65.

Provart SJ, Carmichael CL. The relationship between caries, fluoridation and material deprivation in five-year-old children in County Durham. *Community Dent Health* 1995; **12**: 200–3.

Richards A, Banting DW. Fluoride toothpastes. In: Fejerskov O, Ekstrand J, Burt BA, eds. *Fluoride in dentistry.* Copenhagen Munksgaard, 1996: 328–46.

Richards A, Larsen MJ, Fejerskov O, Thylstrup A. Fluoride content of buccal surface enamel and its relation to caries in children. *Arch Oral Biol* 1977; **22**: 425–8.

Richards A, Kragstrup J, Josephsen K, Fejerskov O. Dental fluorosis developed in post-secretory enamel. *J Dent Res* 1986; **65**: 1406–9.

Richards A, Larsen MJ, Hovgaard O, Fejerskov O. Toothpastes containing fluoride and the concentration of fluoride in saliva. *Tandlaegebladet* (Dan Dent J) 1988; **92**: 146–50.

Richards A, Fejerskov O, Baelum V. Enamel fluoride in relation to severity of human dental fluorosis. *Adv Dent Res* 1989; **3**: 147–53.

Richards LF, Westmoreland WW, Tashiro M, McKay CH, Morrison JT. Determining optimum fluoride levels for community water supplies in relation to temperature. *J Am Dent Assoc* 1967; **74**: 389–97.

Riley JC, Lennon MA, Ellwood RP. The effect of water fluoridation and social inequalities on dental caries in 5-year-old children. *Int J Epidemiol* 1999; **28**: 300–5.

Riordan PJ. Dental fluorosis, dental caries and fluoride exposure among 7-year-olds. *Caries Res* 1993; **27**: 71–7.

Ripa LW. A critique of topical fluoride methods (dentifrices, mouthrinses, operator-, and self-applied gels) in an era of decreased caries and increased fluorosis prevalence. *J Public Health Dent* 1991; **51**: 23–41.

Rock WP, Sabieha AM. The relationship between reported toothpaste use in infancy and fluorosis of permanent incisors. *Br Dent J* 1997; **183**: 165–70.

Rolla G, Saxegaard E. Critical evaluation of the composition and use of topical fluorides, with emphasis on the role of calcium fluoride in caries inhibition. *J Dent Res* 1990; **69** (Special No.): 780–5.

Schioth JT. Effect of fluoride lacquering on the need of dental care in a group of adolescent school pupils. *Nor Tannlaegeforen Tid (Nor Dent J)* 1981; **91**: 123–6.

Schulz EM, Epstein JS, Forrester DJ. Fluoride content of popular carbonated beverages. *J Prev Dent* 1976; **3**: 27–9.

Seppa L, Pollanen L. Caries preventive effect of two fluoride varnishes and a fluoride mouthrinse. *Caries Res* 1987; **21**: 375–9.

Simard PL, Lachapelle D, Trahan L, Naccache H, Demers M, Brodeur JM. The ingestion of fluoride dentifrice by young children. *ASDC J Dent Child* 1989; **56**: 177–81.

Sjögren K, Birkhed D. Factors related to fluoride retention after toothbrushing and possible connection to caries activity. *Caries Res* 1993; **27**: 474–77.

Sjögren K, Birkhed D, Rangmar B. Effect of modified toothpaste technique on approximal caries in pre-school children. *Caries Res* 1995; **29**: 435–41.

Smith FA, Ekstrand J. The occurrence and the chemistry of fluoride. In: Fejerskov O, Ekstrand J, Burt BA, eds. *Fluoride in dentistry*, 2nd edn. Copenhagen: Munksgaard, 1996: 17–26.

Spak CJ, Hardell LI, De Chateau P. Fluoride in human milk. *Acta Paediatr Scand* 1983; **72**: 699–701.

Spak CJ, Ekstrand J, Ericsson S, Leksell LG. Distribution of fluoride to the central nervous system [Abstract]. *Caries Res* 1986; **20**: 157.

Stamm JW. Milk fluoridation as a public health measure. *J Can Dent Assoc* 1972; **38**: 446–8.

Steiner M, Marthaler TM, Wiesner V, Menghini G. Caries incidence in schoolchildren in the canton of Glarus 9 years after the introduction of highly fluoridated table salt (250 mg F/kg). *Schweiz Monatsschr Zahnmed* 1986; **96**: 688–99.

Steiner M, Menghini G, Marthaler TM. The caries incidence in schoolchildren in the Canton of Glarus 13 years after the introduction of highly fluoridated salt. *Schweiz Monatsschr Zahnmed* 1989; **99**: 897–901.

Stephen KW, Creanor SL, Russell JI, Burchell CK, Huntington E, Downie CF. A 3-year oral health dose–response study of sodium monofluorophosphate dentifrices with and without zinc citrate: anti-caries results. *Community Dent Oral Epidemiol* 1988; **16**: 321–5.

Stephen KW, Banoczy J, Pahkamov GN. *Milk fluoridation for the prevention of dental caries.* Geneva: World Health Organization/Borrow Milk Foundation, 1996.

Szwejda LF. Fluorides in community programs: results after two years from a fluoride gel applied topically. *J Public Health Dent* 1971; **31**: 241–2.

Szwejda LF, Tossy CV, Below DM. Fluorides in community programs; results from a fluoride gel applied topically. *J Public Health Dent* 1967; **27**: 192–4.

Tavener JA, Davies GM, Davies RM, Ellwood RP. The prevalence and severity of fluorosis in children who received toothpaste containing either 440 or 1,450 ppm F from the age of 12 months in deprived and less deprived communities. *Caries Res* 2006; **40**: 66–72.

Taves DR. Dietary intake of fluoride ashed (total fluoride) v. unashed (inorganic fluoride) analysis of individual foods. *Br J Nutr* 1983; **49**: 295–301.

Tewari A, Chawla HS, Utreja A, caries preventive effect of three topical fluorides ($1^1/_2$ years clinical trial in Chandigarh school children of North India). *J Int Assoc Dent Child* 1984; **15**: 71–81.

Thylstrup A, Fejerskov O. Clinical appearance of dental fluorosis in permanent teeth in relation to histologic changes. *Community Dent Oral Epidemiol* 1978; **6**: 315–28.

Thylstrup A, Fejerskov O. A scanning electron microscopic and microradiographic study of pits in fluorosed human enamel. *Scand J Dent Res* 1979; **87**: 105–14.

Thylstrup A, Fejerskov O, Bruun C, Kann J. Enamel changes and dental caries in 7-year-old children given fluoride tablets from shortly after birth. *Caries Res* 1979; **13**: 265–76.

Thylstrup A, Bille J, Bruun C. Caries prevalence in Danish children living in areas with low and optimal levels of natural water fluoride. *Caries Res* 1982; **16**: 413–20.

Toumba KJ, Curzon ME. Slow-release fluoride [review]. *Caries Res* 1993; **27** (Suppl 1): 43–6.

Triol CW, Mandanas BY, Juliano GF, Yraolo B, Cano-Arevalo M, Volpe AR. A clinical study of children comparing anticaries effect of two fluoride dentifrices. A 31-month study. *Clin Prev Dent* 1987; **9**: 22–4.

Tveit AB, Lindh U. Fluoride uptake in enamel and dentin surfaces exposed to a fluoride-containing amalgam *in vitro*. A proton microprobe analysis. *Acta Odontol Scand* 1980; **38**: 279–83.

Volpe AR, Petrone ME, Davies R, Proskin HM. Clinical anticaries efficacy of NaF and SMFP dentifrices: overview and resolution of the scientific controversy. *J Clin Dent* 1995; **6** (Special No.): 1–28.

Vrbic V. Retention of a fluoride-containing sealant on primary and permanent teeth 3 years after placement. *Quintessence Int* 1999; **30**: 825–8.

Walker A, Gregory J, Bradnock G, Nunn J, White D. *National Diet and Nutrition Survey: young people aged 4–18 years*, Vol. 2; *Report of the oral health survey 2000*. London: The Stationery Office, 2000.

Watson PS, Pontefract HA, Devine DA, *et al*. Penetration of fluoride into natural plaque biofilms. *J Dent Res* 2005; **84**: 451–5.

Weatherell JA, Deutsch D, Robinson C, Hallsworth AS. Assimilation of fluoride by enamel throughout the life of the tooth. *Caries Res* 1977; **11** (Suppl 1): 85–115.

Whitford GM. *The metabolism and toxicity of fluoride*, 2nd rev. edn. *Monographs in oral science*, Vol. 16. Basel: Karger, 1996.

Winter GB, Holt RD, Williams BF. Clinical trial of a low-fluoride toothpaste for young children. *Int Dent J* 1989; **39**: 227–35.

19

The role of dietary control

D.T. Zero, P. Moynihan, P. Lingström and D. Birkhed

Introduction

Of the many factors that contribute to the development of dental caries, diet plays an important role. In conjunction with oral hygiene and other measures such as widespread use of fluoride, dietary control makes an important contribution to the multifaceted strategy for caries control. The aim of this chapter is to summarize the evidence base for current dietary measures for caries control. The association between components of the modern-day diet and disease levels is discussed, and groups of people who are at increased dietary risk are considered. Fifty years ago dietary issues relevant to dental caries were largely concerned with dietary sugars. Although sugars are undoubtedly the most important dietary factors in the etiology of dental caries, today's diet contains an increasing range of fermentable carbohydrates, including highly processed starch-containing foods, and foods that contain novel synthetic carbohydrates such as oligofructose, sucralose and glucose polymers. Coupled with this, there now exists a wide range of non-cariogenic sweeteners that have an important role to play in caries control. Research continues to identify foods and factors that protect against dental caries and those that have a practical dietary application can help to make dietary advice more positive, which aids compliance. However, dietary control is not limited to advice at the level of the individual. Continued action at a national level is necessary to promote safe dietary practices for dental as well as general health. The following paragraphs consider these issues and provide an overall insight into the important role of dietary control for the management of dental caries. The role of diet in the increasingly prevalent problem of dental erosion will also be discussed.

Diet and dental caries in humans

There is today overwhelming evidence that frequent consumption of fermentable carbohydrates is associated with the prevalence of dental caries. Evidence is mainly found in a wide range of human epidemiological (observational) and experimental (interventional) studies, where each one adds important information to the overall picture. However, during evaluation, the strengths and weaknesses of each study need to be borne in mind. An overall important factor is that dental caries and food consumption are events that occur at widely differing time-points: to determine fully the effect of diet, the assessment of frequency and form of carbohydrate intake should be made years earlier than the clinical examination of caries. Another problem in evaluating diet and caries is the large intraindividual and interindividual variations that are found. The diet–caries relationship therefore needs to be evaluated not only against the quantity and type of fermentable carbohydrate consumed, but also against several background factors, including:

- intake pattern
- total food intake
- salivary secretion rate
- plaque composition
- use of fluoride
- socioeconomic variables.

It is also important to remember that several of the studies have been conducted in another era and in special groups of subjects. This does not imply that the results obtained are invalid, but a healthy skepticism about some of these findings should be maintained.

Several issues affect the reliability and validity of data from national surveys attempting to link the consumption of sugars to caries. The discrepancies encountered in correlating data on sugars consumption with caries in humans may be due more to uncertainties in the collection of the data than to conceptual problems. Estimations of consumption based on supply data do not take into account such factors as age distribution and socioeconomic, ethnic and cultural differences within a country, which may affect the actual sugar consumption. In spite of this, a positive correlation between international data on the sugar consumption for 47 countries and caries development [expressed as decayed missing and filled teeth (DMFT)] of 12-year-olds has been demonstrated (Sreebny, 1982) (Fig. 19.1). The same strong correlation was not found when a similar comparison was made for 6-year-old children in 23 nations; however, for both groups, the availability of less than 50 g sugar per person per day in a country was associated with dmft or DMFT scores less than 3.

The relation of starch to dental caries has long been under debate and we have relatively little information about the possible relationships of starch to dental caries in humans, in comparison with the extensive knowledge about the relationship of sugars and sugar-containing items to dental

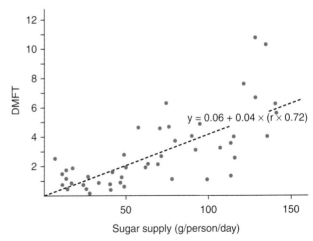

Figure 19.1 Dental caries (DMFT) in 12-year-old children and sugar supplies (g/person/day) in 47 countries. Each dot represents one country. (From Sreebny, 1982.)

caries (Sreebny, 1983). When evaluating starch in animal, human plaque pH response and *in situ* caries model studies, there is no doubt that processed food starches in modern diets possess a significant cariogenic potential (Lingström *et al.*, 2000). However, studies on humans do not provide unequivocal data on their actual cariogenicity. Historical data suggest that starch has no or low caries-inducive effect, whereas data from modern societies have shown that starch may indeed contribute to caries development (Lingström *et al.*, 2000).

Epidemiological human studies

The relation between the diet and dental caries can best be demonstrated by situations in which refined carbohydrates (processed white flour foods, bread, crackers, rice, noodles, cereal, etc.) are either almost completely absent from the diet, as in ancient humans (Hardwick, 1960), or abundantly present. In ancient times, both sugar and processed starch were almost completely absent from the diet, which consisted of raw grains, berries, roots and herbs. While dental caries did occur in ancient humans, the prevalence was low. Epidemiological studies have shown that the same holds for contemporary isolated populations with a primitive way of life and consistently low sugar intake. A shift towards habits and diets associated with urban living has almost invariably led to a pronounced increase in dental caries. Such observations have been conducted among, for example, North American Inuits, Greenlanders, Native Americans and the inhabitants of the Island of Tristan da Cunha (Fisher, 1968). The food consumed in a modern society is, compared with earlier periods, characterized by manufactured and more processed foods, a high intake of refined flour and a softer food consistency. The starch consumed during earlier periods differed from the highly gelatinized processed starches that constitute a majority of the modern diet. Thus, it may be unwise to extrapolate results of older epidemiological studies, with respect to the starch–caries relationship, to contemporary society.

More recent data show an increase in caries among the rural populations of developing countries. In spite of the fact that the main focus has been on fermentable sugars, it is important to remember that the differences between native diets and diets associated with urban living involve more than just a change in sugar consumption. An example of this is the studies of the population on the isolated island of Tristan da Cunha (Fisher, 1968). The overall increased consumption of refined carbohydrates makes it difficult to make a clear distinction between the effects of sugar and starch. Although several studies point to a low caries prevalence during the consumption of starch (Rugg-Gunn, 1986), occasionally, an increased caries rate has been observed in relation to certain starches such as a diet consisting of frequent consumption of sago starch in a group of people in Papua New Guinea (Schamschula *et al.*, 1978).

It has also been shown that caries prevalence can fall as the refined carbohydrate intake is reduced. As an example, during World War II there were marked changes in the intake of refined carbohydrates in Europe and Japan. A great reduction in caries prevalence, corresponding to a similar reduction in sugars and sugary products and refined flour, was observed (Toverud, 1957; Takeuchi, 1961) (Fig. 19.2).

In a longitudinal study of children aged 6–13 years living in an Australian children's home, Hopewood House, where the diet was mainly lactovegetarian with minimal amounts of sugar and refined flour, the children showed a low caries prevalence compared with a control group. However, caries levels rose to those found in the general population when the children left the home (Harris, 1963). The relation between sugar consumption and the prevalence of dental caries has also been studied in subjects with hereditary fructose intolerance (H), who are unable to eat fructose and sucrose. These individuals have low caries levels (Marthaler, 1967; Newbrun *et al.*, 1980). In a study of 17 H subjects, the sugar intake was 2.5 g for the H and 48.2 g for the control group. The corresponding DMFT levels were 2.1 and 14.3. Both groups ate high levels of starch (160 g/day in the H group and 140 g/day in the control group), indicating that consumption of starch did not appear to be conducive to caries development (Newbrun *et al.*, 1980).

Experimental human studies

Most intervention studies have evaluated either a total replacement or a reduction in the intake of sugars. There are few studies where the relation between diet and dental caries has been studied via an excess of sugar. The Vipeholm study is one of the few where sugar consumption was increased and the relationship between a variety of sugar intakes and caries increment was noted (Gustafsson *et al.*, 1954). It was conducted over a 5-year period (1946–1951) in Sweden, on a population of adult mentally handicapped patients. The main findings were as follows (see also Fig. 19.3):

- A low caries incidence was found when a diet that was almost free of sugars was consumed.
- Caries activity increased with the addition of sugars to the diet, but to a varying degree depending on the manner of consumption.
- Sugars consumed with meals, as sweet drinks or in bread, resulted in a minor increase in caries rate.
- A moderate caries increase was observed for the groups receiving chocolate four times daily, and a dramatic increase for the groups receiving 22 caramels, eight toffees or 24 toffees at and between meals.
- Sugars consumed between meals in a highly retentive (sticky) form resulted in the highest caries activity.

Although a classic study, it has some serious drawbacks, including a complex design where numerous modifications were made during the course of the study. It was carried out

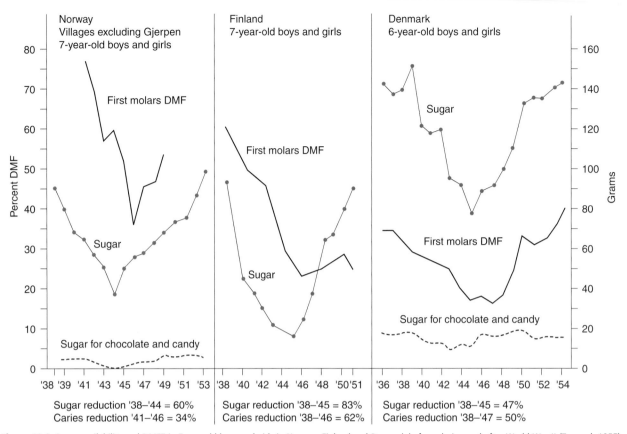

Figure 19.2 Sugar availability and DMFT in 7-year-old boys and girls in Norway, Finland and Denmark before, during and after World War II (Toverud, 1957).

in an institution in a population that is not representative of modern society. Today, the ethics of the Vipeholm study would be unacceptable, but it is important to bear in mind that the link between sugar and caries was not established at the time the study commenced. Nevertheless, the data show that the caries risk is greatest if the sugar is consumed frequently in a form that tends to adhere to the teeth.

Clinical trials of products that are low in sugars or sugar free, which are designed to replace sugar-containing products, are difficult to conduct as the study design would ideally require a sugar-containing control group, which would now be deemed unethical. For this reason, information on the cariogenicity of new products is restricted to data from experimental studies, such as plaque pH studies that measure the acidogenic potential of different foods using pH electrodes placed in dental plaque, and *in situ* caries model experiments that measure the amount of demineralization occurring on enamel or dentin specimens held on intraoral appliances. However, these types of studies are limited in that they do not study the dental health effects of such products as habitually consumed.

In other clinical studies, where different sugar substitutes have been evaluated, caries development in the control group can be used as indirect evidence for the impact of sugars on caries. The Turku sugar study, a controlled longitudinal human study, involved three groups of adult subjects who over 25 months consumed a diet sweetened with sucrose, fructose or xylitol (Scheinin & Mäkinen, 1975). An 85% reduction in caries was found for the individuals in the xylitol group and a 32% reduction for the fructose group, compared with the sucrose group (Fig. 19.4). It should be noted that consumption of starch was high and similar in all three groups. Caries development was virtually eradicated in the xylitol group, indicating the importance of removal of sugar from the diet, rather than starch, in caries control.

The caries increment from either sucrose- or sorbitol-containing sweets has been compared in children aged 3–12 years in a 3-year longitudinal study (Bánóczy *et al.*, 1981). Although there was a high drop-out rate (52%) and the children were living under special conditions, the daily intake of products sweetened with sorbitol resulted in a 45% reduction in caries increment. In one of the few short-term experimental studies conducted, six dental students rinsed with 10 ml of a 50% sucrose solution nine times a day (von der Fehr *et al.*, 1970). After 23 days, a higher mean

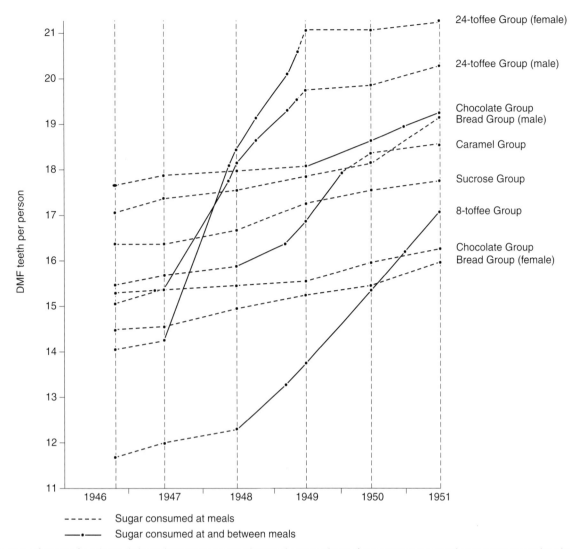

Figure 19.3 Information from the Vipeholm study: DMFT per person relative to the type and time of eating various sugars and sugar-containing products (Gustafsson *et al.*, 1954).

caries index and a greater number of early caries lesions were found compared with six control subjects. The study was interrupted before frank cavitations occurred, but it clearly showed the effect of frequent sugar exposure on the development of caries. The white spots were reversed after cessation of the sucrose rinses. Chewing gum sweetened with 60% sucrose and 20% glucose chewed twice a day for 2 years, by children 7–11 years of age, has been compared with no gum (Glass, 1981). A statistically significant higher caries increment was observed in the group receiving sugared gum.

Influence of different intake patterns

The relative importance of frequency versus the total amount of fermentable carbohydrate consumption is difficult to evaluate. Most studies point to the frequency of eating as being of greater etiological importance for caries than the total consumption of sugars (Karlsbeek & Verrips, 1994). The primary evidence comes from the Vipeholm study discussed above. A positive correlation between the frequency of consumption of confectionery and sugar-containing gum and the DMF rate was also found in a study conducted on 14-year-old Caucasian, Hawaiian and Japanese schoolchildren in Hawaii (Hankin *et al.*, 1973). A range in intake from zero to five or more sweets per day was followed by a corresponding increase in DMF scores.

Against the general perception that frequency of intake is more important than the amount of sugars eaten, two longitudinal studies reported the amount of sugars intake to be more important than frequency (Burt *et al.*, 1988; Rugg-Gunn, 1993; Szpunar *et al.*, 1995); there is, however, undoubtedly a strong correlation between the two variables (Rugg-Gunn, 1993) with an increase in one factor often leading to an increase in the other. Although a high intake

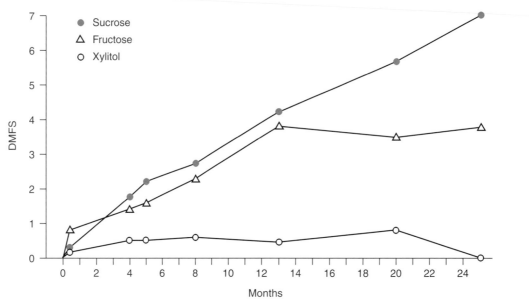

Figure 19.4 Increase in DMFS in the three groups in the Turku experiment based on clinical and radiographic findings and including white spots. (From Scheinin & Mäkinen, 1975.)

frequency increases the overall length of time that the teeth are exposed to sugar-containing foods, it does not give complete information on the total time of exposure. The total cariogenic load is also determined by the form of the food product, i.e. the physical consistency of the sugars-containing foods affects their retention time in the mouth. Distinctions can be made between liquids that are cleared rapidly and adhesive (sticky) foods that vary widely in retentiveness. Particularly high retention rates have been found for products such as sweet biscuits, crackers and potato chips (crisps) (Kashket *et al.*, 1991) (Table 19.1).

Other aspects of intake pattern are also believed to be of importance. The sequence of eating a cariogenic food product during a meal or snack can alter its cariogenic properties (Rugg-Gunn & Nunn, 1999). Both cheese and peanuts can reduce the acid production after a previous intake of sucrose-containing foods. Conversely, starches can increase the cariogenic properties of sugars if they are consumed at the same time. The stickiness of starch enhances the retention time of sugars, resulting in a prolonged pH fall, as occurs in breakfast cereals with added sugars. Another important issue that is difficult to account for in determining the relationship between the dietary intake and caries is that many food products contain hidden sugars. Examples of such sugars-containing products may vary from one country to another. It is not obvious to most people that sugars may be a major constituent in products such as marmalade, breakfast cereals, flavored crisps (chips), caviar, ketchup and, in many countries, bread. Thus, just focussing on confectioneries may have little impact on reducing caries activity if an individual is exposed to many other sugary products per day.

Influence of fluoride on the relationship between sugars and caries

Together with plaque control and the intake of fermentable carbohydrates, the use of fluoride is considered to be the most important factor influencing caries experience. Fluoride has played a major role in the caries decline, mainly due to its effect on inhibiting demineralization and enhancing remineralization, but an effect of fluoride on plaque acidogenicity and cariogenicity has also been suggested. The administration of fluoride in combination with sugar has been suggested as an approach to reduce the cariogenic potential of sugars. The exact mechanisms behind the influence of fluoride on plaque acidogenicity have not been fully evaluated, but it has been conjectured that fluoride may alter different enzymic functions, influence the phosphotransferase system and change the proton-motive force across the cell membrane of oral streptococci.

It is important to note that earlier epidemiological studies were conducted before the widespread use of fluoride. The increased use of fluoride influences the relationship between sugars and dental caries. The relationship between sugar intake and caries levels is thought to be sigmoid (Sheiham, 1983) and the introduction of fluoride has shifted the sugars/caries curve to the right, increasing the 'margin of safety' of sugar intake (Sheiham, 1991). The dramatic decline in dental caries prevalence that has occurred since the 1970s in most Western industrialized countries can be attributed mainly to the widespread use of fluoride and not to changes in diet. In Denmark, where sugar consumption remained at about the same level between 1974 and 1997, there was a sharp decrease in caries experience

Table 19.1 Variation in dry weights of retained food particles in five healthy subjects just after the last bolus of food was swallowed (0 min) and after 5 min; the clearance rates (presented as regression coefficients) are also shown

Food	0 min	5 min	Regression coefficient
Apples	31 ± 46	0	–[a]
Bananas	4 ± 2	0	–
Caramels	64 ± 47	0	–0.99
Chocolate–caramel bars	223 ± 138	0.1 ± 0.2	–0.63
Chocolate–caramel–peanut bars	155 ± 96	1 ± 1	–0.41
Cream-filled sponge cake	116 ± 95	0	–1.00
Cream sandwich cookies	298 ± 50	13 ± 12	–0.26
Dried figs	82 ± 27	2 ± 3	–0.32
Granola bars	151 ± 82	22 ± 20	–0.15
Hot fudge sundaes	–0.1 ± 1	0	–
Jelly beans	46 ± 17	1 ± 2	–0.33
Milk chocolate bars	34 ± 22	0	–
Oatmeal cookies	339 ± 127	44 ± 45	–0.15
Peanut butter crackers	265 ± 105	9 ± 5	–0.27
Plain doughnuts	120 ± 92	1 ± 1	–0.33
Potato chips (crisps)	186 ± 87	21 ± 16	–0.17
Puffed oat cereal	134 ± 129	6 ± 5	–0.24
Raisins	35 ± 15	0.2 ± 0.3	–0.41
Salted crackers	190 ± 39	11 ± 7	–0.23
Sugared cereal flakes	171 ± 67	24 ± 11	–0.16
White bread	49 ± 43	0	–0.91

Data from Kashket *et al.* (1991).
Data are shown as means ± SD.
[a] Foods cleared too rapidly to permit calculation of the coefficients.

(Nyvad, 2003) (Fig. 19.5). The relationship among the frequency of carbohydrate consumption, the use of fluoridated toothpaste and enamel demineralization has been studied using an *in situ* caries model (Duggal *et al.*, 2001). Demineralization was found to occur after seven or more intakes/day when the subjects used a fluoride-containing toothpaste, while demineralization was observed after only three intakes/day during the use of fluoride-free toothpaste.

However, despite the more widespread use of fluoride, the frequency and amount of sugars intake remain important determinants of caries levels. In both longitudinal studies of diet and dental caries, the association between the amount of sugars consumed and dental caries increment was little changed when controlling for oral hygiene practices (e.g. use of fluoride toothpaste) (Rugg-Gunn *et al.*, 1984; Burt *et al.*, 1988). In the National Diet and Nutrition Survey of children aged 1.5–4.5 years (Hinds & Gregory, 1995) and in a study of Swedish school-aged children (Stecksen-Blinks *et al.*, 1985), the use of fluoride only partially dampened the positive relationship between frequency of snacking and caries levels. A systematic review of the evidence for an association between sugars intake and dental caries in modern society has concluded that restriction of consumption of sugars still has a role to play in the

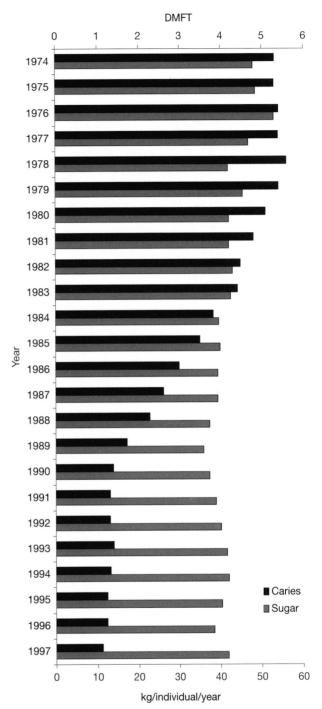

Figure 19.5 Comparison between sugar consumption (kg/individual/year) in Denmark and caries experience (DMFT) in 12-year-old school children between 1974 and 1997. (From Nyvad, 2003.)

control of caries, but that this role is not as strong as it was in the prefluoride era (Burt & Pai, 2001). Therefore, although fluoride has a dramatic effect on caries, it has not eliminated caries, and the optimum use of fluoride, even when achieved, does not remove the underlying cause of caries: dietary sugars.

Groups at increased risk of dental caries in relation to diet

It is likely that protective factors or certain preventive behaviors are present in caries-free subjects, whereas individuals who lack these factors or behaviors may have an increased risk of developing disease. Social and biological factors, as well as dietary risk behaviors, that have a large impact on the development of caries have been identified. If the negative factors are not balanced by positive factors, such as optimum fluoride intake and good oral hygiene, caries may develop. Different diet-related factors that may give an increased caries risk are found in different groups such as infants and toddlers, younger children, people suffering from different diseases, individuals with low socioeconomic status, elderly people, who may have a lower resistance against disease, subjects in different work environments and athletes (Table 19.2).

Infants and toddlers

The dental decay in infants and toddlers collectively known as early childhood caries (ECC) or nursing-bottle caries, where primary maxillary incisors are mainly affected, constitutes a complex problem. The etiology is thought to be night-time bottle feeding or prolonged, on-demand breast feeding (Seow, 1998). However, the evidence for the cariogenic potential of breast milk and milk formula varies and is still inconclusive. Other sweet drinks given to babies in feeding bottles at bedtime or during the night are also associated with increased caries levels. Frequency and duration of exposure are critical in this respect, but the caries experience also often correlates with social and other behavioral factors within the family (Wendt et al., 1995).

Children and adolescents

Based on fluid intake data from the Third National Health and Nutrition Examination Survey (NHANES III, 1988–1994), children in the USA aged 2–10 years with high carbonated soft drink consumption were found to have a significantly higher caries experience in their primary dentition, while consumption of mainly milk, water or juice was less likely to be associated with caries (Sohn et al., 2006). Higher caries prevalence can also be found among older children and adolescents, often associated with lifestyle factors, including an increased intake frequency of candy and soft drinks and snacking at school breaks (Flinck et al., 1999).

Individuals with low socioeconomic status

There is increasing recognition that in many developed countries disparities in health exist among groups with different socioeconomic status (SES), with a disproportionate burden falling on the most disadvantaged people. Poor-quality diets have been associated with increased obesity in the US population, particularly in certain minority groups (Flegal et al., 2002). Reisine and Psoter (2001), based on the findings from a systematic review, found fairly strong evidence for an inverse relationship between SES and the prevalence of caries among young children. The frequency of soft drink consumption has also been shown to be a major determinant of caries experience in low-income African–American adults (Burt et al., 2006).

Elderly and medically compromised people

For adults and elderly people, higher caries rates are often related to medical issues. Today, dietary advice, together with more traditional methods, plays an important role in the medical treatment of many diseases and keeps the symptoms at a low level. A change in the pattern of intake towards a higher frequency is often found in accordance with different gastrointestinal diagnoses, some eating disorders and diabetes. For people suffering from chronic renal failure a low-protein diet must be followed and an adequate intake of non-protein calories must be achieved. Low-protein and protein-free foods tend to be high in refined carbohydrate, which will increase the cariogenic load. Patients requiring dietary energy supplements (e.g. children with failure to thrive, malnourished hospital patients, patients with Crohn's disease) may have an increased risk of caries as energy supplements are high in sucrose, other sugars and glucose

Table 19.2 Examples of individuals with increased caries risk in relation to a high intake of fermentable carbohydrates

Infants and toddlers
  Prolonged breast feeding
  Feeding with bottle at bedtime or night

Children, adolescents
  Frequent intake of soft drinks, confectionery and sugary snacks

Medically compromised people
  Increased intake frequency
  (gastrointestinal diseases, eating disorders, diabetes)

  Increased carbohydrate intake due to total or partial dietary supplementation
  (Crohn's disease, chronic renal failure, chronically ill, malnutrition, failure to thrive)

  Prolonged clearance rate due to reduced salivary secretion rate (Sjögren's syndrome, irradiation, medication)

Athletes
  Sport supplement drinks

In relation to work
  Food sampling
  Work in confectionery industry, bakery
  Monotonous job, night shift

Drug abusers
  Craving for sugar
  Prolonged clearance rate due to reduced salivary secretion rate

polymers. A significantly greater number of decayed, missing and filled teeth have been found in patients with Crohn's disease when compared with matched controls (Rooney, 1984).

A dramatic health change is not necessary to have an increased caries risk. Saliva plays a major role in protecting the teeth, owing to its cleaning actions as well as its acid-neutralizing, antisolubility and antimicrobial properties. A high secretion rate, together with mastication, helps to eliminate sugars and food particles from the oral cavity. A short clearance time reduces the length of time that sugar is available for acid production by the bacteria in the dental plaque. During hyposalivation, which can be found in relation to irradiation in the head and neck area, Sjögren's syndrome, surgery or medication, or in older age groups in poor health, an increased caries rate is often found. Swenander Lanke (1957) performed studies on the clearance of sugar from saliva, to relate the intake of sugar to its availability for bacterial degradation. It was demonstrated that food factors such as sugar concentration, rate of solubilization, rate of enzymic degradation, ability to adhere to the teeth and ability to stimulate salivary flow all affected the rate at which sugar is cleared from saliva. More recent studies have supported this view, revealing slower clearance rates resulting in increased risk for caries in the elderly (Hase *et al.*, 1987), during an artificially induced low secretion rate (Lingström & Birkhed, 1993), and for individuals with normally low secretion rates (Crossner *et al.*, 1991). The clearance rate is believed to be of great importance for today's elderly population, where medically induced low secretion rates are often found in combination with a high number of teeth remaining well into old age. This is of particular importance for the relationship of diet to root caries (Papas *et al.*, 1995).

In all age groups, different medical conditions such as depression, eating disorders, dementia and malnutrition may directly, or via medication, influence salivary properties, resulting in increased caries rates.

Athletes

An effect of sport supplement drinks on dental caries has been discussed. Although no clear evidence of a diet–caries relationship among athletes exists in the literature, such a link cannot be ruled out (Borg & Birkhed, 1987). The specific dietary patterns and increased frequency of sport supplement drinks, often consumed during periods when lower salivary secretion rates may occur, are to be considered as risk factors for dental caries and also dental erosion owing to their acid content (Lussi & Jaeggi, 2006).

Work environment

Working environments that can enhance caries risk can be of two kinds: the job itself is directly linked to an increased intake, or the work environment may promote an increased intake of fermentable carbohydrates. The first category can be exemplified by people working in the catering business or those in industrial food laboratories. For both categories frequent food sampling may occur. The latter risk category may involve subjects working in the confectionery industry or bakeries, where easy access to sugary foods promotes frequent intake. For people working night shifts or those with monotonous jobs, frequent intake of sugary products and snacks is common to 'keep them going'.

Unhealthy lifestyle

Oral effects of the diet in relation to drug abuse are also well known (Rees, 1992). A craving for sugars is felt soon after the intake of drugs such as cannabis and amphetamines. Certain drugs with a sticky consistency may increase the retention time of sugars and many of them also cause dry mouth symptoms. These effects are often enhanced by general bad oral hygiene and an increased intake of pastilles to cover a bad taste.

Multifaceted disease process

The multifaceted nature of the caries process is relevant to any consideration of diet and caries. It may be an oversimplification to attempt to relate the two without also considering the other factors. This has been demonstrated by Sundin *et al.* (1992), who found a low correlation when only caries incidence and consumption of sweets were compared in 69 people aged 15–18 years. The correlation increased when various other factors were combined and the subjects also had poor oral hygiene, a high intake of other sugary products or a low salivary flow rate (Table 19.3). It was concluded that consumption of sweets could still be considered an important caries-related factor, and is particularly harmful when oral hygiene is poor and consumption of other sugary products is high. It is important to keep in mind that one cannot, in a complex disease such as the development

Table 19.3 Results of simple linear correlation analyses between 3-year caries incidence and caries-related factors in 69 18-year-olds

Caries-related factor	*r*
Single factors	
Sweets	0.246
Mutans streptococci count	0.239
Lactobacilli count	0.263
Salivary flow rate	−0.169
Other sugary products	0.164
Combination of factors	
Other sugary products + oral hygiene	0.685
Other sugary products + salivary flow rate	0.672
Other sugary products + oral hygiene + salivary flow rate	0.703
Other sugary products + oral hygiene + lactobacilli count	0.680
Other sugary products + oral hygiene + mutans streptococci count	0.675

Data from Sundin *et al.* (1992).

of caries, look exclusively at one single factor – the diet – without relating it to other factors.

Relative cariogenicity of different carbohydrates

Comparison of different sugars

The monosaccharides (glucose, fructose and galactose) and the disaccharides (sucrose, maltose and lactose) are commonly referred to as sugars, while the term 'sugar' is used synonymously with sucrose. Sugars can be readily metabolized by many bacteria involved in dental biofilm formation, generating acid by-products that can lead to demineralization of the tooth structure. Lactose (milk sugar) has been shown to be less acidogenic than other sugars and less cariogenic, based on animal studies (Rugg-Gunn, 1993). Sucrose has been given special consideration as a cariogenic substrate owing to its unique ability to support the synthesis of extracellular (water-soluble and water-insoluble) glucans by mutans streptococci, enhancing its accumulation in the plaque. Some animal studies in rats superinfected with *Streptococcus mutans* have reported increased cariogenicity of sucrose compared to other sugars; however, this effect appears to be bacterial strain-specific and not consistent across different animal models. More recent clinical studies have indicated that the caries-associated virulence of glucan may have more to do with an alteration in plaque ecology by increasing the porosity of plaque, permitting deeper penetration of dietary sugars and greater acid production adjacent to the tooth surface (Zero, 2004).

Starches

Starch constitutes a heterogeneous food group, which can be divided into starches of different botanical origin. Starches are polymers of glucose that vary in length and branching, e.g. amylose (straight chain, α-1,4 linked glucose) and amylopectin (branched chain, α-1,4 and α-1,6 linked glucose). The starch cariogenicity differs considerably, not only with botanical origin, amount and frequency consumed, but also in relation to food preparation. The starch molecules, which are located within granules can, during heat and mechanical processes, undergo a series of changes in a process called gelatinization (Winter *et al.*, 1971). Products with increased gelatinization are more susceptible to enzymic breakdown, resulting in a higher acidogenic potential (Lingström *et al.*, 1993, 2000). The relative cariogenicity of starch and sugars was evaluated in a 2-year longitudinal dietary study of English schoolchildren in which both dietary intake and dental caries increment were monitored (Rugg-Gunn *et al.*, 1987). When divided according to carbohydrate intake, a lower mean caries increment was found for the high-starch/low-sugars group compared with the low-starch/high-sugars group. The influence of starch on dental caries is likely to be minimal if it is con-

sumed in conjunction with a low-sugar diet and limited eating frequency. In contrast, the cariogenic effect may be amplified when starch is consumed in combination with increased consumption of sugars and high intake frequency. An interaction between starches and sugars can result in prolonged retention on the teeth as well as a shift in plaque ecology towards more caries-inducing plaque properties. These factors may play a particularly important role in patients with hyposalivation and in relation to the development of root caries.

Novel carbohydrates and dental health

Commercially produced novel carbohydrates, including polymers of glucose and oligosaccharides of glucose, fructose and galactose, are increasingly being used in everyday food products owing to their potential health benefits. Information on the dental health effects of these carbohydrates is therefore of great importance.

Glucose syrups and maltodextrins are collectively known as glucose polymers. They are produced by acid hydrolysis of starch and comprise a mixture of mono-, di-, tri-, tetra-, penta-, hexa- and heptasaccharides and alpha limit dextrins (short branched-chain saccharides). Glucose polymers are used to increase the energy content of foods; being virtually tasteless and odorless they may be added to a variety of products without a major influence on the taste and smell of the product. Glucose polymers are frequently added to soft drinks, infant food and drinks, sports drinks, desserts, confectionery and energy supplements.

Streptococcus mutans is capable of intracellular uptake of oligosaccharides composed of three or four glucose units. Salivary amylase may also hydrolyze glycosidic chains, resulting in shorter chains that are readily metabolized by the oral bacteria. The extent of hydrolysis by amylase will be determined by the retention time in the oral cavity. In theory, therefore, glucose polymers are potentially cariogenic; however, evidence to demonstrate this is sparse, with most data from animal, plaque pH and *in vitro* laboratory studies. No difference in caries development was shown between rats fed a diet containing glucose syrups and rats fed a sucrose-containing diet. However, glucose syrups were significantly less cariogenic than sucrose when added to the drinking water of caries-active rats (Grenby & Lear, 1974). In humans, substitution of sucrose with glucose syrups resulted in markedly reduced plaque scores (Fry & Grenby, 1972). There is, however, no strong evidence that the amount of plaque present is related to caries development. Glucose syrups are present, in place of lactose, in soy infant formula, raising concern about the cariogenic potential of these formulae. Although plaque pH studies in human volunteers have shown no significant difference in acidogenic potential between soy infant formula and standard infant milk, no clinical trials have been conducted.

Consumption of maltodextrins depresses plaque pH, but to a lesser extent than sucrose (Moynihan *et al.*, 1996). In the absence of evidence from human clinical trials, advice for the use of glucose polymers should be the same as that for free sugars, and they should not be recommended as sugar substitutes.

Manufactured oligosaccharides

There is increasing interest in the synthesis of novel oligosaccharides and in isolating the transglucosylase enzymes that enable their production. This is not only for economical reasons: their consumption may have potential health benefits. For instance, many of these oligosaccharides are resistant to digestion and pass to the large bowel, where they encourage the growth of lactobacilli and bifidobacteria, which are known to reduce the growth of pathogenic microorganisms. However, many of the species of bacteria found in the colon are also present in dental plaque (e.g. bifidobacteria and lactobacilli), and therefore the dental health effects of these novel carbohydrates warrants investigation.

Isomaltooligosaccharides (IMO), also known as glucosyloligosaccharides, contain monosaccharides that are α1-6 linked (but may contain α1-4) and include isomaltose (glucose α1-6-glucose), isomaltulose (glucose α1-6-fructose, also known as palatinose) and panose (glucose α1-6-glucose α1-4-glucose). They are produced commercially from starch or sucrose by transglucosylation reactions using transglucosylase enzymes.

Plaque pH studies have shown that IMO are less acidogenic than glucose or sucrose, but may nevertheless result in a pH fall to below 5.0. Experimental studies have demonstrated that IMO inhibit glucan synthesis from sucrose and inhibit the sucrose-dependent adherence of *S. mutans* on the tooth surface *in vitro* (for a review see Moynihan, 1998).

Fructooligosaccharides (FOS) are also resistant to digestion in the upper gastrointestinal tract and increase the growth of bifidobacteria. Profeed is an FOS that is marketed as Neosuga, Meioligo, Actilight and Nutraflora. Raftilose (also known as oligofructose) is also widely used in food, especially in Japan. Experimental studies suggest that FOS are potentially as cariogenic as sucrose; however, further studies in animals and human plaque pH studies are required to confirm this.

Some structural isomers of sucrose have similar organoleptic properties to sucrose but have a reduced cariogenic potential. Trehalulose (glucose α-1-1-fructose) is a digestible disaccharide that is 60% as sweet as sucrose and is used in the confectionery industry in Japan. *Streptococcus mutans* and *S. sobrinus* do not utilize trehalulose, it is not a substrate for glucan synthesis (Ooshima *et al.*, 1991) and it does not induce significant caries in rats superinfected with *S. mutans* or *S. sobrinus*. Leucrose (glucose α-1-5-fructose) has also been shown to be non-cariogenic in rats. Sucralose (1′,4′,6′ trideoxy-trichloro-galactosucrose), a chlorinated derivative of sucrose, is now widely available as a sugar alternative, and has been shown to be non-cariogenic in rats (Bowen *et al.*, 1990).

Dental health professionals should be aware and alert their patients that non-digestible oligosaccharides are fermentable carbohydrates, but despite this, products that contain them may be labeled as sugar-free (e.g. chewable sugar-free vitamin tablets).

High-fructose corn syrup

High-fructose corn syrup (HFCS) is produced mainly for economic reasons for use in beverages in the USA. It is chemically similar to invert sugar (50% fructose plus 50% glucose). HFCS, as well as invert sugar, may have slight advantages from a cariological point of view. These sugars do not cause any production of extracellular polysaccharides in the oral cavity and the cariogenicity of invert sugar is slightly less than that of sucrose (Frostell *et al.*, 1991).

Sugars in medicines

Consumption of sugar-containing medicines (cough drops, vitamin preparation and antibiotic syrups) results in a very low pH in dental plaque. Many medicines, particularly those prepared for children, are provided in the form of syrup that is sucrose based, containing up to 70% sugar. Syrups are easier for children to swallow and the dosage is more easily adjusted compared with medications in tablet form, although the latter should be encouraged where possible. Some medicines have to be taken several times a day and often before bedtime, thereby exposing the teeth to sucrose frequently and at night, when there is less saliva available to buffer plaque acids. For a short course of medicine, this should not cause any severe threat to dental health, but for children prescribed medicines on a long-term basis for chronic illness such as epilepsy and chronic infection, there is cause for concern. Control of dental disease in children with chronic illnesses is important to reduce the burden of ill-health. In some conditions such as heart disease, dental caries can predispose to infective endocarditis, increasing morbidity. The issue of sugary medicines damaging teeth was raised as long ago as 1953 and this has been confirmed in several studies showing higher levels of dental caries in young children taking sugared medicines on a long-term basis, a condition sometimes termed 'medication caries'. In chronically ill children, sugared medicine consumption provides approximately 17 g of free sugars/day.

In 1994, the Department of Health in England COMA report, *'Weaning and the weaning diet'* (Department of Health, 1994), highlighted the problem of sugared medicines and recommended that all pediatric medicines were made sugar-free. Children taking long-term sugar-free medicines have been shown to have lower caries than children taking sugared medicines (Maguire *et al.*, 1996). Today, more and more of the manufacturers produce sugar-free medicine and the prescribing of sugar-free formulations should be encouraged by health professionals.

Sugars in medicines pose a threat to the dental health not only of children but also of other groups. Elderly people consume more medication than any other age group and often take long-term medicines with prolonged oral clearance (Maguire & Baqir, 2000). With an increasing trend towards retaining teeth in older age, it is important that sugar-free medications are promoted for use by elderly people, especially when taken frequently, since frequency of sugars intake is an independent risk factor associated with root caries in this age group (Steele *et al.*, 1998).

Some medicines cannot be provided in a sugar-free form, since the sugars present are the active ingredient (e.g. lactulose in the laxative preparation Lactulose BP). Lactulose is composed of lactose and fructose and is resistant to digestion in the upper intestine, but is metabolized by bacteria (e.g. lactobacilli) in the colon. Experiments carried out *in vitro* have shown that lactulose is metabolized by both *S. mutans* and lactobacilli. However, plaque pH studies in human volunteers showed lactulose to pose only a small acidogenic challenge to teeth and, under normal conditions of use, lactulose is unlikely to cause caries (Moynihan *et al.*, 1998).

The sweeteners commonly used in sugar-free liquid oral medicines are sorbitol, hydrogenated glucose syrups (Lycasin) and saccharin (for cariogenicity, see below).

Non-cariogenic sweeteners

One of the main conclusions from the aforementioned Vipeholm study was that sugars in sticky foods consumed between meals was associated with high caries activity. These findings stimulated research on non-acidogenic sugar substitutes (sweeteners) that do not cause pH falls in dental plaque (Birkhed, 1989). It was not until 20 years later, however, that systematic studies carried out in Europe on alternate sweeteners for caries control were published (Mühlemann, 1969; Frostell *et al.*, 1974; Scheinin & Mäkinen, 1975). It is imperative to remember that the usefulness of a sugar substitute has to be looked upon not only from a cariological, but also from a nutritional, toxicological, economic and technical point of view.

When evaluating a non-sugar sweetener in relation to dental caries, it is important to consider the potential for metabolism by oral microorganisms and dental plaque, the influence of consumption on cariogenic microorganisms, and the risk of microbial adaptation to the sweetener. Sugar substitutes can be separated into two major groups: intense sweeteners (non-caloric) and bulk sweeteners (caloric) (Table 19.4).

Intense sweeteners

There are many natural and chemically synthesized intense sweeteners on the market. Some are several thousand times as sweet as sucrose. Glyrrihizin (obtained from licorice root), monellin, thaumatin and mirakulin are examples of naturally occurring intense sweeteners. The latter three are extracted from various fruits. The sweeteners alitame and aspartame are based on amino acids or peptides, while acesulfame-K, cyclamate and saccharin are all chemically synthesized sweeteners. Neohesperdine DC is a modified glycoside, extracted from lemon peel. Intense sweeteners are used in a variety of food products, including soft drinks, beer, confectionery, desserts, ice cream, marmalade and jam. They are also used in dentifrices and in sweetening drops and tablets for use in food, coffee, tea, etc. Currently, about 30% of the carbonated beverages consumed in the USA are sweetened with aspartame.

For safety reasons, there are strict regulations on the use of intense sweeteners, which vary between countries. It should be pointed out, however, that few side-effects of intense sweeteners have been reported in humans. Food labels must declare if a product contains a sweetener and, in the case of aspartame, the label must also say that the product contains a source of phenylalanine, because some individuals are unable to metabolize this amino acid (i.e. those with phenylketonuria).

Intense sweeteners are not metabolized to acids by oral microorganisms, thus they cannot cause dental caries. However, it is important to remember that other ingredients, such as citric or phosphoric acids in beverages, may cause dental erosion. In some food products, intense sweeteners are added as well as sugars, e.g. to fruit-flavored soft drinks, and the naturally occurring sugars in the drink (fructose, glucose and sucrose) may cause caries.

Bulk sweeteners

Among the bulk sweeteners (Table 19.4), sugar alcohols such as sorbitol and xylitol play an important role because of their good technological properties (sweetness, hygroscopity and solubility) and their well-established safety and regulatory acceptance. They are currently used in confectionery, chewing gum, chocolate, jellies and other sweets.

Table 19.4 Examples of intense (non-caloric) sweeteners and bulk (caloric) sweeteners

Intense sweeteners	Bulk sweeteners
Acesulfame-K	Lycasin
Alitame	Maltitol
Aspartame	Mannitol
Cyclmate	Sorbitol
Glyrrihizi	Xylitol
Mirakulin	Isomalt
Monellin	
Neohesperdine DC	
Saccharin	
Sucralose	
Thaumatin	

One of the disadvantages of the bulk sweeteners is that they are only partially absorbed in the small intestine and pass to the colon, where they may induce osmotic diarrhea. For this reason food and drinks containing bulk sweeteners are not recommended for children under 3 years of age, and they may also cause stomach problems when used in sugar-free medicine if the daily intake is high.

Sorbitol

Sorbitol, a six-carbon sugar alcohol, cannot be utilized by the microorganisms that dominate in dental plaque. However, the majority of the strains of mutans streptococci, lactobacilli and some other less frequently encountered oral microorganisms do ferment sorbitol. Concern has been expressed that the observed fermentability of sorbitol, in particular by mutans streptococci, may limit its value as a non-cariogenic sugar substitute. It is essential to bear in mind that there are fundamental differences between the fermentation of sucrose and that of sorbitol by *S. mutans* and other sorbitol-fermenting microorganisms (Birkhed & Bär, 1991). First, the fermentation of sorbitol proceeds at a rather slow rate, and the final pH in liquid cultures normally does not reach such low levels as are regularly seen with glucose or sucrose. Secondly, sorbitol is metabolized by inducible enzymes (enzymes that are usually inactive and only activated if exposed to a substrate), which are synthesized only when the bacteria are exposed to sorbitol for a sufficient period. This means that in the presence of glucose, the bacterial metabolism is rapidly switched back to the metabolic utilization of this more easily available energy source. The constant presence of low levels of glucose in

saliva and the intermittent release of larger amounts of glucose from dietary starch by salivary amylase mean that it is questionable whether dental plaque maintains high sorbitol metabolism. Thirdly, the degradation of sorbitol yields a quantitatively different profile of fermentation endproducts than the catabolism of sucrose. Under anaerobic conditions, lactic acid is the major product of sucrose fermentation, whereas sorbitol yields considerable amounts of ethanol and formic acid, but a smaller proportion of lactic acid. This observation is relevant because lactic acid exerts a stronger demineralizing effect on tooth enamel and dentin than the other volatile fermentation endproducts.

Many studies in which changes in plaque pH have been measured after rinsing with sorbitol solution (Fig. 19.6), or after consumption of sorbitol-based sweets, have concluded that plaque pH drops only marginally and that a critical pH of less than 5.7 is very seldom obtained in dental plaque following sorbitol consumption. It has been argued that there may be adaptive changes in dental plaque upon prolonged exposure, e.g. in a person with a dry mouth, and that this may lead to a possible caries risk on exposed root surfaces (Kalfas *et al.*, 1990). Some studies suggest that prolonged or frequent exposure to sorbitol results in changes in plaque ecology in favor of sorbitol-fermenting bacteria. However, there is no evidence that these adaptive changes will result in dental plaque that metabolizes sorbitol as rapidly as sucrose or glucose (Fig. 19.7). In relation to potential increases in *S. mutans*, there is no doubt that frequent sucrose exposure provides an ecological advantage to this acidogenic and cariogenic microorganism, whereas frequent exposure to sorbitol has hardly any clinically relevant

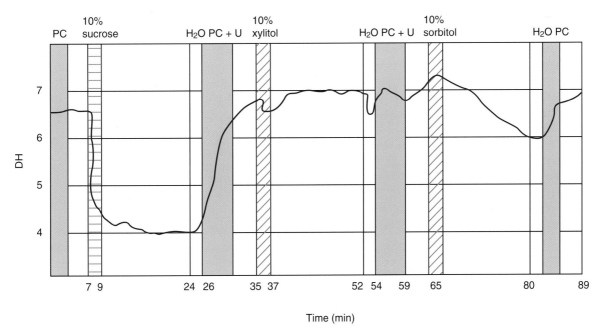

Figure 19.6 Telemetrically recorded interproximal plaque pH after a 10% sucrose rinse; water rinse (H₂O); paraffin chewing (PC) and urea rinse (PC + U); 10% xylitol and 10% sorbitol rinse. (From Mühlemann *et al.*, 1977.)

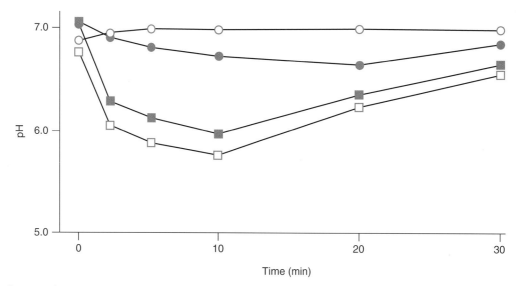

Figure 19.7 Plaque pH after a 30 s mouth rinse with 10% solutions of glucose (□) and sorbitol (○) before and with glucose (■) and sorbitol (●) after a 6-week period with frequent daily mouth rinses with sorbitol (means of 18 subjects). (From Birkhed & Bär, 1991.)

effect. Therefore, it appears that the potential hypoacidogenic properties of sorbitol do not pose a cariogenic threat to the majority of people.

Xylitol

Xylitol is a pentitol, a sugar alcohol with five carbons. Several studies have shown that most oral streptococci and other microorganisms do not ferment xylitol. In contrast to sorbitol, xylitol exerts a bacteriostatic effect on mutans streptococci. The inhibitory effect is apparently due to the entry of xylitol into the bacterial cell resulting in an intracellular accumulation of xylitol 5-phosphate. Ultrastructural studies of *S. mutans* and *S. sobrinus* have shown that the presence of xylitol results in cell degradation, intracellular vacuoles and other damage to the cell. It is well established that xylitol does not lower the pH of dental plaque *in vivo* (Fig. 19.6) or *in vitro* (Mühleman *et al.*, 1977). It has been speculated that xylitol may have an inhibitory effect on the acid production from sucrose and glucose in dental plaque. However, the data are conflicting, as some studies *in vitro* have shown such an effect (Wåler & Rölla, 1983), whereas *in vivo* studies have failed to demonstrate a direct inhibitory action of xylitol on the acid production from sugars (Mühlemann *et al.*, 1977). This means that it is questionable to mix xylitol with sugars in the same product and then market them as 'low cariogenic'. Nevertheless, the non-acidogenicity of xylitol in dental plaque is well documented and probably one of the most important factors related to its non-cariogenicity. When xylitol is consumed frequently and for a long period, the metabolism of dental plaque has been found to be altered, resulting in less acid formation from sucrose (Aguirre-Zero *et al.*, 1993). This may be due to ecological changes in the microflora or reduced produc-

tion of dental plaque. Another possible mechanism is the accumulation of xylitol 5-phosphate in plaque bacteria after exposure to xylitol.

One of the most interesting effects of xylitol, besides being non-acidogenic, is its ability to reduce the population of mutans streptococci. This has been found in several short- and long-term studies. The effects of sorbitol, xylitol, and a mixture of xylitol and sorbitol in chewing gums were compared in adults (Söderling *et al.*, 1989). The plaque and salivary levels of *S. mutans* generally increased in the sorbitol group, but decreased in the two groups using xylitol. A clear dose–response effect in this respect was found in a 3-week cross-over study by Wennerholm *et al.* (1991). Four types of chewing gum containing 70% xylitol, 35% xylitol + 35% sorbitol, 17.5% xylitol + 52.5% sorbitol, or 70% sorbitol were compared. The gum with the highest xylitol content resulted in the lowest *S. mutans* count. The inhibitory effect of xylitol on *S. mutans* has been evaluated in other studies and in other types of products. For example, when 10–20% xylitol was added to a fluoride dentifrice, the level of mutans streptococci in saliva was reduced (Svanberg & Birkhed, 1991). However, Petersson *et al.* (1991) did not find reduced *S. mutans* when using a dentifrice containing only 3% xylitol.

Habitual xylitol consumption by mothers over several years may reduce the mother–child transmission of mutans streptococci (Söderling *et al.*, 2001), which may prevent caries in the primary dentition (Isokangas *et al.*, 2000).

Lycasin, maltitol and mannitol

Other polyols beside sorbitol and xylitol are currently used as bulk sweeteners, especially in confectionery products. The best known are Lycasin, maltitol and mannitol (Table 19.4).

Although these sweeteners have not been evaluated as extensively as sorbitol and xylitol, animal studies, plaque pH studies *in vivo* and incubation studies *in vitro* have indicated that they have a low cariogenic potential.

Lycasin (which is a trade name) is a hydrogenated starch hydrolysate. It is produced from potato or corn starch by partial acid or enzymic hydrolysis and subsequent hydrogenation at high pressure and high temperature. Thus, the final product contains a mixture of hydrogenated mono-, di-, tri- and tetrasaccharides (i.e. sorbitol, maltitol, maltotriitol and maltotetraitol) and higher chain-length hydrogenated saccharides. Various types have been manufactured, but currently, most Lycasin products contain over 50% maltitol and a relatively low proportion of higher molecular weight carbohydrates. This lower latter proportion is an advantage from a cariological point of view because salivary α-amylase can split the higher hydrogenated saccharides to form glucose, maltose and maltotriose, which may be metabolized by dental plaque bacteria. Both animal and bacteriological studies have shown that Lycasin has a low to medium cariogenic potential depending on which type of Lycasin has been used. Hard sugared confectionery sweetened with Lycasin, with a high content of maltitol and a low content of higher saccharides, causes a relatively small decrease in plaque pH (Imfeld & Mühlemann, 1978).

Maltitol is a 12-carbon polyol, which is produced by hydrogenation of maltose. This sugar alcohol cannot be metabolized by most oral microorganisms. However, mutans streptococci, *Actinomyces* and some species of lactobacilli can ferment it at a slow rate (Edwardsson *et al.*, 1977). Both animal experiments and plaque pH studies in human volunteers have suggested that maltitol is virtually noncariogenic. Maltitol lozenges eaten four times a day for 3 months did not affect plaque formation, acid production or the number of mutans streptococci and lactobacilli in dental plaque (Birkhed *et al.*, 1979).

Mannitol, like sorbitol, is a hexitol. It is industrially prepared by hydrogenation of invert sugar, sucrose or monosaccharides. Lactobacilli and *S. mutans* are unique among the dental plaque microflora in their ability to ferment the two-sugar alcohols mannitol and sorbitol. The enzymes mannitol 6-phosphate dehydrogenase and sorbitol 6-phosphate dehydrogenase involved in hexitol catabolism are, however, inducible and their synthesis is inhibited by the presence of glucose in saliva (Brown & Wittenber, 1973). Accordingly, mannitol is of low acidogenicity (Ahldén & Frostell, 1975; Imfeld, 1977).

Use of non-sugar sweeteners for caries control

Several field studies on xylitol, carried out in Russia, Polynesia, Hungary and Estonia (Mäkinen, 2000), have demonstrated that xylitol is non-cariogenic. Moreover, four long-term trials of xylitol in chewing gum have been conducted: the Turku chewing-gum study (Scheinen *et al.*, 1975),

the Ylivieska study (Isokangas *et al.*, 1988), the Montreal study (Kandelman & Gagnon, 1990) and, most recently, the Belize study (Mäkinen *et al.*, 1995).

In the Turku chewing-gum study, young adults were assigned to either a xylitol or a sucrose gum group (Scheinen *et al.*, 1975). The mean caries increment after 1 year, assessed independently by clinical and radiographic means, was 2.9 DMFS in the sucrose and −1.0 in the xylitol group. The corresponding values when also considering recurrent caries were 3.8 and 0.3. However, since there was not a control group chewing a placebo gum, the reduction in caries may not be solely attributed to xylitol. The protective effect of increased salivary flow may, as a result of chewing, have contributed to or accounted for the caries reduction.

The schoolchildren in the Ylivieska study (Isokangas *et al.*, 1988) were all participating in organized dental health programs on an annual basis. They were randomly divided into two test groups using a xylitol gum and a control group which chewed no gum. The authors concluded that xylitol gum, used two to three times/day in combination with basic fluoride use, constitutes a strong instrument in caries control. Two to three years later, the children were re-examined for a possible long-term preventive effect. A significant caries reduction was found, especially among the girls. The authors speculated that the probable explanation for the difference between the xylitol and control groups was the occurrence of microbiological changes in the mouth and/or the maturation of the erupting teeth under favorable physicochemical conditions. The latter hypothesis was partly confirmed in a microbiological study of proximal tooth surfaces in a group of former habitual xylitol gum users (Isokangas *et al.*, 1993). However, neither the influence of the chewing action nor the specific effect of xylitol on caries reduction can be measured from this study, as it did not include a control group on a placebo gum or a gum containing a sugar substitute other than xylitol. It should also be noted that the dental examination was not carried out blind to the group identity of the children.

The subjects in the Montreal study (Kandelman & Gagnon, 1990), like those in the Ylivieska study, participated in an ongoing preventive dental school program. The participants were assigned to one of three groups, two xylitol groups and one control group, which chewed no gum. The gum was distributed three times a day by the teacher supervising the 5 min chewing period. After 12 months, there was a significantly lower DMFS increment in the two xylitol groups than in the control group. Children who used chewing gum with 65% xylitol had less caries than those who used a gum with 15% xylitol. After 24 months, the caries incidence remained lower in the two test groups than in the control group, but no statistically significant difference existed between the 65% and the 15% xylitol groups. A review of clinical trials of xylitol (Imfeld, 1994) states that the similarity in caries levels between the 65% and 15%

xylitol groups suggests that the caries-preventive effect is due to the frequency of chewing rather than the xylitol content of the gum, but no firm conclusion may be drawn as the control group, as in the Turku and Ylivieska studies, did not chew a placebo gum.

The fourth chewing-gum study, the Belize study, was carried out in Central America in children initially aged 10 years, whose caries levels were moderate to high (Mäkinen et al., 1995). Altogether, 1277 children were divided into nine groups, one of which received sugared gum. In seven other groups either xylitol or sorbitol gums, or gums that contained mixtures of these two polyols, were consumed. The children in the ninth group received no gum. The use of gum was supervised by teachers on about 200 schooldays/year and unsupervised on about 165 days/year. The chewing time at school was 5 min, normally in the form of five chewing episodes/day (i.e. 5 × 5 min a day). After 28 months of intervention, the highest mean DMFS scores were found in the two groups using either sugar gum or no gum. The lowest DMFS scores were observed in groups using 100% xylitol gum. The sorbitol gum and the gums containing mixtures of xylitol and sorbitol resulted in higher DMFS scores compared with gum containing only xylitol.

Beside these four chewing-gum studies there is also clinical evidence that xylitol candies are as effective as xylitol gum in caries prevention and that it is economically feasible to include xylitol in school-based caries control programs (Alanen et al., 2000).

The Belize study is the first clinical trial of xylitol that enables a comparison of the caries-preventive action of xylitol to be compared with sorbitol, and the results indicate that xylitol is superior in reducing caries. These findings should now be validated in randomized studies that account for dietary habits, oral hygiene practice and socioeconomic status in other populations. Despite promising findings, there is at present no strong evidence from clinical studies of a superior cariostatic action of xylitol compared with other polyols (Imfeld, 1994; Scheie & Fejerskov, 1998).

The most important goal of preventive dentistry is to reduce the consumption of sweet products to a minimum. However, this may be difficult to achieve. Therefore, if intense and bulk sweeteners can be accepted from a nutritional and toxicological point of view, they may be recommended in certain risk products that are used very frequently, e.g. chewing gum, confectionery, medicine and beverages. The impact of using non-cariogenic sugar substitutes in medicine and beverages is not known since controlled clinical studies are lacking, but the caries-preventive effect can expected to be considerable. In chewing gums and confectionery, the caries-reducing effect can be expected to be 20–40% depending on the intake frequency of the sugar-free products and on the caries activity.

A recent 3-year community intervention trial in Lithuania on the caries-preventive effect of sugar-substituted chewing gum showed that the effect was more related to the chewing process itself, rather than being an effect of gum sweeteners, such as polyols (sorbitol and xylitol) and carbamide (Machiulskiene et al., 2001).

Protective factors in foods

Foods and food components that have anticariogenic properties are sometimes referred to as 'cariostatic factors'. Fluoride is undoubtedly the most effective of these factors and has been discussed previously. Here, an overview of other protective factors and the implications of their consumption for dental health are given.

Despite being one of the main sources of sugars in the diet of young children, cow's milk is non-cariogenic. The sugar in milk is lactose, which is the least cariogenic sugar, and milk is also known to contain protective factors. In situ caries model experiments have shown that cow's milk causes less enamel solubility than lactose or sucrose solutions and reduces the cariogenic potential of sugar-containing foods. The non-cariogenic nature of milk can be attributed to the presence of calcium, phosphate and casein, and plaque pH and animal studies have confirmed its caries-preventive nature. Recent epidemiological studies indicate a positive or neutral effect of cow's milk consumption on caries (Levy et al., 2003; Marshall et al., 2003).

Compared with cow's milk, breast milk contains more lactose (~7% vs 4–5%) and lower concentrations of calcium and phosphate and so, in theory, may be more cariogenic. However, epidemiological evidence indicates that breast feeding is associated with lower dental caries (Holt et al., 1982; Silver, 1987). This could be a secondary effect due to socioeconomic status, which is linked to both breast feeding and lower consumption of sugars. However, there is no opportunity to add additional sugars to breast milk feeds, and breast-fed infants are less likely to use reservoir feeders containing sugary liquids (Rugg-Gunn & Nunn, 1999). There have been reports of cases of severe dental caries associated with prolonged (usually over 2 years) on-demand breast feeding, often when infants have suckled during the night (Hackett et al., 1984). However, these cases are rare and associated with unusual feeding practices. Breast feeding should be promoted since it provides the best infant nutrition.

Numerous animal studies and experimental studies have indicated that cheese is anticariogenic (for a review see Moynihan, 2000). Consumption of cheese increases oral pH by stimulating salivary flow and raises plaque calcium concentrations, both of which protect against demineralization. Cheese also contains casein phosphopeptides, amorphous calcium phosphate nanocomplexes which play an important role in the remineralization process (Reynolds et al., 2003). Meals containing cooked cheese have also been shown to increase plaque calcium concentrations, which is important as a strong relationship exists between calcium concentrations in dental plaque and dental caries increments (Fig. 19.8). Cheese intake was shown to be higher in children who remained caries free over a 2-year period than in children who developed most caries (Rugg-Gunn *et al.*, 1984), and children who consumed 5 g of Edam daily following breakfast for a period of 2 years had a significantly lower caries increment than controls (Gedalia *et al.*, 1994).

A lower than expected caries level in groups of people known to have high carbohydrate diets, such as the Bantu tribe of South Africa and sugarcane cutters, led to an interest in the presence of protective factors in foods of plant origin. Protective factors in plants include organic phosphates, inorganic phosphates, polyphenols and phytate. It has been postulated, from the results of animal studies, that organic phosphates protect the teeth by adsorbing to the enamel, forming a protective coat. However, organic phosphates have not been found to be effective in humans.

Phytate is anticariogenic and acts by adsorbing to the enamel surface to form a physical barrier that protects against plaque acids. Phytate naturally present in food is, however, unlikely to be released from the food structure before being swallowed. Phytate is unsuitable as a cariostatic food additive because it is known to reduce the absorption of iron, magnesium, calcium and zinc. One of the main reasons why people who consume diets high in unrefined plant foods have fewer carious lesions is probably the stimulation of saliva flow that occurs on consumption of fibrous foods. Saliva not only helps to clear food debris from the mouth, but also buffers plaque acid and therefore promotes remineralization of tooth enamel.

Inorganic phosphates prevent demineralization of enamel, although much of the evidence comes from animal studies and studies in humans have produced equivocal results. The most effective inorganic phosphate in preventing dental caries is sodium trimetaphosphate (Na-TMP), which was shown to be effective when added to chewing gum and chewed by children three times a day (Finn *et al.*, 1978). However, the levels of Na-TMP required to prevent dental caries may result in undesirably high sodium intakes.

There is increased interest in foods that contain polyphenols, as animal and experimental studies have shown these compounds to have antibacterial properties. Apples contain polyphenols and are a good stimulus to salivary flow. However, they are acidic in nature and contain sugars; clinical trials conducted several decades ago on the dental health effects of apples produced equivocal results. Tea also contains polyphenols, in addition to fluoride and flavanoids. Tea extracts have also been shown to inhibit salivary amylase activity (Kashket & Paolino, 1998). Animal studies have found that infusions of black tea reduce dental caries (Rosen *et al.*, 1984). Epidemiological studies of caries levels in tea drinkers compared with non-drinkers have produced mixed results. Findings of recent studies suggest that cranberries may act cariostatically through reducing bacterial adherence and glucosyltransferase activity of *S. mutans* (Koo *et al.*, 2006).

Consumption of foods with cariostatic properties that are also healthy in terms of the diet in general, e.g. milk, cheese and unrefined plant foods, should be encouraged. However, some of the cariostatic factors identified in foods have limited application in their natural source and these

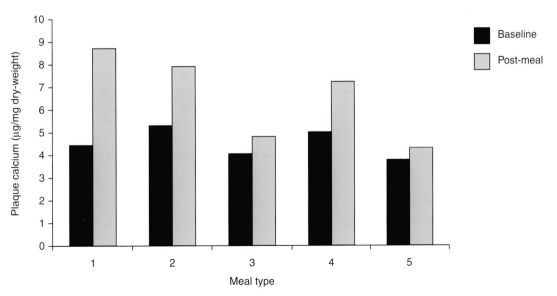

Figure 19.8 Plaque calcium concentration before and after consumption of cheese and cheese-containing meals. Mean values of 16 subjects. 1: 15 g cube of cheese; 2: test meal, pasta in cheese sauce; 3: control meal: pasta in mushroom sauce; 4: test meal: chicken breast with cheese and ham filling; 5: control meal: chicken breast with mushroom and ham filling. (Based on data from Moynihan *et al.*, 1999.)

include esters in honey, cocoa factor in chocolate, gly-cyrrhizinic acid in licorice and phytate. There is a potential for cariostatic factors to be isolated from foods for use as anticariogenic food additives; however, the effectiveness of these 'additives' would need to be confirmed in human clinical trials.

Sugar-free chewing gum, in addition to being sweetened with non-cariogenic sweeteners, provides a gustatory and mechanical stimulus to salivary flow and therefore may be considered as cariostatic. Chewing sugar-free gum for 20 min following a meal or snack has been shown to accelerate the return to resting oral pH. The results of clinical trials of sugar-free gums have already been discussed.

Diet and dental erosion

In addition to being the main driver of dental caries, diet plays an important role in another destructive process, dental erosion, which results in the surface dissolution of dental hard tissues. While there are similarities between dental caries and erosion in that both result from the demineralization of tooth mineral by acids, the major difference is that dental erosion occurs in the absence of the dental biofilm. Dental erosion is the main pathological factor leading to tooth wear, which along with abrasion and attrition contributes to the multifactorial nature of this condition.

The process of dental erosion is reasonably straightforward. However, the clinical expression of dental erosion is fairly complex and is modified by the chemical and physical properties of a food or beverage (Lussi et al., 1993; Larsen & Nyvad, 1999), and biological and behavioral factors (Zero & Lussi, 2000). While dental erosion is recognized as an increasingly important problem in most European countries, it is not receiving much attention in the USA (Derry et al., 2000). Changes in lifestyle and the increasing availability of acidic beverages and juices are considered to be responsible for an increase in the prevalence of dental erosion, primarily in young children and adolescents (Millward et al., 1994; Al-Dlaigan et al., 2001). In addition, the improvement in oral hygiene and obsession with whiter teeth may be having an unintended negative consequence by rendering teeth more susceptible to acids of extrinsic and extrinsic origin, because, counter-intuitively, plaque and stains on teeth actually provide protection against dental erosion (Zero, 1996).

The potential of acidic foods and beverages to cause erosion has been known for some time (Miller, 1907). A wide range of acidic food substances has been implicated by varying degrees of scientific evidence, including citrus fruit juices and other acidic fruit juices, acidic carbonated beverages, acidic uncarbonated beverages, acidic sport drinks, wines, cider, acidic herbal teas, citrus fruits and other acidic fruits and berries, salad dressing, vinegar conserves and acidic fruit-flavored candies (for a review see Zero, 1996).

Of particular dietary concern is the high and increasing intake of acidic beverages, especially juices and soft drinks, which in addition to adding low- or non-nutritive calories, may be contributing to dental erosion. In the USA the consumption by adolescences of fruit juices and soft drinks has more than doubled over the past 30 years, while over the same period the consumption of milk decreased by 36% (Cavadini et al., 2000).

The erosive potential of dietary sources of acids, namely citric (citrus juices), phosphoric (soft drinks), malic (apple juice), tartaric (grape juice and wine), acetic (vinegar) and other acids found in beverages and foods has been shown in many in vitro, in situ and in vivo studies (for reviews Zero, 1996; Lussi et al., 2004). The erosive potential of an acidic food or drink is not entirely dependent on its pH, but is also strongly affected by its titratable acid content (buffering capacity) and by the calcium-chelation properties (Zero & Lussi, 2005). Citric acid is considered to have greater ability to cause erosive tooth wear than other dietary acids owing to its calcium-chelating properties. The ultimate erosive potential of a food or drink depends on an interaction among its chemical properties (pH, total acid content, calcium, phosphate and fluoride content, and adhesiveness), biological factors (salivary flow rate, buffering capacity and composition, pellicle formation, tooth composition, and dental and soft-tissue anatomy) and behavioral (lifestyle) factors (eating and drinking habits, especially the frequency, duration and timing of exposure). The interplay of these factors at a given tooth surface determines the degree of saturation in relationship to tooth mineral and whether erosion will occur or not.

Promoting good dietary habits for dental health

Factors that influence diet at a national level

The availability and range of foods have increased substantially over the past 50 years in industrialized countries and as advances in food technology progress, diet will continue to change. It is therefore important that action on dietary advice is taken at a national level to ensure that dietary changes are changes for the better. The most obvious expression of the recent changes in dietary patterns is the increasing number of overweight and obese individuals. Obesity and its consequences have become a major global health problem in most industrialized and developing countries. While a link between the consumption of sugars and obesity has been established (Ludwig et al., 2001) and the role of sugars in caries development is beyond refute, the relationship between dental caries and obesity remains inconclusive owing to the limited number of high-quality studies supporting this contention (Kantovitz et al., 2006). Willershausen et al. (2004) reported an association between an increase in dental caries and overweight schoolchildren (6–11 years old); however, other studies have not been able to support a relationship (Chen *et al.*, 1998; Macek & Mitola, 2006). Strategies intended to limit consumption of sugars will also be likely to have a positive impact on caries control.

International organizations such as the World Health Organization (WHO) and Food and Agricultural Organization (FAO) periodically hold expert consultations on matters relating to diet and health, which help to guide governments in the formation of country-specific recommendations. The recent WHO/FAO (2003) consultation 'Diet, Nutrition and the Prevention of Chronic Diseases' has made recommendations that are globally applicable. With respect to sugars intake, the report stated:

The best available evidence indicates that the level of dental caries is low in countries where the consumption of free sugars is below 15–20 kg per person per year. This is equivalent to a daily intake of 40–55 g per person and the values equate to 6–10% of energy intake. It is of particular importance that countries with low consumption levels do not increase consumption levels. For countries with high consumption levels it is recommended that national health authorities and decision-makers formulate country-specific and community-specific goals for reduction in the amount of free sugars aiming towards the recommended maximum of not more than 10% energy intake.

The report also stated that to minimize the risk of dental erosion the amount and frequency of intake of soft drinks and juices should be limited.

Government food policy

Governments publish reports on diet and health that inform food policies. In the UK, the Department of Health Committee on Medical Aspects of Food Policy has produced reports on issues related to diet, such as the 1989 report *Dietary sugars and human disease*. Such reports inform food policy and help to direct health education. The governments of many countries have produced oral health strategies which emphasize diet and the need to reduce consumption of sugars. The consistent nutritional public health message is to increase the intake of starch-rich staple foods (in particular wholegrain varieties), fruits and vegetables, and reduce the intake of fat, non-milk extrinsic sugars (free sugars) and alcohol. These dietary messages should be promoted by all health professionals, including dietetic, medical and dental professionals, and all government departments (health, agriculture, education and industry).

Government-funded health education bodies, such as the National Institutes of Health (NIH) in the USA, produce leaflets and booklets on issues relating to diet and dental health. In the UK the booklet *The scientific basis of dental health education* (Levine & Stillman-Lowe, 2003) is now in its fifth edition and is widely referred to by dental health professionals and other medical professionals alike.

Such documents are important in order that health professionals give advice that is accurate and consistent.

Governments also have a strong influence on schools, with respect to both curriculum content and food provision. It is important that governments are informed on current issues regarding goals to reduce the sugars intake of children and on the importance of nutrition education, so that it remains an important part of the curriculum in schools. Governments also have a role to play in ensuring that health professionals are adequately qualified with respect to dietary issues, and should provide funding for primary and continued education in this area. There is both the need and opportunity for increased training of nutritionists in dental health issues and for more training of dentists in dietary issues.

Governments have an important role to play in both health education and funding research. It is important that they continue to fund ongoing and comprehensive nutritional surveillance of populations, so that the sugars-eating habits and nutrition of population groups are monitored, and the relationship between diet and dental caries is re-examined periodically. In the UK, the Food Standards Agency conducts ongoing national nutritional surveys of different population age groups, 'The National Diet and Nutrition Surveys', which include a dental examination, and thereby enable examination of relationships between diet and oral health. Similarly in the USA, the NHANES provides data on dietary patterns and oral health of adults. It is also important that government funding is available for research in primary care as the emphasis on evidence-based practice increases.

Government legislation and regulation

Food labeling is carefully controlled and nutrition labeling is an important component of this. There is much debate as to whether nutrition labeling should be compulsory or voluntary, but at present in Europe it is voluntary and a product only has to have a nutrition label if a health or nutrition claim is made. For example, if a soft drink claims to have 'no added sugar', then the sugar content must be labeled (Table 19.5a). The problem with this system is that high-sugar foods do not tend to make health claims, and therefore the manufacturer need not label them. If the manufacturer voluntarily labels the product, sugars may be included under the wider umbrella of carbohydrate, along with starch (Table 19.5b). This is unhelpful to consumers, who know that they should reduce their intake of sugars but increase their intake of starch. There is still a wide scope for improvement in nutritional labeling systems for content of sugars in foods.

Advertising on television is expensive and out of reach of most health promotion campaigners. However, the food industry spends millions on television advertising to promote food products that are often of low nutritional value,

Table 19.5 Examples of how foods are labeled: (a) giving sugar content; (b) not specifying sugar content

(a)	Nutrition information
Typical values	Per 100 g of product
Energy	1410 kJ
	335 kcal
Protein	11.5 g
Carbohydrate of which sugars	66.8 g
	0.7 g
Fat of which saturates	2.2 g
	0.5
Fiber	12.5
Sodium	trace

(b)	Nutrition information
Typical values	Per 100 g of product
Energy	2039 kJ
	468 kcal
Protein	4.4 g
Carbohydrate	66.8 g
Fat	22.4 g

and high in sugars and fat (Dibb & Castell, 1995). Such advertising is in strong opposition to health promotion, and unless television authorities and governments in all countries impose stricter codes of conduct, television advertising will continue to promote the consumption of high-sugar foods by children. All countries should follow the example of Canada, Belgium and Sweden, where all advertising during children's viewing times is restricted.

Professional organizations and national campaigns

National professional organizations of dentists, doctors and nutritionists may influence national policy, and most have policy documents concerning diet and dental health. Such bodies inform governments with unbiased information on sugars, diet and dental caries. It is highly desirable, however, that all such professional bodies are promoting the same messages, and professional liaison between disciplines is therefore essential.

Pressure groups and consumer organizations have been known to initiate and promote campaigns on dental and diet-related issues. For example, the group Action and Information on Sugars launched a 'Chuck the Sweets off the Checkout' campaign in the UK. As a result of this campaign, the majority of supermarkets in the UK removed sweets from the checkout, resulting in a 30% decrease in supermarket confectionery sales.

Food industry

A lot of information on diet and health is generated by the sugar-related industries; they may wish to be seen as being concerned about health, but their main objectives are to promote the consumption of sugar and sugar-rich foods and generate profits for shareholders. Educational information produced by the food industry keeps its interests at heart; some of it is good, but with respect to sugars and dental caries, the information presented is quite different from that being promoted by governments and health education bodies. Since the 1980s, supermarkets have responded to consumer demand for information on diet and health and many produce good information leaflets. Those concerned with dental health education must ensure that the information distributed is scientifically correct.

It is important that health professionals work with the food industry and encourage the increased production of low-sugars and sugars-reduced foods. There has been a sharp rise in the use of convenience foods over the past few decades. The shift towards reliance on convenience foods away from home food preparation means that the consumer has little control over how much sugar is added. Sugar is often hidden, so people are unaware of how much they are consuming. Positive actions by the food industry in terms of dental health have been the production of sugar-free sweets and sweeteners and also the development of soft drinks with lower erosive and cariogenic potential.

Advice at a group level

Much can be achieved at a local community level to promote good dietary habits for dental health. In the past many initiatives took place but were not evaluated. It is important that health promotion initiatives are evaluated to ensure that the findings of projects can contribute to evidence-based health care. Health promotion related to diet and dental health can take place in health centers, dental practices, schools and the workplace. Health professionals involved in antenatal care, such as midwives and health visitors, are an important source of information for parents and it is vital that they receive adequate and ongoing training in diet and related issues. School governors are important in determining health policies in UK schools that cover areas such as tuck shops. There is evidence from Australia and England that banning sweets in schools reduces the development of dental caries in children (Rugg-Gunn & Nunn, 1999).

Community dental officers have an important role to play in promoting the importance of diet and oral health, and in educating other community-based health professionals in the topic, e.g. by working with community dietitians, practice nurses and pharmacists. Community health programs have existed in Scandinavia for a number of years; these include dietary advice for dental health at both the individual and group level. In Finland such advice has focussed on avoiding frequent consumption of sugar and using xylitol gum at least once a day. In Switzerland there has been much success with programs to encourage the use of sugar-free confectionery under the logo 'safe for teeth' (*Zahnfreundlich*), which now amounts to almost a quarter of confectionery sold. Scandinavian preventive dentists promoted Saturday Sweets Day, a system whereby children accumulate sweets and confectionery given to them over the week and consume them in one go on a Saturday. This means that frequency of consumption is decreased considerably without inflicting deprivation.

Advice at an individual level

The details of dietary advice to individuals will be dealt with in Chapter 27. Here, some general considerations for advice at the level of the individual are presented. Dietary control is an important part of caries prevention. Some may argue that diet is unimportant because you cannot change what people eat. However, diets do change and have done so considerably over the last half century; it is important that there is continued effort to ensure that changes are desirable in terms of dental health. There is scientific support that dietary interventions can have a positive impact on dietary behaviors (Bradbury *et al.*, 2006; Knai *et al.*, 2006). While the evidence is dated, studies have shown that dietary advice to restrict sugar consumption can be effective in reducing dental caries (Becks, 1950; Nikiforuk, 1985). Despite its importance, statistics indicate that the provision of dietary advice in dental practice is lacking. In the UK, the Dental Survey of the National Diet and Nutrition Survey indicated that less that 50% of parents of preschool children had received any advice from their dentist regarding diet and dental health (Hinds & Gregory, 1995). It is known that many dental practices do not follow set protocols for the provision of dietary advice, are not in agreement over whose role it is to provide this advice, and think that there are inadequate provisions for delivering this important part of patient care. Many factors influence individual food choice, which is why it is often difficult to try to get patients to change what they eat. Physiological, psychological, behavioral, socioeconomic and cultural factors all influence food choice, and all must be considered when facilitating dietary change. There have been far too few studies into the effectiveness of dietary advice in dental practice and this area warrants further research.

Preventive dentistry often focusses on the level of the individual, and governments argue that individuals, with support from health professionals, should be responsible for their own actions. Whether all individuals should receive preventive dietary advice is not a straightforward question (as discussed by Rose, 1993). If all patients were to be given dietary advice, this would leave limited time to conduct the task to a satisfactory level. It has also been argued that providing preventive advice to low-risk patients may cause unnecessary inconvenience (to the patient) and cost (to the dentist) for little benefit. An alternative approach is to screen patients who are at high risk. However, this requires a robust screening process, and screening is not foolproof and inevitably leads to some high-risk patients being undetected. All individuals need to be made aware of the factors that contribute to dental caries. A sensible approach would be to provide advice at two levels: general advice to all patients (verbal, written and visual information in the waiting room and practice to reinforce messages) and individual customized advice to those patients who are at higher risk. Leaflets are useful for providing general advice, especially if tailored to the age group and level of literacy of the patient. Failure to provide dietary advice as part of total patient care could be seen to be negligent, as the disease will progress if dietary changes are not made. To succeed in individual dietary intervention, one must do far more than provide knowledge. Dietary intervention needs accurate appraisal of needs, circumstances, and the ability and willingness of the patient to change (Lake, 2006). The dentist is largely a facilitator and the motivation for change must come from within the patient. Dentists should be adequately qualified and confident to provide advice to the majority of their patients; however, in some instances the dentist may require the help and expertise of a registered dietitian. Such cases may include patients on special therapeutic diets and those with unusual eating habits and eating disorders.

Successful dietary advice at the level of the individual (advice that leads to caries reduction) requires effective advice, adequate provision and resources to provide advice, and patient compliance. However, efforts at this level need to be reinforced with population-based strategies for caries control.

References

Aguirre-Zero O, Zero DT, Proskin HM. Effect of chewing xylitol chewing gum on salivary flow rate and the acidogenic potential of dental plaque. *Caries Res* 1993; **27**: 55–9.

Ahldén M-L, Frostell G. Variation of pH of plaque after a mouth rinse with a saturated solution of mannitol. *Odontol Rev* 1975; **26**: 1–6.

Alanen P, Isokangas P, Gutmann K. Xylitol candies in caries prevention: results of a field study in Estonian children. *Community Dent Oral Epidemiol* 2000; **28**: 218–24.

Al-Dlaigan YH, Shaw L, Smith A. Dental erosion in a group of British 14-year-old school children. Part II: Influence of dietary intake. *Br Dent J* 2001; **190**: 258–61.

Bánóczy J, Hadas E, Esztary I, Marosi I, Nemes J. Three-year results with sorbitol in clinical longitudinal experiments. *J Int Assoc Dent Child* 1981; **12**: 59–63.

Becks H. Carbohydrate restriction in the prevention of dental caries using the LA. count as one index. *J Cal State Dent Assoc* 1950; **26**: 53–8.

Birkhed D. Sugar substitutes – one consequence of the Vipeholm study? *Scand J Dent Res* 1989; **97**: 126–9.

Birkhed D, Bär A. Sorbitol and dental caries. *World Rev Nutr Diet* 1991; **65**: 1–37.

Birkhed D, Edwardsson A, Ahldén M-L, Frostell G. Effects of 3 months consumption of hydrogenated starch hydrolysate (Lycasin), maltitol, sorbitol and xylitol on human dental plaque. *Acta Odont Scand* 1979; **37**: 103–15.

Borg A, Birkhed D. Dental caries and related factors in a group of young Swedish athletes. *Int J Sports Med* 1987; **8**: 234–5.

Bowen WH, Young DA, Pearson SK. The effects of sucralose on coronal and root-surface caries. *J Dent Res* 1990; **69**: 1485–7.

Bradbury J, Thomason JM, Jepson NJA, Walls AWG, Allen PF, Moynihan PJ. Nutrition counseling increases fruit and vegetable intake in the edentulous. *J Dent Res* 2006; **85**: 463–8.

Brown AT, Wittenber CL. Mannitol and sorbitol catabolism in *Streptococcus mutans*. *Arch Oral Biol* 1973; **18**: 117–26.

Burt B, Pai S. Sugar consumption and caries risk: a systematic review. *J Dent Educ* 2001; **65**: 1017–23.

Burt BA, Eklund SA, Morgan KJ, *et al.* The effects of sugars intake and frequency of ingestion on dental caries increment in a three-year longitudinal study. *J Dent Res* 1988; **67**: 1422–9.

Burt BA, Kolker JL, Sandretto AM, Yuan Y, Sohn W, Ismail AI. Dietary patterns related to caries in a low-income adult population. *Caries Res* 2006; **40**: 473–80.

Cavadini C, Siega-Riz AM, Popkin BM. US adolescent food intake trends from 1965 to 1996. *Arch Dis Child* 2000; **83**: 18–24.

Chen W, Chen P, Chen SC, Shih WT, Hu HC. Lack of association between obesity and dental caries in three-year-old children. *Zhonghua Min Guo Xiao Er Ke Yi Xue Hui Za Zhi* 1998; **39**: 109–11.

Crossner C-G, Hase JC, Birkhed D. Oral sugar clearance in children compared to adults. *Caries Res* 1991; **25**: 201–6.

Department of Health. *Dietary sugars and human disease.* Report on Health and Social Subjects No. 36. London: HMSO, 1989.

Department of Health. *Weaning and the weaning diet.* Report on Health and Social Subjects No. 45. London: HMSO, 1994.

Derry C, Wagner ML, Longbotton C, Simon R, Nugent ZJ. The prevalence of dental erosion in a United States and a United Kingdom sample of adolescents. *Pediatr Dent* 2000; **22**: 505–10.

Dibb S, Castell A. *Easy to swallow, hard to stomach: the results of a survey of food advertising on television.* London: National Food Alliance, 1995.

Duggal MS, Toumba KJ, Amaechi BT, Kowash MB, Higham SM. Enamel demineralization *in situ* with various frequencies of carbohydrate consumption with and without fluoride toothpaste. *J Dent Res* 2001; **80**: 1721–4.

Edwardsson S, Birkhed D, Mejáre B. Acid production from Lycasin, maltitol, sorbitol and xylitol by oral streptococci and lactobacilli. *Acta Odontol Scand* 1977; **35**: 257–63.

von der Fehr FR, Löe H, Theilade E. Experimental caries in man. *Caries Res* 1970; **4**: 131–48.

Finn SB, Frew RA, Leibowitz R, *et al.* The effect of sodium trimetaphosphate (TMP) as a chewing gum additive on caries increments in children. *J Am Dent Assoc* 1978; **96**: 651–5.

Fisher FJ. A field survey of dental caries, periodontal disease and enamel defects in Tristan da Cunha. 2. Methods and results. *Br Dent J* 1968; **125**: 447–53.

Flegal KM, Carroll MD, Ogden CL, Johnson CL. Prevalence and trends in obesity among US adults, 1999–2000. *JAMA* 2002; **288**: 1772–3.

Flinck A, Källestål C, Holm AK, Allebeck P, Wall S. Distribution of caries in 12-year-old children in Sweden. Social and oral health-related behavioural patterns. *Community Dent Health* 1999; **16**: 160–5.

Frostell G, Blomlöf L, Blomqvist T, *et al.* Substitution of sucrose by Lycasin in candy. 'The Roslagen study'. *Acta Odontol Scand* 1974; **32**: 235–54.

Frostell G, Birkhed D, Edwardsson S. Effect of partial substitution of invert sugar for sucrose in combination with Duraphat treatment on caries development in preschool children. The Malmö study. *Caries Res* 1991; **25**: 304–10.

Fry AJ, Grenby TH. The effects of reduced sucrose intake on the formation and composition of dental plaque in a group of men in the Antarctic. *Arch Oral Biol* 1972; **17**: 217–26.

Gedalia I, Ben-Mosheh S, Biton J, Kogan D. Dental caries protection with hard cheese consumption. *Am J Dent* 1994; **7**: 331–2.

Glass RL. Effects on dental caries incidence of frequent ingestion of small amounts of sugars and stannous EDTA in chewing gum. *Caries Res* 1981; **15**: 256–62.

Grenby TH, Lear CJ. Reduction in smooth surface caries and fat accumulation in rats when sucrose in drinking water is replaced by glucose syrup. *Caries Res* 1974; **8**: 368–72.

Gustafsson BE, Quensel C-E, Swenander Lanke L, *et al.* The Vipeholm Dental Caries Study. The effect of different levels of carbohydrate intake on caries activity in 436 individuals observed for five years. *Acta Odontol Scand* 1954; **11**: 232–64.

Hackett AF, Rugg-Gunn AJ, Murray JJ, Roberts GJ. Can breast feeding cause dental caries? *Hum Nutr Appl Nutr* 1984; **38A**: 23–8.

Hankin JH, Chung CS, Kau MCW. Genetic and epidemiological studies of oral characteristics in Hawaii's school children: dietary patterns and caries prevalence. *J Dent Res* 1973; **52**: 1079–86.

Hardwick JL. The incidence and distribution of caries throughout the ages in relation to the Englishman's diet. *Br Dent J* 1960; **108**: 9–17.

Harris R. Biology of the children of Hopewood House, Bowral, Australia. 4. Observations of dental caries experience extending over five years (1957–1961). *J Dent Res* 1963; **42**: 1367–99.

Hase JC, Birkhed D, Grennert M-L, Steen B. Salivary glucose clearance and related factors in elderly people. *Gerodontics* 1987; **3**: 146–50.

Hinds K, Gregory JR. *National Diet and Nutrition Survey: children aged 1.5 to 4.5 years*, Vol. 2, *Report of the dental survey.* London: HMSO, 1995.

Holt RD, Joels D, Winter GB. Caries in preschool children, the Camden study. *Br Dent J* 1982; **153**: 107–9.

Imfeld T. Identification of low caries risk dietary components. *Monogr Oral Sci* 1977; **11**: 1–198.

Imfeld T. Clinical caries studies with polyalcohols: a literature review. *Schweiz Monatsschr Zahnmed* 1994; **104**: 941–5.

Imfeld T, Mühlemann HR. Addendum to: Acid production from Swedish Lycasin (candy quality) and French Lycasin (80/85) in human dental plaque. *Caries Res* 1978; **12**: 256–63.

Isokangas P, Alanen P, Tiekso J, Mäkinen KK. Xylitol chewing gum in caries prevention: a field study in children. *J Am Dent Assoc* 1988; **117**: 315–20.

Isokangas P, Mäkinen KK, Tiekso J, Alanen P. Long-term effect of xylitol chewing gum in the prevention of dental caries; a follow-up 5 years after termination of prevention program. *Caries Res* 1993; **27**: 495–8.

Isokangas P, Söderling E, Pienihakkinen K, Alanen P. Occurrence of dental decay in chldren after maternal consumption of xylitol chewing gum, a follow-up from 0–5 years of age. *J Dent Res* 2000; **79**: 1885–9.

Kalfas S, Svensäter G, Birkhed D, Edwardsson S. Sorbitol adaptation of dental plaque in people with low and normal salivary secretion rates. *J Dent Res* 1990; **69**: 442–6.

Kandelman D, Gagnon G. A 24-month clinical study of the incidence and progression of dental caries in relation to consumption of chewing gum containing xylitol in school preventive programs. *J Dent Res* 1990; **69**: 1771–5.

Kantovitz KR, Pascon FM, Rontani RM, Gaviao MB. Obesity and dental caries – a systematic review. *Oral Health Prev Dent* 2006; **4**: 137–44.

Karlsbeek H, Verrips GH. Consumption of sweet snacks and caries experience of primary school children. *Caries Res* 1994; **28**: 477–83.

Kashket S, Paolino VJ. Inhibition of salivary amylase by water-soluble extracts of tea. *Arch Oral Biol* 1998; **33**: 845–6.

Kashket S, van Houte J, Lopez LR, Stocks S. Lack of correlation between food retention on the human dentition and consumer perception of food stickiness. *J Dent Res* 1991; **70**: 1314–19.

Knai C, Pomerleau J, Lock K, McKee M. Getting children to eat more fruit and vegetables: a systematic review. *Prev Med* 2006; **42**: 85–95.

Koo H, de Guzman N, Schobel BD, Vacca Smith AV, Bowen WH. Influence of cranberry juice on glucan-mediated processes involved in *Streptococcus mutans* biofilm development. *Caries Res* 2006; **40**: 20–7.

Lake A. Changing dietary behaviour. *Quintessence Int* 2006; **37**: 788–91.

Larsen MJ, Nyvad B. Enamel erosion by some soft drinks and orange juices relative to their pH, buffering effect and contents of calcium phosphate. *Caries Res* 1999; **33**: 81–7.

Levine R, Stillman-Lowe C. The scientific basis of oral health education, 5th edn. London: BDA Books, 2003.

Levy S, Warren JJ, Broffitt B, Harris SL, Kanellis MJ. Fluoride, beverages and dental caries in the primary dentition. *Caries Res* 2003; **37**: 157–65.

Lingström P, Birkhed D. Plaque pH and oral retention after consumption of starchy snack products at normal and low salivary secretion rate. *Acta Odontol Scand* 1993; **51**: 379–88.

Lingström P, Birkhed D, Granfeldt Y, Björck I. pH measurements of human dental plaque after consumption of starchy foods using the microtouch and the sampling method. *Caries Res* 1993; **27**: 394–401.

Lingström P, van Houte J, Kashket S. Food starches and dental caries. *Crit Rev Oral Biol Med* 2000; **11**: 366–80.

Ludwig DS, Peterson KE, Gortmaker SL. Relation between consumption of sugar-sweetened drinks and childhood obesity: a prospective, observational analysis. *Lancet* 2001; **357**: 505–8.

Lussi A, Jaeggi T. Occupation and sports. *Monogr Oral Sci* 2006; **20**: 106–11.

Lussi A, Jaggi T, Scharer S. The influence of different factors on *in vitro* enamel erosion. *Caries Res* 1993; **27**: 387–93.

Lussi A, Jaeggi T, Zero D. The role of diet in the aetiology of dental erosion. *Caries Res* 2004; **38** (Suppl 1): 34–44.

Macek MD, Mitola DJ. Exploring the association between overweight and dental caries among US children. *Pediatr Dent* 2006; **28**: 375–80.

Machiulskiene V, Nyvad B, Baelum V. Caries preventive effect of sugar-substituted chewing gum. *Community Dent Oral Epidemiol* 2001; **29**: 278–88.

Maguire A, Baqir W. Prevalence of long-term use of medicines with prolonged oral clearance in the elderly: a survey in northeast England. *Br Dent J* 2000; **189**: 267–72.

Maguire A, Rugg-Gunn AJ, Butler TJ. Dental health of children taking antimicrobial and non-antimicrobial liquid oral medication long-term. *Caries Res* 1996; **30**: 16–21.

Mäkinen K. The rocky road of xylitol to its clinical application. *J Dent Res* 2000; **79**: 1352–5.

Mäkinen KK, Bennett CA, Hujoel PP, Isokangas PJ, Isotupa KP, Pape HR Jr. Xylitol chewing gums and caries rates, a 40-month cohort study. *J Dent Res* 1995; **74**: 1904–13.

Marshall T, Levy SM, Broffitt B, *et al*. Dental caries and beverage consumption in young children. *Pediatrics* 2003; **112**: 184–91.

Marthaler TM. Hereditary fructose intolerance. *Br Dent J* 1967; **120**: 597–9.

Miller WD. Experiments and observations on the wasting of tooth tissue erroneously designated as erosion, abrasion, denudation, etc. *Dent Cosmos* 1907; **49**: 109–24.

Millward A, Shaw L, Smith AJ, Rippin JW, Harrington E. The distribution and severity of tooth wear and the relationship between erosion and dietary constituents in a group of children. *Int J Paediatr Dent* 1994; **4**: 152–7.

Moynihan PJ. Update on the nomenclature of carbohydrates and their dental effects. *J Dent* 1998; **26**: 209–18.

Moynihan P. Foods and factors that protect against dental caries. *Br Nutr Found Nutr Bull* 2000; **25**: 281–6.

Moynihan PJ, Gould MEL, Huntley N, Thorman S. Effect of glucose polymers in water, milk and a milk substitute (Calogen) on plaque pH *in vitro*. *Int J Paediatr Dent* 1996; **6**: 19–24.

Moynihan PJ, Ferrier S, Blomley S, Russell RRBR. Acid production from lactulose by dental plaque bacteria. *Lett Appl Microbiol* 1998; **27**: 173–7.

Moynihan PJ, Ferrier S, Jenkins GN. The cariostatic potential of cheese: cooked cheese-containing meals increase plaque calcium concentration. *Br Dent J* 1999; **187**: 664–7.

Mühlemann HR. Zuckerfreie, zahnschonende und nich-kariogene Bonbons und Süssigkeiten. *Schweiz Monatsschr Zahnmed* 1969; **79**: 117–45.

Mühlemann HR, Schmid R, Noguchi T, Imfeld T, Hirsch RS. Some dental effects of xylitol under laboratory and *in vivo* conditions. *Caries Res* 1977; **11**: 263–76.

Newbrun E, Hoover C, Mettraux G, Graf H. Comparison of dietary habits and dental habits of subjects with hereditary fructose intolerance and control subjects. *J Am Dent Assoc* 1980; **101**: 619–26.

Nikiforuk G. Reducing the cariogenicity of the diet. In: *Understanding dental caries, 2. Prevention*. Basel: Karger, 1985: 174–203.

Nyvad B. Sukker og caries. In: Mølgaard C, Lyhne Andersen N, Barkholt V, *et al*. *Sukkers sundhedsmæssige betydning*. Copenhagen: Danish Board of Nutrition, 2003; 59–67 (in Danish).

Ooshima T, Izumitani A, Fujiwara T, Nakajima Y, Hamada S. Trehalulose does not induce dental caries in rats infected with mutans streptococci. *Caries Res* 1991; **25**: 277–82.

Papas AS, Joshi A, Palmer CA, Giunta JL, Dwyer JT. Relationship of diet to root caries. *Am J Clin Nutr* 1995; **61** (Suppl): 423–9S.

Petersson LG, Birkhed D, Gleerup A, Johansson M, Jönsson G. Caries-preventive effects of dentifrices containing various types and concentrations of fluorides and sugar alcohols. *Caries Res* 1991; **25**: 74–9.

Rees TD. Oral effects of drug abuse. *Crit Rev Oral Biol* 1992; **3**: 163–84.

Reisine ST, Psoter W. Socioeconomic status and selected behavioral determinants as risk factors for dental caries. *J Dent Educ* 2001; **65**: 1009–16.

Reynolds EC, Cai F, Shen P, Walker GD. Retention in plaque and remineralization of enamel lesions by various forms of calcium in a mouthrinse or sugar-free chewing gum. *J Dent Res* 2003; **82**: 206–11.

Rooney TP. Dental caries prevalence in patients with Crohn's disease. *Oral Surg Med Oral Pathol* 1984; **57**: 623–4.

Rose G. *Prevention for individuals and the high-risk strategy*. Oxford: Oxford University Press, 1993.

Rosen S, Elvin-Lewis M, Beck FM, Beck EX. Anti-cariogenic effects of tea in rats. *J Dent Res* 1984; **63**: 658–60.

Rugg-Gunn AJ. *Starchy foods and fresh fruits: their relative importance as a source of dental caries in Britain. A review of the literature*. Report of the Health Education Authority, Occasional Paper No. 3. London: HEA, 1986: 5–32.

Rugg-Gunn AJ. *Nutrition, diet and oral health*. Oxford: Oxford University Press, 1993.

Rugg-Gunn AJ, Nunn JH. *Nutrition, diet and oral health*. Oxford: Oxford University Press, 1999.

Rugg-Gunn AJ, Hackett AF, Appleton DR, Jenkins GN, Eastoe JE. Relationship between dietary habits and caries increment assessed over two years in 405 English adolescent schoolchildren. *Arch Oral Biol* 1984; **29**: 983–92.

Rugg-Gunn AJ, Hackett AF, Appleton DR. Relative cariogenicity of starch and sugars in a two-year longitudinal study of 405 English schoolchildren. *Caries Res* 1987; **21**: 464–73.

Schamschula RG, Adkins BL, Barmes DE, Charlton G, Davey BG. *WHO study of dental caries etiology in Papua New Guinea*. WHO Offset Publication 40. Geneva: World Health Organization, 1978: 18–40.

Scheie AA, Fejerskov O. Xylitol in caries prevention: what is the evidence for clinical efficacy? *Oral Dis* 1998; **4**: 268–78.

Scheinin A, Mäkinen KK. Turku sugar studies I–XXI. *Acta Odontol Scand* 1975; **33** (Suppl 70): 1–351.

Scheinin A, Mäkinen KK, Tammisalo E, Rekola M. Turku sugar studies. XVIII. Incidence of dental caries in relation to 1-year consumption of sucrose and xylitol chewing gum. *Acta Odontol Scand* 1975; **33**: 269–78.

Seow WK. Biological mechanisms of early childhood caries. *Community Dent Oral Epidemiol* 1998; **26** (Suppl 1): 8–27.

Sheiham A. Sugars and dental decay. *Lancet* 1983; **1**: 282–4.

Sheiham A. Why sugar consumption should be below 15 kg per person per year in industrialised countries, the dental evidence. *Br Dent J* 1991; **167**: 63–5.

Silver DH. A longitudinal study of infant feeding practice, diet and caries, related to social class in children aged 3 and 8–10 years. *Br Dent J* 1987; **163**: 296–300.

Söderling E, Mäkinen KK, Chen CY, Pape HR Jr, Loesche W, Mäkinen PL. Effect of sorbitol, xylitol, and xylitol/sorbitol chewing gums on dental plaque. *Caries Res* 1989; **23**: 378–84.

Söderling E, Isokangas P, Pienihakkinen K, Tenovuo J, Alanen P. Influence of maternal xylitol consumption on mother–child transmission of mutans streptococci: 6-year follow up. *Caries Res* 2001; **35**: 173–7.

Sohn W, Burt BA, Sowers MR. Carbonated soft drinks and dental caries in the primary dentition. *J Dent Res* 2006; **85**: 262–6.

Sreebny LM. Sugar availability, sugar consumption and dental caries. *Community Dent Oral Epidemiol* 1982; **10**: 1–7.

Sreebny LM. Cereal availability and dental caries. *Community Dent Oral Epidemiol* 1983; **11**: 148–55.

Stecksen-Blinks C, Arvidsson S, Holm A-K. Dental health, dental care and dietary habits in children in different parts of Sweden. *Acta Odontol Scand* 1985; **43**: 59–67.

Steele JG, Sheiham A, Marcenes W, Walls AWG. *National Diet and Nutrition Survey: people aged 65 years and over*, Vol. 2, *Report of the oral health survey*. London: The Stationery Office, 1998.

Sundin B, Granath L, Birkhed D. Variation of posterior approximal caries incidence with consumption of sweets with regard to other caries-related factors in 15–17-year-olds. *Community Dent Oral Epidemiol* 1992; **20**: 76–80.

Svanberg M, Birkhed D. Effect of dentifrices containing either xylitol and glycerol or sorbitol on mutans streptococci in saliva. *Caries Res* 1991; **25**: 449–53.

Swenander Lanke L. Influence on salivary sugar of certain properties of foodstuffs and individual oral conditions. *Acta Odontol Scand* 1957; **15** (Suppl 23): 5–156.

Szpunar SM, Eklund SA, Burt BA. Sugar consumption and caries risk in schoolchildren with low caries experience. *Community Dent Oral Epidemiol* 1995; **23**: 142–6.

Takeuchi M. Epidemiological study on dental caries in Japanese children before, during and after World War II. *Int Dent J* 1961; **11**: 443–57.

Toverud G. The influence of war and post war conditions on the teeth of Norwegian school children II and III. *Millbank Mem Fund Q* 1957; **35**: 127–96.

Wåler SM, Rölla G. Effect of xylitol on dental plaque *in vivo* during carbohydrate challenge. *Scand J Dent Res* 1983; **91**: 256–9.

Wennerholm K, Emilson CG, Birkhed D. Sweeteners and dental health. In: Marie S, Piggott JR, eds. *Handbook of sweeteners*. Glasgow: Blackie and Son, 1991: 205–24.

Wendt LK, Svedin CG, Hallonsten AL, Larsson IB. Infants and toddlers with caries. Mental health, family interaction, and life events in infants and toddlers with caries. *Swed Dent J* 1995; **19**: 17–27.

Willershausen B, Haas G, Krummenauer F, Hohenfellner K. Relationship between high weight and caries frequency in German elementary school children. *Eur J Med Res* 2004; **9**: 400–4.

WHO/FAO. *Diet, nutrition and the prevention of chronic diseases*. WHO Technical Report Series, 916. Geneva: World Health Organization/Food and Agricultural Organization, 2003.

Winter GB, Rule DC, Mailer GP, James PMC, Gordon PH. The prevalence of dental caries in pre-school children aged 1 to 4 years. *Br Dent J* 1971; **130**: 271–7.

Zero DT. Etiology of dental erosion – extrinsic factors. *Eur J Oral Sci* 1996; **104**: 162–77.

Zero D. Sugars – the arch criminal? *Caries Res* 2004; **38**: 277–85.

Zero DT, Lussi A. Etiology of enamel erosion – intrinsic and extrinsic factors. In: Addy M, Embery G, Edgar M, Orchardson R, eds. *Tooth wear and sensitivity*. London: Martin Dunitz, 2000; 121–39.

Zero DT, Lussi A. Erosion – chemical and biological factors of importance to the dental practitioner. *Int Dent J* 2005; **55** (Suppl 4): 285–91.

Part V
Operative intervention

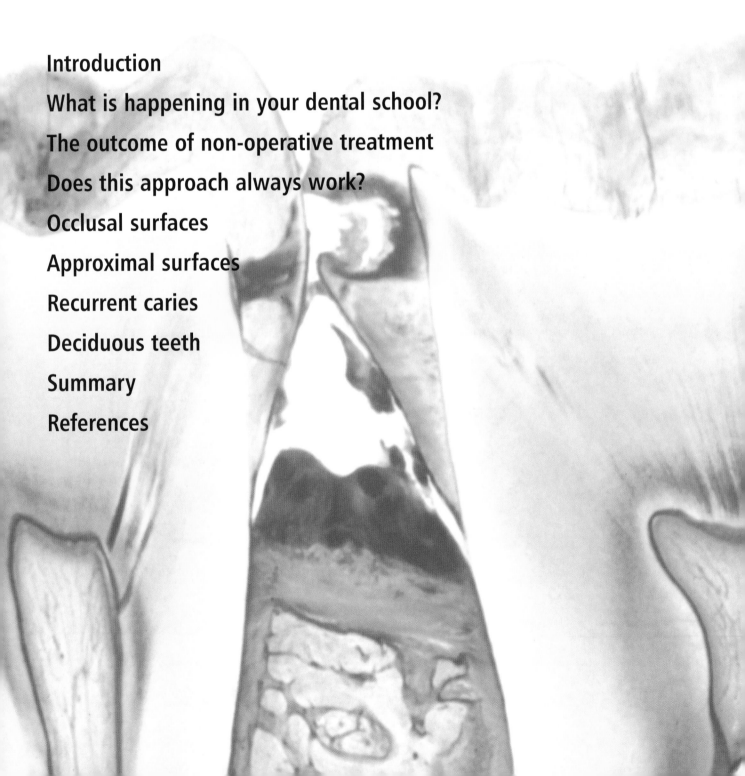

20

The role of operative treatment in caries control

E.A.M. Kidd, J.P. van Amerongen and W.E. van Amerongen

Introduction

In the past, and sometimes even now, a radiograph showing demineralization in enamel or demineralization up to the enamel–dentin junction, for example on the distal surfaces of the lower molar and premolars in Fig. 20.1, led to the decision to place a restoration. However, recent research has shown that this approach is now outdated and incorrect. The radiograph shows that demineralization is present, but what also matters is the activity of the lesion. If the lesion is arrested it requires neither non-operative nor operative treatment. In contrast, the management of an active lesion requires modification of the processes in the biofilm so that mineral loss is arrested. Earlier chapters have discussed the roles of plaque control, fluoride, dietary control and salivary stimulation in these processes. Notice that the carious process is multifactorial and therefore the management strategies will reflect this. This chapter will discuss the role of operative treatment in caries management, but it will also point out when it is not required. Restorations form part of a local treatment strategy to facilitate plaque control. In some situations they are very important, but they are neither the beginning nor the end of the story.

What is happening in your dental school?

Take a few moments to consider what is happening in your dental school. For many years operative dentistry has been synonymous with caries treatment. Caries is 'treated' by filling holes in teeth. This approach is not valid scientifically, but many of your teachers will have been brought up under

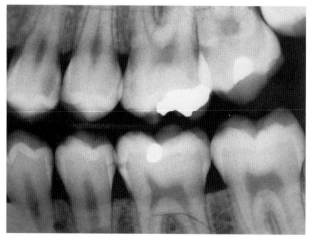

Figure 20.1 Radiograph showing demineralization in the outer enamel on the distal aspects of both lower premolars. It would be incorrect to place restorations here. These lesions should be treated non-operatively and reassessed. The lesions on the mesial and distal aspects of the lower first molar should also not be treated operatively. However, the distal lesion on the upper right first premolar extends well into the dentin. It will be cavitated and operative treatment is required because it is impossible for the patient to remove plaque from this cavity.

this regimen and it is surprisingly difficult to shed this misconception.

It may be useful to consider the following questions in relation to your school and discuss them with your teachers. You are then in a position to assess the attitudes of those who teach you and assess how you are responding.

1. How is cariology taught? Is the course purely lecture based or do those who supervise your clinical work with patients show you how to put science into practice?
2. Are you taught to distinguish between active and arrested caries and consider the consequences?
3. Are you routinely expected to assess the risk of your patients developing caries lesions? If you do this, how does it modify your treatment plan?
4. Are you expected to show your patients how to institute effective plaque control? Are toothbrushes and floss available so that you can provide them with cleaning aids appropriate to their needs? Do your teachers encourage this and give you credit for it?
5. Are you encouraged to advise patients on appropriate use of fluoride?
6. Are diet sheets available in your clinic?
7. Do you ever measure salivary flow in your patients? If you do, what do you do with the information?
8. Are all your clinical teachers committed to non-operative treatment? Do you enjoy doing this form of dentistry or would you rather be doing operative treatment?
9. Is there a points system in your school to assess the quantity of work you carry out? If there is, are points awarded for non-operative as well as operative treatment?
10. If only operative treatment counts towards these requirements, does this influence your attitude towards non-operative treatment? Do you feel it is a waste of time?
11. Do you recall your patients over a period of years so that you can assess the success or otherwise of the treatment?
12. How do your patients react when you suggest that a filling is not needed but that you can help them arrest an active carious lesion? Are they pleased? Do you get the impression they wish you to take the responsibility and fill the tooth? What are they expecting from you?

The outcome of non-operative treatment

What effects does non-operative treatment have on initial demineralized lesions and on cavities? Can they be cured (healed) or just stopped in their tracks (arrested)?

Initial lesions

In early experiments, von der Fehr *et al.* (1970) and Koch (1988) showed that normal individuals can be turned into individuals with high caries risk. Within a short period numerous lesions can develop when oral hygiene is withdrawn and a sugar-rich diet is offered. However, when effective oral hygiene and application of topical fluoride is instituted, and a normal, less sugar-containing diet is consumed, reversal of the situation seems possible; at least, after some time, the initial lesions are not visible any more. Thylstrup *et al.* (1993) have shown that in the very early lesion only the external microsurface is dissolved by plaque. When the plaque is removed mechanically at this stage, the eroded area will change into a hard and shiny surface instead of the chalky and white aspect of the earlier active lesion. It is suggested this phenomenon is caused by wear and polishing, rather than by recovery of the carious surface.

Further progression of the lesion leads to deeper surface and subsurface dissolution. Once again, intervening by removal of plaque, fluoride application and better diet, leads to wear and a polished surface, and an arrested subsurface lesion.

These lesions remain visible as shiny white or brown lesions, often seen on buccal surfaces. The carious process has stopped but the arrested lesion may be seen throughout life as whitish or brownish scar tissue (Fig. 20.2). Research has shown these areas are more resistant to a subsequent carious attack than sound enamel (Koulourides *et al.*, 1980).

There is little dispute about the management of lesions that are not cavitated. Few dentists would attack these with a dental drill although, as will be shown later, it is not always easy to know on an approximal surface whether a lesion is cavitated. But what should be done when further progression has led to a cavity?

Cavitated lesions

Several authors have shown that when an occlusal lesion has turned into a cavity, the dentin is always involved in the process (van Amerongen *et al.*, 1992; Ekstrand *et al.*, 1995). Most of these lesions are detectable on a radiograph and they contain many microorganisms. They can be considered as active (Espelid *et al.*, 1994; Ekstrand *et al.*, 1997, 1998a) because measures directed at removing plaque are ineffective on the cavitated occlusal surface; the brush cannot get into the undermined cavity. Approximal cavities, where an adjacent tooth is present, are also difficult to reach. Dental floss will skim the surface, but not access the cavity (Fig. 20.1).

Free smooth surfaces

However, where a cavity is on a free smooth surface, the situation is different. Now the area is easily reached by a toothbrush, although where the process is undermining the enamel, removal of the overhanging enamel margins by grinding and polishing should be considered to aid cleaning the whole area (Fig. 20.3a, b). Cavities in these surfaces, cleaned twice daily with a fluoride toothpaste, can be

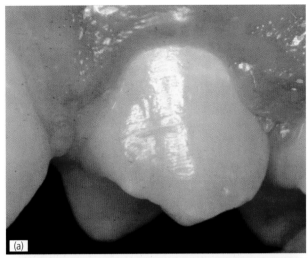
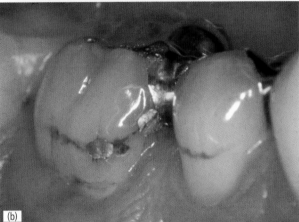
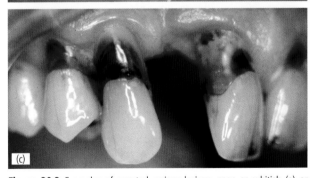

Figure 20.2 Examples of arrested carious lesions, seen as whitish (a) or brownish (b) scar tissue on enamel surfaces. In (c) arrested lesions are on root surfaces.

arrested and converted into leathery or hard lesions. In time, even extensive soft lesions can turn into hard, shiny, but still discolored, surfaces.

The same argument pertains to lesions developing on root surfaces (Nyvad & Fejerskov, 1986). Active root carious lesions can be converted into inactive stages by daily plaque removal with a fluoride-containing toothpaste (Figs 2.42–2.57, 20.4). The surface of the active lesion is heavily infected by microorganisms. When the activity is decreased and finally arrested it has been shown that the carious

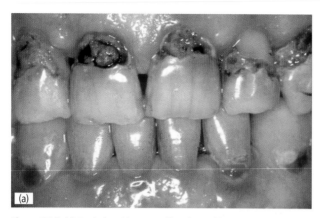

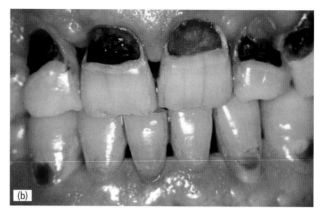

Figure 20.3 (a) Cervical cavities covered by plaque. (b) Same cavities 14 days later after removing overhanging enamel with a diamond finishing bur and instruction in cleaning. The teeth were brushed twice a day with fluoride toothpaste.

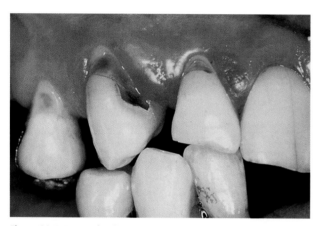

Figure 20.4 Root-surface lesions on smooth surfaces. Lesions arrest following plaque removal with a fluoridated toothpaste.

lesions contain few bacteria that can be cultivated (Parikh *et al.*, 1963; Sarnat & Massler, 1965; Nyvad & Fejerskov, 1990; Schüpbach *et al.*, 1992).

Does this approach always work?

It should be noted that not all clinical studies that have focussed on lesion arrest through improved dental hygiene have been entirely successful. A study in young Swedish people showed that even under strict caries preventive control many initial approximal lesions slowly progress (Mejàre *et al.*, 1999, 2004). In a Swedish study of periodontal patients subject to an intensive prophylactic program only about half of 99 active root carious lesions were converted into inactive lesions on buccal and lingual surfaces within 12 months (Emilson *et al.*, 1993). The results on approximal surfaces, which are often more difficult to clean, were less favorable. Analysis of the plaque scores showed substantially more plaque on surfaces with active caries than on surfaces with inactive caries. These findings imply that the quality of plaque removal is crucial for arresting active carious lesions. They also imply that where a patient

is unable to access and remove plaque, operative dentistry has a role to play to restore the integrity of the tooth surface and allow the patient to clean.

Occlusal surfaces

The anatomy of the fissure can favor plaque stagnation and this is particularly likely during eruption of the tooth (Carvalho *et al.*, 1992). This happens because the tooth is below the occlusal plane and its surface tends to be missed by the toothbrush. Children often need assistance to brush the occlusal surfaces of erupting teeth, with a parent standing behind the child and holding the brush at right angles to the arch, so that the occlusal surface is brushed individually.

When an active enamel lesion is diagnosed in a fissure, or if a high risk is established and fissures are sound, a fissure sealant could be indicated. An unfilled or lightly filled resin is used to penetrate the fissures and prevent plaque accumulation on the occlusal surface.

A fissure sealant has the advantage that the tooth does not have to be cut and no irreversible intervention is involved. Active lesions covered by the resin do not progress further and the possible development of new lesions at other sites in the fissure is prevented.

Sealants have been used preventively for many years (Simonsen, 1991). Concern has been expressed about placement of sealants over undiagnosed dentin caries. However, there is ample evidence that caries does not progress as long as the fissure remains sealed (Handleman *et al.*, 1976; Handleman, 1982; Mertz-Fairhurst *et al.*, 1986). Even obvious caries in dentin on a radiograph has been shown not to progress over a 10-year period (Mertz-Fairhurst *et al.*, 1998) provided it is sealed off from the oral environment with a composite restoration. Thus, sealing appears to be very effective in conserving the tooth.

However, this conservative approach to occlusal lesions that are radiographically in dentin inevitably seals over infected dentin. This approach is not the usual one, and many schools will teach that a cavitated occlusal lesion should be treated operatively. This involves accessing the demineralized soft dentin, removing most of the infected dental tissue and adjusting the remaining cavity so that the filling material of choice can be applied. The concerns about sealing over infected dentin will be discussed further in Chapter 21.

Approximal surfaces

Where a cavitated carious lesion is present on an approximal surface the adjacent tooth may prevent plaque removal by either a brush or dental floss (Fig. 20.1). Now the lesion is likely to progress, albeit slowly (Mejàre *et al.*, 1999, 2004).

As discussed in Chapter 5, the radiograph is important in detecting demineralization, although a single radiograph will not give information on the activity of a lesion. However, a series of reproducible radiographs, taken over years, will give a clear picture of progression or arrest (Fig. 20.5). The presence or absence of cavitation cannot be seen on a radio-

graph, but several clinical studies conducted since the early 1970s have related radiographic appearance to cavitation in permanent teeth. These studies are listed in Table 20.1. Figure 20.6 shows the radiographic appearances.

This research assists the dentist in knowing when a lesion may be cavitated and therefore when operative intervention may be a necessary part of caries control. R4 lesions should always be treated operatively. R3 lesions may or may not be cavitated. Cavitation is more likely in a high-risk patient (Lunder & von der Fehr, 1996) and when the adjacent gingival papilla is inflamed (Ekstrand *et al.*, 1998b; Ratledge *et al.*, 2001). Separating the teeth (see Fig. 4.28) will allow gentle use of a probe to confirm whether a cavity is present.

Recurrent caries

In posterior teeth the bitewing radiograph is the salient diagnostic tool for the diagnosis of new caries at the margin of a restoration. The lesion usually forms cervically because this is the area of plaque stagnation (Kidd *et al.*, 1992).

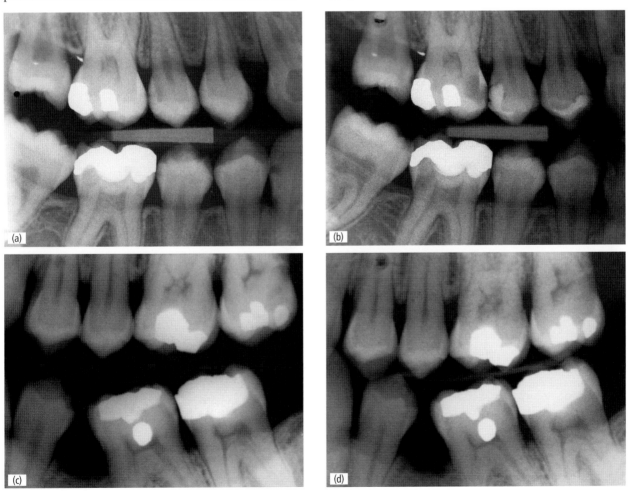

Figure 20.5 Radiographs showing lesion progression and lesion arrest. (a, b) Look particularly at the mesial surface of the upper first molar. The radiographs were taken 18 months apart and caries progression is rapid. (c, d) Look at the distal surface of the first lower molar. The radiographs were taken 3 years apart and the lesions are similar in size.

Table 20.1 Clinical studies relating radiographic appearance to cavitation in permanent teeth

Study	Number and characteristics of subject in sample group	Study design	Percentage of approximal cavitated surfaces found, increasing radiographic depth scores with number in parentheses				
			RO	R1	R2	R3	R4
Rugg-Gunn (1972)	370 approximal surface with open contacts in 13-year-old children	Standardized bitewing radiographs taken followed by direct visual assesssment of open contacts (one observer)	0.8% (283)	20.7% (58)	47% (17)	100% (12)	–
Bille & Thylstrup (1982)	Children aged 8–15 years 158 surfaces restored	Clinical assessment during cavity preparation recorded by seven observers	0% (6)	14% (50)	20% (35)	52% (58)	100% (9)
Mejàre et al. (1985)	63 teenagers, 598 surfaces in premolar and molar teeth	Teeth radiographed before orthodontic extraction followed by direct visual inspection (three observers)	1% (463)	11% (16)	31% (13)	100% (6)	–
Thylstrup et al. (1986)	660 approximal lesions restored in adults and children	Clinical tissue changes at time of operative treatment recorded by 263 observers	30% (13)	7% (72)	11% (143)	52% (330)	88% (102)
Mejàre & Malmgren (1986)	43 children aged 7–18 years	Clinical tissue changes recorded during cavity preparation following tooth separation (one observer)	–	–	61% (28)	78% (32)	–
Pitts & Rimmer (1992)	211 children, aged 5–15 years, 1468 surfaces assessed	Visual inspection following tooth separation	0% (1323)	0% (100)	10.5% (19)	40.9% (22)	100% (4)
de Araujo et al. (1992)	168 high-school students; standardized radiographs taken	Direct visual examination following tooth separation	–	13% (19)	26% (27)	90% (19)	–
Seddon (1995)	Patients aged 6–22 years	Cavity recorded on impression following separation (one observer)	7% (44)	6% (48)	15% (97)	48% (52)	100% (10)
Lunder & von der Fehr (1996)	Patients aged 17–18 years	Cavity recorded on impression and stone die made (two observers)	–	–	30% (23)	65% (23)	–
Akpata et al. (1996)	108 molar and premolar teeth in patients aged 17–48 years; two adjacent carious surfaces were chosen and the deeper was restored	Direct visual assessment of adjacent surface following tooth separation (two observers)	–	0% (16)	19% (31)	79% (43)	100% (18)
Hintze et al. (1998)	390 approximal surfaces in 53 young adults aged 20–37 years	Direct visual assessment of adjacent surface following tooth separation (four observers). Only 16–25 found to be cavitated	3%	5%	8% (n values not given)	35%	78–100%
Ratledge (1999)	54 approximal surfaces in 32 adult patients aged 19–76 years, referred for operative treatment	Cavity recorded on impression following separation (one observer)	–	–	–	85% 54	

Two particular phenomena are worthy of comment with respect to amalgam restorations: ditching and discoloration around the restoration (Fig. 20.7). Ditching usually occurs on the occlusal surface of an amalgam filling and both laboratory and clinical studies have shown that this appearance is neither synonymous with nor indicative of recurrent caries (Kidd & O'Hara, 1990; Kidd et al., 1995; Rudolphy et al., 1995). Similarly, a clinical study has shown that discoloration around an amalgam restoration with clinically intact margins is a poor predictor of infected dentin beneath the restoration (Kidd et al., 1995). Thus, an amalgam filling should not be replaced simply because of ditching or staining around it. A cavitated carious lesion at the margin of the restoration, which cannot be cleaned, is an indication for repairing or replacing the restoration.

The same argument applies to tooth-colored fillings. Staining and color change at the margin of the restoration do not reliably predict soft infected dentin beneath the filling (Kidd & Beighton, 1996). If these color changes were routinely to trigger replacement of restorations, many fillings would be removed unnecessarily. Recurrent caries is primary caries next to a filling (Mjör & Toffenetti, 2000) (Fig. 20.7c) and this means that the lesion can be diagnosed by careful clinical–visual and radiographic examination.

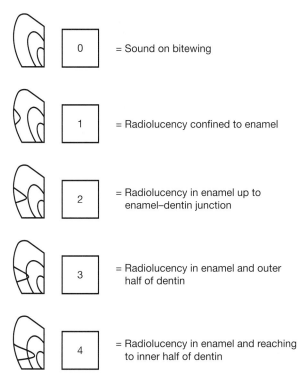

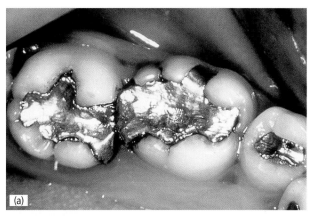

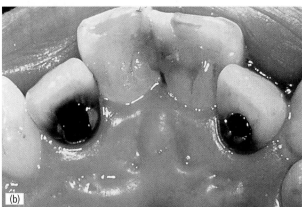

0 = Sound on bitewing

1 = Radiolucency confined to enamel

2 = Radiolucency in enamel up to enamel–dentin junction

3 = Radiolucency in enamel and outer half of dentin

4 = Radiolucency in enamel and reaching to inner half of dentin

Figure 20.6 Diagrammatic representation of approximal demineralization as seen on bitewing radiographs.

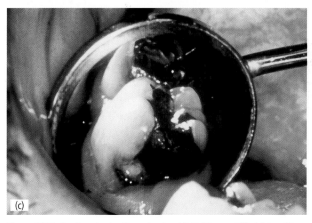

Figure 20.7 Amalgam restorations showing (a) ditching and (b) staining. These appearances are not synonymous with recurrent caries. (c) Operative dentistry is required where a cavity is present next to an amalgam (recurrent caries) that is difficult to clean.

Deciduous teeth

The discussion so far has concerned permanent teeth. It is suggested that the role of operative dentistry in caries control is to facilitate plaque control in uncleanable areas. Do these arguments pertain in deciduous teeth? Is it relevant that these teeth are only in the mouth for 6–9 years (Table 20.2)?

There are some obvious anatomical differences between deciduous and permanent teeth (Fig. 20.8).

- Deciduous teeth are smaller.
- The enamel and dentin are thinner.
- The pulp is relatively larger.
- The pulp horns are nearer to the surface.
- The contact points are flatter and wider.
- There is a clear constriction at the transition from crown to roots in deciduous molars.
- The occlusal surface is small in relation to the rest of the crown, particularly with the first deciduous molar.

Children under 3 years of age may find it difficult to co-operate with operative procedures, and from the dentist's perspective the mouths are small, wet and potentially wriggling! So, is it necessary to carry out operative procedures in these diminutive and difficult conditions?

Why restore deciduous teeth?

The carious process will progress to involve pulpal tissues more rapidly in deciduous than in permanent teeth (Shwartz *et al.*, 1984). This is a simple consequence of the smaller width of dental hard tissue and larger dimensions of the pulp (Fig. 20.8). When caries rates for the mesial surface of

Table 20.2 Eruption times and lifespan of deciduous teeth (in years)

	Deciduous eruption times	Permanent eruption times	Lifespan
Central incisor	0.5	7	6.5
Lateral incisor	0.75	8	7.25
Canine	1.5	9/12[a]	7.5/10.5[a]
First molar/premolar	1	10	9
Second molar/premolar	2	11	9

[a] Upper/lower arch.

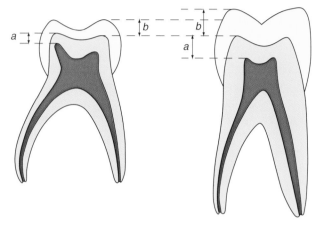

Figure 20.8 Anatomical differences between a deciduous (left) and a permanent (right) molar: *a* is the difference in dentin thickness; *b* is the difference in enamel thickness.

the first permanent molar and the distal surface of the second primary molar were compared, the enamel caries rate in the deciduous tooth was more than twice that for the permanent tooth. For both dentitions once the lesion has reached the inner half of the enamel on a radiograph, caries rates were three to six times higher in dentin than in enamel (Mejàre & Stenlund, 2000). Thus, despite the temporary nature of the deciduous dentition it would seem prudent to restore teeth where cavities (occlusal and approximal) preclude plaque removal as these lesions seem destined to progress (Fig. 20.9). Sometimes the undermined enamel breaks down and then, because the cavity is now cleanable, the caries process arrests (Fig. 20.10). However, on occasions the dentist can aid plaque control and avoid restoration by removing overhanging enamel (Fig. 20.11). The management seen in this picture is controversial and may result in some heated discussion with your teachers.

Caries progression and pulpal pathology will result in pain, which may be acute and distressing for all involved, young children and their parents. Chronic pain may be more insidious, but may result in loss of sleep, behavioral changes, uncomfortable eating and loss of appetite.

Consequences of not restoring deciduous teeth

Many practitioners working within the general dental services in the UK are not restoring deciduous teeth. The care index, which measures the proportion of carious teeth treated by restoration, has fallen in the 5-year-old child population in England from 24% in 1987 to 13% in 1996 (Nugent & Pitts, 1997). This situation has given an opportunity to assess the consequences of not restoring deciduous teeth.

Results of a retrospective analysis of the dental records of 677 children from the north-west of England who were regular dental attenders of 50 general dental practitioners have yielded some challenging results. To be included in the study, the children had to have approximal caries in their

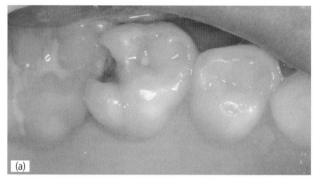

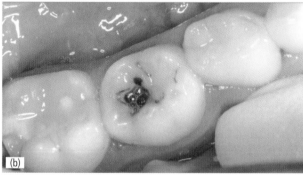

Figure 20.9 Occlusal and approximal lesions in deciduous teeth. (a) The approximal lesion is difficult to clean and would benefit from restoration. (b) The occlusal lesion can be cleaned. It is arrested and does not require restoration.

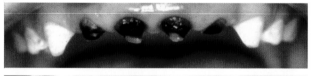

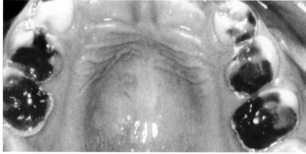

Figure 20.10 Arrested caries lesions in the primary dentition.

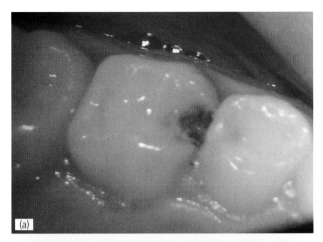

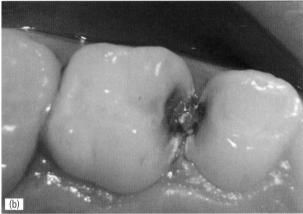

Figure 20.11 (a) Carious lesions in deciduous molars. (b) A bur has been used to remove overhanging enamel in the second molar and slice the distal aspect of the first molar. There is now a V-shaped space between the two teeth that will not trap food and allows cleaning. (Courtesy of R.J.M Gruythuysen.)

primary teeth, making this a high caries risk group. Some 4000 carious teeth were included (Tickle *et al.*, 2002; Milsom *et al.*, 2002). It may be important to note that diagnosis of caries was purely clinical; there is no mention of radiographs in these papers.

Over 80% of carious primary molars and 40% of carious anterior teeth were restored by these 50 practitioners. Twelve per cent of the teeth were extracted owing to pain or infection and the earlier caries was recorded in a tooth, the more likely was extraction owing to pain or infection. Over 80% of the primary teeth with caries exfoliated painlessly whether filled or unfilled. Of particular interest was the finding that restoration status, filled or unfilled, had no effect on whether the tooth was extracted due to pain and infection. This would appear to indicate that, in these patients, restoration of deciduous teeth did not necessarily prevent pain and infection.

A particularly disturbing finding was that on a patient basis, 48% of the children experienced at least one episode of pain and the more teeth affected by decay, the more likely it was that pain would be recorded. This result seems

really shocking and appears to represent a major failure of dental care. It has been suggested (Duggal, 2002) that by the time most proximal caries is manifest clinically, pulp inflammation is irreversible. Thus, large restorations in primary molars carried out without due consideration of the state of the pulp are bound to fail. The use of radiographs to indicate lesion depth and aid diagnosis is not mentioned in these papers. It is possible that the dentists were doing fillings on lesions so deep that their pulps were irretrievably damaged (M. Tickle, personal communication, 2005; Bandlish, 2002). In Chapter 4 it is noted that clinical diagnosis of approximal caries can be difficult in deciduous teeth.

The analysis of the dentists' records appeared to show that they were providing appropriate preventive care, including oral hygiene instruction, dietary advice and fluoride varnish application (Tickle *et al*, 2003). It was suggested that the preventive care was reactive to a very poor dental state and perhaps not very effective at this late stage of disease progression.

A retrospective analysis of the records of 481 children treated by a single practitioner in Leeds and Halifax, northern England, is also of interest in this discussion. This dentist's policy was to concentrate on preventive treatment but not to restore deciduous teeth (Levine *et al.*, 2002). Of the 1409 carious teeth analyzed, 18% gave pain and were extracted or treated restoratively and the remaining 82% exfoliated without problem. The risk factors for pain and infection were shown to be the development of multisurface lesions in younger patients, disease extending beyond single surfaces and disease in the lower deciduous molars (Levine *et al.*, 2003). The age at which a subject first presented with decay was a good predictor of outcome, representing the time available, before exfoliation, for decay to progress and cause symptoms.

Collectively, these retrospective studies show that it is not inevitable that unrestored deciduous teeth will cause pain. There is now an urgent need for prospective research, in the form of randomized controlled clinical trails, to compare the outcome of appropriate restoration (including pulp therapy where indicated) with no restorative treatment.

In the meantime, the authors of this chapter would suggest that radiographs, to assess the depth of lesion penetration, are an important part of diagnosis before treatment planning. Further, cavitated lesions, where plaque removal is impossible, are likely to progress, irrespective of non-operative treatments, and should be restored or sealed unless the tooth is close to exfoliation.

Summary

The most important reason for placing a restoration is to aid plaque control. The caries process is sent back to the tooth surface to start again. This also gives the dentist and patient time to institute measures that may control future lesion progression. The other reasons for recommending restorative treatment are (Elderton & Mjör, 1988):

- where the integrity of the tooth is restored before demineralization causes so much destruction that restoration is difficult
- where the tooth is sensitive to hot, cold and sweet
- where the pulp is endangered
- if previous attempts to arrest the lesion have failed and there is evidence that the lesion is progressing (this requires an observation period)
- where function is impaired
- where drifting is likely to occur through loss of a contact point
- for aesthetic reasons.

The dentist will enjoy restoring teeth – the technical and aesthetic challenges can be thrilling. However, before reaching for the bur the dentist must have considered the non-invasive options. Restorative dentistry is but a part of plaque control – non-operative treatment is also important.

References

Akpata ES, Farid MR, Al-Saif K, Roberts EAU. Cavitation at radiolucent areas on proximal surfaces of posterior teeth. *Caries Res* 1996; **30**: 313–16.

van Amerongen JP, Penning C, Kidd EAM, ten Cate JM. An *in vitro* assessment of the extent of caries under small occlusal cavities. *Caries Res* 1992; **26**: 89–93.

de Araujo FB, Rosito DB, Toigo R, dos Santos CK. Diagnosis of approximal caries: radiographic versus clinical examination using tooth separation. *Am J Dent* 1992; **5**: 245–8.

Bandlish LK. Carious primary teeth [letter]. *Brit Dent J* 2002; **192**: 669.

Bille J, Thylstrup A. Radiographic diagnosis and clinical tissue changes in relation to the treatment of approximal carious lesions. *Caries Res* 1982; **16**: 1–6.

Carvalho JC, Thylstrup A, Ekstrand K. Results after 3 years non-operative occlusal caries treatment of erupting permanent first molars. *Community Dent Oral Epidemiol* 1992; **20**: 187–92.

Duggal MS. Carious primary teeth: their fate in your hands. *Br Dent J* 2002; **192**: 215.

Ekstrand KR, Kuzmina I, Björndal L, Thylstrup A. Relationship between external and histologic features of progressive stages of caries in the occlusal fossa. *Caries Res* 1995; **29**: 243–50.

Ekstrand KR, Ricketts DNJ, Kidd EAM. Reproducibility and accuracy of three methods for the assessment of demineralization depth on the occlusal surface: an *in vitro* examination. *Caries Res* 1997; **31**: 224–31.

Ekstrand KR, Ricketts DNJ, Kidd EAM, Qvist V, Schou S. Detection, diagnosing, monitoring and logical treatment of occlusal caries in relation to lesion activity and severity. An *in vivo* examination with histological validation. *Caries Res* 1998a; **32**: 247–54.

Ekstrand KR, Bruun C, Bruun M. Plaque and gingival status as indicators for caries progression on approximal surfaces. *Caries Res* 1998b; **32**: 41–5.

Elderton RJ, Mjör IA. Treatment planning. In: Hörsted-Bindslev P, Mjör IA, eds. *Modern concepts in operative dentistry.* Copenhagen: Munksgaard, 1988. pp. 59–88.

Emilson CG, Ravald N, Birkhed D. Effects of 12 month prophylactic programme on selected oral bacterial populations on root surfaces with active and inactive carious lesions. *Caries Res* 1993; **27**: 195–200.

Espelid I, Tveit AB, Fjelltveit A. Variation among dentists in radiographic detection of occlusal caries. *Caries Res* 1994; **28**: 169–75.

von der Fehr ER, Löe H, Theilade E. Experimental caries in man. *Caries Res* 1970; **4**: 131–6.

Handleman S. Effect of sealant placement on occlusal caries progression. *Clin Prev Dent* 1982; **4**: 11–16.

Handleman S, Washburn F, Wopperer P. Two-year report of sealant effect on bacteria in dentine caries. *J Am Dent Assoc* 1976; **93**: 967–70.

Hintz H, Wenzel A, Danielsen B, Nyvad B. Reliability of visual examination, fibreoptic transillumination, and bitewing radiography, and reproducibility of direct visual examination following tooth separation for the identification of cavitated carious lesions in contacting approximal surfaces. *Caries Res* 1998; **32**: 204–9.

Kidd EAM, Beighton D. Prediction of secondary caries around tooth-coloured restorations: a clinical and microbiological study. *J Dent Res* 1996; **75**: 1942–6.

Kidd EAM, O'Hara JW. The caries status of occlusal amalgam restorations with marginal defects. *J Dent Res* 1990; **60**: 1275–7.

Kidd EAM, Toffenetti F, Mjör IA. Secondary caries. *Int Dent J* 1992; **42**: 127–8.

Kidd EAM, Joyston-Bechal S, Beighton D. Marginal ditching and staining as a predictor of secondary caries around amalgam restorations: a clinical and microbiological study. *J Dent Res* 1995; **74**: 1206–11.

Koch G. Importance of early determination of caries risk. *Int Dent J* 1988; **38**: 203–10.

Koulourides T, Keller SE, Manson-Hing L, *et al.* Enhancement of fluoride effectiveness by experimental cariogenic priming of human enamel. *Caries Res* 1980; **14**: 32–9.

Levine RS, Pitts NB, Nugent ZL. The fate of 1,587 unrestored carious teeth: a retrospective general dental practice based study from northern England. *Br Dent J* 2002; **193**: 99–103.

Levine RJ, Nugent ZL, Pitts NB. Pain prediction for preventive non-operative management of dentinal caries in primary teeth in general dental practice. *Br Dent J* 2003; **195**: 202–6.

Lunder N, von der Fehr FR. Approximal cavitation related to bitewing image and caries activity in adolescents. *Caries Res* 1996; **30**: 143–7.

Mejàre I, Malmgren B. Clinical and radiographic appearance of proximal carious lesions at the time of operative treatment in young permanent teeth. *Scand J Dent Res* 1986; **94**: 19–26.

Mejàre I, Stenlund H. Caries rates for the mesial surface of the first permanent molar and the distal surface of the second primary molar from 6 to 12 years of age in Sweden. *Caries Res* 2000; **34**: 454–61.

Mejàre I, Grondahl HG, Carlstedt K, Grever AC, Ottosson E. Accuracy at radiography and probing for the diagnosis of proximal caries. *Scand J Dent Res* 1985; **93**: 178–84.

Mejàre I, Källestål C, Stenlund H, Johansson H. Caries development form 11 to 22 years of age: a prospective radiographic study. *Caries Res* 1999; **33**: 93–100.

Mejàre I, Stenlund H, Zelezny-Holmlund C. Caries incidence and lesion progression from adolescence to young adulthood: a prospective 15-year cohort study in Sweden. *Caries Res* 2004; **38**: 130–41.

Mertz-Fairhurst E, Schuster G, Fairhurst C. Arresting caries by sealants: results of a clinical study. *J Am Dent Assoc* 1986; **112**: 194–7.

Mertz-Fairhurst EJ, Curtis JW, Ergle JW, Rueggeberg FA, Adair SM. Ultra conservative and cariostatic sealed restorations: results at year 10. *J Am Dent Assoc* 1998; **129**: 55–66.

Milsom KM, Tickle M, Blinkhorn AS. Dental pain and dental treatment of young children attending the general dental service. *Br Dent J* 2002; **192**: 280–4.

Mjör IA, Toffenetti F. Secondary caries: a literature review with case reports. *Quintessence Int* 2000; **31**: 165–79.

Nugent ZJ, Pitts NB. Patterns of change and results overview 1985/6–1995/6 from the British Association for the Study of Community Dentistry (BASCD) co-ordinated National Health Service surveys of caries prevalence. *Community Dent Health* 1997; **14**(Suppl 1): 30–54.

Nyvad B, Fejerskov O. Active root surface caries converted into inactive caries as a response to oral hygiene. *Scand J Dent Res* 1986; **94**: 281–4.

Nyvad B, Fejerskov O. An ultrastructural study of bacterial invasion and tissue breakdown in human experimental root surface caries. *J Dent Res* 1990; **69**: 2218–25.

Parikh SR, Massler M, Bahn A. Microorganisms in active and arrested carious lesions of dentine. *NY State Dent J* 1963; **29**: 347–55.

Pitts NB, Rimmer PA. An *in vivo* comparison of radiographic and directly assessed clinical caries status of posterior approximal surfaces in primary and permanent teeth. *Caries Res* 1992; **26**: 146–52.

Ratledge DK. A clinical and laboratory investigation of the tunnel restoration. Thesis, University of London, 1999.

Ratledge DR, Kidd EAM, Beighton D. A clinical and microbiological study of approximal carious lesions. Part 1: The relationship between cavitation, radiographic lesion depth, the site-specific gingival index and the level of infection of the dentin. *Caries Res* 2001; **35**: 3–7.

Rudolphy MP, van Amerongen JP, Penning C, ten Cate JM. Grey discoloration and marginal fracture for the diagnosis of secondary caries in molars with occlusal amalgam restorations: an *in vitro* study. *Caries Res* 1995; **29**: 371–6.

Rugg-Gunn AJ. Approximal carious lesions. A comparison of the radiological and clinical appearances. *Br Dent J* 1972; **133**: 481–4.

Sarnat H, Massler M. Microstructure of active and arrested dentinal caries. *J Dent Res* 1965; **44**: 1389–401.

Schüpbach P, Guggenheim B, Lutz F. Human root caries: histopathology of arrested lesions. *Caries Res* 1992; **26**: 153–64.

Seddon RP. The detection of cavitation in carious approximal surfaces *in vivo* by tooth separation and impression techniques. Thesis, University of London, 1995.

Shwartz M, Grondahl H-G, Pliskin JS, Boffa J. A longitudinal analysis from bitewing radiograph of the rate of progression of approximal carious lesions through human dental enamel. *Arch Oral Biol* 1984; **29**: 529–36.

Simonsen R. Retention and effectiveness of dental sealant after 15 years. *J Am Dent Assoc* 1991; **122**: 34–42.

Thylstrup A, Bille J, Qvist V. Radiographic and observed tissue changes in approximal carious lesions at the time of operative treatment. *Caries Res* 1986; **20**: 75–84.

Thylstrup A, Brunn C, Holmen L. *In vivo* caries models – mechanisms for caries initiation and arrestment. *Adv Dent Res* 1993; **8**: 144–57.

Tickle M, Milsom K, King D, Kearney-Mitchell P, Blinkhorn A. The fate of the carious primary teeth of children who regularly attend the general dental service. *Br Dent J* 2002; **192**; 219–23.

Tickle M, Milsom KM, King D, Blinkhorn AS. The influence on preventive care provided to children who frequently attend the UK general dental service. *Brit Dent J* 2003; **194**: 329–32.

21

Caries removal and the pulpo-dentinal complex

E.A.M. Kidd, L. Bjørndal, D. Beighton and O. Fejerskov

Introduction

The complete divorcement of dental practice from studies of the pathology of dental caries, that existed in the past, is an anomaly in science that should not continue. It has the apparent tendency to make dentists mechanics only (Green Vardiman Black, 1908).

When Black wrote his textbook *Operative dentistry* in 1908, he based it on his observations and understanding of the disease processes at that time, and indeed devoted one of two volumes to describing dental caries in detail.

Over the past century something has gone strangely wrong, as implied in the Preface to this book. In many dental schools the science of cariology and the technicalities of operative dentistry are taught and researched separately from each other. Generations of students have passed through operative technique courses and phantom-head exercises restoring natural caries-free teeth or, even worse, plastic counterfeits. This use of plastic may be essential if natural teeth are not available, but it is less than ideal because it encourages a template, mechanical approach to a subject that should be taught biologically.

When caries-free natural or plastic teeth are used, the eventual appearance of caries lesions in patients is a considerable inconvenience, ruining stereotyped preconceptions of outline forms, appropriate depths, widths and angles taught in classical phantom-head courses. It is hoped that readers will follow the logic of what follows and forgive the apparently endless questioning and trawling of the literature in search of evidence to confirm or refute current practice and look at operative treatment in biological terms.

This chapter will try to assemble the biological evidence behind caries removal to suggest a more conservative treatment based on sound biological principles. The discussion begins by considering what drives the demineralization process on various tooth surfaces.

Summary of caries lesion progression in dentin

In Chapters 1–3 it was emphasized that in principle any caries lesion can be arrested by plaque control alone if the cariogenic challenge at a tooth site is kept low. Indeed, plaque removal alone will arrest lesions that appear active, even when the outer enamel surface has broken down, provided the cleaning aid can access the cavity (see the clinical evidence in Chapter 2). The premise that operative intervention is not always required was implied in 1908 by G.V. Black, who suggested that simple cleaning of buccal surfaces would arrest decay in the enamel.

Decades later the interpretation of the early histopathological pattern of the caries progression as a spread along the enamel–dentin junction subjacent to uncavitated enamel lesions (Silverstone & Hicks, 1985) gave an opposite signal in relation to the clinical management. In reality, a need for early operative intervention could be argued, if an uncontrolled caries progression in dentin was believed to take place, undermining sound enamel. However, more recent analyses of the non-cavitated lesion disclosed a close structural interrelation with no spread of demineralization along the enamel–dentin junction (Fig. 21.1a). The clinical impact of this is important and can be summarized as follows: the early dentin reaction beneath enamel lesions is not an uncontrolled spreading phenomenon, but is related

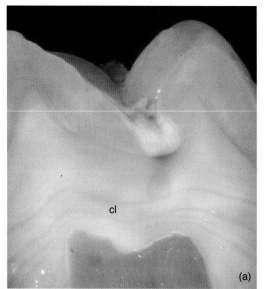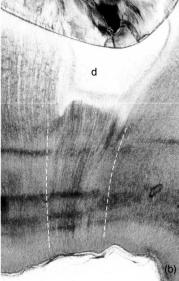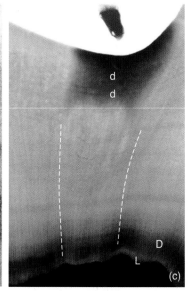

Figure 21.1 Example of the close interrelation between the non-cavitated enamel lesion and the pulpo-dentinal complex with no spread along the enamel–dentin junction and the formation of tubular sclerosis/hypermineralized dentin. (a) Macroscopic and (b, c) histological overviews of the lesion. Zones of dentin demineralization (dd) and hypermineralized dentin (within the white dotted line, c). cl: Owen's contour lines. The non-pathological occurrence of dark zone (D) and light zone (L). (Modified from Bjørndal *et al.*, 1998. Figures reproduced with permission from S. Karger AG, Basel.)

to the spread of the non-cavitated enamel lesion. Early dentin reactions per se should not, therefore, be regarded as a problem justifying an operative intervention. Following the non-operative line by G.V. Black, the early dentin reactions can be arrested by means of plaque removal at the enamel surface.

Likewise, Chapter 3 showed that just as in the case of an enamel lesion, the root surface is reacting to the dynamic process that occurs in the microbial biofilm at the tooth surface by developing a subsurface type of lesion (Figs 3.65–3.68). From a microbiological point of view there are substantial differences in how early during caries lesion formation the bacteria invade the tissues between enamel on the one hand and cementum and dentin on the other. Thus, as shown in Fig. 3.64, cementum and dentin are invaded by microorganisms very early during lesion formation, but for the following discussion it is important to remember that with time, regular plaque removal and fluoride exposure, active lesions become arrested and convert to inactive lesions (Nyvad & Fejerskov, 1986). The majority of root lesions undergo natural reversal and repair as the gingival tissues recede and biofilm accumulation over the lesion is reduced. For clinical evidence see Figs 2.42–2.51.

To extend the argument, it is important to consider the different levels of infection in both active and arrested root-surface lesions (Beighton *et al.*, 1993). Active root caries lesions are heavily infected with bacteria that enter the demineralized dentin along the collagen fibers of the exposed cementum and dentin, and along and within the dentinal tubules. Yet, arrested lesions are minimally infected as tooth brushing and other methods of plaque control remove not only the microbial biofilm at the surface, but also part of the softened infected dentin (Fig. 3.69). However, many microorganisms are left within the dentin without this resulting in further lesion progression or pulpal reactions.

Leaving infected dentin in this situation is not deleterious to the tooth. This argument may be especially hard for clinicians to accept, as they have often been taught that caries management necessitated removal of all soft and infected dentin. The discussion must now be extended to consider caries lesions that have penetrated the enamel with active cavitated lesions established in the subjacent dentin.

In a cavitated coronal lesion, the cavity is often filled with large accumulations of microorganisms (Fig. 21.2a) that may even grow in large colonies resembling isolates in a laboratory dish. If these are removed with a toothbrush the underlying, partly softened dentin is exposed. However, if the microorganisms cannot be removed with tooth brushing or dental floss, then the lesion cannot be arrested. In contrast to the non-cavitated lesion, a spread of demineralization in both the enamel and dentin is noted along the enamel–dentin junction (Figs 21.2b, c, 21.3).

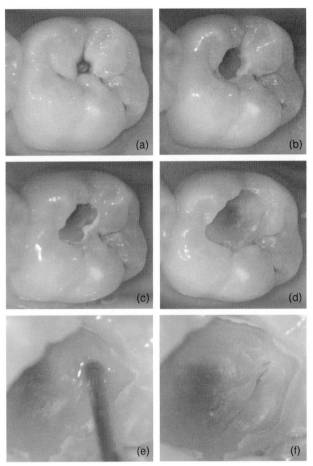

Figure 21.2 The cavitated coronal lesion with accumulations of microorganisms, and with a change in enamel translucency around the cavity (a) demonstrating that enamel demineralization at this stage develops along the enamel–dentin junction (EDJ) and creates a retrograde pattern of enamel demineralization (b, c). The clinical removal of overhanging and undermined enamel is here guided by the retrograde pattern of enamel demineralization (d). The opening of the closed ecosystem along the EDJ shows a brown discolored demineralized dentin related to the exposed central and oldest part of the lesion, whereas the peripheral and outermost area has a more light yellow discoloration. A probe penetrates with easy fragment loss of the tissue, which is very soft and oozing moisture (d–f). Note the gap is visible in the clinic between the enamel and the dentin, owing to extensive dentin demineralization (e, f).

The microbial plaque in a cavity maintains a particular ecological environment as pH is kept low over a much longer period than in microbial biofilms on the enamel surface (Fejerskov *et al.*, 1992; Larsen & Pearce, 1992).

At this stage, operative dentistry may have a role to play. However, a question must be asked: what are the relative roles, as far as lesion progression is concerned, of the microbial plaque in the cavity and the microbial populations within the infected dentin? In 1938, Anderson demonstrated that large, active occlusal lesions of first molars became arrested by opening up the overlying enamel and allowing the patient access to the cavity. After removing the undermined enamel to allow self-cleaning of the lesion, he

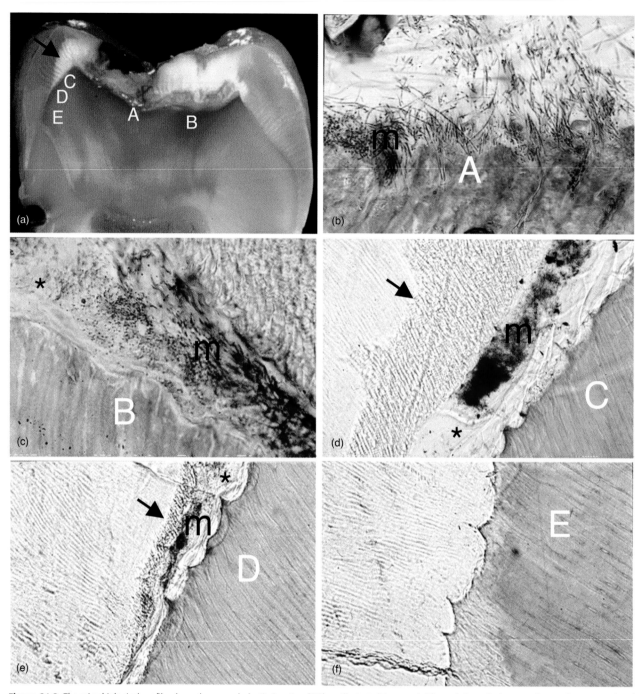

Figure 21.3 The microbiological profile along the enamel–dentin junction (EDJ) as illustrated in a tooth bisected through the central part of a cavitated and closed lesion environment (a). Note the undermined enamel (arrow). Sites A–E along the EDJ are histologically detailed in b–f. The microorganisms (m) penetrate the dentinal tubules (b). Heavy microbial (m) accumulation is shown along the EDJ gap (*, c). Both the microbial (m) accumulation and the size of the EDJ gap (*) decrease (d, e). Arrows show a pattern of the demineralized enamel rod structure. At the outermost affected EDJ area, only the dentin shows alterations in terms of stained demineralization (f). [From Bjørndal & Kidd, 2005, reproduced from *Dental update*, by permission of George Warman Publications (UK) Ltd, Guildford.]

observed that the soft surface layer of the lesion became worn away, leaving a hard, darkly pigmented, eburnated surface. This is the explanation behind large, occlusal, black cavities, which are hard on probing and are often found in children and adults where functional occlusion and attri-

tion break down the undermined enamel and eliminate most of the plaque in the cavity (Fig. 2.37). This scenario is the same as seen in arrested root-surface caries and documented both clinically (Nyvad & Fejerskov, 1986) and experimentally *in situ* (Nyvad *et al.*, 1997). Logically and scientifically, there are no reasons why the process of treating root caries and occlusal caries should be any different.

The pulpo-dentinal complex and caries

Dentin is a vital tissue containing odontoblast processes, and therefore dentin and pulp must be considered as one unique functional entity (Ogawa *et al.*, 1983). Exposure of dentin to the oral environment as a result of occlusal attrition or gingival recession inevitably results in a cellular response in the pulpo-dentinal organ. The metabolic activities in the oral biofilm are also an assault on this complex vital tissue. However, as most lesions develop and progress slowly over months and years, dentin is capable of mounting a cellular-driven defence (Bjørndal & Mjör, 2001) through the physiological mechanism of tubular sclerosis (Fig. 21.1b, c). This plugging of the tubules by minerals (Figs 3.52–3.56) reduces or blocks the fluid movement in the tubules, and hence reduces hypersensitivity to stimuli such as cold and rapid air movement. Previous restorations in the tooth may also have altered the dentin significantly (Mjör & Ferrari, 2002).

In slowly progressing or chronic lesions, the obturation of the tubules continues, not only by growth of the peritubular dentin but also as a result of reprecipitation of mineral salts within the tubules. The growth of peritubular dentin is a physiological process which with age may almost obliterate the tubular space and render the dentin brittle. The mechanism behind the precipitation of mineral crystals within the tubules is thought to be a physicochemical process. The mineral salts are most likely to be derived from the dissolved hydroxyapatite crystals as part of the carious process. These precipitated crystals may make the dentin more mineralized and less permeable. The permeability of dentin subjacent to caries lesions has been shown to be only 14% of that in unaffected dentin in the same age group of young adults (Tagami *et al.*, 1992). It is important to appreciate that there is a substantial variation in this physiological defense mechanism whereby the odontoblasts, through yet unknown mechanisms, gradually occlude the tubules and hence block the immediate pathways between the oral environment and the pulp.

Inflammatory reactions in the pulp have been shown to occur while the caries process is still in enamel (Brännström & Lind, 1965). However, knowledge about rates of caries progression is relevant and necessary in order to interpret the histological picture (Bjørndal *et al.*, 1998). Cellular proliferations in the subodontoblastic region have been noted in the active enamel lesion. Dendritic cells, similar to macrophages, are found at an early stage in this area; these are immunocompetent cells that play an active role in the defense of the pulp (Jontell *et al.*, 1998). Beneath a slowly progressing enamel lesion there is no cellular proliferation. Thus, the metabolic activities in the oral biofilm are mir-rored along the pulp–dentin interface at a very early stage of lesion formation (Bjørndal *et al.*, 1998).

In the rapidly progressing enamel lesion, the odontoblasts may be destroyed and replaced with non-odontoblastic cells which lay down atubular dentin also described as fibrodentin. Occasionally, the odontoblasts degenerate and are not replaced, and the tubules are left partly empty. In the old literature these are called 'dead tracts' (Fish, 1932). However, in addition to these protective mechanisms, the primary odontoblasts corresponding to the affected parts of the dentin respond by enhancing the otherwise slowly ongoing secondary dentin formation, and a patch of reactionary (tertiary) dentin, containing fewer and irregular tubules, is formed along the pulp wall (Fig. 3.38, parts 3–6).

Since the caries often progresses in an intermittent fashion with periods of demineralization and remineralization, the pulp and dentin reactions are also likely to modulate through active and reparative phases. This could happen owing to sudden changes occurring in the local lesion environment, as noted for example when a cavitated deep lesion arrests because the overlying, undermined enamel breaks away and the lesion becomes cleanable. The histological examination of deep, untreated lesions shows that the quality of the tertiary dentin can be related to lesion activity. In slowly progressing lesions the tertiary dentin contains tubules and resembles normal dentin (Fig. 21.4), whereas in rapid lesion progression there is either an atubular dentin formation (Fig. 21.5) or no tertiary dentin (Bjørndal & Darvann, 1999).

Pulp inflammation may or may not be associated with toothache. Acute and chronic pulpitis are recognized. These conditions are based on histopathological examination of stained sections of demineralized teeth with caries lesions (Reeves & Stanley, 1966; Massler, 1967; Shovelton, 1968) without any knowledge of the history of the tooth, for instance why it was extracted. These terms do not provide any information about the progression of the lesion (active or arrested) at the time when the tooth was extracted. Perhaps this explains why it has not been possible to establish a good correlation between clinical symptoms and the histopathological conditions of the pulp.

Pulp reactions to deep caries lesions exhibit chronic inflammatory exudates with lymphocytes, macrophages and plasma cells, and tertiary dentin formation. Polymorphonuclear leukocytes predominate in acute pulpitis, as in inflammation of connective tissue elsewhere in the body. The cellular infiltration subjacent to the caries lesion varies in intensity, and the leukocytes may infiltrate the odontoblastic layer and the subodontoblastic area to the extent that they destroy the odontoblasts. This is followed by atubular dentin formation. As the acute response settles, new dentinal matrix can be laid down. The combination of atubular dentin and new dentinal matrix, also described as reparative dentinogensis,

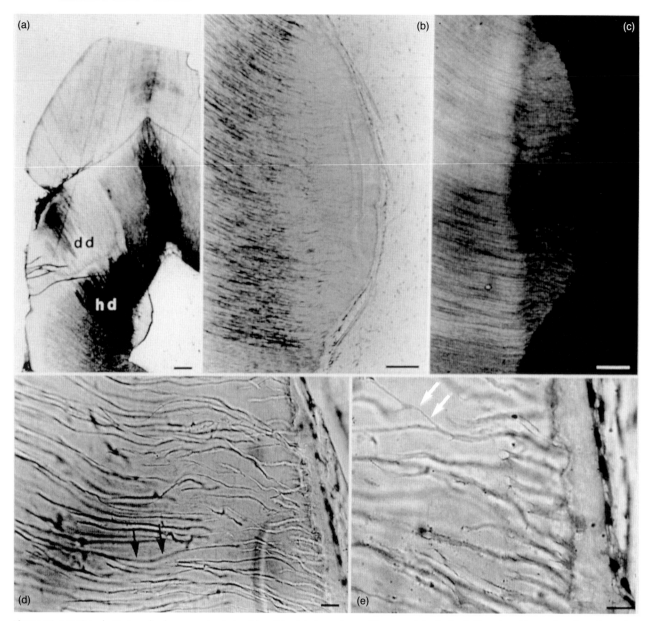

Figure 21.4 Tertiary dentin in a slowly progressing lesion (a) contains tubules and resembles normal dentin (b–e). The odontoblast region along the tertiary dentin is associated with orthodentinal tubules (black arrows, d) as well as new tubules indicating the 'footprints' of new secondary odontoblast cells (white arrows, e). dd = dentin demineralization, hd = hypermineralized dentin. (Bjørndal & Darvann, 1999.)

is recognized clinically as dentin bridge formation following pulp capping procedures. Even if a local abscess is formed, this healing is a likely outcome, although microorganisms must not be involved if this is to take place. The reparative dentin is particularly irregular in structure and the tubules will not be a continuation of the primary dentinal tubules. This situation will affect the permeability of the dentin, and in that way it provides a barrier against future influx of toxic, allergenic components and bacterial antigens.

However, it is important to realize that tertiary dentin per se cannot protect the tooth from complete destruction.

If the caries process continues, the pulp will eventually degenerate. Inflammation as a tissue response is a major defense mechanism against trauma, noxious agents and immunological challenges. It was long believed that inflammation in the pulp was destructive, because the swelling that accompanies it may result in compression of the blood vessels in the non-compliant location of the pulp within the tooth. However, since this occurs only in advanced cases, pulp inflammation must also be regarded as an important defense mechanism of the dental pulp (Heyeraas et al., 2001). The localized increase in tissue fluid pressure that is found associated with pulpitis can result in toothache.

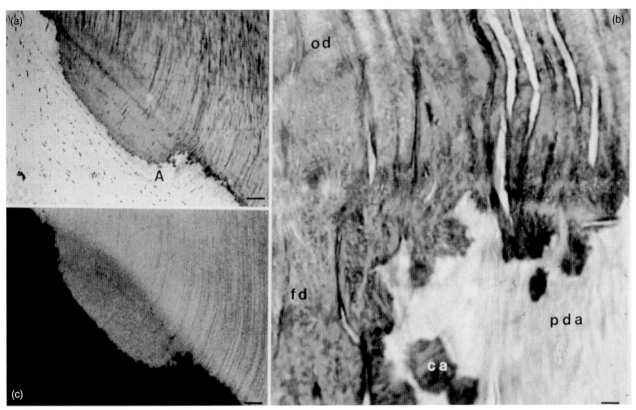

Figure 21.5 Atubular or fibrodentin formation (fd) is noted subjacent to rapid lesion progression (a–c). Site A is detailed (b) and discloses the termination of the tubules in the orthodentin (od) as well as a well-defined pattern of a calcospheritic (ca) mineralization of the predentin area (pda). (From Bjørndal & Darvann, 1999, reproduced with permission from S. Karger AG, Basel.)

Clinical diagnosis of pulpitis

A chronically inflamed pulp is usually symptomless. However, the localized increase in tissue fluid pressure associated with acute inflammation usually results in toothache. The painful response may be initiated by hot, cold or sweet stimulae. Unfortunately, the pain is often not well localized to the offending tooth, and the patient may not even be able to indicate which quadrant is involved.

What matters to the clinician is whether or not the pulp is likely to survive. Since clinical symptoms relate so poorly to pulp pathology, there is an obvious problem here. A useful rule of thumb is to divide clinical pulpitis into reversible and irreversible pulpitis. In reversible pulpitis the clinician hopes to be able to preserve a healthy vital pulp. The clinical diagnosis of reversible pulpitis is made when the pain evoked by a hot, cold or sweet stimulus is of short duration, disappearing when the stimulus is removed. In contrast, if pain persists for minutes or hours after removal of the stimulus, a clinical diagnosis of irreversible pulpitis may be made, and the pulp removed and replaced by a root filling. Alternatively, the tooth may be extracted. It is important to realize that these are relatively crude, clinical guidelines. There is no clinical device that can measure the degree of

pulp inflammation and inform the dentist whether it is reversible or irreversible.

The relevance of pulpo-dentinal reactions to operative management

It is the pulpo-dentinal complex, already under stress from the caries process, that the clinician then interferes with when suddenly instituting extensive operative treatment. At this point, the reader may conclude that the pulpo-dentinal complex may fare better with minimal intervention rather than the traditional operative approach, which focusses on removing infected dentin before restoring the tooth.

In 1967 Massler elegantly distilled current scientific knowledge on this subject. His biological sense of frustration at some of his clinical colleagues jumps from the pages: 'it is somewhat disturbing to the biologically orientated clinical teacher to witness the overly focussed attention of some dentists upon the operative and restorative phases of dentistry, the "drilling and filing" of teeth, to the neglect of the disease process which causes the lesion (cariology) and the preoperative treatment of the wounded tooth-bone'. These words are the reincarnation of G.V. Black's plea, written some 60 years earlier than Massler and reproduced at the beginning of this chapter.

From this statement and the present understanding of the caries process as outlined in Chapters 1, 2, 3 and 20, logical clinical management should follow, i.e. to convert active lesions into inactive or arrested lesions, thus aiding the defense and healing processes in dentin and pulp before restoration procedures are attempted (Bjørndal & Mjör, 2001).

The current operative tradition

Nevertheless, current clinical practice is immediately to perform operative intervention in order to:

- remove softened (Fig. 21.6a–d), infected carious dentin (because, according to present paradigms, the infected

tissue should be eliminated until dentin that is hard to touch has been obtained)
- extend the removal of enamel and dentin to obtain a cavity suitable for insertion of the restorative material of choice
- apply some agent, e.g. calcium hydroxide or zinc oxide eugenol cement, to protect the pulpo-dentinal complex from:
  - toxic effects of restorative materials
  - microorganisms penetrating owing to leakage at the tooth–restoration interface
  - thermal fluctuations.

The question is, however, whether this is appropriate with the present knowledge about the disease and the way in which lesions progress. Is it necessary to remove infected soft dentin mechanically (Fig. 21.6a–d) to arrest further lesion progression? If it is, how best should this be done without further compromising the survival of the tooth?

The infected dentin concept and its clinical consequence

Thus far, the evidence presented in most of the chapters has strongly argued that the bacterial load in the biofilm and the microbiological mass in the cavity drive the caries process. Hence, the plaque should be removed to arrest any lesion. Once the microorganisms start invading the tissues, the dentist is faced with the dilemma of whether all of the infected dentin can be removed. The simple answer is that it is not possible.

As emphasized in the schematic illustration in Fig. 21.7, softening of dentin precedes the organisms responsible for it (MacGregor *et al.*, 1956; Fusayama, 1979, 1988; Ogawa *et al.*, 1983). However, microorganisms may invade any open, empty tubule in dentin exposed to the oral environment without necessarily demineralizing the tissue. A few organisms will remain even if all soft dentin is removed. These organisms remain viable beneath restorations without apparently causing any detrimental effect. Little evidence has been produced to support the concept of removing infected dentin. Indeed, it is not possible to do this. However, these traditional operative drilling and filling procedures (Fig. 21.6a–d) are still being taught and practiced (Kidd *et al.*, 1996, 2003). Maybe the appreciation of dental caries as an infectious disease led the profession to think that all infected tissues should be eliminated.

Still today, the most commonly used approach to the removal of infected dentin is to remove all soft tissue with a bur (Fig. 21.6a) or an excavator (Fig. 21.6c, d). Some dental schools teach that the enamel–dentin junction should be rendered hard and stain free. Other schools teach students to remove everything to the hard substrate and ignore the stain. Since the degree of discoloration alone is a subjective

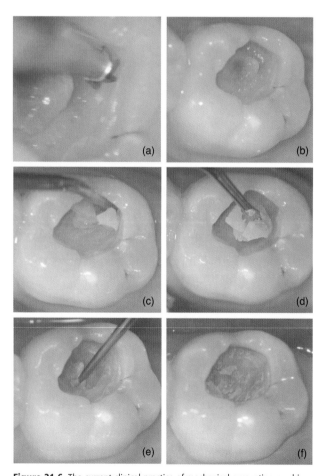

Figure 21.6 The current clinical practice of mechanical excavation combines a peripheral dentin excavation, carried out using a round burr (a, b), with elimination of the centrally infected tissue using an excavator (c, d). The probe is used to assess clinical consistency, and here dentin that is hard to the touch has not yet been obtained (e). Note that the deeper and soft carious dentin is a fragmented tissue (f). An excavation close to the pulp represents a risk, because cracks along the fragments may lead to pulp exposure.

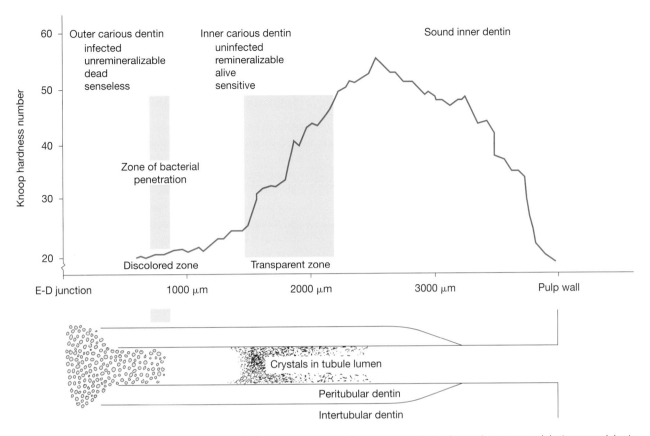

Figure 21.7 Schematic drawing of the relation between the Knoop hardness curve, the outer carious dentin, the translucent zone and the inner sound dentin. Underneath is shown the relation to bacterial invasion, and mineralization phenomena in the dentinal tubules. (Modified from Ogawa *et al.*, 1983.)

and rather unreliable guide to gauge the level of dentin infection, and since a few bacteria remain whatever restorative approach is adopted and practiced, it seems logical to leave stain as the more conservative approach (Kidd *et al.*, 1996). This statement can be underlined when viewing the microbiological profile along the enamel–dentin junction. A systematic decrease in bacteria is observed laterally along the gap (see Fig. 21.3b–e). At the outermost affected area, only stained demineralized dentin is noted with no gap and hence no appearance of bacteria (see Fig. 21.3f).

Over the pulpal surface, discolored dentin should be left untouched, provided that it is 'reasonably hard', and the tooth is symptomless and responds as vital to pulp testing. Vigorous hand excavation over the pulpal surface is positively contraindicated, once the cavity floor is 'reasonably firm', because the clinical nature of deeper and soft carious dentin discloses a fragmented tissue (Fig. 21.6e–f). Now excavation close to the pulp represents a risk, because cracks along the fragments may lead to pulp exposure. However, the student may find that one teacher's subjective definition of 'reasonably firm' is another's 'rather soft' definition of firmness. Since there is no evidence to support or refute either approach, it is difficult to be more specific regarding the degree of firmness. Soft dentin is usually wet (Fig. 21.2e)

but sometimes, particularly when an old restoration has been removed, the dentin may appear dry and friable. This dentin has been shown to be lightly infected (Kidd *et al.*, 1996) and it may represent residual caries that a previous dentist left during cavity preparation. It may not require vigorous excavation.

The subjective clinical assessment of carious dentin led Fusayama to develop a caries dye (acid red in propylene glycol) (Fusayama & Terachima, 1972; Fusayama, 1979, 1988) to differentiate clinically 'infected' from 'affected' dentin (Hosoda & Fusayama, 1982; Kuboki *et al.*, 1984; Fusayama, 1988). He reported that the more superficial zone of infected dentin was an irreversibly damaged, bacterially infected layer that would never remineralize. The deepest affected dentin has been claimed to harden as a result of remineralization (Eidelman *et al.*, 1965) (Fig. 21.7). Fusayama's group tentatively suggested that the dye staining front coincided with the bacterial invasion of the dentin. However, several studies have reported that the dye does not discretely discriminate the bacterially infected from softened affected tissues (Anderson *et al.*, 1985; Boston & Graver, 1989; Kidd *et al.*, 1993). Consequently, its injudicious use may lead to the overpreparation of tissues, encouraging excess removal at the enamel–dentin junction

(Kidd *et al.*, 1993), despite absence of bacteria at the outermost area (Fig. 21.3f), as well as unnecessary removal of dentin over the pulpal surface (Yip *et al.*, 1994).

Others have recommended the chemical removal of carious (infected) dentin (Beeley *et al.*, 2000) based on the philosophy that sodium hypochlorite, which is a non-specific proteolytic agent, can remove partly demineralized dentin. This concept has been further developed, and a gel is presently marketed that can be applied in the carious cavity and left for a while to dissolve the dentin matrix components, which contain partly degraded collagen. It would, however, be unfortunate if dentists started to apply this on, for example, root-surface lesions that are accessible to arrest by plaque control alone. Not only would this be unnecessary with the knowledge about how to arrest such lesions (Nyvad & Fejerskov, 1986), but it would result in an increased need for restorations. The question is, again, does this part of the dentin need to be removed? To answer this question it is now important to examine that literature that has investigated the consequences of leaving infected dentin.

Studies placing fissure sealants over carious dentin

Several studies have examined the consequences of simply sealing over carious dentin. Table 21.1 gives a chronological overview of this work. All studies, with the exception of Weerheijm *et al.* (1992), were prospective and in many there were unsealed, control, lesions. Caries activity was assessed in a number of ways including clinical observation, lesion depth measurement, radiographic lesion depth measurement and microbiological sampling. Observation periods varied from 2 weeks to 5 years.

The disparity of methodologies militates against a systematic review of the studies, but some uniform themes emerge. Sealed lesions appeared to arrest both clinically and radiographically. Investigations of the fate of the sealed bacteria showed a decrease in microorganisms with time or their complete elimination. No pulpitis was reported in sealed teeth. In contrast, lesions progressed where sealants were lost and in unsealed, control teeth.

The study by Weerheijm *et al.* (1992) is an interesting outlier. This work was a retrospective examination of sealed teeth where radiographs showed radiolucency in dentin beneath a sealant that was clinically intact. This methodology precluded microbiological sampling before the sealant was placed, which is unfortunate because there can be no comparison of microbial counts before and after sealing. Nevertheless, it is worrying that cariogenic microorganisms were found in 50% of the teeth and the dentin was often soft and moist, rather than leathery or dry. This would seem to indicate active lesions. The microbiological examination in this work was more detailed than in many other studies examining for lactobacilli, mutans streptococci and non-mutans streptococci. Since there was no preoperative sample, it is impossible to know whether sealing had changed the numbers or the distribution of the microflora.

Stepwise excavation studies

In stepwise excavation, first described by Bodecker in 1938, only part of the soft, dentin caries is removed at the first visit during the acute phase of caries progression. The cavity is restored and reopened after a period of weeks. Further excavation is now carried out before a definitive restoration. The objective of the exercise is to arrest lesion progression and allow the formation of tertiary dentin before final excavation, making pulpal exposure less likely.

This procedure has been investigated scientifically for more than 30 years. These studies have involved baseline investigations of carious dentin and then a reanalysis after a period of sealing it in the tooth. This work is important evidence of the consequences of sealing infected dentin into teeth (Fig. 21.8).

Table 21.2 gives a chronological overview of stepwise excavation studies. The majority of these studies have no control. Most have been done on permanent teeth with deep lesions (Fig. 21.9). The amount of carious dentin removed at the initial excavation varies from access to caries only (Fig. 21.2d) to removing the bulk of the carious dentin (Fig. 21.6f).

The restorative materials are also very variable. They include calcium hydroxide, zinc oxide and eugenol, amalgam, glass-ionomer cement and composite resin. Times to re-entry are also very variable, the shortest being 3 weeks, the longest 2 years.

Caries activity has been assessed clinically, radiographically and often by microbiological examination at initial entry and on re-entry. With such differing methodologies, a systematic review is not possible, but some themes emerge.

- The clinical success rate appears high. Exposure is usually avoided using the stepwise technique and symptoms rarely arise between excavations. Control lesions are often exposed by conventional excavation.
- Some studies report that the dentin is altered on re-entry, being dryer, harder and darker (Fig. 21.8d).
- Microbiological monitoring indicates substantial reductions in cultivable flora. Some teeth appear sterile, but in most some microorganisms survive. The nutrients available for the growth of these bacteria are very different from those available to the bacteria above and within the cavity. No longer do they have access to dietary carbohydrates. The major source of nutrients to support bacterial persistence and growth are the proteins and glycoproteins passing through the dentinal tubules from the dental pulp. Several studies (Bjørndal & Larsen, 2000; Maltz *et al.*, 2002; Paddick *et al.*, 2005) suggest that the cultivable

Table 21.1 Chronological overview of studies placing sealants over carious dentin

Study	Treatment (n)	Period	Control (n)	Indication of caries activity	Results and conclusions
Jeronimus et al. (1975)	Occlusal lesions of varying depths on bitewing Etching, sealant (33) Etching, sealant (33) Etching, sealant (30) Etching, sealant (25)	10 min 2 weeks 3 weeks 4 weeks		Gross observation carious dentin Microorganisms: % positive cultures	Many sealants lost Where sealant was intact, dentin became dry, dark, leathery Decrease in microorganisms in shallow lesions, but persisted in deeper lesions
Handelman et al. (1976)	Etching, sealant (60)	0–2 years	Untreated (29)	Clinical observation Radiography Microorganisms	No increase in radiographic lesion depth Large reduction in microorganisms in comparison to controls, increased with time
Going et al. (1978)	Etching, sealant (46)	5 years	Untreated (21)	Clinical observation Microorganisms	Sealed teeth caries arrested On re-entry either sterile or large reduction in microorganisms in comparison to controls, but S. mutans and lactobacilli survived
Mertz-Fairhurst et al. (1979a)	Occlusal lesions at EDJ on X-ray Etching, sealant (4)	6–12 months	Untreated (4)	Lesion depth measurements Microorganisms	No increase in lesion depth in test. Control lesions increased in depth Absence of microorganisms in test sealed teeth
Mertz-Fairhurst et al. (1979b)	Occlusal lesions at EDJ on X-ray Etching, sealant (4)	6–12 months	Untreated (6)	Clinical observations Radiographs	Under sealant dentin powdery, dry, white, with hard, glassy, smooth dentin beneath Control dentin spongy, soft, yellow Sealed teeth: no or small increase in depth. Control: increase in depth
Jensen & Handelman (1980)	Etching, sealant (106)	0–12 months	Unsealed Unsealed and etched	Microorganisms	Etching alone reduced microorganisms by 75% In sealed teeth, bacterial counts reduced with time
Handelman et al. (1981)	Etching, sealant (108)	2–5 years	Contralateral routine amalgam	Radiographic lesion depth	Decrease in lesion depth provided sealant intact
Mertz-Fairhurst et al. (1986)	Etching, sealant (14)	1–17 months	Unsealed (14)	Direct lesion depth measurements and radiographs Microorganisms	Unsealed lesions got deeper, but sealed lesions did not All but one sealed lesion, no microorganisms
Weerheijm et al. (1992)	Teeth already etched and sealed, but occlusal radiolucency in dentin (30)			Microorganisms: total colony-forming units, lactobacilli, mutans streptococci, non-mutans streptococci Clinical observation of dentin	Cariogenic microorganisms found in 50% of teeth despite sealant Dentin soft, moist, dark (not leathery, dry)

EDJ, enamel–dentin junction.

flora is altered on re-entry to a less cariogenic flora. Paddick et al. (2005) showed that the caries-associated bacteria, mutans streptococci and lactobacilli, failed to persist and the flora was dominated by *Streptococcus oralis* and *Actinomyces naeslundii*, two species able to liberate and utilize the sugars from glycoproteins present in the tubules. The supply of nutrients will diminish as the tubules become sclerosed and even these bacteria may die. It is entirely reasonable that as the pH falls, and the supply of nutrients decreases within the lesion, the ecol-ogy will alter. This concept was presented with respect to plaque in Chapter 10.

- There is a possibility that there may be an effect from the dental material on the outcome, but very few studies have addressed this in a controlled manner.

Why re-enter?

The studies in Table 21.2 seem to show that the depth of the first excavation is not relevant to the level of infection of

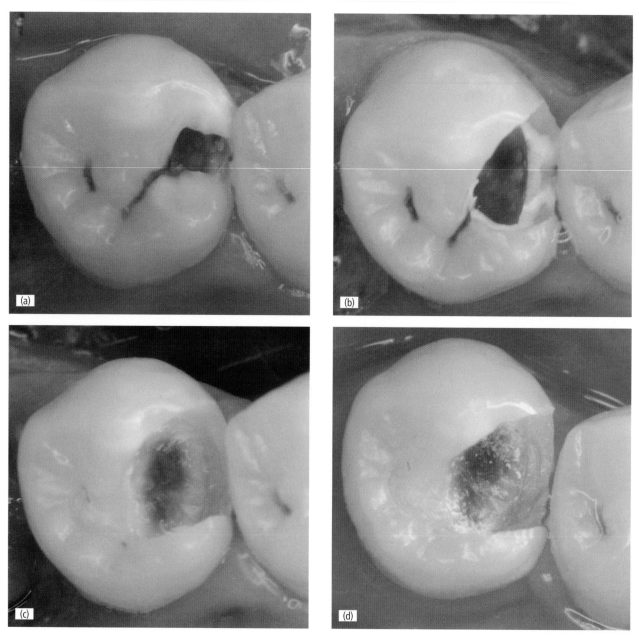

Figure 21.8 Deep caries lesion in a lower premolar during sequences of stepwise excavation (a–d). Undermined enamel along the enamel–dentin junction can be noted clinically as a white zone around the cavity (a). During removal of undermined enamel a clear pattern of demineralized enamel (b) is noted along the enamel–dentin junction. In the first excavation procedure the superficial and central pattern of demineralized dentin is removed, including the peripheral parts of the lesion. The exposed soft dentin is light brown (c). Following temporary filling and a treatment interval of 6 months, and before final excavation, the central exposed dentin is dark brown (d). (From Bjørndal, 1999, reproduced with permission from the *Danish Dental Journal*.)

the soft, dry dentin that is found on re-entry. The final excavation allows the dentist to be sure that there is no exposure and removes the remaining infected dentin. The logic here is that the carious process may continue, albeit slowly, in this infected tissue. So, perhaps, the final excavation is needed to ensure the survival of the restoration.

However, perhaps there is no need to re-enter, and this is the basis of the indirect pulp capping technique (Prader, 1958; Eidelman *et al.*, 1965; Hilton & Summitt, 2000),

although most of the demineralized tissue is removed in this procedure. In stepwise excavation, in contrast, soft, wet dentin is left in place. Is it now necessary to re-enter? After all, if the caries process is driven by the activity in a biofilm exposed to the oral cavity, the process should be arrested simply by sealing the cavity. The persistence of a few microorganisms may be irrelevant. Perhaps they are just opportunistic squatters adapted to the new environment in which they find themselves.

Table 21.2 Chronological overview of stepwise excavation studies

Study	Tooth type; lesion depth	Treatment	Control	Time to re-entry	Indication of carious activity	Results and conclusions
Law & Lewis (1961)	Deciduous and permanent; deep lesions	Access to caries then Ca(OH)$_2$ + H$_2$O on dentin; amalgam (n = 66), re-entry at 6 months, excavation completed (n = 57)		6–24 months	Clinical observation; observation of dentin on re-entry radiographs	76% clinically (no exposure) and radiographically (no pathology) successful
Schouboe & MacDonald (1962)	Molars with occlusal caries	Access, carious dentin sampled. Gold plate over dentin, then amalgam (n = 17)		69–139 days	Microorganisms	Positive cultures in 14 cases; a different flora on re-entry
King et al. (1965)	? Deciduous; deep lesions; no pulpitis	Only deepest layer of decayed dentin left; capped with Ca(OH)$_2$ or ZnO/Eug or amalgam. Restored amalgam (n = 51)		25–206 days	Observation of dentin on re-entry microorganisms	Initial samples of deep, soft, dentin, infected dentin harder on re-entry with Ca(OH)$_2$ and ZnO/Eug but not with amalgam; 3/8 teeth exposed after further caries removal with amalgam. Microorganisms on re-entry: Ca(OH)$_2$ teeth 61.4% sterile, ZnO/Eug teeth 81.8% sterile, amalgam teeth 0% sterile but number of organisms reduced
Kerkhove et al. (1967)	Deciduous and permanent; deep lesions	Only deepest layer decayed dentin left. 41 teeth Ca(OH)$_2$ and amalgam; 35 teeth ZnO/Eug and amalgam		3–12 months	Observation of dentin on re-entry; radiopacity relative to control area assessed visually and densitometrically	92% clinical success. On re-entry dentin dry, hard, brownish yellow; increased radiopacity; very slight time but not material dependent
Magnusson & Sundell (1977)	Deciduous; deep lesions; no pulpitis	Partial excavation; Ca(OH)$_2$, ZnO and Eug cement. At entry all soft carious dentin excavated (n = 55)	Full excavation (n = 55)	4–6 weeks	Clinical observation; observation of dentin on re-entry	15% treatment group pulp exposed; 53% control group pulp exposed
Weerheijm et al. (1993)	Permanent molars; small, visible; occlusal lesions	Part of lesion opened to dentin; this filled with GIC; remainder sealed with GIC. At re-entry all caries removed and composite placed (n = 20)	As treatment but Delton sealant used (n = 4)	7 months	Clinical observation of dentin on re-entry; microorganisms	Poor retention of GIC sealant; microorganisms 100 times less in re-entry sample, but still found in 90% of second samples
Leksell et al. (1996)	Permanent; deep; no pulpitis	Bulk carious dentin excavated. Ca(OH)$_2$, ZnO and Eug cement. At re-entry all soft dentin removed with excavators or burs (n = 57)	All soft caries removed. Ca(OH)$_2$ ZnO/Eug cement, then GIC composite or amalagam (n = 57)	8–24 weeks	Clinical observation	17.5% treatment group exposed; 40% control group exposed
Kreulen et al. (1997)	Permanent molars; occlusal caries on radiograph	Lesions opened to dentin. Filled with resin modified glass-ionomer (n = 40)	As treatment but filled amalgam (n = 40)	6 months	Clinical observation of dentin on re-entry; microorganisms	Dentin darker and harder on re-entry. Substantial decrease in total viable count, mulans streptococci and lactobacilli; more reduction with resin-modified glass ionomer than amalgam

continued

Table 21.2 Chronological overview of stepwise excavation studies (continued)

Study	Tooth type; lesion depth	Treatment	Control	Time to re-entry	Indication of carious activity	Results and conclusions
Weerheijm et al. (1999)	Permanent molars; occlusal caries on radiograph	Lesions opened to dentine. Filled with resin modified glass-ionomer (n = 33)	As treatment but filled amalgam (n = 33)	2 years	Microorganisms	25 patients reviewed. Substantial decrease in total viable count, mutans streptococci and lactobacilli. More decrease in glass-ionomer than amalgam. Microorganisms not cultured in 11 out of 50 cases
Bjørndal et al. (1997)	Permanent; no pulpitis; deep lesions	Peripheral excavation and excavation of 'cariogenic biomass' and superficial demineralized dentin. Ca(OH)₂ and temporary filling. At re-entry, complete excavation (n = 31)		6–12 months	Clinical observation of dentin on re-entry; microorganisms	No pulpal exposures at final excavation. At re-entry dentin darker, harder, dryer

Substantial reduction in colony-forming units, not time dependent |
Bjørndal & Thylstrup (1998)	Permanent; no pulpitis; deep lesions	Peripheral excavation and excavation of 'cariogenic biomass' and superficial demineralized dentin. Ca(OH)₂ and temporary restoration (n = 94)		2–9 months	Clinical observation of dentin on re-entry; follow-up clinical and radiographic examination 1 year after final restoration	Dentin harder and darker on re-entry. Five exposures on final excavation (two sensitive to pressure, two inadequate seal); 88 cases symptomless at 1 year, one case lost temporary and needed root treatment
Bjørndal & Larsen (2000)	Permanent; no pulpitis; deep lesions	As above plus microbiological sampling (n = 9)		4–6 months	Clinical observation of dentin on re-entry; microorganisms	Dentin harder and darker on re-entry. Colony-forming units and proportion of lactobacilli substantially reduced; Gram-negative rods declined; flora dominated by A. naeslundii and various streptococci
Maltz et al. (2002)	Permanent; no pulpitis; deep lesions	Cavity walls made hard, incomplete caries removal pulpally. Ca(OH)₂ and ZnO/Eug cement		6–7 months	Clinical observation of dentin before and after re-entry; radiographic examination; microorganisms	Dentin dryer, harder, darker on re-entry. Increase in radiopacity during study period; bacterial counts decreased significantly
Paddick et al. (2005)	Permanent; no pulpitis, lesions in dentin on radiograph	Cavity walls made hard, very little caries removed over pulp. Bonded composite (n = 10)		5 months	Microbiological examination before sealing and on re-entry	Less diverse microbiota on re-entry. Proposed that the change in available nutrients was responsible for change in microbiota

Ca(OH)₂: calcium hydroxide; Eug: eugenol; GIC: glass-ionomer cement; ZnO: zinc oxide.

Randomized controlled clinical trials

Are there deleterious consequences after incomplete caries removal? Only randomized controlled clinical trials will answer this question. There are some important rules to be followed in these trials, including:

- well-defined inclusion criteria
- a calculation of the number of treatments needed to show a difference between control and experimental groups
- a central randomization of patients to control or experimental groups

- a follow-up examination by an examiner who is not aware of which group the patient belongs to.

Ideally, these trials should be carried out in a number of centers. A randomized, controlled, multicenter clinical trial has been set up in Sweden and Denmark (Bjørndal et al., unpublished results). Final excavation is being compared with stepwise excavation in deep caries lesions and the rules defined above are being followed. Table 21.3 documents four existing studies where randomization has been part of the design. Two of these selected deep lesions in deciduous

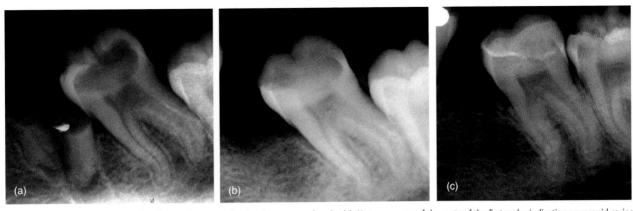

Figure 21.9 A deep lesion treated with stepwise excavation in a lower second molar (a). Note remnants of the roots of the first molar indicating very rapid caries progression. The second molar was permanently restored with a composite inlay. After 1 year, pulp vitality was confirmed, and a new radiograph showed no apical radiolucency (b). Four-year recall confirmed the vitality of the pulp as well as the absence of apical radiolucency (c). However, complete arrest of caries activity has not been achieved; a new proximal lesion has progressed in the third molar. (Modified from Bjørndal, 1999, reproduced with permission.)

Table 21.3 Randomized controlled clinical trials of 'complete' versus 'incomplete' caries removal

Study	Tooth type; lesion depth	Treatment	Control	Observation period	Results and conclusions
Magnusson & Sundell (1977)	Deciduous; deep but no pulpitis	Cavity washed with microbiocidal solution. Partial excavation, calcium hydroxide, zinc oxide and eugenol cement At re-entry, all soft carious dentin excavated ($n = 55$)	All softened dentin excavated regardless of risk of exposure ($n = 55$)	Re-entry 4–6 weeks in treatment group	Treatment: two cases pulpitis between visits, dentin 'altered' on re-entry, 15% pulps exposed Control: 53% pulps exposed
Leksell et al. (1996)	Permanent; deep but no pulpitis	Bulk carious tissue excavated, calcium hydroxide, zinc oxide and eugenol cement At re-entry all soft dentin removed with excavator or burs ($n = 57$)	All softened dentin removed. If no exposure, calcium hydroxide, zinc oxide and eugenol cement, glass-ionomer cement. In some teeth composite or amalgam on top of this ($n = 70$)	Re-entry 8–24 weeks in treatment group	Treatment: 17.5% pulps exposed, easy to distinguish between 'soft' and 'hard', dentin on re-entry Control: 40% pulps exposed
Mertz-Fairhurst et al. (1998)	Permanent; occlusal lesions no deeper then halfway into dentin on radiograph	EDJ not made caries free. Moist, soft, infected dentin left at EDJ and over pulp Restored bonded, sealed, composite ($n = 156$)	Complete caries removal Amalgam and sealant group ($n = 77$) Conventional amalgam group ($n = 79$)	No re-entry 10-year follow-up	No exposure during caries removal Treatment: 85 teeth reviewed at 10 years, caries apparently arrested, one lesion 'caved in' Control: some conventional amalgam, rest failed with new caries at margin
Ribeiro et al. (1999)	Deciduous; no pulpitis; no exposure expected	EDJ made caries free with round bur, but moist, soft, infected dentin left over pulp Restored dentin bonding agent and composite ($n = 24$)	Caries removal with slow round bur guided by caries dye. All dye-stained dentin removed. Restored dentin bonding agent and composite ($n = 24$)	No re-entry Followed for 1 year; assessed on radiograph and histology	Treatment: all restorations retained, excellent marginal integrity after 1 year On radiograph: 46% regressed, 25% progressed, 29% unchanged; adhesive system formed altered hybrid layer histologically Control: pulpal necrosis in one tooth, all other restorations retained, excellent marginal integrity, adhesive system formed hybrid layer

EDJ: enamel–dentin junction.

(Magnusson & Sundell, 1977) or permanent (Leksell *et al.*, 1996) teeth where exposure seemed likely following conventional caries removal. Both studies strongly support a stepwise approach (using calcium hydroxide after initial excavation) if pulp exposure is to be avoided. In these cases, conventional caries removal was deleterious; both studies re-entered.

The other two studies in Table 21.3 selected less advanced lesions and did not re-enter to remove the remaining soft dentin in the treatment groups. Both studies sealed incompletely excavated cavities with dentin bonding agents and composite resins. The work of Ribeiro *et al.*, (1999) on deciduous teeth concluded that the clinical performance of the restorations was not adversely affected by the incomplete caries removal after 1 year. The study by Mertz-Fairhurst *et al.* (1998) was remarkable for a 10-year follow-up of occlusal restorations placed over moist, soft, infected dentin left both at the enamel–dentin junction and over the pulp. Remarkably, half of the patients were still available for recall after 10 years. Lesion progression was arrested and there were no more clinical failures in this group than in control groups with conventional caries removal, although it is not known whether this observation would have changed if all the patients had been available for recall.

On the basis of four enrolled studies, a systematic review of complete or ultraconservative removal of decayed tissue in unfilled teeth (Ricketts *et al.*, 2006) drew the following conclusions:

- Partial caries removal in symptomless, primary or permanent teeth reduces the risk of pulpal exposure.
- No detriment to the patient in terms of pulpal symptoms was found.
- Partial caries removal would appear preferable in the deep lesion to reduce the risk of carious exposure.
- There is insufficient evidence to know whether it is necessary to re-enter and excavate further in the stepwise excavation technique, but studies that did not re-enter reported no adverse consequences.
- There is a need for further randomized, controlled clinical investigation of the need to remove demineralized tissue before restoring the tooth.

Conclusions

Based on the discussions presented herein, there appears to be little logic in the current practice of caries removal. Biologically, it would appear to be potentially damaging even to attempt to remove all infected dentin. It is not even possible to achieve this. The evidence shows that provided either the cavity is sufficiently accessible to regular plaque removal, or a restoration is placed that seals the cavity, then infected and partially softened dentin may be left. It does not prejudice pulpal health and the caries process does not

continue. These statements appear logical and predictable, when seen in the light of the knowledge about the nature of dental caries as presented throughout this textbook.

These arguments will have a strong bearing on the future of restorative dentistry. Well-controlled clinical studies need to be conducted in combination with various laboratory and microbial studies to explain these very intriguing observations. However, it is interesting that Black (1908) and Massler (1967) came to similar conclusions so many years ago, but it is only now that there is a broader appreciation of the need to rethink the most appropriate way of controlling dental caries and its lesion progression. So far, many dentists have been performing a variety of often unnecessary operative procedures which all too often may have added to loss of teeth with time. A range of restorative treatment alternatives will appear, but it should be demanded that all new treatments are based on carefully designed clinical studies before being uncritically implemented in daily dental practice.

References

Anderson BG. Clinical study of arresting dental caries. *J Dent Res* 1938; **17**: 443–52.

Anderson MH, Loesch WJ, Charbeneau GT. Bacteriologic study of a basic fuchsin caries-disclosing dye. *J Prosth Dent* 1985; **54**: 51–5.

Beeley JA, Yip HK, Stevenson AG. Chemomechanical caries removal: a review of the techniques and latest developments. *Br Dent J* 2000; **188**: 427–30.

Beighton D, Lynch E, Heath MR. A microbiological study of primary root-caries lesions with different treatment needs. *J Dent Res* 1993; **72**: 623–9.

Bjørndal, L. Behandling af profunde carieslæsioner med gradvis ekskavering. En praksisbaseret undersøgelse. *Tandlaegebladet* 1999; **103**: 498–506 (English summary).

Bjørndal L, Darvann T. A light microscopic study of odontoblastic and non-odontoblastic cells involved in tertiary dentinogenesis in well-defined cavitated carious lesions. *Caries Res* 1999; **33**: 50–60.

Bjørndal L, Kidd EAM. The treatment of deep dentine caries lesions. *Dental Update* 2005; **32**: 402–13.

Bjørndal L, Larsen T. Changes in the cultivable flora in deep carious lesions following a stepwise excavation procedure. *Caries Res* 2000; **34**: 502–8.

Bjørndal L, Mjör IA. Pulp–dentin biology in restorative dentistry. Part 4: Dental caries – characteristics of lesions and pulpal reactions. *Quintessence Int* 2001; **32**: 717–35.

Bjørndal L, Thylstrup A. A practice-based study of stepwise excavation of deep carious lesions in permanent teeth: a 1-year follow-up study. *Community Dent Oral Epidemiol* 1998; **26**: 122–8.

Bjørndal L, Larsen T, Thylstrup A. A clinical and microbiological study of deep carious lesions during stepwise excavation using long treatment intervals. *Caries Res* 1997; **31**: 411–17.

Bjørndal L, Darvann T, Thylstrup A. A quantitative light microscopic study of odontoblast and subodontoblastic reactions to active and arrested enamel caries without cavitation. *Caries Res* 1998; **32**: 59–69.

Black GV. *Operative dentistry*, Vol. 1, *Pathology of the hard tissues of the teeth*. Chicago, IL: Medico-Dental Publishing Co., 1908.

Bodecker CF. Histologic evidence of the benefits of temporary fillings and successful pulp capping of deciduous teeth. *J Am Dent Assoc* 1938; **25**: 777–86.

Boston DW, Graver HT. Histological study of an acid red caries-disclosing dye. *Op Dent* 1989; **14**:186–92.

Brännström M, Lind PO. Pulpal response to early caries. *J Dent Res* 1965; **44**: 1045–50.

Eidelman E, Finn SB, Koulourides T. Remineralization of carious dentin treated with calcium hydroxide. *J Child Dent* 1965; **32**: 218–25.

Fejerskov O, Scheie AA, Birkhed D, Manji F. Effect of sugar cane chewing on plaque pH in rural Kenyan children. *Caries Res* 1992; **26**: 286–9.

Fish EW. *An experimental investigation of enamel, dentin and the dental pulp*. London: John Bale Sons and Danielsson, 1932.

Fusayama T. Two layers of carious dentin: diagnosis and treatment. *Op Dent* 1979; **4**: 63–70.

Fusayama T. Clinical guide for removing caries using a caries-detecting solution. *Quintessence Int* 1988; **19**: 397–401.

Fusayama T, Terachima S. Differentiation of two layers of carious dentin by staining. *J Dent Res* 1972; **51**: 866.

Going RE, Loesch WJ, Grainger DA, Syed SA. The viability of microorganisms in carious lesions four years after covering with a fissure sealant. *J Am Dent Assoc* 1978; **97**: 455–62.

Handelman SL, Washburn F, Wopperer P. Two-year report of sealant effect on bacteria in dental caries. *J Am Dent Assoc* 1976; **93**: 967–70.

Handelman SL, Leverett DH, Solomon ES, Brener CM. Radiographic evaluation of the sealing of occlusal caries. *Community Dent Oral Epidemiol* 1981; **9**: 256–9.

Heyeraas KJ, Sveen OB, Mjör IA. Pulp–dentin biology in restorative dentistry. Part 3: Pulpal inflammation and its sequelae. *Quintessence Int* 2001; **32**: 611–25.

Hilton TJ, Summitt JB. Pulpal considerations. In: Summitt JB, Robbins JW, Schwartz RS, eds. *Operative dentistry*. Chicago, IL: Quintessence, 2000: 103.

Hosoda H, Fusayama T. A tooth substance saving restorative technique. *Int Dent J* 1982; **34**: 1–12.

Jensen ØE, Handelman SL. Effect of an autopolymerizing sealant on viability of microflora in occlusal dental caries. *Scand J Dent Res* 1980; **88**: 382–8.

Jeronimus DJ, Till MJ, Sveen OB. Reduced viability of microorganisms under dental sealants. *J Dent Child* 1975; **42**: 275–80.

Jontell M, Okiji T, Dahlgren U, Bergenholtz G. Immune defence mechanisms of the dental pulp. *Crit Rev Oral Biol Med* 1998; **9**: 179–200.

Kerkhove BC, Herman SC, Klein AI, McDonald RE. A clinical and television densitometric evaluation of the indirect pulp capping technique. *J Dent Child* 1967; **34**: 192–201.

Kidd EAM, Joyston-Bechal S, Beighton D. The use of a caries detector dye during cavity preparation: a microbiological assessment. *Br Dent J* 1993; **174**: 245–8.

Kidd EAM, Ricketts D, Beighton D. Criteria for caries removal at the enamel–dentin junction: a clinical and microbiological study. *Br Dent J* 1996; **180**: 287–91.

Kidd EAM, Smith BGN, Watson T. *Pickard's manual of operative dentistry*. Oxford: Oxford University Press, 2003: 63.

King JB, Crawford JJ, Lindahl RL. Indirect pulp capping: a bacteriologic study of deep carious dentin in human teeth. *Oral Surg Oral Med Oral Pathol* 1965; **20**: 663–71.

Kreulen CM, de Soet JJ, Weerheijm KL, Van Amerongen WE. In vivo cariostatic effect of resin modified glass ionomer cement and amalgam on dentine. *Caries Res* 1997; **31**: 384–9.

Kuboki Y, Liu CF, Fusayama T. Mechanism of differential staining in carious dentin. *J Dent Res* 1984; **62**: 713–14.

Larsen MJ, Pearce EIF. Some notes on the diffusion of acidic and alkaline agents into natural human caries lesions *in vitro*. *Arch Oral Biol* 1992; **37**: 411–16.

Law DA, Lewis TM. The effect of calcium hydroxide on deep carious lesions. *Oral Surg Oral Med Oral Pathol* 1961; **14**: 1130–7.

Leksell E, Ridell K, Cvek M, Mejàre I. Pulp exposure after stepwise versus direct complete excavation of deep carious lesion in young posterior permanent teeth. *Endod Dent Traumatol* 1996; **12**: 192–6.

MacGregor AB, Marsland EA, Batty I. Experimental studies of dental caries. The relation of bacterial invasion to softening of the dentin. *Br Dent J* 1956; **101**: 230–5.

Magnusson BO, Sundell SO. Stepwise excavation of deep carious lesions in primary molars. *J Int Assoc Dent Child* 1977; **8**: 36–40.

Maltz M, de Oliveira EF, Fontanella V, Bianchi R. A clinical, microbiologic, and radiographic study of deep caries lesions after incomplete caries removal. *Quintessence Int* 2002; **33**: 151–9.

Massler M. Pulpal reactions to dental caries. *Int Dent J* 1967; **17**: 441–60.

Mertz-Fairhurst EJ, Schuster GS, Williams JE, Fairhurst CW. Clinical progress of sealed and unsealed caries. I. Depth changes and bacterial counts. *J Prosthet Dent* 1979a; **42**: 521–6.

Mertz-Fairhurst EJ, Schuster GS, Williams JE, Fairhurst CW. Clinical progess of sealed and unsealed caries. II. Standardized radiographs and clinical observations. *J Prosthet Dent* 1979b; **42**: 633–7.

Mertz-Fairhurst EJ, Schuster GS, Fairhurst CW. Arresting caries by sealants: results of a clinical study. *J Am Dent Assoc* 1986; **112**: 194–8.

Mertz-Fairhurst E, Curtis JW, Ergle JW, Rueggeberg FA. Ultraconservative and cariostatic sealed restorations: results at year 10. *J Am Dent Assoc* 1998; **129**: 55–66.

Mjör IA, Ferrari M. Pulp–dentin biology in restorative dentistry. Part 6: Reactions to restorative materials, tooth-restoration interfaces, and adhesive techniques. *Quintessence Int* 2002; **33**: 35–63.

Nyvad B, Fejerskov O. Active root-caries converted into inactive caries as a response to oral hygiene. *Scand J Dent Res* 1986; **94**: 281–4.

Nyvad B, ten Cate JM, Fejerskov O. Arrest of root surface caries *in situ*. *J Dent Res* 1997; **76**: 1845–53.

Ogawa K, Yamashita Y, Ischijo T, Fusayama T. The ultrastructure and hardness of the transparent layer of human carious dentin. *J Dent Res* 1983; **62**: 7–10.

Paddick JS, Brailsford SR, Kidd EAM, Beighton D. Phenotypic and genotypic selection of microbiota surviving under dental restorations. *Appl Environ Microbiol* 2005; **71**: 2467–72.

Prader F. Conservative treatment of the floor of the carious cavity – carious dentine near the pulp. *Int Dent J* 1958; **8**: 627–38.

Reeves R, Stanley HR. The relationship of bacterial penetration and pulpal pathosis in carious teeth. *Oral Surg* 1966; **22**: 59–65.

Ribeiro CCC, Baratieri LN, Perdigao J, Baratieri NMM, Ritter AV. A clinical, radiographic, and scanning electron microscope evaluation of adhesive restorations on carious dentin in primary teeth. *Quintessence Int* 1999; **30**: 591–9.

Ricketts DNJ, Kidd EAM, Innes N, Clarkson J. Complete or ultraconservative removal of decayed tissue in unfilled teeth. *Cochrane Database of Systematic Reviews* 2006 (Issue 3). Art. No. CD003808. DOI 10.1002/14651858. pub. 2.

Schouboe T, MacDonald JB. Prolonged viability of organisms sealed in dentinal caries. *Arch Oral Biol* 1962; **7**: 525–6.

Shovelton DS. A study of deep carious dentin. *Int Dent J* 1968; **18**: 392–405.

Silverstone LM, Hicks MJ. The struture and ultrastructure of the carious lesions lesions in human dentin. *Gerodontics* 1985; **1**: 185–93.

Tagami J, Hosoda H, Burrow MF, Nakajima M. Effect of ageing and caries in dentin permeability. *Proc Finn Dent Soc* 1992; **88** (Suppl 1): 149–54.

Weerheijm KL, de Soet JJ, van Amerongen WE, de Graaf J. Sealing of occlusal caries lesions: an alternative for curative treatment? *J Dent Child* 1992; **59**: 263–8.

Weerheijm KL, de Soet JJ, van Amerongen WE, de Graaff J. The effect of glass ionomer cement on carious dentin. *Caries Res* 1993; **27**: 417–23.

Weerheijm KL, Kreulen CM, de Soet JJ, Grown HJ, van Amerongen WE. Bacterial counts in carious dentin under restorations; 2 year *in vivo* effects. *Caries Res* 1999; **33**: 130–4.

Yip HK, Stevenson AG, Beeley JA. The specificity of caries detector dyes in cavity preparation. *Br Dent J* 1994; **176**: 417–21.

22

Restoring the tooth: 'the seal is the deal'

J.P. van Amerongen, W.E. van Amerongen, T.F. Watson,
N.J.M. Opdam, F.J.M. Roeters, D. Bittermann and E.A.M. Kidd

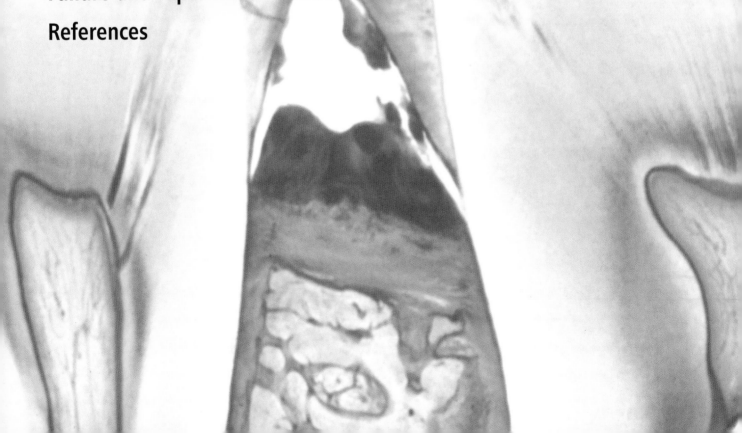

Introduction

From the preceding chapters it is clear that invasive (i.e. surgical or restorative) intervention should be avoided for as long as possible. An important reason is that non-operative treatment can result in arrest of lesions. Not only early carious lesions can be treated in this way: cavitated lesions, especially those occurring in smooth, free surfaces can be arrested by non-invasive procedures (Figs 20.2c and 22.1). This preserves the surrounding hard tissues. Another reason to postpone restorative intervention is that the decision to restore a tooth is the start of a restorative cycle in which restorations will be replaced several times, especially when the clinical work is poor (Elderton, 1990), finally resulting in serious destruction of the dental hard tissues (Fig. 22.2). This may ultimately lead to extraction (Lutz *et al.*, 1998) because every time the dentist takes the bur it is almost inevitable that sound tooth substance is cut away next to the carious lesion. This is particularly easy to do with ultraspeed rotary equipment. Research has shown every replacement of an amalgam restoration will increase the width of the cavity (Elderton, 1977). Tooth-colored adhesive restorations are much more difficult to remove than amalgam without sacrificing sound tooth structure. There are two reasons for this: the filling looks like the tooth, especially when covered with water from the high-speed handpiece, and because the filling is adhesive it cannot be pushed away from the cavity margin. After a number of repeat restorations, the dentist simply runs out of occlusal surface. During the preparation of proximal surfaces, iatrogenic damage will occur in the neighboring surface almost every time, in spite of very careful operating procedures (Lussi & Gygax, 1998; Lenters *et al.*, 2006). For these reasons, the dentist should be careful in making decisions regarding restorative intervention. Watchful waiting and non-operative treatment should always be the first options.

Unfortunately, however, the general practitioner is confronted daily with cavities that cannot be treated just by non-operative measures, e.g. occlusal or proximal cavities where it is impossible to facilitate effective biofilm removal. The cavity needs to be filled up and recontoured first to facilitate plaque control. Other conditions indicative for restorative treatment were given in Chapter 20.

As early as 1908, G.V. Black published a classification for caries related to its position on the tooth. Subsequently, the same classification was and is used to point out the location of the preparation (Black, 1908). The classification is:

- class 1: lesions beginning in pits and fissures in any part of the teeth in which these occur
- class 2: lesions beginning in the proximal surfaces of the bicuspids and molars
- class 3: lesions beginning in the proximal surfaces of the incisors and cuspids, which do not require the removal and restoration of the incisal angle
- class 4: lesions beginning in the proximal surfaces of the incisors, which require the removal and restoration of the incisal angle
- class 5: lesions beginning in the gingival third – not pit or fissure related – of the labial, buccal or lingual surfaces of the teeth.

The principles for cavity preparation have changed since the 1970s. The emphasis now is on making preparations as small as possible and the principle 'extension for prevention' as postulated by Black is rarely applied as a routine action. Extension for prevention meant the placing of cavity margins at points, or along lines, that would be cleaned by the excursions of food in chewing. The aim was to prevent the recurrence of decay at the margins of fillings by positioning the margins to obtain this cleaning effect.

Now it is known that extension of the cavity will not invariably prevent the development of recurrent caries and indeed it turns out that the longevity of a tooth is better when a preparation is kept small (Walls *et al.*, 1988). This

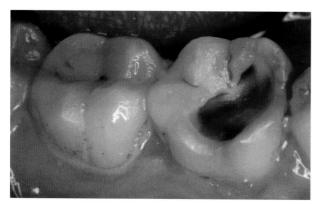

Figure 22.1 Arrested occlusal lesion.

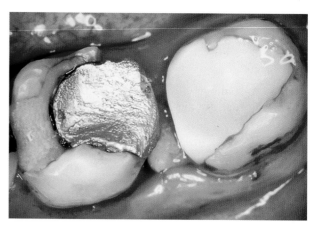

Figure 22.2 Iatrogenic damage caused by repeated treatment procedures. These are poor restorations and this makes it likely that a new dentist will wish to replace them.

knowledge has led to a more conservative approach during cavity preparation. The outline will be determined by the location and the extent of the carious process rather than the old adages as described by our famous ancestors. There is now no such thing as a 'standard preparation'.

The 'extension for prevention' principle has largely been abandoned, and stereotyped outlines should be avoided. The contemporary approach is to remove the appropriate amount of demineralized tissue and then design what is left to receive the appropriate restorative material.

This has some important implications for the preclinical teaching of operative dentistry. It is obvious that this must precede work on patients, but it needs to be carried out on natural carious and filled teeth. Caries-free, or worse still, plastic counterfeits will not do because the student can only prepare a stereotyped outline on these and that is the exact opposite of contemporary teaching. In addition, developments with dental simulations using virtual reality do not yet include natural carious teeth and are therefore inevitably stereotyped preparations.

These days, adhesive restorative materials have allowed dentists to make smaller preparations, leading to the preservation of hard dental tissues. The adhesive materials may also support tooth tissue undermined by demineralization. These materials are usually tooth-colored so that satisfying aesthetic results can be achieved.

To obtain a functional, aesthetic and durable restoration it is necessary to design a proper cavity form, taking into account pulpo-dentinal biology, and to choose the right dental filling material. To fulfill these requirements the restorative procedure should facilitate a very close contact between filling and tooth: 'the seal is the deal'. This sealed tooth is cleanable and protects the dentin–pulp complex.

From the preceding chapters and this paragraph it can be concluded that the following principles have to be considered before taking a bur and starting an operative procedure.

Principles

- diagnosis of pulp state, preoperative
- avoidance of damage to sound tooth structure
- cleanability of the restoration
- restorations, preferably with adhesive materials (from a cariological point of view), which:
  - seal the cavity (so that the pulp is protected and cariogenic organisms die)
  - support and strengthen weakened tissue
  - aid retention
  - other considerations concerning the material such as appearance, toxicity, strength, wear, handling characteristics and radiopacity (for caries diagnosis).

Before describing restorative procedures for different caries classifications, an extended section on adhesive filling materials is presented below. Other principles are not fur-

ther discussed here because they are described above or in several other places in this book.

Materials

Minimally invasive dentistry and the materials to support this concept have become a major driver for the manufacturers of dental materials. Both cariology and materials science have contributed to a new form of dentistry. Materials have been developed and can now be used in ways that may, at first sight, seem imprecise and careless in their application to the management of a complex disease process, preserving as much tooth structure as possible. The role of operative treatment is to restore the tooth after damage due to disease or trauma. The goal of the treatment for tissue damage due to caries is to encourage recovery of the pulp–dentin complex, perhaps by sealing the cavity, and also to restore the tooth's functional anatomy with tough materials that can be kept clean and plaque free by the patient.

Requirements for a satisfactory material are no longer just high strength and low wear, but a complex set of inter-related properties dominated by biocompatibility and aesthetics. Appropriate mechanical characteristics are still required but, thanks to the use of adhesive techniques, restorations can be integrated with the remaining tooth structure. This should contribute significantly to the longevity of the restored tooth. The introduction of bonding made possible great achievements in the restoration of teeth. In addition to the benefits of adhesive techniques, the impact of aesthetics has been considerable, with new materials able to mimic the optical characteristics of the tooth. The patient is increasingly aware of such possibilities, often demanding aesthetic restorations.

Patients are now also aware of the potential adverse effects of dental materials on the environment and health. In this respect it is strange that patients tend to have more distrust of the well-established and relatively uncomplicated material, silver amalgam, than the chemically complex resin-based composites. This is despite a wealth of scientific literature that disproves any serious association between health problems and the mercury-containing filling material (Leinfelder, 1991; Flanders, 1992). The widespread acceptance of resin systems is perhaps surprising since the components have been shown to affect biological reactions (Hengsten-Pettersen & Jacobsen, 1990). The demise of silver amalgam is, in fact, more likely to be due to increasing concerns regarding the safe disposal of the waste products rather than issues that may relate to its clinical usage. As a material, amalgam is quite forgiving of clinical mishandling: it is often stated by older dentists that it is less technique sensitive than resin composites. This reflects on the training of these individuals, as it is increasingly clear that newer generations of dental graduate are perfectly capable of producing adequate resin composite restorations in a wide range of clinical situations.

However, the majority of problems associated with resin-based materials are due to the material's dimensional change during its transition from the viscous into the solid state. To be more specific, a shrinking restorative material may have problems sealing the cavity against bacterial invasion and, in the case of bonding, the restrained contraction may cause mechanical stress in the restored tooth. The phenomenon of adhesion plays such a dominant role in dentistry that a short discussion on the principles is appropriate.

Adhesives

Adhesion bonds two materials in intimate contact across an interface. In physics, adhesion refers to attraction forces between particles at atomic distances. However, the term is now used to quantify the resistance of a joint between two materials against separation in a certain loading test (O'Brien, 1989; Allen, 1992; Packham, 1992). In the dental literature, the word adhesion is usually used for three different mechanisms of bonding or a combination of the three. These mechanisms are:

- chemical adhesion, which is based on primary valence forces; charged particles are exchanged between the two materials, e.g. ionic, covalent and metallic bonds
- physical adhesion, which relies on secondary valence forces; attraction forces occur at the interaction of dipoles or at the interaction of unshielded electron clouds
- mechanical adhesion, which refers to penetration of one material into the other at a microscopic level.

Adhesion in dentistry

Chemical (and physical) adhesion is the mechanism responsible for the porcelain-to-metal bonds and soldering joints. In addition, the adhesion of glass-ionomers to mineral tissues is believed to be mainly of a chemical nature. Physical adhesion is responsible for the retention of plaque and calculus and the retention of a full denture. Most of the resin systems only adhere to dental hard tissues by mechanical adhesion, a micromechanical attachment. Micropores are created in the tissue surface by acid etching after which, under certain circumstances, the monomers can penetrate into the substrate. After polymerization, the two materials are connected through the interlocking of resin-impregnated tooth enamel or dentin.

To obtain any of these forms of adhesion, a close contact between the two substances is a prerequisite. When molecular forces are involved, the distance between the surfaces has to be in the order of 1 nm ($= 10^{-9}$ m). It is almost impossible for two solid surfaces to approach each other like this for a substantial surface area. The most common way to achieve such a close contact is to bring one of the materials into the plastic–liquid state and let it flow over the second one. The liquid is now called the adhesive and the solid the substrate. The bond is achieved after solidification of the adhesive. The adhesive can also be used to fill the gap between two different substrates, as in the luting of crowns and inlays. In principle, solidification is not required to obtain such adhesion. An example is when a drop of water is applied between two plates of glass; it is now almost impossible to separate the plates in a transverse direction. Water is now the adhesive. However, the bond strength in shear loading of such a system is negligible. In practice it is essential that the adhesive will solidify.

In modern direct filling techniques, the aim is to have restorative materials with adhesive properties. This has yet to be achieved with a material that is clinically satisfactory in all respects and so a separate adhesive–restoration phase is usually implemented. To understand the various problems associated with bonding, some basic physical laws have to be defined.

Surface conditions and wetting

Surface energy comes from the greater mobility of atoms at the outer surface of a material. These surface atoms are not completely compensated in charge by neighboring atoms, as is the case in the interior of the material. The atoms at the surface are attracted to the bulk of the substance, causing a contractile force called surface tension. In the case of a liquid, the surface tension causes the formation of a drop, because a sphere requires the smallest outer surface of all possible shapes at one certain volume. Effective close contact over a wide area of the substrate by the adhesive can only proceed when certain criteria are fulfilled. First of all, the substrate should be wetted. Wetting is the degree of spread by which a drop of fluid flows over a solid surface. The measure for wetting is the contact angle. This is the angle between the drop-sphere and the plane of the substrate. If this angle is small wetting is good, whereas when the angle is more than 90° wetting of the substrate by the fluid is poor. Hydrophilic substrates can easily be wetted by water. A hydrophobic surface is hard to wet by water. Good wetting means that there is a strong attraction between the molecules of the substance and the liquid. This attraction is influenced by the surface energy.

Conditioning of the surface can affect the wettability. The contact angle of the usual Bis-GMA-TEGDMA sealants on clean tooth enamel is approximately 55°. After etching with phosphoric acid, the contact angle decreases to approximately 0°, which means that acid conditioning of tooth enamel not only creates microcrevices for mechanical retention, but also promotes the wettability of the substrate by the adhesive. Apparently, the acid etching causes polarity at the enamel surface to accept the polar monomer. In this context it is worth noting that a fluoride application decreases the polarity of the surface. Therefore, fluoride should not be applied to the substrate before application of the monomer. The acid-etched enamel surface should be protected from contamination with saliva for a similar reason.

Capillary penetration

The surface energy of a liquid creates pressure that drives the liquid into narrow crevices and thin tubes. Dependent on the surface tension of a liquid, it rises or sinks within a crevice. The degree of capillary elevation or depression is proportional to the surface energy and inversely proportional to the contact angle and the capillary radius or the width of the crevice. That is one of the reasons why plaque accumulates preferentially in fissures and at the narrowest interdental sites. If the supply of liquid is limited, negative pressure cannot be balanced by capillary rise and the liquid will exert contractile stress on the walls of the tube or the crevice. This is the mechanism responsible for the clinging together of two wet, flat glass plates. The retention of a complete denture relies partly on the contractile pressure of saliva between the denture and the mucosa.

Whether a fluid can infiltrate pores or crevices also depends on its viscosity. The viscosity or internal friction of a fluid is defined as the ratio between the shearing stress and the rate of shear. For optimal infiltration of conditioned enamel or dentin, the adhesive should be of low viscosity and exhibit high surface tension and good wettability. The surface tension of the substrate should be superior to that of the adhesive. The viscosity is determined by the interaction of the molecules with each other as well as their size. Moreover, viscosity is temperature dependent.

Dimensional stability

If the molecules of a certain monomer system are small, penetration into the substrate will be promoted. However, this will bring about greater setting shrinkage than larger sized monomer molecules. If the adhesive is not dimensionally stable during setting and not dimensionally compatible with the substrate during thermal or mechanical loading, the stresses at the interface may damage the joint. The nature of failure can be adhesive, cohesive or a combination of the two. Proper adhesion is said to be achieved when the joint is stronger than the cohesive strength of either material alone. The nature of failure may also be dependent on anomalous stress distributions inherent in the mode of loading. Dependent on the way of conditioning and the properties of the adhesive, bonding to tooth structure can be obtained by:

- chemical bonding to the inorganic and organic components of the tissue
- penetration of low-viscosity materials into microcrevices and pores of the substrate and subsequent solidification to form an interdiffusion or hybrid zone with the tissue.

Hydrophilic resins

A low molecular weight hydrophilic resin (e.g. hydroxyethyl methacrylate: HEMA), in a suitable solvent (e.g. water, alcohol, acetone), will flow into the dentinal tubules and the porous intertubular dentin between them. The type of solvent in use is critical for the method of handling the bonding agent.

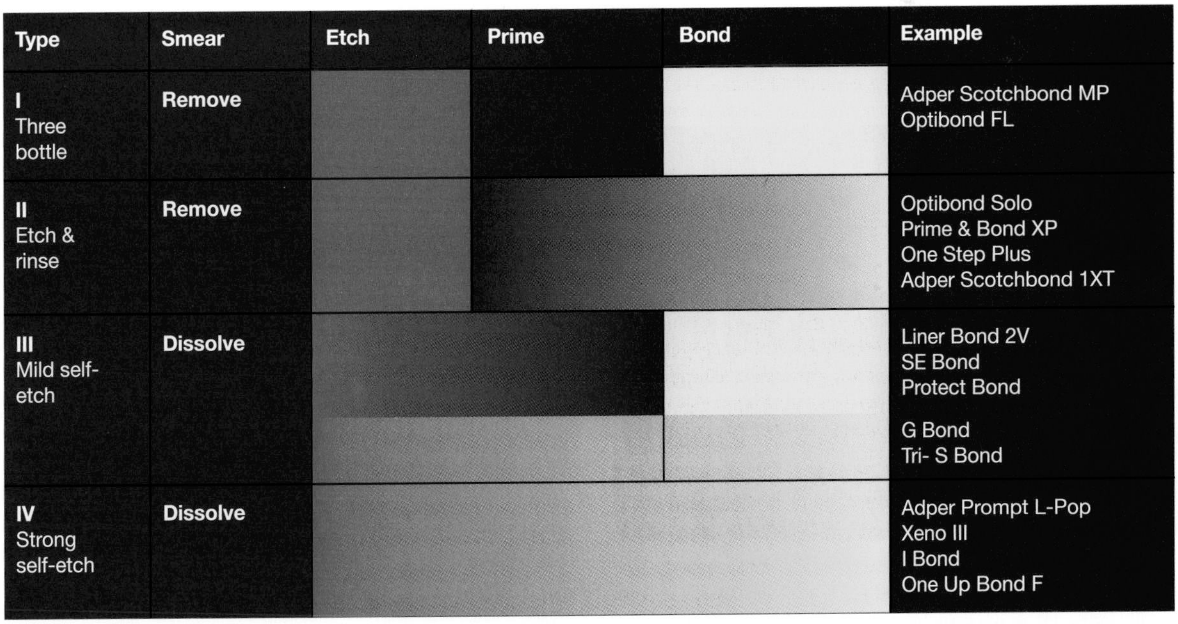

Type	Smear	Etch	Prime	Bond	Example
I Three bottle	Remove				Adper Scotchbond MP Optibond FL
II Etch & rinse	Remove				Optibond Solo Prime & Bond XP One Step Plus Adper Scotchbond 1XT
III Mild self-etch	Dissolve				Liner Bond 2V SE Bond Protect Bond
					G Bond Tri- S Bond
IV Strong self-etch	Dissolve				Adper Prompt L-Pop Xeno III I Bond One Up Bond F

Figure 22.3 Classification of dentin bonding agents based on mechanism of action and number of bottles/stages (One Step Plus: Bisco Corporation Schaumburg, IL, USA; Prime & Bond XP, Xeno III: Dentsply De Trey, Konstanz, Germany; Adper Scotchbond, MP, 1XT, Prompt L-Pop: 3M ESPE, St Paul, Minnesota, USA; Fuji Bond LC: G Bond GC Corporation, Itabashi-ku, Tokyo, Japan; I Bond: Heraeus-Kulzer, Hanau, Germany; Optibond FL: Kerr Corporation, Orange, CA, USA; Liner Bond 2V, SE Bond, Protect Bond; Tri S Bond: Kuraray Dental, Chiyoda-ku, Tokyo, Japan; One Up Bond F Plus: Tokuyama Dental Corporation, Tsukuba, Japan).

Classifications of adhesives

There have been many different classifications of dentin bonding agents: based on when they were introduced ('generations'), how many stages, how many bottles, etc. (Van Meerbeek *et al.*, 2003). Figure 22.3 gives a good summary of the different types currently available.

Bonding to enamel

Enamel is a substrate that can be dried relatively easily, and the use of hydrophobic resins such as conventional fissure sealants dictates such an approach, even though vigorous postetch drying for 10–20 s will cause collapse of the exposed hydroxyapatite crystals. In this way, the ideal enamel etch pattern would show clinically as a 'frosty' appearance awaiting these resin intermediaries. Many bonding systems are now designed to work in a moist environment using hydrophilic (water-liking) resins dissolved in water miscible solvents: these displace the water from the tooth surface. When using these materials profound drying of the tooth is contraindicated.

Bonding to dentin

Although it is possible to dry out dentin after etching, in the same way as enamel, the net result may prevent satisfactory resin penetration for some of the bonding agents in use. This is because the drying causes the fragile, exposed collagen network to collapse and the resin cannot penetrate this collapsed structure.

The main problem with dentin bonding is that a hydrophobic resin composite is required to stick to a 'watery' substrate. Resin technology has now developed such that it is possible to produce a bonding agent in a solvent that will infiltrate and stick to wet dentin (Fig. 22.4) and maintain the bond over a significant period.

Bonding to wet dentin (and enamel)

Most dentin bonding agents require smear layer removal with weak acids. This smeared structure is a layer of disaggregated tissue impacted into the surface of the tooth by the action of any mechanical preparation technique. There are two common ways of achieving smear layer removal. The more established systems use a separate etch stage with phosphoric acid followed by the bonding agent, while others combine acid and the bonding agent and are therefore called 'self-etching'.

Separate etching stage

The smear layer is removed with acid (Fig. 22.5) and then the bonding agent is applied. The type I adhesives use alcohol and water as the solvent base for the hydrophilic resin primer; these materials will be capable of rewetting a dried collagen surface, although their penetration time into the substrate may be slightly longer than for the more volatile solvent bases such as acetone. A second layer of more hydrophobic resin is then applied and polymerized.

In the type II adhesives, all the adhesive components are included in one bottle, normally with a solvent such as acetone, and are applied as multiple layers. The acetone will mix freely with water and therefore requires a moist tooth surface for thorough dentin penetration in the technique described as 'wet bonding'. This means that the tooth surface should not be dried out too much as this will cause collapse of the exposed collagen network, and enamel crystallites, with grossly inadequate penetration of the bonding agent. Judging the correct degree of wetness in these situations is a problem. Some suggest that surplus water should

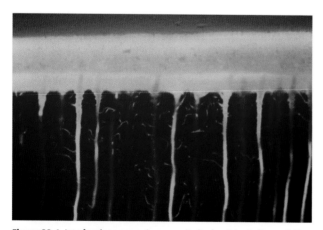

Figure 22.4 Interface between resin composite (top) and dentin (bottom). Type II adhesive has been labeled with rhodamine B dye and imaged using a confocal microscope. Dark band at top is composite. Orange band with fillers present is the air-inhibited layer between the composite and the adhesive. Yellow band immediately above the dentin is the hybrid zone of resin infiltration. Resin tags are very prominent within the dentin tubules and these can also be seen within the lateral branches. Field width 100 μm.

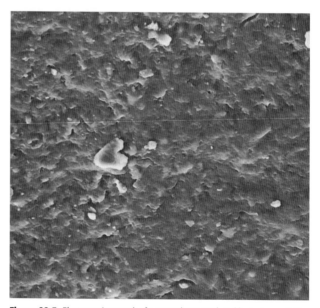

Figure 22.5 Electron micrograph of a smear layer produced by instrumentation with an excavator of the dentin surface. The way in which the smear layer is managed is still a contentious issue in the development and handling of adhesive materials. Resin replica of dentin surface, field width 100 μm.

be removed by the use of a cotton-wool pledget. For these materials, the desiccating effect of an air blast and the frosted appearance of etched enamel should be avoided.

Having acted as a good wetting agent on the dentin and enamel, multiple coats of adhesive are applied and the relative stiffness of the resin component is increased by evaporation of solvent; this solvent evaporation is most often overlooked by practioners (Jacobsen *et al.*, 2003). The region between the unaffected dentin and the restoration is a mixture of both and so is called the hybrid zone (Fig. 22.4). Another name for it is the interdiffusion zone, which also indicates the 5–10 μm penetration of the resins into the intertubular dentin.

Self-etching adhesives

A problem with bonding agents that have a separate etching stage is that successful bonds will only be achieved if the adhesive resin penetrates to the depth of demineralization caused by the acid etching. If this fails to occur then nanoleakage or micropermeability will develop in the interface and expose the resin to more rapid hydrolytic breakdown. Materials that use a self-etching combination are less likely to suffer from this problem because the two components are already combined (Fig. 22.3). They will also not require a separate washing and drying stage before the application of the bonding agent, so helping to reduce the risk of contamination. Self-etching adhesives would therefore appear to offer the ideal solution of simple handling and technique insensitivity, giving excellent dentin bonds. However, the evidence for successful enamel bonding with these materials has been less convincing. These materials may be applied as two separate stages or alternatively as one component (Fig. 22.3).

The materials applied in two stages (type III adhesives), have well-recognized advantages for bonding to dentin, but the materials that combine all of the components (type IV) may be more at risk of hydrolytic breakdown because of the presence of residual water in the adhesive at polymerization and problems of residual adhesive acidity affecting overlying composite polymerization (Tay & Pashley, 2003). Placement of an intermediate layer of resin is of some help in reducing these problems, but one has then returned to the type III format. It is evident that the type IV adhesives are currently separating into two subgroups: those with a very low pH and those that are less aggressive in their etching rate.

Bonding to carious dentin with resin-based materials

Carious dentin consists of two layers: the outer layer, consisting of highly infected and demineralized dentin, and the inner layer, which may not be infected, but shows a degree of demineralization (see Chapter 21). This is due to the action of the acids produced by the metabolic activity of the bacteria located in the outer layer, and this layer has the potential to be remineralized (Fusayama, 1979). In clinical situations, the bonding surface most frequently encoun-

tered after thorough caries excavation consists of caries-affected dentin (Harnirattisai *et al.*, 1992). Thus, adequate bonding to caries-affected dentin may contribute to the longevity of the restoration.

The type of dentin may have an effect on the bond strength of any dental adhesive (Nakajima *et al.*, 1999a, b, 2000; Arrais *et al.*, 2004). Laboratory testing by the Knoop-hardness method shows that the hardness of caries-affected dentin is about half that of normal dentin (Marshall *et al.*, 1997, Nakajima *et al.*, 1995, 1999a, b, 2000; Ceballos *et al.*, 2003), measured in the laboratory. Caries-affected dentin is also more porous than normal dentin. The weakest link in the resin-caries-affected dentin assembly may be the cohesive strength of caries-affected dentin (Tagami *et al.*, 1992, Yoshiyama *et al.*, 2000a; Sonoda *et al.*, 2005). However, this soft nature allows deeper penetration of the monomers, and allows the establishment of a thicker hybrid layer (Nakajima *et al.*, 1995, 1999a, b, 2000; Marshall *et al.*, 1997; Ceballos *et al.*, 2003). It has, however, been shown that the thickness of the hybrid layer is unrelated to the bond strength measured in the laboratory (Nakajima *et al.*, 1995, 1999a, b, 2000; Marshall *et al.*, 1997; Ceballos *et al.*, 2003). Caries-affected dentin contains dentinal tubules that are filled with acid-resistant B-octocalciumphosphate (whitlockite) minerals (Ogawa *et al.*, 1983; Harnirattisai *et al.*, 1992; Versluis *et al.*, 1997; Cardoso *et al.*, 1998; Montes *et al.*, 2001; Arrais *et al.*, 2004) that interfere with the infiltration of adhesive resins and the formation of resin tags (Harnirattisai *et al.*, 1992; Finger *et al.*, 1994). This may explain why most of the studies on bonding to carious dentin show lower bond strengths to caries-affected dentin than to normal dentin (Nakajima *et al.*, 1995, 1999a, b; Yoshiyama *et al.*, 2000a, b, 2002; Arrais *et al.*, 2004).

Another important factor that contributes to the bond strength to caries-affected dentin is the type of adhesive system used (Yoshiyama *et al.*, 2000b, 2002). Nakajima (1999b) indicated that the benefit of moist bonding over dry bonding extended to caries-affected dentin. Furthermore, the total-etch type I and II adhesives tended to produce higher bond strength values than the type III self-etch adhesives (Yoshiyama *et al.*, 2000a; Inoue *et al.*, 2001; Ceballos *et al.*, 2003). The application of 32–37% phosphoric acid in total-etch adhesives (types I and II) seems to solubilize the intratubular mineral deposits in caries-affected dentin (Nakajima *et al.*, 1999a, 2000; Yoshiyama *et al.*, 2000b) better than weaker acids in self-etch adhesives, thereby contributing to better resin retention (Pashley & Carvalho, 1997). Arrais *et al.* (2004) claimed that additional, extended, acid etching could increase dentinal permeability of the caries-affected dentin by partial removal of intratubular deposits, thus improving the bond strength. However, unless there is an excellent tubular seal, this may make the tubules more permeable to fluid exudate which may, in turn, act as a substrate for the remaining bacteria.

Alternative caries excavation techniques may lead to differences in the quality and quantity of dentin remaining and of the smear layer remaining after cavity preparation. These differences may be clinically significant when considering the surface bonding with many adhesive restorative materials (Banerjee *et al.*, 2000). Sonoda *et al.* (2005) indicated that remnants of carious dentin after conventional hand excavation would no doubt contain a caries-infected smear, which may affect bonding, especially with the type III self-etch systems. Moreover, the smear layer formed on caries-affected dentin includes acid-resistant crystals that may hamper the diffusion of the self-etching primer into the underlying intact dentin (Yoshiyama *et al.*, 2000b). With the use of Carisolv™ gel (containing sodium hypochlorite and three amino acids – lysine, leucine and glutamic acid – together with carboxymethylcellulose), as an alternative method to prepare the cavity, it may be possible to achieve the same bond strengths to normal and caries-affected dentin, using the total-etch or self-etching technique. The effect of Carisolv on reducing the smear layer may be a factor influencing the bond strengths to caries-affected dentin. In contrast to the relative homogeneous topography of the smear layer's surface after rotary preparation, caries removal with Carisolv gel shows a more rough, irregular surface with some open tubules, which may improve bonding between the restoration and the tooth (Wennerberg *et al.*, 1999; Banerjee *et al.*, 2000; Fure *et al.*, 2000, Sonoda *et al.*, 2005). In contrast, Cehreli *et al.* (2003) claimed that the use of Carisolv does not improve the bonding to caries-affected dentin compared with other more traditional caries-removal methods.

It should be noted that the clinical relevance of bond strength is unknown. Since most carious cavities are undercut once prepared, the bond may be more relevant to cavity seal than retention of the restoration. Furthermore, there seems to be no information on the possibility of bonding to heavily infected, wet, soft dentin, as discussed in Chapter 21.

Restorative materials

New products are often launched on the market before relevant research findings are published and much of this research is laboratory based rather than using randomized controlled clinical trials. Both scientists and practitioners are confused about new nomenclature, compositions, properties, clinical performance and biocompatibility. The current materials for direct restorations can be summarized in three categories: amalgam, resin-based composites and glass-ionomers. They are similar in that they can set from a viscous into a non-homogeneous solid state of harder particles embedded in a softer matrix. However, they differ substantially in their properties. For this reason appropriate understanding of the composition and properties of materials is required to select and handle them appropriately.

Amalgam

Amalgam is an alloy of mercury with one or more other metals. Dental amalgam is made by mixing mercury with a powdered silver and tin alloy. There may be additions of copper, zinc, palladium, indium and selenium to the alloy. The powder particles can be composed of irregular filings, spherical particles or a combination of both types. The spherical particles are easier to wet and therefore require less mercury to form a consistent mix. The fresh mix has a plasticity that permits it to be conveniently packed into a tooth cavity. A correct mix, resulting in a shiny and coherent sample, will optimize the working time and coherence between the subsequent layers. This reduces the number of voids inside the filling. During condensation, excess mercury has to be squeezed out. It is more difficult to condense 'spherical amalgam' because the smooth, slippery spherical particles offer little frictional resistance.

As a result of chemical reactions, the plastic mass hardens into a strong, but brittle material. This reaction is fast initially, but may last for several hours and days until it reaches the equilibrium of partly reacted original particles, embedded in two newly formed solid-state phases, one of silver–tin (gamma-1) and one of mercury–tin (gamma-2). The surface layer of the alloy powder reacts with mercury, whereas the alloy core remains intact. The alloy core exists as filler in the amalgam matrix.

Amalgam was introduced in dentistry in 1835 and was not essentially altered until the late 1960s, when the high-copper alloys were introduced. Here, the copper content is around 10–30 wt%. From both *in vitro* and *in vivo* tests it became clear that an increased copper content resulted in an increased resistance to corrosion and an improvement in certain mechanical properties. The copper prevents the formation of the mercury–tin phase. This phase (gamma-2) is the weakest and most corrosive phase in the amalgam. By reducing this corrosion-prone component, marginal degradation is less frequent and the black tattooing of the adjacent tissue by tin is less apparent. For many years sealing of the dentin tubules with a varnish was recommended to reduce marginal leakage and discoloration. Amalgam does not adhere to tooth structure. The amalgam restoration is retained by macromechanical devices, such as undercuts, which may have to be prepared at the cost of sound tooth structure.

The bonding of an amalgam mix to the cavity walls with tooth structure impregnating resins was introduced recently. The bonding of amalgam improves the marginal adaptation and reduces the marginal leakage (Torii *et al.*, 1989). The fracture resistance of teeth restored with amalgam-bonded mesio-occlusal-distal (MOD) restorations was more than twice that of those containing unbonded amalgams (Eakle *et al.*, 1992). During hardening, amalgam shows a volume contraction of a maximum 0.2%, which is far less than that of resin-based composites. After some time the material expands to some extent and corrosion products may also seal these margins.

Amalgam is considered to be the least technique sensitive of all permanent restorative materials (Leinfelder, 1991; Craig, 1997). Restorations with satisfactory mechanical properties can be provided under a wide range of operating conditions and variation in the skill levels of clinicians.

Resin-based composites

Not long after synthetic polymers were introduced for industrial use, the first efforts were made to find dental applications for these easy-to-process and inexpensive materials, which are generally made to adhere to tooth structure via micromechanical retention (see above). The main disadvantage is that their setting (see above) is accompanied by considerable shrinkage. Much work is currently underway to develop composites with low shrinkage (Weinmann et al., 2005), but these materials often present challenges in other ways with respect to their bonding to tooth tissue.

Substantial improvements in reducing the curing contraction and increasing mechanical properties have been achieved in modern resin-based composites. Composites are compound materials, which consist of two or more different materials (i.e. resin plus filler) with greatly diverging properties (mechanical, physical, chemical or biological) and excellent coherence. A composite unites the properties of the combined materials. Bone and dentin are examples of a composite, where ultrafine crystallites of inorganic hydroxyapatite, $Ca_{10}(PO_4)_6.2H_2O$, surround the organic material, collagen, to form a coherent, strong material. Taken individually, the components would be unsuitable for the function of bone or dentin; isolated fine crystals would lack coherence, while the collagen (without the crystals) would act as a rubbery material. Concrete is another example of a composite, consisting of three different materials, namely gravel, sand and cement, coherently bound together into a very strong construction material. Structurally, dental composites resemble concrete. Like concrete, the surface of a dental composite roughens with time owing to erosion of the resin matrix, which is substantially softer than the filler component. Only when the filler particle size is below 0.5 μm can the surface be polished and then remain so smooth that light (wavelength 0.4–0.8 μm) will be reflected and the surface appear glossy. It is hard for a manufacturer to mix the finely powdered filler component into the viscous resin. For this reason, the first generation dental composites, called conventional composites, had relatively large filler particles (~20 μm) of glass or quartz. To obtain radiopacity, heavy metals, such as zinc, barium, strontium or yttrium, are incorporated into the glass. However, 20 μm is the average diameter of human hair, and this can be seen with the naked eye, making it unacceptable as a dental filling material. To obtain smooth-surface composites, colloidal silica (0.04 μm) was mixed in

the resin and the polymerized material milled into small particles (10–50 μm). These prepolymerized particles were mixed with low-filled monomer and this mix was supplied to the clinician. These 'microfill' composites are easily polished, but suffer from inferior mechanical properties because of the relatively high resin content. Subsequently, mixtures of coarse filler particles with a matrix of microfilled resin were developed and called hybrid composites. Nowadays, industry is able to manufacture highly filled (hybrid) composites, where the 'coarse' filler particle size is below 0.5 μm: the submicron hybrids.

To obtain a real composite, the filler particles have to be bound to the matrix. This is usually achieved by coating the inorganic filler particles with a thin film of vinyl-silane, to obtain a chemical bond between the two components. Thus, a resin-based dental composite contains at least three components. In contrast to amalgam and glass-ionomers, the silanized filler particles in resin-based composites do not take part in the reaction process. It should also be understood that the silane coupling is hydrolyzable and therefore the material may degrade.

Modern composites are strong and stable materials, with stiffness values similar to tooth structure. Unfortunately, their curing is still accompanied by shrinkage. This affects the marginal integrity of the restoration because the material will potentially pull away from the cavity wall as it sets. The polymerization stress in the adhesive restoration is proportional to the polymerization shrinkage and to the stiffness (module) of the material. However, these materials are adhesively bonded to the cavity walls. Unfortunately, contractile forces exceed the bond strength of the dental adhesives. Shrinkage stress-compensating flow is only possible from free, unbound surfaces. Therefore, the stress in adhesive restorations is also dependent on the configuration of the restoration. The configuration factor (C) is defined as the ratio between the bound and unbound surfaces of the restoration (Davidson, 1986; Feilzer et al., 1987). For unrestrained contraction, the configuration factor is low for class IV and high for class I, II, III and occasionally, class V restorations. Porosity may also contribute to stress relief by flow: the interstices of the bubbles effectively increase the free surface area of the porous material. To offset the high polymerization stresses in the rigid hybrid composite restorations, linings or bases of more flexible materials, such as the lightly filled 'flowable' composites or glass-ionomers, have been proposed (McLean et al., 1985; Davidson et al., 1991).

In the late 1970s and early 1980s photo-polymerizable resin-based composites were introduced. These materials succeeded because of their advantages in handling and storage. Yet, this apparently simple technique created new pitfalls. In deep cavities, it has to be remembered that light-cured materials can only be completely polymerized in thin increments (1.5–2 mm). The tip of the polymerization unit has to be placed as close to the restorative material as possible to obtain a sufficient light intensity for the initial setting process. In some areas of the mouth it is difficult to gain this access for light polymerization. In addition, the sudden stiffening of the light-curing composite brings about a sudden polymerization stress, which usually is more harmful to the marginal integrity than the slowly developing stress in autocuring composites (Davidson-Kaban *et al.*, 1997).

Glass-ionomers

The first glass-ionomer cement was developed by Wilson and Kent (1972). The setting reaction of the conventional glass-ionomers starts when an acid-soluble glass powder and an aqueous solution of a poly-acid are brought into contact with each other, producing an acid–base reaction. The powdered fluoro-alumino-silicate glass works as the base.

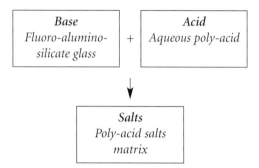

The acid attack of the glass particles releases calcium, strontium and aluminum ions. The metal ions combined with the carboxylic acid groups of the poly-acid (usually a poly-carboxylic acid) form the poly-acid salts matrix, while the glass surface is initially changed into a silica hydrogel structure (Matsuya *et al.*, 1996). Although the aluminum ion in the aluminum oxide does not react with acid, it does react when present in the silicate glass. When these materials are presented to the dentist, the poly-acid is either part of the liquid as an aqueous solution or incorporated into the cement powder as a freeze-dried powder. In the latter case, the liquid is simply water in which the freeze-dried poly-acid dissolves on mixing. The set cement is an organic–inorganic complex with high molecular weight. Glass-ionomer cements are also defined as a polyalkenoate; however, the term glass-ionomer cement has been more widely accepted by the dental professionals, and describes this kind of cement accurately. Thanks to the presence of poly-acids, the glass-ionomer cement has the ability to adhere under wet conditions to tooth structures or metals without a special substrate treatment (Akinmade & Nicholson, 1993). The mechanism of adhesion to the tooth structure and to metal has not been elucidated completely, but it is thought that the reaction of the carboxyl group in the acid with the calcium ions in the apatite is of prime importance. There is still the possibility that a chelating

linkage exists, since glass-ionomer cements can adhere to metal. Like the resin-based composites, glass-ionomers also shrink during their setting process. However, the accompanying stress is less destructive, because the gradual reaction leads initially to a rubbery material (Davidson, 1991). In addition, the intrinsic porosity allows more stress-relieving flow and there is a compensating uptake of water from the tooth tissue that allows immediate swelling to occur (Watson *et al.*, 1998).

The glass was developed on the basis of the already existing dental silicate cements, and is prepared by melting Al_2O_3, SiO_2, metal oxides, metal fluorides and metal phosphates at high temperatures (Saito *et al.*, 1999). The surface layer of the glass powder reacts with acid, whereas the glass core remains intact. The glass core exists as filler in the cement matrix. The reactivity of the glass surface controls the nature of the set cement. However, the intersurface condition in glass-ionomer cement is different from the inner surface of fillers in a resin composite. This silica gel layer matures over a period of weeks or even months. In any state of the reaction and also in the setting process, all of these materials are sensitive to dehydration, but also to water uptake. The freshly set material would be adversely affected if it dried out, but the surface is also weakened by getting wet. This means that the dentist must take great care that the freshly set material is neither contaminated with water nor allowed to dry out.

The compressive strength of glass-ionomer cement is known to increase over 1 year. Newer generations of glass-ionomers have a faster setting process, resulting in reduced moisture sensitivity at the critical initial reaction period. In the search for greater strength, the formulation of conventional glass-ionomers has been, and is still being, modified. Efforts have been made to improve the properties of conventional glass-ionomer cements by mixing metal alloy powder with the glass-ionomer powder. Commercial examples are Miracle mix (Simmons, 1990), where amalgam alloy is mixed with the glass powder, and Cermet (ceramic and metal), where silver particles are fused to the glass powder (McLean & Gasser, 1985). These materials are also called metal-modified glass-ionomer cements: they have mainly been superseded by tooth-colored, high-viscosity glass-ionomers with equivalent or better mechanical properties. Another option to improve the initial strength of glass-ionomers is to apply gentle heat via a composite curing lamp or to use ultrasonic instruments to impart energy to the immature, unset cement, so accelerating the chemical reaction (Towler *et al.*, 2001).

A potential advantage of conventional glass-ionomers is that they release fluoride. Laboratory studies encouraged the belief that this fluoride would make the development of recurrent caries less likely (Hicks *et al.*, 1986; Swift, 1989; Forss & Seppa, 1990; Svanberg *et al.*, 1990; Tyas, 1991; ten Cate & Van Duinen, 1995; Williams, *et al.*, 1996; Nagamine *et al*, 1997). However, there is contradiction in the literature (Tyas, 1991; Mount, 1999; Mjör & Toffenetti, 2000) on the clinical reality of the laboratory promise. Dentists replace as many glass-ionomer restorations with composites because they diagnose recurrent caries, although the reason the dentist selected the material in the first place is not known. Glass-ionomer may have been selected for patients considered at high risk for caries. To serve those dentists who have problems deciding between composite and glass-ionomer, a real hybrid restorative material was introduced. Here, the industry has tried to combine the properties of resin-based composites and conventional glass-ionomers into one, the light-curing glass-ionomer.

Resin-modified glass-ionomer cements

Light-curable glass-ionomers were developed with the aim of combining the advantages of immediate light curing with some of the properties of conventional glass-ionomer cements. They can be described as hybrid ionomers or resin-modified glass-ionomers. The setting reaction of resin-modified glass-ionomers should have a light-curing mechanism in addition to the acid–base reaction of the glass-ionomer part. The slow acid–base reaction allows the bulk of the cement to mature, to obtain the final strength, while the initial setting is by the light-mediated polymerization of methacrylate monomers (Anstice & Nicholson, 1995).

Some of the mechanical properties of the resin-modified glass-ionomers, such as flexural strength, have been improved by the addition of polymerizable monomers. The fluoride release rate of these materials is in the same order as conventional glass-ionomers. Owing to the usefulness of light polymerization, many dentists changed from conventional to resin-modified glass-ionomers. These materials became quite popular and are still widely used as lining materials under a composite restoration in some countries (notably the USA). Besides the ease of handling, a possible advantage over conventional glass-ionomer cements is their reduced susceptibility to crazing and cracking as a result of desiccation. However, the hydrophilic nature of the incorporated monomer (HEMA) certainly causes rapid water uptake to compensate for setting shrinkage (Sidhu & Watson, 1998) and leads to the formation of an interfacial region called the 'absorption layer' that helps to maintain the interfacial integrity of these materials (Tay *et al*, 2004). Water uptake by these materials also, unfortunately, may lead to staining from dietary sources and so the color stability of these cements may be less than ideal.

Poly-acid-modified composites and compomers

Poly-acid-modified composites, commonly called 'compomers', show, in contrast to conventional glass-ionomers and resin-modified glass-ionomers, a minimal acid–base reaction during their setting process. As a result of water sorption of the filling during the time of clinical service, a further minimal acid–base reaction can occur. This class of restorative materials combines some of the material properties of resin-based composites with some of glass-ionomer cements (McLean *et al*, 1994). Poly-acid-modified composites are chemically similar to resin-based composites, but they include reactive, ion-leachable glass particles and polymerizable acidic monomers. In contrast to glass-ionomers, they contain no water in their formulation.

With regard to the mechanical properties, in particular tensile strength and flexural strength, as well as wear resistance, compomers are superior to glass-ionomers and resin-modified glass-ionomers. However, they do not quite achieve the material properties of composite resins. In contrast to glass-ionomer cements, which bond chemically to the tooth structure, before application of the compomer, the enamel and dentin need to be primed by a bonding agent, to obtain optimum adhesion (Hickel & Manhart, 1999). As with resin-based composites, bonding to tooth structure of compomers is primarily mediated by micromechanical retention (resin tags and resin–dentin interdiffusion). Indeed, compomers are chemically closer to resin composites than to conventional glass-ionomers. Their prime advantage is the ease of handling; therefore, the compomers have rapidly gained a big share of the market. Concerning aesthetics and finishing/polishing procedures, compomers are superior to conventional and resin-modified glass-ionomer cements. They match almost perfectly with the surrounding tooth structure, unlike glass-ionomers, which sometimes look chalky and opaque. Considerably less fluoride is released from the polyacid-modified composites than from resin-modified and conventional glass-ionomers, although in an acidic environment, as would be found underneath plaque, the release of fluoride increases (Marks *et al*, 2000).

Overview on choice of materials

The choice between cement-based or resin-based materials is a difficult one for the clinician to make and, as has been seen, there are materials that are hybrids of both systems. Many of the reasons for choice will depend on the particular preferences of an individual operator and the types of patient that they see. Someone who is dealing with patients with rampant caries in large cavities may be more likely to use glass-ionomer cements as a means of stabilizing the mouth with long-term provisional restorations such as quick-to-use and relatively easily handled glass-ionomer cements. Conversely, if there is more of an aesthetic concern and perhaps the need for high immediate strength, then a resin-based system may be the first choice for use. Another factor that will probably have the biggest impact on the choice of materials is what the clinician has been trained to use and what the health-care economics of their geographic niche dictates that they use. While materials such as glass-ionomer cements and their derivatives have a number of properties that lead to chemical and therapeutic interactions with tooth tissue, there is no doubt that there is a need for the provision of restorative materials that have a far greater potential for bioactivity within the operative dental context. Bioactivity could be defined as the interaction of a material to foster repair and regeneration of the tissue to which it is applied. Clearly, researchers should be striving to make all of these biomaterials capable of such properties, whatever their background chemistry.

Treatment of pit and fissure caries

When pit or fissure caries is observed dental practitioners have a strong tendency to take the bur just to be sure that no (active) caries will be missed. However, to prevent iatrogenic damage, the selection of a treatment option should be as conservative as possible. Figure 22.6 showes a decision-making tree for occlusal fissure lesions with different features leading to different treatment options dependent on lesion activity and risk assessment. From the diagram it appears evident that most of the treatment options are pre-

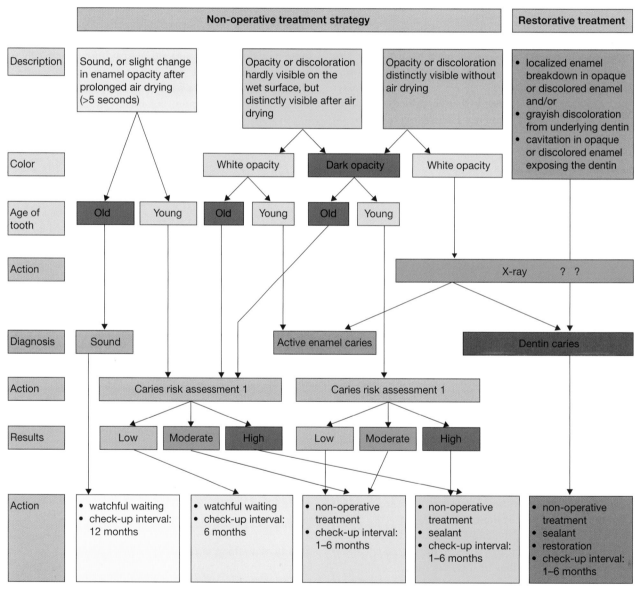

Figure 22.6 Flow diagram for occlusal fissure lesions leading to different treatment options. (1) Low caries risk: no caries development during the past 12 months; shallow and sealed pits and fissures; adequate oral hygiene; adequate use of fluorides; regular dental check-ups. Moderate caries risk: deep pit and fissures; inadequate oral hygiene; inadequate use of fluorides; initial caries lesions; irregular dental check-ups; orthodontic treatment. High caries risk: new caries lesions during the past 12 months; smooth-surface caries; deep pits and fissures; little or no fluoride use; bad oral hygiene; dietary habits favoring caries risk; irregular dental check-ups; low salivary flow. (2) Non-operative treatment: identification and preventive management of risk factors, which may include fissure sealing. (3) Check-up interval depends on the presence of risk factors and an estimate of the extent to which the patient will comply with the dentist's advice.

ventive, non-operative. In contrast, a lesion that has progressed to the stage of a cavity is heavily infected (Ricketts *et al.*, 1995, 2002) and not easy to arrest by cleaning alone owing to the anatomy of the surface. On an occlusal surface the cavity tends to be undercut because the walls of the cavity follow the direction of the enamel prisms. This means that a toothbrush can hardly remove plaque from those undercuts, resulting in an inevitable lesion progression. So, in these cases some enamel and dentin must be removed, and a preparation designed for the chosen restorative material. There are several ways of restoring the tooth. Nowadays composite filling materials that adhere to etched dentin and enamel are the most common restorative materials. The method by which the material is applied is called the all-etch technique.

Alternately, the sandwich technique could be chosen, in which the composite does not adhere directly via an adhesive resin to the dentin. A first layer (of glass-ionomer cement) covers the dentin and the second (composite layer) adheres to the first. It should be mentioned that a special preference for either the all-etch or the sandwich technique cannot be adopted because there is no clear evidence from clinical trials that one technique is superior to the other. Here, the all-etch technique is described as being the most current and appropriate method for permanent molars and premolars.

In primary molars the making of restorations can sometimes be avoided if the circumstances in the mouth are improved. If a patient is able, after instruction and removal of retention places, to keep the lesions plaque free the carious process will be arrested. Under these circumstances restoration is not necessary (Fig. 22.7). When the process cannot be arrested a filling is required. Because of the physiological wear of primary molars, other adhesive materials with less wear resistance are preferred. Certain brands of compomers and the highly viscous glass-ionomer cements have less wear resistance than composites. To be able to follow the wear pattern of primary teeth, these materials are to be preferred above composites. Both are suitable for restoring pit and fissure lesions.

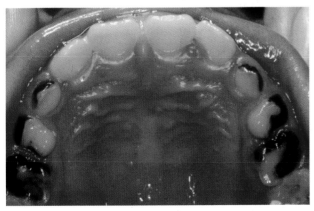

Figure 22.7 Arrested lesions in primary teeth.

Amalgam, the traditional plastic material of choice, is still an option and will be mentioned, although its use is outdated in occlusal restorations, for the following reasons:

- the positive developments in physical properties of tooth-colored materials
- the abandoning of traditional preparation forms in favor of smaller, tissue-preserving preparations
- adhesive, tooth-colored materials support weakened dental tissue
- the good appearance of tooth-colored materials
- the increasing resistance to amalgam, and especially against putative toxic and allergic effects of the mercury component.

When active, initial caries has been diagnosed in pits or fissures, or if a high risk has been established, e.g. in erupting molars, where good plaque removal is not established, sealants may be indicated (Fig. 22.8). The application of a sealant is a procedure in which fissures are covered with a flowable resin or a highly viscous glass-ionomer cement to prevent the development or the progression of caries. This procedure is sometimes described as a preventive measure and at other times as a restorative treatment. Therefore, before taking a bur and initiating real filling activities, the application of a sealant should be seriously considered.

Fissure sealants

Indications

Fissures are susceptible to caries (Ripa, 1993) because of their anatomy, favoring plaque maturation and retention. This could imply that fissures should be sealed as early as possible during the stage of eruption to prevent lesion development. However, many fissures remain caries free throughout life and lesions can be prevented by tooth brushing. Thus, this automatic approach would constitute overtreatment. The indications for fissure sealants are (Ekstrand & Christiansen, 2005):

- active fissure caries has been diagnosed
- a high risk has been established
- fissures are deep and the patient or parent either cannot, or will not, remove plaque effectively.

Sealant application may be advised in young children with erupting teeth and sometimes in older patients (Ripa *et al.*, 1988).

Effectiveness

As described previously (Chapter 20), sealants have been used successfully for many years (Simonsen, 1991). Even when active dentin lesions are inadvertently covered by a sealant, the carious process does not progress further, and the possible development of new lesions in other sites of the fissure is prevented. Sealed lesions that are radiographically evident have been shown not to progress over a

10-year period (Handelman *et al.*, 1976; Handelman, 1982; Mertz-Fairhust *et al.*, 1986, 1995; Briley *et al.*, 1994).

Sealed restorations, placed directly over frankly cavitated lesions, arrested the progression of these lesions. These restorations appear effective in conserving sound tooth structure and preventing recurrent caries (Mertz-Fairhust *et al.*, 1998).

Materials

Both lightly filled resins and glass-ionomer cements have been used. Resins flow better into deep fissures and are better retained than glass-ionomer cements. Despite this, it was not possible to demonstrate a significant difference between the two materials when caries incidence was compared after 2 years (Mejàre & Mjör, 1990; Forss *et al.*, 1994). It is possible that the glass-ionomer cement released fluoride deep in the fissures (Karlzen-Reuterving & van Dijken, 1995). Since glass-ionomer cement is less affected by the presence of a small amount of moisture during placement, the material should be chosen when moisture control is a problem, for instance in a young child with erupting first molars. In other cases, lightly filled or flowable composite resins are usually selected.

Treatment procedure (Figs 22.9–22.15)

An advantage of the application of a fissure sealant is that no irreversible interventions are necessary. After acid etching, a lightly filled resin fissure sealant or a flowable resin is used to penetrate the fissures and prevent plaque accumulation.

Cleaning

The surface to be sealed may be cleaned with a toothbrush and toothpaste and a probe which is dragged carefully through the fissures, or with a bristle brush in a handpiece and pumice and water slurry (Pope *et al.*, 1996). Other dentists prefer to use a high-pressure spray of salt solution (sodium hydrogen carbonate); this is called air polishing.

Isolation

Research has not been able to demonstrate a significant difference between the retention of sealants that were applied under rubber dam isolation and those that were applied just with the help of cottonwool rolls. Nevertheless, it is advisable to use a rubber dam, if possible, because this makes it easier to prevent salivary contamination of the cleaned and etched surfaces. Another advantage is that a direct contact between mucous membranes and unpolymerized resin can be prevented.

Etching

After rinsing, the surface is dried. Then an etchant, mostly a coloured 37% phosphoric acid gel, is applied over the whole occlusal surface. If necessary, the application is extended onto the lingual or buccal surface where grooves and pits require sealing. The acid gel can be applied with a brush or with a disposable syringe and blunt needle. Once the surface is covered with the gel, the enamel is etched for 15 s. Then, the gel is thoroughly rinsed; initially with water from the three-in-one syringe, then with water–air spray for at least 20 s to remove the colored gel and precipitates that might be formed from the etch pits. Subsequently, the surface should be dried carefully. Now the surface appears as a matt, white and frosty area (Fig. 22.11). If application of rubber dam was not possible and the surface is contaminated by saliva, just rinsing and drying is not sufficient; a re-etching procedure is required.

Sealant application

Light-curing fissure sealant is now applied to the etched surface using a small disposable brush or an applicator supplied by the manufacturer. Care should be taken that no air bubbles are included. If air bubbles are seen they can be moved away by gentle use of an explorer. The tip of the curing light is placed close to the occlusal surface for 20 s to polymerize the sealant. When the sealant is cured, the surface has to be wiped with a cotton roll to remove the superficial layer that is not polymerized owing to the inhibiting effect of oxygen in the atmosphere.

The next step is a check that all fissures are covered and that the sealant has adhered to the enamel. If the dentist is unsure of the bond, a periodontal scaler can be gently used at its edge to check that it cannot be lifted off the enamel surface. After removal of the rubber dam, the occlusion and articulation are checked with articulating paper and corrected with fine diamond finishing burs if necessary.

Glass-ionomer cement sealant, press-finger technique

As mentioned earlier, the application of a glass-ionomer cement sealant may be indicated, especially during the eruption period of first and second permanent molars, when moisture control is difficult. In those cases the newly developed press-finger technique may be a good alternative for the resin sealant (see also Chapter 23).

Composite–fissure sealant restoration

Simonsen (1977) was the first to describe the combination of a composite restoration and a sealant. He called this 'preventive resin restoration' (PRR) and others subsequently renamed it 'sealant restoration'. An enormous advantage of the concept was that hard tissue was preserved, especially when compared with traditional amalgam preparations where every fissure in an occlusal surface was cut and restored following Black's principles of 'extension for prevention' (Ripa & Wolff, 1992). In the composite–fissure sealant technique, demineralized tissue is only removed from the cavitated part of the fissure. This is repaired by placing a composite restoration, after which the remaining fissure is covered and protected by a sealant. The concept is the application of Black's original principles of extension

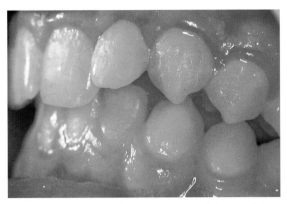

Figure 22.8 Patient, 15 years of age, showing a lot of plaque and gingivitis. The molars of this patient are seen in Figs 22.9–22.16.

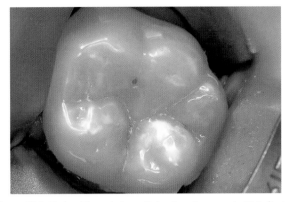

Figure 22.9 Occlusal fissure in lower first molar, where a sealant is indicated.

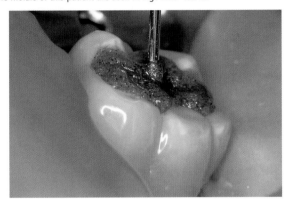

Figure 22.10 Etching of the occlusal surface with a 37% phosphoric acid gel.

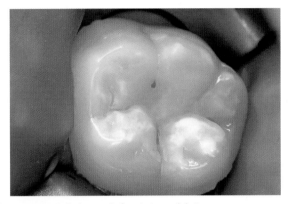

Figure 22.11 Etched enamel after rinsing and drying.

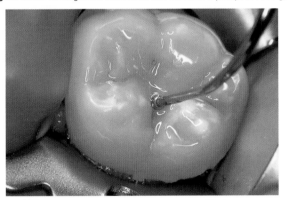

Figure 22.12 Application of fissure sealant to the whole occlusal surface.

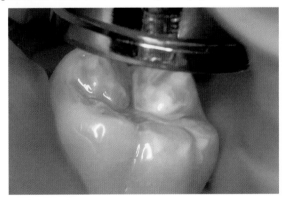

Figure 22.13 Sealant being light-cured.

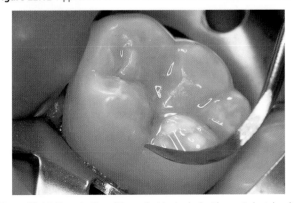

Figure 22.14 The retention of the sealant is checked with a periodontal scaler.

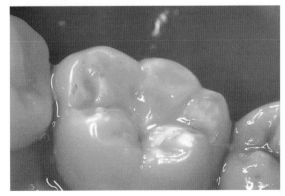

Figure 22.15 The occlusion is checked with articulating paper, which will locate areas of occlusal contact with a colored mark.

for prevention using modern materials. It may be questioned whether it is actually necessary to do this, because it may be obvious that some parts of the fissure system are kept plaque free and are not at risk. However, in practice it is easier to seal the entire area than selected parts of it and the technique does not involve tooth destruction.

Treatment procedure (Figs 22.16–22.27)
Cavity preparation

The preparation should be confined to the removal of demineralized enamel and soft dentin, although sometimes it appears necessary to take away some sound enamel to gain access to soft, demineralized dentin. Preparation of an

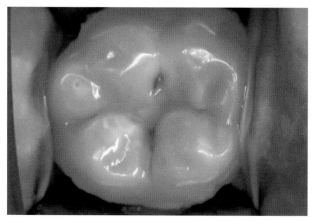

Figure 22.16 Occlusal surface of first molar isolated with rubber dam after cleaning, showing carious lesions to be restored by composite-fissure sealant technique.

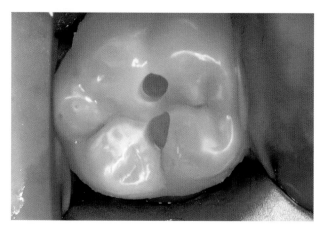

Figure 22.17 Carious lesions in two different locations are opened to facilitate caries excavation.

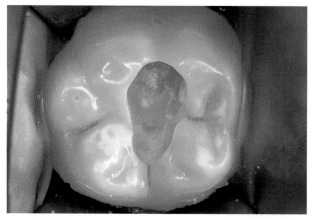

Figure 22.18 Soft caries is removed.

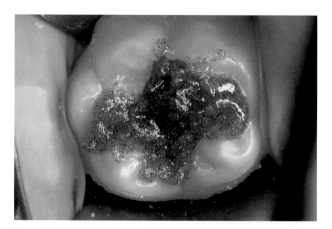

Figure 22.19 Dentin and enamel walls of the cavity, and the occlusal surface of the tooth are etched with acid gel.

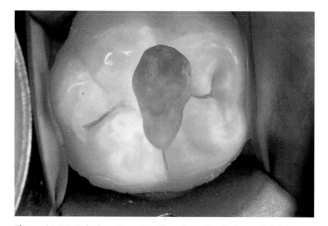

Figure 22.20 Etched cavity and tooth surface after rinsing and drying.

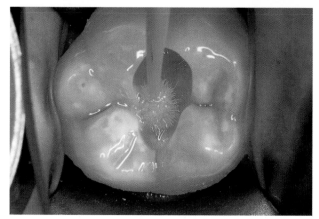

Figure 22.21 Application of primer-bond to the cavity walls.

occlusal bevel is not necessary (Isenberg & Leinfelder, 1990). Thus, the preparation tends to be shallow, with a narrow outline form and rounded internal line angles (Hilton, 2001).

Filling

The all-etch technique will be described. Rubber dam is applied to isolate the tooth. The tooth and the cavity are cleaned, then the enamel and the dentin are etched for 15 s, washed and dried. Subsequently, a primer and a bonding agent are applied following the exact descriptions of the manufacturer. Either a specifically designed composite resin for use in posterior teeth or a universal composite is then used. The material must be placed in incremental layers not exceeding 2 mm in depth. Each increment should be

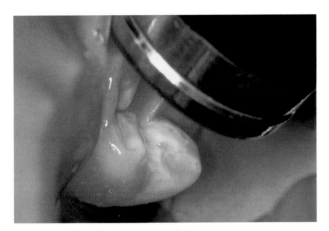

Figure 22.22 Primer-bond being light cured.

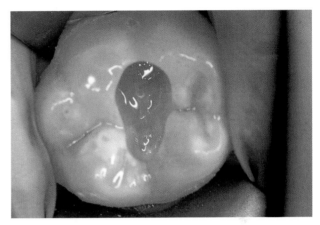

Figure 22.23 Primer-bond polymerized.

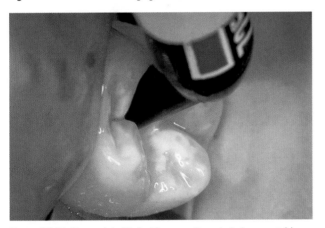

Figure 22.24 The tooth is filled with composite resin in incremental layers not exceeding 2 mm.

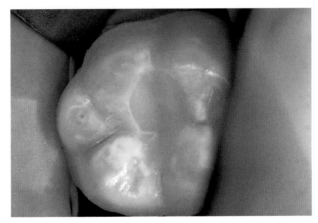

Figure 22.25 Composite polymerized and finished.

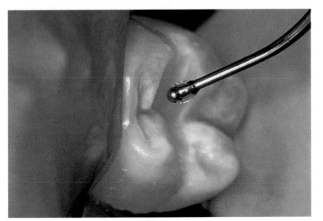

Figure 22.26 A fissure sealant is applied to the whole occlusal surface.

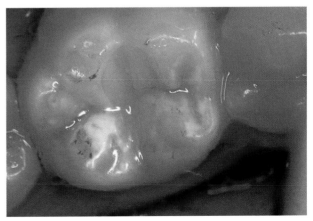

Figure 22.27 After polymerization and checking of the sealant with a periodontal scaler, the occlusion is checked with articulating paper.

cured before the next is syringed into the cavity or applied with a small non-stick instrument. After the final polymerization a sealant is applied to cover the fissures and the restoration. The rubber dam is removed and the retention of the sealant checked. The occlusal contacts are checked with articulating paper, and excess resin is carefully removed with fine diamond or multifluted tungsten carbide finishing burs. Final polishing can be carried out with rubber polishing cups or points.

Extended occlusal composite restoration

The same procedure as described above can be applied to extensive occlusal lesions. Even when a cusp has fractured or when it is completely undermined by extensive caries progression, as much sound tissue should be preserved as possible. Undermined and overhanging enamel can be supported with adhesive posterior composite materials and glass-ionomer cements. Where the outline of the preparation is placed beyond the occlusal surface, a bevel should be prepared to optimize the adaptation of the composite to the enamel. It should be kept in mind that on those places where mastication pressure is obvious a minimum thickness of 2 mm composite material is required.

The restorative procedure, isolation, etching, primerbonding, incremental application of composite, polymerization and finishing, is carried out as described before.

Amalgam class I restoration

Amalgam would not now be chosen as the restorative material for a primary occlusal carious lesion. When an occlusal amalgam has failed and is to be replaced, a composite or glass-ionomer sandwich will often be chosen in preference to amalgam. However, some dentists regard amalgam as the material of choice in larger cavities if the restorative material must take considerable occlusal force. The suggestion here is that amalgam may cause less wear to opposing teeth than composite resin, but evidence for this argument is lacking. Extensive information about the working method to be used with amalgam restorations can be found in several handbooks on operative dentistry (e.g. Overton *et al.*, 2006).

Treatment of approximal caries

Class II restorations (Figs 22.28–22.53)

Cavity preparation

Once it has been decided that a carious lesion must be restored, this should be preferably done with an adhesive technique, because then it is possible to preserve and reinforce undermined and weakened parts of the tooth by the bonded restoration. After achieving adequate access to the carious dentin, soft, infected dentin is removed. To achieve a good bonding to the dentin, further preparation of the dentin inside the enamel–dentin junction should be considered. As previously stated, although it is not necessary to

remove infected dentin to stop lesion progression, it has reduced adhesive properties that may jeopardize the longevity of the restoration. Especially when larger stressbearing restorations have to be placed, optimal adhesion may be important, although there is no experimental proof of this. However, central excavation of affected and discolored carious dentin over the pulp should be avoided at all times to limit the risk of pulpal damage and exposure. The excavation procedure is finally followed by an adjustment of the cavity outline.

Preparation concepts

For the restoration of class II carious lesions the following preparation designs are available.

- *Box-only class II preparations*: Such preparations are simple, allow good access to the carious lesion and enable a controlled restorative procedure. Box-only restorations show a good survival rate in clinical studies (Kreulen *et al.*, 1995; Nordbø *et al.*, 1998) (Figs 22.48–22.50).
- *Tunnel preparations*: Tunnel preparations allow the marginal ridge to stay intact. However, visibility and access in a tunnel preparation are difficult, and the area of primary cavitation in particular is difficult to gain access to. This may result in improper seal of the cavity, because carious enamel and small areas of cavitation may stay behind proximally. As a proper adaptation in the narrow-shaped tunnel is difficult to achieve this may lead to an incomplete restored cavity and hence an ongoing carious process at the site of the primary lesion (Ratledge *et al.*, 2001). In clinical studies, tunnel restorations have shown many failures owing to fracture of the marginal ridge and recurrent caries (Strand *et al.*, 1996; Pilebro *et al.*, 1999; Nicolaisen *et al.*, 2000). For this reason, this technique should not be used routinely for class II defects.
- *Traditional class II preparations according to Black*: These preparations are never the first choice when a primary carious lesion is present. However, a design according to Black's principles is often the result after removal of an existing amalgam restoration. When an adhesive restoration is chosen in this situation, weakened cusps can stay intact, whereas they should be removed when amalgam is the restorative material of choice.

Finishing the outline

Traditionally, the enamel margins of a composite preparation are finished with a bevel. Claimed advantages of a bevel are the reduction of microleakage and the prevention of fracture of enamel prisms, as shown by a number of *in vitro* studies (Lösche *et al.*, 1993; Opdam *et al.*, 1998). However, in the few clinical studies comparing beveled and butt-joint restorations, no differences could be demonstrated (Wilson, 1991; Qvist & Strøm, 1993).

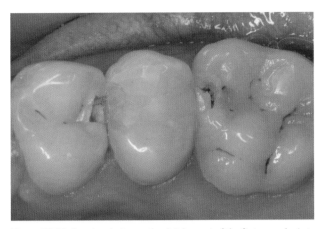

Figure 22.28 A carious lesion on the distal aspect of the first premolar is to be restored. Note the presence of old composite restorations in the second premolar and another lesion mesially in the upper first molar.

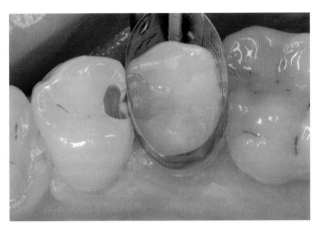

Figure 22.29 A band is placed around the second premolar to protect its approximal surface, while the carious lesion on the distal aspect of the first premolar is opened with a diamond bur.

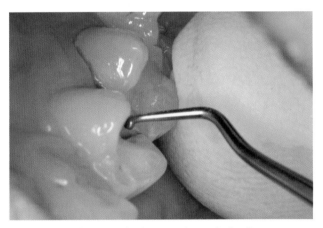

Figure 22.30 Soft dentin is hand excavated. Note the firm finger rest.

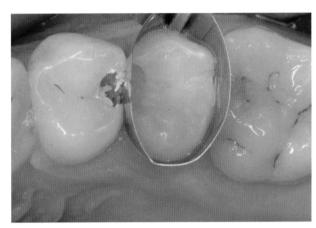

Figure 22.31 Partially excavated cavity. Note the soft, wet dentin.

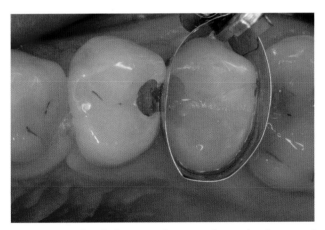

Figure 22.32 After further excavation, note the overhanging enamel buccally and lingually.

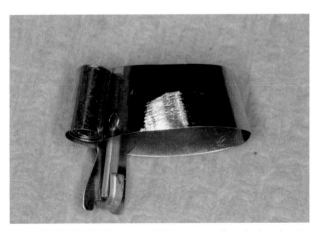

Figure 22.33 The band is removed. Note the scores from the bur, showing that it has performed its protective function.

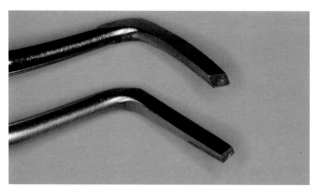

Figure 22.34 Enamel hatchet (bottom) and cervical margin trimmer (top).

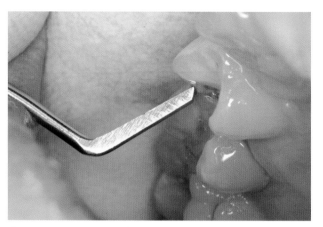

Figure 22.35 Removing overhanging enamel with a hatchet.

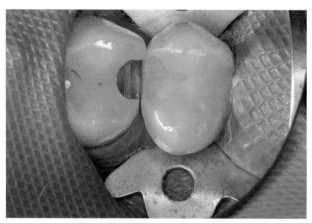

Figure 22.36 A rubber dam is applied.

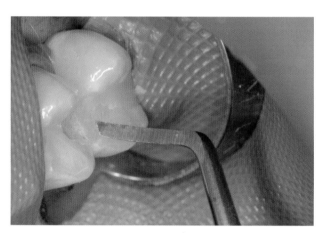

Figure 22.37 A cervical margin trimmer is to be used for the preparation of the cervical bevel.

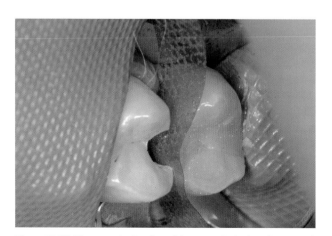

Figure 22.38 The approximal surface of the composite in the adjacent tooth is polished.

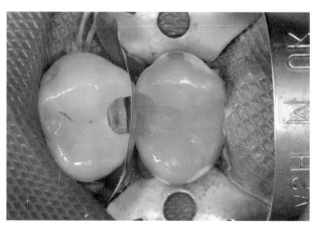

Figure 22.39 The completed preparation with a matrix band in place, but note the large gap between the band and the cervical margin of the tooth.

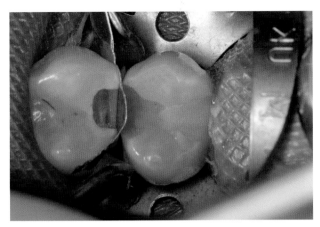

Figure 22.40 A wedge has been inserted to close the gap.

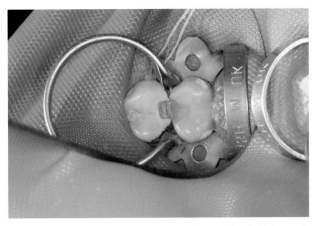

Figure 22.41 A ring sectional matrix (Danville) is placed to hold the matrix in position and slightly separate the teeth.

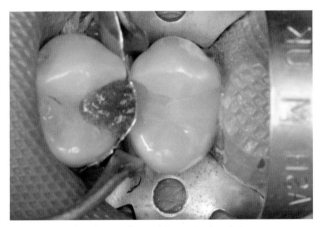

Figure 22.42 Phosphoric acid is used for total etch technique.

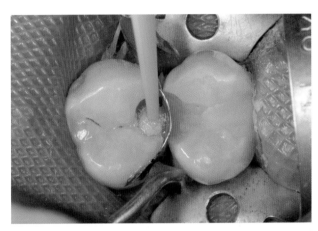

Figure 22.43 After washing and careful drying, the adhesive is applied and the solvent of the adhesive is gently evaporated by air.

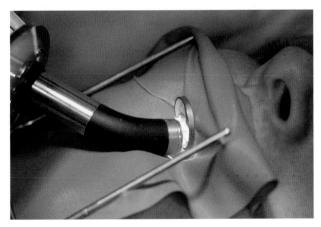

Figure 22.44 Light-curing of the adhesive.

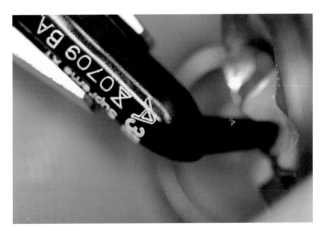

Figure 22.45 Placement of the hybrid resin composite in increments using a tip. The composite is in a compule and injected through a small tip.

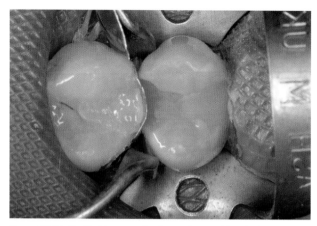

Figure 22.46 The final increment has been polymerized but the filling requires finishing.

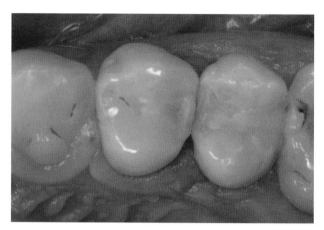

Figure 22.47 Finished restoration. Enough space is left for a properly contoured restoration in the second premolar.

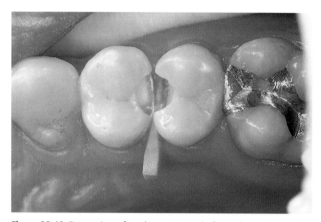

Figure 22.48 Preparations of two box cavities in the first and second premolars. Note that a glass-ionomer liner is placed, which was common practice at the time of treatment (December 1988).

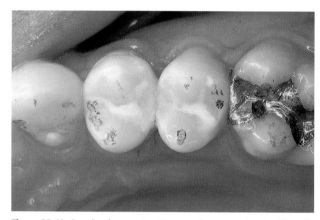

Figure 22.49 Completed restoration. Fissure sealants were placed additionally.

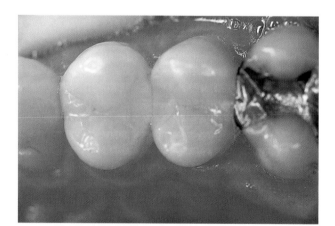

Figure 22.50 Both restorations were functioning adequately 11 years later. Note that the sealants have been lost almost completely owing to wear.

Protecting the adjacent tooth

Damage to adjacent teeth occurs often during class II preparation, as shown by several studies (Lussi & Gygax, 1998; Medeiros & Seddon, 2000; Lenters *et al.*, 2006).

During a 7-year observation period by Qvist *et al.* (1992), approximal damage in originally sound adjacent teeth resulted in a 3.5- and 2.5-fold increase in the perceived need for restorative therapy of adjacent primary and permanent surfaces, respectively. Placement of a bevel with a bur is an additional risk for iatrogenic damage to the adjacent tooth surface. Therefore, a special protocol to protect the neighboring tooth should be mandatory when it has a sound proximal surface. To avoid damage to the adjacent teeth, metal matrices – full matrix (e.g. Automatrix, Tofflemire) or sectional (e.g. Interguard) – can be placed for protection, but handling such devices is often difficult and not well appreciated by dentists. A practical and predictable way to avoid damage to the adjacent tooth when a box-type preparation is made, is to gain access to the carious lesion from the occlusal surface, with the bur entering just inside the marginal ridge (Fig. 22.51). Then, excavation of the carious dentin can take place, while the remaining enamel wall can stay intact and serve as a protection for the rotary instruments. Once excavation is finished, this small

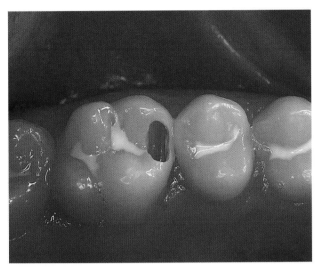

Figure 22.51 To prevent damage to the adjacent tooth a carious lesion in the mesial aspect of the first molar is prepared and excavated before the thin enamel wall next to the approximal contact area is removed.

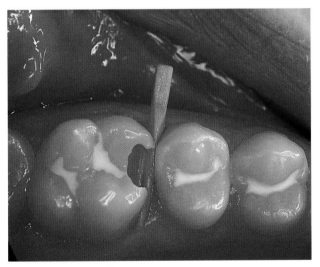

Figure 22.53 Completed preparation.

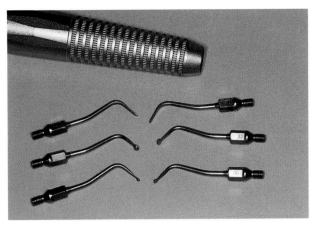

Figure 22.52 The enamel is removed using a sonic preparation device (Sonicsys, KAVO).

and thin wall of enamel is broken away with hand instruments, after which the outline can be finished using specially designed sonic preparation devices (Figs 22.52, 22.53). These sonic devices allow the dentist to keep the bur away from the adjacent approximal surface, thus saving the adjacent tooth (Opdam *et al.*, 2002b).

Material selection

Resin composites

Resin composites are the most favorable materials for restoring class II cavities. Combined with an adhesive technique, they enable the preparation to be as small as possible (Walls *et al.*, 1988) and strengthen the remaining tooth after the restoration (Ausiello *et al.*, 1997). Submicrometer

hybrid composites are suitable to restore the smaller defects. For larger restorations in stress-bearing areas a hybrid composite with a higher filled load has the advantage of better strength and wear resistance.

To achieve a good adaptation requires not only a proper adhesive technique but also placement of the composite resin in the cavity without voids. To achieve this, syringeable materials are preferred. They are inserted with a preloaded tip. The tip should have a small diameter at the end, which gives better access to the cavity, resulting in a better adaptation (Opdam *et al.*, 1996, 2002a). However, the smaller the cavity, the more difficult it will be to obtain a good adaptation of the composite material to the cavity wall (Opdam *et al.*, 2002a).

Flowable composites are frequently used in very narrow cavities, where concern exists about the adaptation of a stiffer composite. However, the material properties of flowable composites are inferior to normal hybrid composites (Bayne *et al.*, 1998). Therefore, the application of normal hybrid should be preferred, while flowable composites should be restricted in their use. In those cases where difficult access hampers the insertion of the composite resin, a small amount of flowable composite resin could be inserted and left uncured, after which the hybrid material is inserted. Hence, the flowable composite will be pressed out of the cavity, meanwhile sealing the outline and reducing the risk for voids and porosities (Opdam *et al.*, 2002a). This 'snow-plough technique' can be used to achieve a good adaptation in narrow-shaped cavities.

Glass-ionomer cements

Glass-ionomer cements gained popularity through their ability to bond directly to enamel and dentin and their continuous fluoride release. However, the clinical relevance of this fluoride release for caries inhibition is still not proven (Randall & Wilson, 1999).

Moreover, owing to their lack of strength and wear resistance these materials are not suitable for restoring class II cavities in permanent teeth (Braem *et al.*, 1995; Wendt *et al.*, 1998). Tunnel restorations made with a glass-ionomer cement show a high incidence of marginal ridge fractures (Strand *et al.*, 1996; Pilebro *et al.*, 1999), which may be related to their lack of support to weakened enamel stuctures.

Newer versions of chemically curing glass-ionomers such as Ketac Molar (ESPE) or Fuji IX (GC) claim improved material properties, but still have not been proven to be class II materials in clinical trials.

Compomers

These materials should be considered as closely related to resin composites. Material properties are poorer than those from resin composites, but better than those from glass-ionomer cements (El-Kalla & Garcia-Godoy, 1998; Meyer *et al.*, 1998). The popularity of compomers can be explained by their simple adhesive technique, which facilitated their use in pediatric dentistry, and their claimed fluoride release. However, the amount of fluoride release is less than that of the glass-ionomer cements, and its clinical relevance should be questioned. Even the clinical relevance of the fluoride release of glass-ionomer cements can be doubted (Randall & Wilson, 1999).

Compomers should not be used to restore class II defects in permanent teeth, as long-term clinical data about these materials are still lacking and the alternative material, resin composite, has been proven to be a suitable material. However, compomers have been proven to be suitable for use in class II preparations in deciduous teeth (see later in this chapter).

Amalgam

Dental amalgam could still be used for the treatment of carious lesions or for replacement of old restorations. However, when primary lesions are to be restored it should be questioned whether amalgam should be chosen. The use of dental amalgam should be restricted to those cases where the skills of the dentist do not allow composite placement in a proper way. Nowadays, in many dental schools, students are trained in handling composite resins and adhesive techniques and, therefore, it can be expected that the use of amalgam will further diminish in the future.

Procedures for placing an amalgam restoration are beyond the scope of this book, and the reader is referred to handbooks on operative dentistry.

Restorative procedure
Moisture control and matrices

To obtain a restoration of high quality there should be absolute moisture control during the restorative procedure. A rubber dam can be placed for this purpose, but in many situations isolation can also be achieved using cottonwool rolls and a saliva ejector. Moreover, properly and firmly placed wooden wedges can be very helpful to control bleeding during the restorative procedure. There is no scientific evidence that a rubber dam is mandatory when placing a composite resin restoration, although it can make operating conditions easier. Moisture control is more dependent on the skills of the operator and the dental nurse than on the chosen technique.

Matrices and wedges are placed before the adhesive procedure is started. Otherwise, the etched and/or bonded surface might be contaminated by blood and saliva when matrices are placed afterwards. This can even happen with a rubber dam in place. The type of matrix and wedges plays an important role in the marginal quality and proximal contour of the class II restoration. Plastic matrices can be used, but are sometimes more difficult to insert than metal matrices. Metal matrices are therefore preferred, also because the theory that composite shrinks towards the light source is not valid anymore (Versluis *et al.*, 1998). Dentists have a choice of circumferential and sectional matrix systems. Both have advantages and disadvantages. Full matrix systems placed around a tooth, such as the Automatrix and Tofflemire retainer, are easy to place, but have to pass the unprepared contact site in cases where only one proximal surface of the tooth has to be restored. A contoured matrix will provide a better shaped proximal surface and should be used preferably. Sectional matrices such as Palodent, Compositight and Contact Matrix have the advantage of a contoured shape (Fig. 22.54).

Approximal contact

The amalgam-trained dentist will seldom have a problem obtaining a good contact because amalgam can be properly condensed. There is no scientific proof that dental composites can be condensed similarly, even when highly viscous, 'packable', materials are used. However, when composites are used proximal contacts can be achieved easily when special separation rings are placed, as delivered with the previously mentioned sectional matrix systems (Figs 22.41

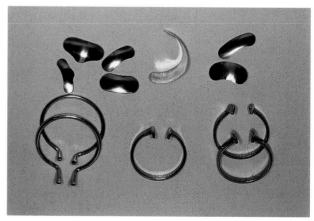

Figure 22.54 Various matrix systems with metal sectional matrix bands including separation rings: GDS (left), Palodent (middle) and Danville (right).

and 22.54). In a clinical study Loomans *et al.* (2006) showed that with these separation rings stronger contacts could be obtained than before the preparation. The prewedging technique, as described by Albers (1985) did result in diminished contact strength. With properly placed separation rings, a tight approximal contact can be created in almost every situation, independent of the type and consistency of restorative material and the matrix system used (Loomans *et al.*, 2007).

Adhesive technique

As mentioned before, a total-etch technique can be used to restore carious class II lesions. A sandwich technique, including the placement of a lining or base of glass-ionomer cement, is also recommended to restore these lesions. Amalgam and composite resin restorations (with either a total-etch or sandwich technique), placed in a general practice, showed comparable longevities in a retrospective study (Opdam, 2007). Clinical studies on closed sandwich restorations, with a glass-ionomer as a liner on the dentin, show favorable results (Gaengler *et al.*, 2001; Da Rosa Rodolpho *et al.*, 2006). Clinical studies on open sandwich restorations, in which the glass-ionomer cement is placed interproximally at the junction between composite and tooth tissue in the cervical area, also show satisfying results, although after 6 years problems with dissolving of the glass-ionomer and fracture are increasing (van Dijken *et al.*, 1999a; Anderson-Wenckert & Leinfelder, 2004). Composite restorations placed without a liner and with a total-etch technique show good results in longevity studies (Wendt *et al.*, 1992; Baratieri *et al.*, 2001; Pallesen & Qvist, 2003; van Dijken & Sunnegardh-Gronberg, 2005). Therefore, both techniques are clinically proven, although the total-etch technique seems the more favorable owing to its simplicity. Etching of enamel as well as dentin should last for only 15 s (Fig. 22.42), after which the dental adhesive is placed according to the manufacturer's instructions (Figs 22.43, 22.44). A total-etch technique including a conditioner, primer and adhesive is preferred to a one-bottle adhesive combining primer and adhesive in one compo-

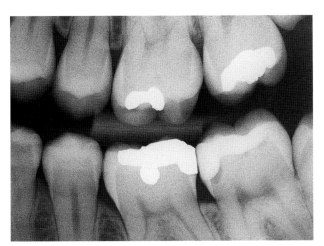

Figure 22.55 Suspect radiographic appearance due to the use of a radiolucent liner under restoration in lower second molar.

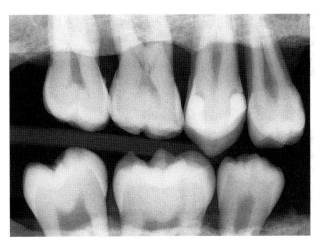

Figure 22.56 The use of a thick adhesive provides a confusing radiographic image, which could be interpreted as recurrent caries in the second upper premolar.

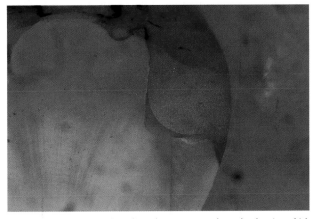

Figure 22.57 Cross-section through an extracted tooth showing thick adhesive pooling at the cervical part of the restoration. Note that the bevel is filled with adhesive resin.

nent, because the latter systems are considered more operator sensitive in laboratory studies (Tay *et al.*, 1996; Frankenberger *et al.*, 2000). This may explain why dentists sometimes report postoperative sensitivity in relation to posterior composite restorations. As a good alternative, two-step self-etching primer systems can be used, as these materials also show good clinical performance (Peumans *et al.*, 2005). Self-etching systems have been shown to result in less postoperative sensitivity (Opdam *et al.*, 1998; Unemori *et al.*, 2004). The available adhesive systems may include a thick or thin viscous adhesive resin. The use of thick adhesives may result in pooling of the resin at the cervical area of the restoration. In the absence of radiopacity, such thick adhesive layers may appear on the bitewing radiograph as a radiolucent zone and may be mistakenly interpreted as recurrent caries (Opdam *et al.*, 1997). This phenomenon may also appear when non-radiopaque liners and base materials are used. Therefore, low-viscosity adhesive resins, resulting in a thin layer (<40 μm), are preferred to enable reliable diagnosis of caries in the future (Figs 22.55–22.57).

Thick layers of adhesive are sometimes recommended to compensate for polymerization shrinkage. A clinical evidence base for this suggestion is lacking, but if any thick layers are used, these materials should be radiopaque.

After the adhesive has been cured, the composite can be placed into the cavity, preferably using a preloaded tip that can be placed on the cavity bottom. Moderately sized and larger class II restorations should be placed in increments less than 2 mm in thickness to reduce polymerization shrinkage stress and to allow proper curing of the composite material.

Finishing of the restoration can be done using fine diamond burs, aluminum oxide disks or rubber polishing cups or points. The latter have the advantage of not being aggressive to enamel and adjacent teeth. During the finishing procedure, the occlusion should be checked to ensure that the restoration is not too high.

Treatment of caries in anterior teeth and the cervical area

Material selection

For restoring anterior teeth, restorative materials should have different material requirements from those used in posterior teeth. For anterior materials and for materials used in the cervical area, strength and wear resistance are less important properties. However, the aesthetics of the restorative material should be excellent and, therefore, a variety of shades should be available. Color stability and translucency are other important properties.

Composite resins

These are the first-choice materials for restoration of class III, IV and V defects. Both modern hybrids and microfilled composites have sufficient strength and wear resistance to function well in class III and V restorations (Van Meerbeek *et al.*, 1994; van Dijken, 1996; van Dijken *et al.*, 1999b), while hybrid composites should be used in class IV cavities where occlusal forces are present and microfills may be not strong enough to prevent 'chipping'. The dentist should select the material on the basis of the desired aesthetic properties and handling characteristics. A suitable anterior composite should be available in different shades and degrees of translucency, as natural teeth are composed of enamel and dentin, which differ in opacity. Therefore, cervical restorations should be more opaque and incisal edges of teeth should be restored with more translucent composites. As in class I restorations with difficult access, an injection technique, using preloaded tips or compules, offers the best opportunity to achieve a good adaptation of the composite (Opdam *et al.*, 1996, 2002a). This technique should also be advised when restoring deeper cavities in the anterior region.

Compomers

In some clinical studies, compomers performed well in class III restorations (van Dijken, 1996). However, the preparation should be etched and a dental adhesive applied as this will improve the quality of the enamel margins (Lösche *et al.*, 1997). The aesthetic properties of compomers are inferior to those of composites, but better than resin-modified glass-ionomer cements. A correct shade match is more difficult to achieve when a compomer is used (Yap *et al.*, 1995). As the benefits of the fluoride release of compomers are in doubt, there seems no advantage in using compomers instead of composites in class III and V restorations. Class IV restorations should preferably not be placed with a compomer, owing to the inferior appearance, strength and wear characteristics.

Glass-ionomer cements

Glass-ionomer cements are not suitable for class IV restorations. For class III preparations restorative cements can be used, but the procedure is time consuming and the appearance of the restoration is not as good as a compomer or resin-composite restoration (van Dijken, 1996). When a resin-modified glass-ionomer is used, the restoration will show discoloration and roughening of the surface in time (Folwaczuy *et al.*, 2000).

Class V restorations can be placed successfully using a restorative glass-ionomer cement, as reported in several clinical studies (Neo *et al.*, 1996; Gladys *et al.*, 1998). A systematic review on class V adhesive restorations showed that glass-ionomer restorations showed high retention rates (Peumans *et al.*, 2005). Although their retention is good, maintenance of the anatomical form is poor (Neo & Chew, 1996). When root caries is treated the possible cariostatic effect of the glass-ionomer cement may play a role in the material selection, but there is no sound clinical evidence for this assumption (Randall & Wilson, 1999).

Restorative procedure class III and IV

The preparation for a class III carious lesion can be restricted to the removal of decayed carious tissue. In case of the presence of a contact with an adjacent tooth surface, access should be labial, palatal or lingual to the lesion. The choice of access depends on the location of the lesion. Care should be taken not to damage the adjacent tooth and, as with class II preparations, sonic preparation devices can be used to finish the preparation outline without damaging the adjacent tooth surface (Figs 22.58–22.60).

A bevel of at least 1 mm in width should be placed, not only to improve marginal adaptation but also to improve aesthetics, as it will make the outline of the restoration less visible. At the incisal edge of a class IV preparation a bevel should be omitted to avoid a thin margin of composite, which is less resistant to fracture when loaded.

Using a mylar strip secured with an interdental wedge, an approximal preparation can be easily restored. For the dentin part of the restoration a more opaque composite should be used, which is covered with a more translucent composite where enamel is normally present. An injection technique can be helpful to achieve good adaptation. The restoration can be finished using tungsten carbide or fine diamond burs and soflex disks or rubber cups and points.

Restorative procedure class V

Resin composite (and compomer) (Figs 22.61–22.75)

Most smooth-surface lesions can be arrested by cleaning alone, but sometimes appearance, a cleaning difficulty or the proximity of the pulp necessitates restoration. In those cases the preparation can be restricted to removal of soft, demineralized dentin. For esthetic reasons brown-stained dentin is sometimes also removed. Subsequently, a bevel can be placed at the enamel margin of the preparation. To avoid moisture contamination during the restorative procedure the gingiva should not be damaged during preparation. When the cervical outline of the preparation is located at or below the gingiva, placing of a rubber dam can be very difficult. Moisture control can also be achieved using

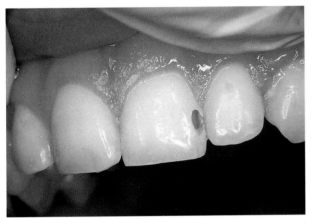

Figure 22.58 A class III lesion is opened from the buccal side. A thin enamel wall is left in place.

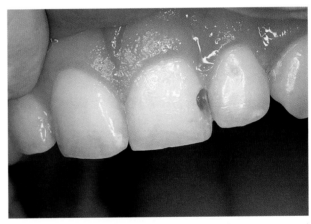

Figure 22.59 A sonic preparation device has removed the remaining enamel and finished the outline.

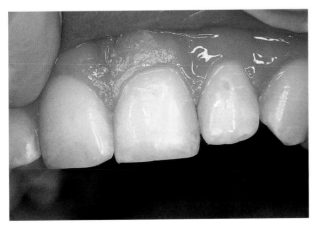

Figure 22.60 Completed restoration.

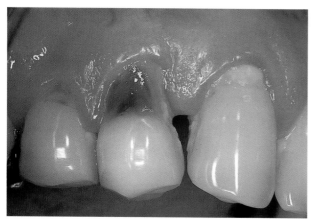

Figure 22.61 Soft carious lesion at the root surface of the first premolar.

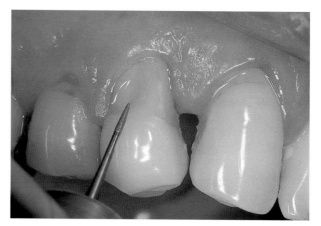

Figure 22.62 After removal of the soft and decayed tissue, a bevel is placed along the occlusal outline.

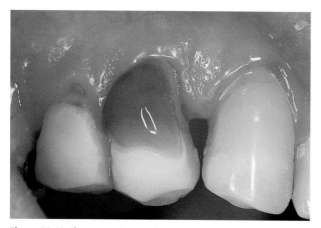

Figure 22.63 The preparation is etched for 15 s.

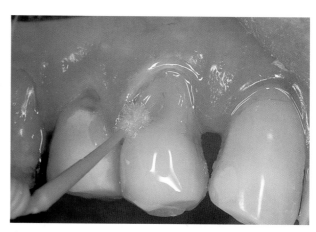

Figure 22.64 After rinsing and gentle air-drying, the adhesive and primer are applied.

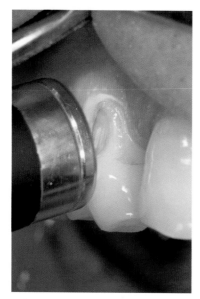

Figure 22.65 Light-curing of the adhesive.

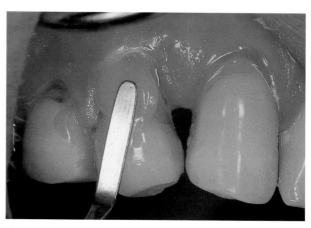

Figure 22.66 Placement of the composite.

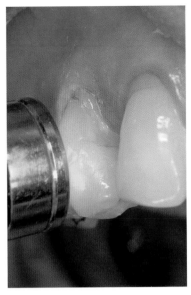

Figure 22.67 Curing of the composite.

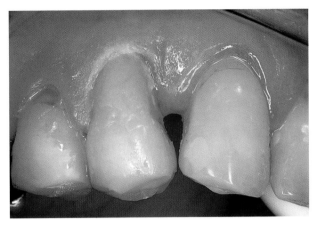

Figure 22.68 After curing of the restoration.

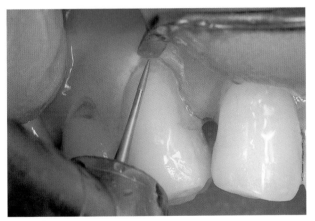

Figure 22.69 Finishing the restoration using a fine-grit diamond bur. A hand instrument is used to protect the gingiva.

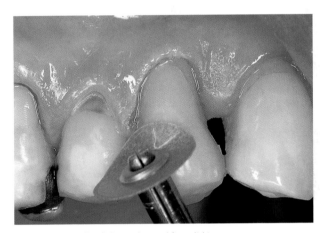

Figure 22.70 Soflex disks can be used for polishing.

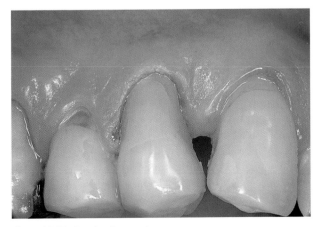

Figure 22.71 Completed restoration.

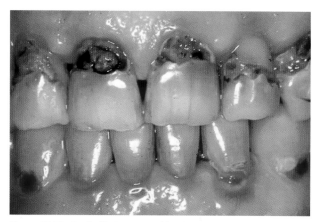

Figure 22.72 Cervical lesions covered by plaque.

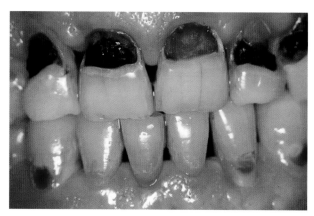

Figure 22.73 Same cavities 14 days later after removing overhanging enamel with a diamond finishing bur (Horico 249/F/014) and instruction. Teeth were brushed twice a day with toothbrush and toothpaste with fluoride. From a cariological point of view these lesions are now stable, but to improve their appearance they are to be restored with composite.

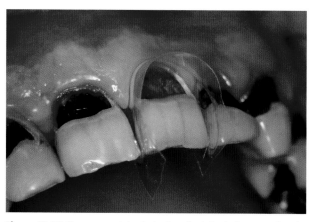

Figure 22.74 Some more stained, demineralized dentin is removed and a matrix strip (Contourstrip-Vivadent) is inserted between the tooth and the gingiva.

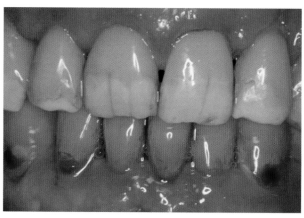

Figure 22.75 Completed restorations directly after placement. The small color difference is due to the teeth being dry, and will disappear after some hours when they are wet with saliva.

cotton rolls and a saliva ejector when no bleeding occurs. When gingival bleeding is present, or is expected to occur during the adhesive procedure, a special matrix strip (Contourstrip-Vivadent) can be inserted between the tooth and the gingiva (Figs 22.72–22.75).

In cases where the tooth to be treated is properly isolated, a restoration can be placed without a matrix. The best results can be achieved by using a medium-viscosity composite which can be shaped using a hand instrument.

In class V restorations, either a three-step total-etch or a two-step self-etching adhesive system is recommended when using a resin composite or a compomer. Clinical studies have reported good results for these class V restorations (Peumans *et al.*, 2005).

The restoration is finished using special composite finishing burs (tungsten carbide or diamond) and aluminum oxide disks or rubber cups and points.

Glass-ionomer cement (Figs 22.76–22.83)

When a class V defect is restored with a chemical-curing glass-ionomer cement, a special metal cervical matrix can be selected and burnished to the contour of the tooth. Depending on the type of cement, the preparation can be cleansed with a conditioner (mostly polyacrylic acid) and rinsed. After gentle drying, the cement is mixed and injected into the cavity. Then the matrix is placed and surplus material removed. When such a cervical matrix is not used, the preparation should be overfilled. The material is then left undisturbed.

It is then necessary to wait for 5–10 min until the restoration is initially set. Setting can be accelerated by using the heat from a light-polymerization unit (Kleverlaan *et al.*, 2004). After setting the restoration can be finished, although it is better to wait for 24 h if possible. During the setting process the material is covered with a varnish or

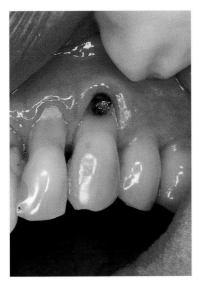

Figure 22.76 Carious lesion present in the upper canine.

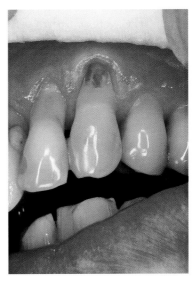

Figure 22.77 After excavation.

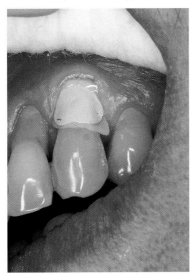

Figure 22.78 After injection of the cement, a special matrix is placed and surplus is removed.

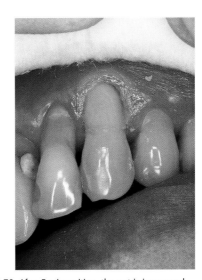

Figure 22.79 After 5 min waiting, the matrix is removed.

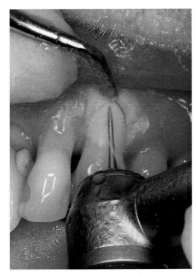

Figure 22.80 Finishing using a fine-grit diamond bur.

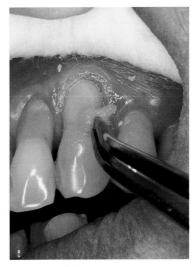

Figure 22.81 Application of the protective varnish.

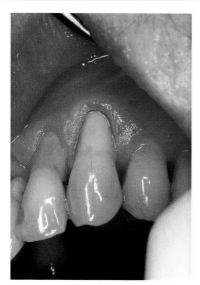

Figure 22.82 Finished restoration.

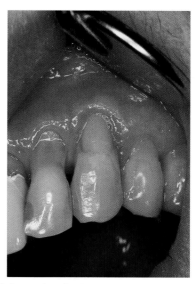

Figure 22.83 Restoration after 3 years.

resin sealant to prevent desiccation or water uptake, as this would disturb the setting reaction of the material. The procedure of restoring the cavity using resin-modified glass ionomer is similar to that for a resin composite. However, the finishing of the restoration can be performed immediately after the light polymerization is completed.

Restorative procedures in the primary dentition

Introduction

There are anatomical and physiological differences between permanent and primary teeth, and this has consequences not only for the shape and size of the preparation, but also for the choice of the restorative material. These differences are (see Fig. 20.8):

- the primary teeth are smaller than the permanent teeth
- the thickness of the enamel is only 1–1.5 mm
- there are fewer pits and fissures in deciduous molars
- the occlusal surface is smaller, in particular with the first primary molar
- the pulp chamber is relatively large
- the dentin layer is relatively thin, except at the occlusal fossa
- the shape of molars, in particular of the second primary molars, is extremely bulbous
- at the transition of crown to root there is a marked constriction
- the path of the prisms in the cervical region is more horizontally oriented
- the occlusal surface abrades more extensively.

Thin enamel and dentin walls can easily lead to fracture of parts of the tooth as well as of the restoration. Owing to a strong physiological wear of enamel, the restoration will be proud of the occlusal surface of the tooth and therefore becomes vulnerable to fracture, in particular when a material is used with a high wear resistance (Villalta & Rodrigues, 2005). By using restorative materials with lower wear values, such as compomers, the risk of fracture can be reduced (Hickel *et al.*, 2005).

Class I

Preparation

Single-surface preparations in primary molars are similar to those in permanent molars and premolars. Only the size and depth are different.

Restoration

The smaller dimensions may lead to smaller occlusal forces. Therefore, the mechanical properties of the restorative material may be of less importance. From this point of view, any restorative material can be used. However, because of the high physiological wear of the teeth, a highly viscous glass-ionomer or a compomer is preferred.

Class II (Figs 22.84–22.87)

Preparation

The differences between deciduous and permanent teeth listed in the introduction to this section necessitate the following modifications to the preparation.

- Owing to the small occlusal surface and bulbous shape of deciduous molars, and because there are usually contact areas rather than contact points, the walls of the box should diverge in a cervical direction.
- Since the pulp chamber is relatively large, the preparation should be kept as small as possible in a mesio-distal direction, to avoid unnecessary pulp exposure.

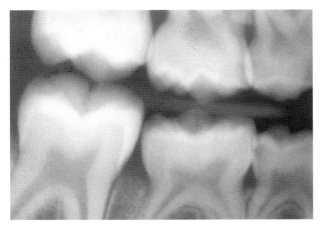

Figure 22.84 Bitewing radiograph showing distal lesion in lower first molar.

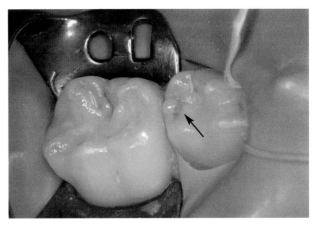

Figure 22.85 Clinical view: note the dark appearance of the lesion shining through the enamel distally (arrow).

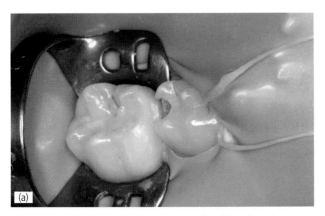

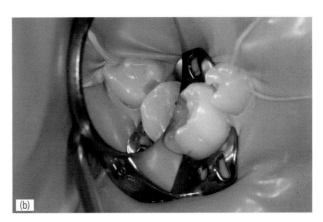

Figure 22.86 (a) The completed cavity preparation; (b) a mirror view.

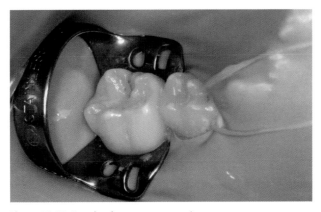

Figure 22.87 Completed compomer restoration.

- Making the preparation deeper than the carious lesion in cervical direction, there is a chance that the size of the cervical wall will decrease dramatically, owing to the bulbous shape of the primary molar.
- There is no need to finish the cervical outline of the preparation with gingival margin trimmers because the path of the prisms in the cervical region is more horizontally oriented than in permanent teeth.

Restoration

Failure of multisurface restorations in primary molars is mainly caused by recurrent caries (composites) or bulk fracture (glass ionomer) (Hickel *et al.*, 2005). Compomer could be the solution. It contains fluoride, which may be released in an acidic environment (acid plaque), and it is strong enough to withstand chewing forces. The wear resistance may be similar to that of enamel, making a compomer the material of choice (Roeters *et al.*, 1998; Marks *et al.*, 1999, 2000).

Class III and IV

Preparation and restoration

As in the permanent dentition, aesthetics play a prominent role in the restoration of front teeth. Compomers and composites are therefore the materials of choice. Beveling does not contribute to the adhesion of the restoration because the enamel layer is thin. To increase adhesion, the surface can be enlarged by completely grinding the enamel surface and then covering it with restorative (Kilpatrick, 1993).

Prefabricated polycarbonate crowns would be an alternative, although they are not very popular because of problems with achieving acceptable marginal adaptation.

The nickel–chromium crown (Figs 22.88–22.92)

Nickel–chromium is a much better material for prefabricated crowns than stainless steel. The crowns are elastic, cervically constricted to fit the primary molars and thin at the margins. Thus, little adaptation of the crown is needed to achieve a good fit. The indications for Ni-Cr crowns are:

- in case of extensive caries or with caries in more than two surfaces
- after a pulp treatment
- in case of molars with developmental disturbances, such as enamel hypoplasia and hypomineralization. With dentinogenesis imperfecta, these crowns can also offer an acceptable solution. Ni-Cr crowns can also be the best means for restoring permanent molars with similar anomalies in young children (Koch & Garcia-Godoy, 2000).

Preparation

After removal of soft carious tissue, the molar is prepared to receive the crown, trying to preserve as much retention as possible. The occlusal part of the crown is reduced by about 1.5 mm. This can be facilitated by making several grooves of this depth, following the slopes of the cusps and then removing the tissue between the grooves. Before slicing the proximal surfaces, wedges should be placed to create space with the adjacent teeth. These adjacent teeth should be protected with a matrix band to avoid damage during preparation. A flame-shaped diamond bur is used to reduce the proximal contours and eliminate undercuts. The cervical outline of the preparation should remain in the enamel for an optimal retention of the crown. Reduction of the buccal and lingual surfaces is not desirable, unless a little removal of the bulbosity is necessary to allow the crown to seat. Finally, all sharp edges have to be rounded off (Savide, 1980; Fayle, 1999).

Selection, preparation and placement of the crown

Measuring the mesio-distal length of the molar or the distance between the surfaces of the adjacent teeth allows selection of the appropriate crown size. The mesio-distal dimension of the molar on the contralateral side can be used for the same purpose. Crowns for lower molars are placed, starting at the buccal surface and then turned over onto the lingual surface. With upper molars the procedure is the reverse. The crown fits properly when a 'snap-on' effect is experienced. If it is still not possible to get the crown seated, a little bit more tooth material has to be removed. If the crown is too long and the surrounding mucosa becomes blanched, the length can be reduced with scissors or an Arkansas stone. However, too much reduction makes the crown wider and the retention less. When the margin of the crown lies about 1 mm past the gingival margin, the right length has been achieved. The margin of the crown should be polished before final placement, especially if scissors have been used.

For cementation, a glass-ionomer cement is the material of choice. The patient can help to seat the crown by biting on it before it has reached its final position. Finally, all excess of cement must be thoroughly removed with a probe or scaler. Interproximally, a piece of floss with a little knot can be used for this purpose (Martens & Dermaut, 1983; Noffsinger *et al.*, 1983; Rector *et al.*, 1985; Fayle, 1999).

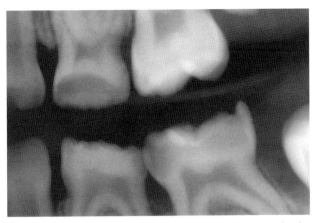

Figure 22.88 Bitewing radiograph showing caries in the lower second molar.

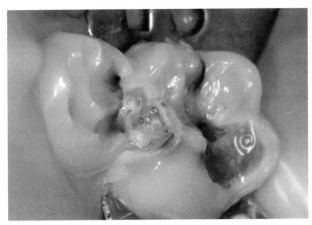

Figure 22.89 Clinical view to show carious lesions. Note they are not cleanable.

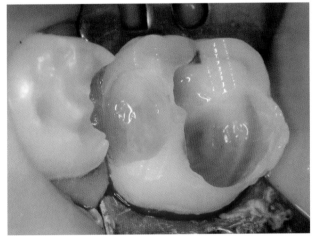

Figure 22.90 After caries removal, reducing occlusal surface and proximal slices, soft, demineralized dentin has been left over pulp (compare with radiograph).

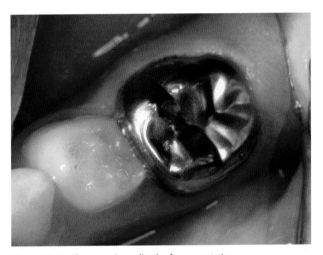

Figure 22.91 The crown immediately after cementation.

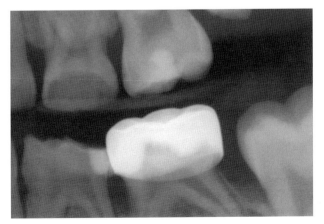

Figure 22.92 Bitewing radiograph showing teeth restored, including the crown.

A novel technique using preformed metal crowns (Figs 22.93–22.95)

In 2006 a new technique using preformed metal crowns was described (Innes *et al.*, 2006) which seems to break every rule in the book. It is called the Hall technique, after its developer. The crown is cemented without any preparation and without caries removal. Having selected a crown of appropriate size, it is filled with glass-ionomer cement, seated on the tooth and bitten into position by the patient. Thus, infected dentin is left and covered by the crown. This restoration is inevitably 'high' on the bite. This is operative sacrilege in every sense! However, results of this longitudinal retrospective study (13 years) demand that the technique should at least be considered seriously.

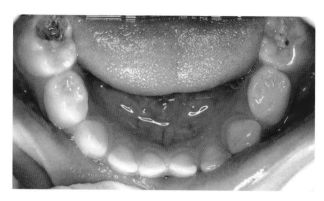

Figure 22.93 Hall technique before cementation; no caries removal and no occlusal or proximal reduction. (Courtesy of N.P.T. Innes.)

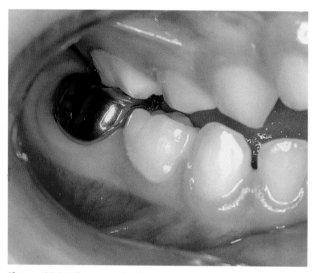

Figures 22.94 The crown directly after cementation. Inevitably the bite is 'high'. (Courtesy of N.P.T. Innes.)

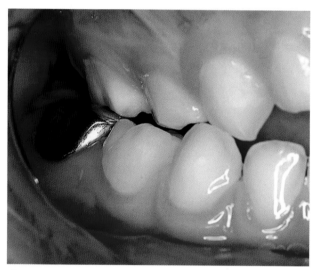

Figures 22.95 Six weeks later. The bite has nearly re-established. (Courtesy of N.P.T. Innes.)

Failure and repair of restorations

Repair, rather than complete replacement, should always be considered as the first option when a restoration is judged to have failed.

Modern adhesive restorations are often simple to repair. In the past, failure or malfunction of restorations, or progressive carious lesions, always led automatically to the complete replacement of the restoration and to further loss of hard dental tissue (Elderton, 1990). Indeed, further loss of tooth tissue is almost inevitable when removing a bonded, tooth-colored restoration. An air rotor must be used to cut the filling material, but the water spray makes it impossible for the dentist to differentiate filling from tooth. On no account should attempts be made to push the filling away from the bonded tooth surface. This technique was the accepted procedure when removing amalgam, which is not bonded to the tooth, but could fracture the bonded tooth surface if it is used with an adhesive restoration. Figures 22.96–22.100 demonstrate examples of different failures or assumed failures, and possible solutions for repair.

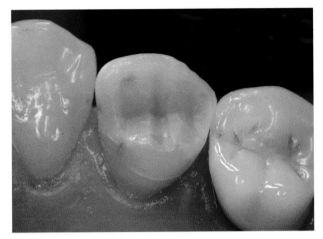

Figure 22.96 Lingual crack caused by polymerization shrinkage of composite. Therapy? None, as long as the patient does not have complaints.

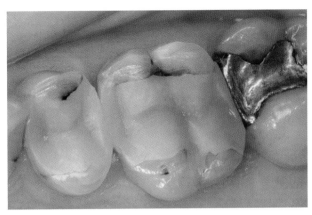

Figure 22.97 Marginal breakdown of composite restorations. Therapy? No cavity preparation required, just local cleaning, etching, adhesive application and composite completion.

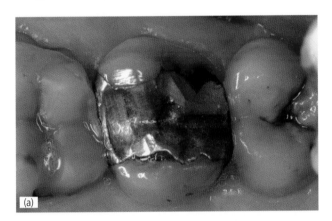

(a)

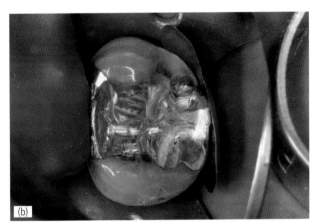

(b)

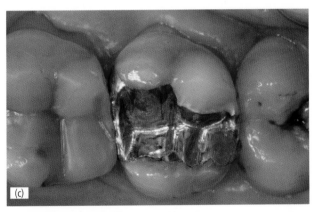

(c)

Figure 22.98 (a) The distobuccal cusp is fractured. (b) A bevel is placed in the enamel and the cusp replaced with composite. (c) The completed and polished restoration.

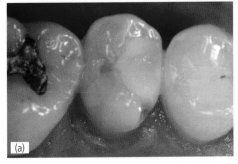

(a)

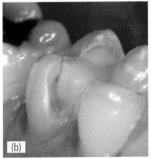

(b)

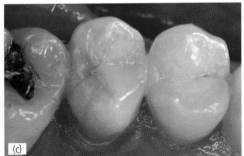

(c)

Figure 22.99 (a) The enamel has fractured on the lingual side of the proximal box. (b) The defect is cleaned, etched, bonded and filled. (c) The completed repair.

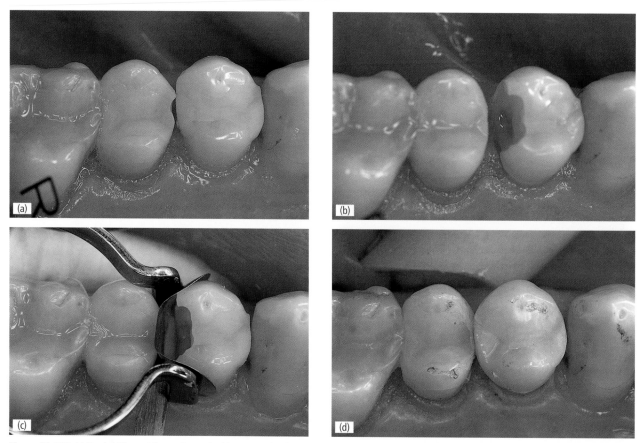

Figure 22.100 (a) Tooth 14 has a 12-year, 3-month-old mesio-occlusal-distal composite resin restoration. On the radiograph a cervical secondary carious lesion is present. Note the small fracture of the marginal ridge of the composite restoration in tooth 15 mesially. (b) A distal box is prepared and the mesial contour of tooth 15 is reshaped. (c) Placement of sectional matrix, wooden wedge and separation ring results in tight approximal contact. (d) A syringeable hybrid composite was used to complete the restoration.

References

Akinmade AO, Nicholson JW. Glass-ionomer cements and adhesives. Part I. Fundamental aspects and their clinical relevance. *J Mater Sci Mater Med* 1993; **4**: 95–101.

Albers HF. *Tooth colored restoratives*, 7th edn. Cotati, CA: Alto Books 1985.

Allen KW. Theores of adhesion. In: Packham DE, ed. *Handbook of adhesion*. Essex: Longman Scientific & Technical, 1992: 473–5.

Andersson-Wenckert IE, van Dijken JW, Kieri C. Durability of extensive class II open-sandwich restorations with a resin-modified glass ionomer cement after 6 years. *Am J Dent* 2004; **17**: 43–50.

Anstice HM, Nicholson JW. Investigation of the post-hardening reaction in glass-ionomer cements based on poly(vinyl phosphonic acid). *J Mater Sci Mater Med* 1995; **6**: 420–5.

Arrais CAG, Giannini M, Nakajima M, Tagami J. Effects of additional and extended acid etching on bonding to caries-affected dentine. *Eur J Oral Sci* 2004; **112**: 458–64.

Ausiello P, De Gee AJ, Rengo S, Davidson CL. Fracture resistance of endodontically-treated premolars adhesively restored. *Am J Dent* 1997; **10**: 237–41.

Banerjee A, Kidd EAM, Watson TF. Scanning electron microscopic observations of human dentine after mechanical caries excavation. *J Dent* 2000; **28**: 179–86.

Baratieri LN, Ritter AV. Four-year clinical evaluation of posterior resin-based composite restorations placed using the total-etch technique. *J Esthet Restor Dent* 2001; **13**: 50–7.

Bayne SC, Thompson JY, Swift EJ, Stamatiades P, Wilkerson MA. Characterization of first-generation flowable composites. *J Am Dent Assoc* 1998; **129**: 567–76.

Black GV. *Operative dentistry*, Vol. 1, *Pathology of the hard tissues of the teeth*. Chicago, IL: Medico-Dental Publishing Company, 1908.

Braem MJA, Lambrechts P, Gladys S, Vanherle G. *In vitro* fatigue behavior of restorative composites and glass ionomers. *Dent Mater* 1995; **11**: 137–41.

Briley JB, Dove SB, Mertz-Fairhurst EJ. Radiographic analysis of previously sealed carious teeth (Abstract 2514). *J Dent Res* 1994; **73**: 416.

Cardoso PEC, Braga RR, Carrilho MRO. Evaluation of micro-tensile, shear and tensile tests determining the bond strength of three adhesive systems. *Dent Mater* 1998; **14**: 394–8.

ten Cate JM, Van Duinen RNB. Hypermineralization of dentinal lesions adjacent to glass-ionomer cement restoration. *J Dent Res* 1995; **74**: 1266–71.

Ceballos L, Camejo DG, Victoria Fuentes M, *et al.* Microtensile bond strength of total-etch and self-etching adhesives *J Dent* 2003; **31**: 469–77.

Cehreli ZC, Yazici AR, Akca T, Ozgunaltay G. A morphological and micro-tensile bond strength evaluation of a single-bottle adhesive to caries-affected human dentine after four different caries removal techniques. *J Dent* 2003; **31**: 429–35.

Craig RG. *Restorative dental materials*, 10th edn. St Louis, MO: Mosby Year Book, 1997.

Da Rosa Rodolpho PA, Cenci MS, Donassollo TA, Loguercio AD, Demarco FF. A clinical evaluation of posterior composite restorations: 17-year findings. *J Dent* 2006; **34**: 427–35.

Davidson CL. Resisting the curing contraction with adhesive composites. *J Prosthet Dent* 1986; **55**: 446–7.

Davidson CL. Glass-ionomer bases under posterior composites. *J Esthet Dent* 1991; **6**: 223–6.

Davidson CL, Van Zeghbroeck L, Feilzer AJ. Destructive stresses in adhesive luting cements. *J Dent Res* 1991; **70**: 880–2.

Davidson-Kaban SS, Davidson CL, Feilzer AJ, de Gee AJ, Erdilek N. The effect of curing light variations on bulk curing and wall-to-wall quality of two types and various shades of resin composites. *Dent Mater* 1997; **13**: 344–52.

van Dijken JWV. 3-Year clinical evaluation of a compomer, a resin-modified glass ionomer and a resin composite in class III restorations. *Am J Dent* 1996; **9**: 195–8.

van Dijken JW, Kieri C, Carlen M. Longevity of extensive class II open-sandwich restorations with a resin-modified glass-ionomer cement. *J Dent Res* 1999a; **78**: 319–25.

van Dijken JWV, Olofsson AL, Holm C. Five year evaluation of class III composite resin restorations in cavities pre-treated with an oxalic- or a phosphoric acid conditioner. *J Oral Rehabil* 1999b; **26**: 364–71.

van Dijken JW, Sunnegardh-Gronberg K. A four-year clinical evaluation of a highly filled hybrid resin composite in posterior cavities. *J Adhes Dent* 2005; **7**: 343–9.

Eakle WS, Staninec M, Lacy AM. Effect of bonding on fracture resistance of teeth restored with amalgam. *J Prosthet Dent* 1992; **68**: 257–60.

Ekstrand KR, Christiansen MEC. Non-operative caries treatment programme for children and adolescents. *Caries Res* 2005; **39**; 45–67.

Elderton RJ. The quality of amalgam restorations. In: Allred H, ed. *Assessment of the quality of dental care*. London: London Hospital Medical College, 1977: 45–81.

Elderton RJ. Principles in the management of dental caries. In: Elderton R, ed. *The dentition and dental care*. Oxford: Heinemann Medical Books, 1990: 237–62.

El-Kalla IH, Garcia-Godoy F. Mechanical properties of compomer restorative materials. *Oper Dent* 1998; **24**: 2–8.

Fayle SA. UK national clinical guidelines in paediatric dentistry. Stainless steel preformed crowns for primary molars. *Int J Paediatr Dent* 1999; **9**: 311–14.

Feilzer AJ, De Gee AJ, Davidson CL. Setting stress in composite resin in relation to configuration of the restoration. *J Dent Res* 1987; **66**: 1636–9.

Finger WJ, Inoue M, Asmussen E. Effect of wettability of adhesive resins on bonding to dentin. *Am J Dent* 1994; **7**: 35–8.

Flanders RA. Mercury in dental amalgam. *J Public Health Dent* 1992; **52**: 303–11.

Folwaczny M, Loher C, Mehl A, Kunzelmann KH, Hickel R. Tooth-colored filling materials for the restoration of cervical lesions: a 24-month follow-up study. *Oper Dent* 2000; **25**: 251–8.

Forss H, Seppä L. Prevention of enamel demineralization adjacent to glass ionomer filling materials. *Scand J Dent Res* 1990; **98**: 173–8.

Forss H, Saarni U-M, Seppä L. Comparison of glass-ionomer and resin-based fissure sealants; a 2-year clinical trial. *Community Dent Oral Epidemiol* 1994; **22**: 21–4.

Frankenberger R, Krämer N, Petschelt A. Technique sensitivity of dentin bonding: effect of application mistakes on bond strength and marginal adaptation. *Oper Dent* 2000; **25**: 324–30.

Fure S, Lingström P, Birkhed D. Evaluation of Carisolv™ for the chemo-mechanical removal of primary root caries *in vivo*. *Caries Res* 2000; **34**: 275–80.

Fusayama T. Two layers of carious dentine: diagnosis and treatment. *Oper Dent* 1979; **4**: 63–70.

Gaengler P, Hoyer I, Montag R. Clinical evaluation of posterior composite restorations: the 10-year report. *J Adhes Dent* 2001; **3**: 185–94.

Gladys S, Van Meerbeek B, Lambrechts P, Vanherle G. Marginal adaptation and retention of a glass-ionomer, resin-modified glass-ionomers and a polyacid-modified resin composite in cervical class-V lesions. *Dent Mater* 1998; **14**: 294–306.

Handelman S. Effect of sealant placement on occlusal caries progression. *Clin Prev Dent* 1982; **4**: 11–16.

Handelman S, Washburn F, Wopperer P. Two-year report of sealant effect on bacteria in dental caries. *Am Dent Assoc* 1976; **93**: 967–70.

Harnirattisai C, Inokoshi S, Shimada Y, Hosoda H. Interfacial morphology of an adhesive composite resin and etched caries-affected dentin. *Oper Dent* 1992; **17**: 222–8.

Hengsten-Pettersen A, Jacobsen N. The role of biomaterials as occupational hazards in dentistry. *Int Dent J* 1990; **40**: 159–66.

Hickel R, Manhart J. Glass-ionomers and compomers in pediatric dentistry. In: Davidson CL, Mjör IA, eds. *Advances in glass-ionomer cements*. Berlin: Quintessence, 1999: 201–26.

Hickel R, Kaaden C, Paschos E, Buerkle V, Garcia-Godoy F, Manhart J. Longevity of occlusally-stressed restorations in posterior primary teeth. *Am J Dent* 2005; **18**: 198–211.

Hicks MJ, Flaitz CM, Silverstone LM. Secondary caries formation *in vitro* around glass ionomer restorations. *Quintessence Int* 1986; **17**: 527–32.

Hilton TJ. Direct posterior esthetic restorations. In: Summitt JB, Robbins JW, Schwartz RS, eds. *Fundamentals of operative dentistry*, 2nd edn. Berlin: Quintessence, 2001: 260–305.

Innes NPT, Stirrups DR, Evans DJP, Hall N, Leggate M. A novel technique using preformed metal crowns for managing carious primary molars in general practice – a retrospective analysis. *Br Dent J* 2006; **200**: 451–4.

Inoue S, Vargas MA, Abe Y, *et al*. Microtensile bond strength of eleven contemporary adhesives to dentin. *J Adhes Dent* 2001; **3**: 237–45.

Isenberg BP, Leinfelder KF. Efficacy of beveling posterior composite resin preparations. *J Esthet Dent* 1990; **2**: 70–3.

Jacobsen T, Soderholm KJM, Yang M, Watson TF. Effect of composition and complexity of dentin-bonding agents on operator variability – analysis of gap formation using confocal microscopy. *Eur J Oral Sci* 2003; **111**: 523–8.

Karlzen-Reuterving G, van Dijken JWV. A three-year follow-up of glass ionomer cement and resin fissure sealants. *J Dent Child* 1995; **62**: 108–10.

Kilpatrick NM. Durability of restorations in primary molars. *J Dent* 1993; **21**: 67–73.

Kleverlaan CJ, van Duinen RN, Feilzer AJ. Mechanical properties of glass ionomer cements affected by curing methods. *Dent Mater* 2004; **20**: 45–50.

Koch MJ, Garcia-Godoy F. The clinical performance of laboratory-fabricated crowns placed on first permanent molars with developmental defects. *J Am Dent Assoc* 2000; **131**: 1285–90.

Kreulen CM, van Amerongen WE, Akerboom HBM, *et al*. Two-year results with box-only resin composite restorations. *J Dent Child* 1995; **62**: 395–400.

Leinfelder KF. Dental amalgam alloys. *Curr Opin Dent* 1991; **1**: 214–17.

Lenters M, van Amerongen WE, Mandari GJ. Iatrogenic damage to the adjacent surfaces of deciduous molars, in three different ways of cavity preparation. *Eur Arch Paediatr Dent* 2006; **7**: 6–10.

Loomans BA, Opdam NJ, Roeters FJ, Bronkhorst EM, Burgersdijk RC, Dorfer CE. A randomized clinical trial on proximal contacts of posterior composites. *J Dent* 2006; **34**: 292–7.

Loomans BAC, Opdam NJM, Roeters FJM, Bronkhorst EM, Plasschaert AJM. The long-term effect of a composite resin restoration on proximal contact tightness. *J Dent* 2007; **35**: 104–8. Epub 9 August 2006.

Lösche GM, Neuerburg CM, Roulet JF. Die adhäsive Versorgung konservativer Klasse II Kavitäten. *Dtsch Zahn Zeitschr* 1993; **48**: 26–30.

Lösche AC, Lösche GM, Roulet J-F. Klasse-III-Füllungen aus lichthärtenden Glasionomerzementen und Kompomeren mit und ohne Schmelzätzung. *Dtsch Zahn Zeitschr* 1997; **52**: 819–23.

Lussi A, Gygax M. Iatrogenic damage to adjacent teeth during classical proximal box preparation. *J Dent* 1998; **26**: 435–41.

Lutz F, Krejci I, Besek M. Konservierende Zahnheilkunde-Restaurationen für wen? *Schweiz Monatsschr Zahnmed* 1998; **108**: 18–26.

McLean JW, Gasser O. Glass cermet cements. *Quintessence Int* 1985; **16**: 333–43.

McLean JW, Prosser HJ, Wilson AD. The use of glass-ionomer cements in bonding composite resins to dentine. *Br Dent J* 1985; **158**: 410–14.

McLean JW, Nicholson JW, Wilson AD. Proposed nomenclature for glass-ionomer dental cements and related materials. *Quintessence Int* 1994; **25**: 587–9.

Marks LAM, Weerheijm KL, van Amerongen WE, Groen HJ, Martens LC. Dyract versus Tytin class II restorations in primary molars, 36 months evaluation. *Caries Res* 1999; **33**: 387–92.

Marks LA, Verbeeck RM, De Maeyer EA, Martens LC. Effect of a neutral citrate solution on the fluoride release of resin modified glass ionomer and polyacid-modified composite resin cements. *Biomaterials* 2000; **21**: 2011–16.

Marshall GW, Marshall SJ, Kinney JH and Balooch M. The dentin substrate: structure and properties related to bonding. *J Dent* 1997; **25**: 441–58.

Martens LC, Dermaut LR. The marginal polishing of Ion Nicro crowns: a preliminary report. *J Dent Child* 1983; **50**: 417–21.

Matsuya S, Maeda T, Ohota M. IR and NMR analyses of hardening and maturation of glass-ionomer cement. *J Dent Res* 1996; **75**: 1920–7.

Medeiros VAF, Seddon RP. Iatrogenic damage to approximal surfaces in contact with class II restorations. *J Dent* 2000; **28**: 103–10.

Mejäre I, Mjör IA. Glass ionomer and resin-based fissure sealants: a clinical study. *Scand J Dent Res* 1990; **98**: 345–50.

Mertz-Fairhust E, Schuster G, Fairhust C. Arresting caries by sealants: results of a clinical study. *J Am Dent Assoc* 1986; **112**: 194–7.

Mertz-Fairhust EJ, Adair SM, Sams DR, *et al*. Cariostatic and ultraconservative sealed restorations: nine-year results among children and adults. *J Dent Child* 1995; **62**: 97–107.

Mertz-Fairhust EJ, Curtis JW, Ergle JW, *et al*. Ultraconservative and cariostatic sealed restorations: results at year 10. *J Am Dent Assoc* 1998; **129**: 55–66.

Meyer JM, Cattani-Lorente MA, Dupuis V. Compomers: between glass-ionomer cements and composites. *Biomaterials* 1998; **19**: 529–39.

Mjör IA, Toffenetti F. Secondary caries: a literature review with case reports. *Quintessence Int* 2000; **31**: 165–79.

Montes MAJR, de Goes MF, da Cunha MRB *et al*. A morphological and tensile bond strength evaluaiton of an unfilled adhesive with low-viscosity composites and a filled adhesive in one and two coats. *J Dent* 2001; **29**: 435–41.

Mount GJ. Glass-ionomers: advantages, disadvantages and future implications. In: Davidson CL, Mjör IA, eds. *Advances in glass-ionomer cements*. Berlin: Quintessence, 1999: 269–94.

Nagamine M, Itota T, Torii Y, Irie M, Staninec M, Inoue K. Effect of resin-modified glass ionomer cements on secondary caries. *Am J Dent* 1997; **10**: 173–8.

Nakajima M, Sano H, Burrow MF, *et al*. Tensile bond strength and SEM evaluation of caries-affected dentin using dentin adhesives. *J Dent Res* 1995; **74**: 1679–88.

Nakajima M, Ogata M, Tagami J, Sano H. Pashley DH. Bonding to caries-affected dentin using self-etching primers. *Am J Dent* 1999a; **12**: 309–14.

Nakajima M, Sano H, Zheng L, Tagami J, Pashley DH. Effect of moist vs dry bonding to normal vs caries-affected dentin with scotchbond multi-purpose plus. *J Dent Res* 1999b; **78**: 1298–303.

Nakajima M, Sano H, Urabe I, Tagami J, Pashley DH. Bond strengths of single-bottle dentin adhesives to caries-affected dentin. *Oper Dent* 2000; **25**: 2–10.

Neo J, Chew C. Direct tooth-colored materials for noncarious lesions: a 3-year clinical report. *Quintessence Int* 1996; **27**: 183–8.

Neo J, Chew CL, Yap A. Clinical evaluation of tooth-colored materials in cervical lesions. *Am J Dent* 1996; **9**:15–18.

Nicolaisen S, Von der Fehr FR, Lunder N, Thomsen I. Performance of tunnel restorations at 3–6 years. *J Dent* 2000; **28**: 383–7.

Noffsinger DP, Jedrychowski JR, Caputto AA. Effects of polycarboxylate and glass ionomer cements on stainless steel crown retention. *Pediatr Dent* 1983; **5**: 68–71.

Nordbø H, Leirskar J, Von der Fehr FR. Saucer-shaped cavity preparation for posterior approximal resin composite restorations: observations up to 10 years. *Quintessence Int* 1998; **29**: 5–11.

O'Brien WJ. Surface phenomena and adhesion. In: O'Brien WJ, ed. *Dental materials, properties and selection*. Chicago, IL: Quintessence, 1989: 71–88.

Ogawa K, Yamashita Y, Ichijo T, Fusayama T. The ultrastructure and hardness of the transparent layer of human carious dentin. *J Dent Res* 1983; **62**: 7–10.

Opdam NJ, Roeters JJM, Peters TCRB. Cavity wall adaptation and voids in adhesive class I resin composite restorations. *Dent Mater* 1996; **12**: 230–5.

Opdam NJM, Roeters FJM, Verdonschot EH. Adaptation and radiographic evaluation of four adhesive systems. *J Dent* 1997; **25**: 391–7.

Opdam NJM, Roeters JJM, Kuijs R, *et al*. Necessity of bevels for box only class II composite restorations. *J Prosthet Dent* 1998; **80**: 274–9.

Opdam NJM, Roeters FJM, Joosten M, Veeke O. Porosities and voids in class 1 restorations placed by six operators using a packable or syringeable composite. *Dent Mater* 2002a; **18**: 58–63.

Opdam NJM, Roeters FJM, Van Berghem E, Eijsvogels E, Bronkhorst E. Microleakage and damage to adjacent teeth when finishing class II adhesive preparations using either a sonic device or bur. *Am J Dent* 2002b; **15**: 317–20.

Opdam NJM, Bronkhorst EM, Roeters FJM, Loomans BAC. Longevity and reasons for failure of sandwich and total-etch posterior composite resin restorations. *J Adhesive Dentistry* 2007 (in press.)

Overton JD, Summitt JB, Osborne JW. Amalgam restorations. In: Summitt JB, Robbins JW, Hilton TJ, Schwartz RS, eds. *Fundamentals of operative dentistry*, 3rd edn. Berlin: Quintessence, 2006: 340–94.

Packham DE. Adhesion. In: Packham DE, ed. *Handbook of adhesion*. Essex: Longman Scientific & Technical, 1992: 18–20.

Pallesen U, Qvist V. Composite resin fillings and inlays. An 11-year evaluation. *Clin Oral Invest* 2003; **7**: 71–9.

Pashley DH, Carvalho RM. Dentine permeability and dentine adhesion. *J Dent* 1997; **25**: 355–72.

Peumans M, Kanumilli P, De Munck J, van Landuyt K, Lambrechts P, Van Meerbeek B. Clinical effectiveness of contemporary adhesives: a systematic review of current clinical trials. *Dent Mater* 2005; **21**: 864–81.

Pilebro CE, van Dijken JWV, Stenberg R. Durability of tunnel restorations in general practice: a three-year multicenter study. *Acta Odont Scand* 1999; **57**: 35–9.

Pope BD, Garcia-Godoy F, Summitt JB, *et al*. Effectiveness of occlusal fissure cleansing methods and sealant micromorphology. *J Dent Child* 1996; **63**: 175–80.

Qvist V, Strøm C. 11-Year assessment of class III resin restorations completed with two restorative procedures. *Acta Odont Scand* 1993; **51**: 253–62.

Qvist V, Johannessen L, Bruun M. Progression of approximal caries in relation to iatrogenic preparation damage. *J Dent Res* 1992; **71**: 1370–3.

Randall RC, Wilson NHF. Glass-ionomer restoratives: a systematic review of a secondary caries treatment effect. *J Dent Res* 1999; **78**: 628–37.

Ratledge DK, Kidd EAM, Beighton D. A clinical and microbiological study of approximal carious lesions part 2. *Caries Res* 2001; **35**: 8–11.

Rector JA, Mitchell RJ, Spedding RH. The influence of tooth preparation and crown manipulation on the mechanical retention of stainless steel crowns. *J Dent Child* 1985; **52**: 422–7.

Ricketts DNJ, Kidd EAM, Beighton D. Operative and microbiological validation of visual, radiographic and electronic diagnosis of occlusal caries in non-cavitated teeth judged to be in need of operative care. *Br Dent J* 1995; **179**: 214–20.

Ricketts DNJ, Ekstrand KR, Kidd EAM, Larsen T. Relating visual and radiographic ranked scoring systems for occlusal caries detection to histological and microbiological evidence. *Oper Dent* 2002; **27**: 231–7.

Ripa LW. Sealants revisited: an update of the effectiveness of pit- and fissure sealants. *Caries Res* 1993; **27**: 77–82.

Ripa LW, Wolff MS. Preventive resin restoratios: indications, technique, and success. *Quintessence Int* 1992; **23**: 307–15.

Ripa LW, Leske GS, Varma OA. Longitudinal study of the caries susceptibility of occlusal and proximal surfaces of first permanent molars. *J Public Health Dent* 1988; **48**: 8–13.

Roeters JJM, Frankenmolen F, Burgersdijk RCW, Peters TCRB. Clinical evaluation of Dyract in primary molars: 3-year results. *Am J Dent* 1998; **11**: 143–8.

Saito S, Tosaki S, Hirota K. Characteristics of glass-ionomer cements. In: Davidson CL, Mjör IA, eds. *Advances in glass-ionomer cements*. Berlin: Quintessence, 1999: 15–20.

Savide NL. The effect of tooth preparation on the retention of stainless steel crowns. *J Dent Child* 1980; **46**: 385–9.

Sidhu SK, Watson TF. Interfacial characteristics of resin-modified glass-ionomer cements. *J Dent Res* 1998; **77**: 1749–59.

Simmons JJ. Silver-alloy powder and glass ionomer cement. *J Am Dent Assoc* 1990; **120**: 49–52.

Simonsen RJ. Acid etch as a preventive technique in dentistry. In: Caldwell RC, Stallard RE, eds. *A textbook of preventive dentistry*. Philadelphia, PA: Saunders, 1977; pp. 325–6.

Simonsen RJ. Retention and effectiveness of a single application of white sealant after 15 years. *J Am Dent Assoc* 1991; **122**: 34–42.

Sonoda H, Banerjee A, Sherriff M, Tagami J, Watson TF. An *in vitro* investigation of microtensile bond strengths of two dentine adhesives to caries-affected dentine. *J Dent* 2005; **33**: 335–42.

Strand GV, Nordbø H, Tveit AB. A three-year clinical study of tunnel restorations. *Eur J Oral Sci* 1996; **104**: 384–9.

Svanberg M, Mjör IA, Yrstavik D. *Mutans streptococci* in plaque from margins of amalgam, composite and glass ionomer restorations. *J Dent Res* 1990; **69**: 861–4.

Swift EJ Jr. Effect of glass ionomers on recurrent caries. *Oper Dent* 1989; **14**: 40–3.ell

Tagami J, Hosoda H, Burrow MF, Nakajima M. Effect of aging and caries on dentin permeability. *Proc Finnish Dent Soc* 1992; **88** (Suppl 1): 149–54.

Tay FR, Pashley DH. Water treeing – a potential mechanism for degradation of dentin adhesives. *Am J Dent* 2003; **16**: 6–12.

Tay FR, Gwinnett AJ, Wei SHY. The overwet phenomenon: a transmission electron microscopic study of surface moisture in the acid-conditioned, resin–dentin interface. *Am J Dent* 1996; **9**: 161–6.

Tay FR, Sidhu SK, Watson TF, Pashley DH. Water-dependent interfacial transition zone in resin-modified glass-ionomer cement/dentin interfaces. *J Dent Res* 2004; **83**: 644–9.

Torii Y, Staninec M, Kawakami M, Imazato S, Torii M. *In vitro* inhibition of caries around amalgam restorations by amalgam bonding. *Oper Dent* 1989; **14**: 142–8.

Towler MR, Bushby AJ, Billington RW, Hill RG. A preliminary comparison of the mechanical properties of chemically cured and ultrasonically cured glass ionomer cements, using nano-indentation techniques. *Biomaterials* 2001; **22**: 1401–6.

Tyas MJ. Cariostatic effect of glass ionomer cement: a five-year clinical study. *Aust Dent J* 1991; **36**: 236–9.

Unemori M, Matsuya Y, Akashi A, Goto Y, Akamine A. Self-etching adhesives and postoperative sensitivity. *Am J Dent* 2004; **17**: 191–5.

Van Meerbeek B, Peumans M, Verschueren M, *et al*. Clinical status of ten dentin adhesive systems. *J Dent Res* 1994; **73**: 1690–702.

Van Meerbeek B, De Munck J, Yoshida Y, *et al*. Buonocore memorial lecture: adhesion to enamel and dentin: current status and future challenges. *Oper Dent* 2003; **28**: 215–35.

Versluis A, Tantbirojn D, Douglas WH, Why do shear bond tests pull out dentin?. *J Dent Res* 1997; **76**: 1298–307.

Versluis A, Tantbirojn D, Douglas WH. Do dental composites always shrink toward the light? *J Dent Res* 1998; **77**: 1435–45.

Villalta P, Rodrigues CR. *In vitro* occlusal wear of restorative materials on primary teeth. *J Clin Pediatr Dent* 2005; **29**: 221–4.

Walls AWG, Murray JJ, McCabe JF. The management of occlusal caries in permanent molars. A clinical trial comparing a minimal composite restoration with an occlusal amalgam restoration. *Br Dent J* 1988; **164**: 288–92.

Watson TF, Pagliari D, Sidhu SK, Nassan M. Confocal microscopic observation of structural changes in glass ionomer cements and tooth interfaces. *Biomaterals* 1998; **19**: 581–8.

Weinmann W, Thalacker C, Guggenberger R. Siloranes in dental practice. *Dent Mater* 2005; **21**: 68–74.

Wendt L-K, Koch G, Birkhed D. Replacements of restorations in the primary and young permanent dentition. *J Adhes Dent* 1998; **22**: 149–55.

Wendt SL, Leinfelder KF. Clinical evaluation of Clearfil Photoposterior: 3-year results. *Am J Dent* 1992; **5**: 121–5.

Wennerberg A, Sawase T, Kultje C. The influence of Carisolv™ on enamel and dentine surface topography. *Eur J Oral Sci* 1999; **107**: 297–306.

Williams B, Laxton L, Holt RD, Winter GB. Fissure sealants; a 4-year clinical trial comparing an experimental glass polyalkenoate cement with a bis glycidyl methacrylate resin used as fissure sealants. *Br Dent J* 1996; **180**: 104–8.

Wilson AD, Kent BE. A new translucent cement for dentistry: the glass-ionomer cement. *Br Dent J* 1972; **132**: 133–5.

Wilson NHF. Performance of Occlusin in butt-joint and bevel-edged preparations: five year results. *Dent Mater* 1991; **7**: 92–8.

Yap AUJ, Bhole S, Tan KBC. Shade match of tooth-colored restorative materials based on a commercial shade guide. *Quintessence Int* 1995; **26**: 697–702.

Yoshiyama M, Tay FR, Doi J, *et al*. Bonding of self-etching and total-etch adhesives to carious dentin. *J Dent Res* 2000a; **81**: 556–60.

Yoshiyama M, Urayama A, Kimochi T, Matsuo T, Pashley DH. Comparison of conventional vs self-etching adhesive bonds to caries-affected dentin. *Oper Dent* 2000b; 25: 163–9.

Yoshiyama M, Tay FR, Doi J, *et al*. Bonding of self-etch and total-etch adhesives to carious dentin. *J Dent Res* 2002; **81**: 556–60.

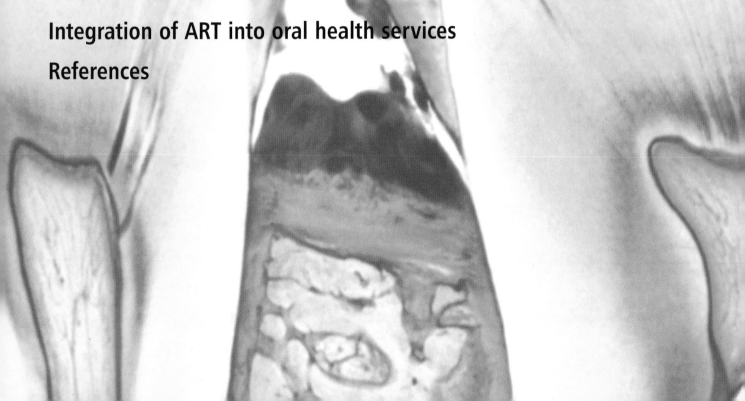

23

The atraumatic restorative treatment approach

J.E. Frencken and W.E. van Amerongen

History of ART

Atraumatic restorative treatment (ART) is a minimally invasive approach both to prevent dental caries and to stop its further progression. It consists of two components: sealing caries-prone pits and fissures and restoring cavitated dentin lesions with sealant restorations (Frencken & Holmgren, 1999). The placement of an ART sealant involves the application of a high-viscosity glass-ionomer that is pushed into the pits and fissures under finger pressure. An ART restoration involves the removal of soft, completely demineralized carious tooth tissue using hand instruments. This is followed by restoration of the cavity with an adhesive dental material that simultaneously seals any remaining pits and fissures that remain at risk.

ART was initially developed in response to the need to find a method of preserving decayed teeth in people of all ages in both developing countries and disadvantaged communities where resources such as electricity, piped water and finance were scarce. Without this intervention, such teeth would decay further until they were lost through extraction. The approach that ultimately became known as ART was pioneered by J.E. Frencken in the mid-1980s as part of a primary oral health-care program of the dental school in Dar es Salaam, Tanzania. To support the newly established dental school, western donors had given 'mobile' cast-iron dental chairs, and drill and suction devices. To become operational in rural Tanzania this equipment required an electrical generator, petrol and a vehicle to transport it. As the aim of a training institution is to train students such that they will be able to implement what they have learnt after graduation, it soon became apparent that the community oral health-care training based on the donated 'mobile' equipment was impractical. Students were frank and told the teaching staff that they would not be able to provide oral care to disadvantaged communities using this mode of treatment if they were to work as dentists in rural areas. This response had nothing to do with students' motivation to work in rural areas or to follow governmental policies. On the contrary, the dental curriculum was designed such that it would prepare students to deal with the oral health problems specific to Tanzania, rather than being a copy of a dental curriculum from a dental school in a Western country, the latter being more the rule than the exception in African countries in the 1970s. The lack of finances to run a mobile program and to purchase spare parts from abroad for the maintenance of the dental equipment, and the absence of a vehicle were reasons cited by the students for hampering the implementation of a community oral health program based on the donated equipment. There were also logistical problems with respect to staffing in certain regions.

So, what should be done? Students needed to be trained in community dentistry and there was much dental decay causing pain and suffering in rural Tanzania. Drastic changes were needed: thinking 'outside the envelope' was required. A small investigation was undertaken as to the kind of instrumentation that was available in dental clinics countrywide. It appeared that hand instruments were available, but that most of the dental equipment was non-functional and that zinc-phosphate cement was the only filling material available. So, the management of cavitated dentin lesions was based on the use of hand instruments and the restorative material available. In practice, this was not found to cause any insurmountable problems since in many cases the cavity opening was big enough to remove its soft content; there was no need to use a powered drill to achieve this. It was possible to fracture thin unsupported enamel to open relatively small cavitated dentin lesions with a hatchet. In the absence of any proper restorative material, the cleaned cavity was then filled with zinc-phosphate cement. The patients preferred this manner of treatment to that provided when using the donated rotary equipment. Following encouraging responses to these early treatments in rural Tanzania, it was decided to start a pilot study using polycarboxylate cement rather than zinc-phosphate cement to fill the cleaned cavities. Evaluation of 28 restorations in children and adults showed only one failure after 9 months. In a number of restorations the polycarboxylate cement was visibly abraded away, but the main outcome was that all people were free of toothache, except for one where the tooth had to be extracted because of pulpitis. However, this cavity was very large before being filled. The enthusiastic patient response and the apparent success of this simple technique were encouraging. The results of the pilot study were presented at the scientific meeting of the Tanzanian Dental Association in 1986, when the ART approach was officially born.

The operators in the pilot study in Tanzania were fourth year dental students and their lecturer. The treatment was performed in health centres. Initially, the patients were treated sitting on a kitchen chair, but this was soon replaced by a more comfortable position. The patient was asked to lie on a table and the operator sat at the end of it. Right from the start, emphasis was placed on comfortable positioning of both the operator and the patient (Fig. 23.1). A specially designed treatment table is not always necessary, but a foam cushion can be placed on a table at the venue and a headrest, with support, clamped to this table. Only the headrest and foam cushion need be taken to the treatment venue.

Based on the encouraging results of the pilot study, a field study was started in Tanzania where a permanent restorative material in the form of glass-ionomer cement was used instead of polycarboxylate cement, which is considered a temporary filling material. Unpublished results indicated a high level of restoration retention and a low level of occlusal abrasion of the glass-ionomer after 3 years. The break-

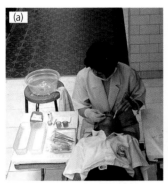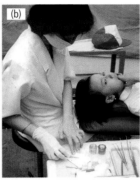

Figure 23.1 ART applied in a school-based oral health program in Indonesia. (a) Note the proper patient to operator position. The treatment table was locally made. (b) The schoolgirl assists the operator by holding the cotton wool roll with her finger, keeping the operation site dry while the operator is mixing the glass-ionomer. (Courtesy of Dr I. Adyatmaka.)

through for ART came during the first major clinical trial in which the ART approach was compared with the traditional amalgam approach in rural Khon Kaen, Thailand, in the early 1990s (Frencken *et al.*, 1994; Phantumvanit *et al.*, 1996). This study gained attention from world leaders in oral health and resulted in the adoption of ART by the World Health Organization (WHO) on World Health Day in 1994.

Reports on other attempts to develop minimal invasive restorative treatment procedures for dental caries suitable for use in field situations are scarce, but have been published, for example, by Smith *et al.* (1990) and McDonald and Sheiham (1994). Many dentists may wonder whether ART is really new, as the individual elements of the ART approach, i.e. the use of hand instruments and the use of adhesive restorative materials, were already available. However, perhaps the potential offered by the combination of these two elements had not been fully appreciated. To make such a potential a reality, there was a determined effort to evaluate ART over long periods, to analyse its strengths and weaknesses, and to set up many trials (in various parts of the world) using improved materials and methods. This was accompanied by courses for oral health-care personnel to ensure the proper implementation of the procedure and matching it to local circumstances.

Since its conception, ART has traveled the world and it is now being used in many countries. It has become part of the dental curriculum in countries as far apart as China, Vietnam, South Africa, Tanzania, the Netherlands, France, the USA, Mexico, Ecuador and Brazil, to name a few. The Fédération Dentaire International (FDI) accepted ART as one of the treatment methods within the concept of minimal intervention dentistry at their annual meeting in Vienna in 2002 (FDI, 2002). ART has gained in popularity among general dental practitioners in developed nations in recent years. Seale and Casamassimo (2003) reported that 44% of US general dental practitioners often used ART as a

restorative procedure to treat children whereas Burke *et al.* (2005) reported that nearly 10% of general dental practitioners in England and Scotland had adopted ART to treat children restoratively. In the Netherlands, ART was used by 26% of general dental practitioners, mainly to treat children and anxious people (Bulut & Sharif, 2004). This information shows that ART is no longer confined to environments where electricity and piped water are unavailable.

The rationale for using ART sealants and ART restorations will now be discussed.

A treatment approach of fissure sealing and minimal operative intervention

ART sealants

The most caries-susceptible period for molars is during eruption, and this can take $1-1^1/_2$ years. The main problem is that the child and parents often do not realize that a new tooth is emerging and it is usually difficult for the child to clean the erupting tooth surface because it is below the level of the arch. Several non-operative measures have been developed. These include cleaning the occlusal surfaces with a toothbrush and fluoridated toothpaste, application of a fluoride varnish, application of a chlorhexidine varnish, sealing pits and fissures with a composite resin and/or a glass-ionomer, and combinations of these. The most appropriate measure very much depends on the ability of the child and parent to co-operate with the cleaning regimen. This approach requires that the dental team regularly examines the child with the parents so that the non-operative care of the erupting tooth can be reinforced. However, in the communities where the ART approach was developed there was no dental team and no opportunity for recall.

The advantage of a sealant over the other non-operative treatments referred to above is its cost-effectiveness in the situation where dental recalls are not possible. If applied properly and retained for a substantial period, sealants may have a long-lasting caries-preventive effect. There are several ways of applying a low-viscosity glass ionomer into pits and fissures. These include the use of a hand instrument, e.g. a ball-ended probe, plugger, ball burnisher or using an explorer to tease the material into fissures, or the use of digital pressure over a thin lead foil to force the material into place. The ART sealants using high-viscosity glass-ionomers are placed under finger pressure. The fissure penetration depth and marginal leakage of ART glass-ionomer sealants were not different from those obtained using a resin-based sealant material (Smales *et al.*, 1997); neither were they different when the glass-ionomer was inserted with a ball-ended burnisher, compared with finger pressure (Beiruti *et al.*, 2006b). The caries-preventive effect and level of retention of ART sealants are presented later in this chapter.

ART restorations

The indications for restorations have been described in Chapter 20. When the lesion has progressed into the dentin and a frank cavity is present that the patient cannot clean, a restoration may be required, facilitating plaque control. In essence, the selection of cases for ART is not different from that described in Chapter 20. A proper diagnosis, in all cases, is of paramount importance. A disadvantage with ART in the field is the absence of radiographs. These may aid lesion detection and also indicate lesion depth and proximity to the pulp. It will be no surprise, therefore, that in communities where ART is being used in the field, the operator needs to have profound knowledge of the clinical symptoms underlying the carious process. The operator must have tooth extraction equipment available to alleviate pain from pulpally inflamed teeth, since root canal treatment is not an option in these conditions and referral to a dental clinic is not possible. Thus, deep cavities may limit the use of ART, but cavities with a very small opening may also pose difficulties. In an adolescent population with a caries prevalence of 41% and a mean DMFT score of 1.1, it was possible to treat 84% of the dentin lesions judged to be in need of a restoration using hand instruments (Makoni *et al.*, 1997). Experience has shown that hand instruments fail to access very small cavities. The approach in these circumstances is to open the cavity as much as possible, remove all debris and the biofilm, and cover the cavity and pits and fissures with a high-viscosity glass-ionomer ART sealant. The success of this management should not come as a surprise having read the discussion in Chapter 21.

Cavity cleaning

The rationale for the use of hand instruments for cavity cleaning with ART is based on tooth anatomy and the nature of the carious process. In enamel caries the demineralization follows the direction of the enamel prisms. It is of particular interest to look at the direction of the enamel prisms in relation to occlusal and approximal surfaces, since these differ. In occlusal lesions, the direction of the enamel prisms results in the carious cavity being narrower at its opening than in its deeper aspects giving it a pyramid-shape (see Fig. 3.46). Further progression of the caries lesion results in demineralized enamel that is either unsupported or poorly supported by the underlying dentin (Fig. 23.2). This enamel can easily be fractured using hand instruments, creating an opening large enough for excavators to enter and removed infected dentin. Knowledge of this process and the recognition of the different stages of enamel and dentin demineralization at the tooth surface are essential in applying the ART approach properly (Fig. 23.3). There is no need to remove all unsupported enamel, only that which is required for access or which is thin and prone to fracture (Fig. 23.4). A dental hatchet, a

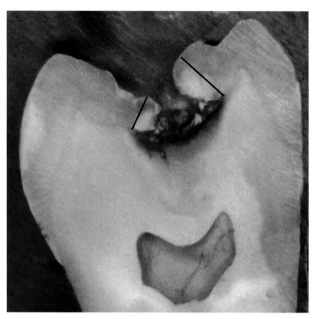

Figure 23.2 A small cavity opening with partly demineralized enamel is presented. The destruction at the enamel–dentin junction is wider than at the cavity opening, giving the lesion a pyramid shape. (Courtesy of Dr E. Verdonschot.)

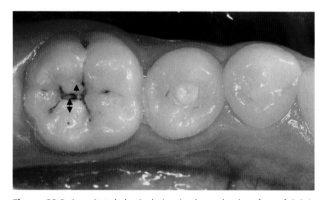

Figure 23.3 A cavitated dentin lesion in the occlusal surface of 3.6 is presented. Note the whitish coloring around the lesion opening (arrows) indicating undermined enamel, cf. Fig. 23.2. This is a sign of partly demineralized enamel that will easily fracture off after slight pressure with a dental hatchet (see lines of cleavage in Fig. 23.2). In doing so, the cavity opening will increase in size and will allow easy access to the excavator for removal of infected dentin. Also note the cavitated lesion in the buccal surface. (Courtesy of Dr B. Monse-Schneider.)

gingival margin trimmer or pyramid-shaped instrument designed specially for this task can be used (Fig. 23.5). In approximal lesions, the direction of the prisms does not lead to a pyramid-shaped lesion and access can sometimes be difficult if attempted through the marginal ridge. For the same reason, it is also difficult to open small cavities in buccal pits and fissures with hand instruments. If too much force needs to be applied to open a cavity further and a rotary handpiece is not available, it is better to place an ART sealant.

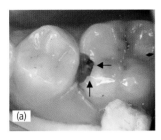
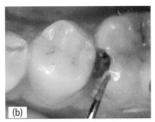
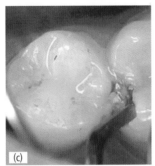

Figure 23.4 Further opening of a cavitated dentin lesion using a hatchet. (a) The enamel buccal to the lesion is demineralized and very thin. (b) The dental hatchet is placed at the edge of the cavity opening and pressed slightly. (c) The enamel is fractured off. The dentist continues to remove enamel that is demineralized.

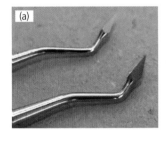
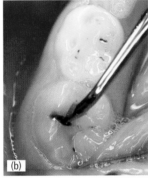

Figure 23.5 Small cavitated dentin lesion in a lower first molar. (a) An enamel access cutter is used to open the cavity further. (b) The end of this pyramid-shaped instrument is placed in the cavity opening and the instrument is turned (anti-)clockwise several times, grinding down the thin enamel that forms the opening.

Efficacy of excavation with hand instruments

Previously, concern has been expressed as to whether hand excavation is as effective as other means at removing infected dentin, although the need to remove infected dentin has been discussed in Chapter 21. An *in-vitro* study showed that hand excavation was the best method in terms of combined efficiency and effectiveness for preparation in permanent teeth. This study used autofluorescence techniques to delineate infected dentin. Removal of caries with a rotating bur was quicker, but overprepared the cavity. Although chemomechanical removal of caries resulted in the most adequate cleaning of cavities, this method was by far the slowest of the methods tested (Banerjee *et al.*, 2000). These results confirm those of an earlier *in vitro* study

showing that in occlusal cavities clinically acceptable excavation of caries at the enamel–dentin junction can be achieved with hand instruments (Smales & Fang, 1999). The efficacy of hand excavation in comparison to chemomechanical removal of caries was also tested in an *in vivo* study showing no difference between the two methods under study: 94% of chemomechanical and 89% of hand-excavated cavities were free of visible caries (Nadanovsky *et al.*, 2001). Recently, another *in vitro* study showed that hand excavation was the most effective and efficient method of removing caries from cavitated lesions in deciduous teeth, in comparison to steel and polymer burs, and the use of a laser (Celiberti *et al.*, 2006). Thus, the evidence shows that hand excavation is the most effective method of removing carious dentin before restoration.

It should be noted that hand instruments can only be used when the dentinal lesion is accessible with respect to both the position of the lesion in the dental arch and access through the enamel. In situations where access cannot be readily achieved with hand instruments, a slowly rotating bur should be used, provided it is available. In summary, it should be noted that there is nothing different or specific about caries removal in the ART as opposed to the 'conventional' technique (Chapter 21).

Atraumatic aspects

Why was the caries management approach using hand instruments termed atraumatic restorative treatment? At the 6-month evaluation of the Thailand study in 1992, it became very apparent that the children who had been treated by ART happily participated, whereas those treated by the traditional rotary handpiece approach were very reluctant to do so. Many of these latter children ran away when they saw the operators, thinking that they needed to be treated again. On asking children of both groups how they had remembered the treatment from 6 months previously, it became clear that there was a high level of acceptance by those treated using ART and an unwillingness to be treated again by those in the traditional rotary handpiece group. Hence the term 'atraumatic' was adopted, not only because of its low level of pain or discomfort, but also because of its minimal destruction of tooth tissue.

Whether ART is 'atraumatic' has been researched by Rahimtoola *et al.* (2000), who investigated the pain aspect during treatment. Two similar groups of patients were treated, either by means of the ART approach or with rotary equipment. Immediately after treatment the patients were asked whether they had felt any pain. Results showed that in the rotary handpiece group there were twice as many complaints about pain as in the ART group (38% versus 19%, respectively). However, the results also showed that atraumatic treatment with respect to pain was not possible in many cases, irrespective of the approach to treatment.

Measuring pain by asking the patient about it is a rather subjective assessment, so an attempt to study this issue more objectively was performed in Indonesia (Schriks & van Amerongen, 2003). Similar treatment groups were investigated by an independent observer. The behavior of the patient and the heart rate were monitored during specific moments in the treatment process. It appeared that with both methods the measure of discomfort was lower in the ART group than in the rotary handpiece group, although the difference was only significant during excavation of the caries in the deeper parts of the lesion.

Although local anesthesia was not used in this particular study, it is still a normal part of contemporary practice, particularly when using rotary equipment. To investigate this further a study was designed where the treatment was preceded by the administration of local anesthesia to half of the patients in both groups. The results showed the most discomfort in the rotary handpiece group with local anesthesia and the least in the ART group without local anesthesia. When the patient was treated again using the same protocol, the effect became even stronger (van Bochove & van Amerongen, 2006). Even uncooperative children referred by private practitioners to specialists of the pediatric department of a university could be treated without the need for local anesthesia when the ART was applied, in contrast to the use of rotary equipment, where local anesthesia was required (Honkala *et al.*, 2003). It is now generally accepted that local anesthesia is seldom required when using hand instruments (ART) to manage dental caries. This is a welcome phenomenon in reducing dental anxiety in children and the population at large, and most probably, also in reducing the level of stress in dentists when treating children.

Hand instruments, unlike rotary instruments, have a limited ability to remove sound tooth tissue. Therefore, single-surface cavities prepared by hand instruments were significantly smaller in size than those prepared through rotary instrumentation (Rahimtoola & van Amerongen, 2002). It has also been reported that surfaces adjacent to cavitated approximal surfaces are usually severely damaged when the cavity is instrumented with a bur without having surface protection (Moopnar & Faukner, 1991; Qvist *et al.*, 1992; Lussi & Gigax, 1998), even to the extent that the iatrogenic damage was considered a caries risk factor (Qvist *et al.*, 1992). Iatrogenic damage to approximal surfaces of neighboring teeth in the process of treating class II lesions has also been reported using hand instruments (Lenters *et al.*, 2006). Scratches were observed which, compared with the damage caused by the use of the bur, were very small. Care should, therefore, be taken when any instruments are used to treat carious lesions.

It can be concluded that the 'atraumatic' of atraumatic restorative treatment implies that it is an approach that causes little or no pain or discomfort to the patient, even without anesthesia, which removes only useless tooth tissue and which minimizes damage to adjacent tooth surfaces when compared with the use of rotary instruments.

The ART approach step-by-step, for use with glass-ionomer restorative material

Equipment required

Unlike traditional dental treatment, only basic dental equipment is required for the ART approach. This means that the approach can be used in many different environments, although the precise equipment may be dictated by the working conditions. These can loosely be divided into the use of ART in a well-equipped dental clinic and ART placed in outreach situations such as in schools or homes. The basic equipment includes an appropriate support for the patient and for the operator, a source of intraoral lighting, dental instruments, restorative materials and other relevant consumable materials (Fig. 23.6).

Dental instruments and consumable materials required

The instruments used in the ART approach have been carefully selected and are based on the steps involved in placing an ART restoration or sealant. No instrument surplus to the essential requirements is used. Almost all the instruments are those commonly found in dental surgeries and are readily available from most dental instrument suppliers. The essential instruments are a mouth mirror, a probe, tweezers, a dental hatchet, an enamel access cutter, excavators and an applier/carver (Fig. 23.7). The consumable materials required include cottonwool rolls, cottonwool pellets, petroleum jelly, tumbler/cup, wooden wedges, matrix bands or plastic strips and articulation paper.

ART procedure

To achieve optimal outcomes with the ART approach it is essential that all the necessary steps be followed (Fig. 23.8a–j):

1. The tooth is isolated.
2. The tooth is cleaned to permit examination of the carious lesion.
3. Access to the carious lesion is achieved using a hatchet or another suitable instrument.
4. Carious tissues are removed with excavators.
5. The cavity and adjacent pits and fissures are further cleaned with a conditioner.
6. The glass-ionomer is mixed according to the manufacturer's instructions.
7. The cavity and pits and fissures are slightly overfilled with the mixed glass-ionomer.
8. A gloved index finger, covered with a thin layer of petroleum jelly, is placed over the top of the restorative

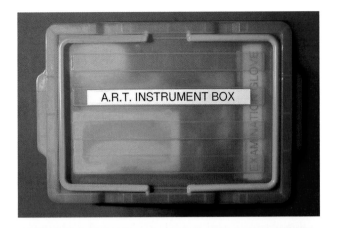

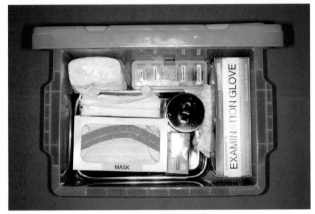

Figure 23.6 All necessary consumables and instruments safely and hygienically placed in a basket ready for transportation to the field. (Courtesy of Dr Y. Songpaisan.)

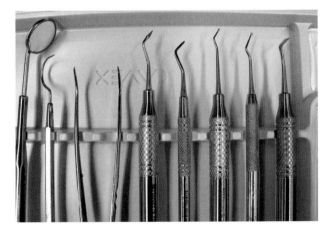

Figure 23.7 A set of ART instruments, consisting of a mouth mirror, an explorer, a pair of tweezers, an enamel access cutter, a dental hatchet, excavators (small and medium-sized) and an applier/carver.

material and pressure is applied to press the restorative material into the cavity and the pits and fissures.

9. The finger is removed carefully sideways.
10. Excess restorative material is removed.
11. The occlusion is checked and the restoration adjusted after initial hardening.

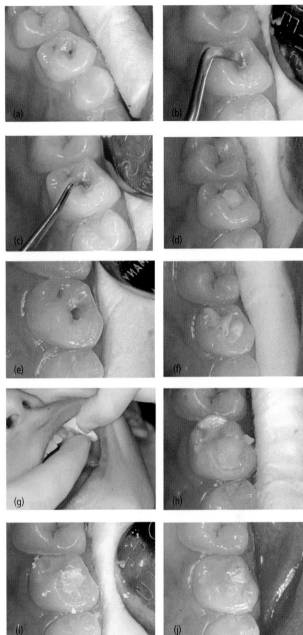

Figure 23.8 (a) Dentinal lesion. Notice the discoloration around the cavity opening, which indicates that the caries has extended under the enamel. This unsupported enamel is demineralized and will break off easily under slight pressure. (b) Opening of cavity further for improved access with the blade of the hatchet. (c) Caries removal using a small excavator. (d) The conditioner is applied to the cleaned cavity, pits and fissures with a cottonwool pellet. (e) The cavity is carefully dried before placing the filling. (f) Incremental cavity and pits and fissures are filled with glass-ionomer. (g) Firm finger pressure is applied over the occlusal surface. This is called the 'press-finger technique'. (h) Excess filling material is visible at the outer margins of the occlusal surface. (i) ART restoration after the bite has been adjusted. The filling material is not yet covered with petroleum jelly. (j) Completed restoration. The cavity has been filled and the pits and fissures have been sealed. (Courtesy of Drs Frencken and Holmgren.)

The ART sealant procedure follows the same steps, except for the cavity excavation part. For a fully detailed description of the steps used in the ART approach the reader is referred to the published textbook on ART (Frencken & Holmgren, 1999) and to a journal (Frencken *et al.*, 1996).

Operators

The reader may have gained an idea that providing ART sealants and ART restorations is simple and easy to learn. However, experience of teaching ART courses to groups of dentists and dental therapists in many countries has shown this not to be the case. There is a profound need for understanding modern cariology and the dynamics of the carious process, in addition to the chemistry and proper handling of glass-ionomers, in order to operate effectively and appreciate the advantages of ART. In addition, many dentists and dental therapists, independent of age, need to practice the techniques under supervision. This boosts their confidence as they learn to treat cavitated lesions that they previously considered unrestorable without the use of a drill and modern surgery. ART courses also contain information on the non-operative management of dental caries, evidence-based results of oral health procedures and how to manage failed ART sealants and ART restorations. Therefore, an ART course can last for 3–5 days, depending on the previous experience of the participants. The WHO Collaborating Centre in Nijmegen, the Netherlands, has developed a manual outlining an ART course (Frencken & Holmgren, 2000).

In certain countries, primary health-care workers have been trained in ART and appear to produce good results (Yee, 2001). The legal system in a country governs the type of personnel allowed to carry out invasive procedures such as ART.

Survival of ART sealants and ART restorations

Since its conception, research has been undertaken to evaluate the ART approach. This resulted in 135 publications available in the electronic library of PubMed that had reported about various aspects of ART, up until September 2007. The majority concern the caries-preventive effect and survival of ART sealants and restorations, since in choosing an intervention it should be evidence based and cost-effective.

Retention and caries-preventive effect of ART sealants

There are basically two families of dental materials in use to seal pits and fissures: composite resins and glass-ionomer cements. It is generally accepted that composite resin sealants are retained longer than low-viscosity glass-ionomer sealants (Simonsen, 2002; Locker *et al.*, 2003).

However, which of the two types of sealant is more able to prevent caries development is less clear. Two structured reviews on the caries-preventive effect of sealants in pits and fissures did not analyze differences between glass-ionomer and resin-based sealants (Mejàre *et al.*, 2003; Ahovuo-Saloranta *et al.*, 2004). Beiruti *et al.* (2006c), in another systematic review, were unable to observe a consistent pattern with respect to the caries-preventive effect of either resin-based or glass-ionomer-based sealants. The authors concluded, therefore, that there is no evidence that either resin-based or glass-ionomer sealant material is superior in preventing dentin lesion development in pits and fissures over time. The glass-ionomer sealants included in this systematic review were of a low- and medium-viscosity consistency.

Many dentists have been taught that resin-based material should be used as the sealant material of choice. These dentists may find themselves in an ethical dilemma working in a field situation where a resin-based material cannot be used because there is no electricity. However, as current evidence shows that glass-ionomer sealants are as good as resin-based sealants in preventing dental caries (Beiruti *et al.*, 2006c), high-viscosity glass-ionomer ART sealants should be used if indicated.

Initially, medium-viscosity glass-ionomers were used as sealant material with ART, but these were succeeded by high-viscosity glass-ionomers in the mid-1990s. A 9-month-long study demonstrated higher retention rates of high-viscosity glass-ionomer sealants applied using the press-finger technique (ART sealants) than for low-viscosity glass-ionomer sealants applied without finger pressure (Weerheijm *et al.*, 1996). Since then, a few longer term studies have been published reporting on the retention and caries-preventive effect of ART sealants. Using the weighted mean to reflect the number of sealants and/or restorations of the individual studies in the final outcome, a meta-analysis was carried out to assess the survival of ART sealants and ART restorations. The analysis showed a weighted mean survival rate of fully and partially retained ART sealants using high-viscosity glass-ionomers after 1, 2 and 3 years of 90%, 82% and 72%, respectively (van't Hof *et al.*, 2006). These relatively high retention rates resulted in a weighted mean annual failure rate (completely lost high-viscosity glass-ionomer ART sealants) in permanent teeth of 9.3% over the first 3 years. The caries-preventive effect of high-viscosity glass ionomers ART sealants appears to be very high. The weighted mean annual caries incidence rate in previously sealed pits and fissures was 1% over the first 3 years (van't Hof *et al.*, 2006).

The high weighted mean retention and caries-prevention rates of high-viscosity glass-ionomer ART sealants that had been reported in the literature led to a comparative study on the caries-preventive effect between these ART sealants and light-cured resin composite sealants (Beiruti *et al.*, 2006a). This study was carried out among children with a mean age of 7.8 years with a low to medium caries risk profile. The authors concluded that the caries-preventive effect of high-viscosity glass-ionomer ART sealants was between 3.1 and 4.5 times higher than that of composite resin sealants after 3–5 years. When analyzing the data for retention of both types of sealant, it appeared that the percentage of sealants that were completely lost annually was almost equal. This unexpected result allowed the study to compare how long each material delayed carious lesion formation. This information is important for dental operating personnel working in societies with limited resources and rudimentary oral health recall systems. In such a situation it would be logical for the dental operator to choose the sealant that has shown the longest caries-preventive effect. The analysis showed that high-viscosity glass-ionomer ART sealants had a four times higher chance of preventing caries development in re-exposed pits and fissures on occlusal surfaces in first molars than is achieved using light-cured composite resin sealant material over a 1–3-year period (Beiruti *et al.*, 2006a).

What could be the reason for the caries-preventive action of glass-ionomer sealants after the material had disappeared? Torppa-Saarinen and Seppä (1990) investigated the pits and fissures of low-viscosity glass-ionomer sealed occlusal surfaces of second molars and premolars that had been clinically scored as having partial or total loss of sealant under the stereomicroscope or scanning electron microscope after 4 months. In most of the cases, glass-ionomer material was still left in the bottom of the fissures. The authors assumed that this finding was in part the reason why glass-ionomer sealants have prevented caries even after they appear to be lost. This assumption is in agreement with the conclusion of studies conducted by other researchers (Mejàre & Mjör, 1990; Övrebö & Raadal, 1990; Williams *et al.*, 1996). It has been reported that glass-ionomers, after proper conditioning, fracture adhesive–cohesively (Inoue *et al.*, 2004) and cohesively within the cement (Papacchini *et al.*, 2005). A cohesive fracture indicates a strong bond of the material to enamel, resulting in the deeper parts of the pits and fissures being covered with glass-ionomer material to various degrees.

The outcomes of the systematic review by Beiruti *et al.* (2006c) and the sealant comparative study referred to above indicate that glass-ionomers, and in particular high-viscosity glass-ionomer, should be the material of choice for sealing caries-prone pits and fissures in field situations. In general, high-viscosity glass-ionomer ART sealants are indicated for use alongside light-cured composite resin sealants when used in a dental practice setting.

Table 23.1 Evaluation criteria used to assess ART restorations

Code	Criterion
0	Present, satisfactory
1	Present, slight deficiency at cavity margin of less than 0.5 mm[a]
2	Present, deficiency at cavity margin of 0.5 mm or more[a]
3	Present, fracture in restoration
4	Present, fracture in tooth
5	Present, overextension of approximal margin of 0.5 mm or more[a]
6	Not present, most or all of restoration missing
7	Not present, other restorative treatment performed
8	Not present, tooth is not present
9	Unable to diagnose
C	Caries present

Using this scoring system, restorations that have survived are coded either 0 or 1, and restoration failure is indicated by codes 2–7 and C.
[a] As assessed using the 0.5 mm ball-end of a metal CPI probe.

Survival of ART restorations

When the survival of restorations is to be studied, criteria of success/failure are required (see Chapter 24). ART restorations have been assessed in two ways: the modified Ryge criteria [United States Public Health Service (USPHS)] (see Tables 24.1 and 24.2) and the ART criteria detailed in Table 23.1. The ART criteria were developed to ensure easy but reliable restoration and sealant assessment in the field. It is unfortunate that the same criteria are not always used in survival studies, because it makes comparison between studies difficult. However, a study of ART restorations that used both criteria claimed that they were comparable (Holmgren *et al.*, 2000), while Lo *et al.* (2001) suggested that the ART criteria may be more stringent than the USPHS criteria. The following discussion is based on a meta-analysis of studies, up to June 2005, that usually used the criteria in Table 23.1 (van't Hof *et al.*, 2006).

Survival of ART restorations in primary molars

Up to 2005, there were seven studies from seven different research groups that fulfilled the inclusion criteria for the meta-analysis on the survival percentages of ART restorations in primary molars (Tables 23.2 and 23.3). The analyses showed that the weighted mean survival rates of single-surface ART restorations using high-viscosity glass-ionomers were statistically significantly higher than those of multiple-surface ART restorations using high-viscosity glass-ionomers in primary molars after 1 and 2 years. This resulted in a weighted mean annual failure rate of single-surface and multiple-surface ART restorations in primary molars over the first 3 years of 4.7% and 17%, respectively (van't Hof *et al.*, 2006).

How do these results relate to those of other restorative treatments? Based on the findings of a systematic review on the longevity of class I and II restorations in primary dentitions over the period 1988–2003 (Hickel *et al.*, 2005), it

Table 23.2 Overview of survival results (%) and 95% confidence interval (CI) of single-surface high-viscosity glass-ionomer ART restorations in primary molars by age and year of survival

Authors	Country	Age (years)	Year of survival		
			1	2	3
			Survival (CI)	Survival (CI)	Survival (CI)
Honkala *et al.*,	Kuwait	<6	99 (92 to 100)	91 (81 to 97)	
Lo & Holmgren	China	<6	87 (77 to 93)	75 (63 to 85)	
Taifour *et al.*	Syria	>6	95 (93 to 97)	91 (88 to 93)	86 (83 to 90)
Yip *et al.* and Yu *et al.* (A)	China	>6	95 (85 to 100)	89 (74 to 100)	
Yip *et al.* and Yu *et al.* (B)	China	>6	94 (82 to 100)	94 (82 to 100)	
Louw *et al.*	South Africa	>6	96 (90 to 99)		
Luo *et al.* and Lo *et al.*	China	>6	93 (83 to 98)	94 (84 to 99)	
Yee	Nepal	>3		67 (43 to 85)	
Weighted mean score			95 (94 to 97)	91 (88 to 93)	86 (83 to 90)

From van't Hof *et al.* (2006), modified with permission.
(A) and (B): same study but different glass-ionomer cement used.

appears that the weighted mean annual failure rate of single-surface ART restorations in primary dentitions is lower than that of comparable amalgam and low- to medium-viscosity glass-ionomer restorations, but higher than for resin-modified glass-ionomer restorations. The situation is different for multiple-surface restorations. The weighted mean annual failure rate of multiple-surface ART restorations using high-viscosity glass-ionomers in primary dentition appears to be higher than that of low- to medium-viscosity glass-ionomer, amalgam and resin-modified glass-ionomer restorations. The systematic review referred to above (Hickel *et al.*, 2005) only provided mean annual failure rates for combined class I and class II resin-based restorations in primary dentition. (Chapter 24 provides further reading on the longevity of restorations.)

Considering the comparison with other restorative materials, it may be concluded that single-surface ART restorations

using high-viscosity glass-ionomers in primary dentitions have a very low mean annual failure rate, but that the mean annual failure rate for multiple-surface ART restorations using high-viscosity glass-ionomers remains rather high. After the meta-analysis had been carried out, Ersin *et al.* (2006) reported a 2-year survival rate of class II ART high-viscosity glass-ionomer restorations of 76.1%. This finding is higher than the results reported in the meta-analysis for comparable restorations produced under rural conditions (Table 23.3).

To improve the survival of multiple-surface ART restorations in primary teeth, one could further consider using resin-modified glass-ionomer, increasing the fracture toughness of current conventional glass-ionomers or changing the restorative technique. An example of the latter option may be to keep the marginal ridge in approximal glass-ionomer restorations in primary teeth out of contact with

Table 23.3 Overview of survival results (%) and 95% confidence interval (CI) of multiple-surface glass-ionomer ART restorations in primary molars by age and year of survival

Authors	Country	Age (years)	Year of survival		
			1	2	3
			Survival (CI)	Survival (CI)	Survival (CI)
Honkala *et al.*	Kuwait	<6	100 (74 to 100)	83 (52 to 98)	
Lo & Holmgren	China	<6	75 (57 to 89)	56 (37 to 76)	
Taifour *et al.*	Syria	>6	72 (68 to 76)	60 (56 to 65)	49 (44 to 54)
Yip *et al.* and Yu *et al.* (A)	China	>6	66 (40 to 91)	49 (22 to 77)	
Yip *et al.* and Yu *et al.* (B)	China	>6	65 (44 to 86)	55 (33 to 77)	
Louw *et al.*	South Africa	>6	73 (65 to 80)		
Luo *et al.* and Lo *et al.*	China	>6	54 (33 to 73)	43 (24 to 63)	
Weighted mean score			73 (70 to 77)	59 (55 to 64)	49 (44 to 54)

From van't Hof *et al.* (2006), modified with permission.
(A) and (B): same study but different glass-ionomer cement used.

the antagonist tooth, thus reducing the possibility of marginal ridge fracture, which was frequently seen in multiple-surface ART restorations. This hypothesis should be tested in a randomized, controlled clinical trial.

In discussing the option of underfilling a cavity in an approximal surface to reduce restoration dislodgment, one should also consider that, towards the end of the life of a primary molar, the tooth will function more as a space maintainer, preventing malalignment of the permanent premolar, than as a full functional unit for chewing food. Orthodontic treatment is not an option in communities where organized oral care is rudimentary and, therefore, a symptom-free primary molar with a less than perfect restoration or no restoration at all can be very acceptable (Tickle *et al.*, 2002; Levine *et al.*, 2002). However, the child should be encouraged to apply a proper cleaning regimen daily.

Survival of ART restorations in posterior permanent teeth

The majority of studies evaluating ART restorations have been conducted on the permanent dentition of adolescents. At this age, dentin caries is most common in the pits and fissures. Hence, the studies presented in Table 23.4 refer only to single-surface ART restorations in posterior perma-

nent teeth. The table shows that the weighted mean annual failure rate of single-surface ART restorations in posterior permanent teeth using high-viscosity glass-ionomers over the first 6 years was 4.7%. The weighted mean survival rates of single-surface ART restorations using high-viscosity glass-ionomers were statistically significantly higher than those of comparable ART restorations using medium-viscosity glass-ionomers after 1, 2 and 3 years (van't Hof *et al.*, 2006). Looking particularly at the first 3 year survival results of single-surface high-viscosity glass-ionomer ART restorations in posterior permanent teeth, it is striking to note the high level of similarity in the survival rates, particularly considering that these studies have been carried out in many different countries by many different researchers and operators, but using almost exclusively the ART evaluation criteria.

How do these results relate to those of other restorative treatments? Based on the findings of a systematic review on restoration survival in posterior teeth in the permanent dentition, covering predominantly the period 1990–2003 (Manhart *et al.*, 2004), it appears that the weighted mean annual failure rate of single-surface ART restorations using high-viscosity glass-ionomers in posterior permanent teeth (van't Hof *et al.*, 2006) is somewhat higher than that of comparable amalgam and composite resin, but lower than

Table 23.4 Overview of survival results (%) and 95% confidence interval (CI) of single-surface ART restorations in posterior permanent teeth by restorative material used and year of survival

| Authors | Country | Year of survival | | | | | |
| | | 1 | 2 | 3 | 4 | 5 | 6 |
		Survival (CI)	Survival (CI)	Survival (CI)	Survival (CI)	Survival (CI)	Survival (CI)
Studies using medium-viscosity glass-ionomers							
Smith *et al.* and Kalf-Scholte *et al.*	Malawi	96 (90 to 99)		81 (72 to 91)			
Phantumvanit *et al.*	Thailand	93 (89 to 96)	83 (77 to 88)	71 (64 to 77)			
Mandari *et al.*	Tanzania		93 (85 to 97)				67[g] (56 to 77)
Frencken *et al.*	Zimbabwe	96 (93 to 98)	92 (89 to 95)	85 (81 to 90)			
Ho *et al.*	China, Hong Kong		91 (78 to 98)				
Weighted mean scores		95[a] (93 to 97)	91[c] (88 to 93)	81[e] (77 to 84)			
Studies using high-viscosity glass-ionomers							
Frencken *et al.*	Zimbabwe	99 (97 to 100)	94 (90 to 97)	88 (84 to 92)			
Ziraps *et al.*	Latvia	100 (92 to 100)	93 (82 to 99)				
Lo *et al.*	China	97 (95 to 99)	94 (91 to 97)	90 (86 to 94)	86 (82 to 90)	82 (77 to 87)	74 (68 to 80)
Ho *et al.*	China, Hong Kong		94 (82 to 99)				
Kikwilu *et al.*	Tanzania	96 (92 to 98)					
Luo *et al.* and Lo *et al.*	China	96 (90 to 99)	96 (90 to 99)				
Rahimtoola *et al.*	Pakistan	98 (93 to 99)	94 (88 to 98)	94 (90 to 99)			
Frencken *et al.*	Syria	93 (90 to 96)	88 (85 to 91)	85 (81 to 89)	80 (76 to 84)	76 (71 to 81)	69 (63 to 75)
Loh	Malaysia	97 (94 to 99)	96 (92 to 98)	96 (92 to 98)	92 (85 to 97)		
Yip *et al.* and Gao *et al.*	China	100 (91 to 100)	94 (71 to 100)				
Mickenautsch *et al.*	South Africa	94 (88 to 98)					
Yee	Nepal		100 (84 to 100)				
Weighted mean scores		97[b] (97 to 98)	94[d] (92 to 95)	92[f] (90 to 93)	85 (82 to 87)	79 (76 to 83)	72[h] (67 to76)

From van't Hof *et al.* (2006), modified with permission.
[a, b] $p = 0.02$; [c, d] $p = 0.03$; [e, f] $p = 0.001$; [g, h] $p = 0.29$.

that for comparable low- to medium-viscosity glass-ionomer restorations. This external validity comparison indicates that the survival rate of single-surface ART restorations in posterior permanent teeth using high-viscosity glass-ionomer is acceptable, particularly when considering that these restorations have generally been produced under field conditions, whereas restorations using the other materials were performed in dental clinics.

Comparison of ART with conventional treatment approaches

Primary dentition

ART restorations placed in the primary dentition have been compared with amalgam restorations, but the number of such studies remains low. The longest study showed a statistically significant difference in cumulative survival rates for single-surface ART restorations in primary molars (86%) in comparison to comparable amalgam restorations (80%) after 3 years. With respect to multiple-surface restorations in primary molars, the study showed a 3-year cumulative survival rate of 49% for ART and 43% for amalgam restorations, a difference that was not statistically significant (Taifour *et al.*, 2002). ART high-viscosity glass-ionomer restorations have also been compared with conventional composite resin restorations in primary molars. Using a split-mouth study design, Ersin *et al.* (2006) found no statistically significant difference between class I ART (96.7%) and comparable composite resin (91%) restorations, and between class II ART (76.1%) and comparable composite resin (82%) restorations after 2 years. Although the number of comparable studies is low, it appears that there is no difference in restoration survival of high-viscosity glass-ionomer ART and those produced conventionally using amalgam or composite resin.

In an attempt to improve the survival rates of multiple-surface ART restorations in primary molars, Eden *et al.* (2006) carried out a study in which self-etch composite resin was used instead of glass-ionomer, in an attempt to eliminate the high fracture rate of glass-ionomer ART restorations. The self-etch composite resin multiple-surface ART restorations in primary molars were produced with hand instruments only and compared to self-etch composite resin restorations produced in the traditional way, using a handpiece. Unfortunately, the 2-year cumulative survival rates of both types of restorations were low, even lower than reported for comparable high-viscosity glass-ionomer ART restorations. The main reason why these self-etch composite resin restorations failed was complete loss of retention (76%).

Permanent dentition

Single-surface ART restorations placed in the permanent dentition have been compared to comparable amalgam,

but not to composite resin restorations. In a meta-analysis based on five studies, Frencken *et al.* (2004) concluded that there appears to be no difference in survival rates between single-surface ART restorations using glass-ionomer and amalgam restorations in permanent teeth over the first 3 years. Subsequently, a study with eight dentists followed restorations for over 6 years in children aged 6–9 years when the restorations were placed (Frencken *et al.*, 2006). The cumulative survival rates of single-surface ART restorations in posterior permanent teeth using high-viscosity glass-ionomer (69%) were statistically significant higher than those of comparable amalgam restorations (60%) at all years except the first (Fig. 23.9). This finding did not change if the relatively few multiple-surfaces ART and amalgam restorations were included. This study shows that, with respect to survival, the ART approach using high-viscosity glass-ionomers produces comparable restorations to the conventional approach using amalgam in posterior permanent teeth.

The same appears to be true for the management of carious cavities in root surfaces of elderly people. Lo *et al.* (2006) investigated the survival of restorations in mainly single-surface carious lesions produced through the ART approach using high-viscosity glass-ionomer and the conventional approach using resin-modified glass-ionomer in institutionalized elderly people in Hong Kong. The researchers reported no statistically significant difference between restorations of the ART (87%) and those of the conventional (91.7%) approach after 1 year.

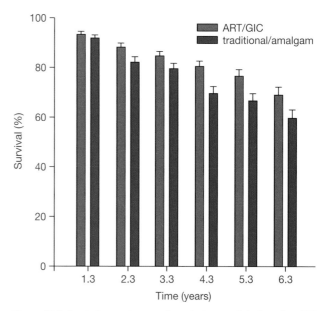

Figure 23.9 Survival percentages and standard error of single-surface ART restorations in posterior permanent teeth using high-viscosity glass-ionomer in comparison to comparable amalgam restorations over time. The difference in restoration survival between the two approaches was statistically significant each year from year 2.3 to 6.3.

Similarly to the comparison between ART and conventional approaches in primary teeth, there appears to be no difference in survival of restorations produced with the new caries management approach (ART) and that of the conventional approach (drill and fill). This result had not been expected when the ART approach was conceived in the 1980s. It shows, however, that the ART approach seems to be a realistic option if one wants to manage dental caries, whether in the dental surgery or in the field.

Causes of failure of ART restorations

ART restorations fail for the same reasons as restorations produced using other materials. Evaluation criteria aim to assess the mechanical condition of the restoration over time as well as the biological condition of the remaining tooth tissue. The mechanical condition is partly dependent on the physical properties of the restorative material and partly on its handling by the operator. The biological condition is largely dependent on the level of cleanliness (oral hygiene) of the restored tooth. Restorations can fail for more than one reason and this will be discussed in detail in Chapter 24.

The preceding text has shown that the survival of ART restorations in single surfaces in primary and permanent teeth is high, but that the survival of multiple-surface ART restorations in primary teeth needs to be improved. Contrary to expectations, recurrent or secondary caries alongside single-surface ART restorations in both primary (Lo & Holmgren, 2001; Lo et al., 2001; Taifour et al., 2002) and permanent teeth after 6 years was rarely observed: 2.4% (Mandari et al., 2003), 3.0% (Lo et al., 2007) and 2.3% (Frencken et al., 2007). These results have been obtained despite the concerns expressed by some critics of ART, who fear that any infected dentin inadvertently left behind in the cavity may lead to recurrence of caries. This fear is unfounded, since recurrent caries appears to be a relatively rare cause of failure of single-surface ART restorations in primary and permanent teeth. The main reported reason for the failure of single-surface ART restorations in primary and permanent teeth is dislodgment of the restoration or part of it (Frencken et al., 1998a, b, 2007; Taifour et al., 2002; Mandari et al., 2003; Lo et al., 2007). This is due to material and operator-related effects. Glass-ionomer material can become dislodged for a number of reasons:

- insufficient removal of caries
- improper mixing of the glass-ionomer powder/liquid
- level of humidity and temperature of mixing glass-ionomer
- incomplete filling of the cavity with hand-mixed glass-ionomer
- saliva and/or blood contamination
- insufficient or no conditioning of the cleaned tooth cavity
- level of co-operation of the child
- skill of the operator.

The effect of insufficient removal of caries was studied using bitewing radiographs (Mhaville et al., 2006). In Tanzania, three different cavity preparations were compared: hand instruments (ART), rotary handpiece and chemomechanical gel. There were no differences in radiologically detected caries beneath class II restorations in primary molars (Mhaville et al., 2006). After 3 years there were no differences in failure rates of these class II glass-ionomer restorations, with or without residual caries. Handling of the glass-ionomer may also influence restoration survival. According to manufacturers, the mixing time (hand-mix versions) of glass-ionomer restoration materials should be between 30 and 45 s, the application time about 90 s and finishing 5 min after starting the mixing. These instructions relate to a room temperature of 21–24°C and the humidity between 40 and 60%. However, the circumstances in which ART restorations have to be made are often quite different: under rather basic conditions, with temperatures much higher than 21°C and a humidity that can reach values of more than 90%.

Insufficient fracture toughness of the glass-ionomer in multiple-surface restorations is thought to be the reason for the high percentage of dislodgment of multiple-surface ART restorations in primary teeth (Lo & Holmgren, 2001; Lo et al., 2001; Taifour et al., 2002). Surprisingly, the level of surface wear of the various glass-ionomer materials used with ART over time was low (Ho et al., 1999; Lo et al., 2001, 2007) and was hardly considered a reason for failure. The effect of preparation size on the survival of class I ART restorations in posterior permanent teeth has also been considered a possible reason for failure. However, in only one of the three studies did small restorations survive better than large ones (Rahimtoola & van Amerongen, 2002; Lo et al., 2007; Frencken et al., 2007).

The operator appears to be a major factor in the survival of ART restorations in studies that have used four or more operators (Frencken et al., 1998a,b, 2007; Rahimtoola & van Amerongen, 2002; Taifour et al., 2003), showing one or more operators to perform worse than their colleagues. The operator effect seems to indicate that, to perform quality ART restorations, the dentists and dental therapists require skill, diligence and comprehension (Grossman & Mickenautsch, 2002), and to achieve these qualifications it is mandatory to follow an ART training course before applying ART in the field and clinic.

Integration of ART into oral health services

It should be realized that organized oral health care is available to only a relatively small proportion of the world's population. Following the development of ART over the years, a reliable caries-management approach has become available for use by a much larger segment of the population. However, the application of ART (a partly operative treatment) without paying attention to non-operative aspects of caries control would only be the work half done. The success of the ART approach led to the development of the Basic Package of Oral Care (BPOC) (Frencken et al., 2002). This package was developed at the WHO Collaborating Centre in Nijmegen and consists of three components:

- pain relief, through extracting non-repairable painful teeth; and other urgent treatment
- prevention of caries and gingivitis, through tooth brushing using affordable fluoride-containing toothpaste
- operative and caries-preventive management, through the use of the ART approach.

Together with oral health promotional activities, the BPOC has the potential to improve the oral health of many communities currently deprived of organized oral care, in a cost-effective manner. The potential of BPOC will be discussed in Chapter 32.

References

Ahovuo-Saloranta A, Hiiri A, Nordblad A, Worthington H, Mäkelä M. Pit and fissure sealants for preventing dental decay in the permanent teeth of children and adolescents (Cochrane Review). In: *The Cochrane Library*, Issue 4. Chichester: John Wiley & Sons, 2004.

Banerjee A, Kidd EAM, Watsen TF. *In vitro* evaluation of five alternative methods of carious dentine excavation. *Caries Res* 2000; **34**: 144–50.

Beiruti N, Frencken JE, van't Hof MA, Taifour D, van Palenstein Helderman WH. Caries-preventive effect of a one-time application of composite resin and glass-ionomer sealants after 5 years. *Caries Res* 2006a; **40**: 52–9.

Beiruti N, Frencken JE, Mulder J. Comparison between two glass-ionomer sealants placed using finger pressure (ART approach) and a ball burnisher. *Am Dent J* 2006b; **19**: 159–62.

Beiruti N, Frencken JE, van't Hof MA, van Palenstein Helderman WH. Caries preventive effect of resin-based and glass ionomer sealants over time: a systematic review. *Community Dent Oral Epidemiol* 2006c; **34**: 403–9.

van Bochove JA, van Amerongen WE. The influence of restorative treatment approaches and the use of local anaesthesia, on the children's discomfort. *Eur Arch Pediatr Dent* 2006; **7**: 11–16.

Bulut T, Sharif S. *Atraumatic restorative treatment in Nederland*. Dissertation, College of Dental Sciences, Nijmegen, 2004.

Burke FJ, McHugh S, Shaw L, Hosy MT, MacPerson L, Delargy S, Dopheide B. UK dentists' attitudes and behaviour towards atraumatic restorative treatment for primary teeth. *Br Dent J* 2005; **199**: 365–9.

Celiberti P, Francescut P, Lussi A. Performance of four dentine excavation methods in deciduous teeth. *Caries Res* 2006; **40**: 117–23.

Eden E, Topaloglu-Ak A, Frencken JE, van't Hof MA. Two-year survival of composite ART and traditional restorations. *Am J Dent* 2006; **19**: 359–63.

Ersin NK, Candan U, Aykut A, Oncag O, Eronat C, Kose T. A clinical evaluation of resin-based composite and glass ionomer cement restorations placed in primary teeth using the ART approach: results at 24 months. *J Am Dent Assoc* 2006; **137**: 1529–36.

Fédération Dentaire International. *FDI policy statement: Minimal intervention in the management of dental caries*. Ferney-Voltaire, France: FDI, 2002.

Frencken JE, Holmgren CJ. *Atraumatic restorative treatment for dental caries*. Nijmegen: STI Book BV, 1999.

Frencken JE, Holmgren CJ. *How to organize and run an ART training course*. Nijmegen: WHO Collaborating Centre of Oral Health Care Planning and Future Scenarios, 2000.

Frencken JE, Songpaisan Y, Phantumvanit P, Pilot T. An atraumatic restorative treatment (ART) technique: evaluation after one year. *Int Dent J* 1994; **44**: 460–4.

Frencken JE, Pilot T, Songpaisan Y, Phantumvanit P. Atraumatic restorative treatment (ART): rationale, technique and development. *J Public Health Dent* 1996; **56**: 135–40.

Frencken JE, Makoni F, Sithole WD, Hackenitz E. Three-year survival of one-surface ART restorations and glass-ionomer sealants in a school oral health programme in Zimbabwe. *Caries Res* 1998a; **32**: 119–26.

Frencken JE, Makoni F, Sithole WD. ART restorations and glass ionomer sealants in Zimbabwe: survival after 3 years. *Community Dent Oral Epidemiol* 1998b; **26**: 372–81.

Frencken JE, Holmgren CJ, van Palenstein Helderman WH. *Basic package of oral care*. Nijmegen: WHO Collaborating Centre for Oral Health Care Planning and Future Scenarios, 2002.

Frencken JE, van't Hof MA, van Amerongen WE, Holmgren CJ. Effectiveness of single-surface ART restorations in the permanent dentition: a meta-analysis. *J Dent Res* 2004; **83**: 120–3.

Frencken JE, Taifour D, van't Hof MA. Survival of ART and amalgam restorations in permanent teeth after 6.3 years. *J Dent Res* 2006; **85**: 622–6.

Frencken JE, van't Hof MA, Taifour D, Al-Zaher I. Effectiveness of the ART and traditional amalgam approach in restoring single-surface cavities in posterior teeth of permanent dentitions in school children after 6.3 years. *Community Dent Oral Epidemiol* 2007; **35**: 207–14.

Grossman ES, Mickenautsch S. Microscope observations of ART excavated cavities and restorations. *S Afr Dent J* 2002; **57**: 359–63.

Hickel R, Kaaden C, Paschos E, Buerkle V, Garcia-Godoy F, Manhart J. Longevity of occlusally-stressed restorations in posterior primary teeth. *Am J Dent* 2005; **18**: 198–211.

Ho TFT, Smales RJ, Fang DKS. A 2-year clinical study of two glass ionomer cements used in the atraumatic restorative treatment (ART) technique. *Community Dent Oral Epidemiol* 1999; **27**: 195–201.

van't Hof MA, Frencken JE, van Palenstein Helderman WH, Holmgren CJ. The ART approach for managing dental caries: a meta-analysis. *Int Dent J* 2006; **56**: 345–51.

Holmgren CJ, Lo ECM, Hu DY, Wan HC. ART restorations and sealants placed in Chinese school children – results after three years. *Community Dent Oral Epidemiol* 2000; **28**: 314–20.

Honkala E, Behbehani J, Ibricevic H, Kerosuo E, Al-Jame G. The atraumatic restorative treatment (ART) approach to restoring primary teeth in a standard dental clinic. *Int J Paediatr Dent* 2003; **13**: 172–9.

Inoue S, Abe Y, Yoshida Y, De Munck J, Sano H, Suzuki K, Lambrechts P, Van Meerbeek B. Effect of conditioner on bond strength of glass-ionomer adhesive to dentin/enamel with and without smear layer interposition. *Oper Dent* 2004; **29**: 685–92.

Lenters M, van Amerongen WE, Mandari GJ. Iatrogenic damage to the adjacent surfaces of primary molars in three different ways of cavity preparation. *Eur Arch Paediatr Dent* 2006; **7**: 6–10.

Levine RS, Pitts NB, Nugent Z. The fate of 1,587 unrestored carious deciduous teeth: a retrospective general dental practice based study from northern England. *Br Dent J* 2002; **193**: 99–103.

Lo ECM, Holmgren CJ. Provision of Atraumatic Restorative Treatment (ART) restorations to Chinese pre-school children – a 30 month evaluation. *Int J Paediatr Dent* 2001; **11**: 3–10.

Lo ECM, Luo Y, Fan MW, Wei SHY. Clinical investigation of two glass-ionomer restoratives used with the atraumatic restorative treatment approach in China: two-year results. *Caries Res* 2001; **35**: 458–63.

Lo ECM, Luo Y, Tan HP, Dyson JE, Corbet EF. ART and conventional root restorations in elders after 12 months. *J Dent Res* 2006; **85**: 929–32.

Lo ECM, Holmgren CJ, Hu D, Wan H, van Palenstein Helderman W. A six-year study of ART restorations placed in Chinese school children. *Community Dent Oral Epidemiol* 2007; **35**: 387–92.

Locker D, Jokovic A, Kay EJ. Prevention. Part 8: The use of pit and fissure sealants in preventing caries in the permanent dentition of children. *Br Dent J* 2003; **195**: 375–8.

Lussi A, Gygax M. Iatrogenic damage to adjacent teeth during classical approximal box preparation. *J Dent* 1998; **26**: 435–41.

McDonald SP, Sheiham A. A clinical comparison of non-traumatic methods of treating dental caries. *Int Dent J* 1994; **44**: 465–70.

Makoni F, Frencken JE, Sithole WD. Oral health status among secondary school students in Harare, Zimbabwe. *S Afr Dent J* 1997; **52**: 491–4.

Mandari GJ, Frencken JE, van't Hof MA. Six-year success rates of occlusal amalgam and glass-ionomer restorations placed using three minimal intervention approaches. *Caries Res* 2003; **37**: 246–53.

Manhart J, Chen HY, Hamm G, Hickel R. Review of the clinical survival of direct and indirect restorations in posterior teeth of the permanent dentition. *Oper Dent* 2004; **29**: 481–508.

Mhaville R, van Amerongen WE, Mandari G. Radiographic assessment of residual caries and marginal integrity after preparation in three different ways and restoration with hand mixed glass-ionomer. *Eur Arch Paediatr Dent* 2006; **7**: 81–4.

Mejàre I, Mjör IA. Glass ionomer and resin-based fissure sealants: a clinical study. *Scand J Dent Res* 1990; **98**: 345–50.

Mejàre I, Lingström P, Petersson LG, *et al.* Caries-preventive effect of fissure sealants: a systematic review. *Acta Odontol Scand* 2003; **61**: 321–30.

Moopnar M, Faulkner KD. Accidental damage to teeth adjacent to crown prepared abutment teeth. *Aust Dent J* 1991; **36**: 136–40.

Nadanovsky P, Cohen Carneiro F, Souza de Mello F. Removal of caries using only hand instruments: a comparison of mechanical and chemomechanical methods. *Caries Res* 2001; **35**: 384–9.

Övrebö RS, Raadal M. Microleakage in fissures sealed with resin or glass ionomer cement. *Scand J Dent Res* 1990; **98**: 66–9.

Papacchini F, Goracci C, Sadek FT, Monticelli F, Garcia-Godoy F, Ferrari M. Microtensile bond strength to ground enamel by glass-ionomers, resin-modified glass-ionomers, and resin composites used as pit and fissure sealants. *J Dent* 2005; **33**: 459–67.

Phantumvanit P, Songpaisan Y, Pilot T, Frencken JE. Atraumatic restorative treatment (ART). Survival of one-surface restorations in the permanent dentition. *J Public Health Dent* 1996; **56**: 141–5.

Qvist V, Johannessen L, Bruun M. Approximal caries in relation to iatrogenic preparation damage. *J Dent Res* 1992; **71**: 1370–3.

Rahimtoola S, van Amerongen E, Maher R, Groen H. Pain related to different ways of minimal intervention in the treatment of small caries lesions. *J Dent Child* 2000; **67**: 123–7.

Rahimtoola S, van Amerongen E. Comparison of two tooth saving preparation techniques for one surface cavities. *J Dent Child* 2002; **69**: 16–26.

Schriks MCM, van Amerongen WE. Atraumatic perspective of ART. Psychological and physiological aspects of treatment with and without rotary instruments. *Community Dent Oral Epidemiol* 2003; **31**: 15–20.

Seale NS, Casamassimo PS. Access to dental care for children in the United States. A survey of general practitioners. *J Am Dent Assoc* 2003; **134**: 1630–40.

Simonsen RJ. Pit and fissure sealants: review of the literature. *Pediatr Dent* 2002; **24**: 393–414.

Smales RJ, Fang DTS. *In vitro* effectiveness of hand excavation of caries with the ART technique. *Caries Res* 1999; **33**: 437–40.

Smales RJ, Gao W, Ho FT. *In vitro* evaluation of sealing pits and fissures with newer glass-ionomer cements developed for the ART technique. *J Clin Pediatr Dent* 1997; **21**: 321–3.

Smith AJE, Chimimba PD, Kalf-Scholte S, Bouma J. Clinical pilot study on new dental filling materials and preparation procedures in developing countries. *Community Dent Oral Epidemiol* 1990; **18**: 309–12.

Taifour D, Frencken JE, Beiruti N, van't Hof MA, Truin GJ. Effectiveness of glass-ionomer (ART) and amalgam restorations in the deciduous dentition – results after 3 years. *Caries Res* 2002; **36**: 437–44.

Taifour D, Frencken JE, Beiruti N, van't Hof MA, Truin GJ, van Palenstein Helderman WH. Comparison between restorations in the permanent dentition produced by hand and rotary instrumentation – survival after 3 years. *Community Dent Oral Epidemiol* 2003; **31**: 122–8.

Tickle M, Milson D, King D, Kearney-Mitchell P, Blinkhorn A. The fate of the carious primary teeth of children who regularly attend the general dental service. *Br Dent J* 2002; **192**: 219–23.

Torppa-Saarinen E, Seppä L. Short-term retention of glass-ionomer fissure sealants. *Proc Finn Dent Soc* 1990; **86**: 83–8.

Weerheijm KL, Kreulen CM, Gruythuisen RJ. Comparison of retentive qualities of two glass-ionomer cements used as fissure sealants. *J Dent Child* 1996; **63**: 265–7.

Williams B, Laxton L, Holt RD, Winter GB. Fissure sealants: a 4-year clinical trial comparing an experimental glass polyalkenoate cement with a bis glycidyl methacrylate resin used as fissure sealants. *Br Dent J* 1996; **180**: 104–8.

Yee R. An ART field study in western Nepal. *Int Dent J* 2001; **51**: 103–8.

24

Longevity of restorations: the 'death spiral'

V. Qvist

Introduction

From a cariological point of view the most important reason for placing restorations is to aid plaque control, and plaque control may be difficult or impossible if a caries lesion has progressed to the stage of a cavitated lesion (see Chapter 20 for further discussion of the role of operative treatment in caries control). Restorations are also undertaken for other reasons such as trauma, wear, erosion and aesthetic demands. Over the past few decades dental health has improved, and the number of restorations placed has declined in the industrialized part of the world, despite the fact that the number of teeth present has increased. However, millions of restorations are still inserted and replaced every year in deciduous and permanent teeth, placing an enormous burden on the resources of the national health-care systems.

Surveys on the reasons for the placement and replacement of restorations have been conducted in various countries. The data indicate that initial restorations, due to primary caries, account for 75–85% of all restorative caries treatment in primary and permanent teeth in children and adolescents (Qvist et al., 1990a, b; Friedl et al., 1994, 1995; Mjör et al., 2002; Forss & Widström, 2003). However, replacement of existing restorations accounts for 60–70% of the restorative interventions carried out in clinical practice on adults in Scandinavia, the UK and the USA (Qvist et al., 1990a, b; Friedl et al., 1994, 1995; Mjör et al., 2000a, b; Forss & Widström, 2004).

Evidence also suggests that the so-called permanent restorations are not permanent in the true sense of the term. Restorations have a limited lifetime and once a permanent tooth has been restored, the filling is likely to be replaced several times in the patient's lifetime in a 'restorative cycle' that eventually may lead to destruction of the tooth: the 'death spiral' (Elderton & Nuttall, 1983; Brantley et al., 1995).

Clinical assessment of restorations

It has been demonstrated that the treatment decisions made by clinicians are subject to a great deal of variation (Nuttall & Elderton, 1983; Bader & Shugars, 1995; Espelid et al., 2001). In clinical dental practice, decisions are often made subjectively with a lack of standardization, as there are no or few valid criteria to decide whether a restoration requires retreatment such as repair or replacement. It is difficult to distinguish between objective and subjective factors in the decision-making process, and it is possible that the subjective influence has a greater impact on longevity of restorations than the clinical properties and biocompatibility of the restorative materials. For example, the clinician may have the opinion that mercury in dental amalgam may be dangerous to the patient and therefore advocate replacement of well-functioning amalgam restorations even in patients who attend with no complaints; or another example: the same marginal discoloration may be interpreted as caries adjacent to a composite resin restoration but not next to a glass-ionomer restoration, owing to different expectations of the cariostatic potential of the restorative materials.

The criteria used for the evaluation of restoration failure vary widely among dentists and may not be explicit (Knibbs, 1997). It is therefore often difficult to determine whether a restoration was replaced because it actually failed, or because a clinician subjectively deemed it to have failed. For example, one clinician may decide to replace an old corroded and 'ditched' amalgam while another may repair or polish it. These important difficulties, and the inevitability of variation between dentists, are discussed further in Chapter 31.

The first standardized method for evaluating the clinical performance of restorations was developed in the 1960s by a Dane, Gunnar Ryge, through the United States Public Health Service (USPHS) (Cvar & Ryge, 1971, 2005). The USPHS system, still widely used today with modifications, bases the evaluation of restorations on three clinical judgments: clinically ideal, clinically acceptable and clinically unacceptable. These judgments are applied to characteristics generally associated with the deterioration process for a given type of restorative material, and each of these characteristics is discussed separately.

Tables 24.1 and 24.2 describe a new and updated modification of the USPHS system, which may be applied for detailed as well as overall clinical assessment of most dental restorations. The modification is based on present knowledge about demands on restorations and actual clinical manifestations of caries in relation to restorations and designated secondary or recurrent caries. The use of the assessment system is exemplified in Figs 24.1–24.4. The examples emphasize the importance of considering alternatives to replacement of restorations such as repair of localized defects, finishing of restorations with superficial staining, smoothing and sealing restorations with marginal discrepancies and staining, and the mere monitoring of defects to examine their progression and sequelae. These simple measures may significantly increase the longevity of restorations and save tooth substance, which is inevitably lost when restorations are replaced (Mjör, 1993; Blum et al., 2003; Gordan et al., 2003). Furthermore, the examples point out the patient's right to participate in decisions where several different treatments are considered professionally justifiable.

Assessment of restoration longevity

The longevity of restorations may be registered in prospective or retrospective longitudinal studies, or it may be assessed in cross-sectional surveys, based on retrospective

Table 24.1 Clinical assessment of restorations

Assessment	Explanation	Intervention
Optimal	The restoration protects the tooth and the surrounding tissues and meets aesthetic demands	None
Acceptable	The restoration exhibits one or more features which deviate from ideal functional and aesthetic conditions, but it protects the tooth and the surrounding tissues	None – *or* Observe – *or* Implement preventive measures – *or* Repair sooner or later
Not acceptable	Aesthetics are obviously compromised or the restoration does not protect the tooth and/or the surrounding tissues. Damage is likely to occur	Observe – *or* Implement preventive measures – *or* Repair sooner or later – *or* Replace sooner or later
Not acceptable	The restoration does not protect the tooth and/or the surrounding tissues. Damage is occurring	Repair immediately – *or* Replace immediately

Modified from Cvar & Ryge (1971, 2005).

Table 24.2 Criteria for clinical assessment of restorations

Category	Assessment	Criteria
Secondary/recurrent caries	Optimal	No evidence of caries contiguous with the margin of the restoration or beyond the restoration
	Acceptable	Evidence of superficial and/or inactive caries, no operative treatment necessary. Preventive measure may be indicated
	Not acceptable	Evidence of deep and/or active caries with cavitation. Preventive measures or operative treatment is indicated
Color match/surface discoloration (tooth-colored restorations)	Optimal	The restoration matches the color, shade and translucency of adjacent tooth tissues
	Acceptable	Slight mismatch in colour, shade or translucency
	Not acceptable	Obvious mismatch outside the normal range of tooth color, shades or translucency
Marginal discoloration	Optimal	No discoloration at the junction of the tooth tissues and the restoration
	Acceptable	Slight superficial or localized marginal staining
	Not acceptable	Obvious deep or extended marginal staining
Marginal integrity	Optimal	No evidence of discrepancies or crevice at the junction of the tooth tissue and the restoration
	Acceptable	Minor or localized marginal discrepancies or crevice
	Not acceptable	Obvious deep or extended marginal discrepancies or crevice and/or mobile or missing restoration
Fracture of restoration or tooth	Optimal	No evidence of surface cracks or fracture of restoration. No evidence of dentinal cracks
	Acceptable	Superficial cracks or minor fractures of restoration or tooth tissues
	Not acceptable	Major fracture of restoration or tooth tissues. Restoration is missing completely or partially, or contact is faulty, or occlusion is affected
Morphology/wear of restoration	Optimal	Restoration restores missing tooth tissues, function and aesthetic
	Acceptable	Morphology compromises plaque removal or aesthetic demands; occlusal or proximal contact is faulty
	Not acceptable	Morphology prevents plaque removal, allows food impaction, overeruption or tooth drifting, or does not meet aesthetic demands
Pulpal complications	Optimal	No dentinal hypersensitivity or pulp pain
	Acceptable	Transient hypersensitivity or pulp pain of minor intensity
	Not acceptable	Frequent or sustained hypersensitivity or moderate/intense pulp pain

Modified from Cvar & Ryge (1971, 2005).

data from dental records, provided records are available to document the complete treatment performed over many years.

The classical longitudinal, randomized controlled trial (RCT) comes close to the ideal test conditions and meets the demands for evidence-based dentistry (Chadwick *et al.*, 2001; Qvist, 2002). The RCT study design has the following characteristics:

- randomised allocation to test and control groups
- 'blinding' of patient as well as therapist if possible
- limited number of restorations of each material or method
- selection of suitable patients and treatments
- treatments and controls performed by one or a few calibrated and skilled clinicians.
- optimal clinical conditions

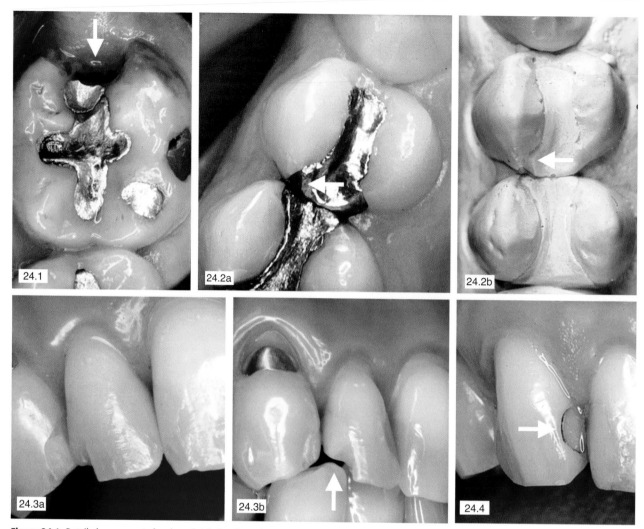

Figure 24.1 *Detailed assessment of occluso-distal, class II amalgam restoration in the lower second molar*: the 28-year-old male patient complains of occasional pain from the region. Fracture and loss of distal part of restoration. Probably minor fracture of disto-lingual cusp, too. Plaque-covered active caries in the cavity. Gingivitis in adjacent gingiva. *Overall assessment and intervention*: damage is occurring in the tooth and the surrounding tissues. The restoration is not acceptable. Replace restoration immediately.

Figure 24.2 *Detailed assessment of occluso-distal, class II amalgam restoration in the first upper premolar [clinical photograph (a) and plaster model (b)]*: minor fracture of buccal part of marginal ridge. No evidence of plaque or caries in the cavity. No evidence of gingivitis in adjacent papilla. No complaints of pain or food impaction. *Overall assessment and intervention*: there is no damage in tooth or surrounding tissues. The restoration is acceptable. No intervention needed.

Figure 24.3 *Detailed assessment of 2-year-old, distal, class III composite resin restoration in the upper lateral (a)*: fracture of disto-incisal corner of the tooth beneath otherwise optimal restoration. *Overall assessment and intervention*: the restoration is not acceptable. Repair or replace restoration sooner or later. However, the 46-year-old female patient did not want the restoration to be repaired. She attended 4 years later with the same unrepaired but now worn restoration, which she still did not want to be repaired. The photograph (b) illustrates that restoration of the incisal tooth fracture would require the reduction of the incisal edge of the lower canine to protect the class IV restoration against fracture and/or loss during occlusion/articulation.

Figure 24.4 *Detailed assessment of 12-year-old, mesial, class III composite resin restoration in the upper canine*: obvious deep and extended marginal staining along the periphery of the restoration. No evidence of secondary or recurrent caries. *Overall assessment and intervention*: the restoration is objectively acceptable. However, the patient may find the restoration not acceptable and in that case it will have to be replaced sooner or later.

- standardized control intervals
- detailed assessments of the quality of the restorations according to well-defined criteria.

In general, the results show what can be obtained with the tested materials and methods under optimal conditions. In other words, they provide dental professionals with the 'gold standard', with which they can compare their everyday results. This is essential for the continuing development of materials and methods. However, it is unrealistic to expect RCT investigations to exceed 10 years, although the requirement for restoration longevity in the permanent dentition may be many times longer to obtain lifelong durability. The reliability of the results may also be contested because the results are based on a few dentists' handling of materials and methods as well as the characteristics of a selected group of patients, and may be challenged by patient drop-outs. When restorative treatment in the primary dentition is studied, another inevitable problem is the high percentage of observations lost at follow-up because of exfoliation of teeth. This makes the presentation and comparison of absolute failure rates questionable. Furthermore, control groups are not always included in longitudinal studies, and the clinical performance of the restorations, therefore, cannot be directly compared with that of another material used for similar purpose. The results of such studies tend to be overoptimistic, especially if manufacturers have directly supported the research.

Contrary to the RCT studies, the practice-based, longitudinal and cross-sectional studies normally have the following characteristics:

- large number of restorations performed without randomization or blinding
- inclusion of all patients in need of treatment
- large number of clinicians with varying clinical experience and skills
- no calibration of clinicians to minimize discrepancy in decision making
- routine daily clinical treatment conditions
- individual follow-ups
- simple assessments of restorations, focussing on the need for repair or replacement.

The lack of randomization and uniform, fixed criteria for decisions to place and replace restorations complicate the studies and the interpretation of the results. Nevertheless, if the clinicians, the patients and the treatments are representative of the actual population, the results from practice-based, longitudinal and cross-sectional studies are of great value because they reflect current dental practice, including the considerable variation in dentists' clinical decision making. In fact, they show what can be expected in daily routine clinical use, although it is likely that the age data in cross-sectional surveys is lacking for 30–40% of the restorations, which probably includes the oldest of the failed restorations (Chadwick *et al.*, 2001; Qvist, 2002; Burke, 2005).

When considering the disparities in the two study designs and their consequences for the results, it is understandable that measurements of restoration longevity are usually shorter in practice-based studies than in RCT studies. It is therefore important to realize that reliable comparisons of the absolute failure rates of different types of restoration presuppose the same study design, although the relative failure rates may be rather independent of the type of study.

The amalgam debate and its consequences for restoration longevity

Until the 1990s, amalgam was the worldwide, all-round material of choice for posterior restorations in primary and permanent teeth. However, changes have occurred for several reasons. The development of alternative tooth-colored restorative materials and the controversy over the potential side-effects of amalgam have had an influence on the selection of restorative materials. The dramatic reduction in caries over recent decades, along with the increased affluence and welfare systems in the industrialized world, has called for treatment with materials other than amalgam.

With a reduced need for operative treatment of caries, the costs of the individual restorations may be relatively less important for the patient and for public dental health-care services as well. Over the past two decades the environmental and health authorities in Scandinavia and a number of other countries have, furthermore, placed increasing pressure on dentists to reduce the use of dental amalgam. The intention is to protect the environment and hence the population from the heavy-metal mercury, and perhaps it is also a response to the emotional debate on the possible injurious effects of amalgam. This has been a debate that has continued in the media without scientific support, in defiance of the fact that health authorities on a worldwide basis confirm that dental amalgam restorations are safe and effective (Danish Environmental Protection Agency, 1987; NHI, 1992; WHO, 1997; Norwegian Board of Health, 1999; Swedish Medical Research Council, 1999).

The result has been a marked phasing-out of the use of dental amalgam, particularly for fillings in primary teeth, but also for fillings in permanent teeth, as illustrated in Fig. 24.5. Since 1992, the altered treatment patterns have been followed up by recommendations and even requirements from

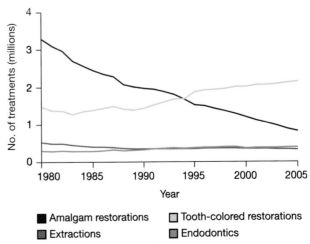

Figure 24.5 Annual number of amalgam restorations, tooth-colored restorations, endodontic treatments and extractions performed in adults in general dental practice in Denmark from 1980 to 2005 (Danish National Health Insurance).

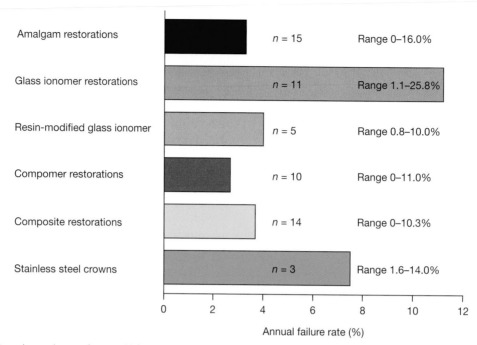

Figure 24.6 Median values and ranges for annual failure rates obtained in longitudinal studies of class I/II restorations in posterior primary teeth using different types of restorative materials. The number of studies (*n*) is given for each material. (Based on Hickel *et al.*, 2005.)

health authorities in some countries not to use amalgam in children below 6 years of age (Germany), not to use amalgam in children and adolescents (Finland, Norway and Sweden), and to limit the use of amalgam to restorations in permanent premolar and molar teeth, where the filling is worn (Denmark). Dentists and authorities have focussed directly and indirectly on the primary dentition because children may potentially be more vulnerable to toxic exposure and because the demands on the clinical properties of the materials and the longevity of the fillings are less here than in the permanent dentition (Bellinger *et al.*, 2006; DeRouen *et al.*, 2006). Although the maximal lifespan for a restoration in a primary tooth is around 8 years, the restorations are usually needed to serve for only 5–6 years, with a median of 2^1/$_2$ years (Qvist *et al.*, 2004a).

Alterations in dental restorative treatment patterns affect the measurements of longevity, especially in cross-sectional studies. As only the age of the failed and replaced fillings is recorded, longevity data on improved and newly introduced materials, such as the whole range of tooth-colored materials, will be encumbered with uncertainty and will probably be too short. In contrast, data on restorative materials or techniques on the decline, such as amalgam, will be relatively too long.

Longevity of restorations in the primary dentition

In the few cross-sectional surveys that include primary teeth, the median longevity of failed and replaced amalgam fill-

ings is only 2–3 years, and this period is even shorter for tooth-colored fillings (Qvist *et al.*, 1990a, b; Friedl *et al.*, 1994, 1995; Mjör *et al.*, 2002; Forss & Widström, 2003). These measurements may, however, be misleadingly short because the majority of restorations inserted in primary teeth will be well functioning until the time for exfoliation and because data on the 20–30% of failed restorations are truncated, owing to the shedding of the teeth. The surveys further indicate that the most frequent reasons for retreatment of restored primary teeth are primary caries in unrestored parts of the teeth, and secondary or recurrent caries in relation to the fillings, although many restorations also fail because of bulk fracture and loss of retention.

Longitudinal studies of posterior restorations in primary teeth have recently been reviewed by Hickel *et al.* (2005). The review includes 57 studies with an observation period of at least 2 years, published from 1971 to 2002/2003. The range and median values obtained for annual failure rates for class I/II restorations in different restorative materials and for stainless steel crowns are given in Fig. 24.6 together with the number of studies incorporated in the calculations. The great disparity in the results for restorations in a given type of material (i.e. the large ranges) is caused by variations in the detailed study design, inclusion criteria, observation period, statement of results, and so on. The disparity and the skewed distribution of the results compromise the reliability of comparisons among different materials and different studies. One way to overcome this problem is to focus on the median failure rates from all studies on a treatment, and by so doing it becomes obvious that posterior restorations in amalgam, composite resin, compomer and resin-modified glass-ionomer have an increased longevity compared with conventional glass-ionomer restorations and stainless steel crowns.

Over the past decade a multicenter project has been carried out in Denmark, aiming to provide a realistic basis for estimation of the consequences for the Danish Public Dental Health Service (PDHS) of using amalgam and alternative restorative materials for restorations in the primary dentition (Qvist *et al.*, 2004a–c). It comprises three longitudinal, prospective and randomized studies with a design that otherwise resembled the design described above for practice-based, longitudinal and cross-sectional studies. The studies include more than 3600 restorations in amalgam, conventional glass-ionomer, resin-modified glass-ionomer, and compomer made in the primary teeth of more than 2200 children and adolescents by 32 PDHS clinicians in everyday practice. The requirements for additional treatment of the restored primary teeth before exfoliation, as well as the need for operative caries treatment of some 2100 adjacent unrestored surfaces in primary and permanent teeth in contact with the restorations, have been assessed.

In accordance with other studies, high frequencies of bulk fractures and loss of retention of class II and even class I conventional glass-ionomer restorations were recorded in the first study in the project (Qvist *et al.*, 2004a; Hickel *et al.*, 2005). This resulted in a two-fold failure rate for restorations in conventional glass-ionomer compared with amalgam, and a $3^1/_2$ year median survival time for restorations in all cavity types in conventional glass-ionomer, versus $6^1/_2$ years for amalgam (Fig. 24.7). The type of restoration

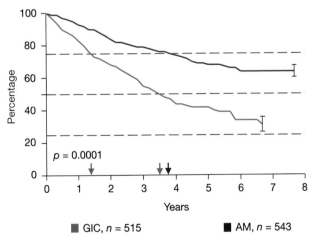

Figure 24.7 Cumulative survival distribution of 515 conventional glass-ionomer (GIC) and 543 amalgam restorations in all cavity types. The curves are drawn as long as at least 10 restorations remained in function. The points at which the curves cross the horizontal, quartile lines are indicated by arrows on the abscissa. It appears that the median or 50% longevity for GIC restorations was $3^1/_2$ years, while more than 75% of the amalgam restorations would still be in function at that time, provided that the teeth have not been exfoliated before then. The difference is highly significant ($p = 0.0001$). The vertical bars represent standard errors of the survival rates (Qvist *et al.*, 2004a).

also influenced the frequencies of retreatments, with by far the shortest longevity for class II restorations in both materials. This is important, as approximately 80% of all restorations in the primary dentition are class II restorations, while only 15% are class I, and 5% are class III and V restorations (Qvist *et al.*, 2004a, b).

The better fracture toughness and wear resistance of resin-modified glass-ionomer cement and polyacid-modified composite resin (compomer), compared with conventional glass-ionomer, were reflected in the findings from early clinical studies, including the second and third parts of the project (Qvist *et al.*, 2004b, c; Hickel *et al.*, 2005). The frequencies of retreatments of teeth filled with the new materials were around 20% for class II restorations, almost the same as for teeth restored with amalgam. Endodontic complication was a major reason for failures of restorations in all restorative materials. This appeared to be a consequence of the inclusion of pulp-capped and pulpotomized teeth in the project. The other major reasons for failure were fracture of the restoration, loss of retention, and degradation and wear. It should be noted that primary and recurrent caries seldom resulted in replacement of restorations, and this finding is in contrast to the results from cross-sectional surveys (Qvist *et al.*, 1990a, b; Friedl *et al.*, 1994, 1995; Mjör *et al.*, 2002; Forss & Widström, 2003). The reasons may be the generally low caries activity in the population studied, along with the numerous class II restorations in the Danish project, as class II restorations seldom fail owing to primary or recurrent caries, but often fail because of fracture of the restoration or tooth.

The median survival times for class II restorations in the resin-modified glass-ionomer cements and the compomers included in the studies all exceeded 5 years, and the 3-year survival rates were almost twice those for conventional glass-ionomers and even higher than for amalgam restorations (Fig. 24.8). However, Fig. 24.8 also shows that the individual clinicians obtained their best result, i.e. their highest survival rates, with different types of restorative materials (Qvist *et al.*, 2004a–c).

Longevity of restorations in the permanent dentition

Another recent survey by Manhart *et al.* (2004) reviewed a large number of longitudinal studies of posterior restorations in permanent teeth performed since 1990 with an observation period of at least 2 years. The longevity of class I/II direct and indirect restorations is illustrated in Fig. 24.9 by the range and median values of the annual failure rates for different types of restorations. The results from different studies on the same restorative material diverge as much as the corresponding results from studies in primary teeth (Fig. 24.6). However, it is notable that the relative longevity of restorations in various materials resembles that for the

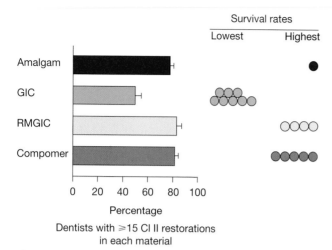

Figure 24.8 Bar graph showing 3-year survival rates (mean, SE) for class II restorations made in amalgam, conventional glass-ionomer (GIC), resin-modified glass-ionomer (RMGIC) and compomer by eight dentists with at least 15 restorations in each type of material. The figure also illustrates that GIC resulted in the lowest 3-year survival rate for all eight dentists, while one dentist received the highest 3-year survival rate with amalgam, two with RMGIC and three with compomer, and two dentists achieved equally superior results with RMGIC and compomer (Qvist *et al.*, 2004a–c).

same type of restorations in primary teeth, although the longevity generally is increased in the permanent dentition. So, the median annual failure rates for posterior restorations in permanent versus primary teeth were 1.5% versus 3.3% for amalgam, 2.0% versus 3.7% for direct composite resin, and 8.8% versus 11.2% for conventional glass-ionomer, respectively (Figs 24.6, 24.9). With these failure rates, it will, in theory, be around 67 years until all posterior amalgam restorations in permanent teeth had failed, compared with 50 years for composite resin restorations and

11 years for glass-ionomer restorations. Although these calculations appear somewhat unrealistic, they indicate the significance of differences in annual failure rates, and give a measure of comparison between materials.

On the basis of the failure rates shown in Fig. 24.9, it may be concluded that indirect composite restorations are not superior to direct composite restorations, and that computer-aided design/manufacture (CAD/CAM) and laboratory manufactured ceramic inlays/onlays have a longevity that approaches that for cast gold and metal–ceramic restorations. Furthermore, it is evident that conventional glass-ionomer is not appropriate for either class I/II or tunnel restorations in permanent teeth, because of wear and bulk fracture of the stress-bearing restorations, fracture of the marginal ridge and recurrent caries of the tunnel restorations.

During the past two decades numerous cross-sectional surveys on restorative treatment behaviors in the permanent dentition have been carried out (Qvist *et al.*, 1990a, b; Friedl *et al.*, 1994, 1995; Mjör *et al.*, 2000a, b; Forss & Widström, 2004). In accordance with longitudinal studies, the surveys clearly point out that resin restorations have a shorter longevity than amalgam restorations in general practice, irrespective of the type of the restoration (Fig. 24.10). However, there has been a gradual increase in the longevity of especially class I and II resin restorations, for which the median age of replaced restorations has doubled from around 3 years in a Danish survey from 1990 (Qvist *et al.*, 1990b) to around 6 years in a recent Norwegian survey (Fig. 24.10) (Mjör *et al.*, 2000a). The increment reflects the development of particular resin materials for stress-bearing restorations with better wear resistance and higher fracture toughness, along with new bonding agents, which have enhanced the marginal adaptation of the restorations. Still,

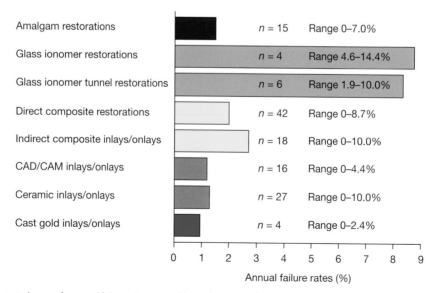

Figure 24.9 Median values and ranges for annual failure rates obtained in longitudinal studies of class I/II restorations in posterior permanent teeth using different types of restorative materials. The number of studies (*n*) is given for each material. (Based on Manhart *et al.*, 2004.)

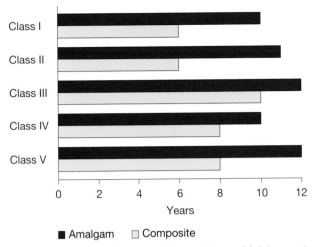

Figure 24.10 Bar graph showing median recorded age of failed composite resin and amalgam restorations in adults in relation to type of restoration. (Based on Mjör *et al.*, 2000a.)

however, recurrent caries and fracture of restorations are major reasons for replacement of direct as well as indirect posterior resin restorations, while occlusal and interproximal wear has diminished significantly. The clinical diagnosis of recurrent caries was the most common reason for replacement of amalgam and even glass-ionomer restorations in all cavity types in the Norwegian survey (Mjör *et al.*, 2000b).

Most practice-based, cross-sectional surveys have recorded the age of restorations at the time they were replaced, whereas few studies have recorded the age of restorations *in situ*, i.e. the age of restorations that have not failed (Jokstad *et al.*, 1994). It appears that the age distributions are similar for failed and acceptable restorations *in situ*, suggesting the validity of using median age of failed restorations as a criterion for restoration performance in practice-based studies, even though patient treatment records often do not extend back to the date of restoration placement.

Factors influencing restoration longevity

Several factors affect the longevity of restorations, including the type and size of the restoration, the type and brand of the restorative material, along with the restorative technique applied, and the quality of the restoration at the time of insertion, together with the dentition, the age of the patient, oral hygiene, the caries activity and the extent to which the patient maintains regular recall appointments in the same dental practice (Letzel *et al.*, 1997; Manhart *et al.* 2004; Hickel *et al.*, 2005). The age of restorations at replacement is, moreover, dependent on the criteria for failure, which vary markedly in general practice. This is especially the case for recurrent caries, because it is clinically difficult to differentiate between discolored marginal discrepancies and active caries lesions (Kidd *et al.*, 1995; Özer, 1997; Mjör & Toffenetti, 2000). The reader should note that in Chapter 20 it is suggested that a cavitated caries lesion, at the margin of the restoration, which cannot be cleaned, is the indication for repairing or replacing a restoration.

The type of failure also influences the longevity in another way (Fig. 24.11). Most failures occur some time after the restorations have been inserted. They are a result of:

- gradual development of recurrent caries
- physical defects such as discoloration of the restoration
- degradation, such as marginal breakdown, 'ditching' or 'chipping'

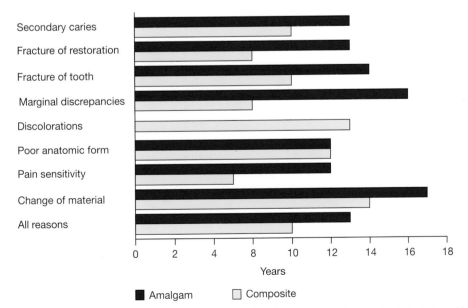

Figure 24.11 Bar graph showing median recorded age of failed composite resin and amalgam restorations in adults in relation to type of failure. (Based on Mjör *et al.*, 2000a.)

Variable	Failures at all	Fracture restoration	Loss of retention	Endodontic complications
Restorative material	★			
Restorative method	★	★		
First-time restoration/replacement	★	★		
Location of restoration: jaw	★			
Location of restoration: tooth				
Location of restoration: surface				★
Base material				
Endodontic treatment of tooth	★			★
Treatment problems				
Age of children	★	★		★
Caries experience at 5 years				
Clinician	★	★	★	★

★ $p < 0.05$.

Figure 24.12 Variables of significance for survival of restorations in the primary dentition and occurrence of the three most frequent types of failure, i.e. bulk fracture of restoration, loss of retention and endodontic complications. (Based on Qvist *et al.*, 2004a–c.)

- continuous detrimental damage to the pulp due to bacterial leakage.

Other failures occur shortly after the restoration is placed, such as:

- bulk fracture due to inadequate dimensions of the restoration or because the occlusion has not been adjusted properly
- loss of restoration due to lack of retention of the restorative material
- pulp complications due to preparation damage, chemical injuries from restorative materials in deep cavities or even pulp capping, regardless of whether it is properly treated or overlooked.

In the above-mentioned Danish project, multivariate survival analyses were used to find the factors that significantly affect restoration failures in the primary dentition (Qvist *et al.*, 2004a–c). Figure 24.12 summarizes the results of the analyses for the important class II restorations for all types of failure and for the three most frequent types, which were bulk fracture, loss of retention and endodontic complications. It is evident that numerous factors related to the patient as well as the treatment, the materials and methods, and the clinician are all decisive for the success of restorative treatments. For example, the risk of failure diminished with increasing age of the child, it was lower for first time than for replacement restorations, and lower for restorations placed in teeth with sound pulps compared with endodontically treated teeth. Furthermore, conventional glass-ionomer showed a higher risk of failure than amalgam and newer restorative materials, and cavity conditioning might further reduce the failure rates for these materials. The significance of the variation among clinicians was

highlighted in the statistical results of the Danish project and has also been shown in a few other investigations on the outcome of dental restorative treatments in primary as well as permanent teeth (Manhart *et al.*, 2004; Hickel *et al.*, 2005). The analyses showed that clinicians using various materials achieve the highest survival rate with one particular material, which may differ from clinician to clinician. Often, the clinicians will not be aware of such differences. Computer-aided evaluations of longevity results may be a valuable tool in the near future. These may help the individual clinician to select optimal restorative materials and

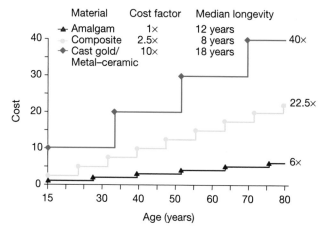

Figure 24.13 Cumulative cost of restorative treatment using amalgam, composite resin or cast gold/ceramic for two- or three-surfaced posterior restorations over a 65-year period. The calculations are based on actual Danish costs: 1× for amalgam restorations, 2.5× for composite and 8× for gold/metal–ceramic restorations, and today's expectations as to the median longevity of the different types of restorations: 8 years for composite, 12 years for amalgam and 18 years for gold/metal–ceramic.

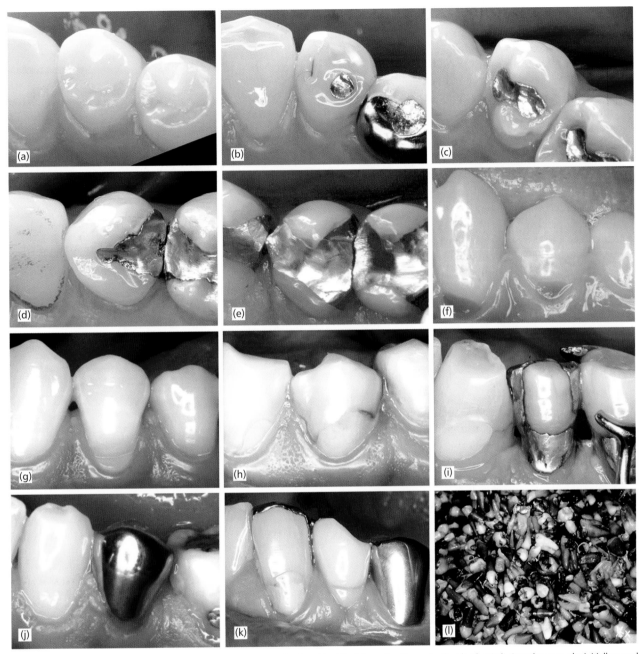

Figure 24.14 Illustration of the detrimental long-term consequences for dental health of the restorative cycle: the 'death spiral'. Over the years, the initially sound first lower premolar (a) has been restored with a localized (b) and then an extended occlusal amalgam restoration (c), a two-surfaced (d) and a three-surfaced occluso-proximal amalgam restoration (e), and because of gingival caries (f) or abrasion (g) a facial composite (h) and amalgam restoration (i), a cast gold crown (j) and eventually a bridge has been made (k) after extraction of the premolar (l).

methods for their specific patient population. They may also help to diminish the clinician's specific restorative shortcomings.

Consequences of restoration longevity for dental health and cost

The cost of restorative therapy, using various materials, differs not only when the tooth is restored, but also over time

owing to differences in longevity (Mjör, 1992; Roulet, 1997; Sjögren & Halling, 2002). Figure 24.13 illustrates the long-term costs for two- and three-surfaced posterior restorations made in the contemporary, improved, composite resin, amalgam and gold/metal–ceramic. The costs are based on updated expectations of the median longevities and actual Danish cost for restorations in the different materials. Over a 65-year period, from 15 to 80 years of age, the cumulative cost of composite restorations would be about 3.5 times that of amalgam restorations, while the similar small gold/metal–ceramic restorations would cost about 6.5 times more than the amalgam restorations.

However, the calculations are unrealistic in the way that they presuppose new restorations to be performed of the same size as the restorations they replace. Successive direct and indirect restorations tend to enlarge the cavity, leading to an increased risk of subsequent tooth fracture (Brantley et al., 1995). Therefore, replacement restorations are likely to be larger, more complex and sometimes more expensive than the initial restorations. Consequently, they may have a shorter longevity and can have an injurious effect on the pulp, occasionally leading to endodontic treatment, involving further expenses. Restorative treatments may, furthermore, involve a risk of iatrogenic damage on adjacent tooth surfaces, which itself will compromise dental health as it often results in caries development and progression (Qvist et al., 1992; Medeiros & Seddon, 2000).

The possible detrimental long-term consequences for the dental health of the 'restorative cycle' or 'the death spiral' are illustrated in the first premolar in the lower jaw in Fig. 24.14.

Concluding remarks

Restorations may be needed to replace lost and defective tissues (see Chapter 20). However, restorations per se will not 'treat away' caries. They have a limited lifetime and most restorations fail owing to clinically diagnosed recurrent caries. The longevity, side-effects, aesthetics and economics of dental restorations are the most important parameters for dentists and patients in the choice of restorative materials (Widström et al., 1992; Forss & Widström, 1996; Burke, 2004; Espelid et al., 2006). Measurements of the longevity of restorations reflect all conditions that affect the restoration from the day of insertion until failure occurs. The longevity of restorations and the cost of placing/replacing restorations are two decisive factors determining the long-term expenses of restorative therapy.

Once a permanent tooth has been restored, the filling is likely to be replaced several times in the patient's life, and repeated replacements of restorations may compromise the survival of the tooth itself, and thus the dental health of the patient. It is therefore important to ensure that a tooth surface is not restored until it is obvious that arrest of the disease is unlikely. Furthermore, it is important to consider all possibilities to prolong the durability of restorations through optimal choice and use of restorative materials, prevention of recurrent disease and improved clinical diagnostics of restoration quality, including minor corrections and repair to postpone replacements.

References

Bader JD, Shugars DA. Variation in dentists' clinical decisions. *J Public Health Dent* 1995; **55**: 181–8.

Bellinger DC, Trachtenberg F, Barregard L, et al. Neuropsychological and renal effects of dental amalgam in children. A randomized clinical trial. *J Am Med Assoc* 2006; **295**: 1775–83.

Blum IR, Mjör IA, Schriever A, Heidemann D, Wilson NFH. Defective direct composite restorations – replace or repair? A survey of teaching in Scandinavian dental schools. *Swed Dent J* 2003; **27**: 99–104.

Brantley CF, Bader JD, Shugars DA, Nesbit SP. Does the cycle of rerestoration lead to larger restorations? *J Am Dent Assoc* 1995; **126**: 1407–13.

Burke FJ. Amalgam to tooth-coloured materials – implications for clinical practice and dental education: governmental restrictions and amalgam-usage survey results. *J Dent* 2004; **32**: 343–50.

Burke FJ. Evaluating restorative materials and procedures in dental practice. *Adv Dent Res* 2005; **18**: 46–9.

Chadwick BL, Dummer PMH, Dunstan F, et al. *The longevity of dental restorations. A systematic review.* York: NHS Centre for Reviews and Dissemination, University of York, 2001.

Cvar JF, Ryge G. *Criteria for the clinical evaluation of dental restorative materials.* USPHS Publication No. 790-244. San Francisco, CA: US Goverment Printing Office, 1971.

Cvar JF, Ryge G. Reprint of criteria for the clinical evaluation of dental restorative materials. 1971. *Clin Oral Investig* 2005; **9**: 215–32.

Danish Environmental Protection Agency. *Statement of mercury. Use – contamination – proposals for solution.* Copenhagen: Notex – Grafisk Service Center, 1987.

Danish National Health Insurance: *Database on dental service patterns in Denmark from 1980 to 2005.* Unpublished statistical data from the Danish Dental Association.

DeRouen TA, Martin MD, Leroux BG, et al. Neurobehavioral effects of dental amalgam in children: a randomized clinical trial. *J Am Med Assoc* 2006; **295**: 1784–92.

Elderton RJ, Nuttall NM. Variation among dentists in planning treatment. *Br Dent J* 1983; **154**: 201–6.

Espelid I, Tveit AB, Mejare I, Sundberg H, Hallonsten AL. Restorative treatment decisions on occlusal caries in Scandinavia. *Acta Odontol Scand* 2001; **59**: 21–7.

Espelid I, Cairns J, Askildsen JE, Qvist V, Gaarden T, Tveit, AB. Preferences over dental restorative materials among young patients and dental professionals. *Eur J Oral Sci* 2006; **114**: 15–21.

Forss H, Widström E. Factors influencing the selection of restorative materials in dental care in Finland. *J Dent* 1996; **24**: 257–62.

Forss H, Widström E. The post-amalgam era: a selection of materials and their longevity in the primary and young permanent dentitions. *Int J Paediatr Dent* 2003; **13**: 158–64.

Forss H, Widström E. Reasons for restorative therapy and the longevity of restorations in adults. *Acta Odontol Scand* 2004; **62**: 82–6.

Friedl KH, Hiller KA, Schmalz G. Placement and replacement of amalgam restorations in Germany. *Oper Dent* 1994; **19**: 228–32.

Friedl KH, Hiller KA, Schmalz G. Placement and replacement of composite restorations in Germany. *Oper Dent* 1995; **20**: 34–8.

Gordan VV, Mjör IA, Blum IR, Wilson NHF. Teaching students the repair of resin based composite restorations: a survey of North American dental schools. *J Am Dent Assoc* 2003; **134**: 317–23.

Hickel R, Kaaden C, Paschos E, Buerkle V, García-Godoy F, Manhart J. Longevity of occlusally-stressed restorations in posterior primary teeth. *Am J Dent* 2005; **18**: 198–211.

Jokstad A, Mjör IA, Qvist V. The age of restorations *in situ. Acta Odontol Scand* 1994; **52**: 234–42.

Kidd EAM, Joyston-Bechal S, Beighton D. Marginal staining and ditching as a predictor of secondary caries around amalgam restorations: a clinical and microbiological study. *J Dent Res* 1995; **74**: 1206–11.

Knibbs PJ. Methods of clinical evaluation of dental restorative materials. *J Oral Rehabil* 1997; **24**: 109–23.

Letzel H, van't Hof MA, Marshall GW, Marshall SJ. The influence of the amalgam alloy on the survival of amalgam restorations: a secondary analysis of multiple controlled clinical trials. *J Dent Res* 1997; **76**: 1787–98.

Manhart J, Chen HY, Hamm G, Hickel R. Buonocore Memorial Lecture. Review of the clinical survival of direct and indirect restorations in posterior teeth of the permanent dentition. *Oper Dent* 2004; **29**: 481–508.

Medeiros VAF, Seddon RP. Iatrogenic damage to approximal surfaces in contact with class II restorations. *J Dent* 2000; **28**: 103–10.

Mjör IA. Long term cost of restorative therapy using different materials. *Scand J Dent Res* 1992; **100**: 60–5.

Mjör IA. Repair versus replacement of failed restorations. *Int Dent J* 1993; **43**: 466–72.

Mjör IA, Toffenetti F. Secondary caries: a literature review with case reports. *Quintessence Int* 2000; **31**: 165–79.

Mjör IA, Dahl JE, Moorhead JE. Age of restorations at replacement in permanent teeth in general dental practice. *Acta Odontol Scand* 2000a; **58**: 97–101.

Mjör IA, Moorhead JE, Dahl JE. Reasons for replacement of restorations in permanent teeth in general dental practice. *Int Dent J* 2000b; **50**: 360–6.

Mjör IA, Dahl JE, Moorhead JE. Placement and replacement of restorations in primary teeth. *Acta Odontol Scand* 2002; **60**: 25–8.

NHI. Effect and side-effects of dental restorative materials. *Adv Dent Res* 1992; **6**: 1–144.

Norwegian Board of Health. *The use of dental filling materials in Norway. IK 2675.* Oslo: Norwegian Board of Health, 1999.

Nuttall NM, Elderton RJ. The nature of restorative dental treatment decisions. *Br Dent J* 1983; **154**: 363–5.

Özer L. *The relationship between gap size, microbial accumulation and the structural features of natural caries in extracted teeth with class II amalgam restorations.* PhD Thesis, University of Copenhagen, 1997.

Qvist V. Longevity of restorations in primary teeth. In: Hugoson A, Falk M, Johansson S, eds. *Consensus conference on caries in the primary dentition and its clinical management.* Stockholm: Förlagshuset Gothia, 2002: 69–83.

Qvist J, Qvist V, Mjör IA. Placement and longevity of amalgam restorations in Denmark. *Acta Odontol Scand* 1990a; **48**: 287–303.

Qvist V, Qvist J, Mjör IA. Placement and longevity of tooth-colored restorations in Denmark. *Acta Odontol Scand* 1990b; **48**: 305–11.

Qvist V, Johannessen L, Bruun M. Progression of approximal caries in relation to iatrogenic preparation damage. *J Dent Res* 1992; **7**: 1370–3.

Qvist V, Laurberg L, Poulsen A, Teglers PT. Eight-year study on conventional glass ionomerand amalgam restorations in primary teeth. *Acta Odontol Scand* 2004a; **62**: 37–45.

Qvist V, Laurberg L, Poulsen A, Teglers PT. Class II restorations in primary teeth: 7-year study on three resin-modified glass ionomer cements and a compomer. *Eur J Oral Sci* 2004b; **112**: 188–96.

Qvist V, Manscher E, Teglers PT. Resin-modified and conventional glass ionomer restorations in primary teeth: 8-year results. *J Dent* 2004c; **32**: 285–94.

Roulet JF. Benefits and disadvantages of tooth-coloured alternatives to amalgam. *J Dent* 1997; **25**: 459–73.

Sjögren P, Halling A. Long-term cost of direct class II molar restorations. *Swed Dent J* 2002; **26**: 107–14.

Swedish Medical Research Council. Novakova V, ed. *Amalgam and health – new perspectives on risk*s. Report 99:1. Göteborg: Novum Grafiska AB, 1999.

Widström E, Birn H, Haugejorden O, Sundberg H. Fear of amalgam: dentist's experience in the Nordic countries. *Int Dent J* 1992; **42**: 65–70.

World Health Organization. Mjör IA, Pakhomov GN, eds. *Dental amalgam and alternative direct restorative materials.* Geneva: WHO, 1997.

Part VI
Caries control and prediction

25

Clinical decision making: technical solutions to biological problems or evidence-based caries management?

V. Baelum

Introduction

The historical bias towards dental mechanics

Appropriate dental care: what is it?

Appropriate caries management: how to get there?

Are we heading towards 'cookbook' dentistry?

Caries-related clinical decision making: what it is not

Caries-related clinical decision making: what it is

Appropriate caries scripts: proposal for a guideline

References

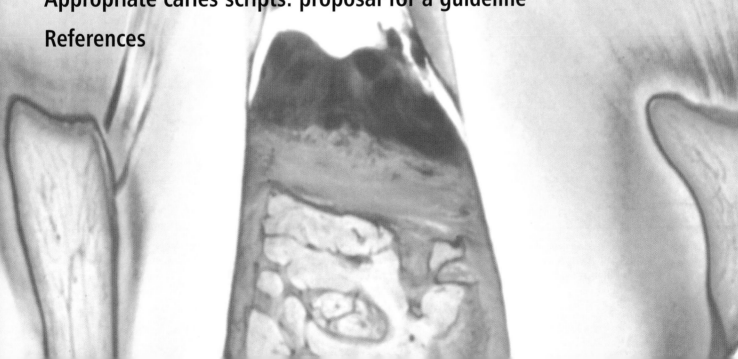

Introduction

Have you ever reflected on the *raison-d'être* of the high-speed drill? Its primary function is to cut away *sound* tooth substance (Elderton, 2003). Thereby, the high-speed drill epitomizes the devotion of much of the dental profession to traditional operative treatment, just as much as it highlights the profession's unjustified confidence in the ability of restorative treatment to bring about oral health.

Already in 1908, G.V. Black noted in his textbook on operative dentistry (Black, 1908) that the 'complete divorce of dental practice from studies of the pathology of dental caries, that existed in the past, is an anomaly in science that should not continue. It has the apparent tendency to make dentists mechanics only.' This quote shows the perception of the day of dentists as technicians, dental surgeons, rather than clinicians exercising evidence-based dental treatment. Regrettably, however, the perception of dentists as dental mechanics still prevails a century later (Niederman & Leitch, 2006): 'For over 100 years, dentists have successfully treated caries and periodontal disease with three metals: silver, gold, and stainless steel. But … we know that caries and periodontal disease are infections. Interestingly, no medical doctor would treat these infections (or any infection) with any of these metals.' Others have found that dental clinicians have a 'collective obsession with all things technical' (Renshaw, 2005), and have noted that dentists are slow to adopt new scientific concepts, but rapidly incorporate new techniques (Niederman & Leitch, 2006). This imbalance has been observed by industry, and most changes in therapy stem from the introduction of new techniques and products to the market (Goldstein & Preston, 2002), often with a notable absence of sound scientific documentation for their efficacy and safety. Dentists' 'enthusiasm for anecdotal information is narcotic in nature' and they feel good when they 'see photographs of these beautiful, bonded restorations, even though they have had a clinical longevity of 30 minutes' (Robbins, 1998).

The historical bias towards dental mechanics

Why does the focus on the technical aspects of dentistry still prevail when we know – and have known for decades now – that caries and periodontal disease are chronic diseases, which will surrender owing to effective control and prevention of biological processes rather than to skillful technical manipulations using high-speed drills and precious metals?

Clearly, a historical bias plays a role (Hume, 1992; Bader & Shugars, 1995b; Niederman & Leitch, 2006). Dentistry, as practiced today, is firmly rooted in a craftsmanship approach, which has become embedded and integrated in pre- and postgraduate education, licensing, insurance, financing and reimbursement systems, and not to forget, also in public opinion. In contrast with many of our pre-

ventive or non-operative services, the technical solutions (e.g. fillings and crowns) constitute tangible and well-defined services. Both dentists and patients therefore consider these services more compatible with the market principles that govern dentistry, than less eye-catching and intangible services, such as sealants, topical fluoride applications, and dietary counseling and oral hygiene instructions.

Financial issues also play a key role. Dentists are remunerated in one of three different ways: fixed salary, per capita remuneration or fee-for-item remuneration (Grytten, 2005). Dental care for adults is almost always based on a fee-for-item remuneration system, and the fees are often higher for the technical solutions than for the preventive and disease-controlling services. This clearly reinforces the bias towards technical interventions against biological problems. In the words of Renshaw (2005): 'Trying to follow this [preventive] philosophy with enthusiasm and working under current financial arrangements, I would be bankrupt in a couple of months. Not an attractive place to be.' However, some dentists, possibly motivated by the prospects of profit, have taken the technical clinical interventions to the other extreme, whereby 'mouths that were frankly only marginally less than perfect' have been subjected to 'high levels of destructive intervention' (Renshaw, 2005). This may happen because competition does not work in the dental market. Patients lack the knowledge and insight necessary to evaluate the extent and the quality of the services offered by the dentists (Grytten, 2005), and this gives the dentists a unique opportunity to influence the amount and type of care provided. This incentive for overtreatment (Wright & Batchelor, 2002), which is called supplier-induced demand, will be directed towards the services with the higher fees and the complex technical solutions, thus once more perpetuating the bias towards operative interventions.

The pregraduate dental education plays a pivotal role in the introduction of the bias towards technical intervention. In pregraduate dental education, emphasis is placed on the mechanistic aspects of dentistry, and in many dental schools there is a notable absence of an evidence-based educational philosophy in the learning process (Robbins, 1998). Robbins (1998) notes that it is 'a long-standing joke around health science centers that the dental students are the only professional students on campus who can't locate the library'. As discussed in Chapter 7, dentistry is taught under the auspices of the master clinician, and the 'art and craft' of clinical decision making is learned mainly through chairside apprenticeship. In this process, focus is placed on the repetition of mechanical and technical procedures, such as cavity preparation and filling placement, in order to refine and disseminate restorative excellence (Thylstrup, 1989; Hume, 1992). Comprehensive dental care is rarely practiced, and often, the procedural repetitions are discipline-limited and practiced in patients purposely selected to represent a need for these particular treatment modalities (Hume, 1992). The result is therefore once again supporting the mental bias towards providing technical solutions to biological problems.

The master clinicians involved in the pregraduate dental education have typically received only limited education in the retrieval, evaluation and synthesis of the scientific information relating to the clinical procedures they teach. Moreover, the time available for such activities may be very limited. The unfortunate result is that the evidence base for the procedures and techniques taught may not receive sufficient attention, and the practices adopted by the dental students may therefore be more influenced by the personal opinions, biases and value judgments of their master clinicians, than by scientific evidence for their efficacy and safety (Ismail & Bader, 2004).

We can therefore foresee two different scenarios for clinical dentistry in the future: one dominated by beauty trade businessmen who sell Hollywood smiles and 'expensive oral trinkets' (Renshaw, 2005) in 'gourmet dentistry' clinics (Boetig, 1987), and one consisting of professional health-care workers who try to maintain an evidence-based approach to the oral health outcomes of patients. As dentistry remains largely unregulated regarding the appropriateness of the treatments and procedures provided (Friedman & Atchison, 1993; Hartshorne & Hasegawa, 2003), the businessman approach stands a good chance of gaining even more ground. However, this is an approach that could engender public distrust (Ecenbarger, 1997), because society at large is increasingly asking for accountability, transparency and high professional standards (Cruess et al., 2000, 2002). Dentists' hard-won status as a profession with a societal responsibility (see Chapters 28 and 32) could very well be at stake here (Neilson, 1998).

Appropriate dental care: what is it?

The bias inherent in clinical dentistry towards providing technical invasive solutions to biological problems gives rise to concerns over the appropriateness of the care provided (Kress, 1980; Hume, 1992). Quality in dentistry has traditionally been associated with technical excellence and mechanical precision (Kress, 1980), and careful inspection of the physical characteristics of restorations has been a key component in outcome assessment (e.g. Cvar & Ryge, 2005). However, the concept of quality in dentistry goes way beyond the 'optimal' physical and functional characteristics of technical solutions (Bader & Ismail, 1999), and addresses the question of whether the procedures provided are indeed the best possible solutions to the problems presented by individual patients. The term 'best' may have many different implications, depending on whose perspective is considered (Table 25.1). The dentists are likely to place emphasis on those aspects of the treatment for which they are directly

responsible, such as the biological properties and mechanical characteristics of the materials used and solutions provided. However, these are usually intangible to the patient, and rather limited in focus. Patients are more likely to focus on the immediately tangible features, such as the aesthetics and comfort of the restorations provided. The long-term outcomes of the treatment, in the form of tooth survival and maintenance of a functional dentition, tend to receive less attention, although it is generally assumed that treatment is better than no treatment (Elderton, 2003). However, the reality is that the best dentistry is no dentistry (Sheiham, 2002).

The appropriateness of the dental care provided has been widely debated over the past few decades (Hume, 1992; Friedman & Atchison, 1993; Sheiham, 2002). It is well documented that there is a substantial variation between dentists in the diagnoses made and the treatments recommended for the same and for similar patients (Ashford, 1978; Rytömaa et al., 1979; Mileman et al., 1982; Espelid & Tveit, 1986, 1987; Tveit & Espelid, 1987; Bader & Shugars, 1992, 1993, 1995a, b; Espelid et al., 1994; Rushton et al., 1996; Kay & Locker, 1996; Kay & Blinkhorn, 1996; Lewis et al., 1996a, b; Blinkhorn & Zadeh-Kabir, 2003). This

Table 25.1 Oral health-care outcomes to consider when discussing the appropriateness of care

Dimension		Example	Primary stakeholder(s)
Biological	Physiological	Salivary flow, inflammation	Dentist
	Microbiological	Oral microbial composition, specific pathogens	Dentist
	Sensory	Presence of pain, paresthesia	Patient Dentist
Clinical	Survival	Tooth loss, survival of restoration	Patient
	Mechanical	Marginal adaptation, contours	Dentist
	Diagnostic	Presence of caries	Dentist
	Functional	Ability to chew, speak	Patient
	Aesthetics	Visibility, color	Patient
Psychosocial	Satisfaction	With treatment, dentist, oral health	Patient
	Perceptions	Aesthetics, oral health rating	Patient
	Preferences	Value of health states and events	Patient
	OHRQoL	Oral health impact on life	Patient
Economical	Direct costs	Out-of-pocket payment, third party payment	Patient Insurance
	Indirect costs	Lost wages, transport	Patient
	Revenues	Income generated	Dentist

Adapted from Bader & Ismail (1999).
OHRQoL: oral health-related quality of life.

results in widely different health outcomes and cost implications for the patients (Shugars & Bader, 1996). The variation in diagnosis and treatment reveals a profound lack of consensus among dental practitioners. The most charitable explanation for this lack of consensus is that insufficient information exists about the oral health outcomes of the treatments provided, and of the causal processes, the pathogenesis, the risk factors, as well as the incidence and progression of the diseases treated, leaving all these factors open to interpretation and personal judgment. However, we should keep in mind that if evidence exists, it is 'unconscionable to proceed or persist with treatments based on nothing more than perceived benefits, subjectively observed "improvements", short-term efficacy based on a very small sample size, old science, poorly done science, good science taken out of context, parts of good science, anecdotal rhetoric, others' opinions, sales pitches, advertising, simple gut-feeling, or, worst of all, knowing charlatanism. These all fall into the category of "it works in my hands", and leave us wide open to the same criticisms that apply to practitioners of alternative medicine' (Neilson, 1998).

The key question is: what to do about it? How can dental professionals ensure that all their patients receive appropriate dental care? A starting point is to consider a useful working definition of appropriate oral health care. In dental health care, the practitioner tries to bring about as many health benefits to the patient as possible, while taking great care that this does not cause damage or introduce adverse effects. Thereby, appropriate dental health care can be defined as the care that maximizes the gap between the expected health benefits and the expected negative consequences of the intended procedures. The dentist seeks to provide a maximum of health benefits at the expense of a minimum of side-effects. Obviously, procedures should only be considered if the expected health benefits exceed the negative consequences by a sufficiently wide margin to make the procedures worthwhile. This definition of appropriate care underlines the fact that knowledge is required not only of the biological, technical and clinical parameters involved, but also of the psychosocial and economic consequences for the patient of different alternatives (Kay & Nuttall, 1995a–e, 2006) (Table 25.1). Importantly, the time-frame considered is a lifetime, and this long-term outcome aspect deserves much more attention than has hitherto been customary. It is thus important to understand that reliance on the restorative approach to the management of caries leads to a spiral of (iatrogenic) damage (Table 25.2) (Elderton, 1993, 2003; Sheiham, 2002).

Appropriate caries management: how to get there?

Most suggestions for a solution to the problem of large variability between dentists and inappropriate dental care bring into discussion the concept of evidence-based care (Grace, 1998; Niederman, 1998; Tinanoff & Douglass, 2001; Marinho *et al.*, 2001; Sheiham, 2002; Goldstein & Preston, 2002; Elderton, 2003; Ismail & Bader, 2004; Pitts, 2004a–c; Gordon & Dionne, 2005; Innes *et al.*, 2005). Evidence-based dental care can be defined as the 'conscientious, explicit, and judicious use of current best evidence in making decisions about the care of individual patients' (Sackett *et al.*, 1996; Niederman, 1998). By 'best evidence' is meant the evidence from clinically relevant research, preferably patient-centered clinical research, into the accuracy and precision of diagnostic tests (including the clinical examination), the power of prognostic markers, and the efficacy and safety of therapeutic, rehabilitative and preventive regimens (Sackett *et al.*, 1996). Most articles on the subject of evidence-based dental care (Pitts, 2004a, b; Gordon & Dionne, 2005) assume that 'all clinicians are … making their own assessments of published work' (Pitts, 2004a). While this might constitute an ideal for the dental academic, it is wholly unrealistic and inefficient in the context of clinical dental practice.

One should be realistic and acknowledge that the task of acquiring and maintaining a solid evidence base for all the interventions and procedures that are carried out by the average dental practitioner is overwhelmingly large. Clinical trial information is published at a rate that makes it practically impossible for anyone to keep up to date in all sub-specialties relevant to general dental practice (Russo *et al.*, 2000; Kim *et al.*, 2001; Yang *et al.*, 2001; Niederman *et al.*, 2002; Park & Niederman, 2002; Nishimura *et al.*, 2002). Moreover, the scientific information provided is often conflicting, leaving it to the users and stakeholders to work out what to believe. This, in turn, necessitates an insight into research designs and scientific methods way beyond what is provided in the introductory courses given during pregraduate dental education. Dentists therefore often lack the know-how to critically appraise and appropriately distill the information (Ismail & Bader, 2004; Niederman & Leitch, 2006), and they therefore resort to doing what they have always done and feel comfortable with (Grace, 1998).

One might indeed wonder whether the duty to distill the evidence should be placed solely with each individual dental practitioner. Clearly, the responsibility for providing appropriate dental health care will always rest with the individual dentist. It is equally clear, however, that the individual dentists should come to the same conclusion about the evidence when retrieving, reading, assessing and distilling the same scientific literature on the basis of the same level of know-how. Placing the responsibility solely with each individual clinical practitioner is therefore an unrealistic and inefficient approach to the problem of providing appropriate, evidence-based dental health care.

This suggests that the responsibility for the implementation of appropriate dental health care rests in two places. First, the dental schools must see to it that the dental curriculum,

Table 25.2 The tooth death spiral

The patient goes to the dentist, but	Clinical examinations are often simplistic and casual Diagnostic tests are largely subjective
So, it is not surprising that	Caries diagnoses are often inaccurate
At the same time	Caries status is not properly taken into account Caries risk factors are not generally considered
Also	Undertaking restorations is considered 'good dentistry'
So, it is no surprise that	Restorative decisions tend to be idiosyncratic and aggressive
However,	Caries etiological factors are not modified Preventive back-up is inadequate Caries is not controlled as a disease
Indeed	Dentists appear to gain fulfillment by cutting sound tooth away The use of outdated concepts of cavity design is commonplace Dentists fail to grasp the exacting nature of restorative procedures
It is no surprise therefore, that	Restorations of mediocre quality are readily placed
In addition,	Bur damage is imparted commonly to the adjacent tooth Inappropriate approximal contours lead to plaque and periodontal disease
In due course the patient is recalled	Recall assessments of restorations tend to be idiosyncratic Ditched margins are commonly assumed to signal restoration failure
Therefore,	Existing restorations are readily deemed to have failed
In particular if	The patient has just changed from a previous dentist
However,	The matter why restorations have failed is not questioned
So, it is not surprising that	Restorations are readily cut out and replaced
Although	The causes of failure remain unidentified
It is almost ubiquitous that	Restorations increase in size when replaced
Thereby,	The teeth become weaker
It is no surprise to find that	Errors in previous restorations are repeated in the new ones The inbuilt cycle of rerestoration is perpetuated
Inevitably, as they increase in size	The restorations become more complex and difficult to carry out Correct chemical treatment of cavity becomes less certain
So, one cannot escape the fact that	Microbial, chemical and mechanical insult to the pulp is more likely
Overall,	The dentist fails to realize the iatrogenic nature of the treatment
Indeed,	The dentist believes that he/she is making the patient more healthy
Sadly,	The patient suffers the same illusion
But, deterioration continues and	Gross fracture of the tooth may occur
So	Crowning is effected as a 'cure-all' procedure
However,	The crown fails to properly fit the margins of the tooth
In due course	The need for endodontic treatment arises
However,	Root canal preparation is inadequate Root canal obturation is incomplete
Not surprisingly,	The periapical lesion persists
This may lead to	Apicectomy and retrograde root filling
Surprisingly, the dentist feels he's	Really saving the patient's dentition
However,	The tooth fails to settle and symptoms continue
Ultimately …	The tooth is extracted!

Adapted from Elderton (2003).

as far as the evidence exists, is based on the principles of evidence-based health care. Competence in acquisition and maintenance of evidence-based knowledge is thus a major issue in the recent document from the Association for Dental Education in Europe, which outlines the future competence profile for European dentists (Plasschaert *et al.*, 2005). Where the evidence does not exist, or is conflicting, the premises used and assumptions made must be explained, so that the emerging practitioners are made aware of the deficiencies in the evidence. The educational philosophy must be changed away from the predominantly mechanistic approach to emphasize the understanding and appreciation of dental literature as the basis for clinical decision making (Robbins, 1998; Clark & Mjör, 2001). Secondly, the pivotal role of professional organizations for continuing professional education would suggest that these organizations might also be expected to carry a considerable responsibility. The professional organizations could engage advisory groups to distill the evidence for the whole range of diagnostic and therapeutic procedures used, and could issue clinical practice guidelines on the basis of such evidence assessments. Finally, it should be noted that a whole range of clinical guidelines based on well-conducted systematic reviews of the available evidence exists already for a number of procedures and therapeutic strategies relevant to clinical dental practice [see, for example, the Cochrane Collaboration (www.cochrane.org), the National Institute for Health and Clinical Excellence (www.nice.org.uk), and the National Guideline Clearinghouse (www.guideline.gov)].

Dentistry still retains the status of a profession, which implies a social contract with society at large to 'be governed by codes of ethics and profess a commitment to competence, integrity and morality, and altruism, and the promotion of the public good' (Cruess *et al.*, 2000, 2002, 2004). In return, the dental profession is 'granted monopoly over the use of its knowledge base, the right to considerable autonomy in practice and the privilege of self-regulation' (Cruess *et al.*, 2004). Dentists' status as a dental profession enjoying these privileges may be in jeopardy if they fail to fulfill this social contract and base their practice on the best evidence.

Are we heading towards 'cookbook' dentistry?

The wish to implement evidence-based dental care by means of clinical practice guidelines may to some be understood as an unwarranted movement towards cookbook dentistry. 'Cookbook' implies a slavish approach to individual care (Sackett *et al.*, 1996), and conflicts not only with the high degree of autonomy that characterizes clinical dental practice, but also with the 'gourmet dentistry' philosophy (Boetig, 1987) now governing significant sections of the dental profession. It is well known that dentists may be reluctant to adhere to clinical practice guidelines (Bahrami *et al.*, 2004; van der Sanden *et al.*, 2005), and there can be little doubt that dentists who understand clinical decision making as an informal and intuitive 'art' optimized through accumulated clinical experience may perceive the implementation of evidence-based guidelines for dental care as an infringement of their professional freedom. What dentists fail to realize is that they are indeed already unconsciously using cookbook thinking in their caries-related clinical decision making. A key problem is that they often use different cookbooks and therefore different recipes for the same course.

Caries-related clinical decision making: what it is not

It is a popular misconception that caries diagnosis can be characterized as a differential diagnostic process, i.e. the assignment of a particular set of signs and symptoms to one of many plausible diagnostic categories (Bader & Shugars, 1997; Baelum *et al.*, 2006). Each dentist knows what he or she is looking for when giving a caries examination to a patient, and this explains the gradual change in terminology away from caries diagnosis towards caries detection (Nyvad, 2004). Although the notion of caries can vary considerably, two major lines of thinking can be identified, which have important consequences for caries-related clinical decision making (Baelum *et al.*, 2006) (see Chapter 7). One line of thinking involves an essentialistic caries concept, according to which caries detection aims to identify the true state of affairs with respect to caries lesion formation, and believes that this can be achieved by the use of increasingly refined high-resolution diagnostic tools. The other line of thinking, which is termed nominalistic, is less concerned with the 'caries truth', but seeks to detect and classify the signs and symptoms of caries in a way that will maximize the health gain for the patient following treatment. The centerpiece of this caries concept is the classification of lesions according to their biologically optimal treatment modality. In nominalistic thinking, focus is therefore on the identification of active versus inactive caries lesions, and cavitated versus non-cavitated lesions. The biological rationale is that cavitated lesions generally necessitate a restoration to facilitate plaque removal and oral hygiene procedures, whereas non-cavitated active lesions may be controlled and arrested using non-operative treatment involving plaque control and fluoride (Nyvad *et al.*, 1999; Baelum *et al.*, 2006). It is important to note that classification of caries lesions according to this scheme can only be achieved by a visual–tactile clinical examination. This contrasts caries detection from the essentialistic perspective, where a multitude of diagnostic tools are typically used, usually including at least a visual–tactile clinical and a bitewing examination.

Another popular misconception in caries-related clinical decision making is that the key issue is the detection of lesions, rather than the exoneration of sound from lesion presence. This continued bias of dentistry towards a focus on caries lesion detection is probably closely related to dentistry being rooted in restorative therapy, which is further perpetuated by the fee-per-service remuneration systems and the profession's perception of dentistry as a high-tech craft. However, appropriate caries-related clinical decision making involves much more than the ability correctly to detect caries lesion presence, as explained in the following.

The technical term used to describe the ability of a diagnostic test, such as our clinical examination, correctly to detect caries lesions is test sensitivity, which expresses the probability that the test detects a caries lesion when a lesion is truly present (see Chapter 7). The test sensitivity has a counterpart, the test specificity, which is the probability that the test indicates no lesion, when there truly is no lesion. It is vital to appreciate that a given diagnostic test, in this example bitewing radiography for the detection of approximal caries cavities, can have very different consequences, depending on the true occurrence of approximal caries cavities in the population where the test is used. (Note that it is clearly not possible to diagnose cavitation on radiographs. Instead, an assumption is invoked, according to which radiographic lesions penetrating, for example, more than halfway through the dentin are deemed cavitated.) This is illustrated in Table 25.3, which makes use of the fairly typical sensitivity and specificity values of 0.66 and 0.95, respectively, estimated in a systematic review of caries diagnostic methods (Bader *et al.*, 2001).

Table 25.3 shows that when the true occurrence of approximal cavities is low, e.g. 0.1%, a total of 506 (7 + 499) surfaces will be diagnosed with cavities. However, only seven of these surfaces are truly cavitated. Conversely, 9494 (9491 + 3) surfaces will be deemed cavity free, although three of these are truly cavitated. Phrased differently, relatively few cavities are overlooked (three out of 10 cavities are overlooked), but this occurs at the expense of considerable overdiagnosis (499 out of 506 positive diagnoses are false). When the true occurrence of approximal cavities is high, e.g. 20%, a total of 1720 surfaces will be diagnosed with cavity, and 1320 of these are truly cavitated. Of the 2000 cavities truly present, 680 will be overlooked. In other words, there is notable overdiagnosis (400 out of 1720 positive diagnoses are false) and a considerable number of cavities (680 out of 2000) is overlooked.

Table 25.3 also shows that when the cavity occurrence is low, most of the diagnostic errors made are false-positive diagnoses, owing to the less-than-perfect test specificity, i.e. the inability of the test to exonerate surfaces as noncavitated. In fact, the table shows that the true cavity occurrence has to be quite high before the imperfect test sensitivity of 0.66 exceeds the imperfect test specificity of 0.95 as the main source of diagnostic errors.

The results presented in Table 25.3 do not take into account the fact that the results of a diagnostic test can be used in different ways. While most dentists, as previously indicated, undoubtedly trust their positive findings, i.e. go for the detection of cavities, it is indeed possible to use a diagnostic test result to exclude diagnoses, i.e. trust the negative findings. The consequences of these two decision strategies are shown in Table 25.4 for the same conditions used to generate the data in Table 25.3. Dentist A is a 'drill–fill–bill' dentist, who performs a restoration in response to a positive bitewing finding; whereas dentist B is a 'preservationist', who trusts negative bitewing findings to exclude the presence of a cavity, and performs non-operative caries treatment for all surfaces with positive findings. Table 25.4 clearly shows that the drill–fill–bill strategy is a rather deleterious response to positive bitewing findings in populations with a low caries occurrence, such as many contemporary populations. For such populations, the preservationist approach is clearly superior from a patient health outcome point of view. Without going into the discussion of where the appropriate cut-point may lie, it is also clear that the preservationist strategy may fail in populations with a high caries occurrence, owing to the non-operative treatment

Table 25.3 Diagnostic consequences, expressed as the number of false-positive and false-negative diagnoses made, when using bitewing radiography with a sensitivity of 0.66 and a specificity of 0.95 (Bader *et al.*, 2001) for the detection of cavitated caries lesions in populations of 10 000 approximal surfaces with different true cavity occurrences

| True cavity occurrence (%) | Correct diagnoses | | Diagnostic errors | | |
	No. of true-positive diagnoses	No. of true-negative diagnoses	No. of false-positive diagnoses	No. of false-negative diagnoses	Total no. of diagnostic errors
0.1%	7	9491	499	3	502
1%	66	9405	495	34	529
5%	330	9025	475	170	645
10%	660	8550	450	340	790
15%	990	8075	425	510	935
20%	1320	7600	400	680	1080

Table 25.4 Who's the better dentist? The clinical consequences of using the bitewing radiographic test from Table 25.3 for each of two dentists with different caries treatment philosophies: dentist A trusts the positive findings and performs a restoration in response to a positive test result; dentist B trusts the negative findings and performs non-operative caries treatment in response to a positive test result

| True cavity occurrence (%) | Dentist A | | | Dentist B | | |
| | No. of surfaces/cavities that are | | | No. of surfaces/cavities that are | | |
	Restored	Overtreated	Undertreated	Treated non-operatively	Insufficiently treated[a]	Undertreated
0.1%	506	499	3	506	7	3
1%	561	495	34	561	66	34
5%	805	475	170	805	330	170
10%	1110	450	340	1110	660	340
15%	1415	425	510	1415	990	510
20%	1720	400	680	1720	1320	680

[a] Non-operative treatment may be insufficient to arrest caries lesion progression in case of cavitation.

provided being insufficient to halt or arrest caries lesion progression. However, populations with high caries occurrence also have high exposure levels to causal factors, whether biological (plaque and carbohydrates), behavioral (oral hygiene and dietary habits), socioeconomic or contextual (environmental). This is exactly why the control of caries in such populations is much better achieved using population strategies based on a common risk factor approach (see Chapter 28). Traditional chairside dentistry, whether using a drill–fill–bill or a preservationist approach to caries management, will achieve little.

The final misconception about caries-related clinical decision making is to think that each patient contact involves a clinical decision analysis, in which the consequences of all the different diagnostic and therapeutic options are subject to an analysis in order to be able to decide the best course of action for the patient in question (Anusavice, 2003). Proponents of this idea often visualize the caries-related clinical decision-making process using decision-flow diagrams, called decision trees (Kay & Nuttall, 1995e; Anusavice, 2003), such as shown in Fig. 25.1. However, this decision tree also shows why it is a misconception that decision analyses are made for individual patients: decision trees are all too complex and cumbersome and difficult to use in daily clinical practice. They require enumeration of all the possible choices faced by the clinician, and of all the courses of action that may be taken when providing dental care to a patient. Their use also necessitates information on the values and utilities attached by the patient to various outcomes of dental treatment, and it is clearly not feasible to obtain such information from each patient. The potential complexity of decision trees is further underscored when it is noted that they may be limited in time to concern a single routine recall visit, or they could be expanded to concern years of patient care, in which case they can become exceedingly complex.

However, decision trees may be used to derive general rules for courses of action under specified circumstances described in terms of the costs of the different options, the probabilities of the different courses of action and outcomes, and the patient values and utilities of the different outcomes.

Decision making involves a choice between different options, as shown in the simplified decision tree in Fig. 25.1. Detection of caries lesions always begins with a visual–tactile clinical examination, whereby tooth surfaces are classified according to the clinical recording system used. This clinical examination means that the patient incurs expenses, designated $Cost_0$. At some point, a decision must be made as to whether the visual examination should be supplemented, e.g. with bitewing radiography, or whether a diagnostic decision can be made without additional information. The probability that bitewing radiographs are added may be designated p, and the probability of proceeding to reach a caries diagnosis is therefore $1 - p$. Choice of the bitewing route means that additional costs ($Cost_A$) are incurred. Having collected the necessary diagnostic information, a diagnosis is reached. In the simple tree shown in Fig. 25.1, the probability of finding a caries lesion based only on a visual–tactile examination is designated q_2, and the probability of finding a caries lesion following the visual–tactile examination supplemented with bitewing radiography is designated q_1. The corresponding probabilities that the surface is deemed sound are therefore $1 - q_2$ and $1 - q_1$, respectively.

Once the caries detection phase is over, it is necessary to enumerate all the treatment options possible for the different types of lesions detected. Again, probabilities can be associated with each choice, e.g. r_1, r_2 and $1 - (r_1 + r_2)$ in Fig. 25.1, just as the costs associated with each treatment option can be listed. In Fig. 25.1 only one outcome is indicated for each treatment option, although the reality is that

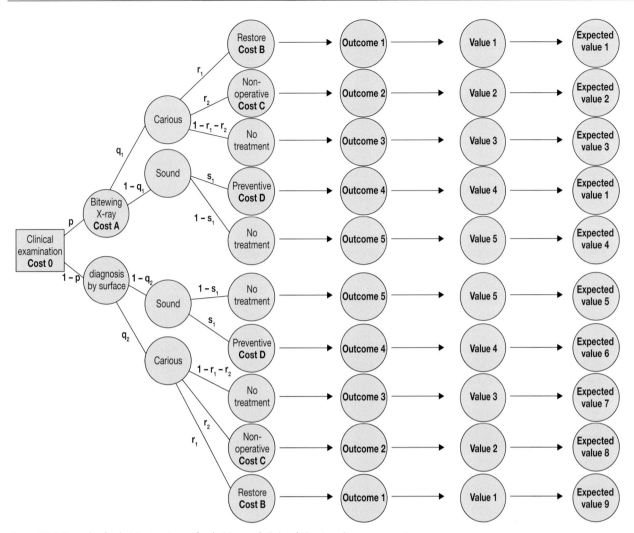

Figure 25.1 Example of a decision tree to use for decision analysis in relation to caries management.

several outcomes exist for each treatment option. As an example, consider what may happen to a restored tooth, say, in the next 5 years. It may develop recurrent caries, it may show ditching, it may fracture, it may become aesthetically unacceptable to the patient, or it may stay as it is. Each of these outcomes will occur with a certain probability, just as each outcome will elicit different treatment options, the costs of which differ.

With the information sketched, it is possible to calculate the expected costs of each treatment option by multiplying the branch probabilities by the costs incurred along the pathway to the option (Raiffa, 1968). If information on the values (preferences or utility) that patients attach to the different outcomes can be obtained, the expected patient value of each outcome can be calculated. These values can be assessed in economic terms by means of the willingness-to-pay assessment (Birch & Ismail, 2002; Birch et al., 2004) or in terms of utility scores (Downer & Moles, 1998; Moles & Downer, 2000; Birch & Ismail, 2002; Mileman & van den

Hout, 2003; Ismail et al., 2004). With information on the expected costs and the expected utilities, formal decision analyses of the best decisions to make can be carried out whenever different options are presented (Raiffa, 1968).

Although the decision-tree methodology described here may be extremely useful for the development and analysis of clinical guidelines, it has very little to do with the kind of thinking used by dental practitioners in their caries-related decision making. It is simply all too cumbersome to be useful in daily clinical practice.

Caries-related clinical decision making: what it is

As alluded to earlier in this chapter, dental practitioners already use cookbook thinking in their caries-related clinical decision making. The decision-tree example in Fig. 25.1 shows that there are all too many decisions and all too many options involved in decision making based on decision trees to allow this process to be repeated *de novo* for each tooth surface in each patient. Instead, dentists resort to the use of caries scripts (Bader & Shugars, 1997). Caries scripts, also described in Chapter 7, can be thought of as mental images of different caries representations stored in the practitioner's memory. These caries scripts contain all the salient features that distinguish the different caries and caries-related representations, and they serve as manuals for the entire clinical decision-making process associated with each representation. The content of the caries script is of the form this-clinical-picture-needs-this-intervention (Bader & Shugars, 1997). Caries scripts are executed automatically and without formal reasoning, drawing on pattern recognition and typical experiences with similar cases (Crespo *et al.*, 2004). Only if an abnormal presentation fails to match an existing caries script will the dentist engage in differential diagnostic considerations.

Clearly, pregraduate dental education plays a crucial role in the formation of individual dentists' caries scripts. Thereby, a pivotal role is once again emphasized for the dental schools in providing their pregraduate dental students with updated and evidence-based caries scripts and a thorough understanding of the scientific underpinnings of diagnosis (Choi *et al.*, 1998; Mileman & van den Hout, 2002). Continuing education also plays a key role. This is illustrated by the dramatic change in the propensity to restore approximal surfaces with various radiographic diagnoses that was observed between 1978/79 and 1984/85 among 17-year-olds in a Danish municipality (Heidmann *et al.*, 1988) (Fig. 25.2). Where 84% of the surfaces with radiographic evidence of a lesion penetrating more than half way into dentin were restored in 1978/79, this was the case for only 47% 6 years later. Translated into absolute numbers of surfaces, it can be shown that 177 surfaces of 217, corresponding to 82%, were spared a restoration as a result of the change in treatment criteria between 1978/79 and 1984/85. This change in treatment criteria was ascribed to the results of studies showing slower progression of the caries process than previously anticipated, as well as studies questioning the outcomes of filling therapy (Heidmann *et al.*, 1988). However, it is important to keep in mind that this knowledge did not diffuse passively among the dental clinicians, but resulted from a series of courses in clinical cariology given by Danish cariology professors during the years 1979–1982, in which the majority of the public health dentists participated. Among other things, these courses pointed to the lower than anticipated frequency of cavitation of radiographically diagnosed approximal caries lesions (Bille & Thylstrup, 1982; Thylstrup *et al.*, 1986). Similar changes in restorative treatment strategies have been described for Norwegian populations (Gimmestad *et al.*, 2003), and were ascribed to an in-service lecture program about the prognosis of approximal caries lesions, as well as an increasing demand for productivity (number of

patients seen per dentist), which may have reduced the propensity to perform restorations. The potential for change is further illustrated by research showing that teaching practitioners about uncertainty in diagnosis and the costs and benefits of action versus no action results in improved consistency and accuracy in caries-related clinical decision making (Choi *et al.*, 1998).

Appropriate caries scripts: proposal for a guideline

The concepts outlined above underline the need for the classification and diagnosis of caries lesions that is keyed to the treatment strategies (Bader & Brown, 1993). Formulation of appropriate treatment strategies necessitates careful consideration of the processes involved in caries lesion formation (Fejerskov & Nyvad, 2003; Fejerskov, 2004; Kidd & Fejerskov, 2004). It is no longer admissible to continue to adhere to old (Black, 1914; Hyatt, 1923), but all-pervading beliefs that the design and preparation of cavities and the use of suitable restorative materials play a role in the cure, let alone the prevention of dental caries (Kidd, 1998, 2004). It has thus been described as a tragic irony of history (Thylstrup, 1989) that the perhaps greatest dental scientist, G.V. Black, is mainly remembered for these cavity design principles, when he in fact was advocating the modern principles of being concerned with interrupting the causal processes, the caries process, that leads to caries lesion formation and progression.

The guideline proposed (Fig. 25.3) is based on the premises detailed in the following text. Current understanding of the etiology and pathogenesis of caries lesion development (see Chapters 10–12) is that caries lesion formation results from a dynamic interaction between the tooth surface minerals and acids produced by the microbial deposits located in stagnation sites with limited salivary access. Caries development (see Fig. 28.2) is the result of a dynamic process that occurs wherever a metabolically active plaque is allowed to form. Very often, this process is self-limiting. Periods characterized by a net mineral loss, corresponding to a drift towards caries lesion formation, may thus alternate with periods characterized by a net mineral gain, corresponding to a drift towards mineral deposition (Manji *et al.*, 1991). Only when the drifts towards demineralization exceed the compensating drifts towards mineral precipitation (remineralization) in either number or duration will the net result over time be the formation of caries lesions in need of intervention.

Caries lesion formation follows a continuum of changes, ranging from minute aberrations in the outermost enamel crystal layers that are only discernible at the ultrastructural level, over the overt cavity to the complete destruction of the tooth crown. Chapters 3 and 4 show that cavity formation constitutes a relatively late stage in the development of caries

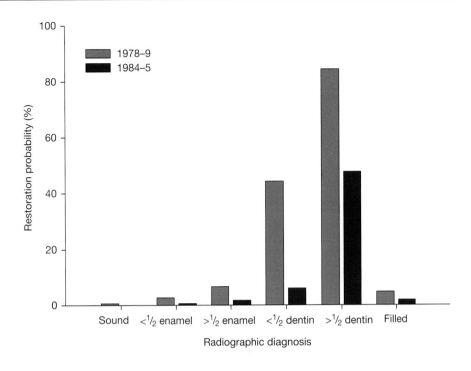

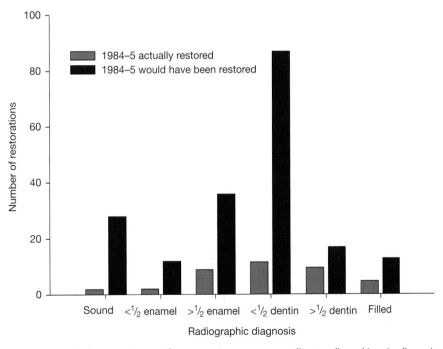

Figure 25.2 (a) The change over 6 years in the propensity to perform restorative treatment according to radiographic caries diagnosis, and (b) the effect of this change on the number of restorations inserted. Data from Heidmann *et al*. (1988).

lesions. Cavity formation is preceded by a whole range of non-cavitated caries lesions. The non-cavitated lesions are histologically characterized by subsurface lesions in the enamel beneath a relatively unaffected surface zone, and demineralization may extend far into dentin before the surface zone begins to break down, leading to cavity formation.

As long as the surface zone has not broken down, it is definitely possible to arrest the lesion formation by non-

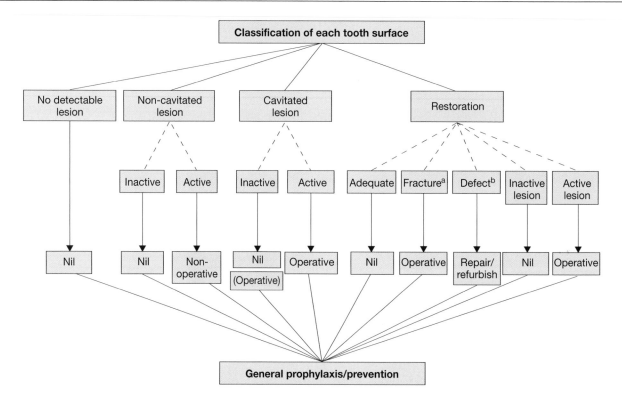

^a Isthumus fractures and large overhangs not amenable to repair/refurbishment.
^b Marginal gaps, fractures, ditching and material surplus.

Figure 25.3 Suggested clinical guideline for the management of dental caries.

operative means (Nyvad & Fejerskov, 1997). As shown in Chapters 14–19 and Chapter 27, dentists have the means and methods to tamper with the caries process: they can remove the microbial deposits and teach their patients oral hygiene procedures to keep these deposits away; they can provide dietary advice to influence the metabolic activity of the plaque; they can use antiplaque chemical agents; and they can apply sealants and topical fluorides, and advice on home use of fluoride toothpaste to control the drift in the demineralization and remineralization process.

Such interventions result in no further lesion progression, but scars, in the form of inactive lesions, may always remain. It is also possible to arrest cavitated lesions (Nyvad & Fejerskov, 1986, 1997; Lo *et al.*, 1998), although the success of this treatment depends on the ability of the patient to keep the lesions clean. That is why the role of restorations in caries management is limited to their ability to facilitate plaque control locally, as stressed in Chapters 20–22. Restorations do not cure caries, and it is a misconception to equate filling carious cavities with caries treatment. It is no such thing. Caries management is what you do when you interfere with the causal processes, e.g. in the form of plaque control, dietary advice and use of topical fluorides. This is what is understood by 'caries control'.

Although the term 'permanent' is often used to describe restorations, the reality is that they are far from permanent. Restorations do not last a lifetime (see Chapter 24), and their longevity is often less than 10 years (Mjör *et al.*, 2000; Mjör & Gordan, 2002). Most of the restorations placed in general dental practice therefore constitute replacements of previous restorations (Deligeorgi *et al.*, 2001), rather than treatment of primary cavities. Each cycle of re-restoration results in increasingly larger restorations (Mjör *et al.*, 1998). This cavity enlargement occurs irrespective of a color difference between the tooth and the replaced restoration, although the increase in cavity size is enhanced when tooth-colored restorations are replaced (Mjör & Gordan, 2002). Therefore, each cycle of re-restoration carries with it an increasing risk of tooth fractures and thereby of crown placement (Wilson *et al.*, 2003).

When asked about the reasons for replacement of restorations, dentists will often cite recurrent (secondary) caries (Deligeorgi *et al.*, 2001; Mjör, 2005). To arrive at a diagnosis of recurrent caries the criteria for diagnosing primary caries must be fulfilled (Mjör & Toffenetti, 2000), the only distinction being that the recurrent caries lesion is located adjacent to an existing restoration. However, the clinical diagnosis of recurrent caries is ill defined and dental practitioners frequently, but mistakenly, diagnose marginal defects and discolorations as recurrent caries (Mjör & Toffenetti, 2000; Mjör & Gordan, 2002; Mjör, 2005). Although most recurrent caries lesions are small lesions localized in the gingival area of the restoration (Mjör & Toffenetti, 2000), the dental practitioners strive towards clinical perfection and technical excellence. This will often urge them to replace restorations rather than attempt the more tooth substance-conserving approaches of repair, refurbishing or 'explorative' cavity preparation (Mjör & Gordan, 2002; Mjör, 2005).

Up-to-date and evidence-based caries management will continue to involve restorations for the foreseeable future, but the limitations of the traditional and rather aggressive restorative approach should be acknowledged (Elderton, 1993). A much more discretionary approach to the caries problem should be taken, which is based on non-operative (causal) treatment (Nyvad & Fejerskov, 1986, 1997; Nyvad et al., 1997) and restricts operative intervention to a minimum (Elderton, 1993; Mjör & Gordan, 2002; Mjör, 2005). Adherence to the clinical guideline shown in Fig. 25.3 will help the dental clinician achieve the goal of delivering appropriate dental health care by maximizing the gap between the expected health benefits and the expected negative consequences of caries-related treatment modalities.

References

Anusavice K. The maze of treatment decisions. In: Fejerskov O, Kidd E, eds. Dental caries. The disease and its clinical management. Oxford: Blackwell Munksgaard, 2003: 251–65.
Ashford JR. Regional variations in dental care in England and Wales. Br Dent J 1978; 145: 275–83.
Bader JD, Brown JP. Dilemmas in caries diagnosis. J Am Dent Assoc 1993; 124(6): 48–50.
Bader JD, Ismail AI. A primer on outcomes in dentistry. J Public Health Dent 1999; 59: 131–5.
Bader JD, Shugars DA. Understanding dentists' restorative treatment decisions. J Public Health Dent 1992; 52: 102–10.
Bader JD, Shugars DA. Agreement among dentists' recommendations for restorative treatment. J Dent Res 1993; 72: 891–6.
Bader JD, Shugars DA. Variation in dentists' clinical decisions. J Public Health Dent 1995a; 55: 181–8.
Bader JD, Shugars DA. Variation, treatment outcomes, and practice guidelines in dental practice. J Dent Educ 1995b; 59: 61–95.
Bader JD, Shugars DA. What do we know about how dentists make caries-related treatment decisions? Community Dent Oral Epidemiol 1997; 25: 97–103.
Bader JD, Shugars DA, Bonito AJ. Systematic reviews of selected caries diagnostic and management methods. J Dent Educ 2001; 65: 960–8.
Baelum V, Heidmann J, Nyvad B. Dental caries paradigms in diagnosis and diagnostic research. Eur J Oral Sci 2006; 114: 263–77.
Bahrami M, Deery C, Clarkson JE, et al. Effectiveness of strategies to disseminate and implement clinical guidelines for the management of impacted and unerupted third molars in primary dental care, a cluster randomised controlled trial. Br Dent J 2004; 197: 691–6.
Bille J, Thylstrup A. Radiographic diagnosis and clinical tissue changes in relation to treatment of approximal carious lesions. Caries Res 1982; 16: 1–6.
Birch S, Ismail AI. Patient preferences and the measurement of utilities in the evaluation of dental technologies. J Dent Res 2002; 81: 446–50.

Birch S, Sohn W, Ismail AI, Lepkowski JM, Belli RF. Willingness to pay for dentin regeneration in a sample of dentate adults. Community Dent Oral Epidemiol 2004; 32: 210–16.
Black GV. A work on operative dentistry, Vol. 1, Pathology of the dental hard tissues of the teeth. Chicago, IL: Medico-Dental Publishing Co., 1908.
Black GV. A work on operative dentistry, Vol. II, The technical procedures in filling teeth, 2nd edn. Chicago, IL: Medico-Dental Publishing Co., 1914.
Blinkhorn A, Zadeh-Kabir R. Dental care of a child in pain – a comparison of treatment planning options offered by GDPs in California and the North-west of England. Int J Paediatr Dent 2003; 13: 165–71.
Boetig D. Dentists polish up their image. Saturday Evening Post, November 1987.
Choi BCK, Jokovic A, Kay EJ, Main PA, Leake JL. Reducing variability in treatment decision-making: effectiveness of educating clinicians about uncertainty. Med Educ 1998; 32: 105–11.
Clark TD, Mjör IA. Current teaching of cariology in North American dental schools. Oper Dent 2001; 26: 412–18.
Crespo KE, Torres JE, Recio ME. Reasoning process characteristics in the diagnostic skills of beginner, competent, and expert dentists. J Dent Educ 2004; 68: 1235–44.
Cruess RL, Cruess SR, Johnston SE. Professionalism: an ideal to be sustained. Lancet 2000; 356: 156–9.
Cruess SR, Johnston S, Cruess RL. Professionalism for medicine: opportunities and obligations. Med J Aust 2002; 177: 208–11.
Cruess SR, Johnston S, Cruess RL. 'Profession': a working definition for medical educators. Teach Learn Med 2004; 16: 74–6.
Cvar JF, Ryge G. Reprint of criteria for the clinical evaluation of dental restorative materials. Clin Oral Invest 2005; 9: 215–32.
Deligeorgi V, Mjör IA, Wilson NHF. An overview of reasons for the placement and replacement of restorations. Prim Dent Care 2001; 8: 5–11.
Downer MC, Moles DR. Health gain from restorative dental treatment evaluated by computer simulation. Community Dent Health 1998; 15: 32–9.
Ecenbarger W. How honest are dentists? Readers Digest 1997; (February): 50–6.
Elderton RJ. Overtreatment with restorative dentistry: when to intervene? Int Dent J 1993; 43: 17–24.
Elderton RJ. Preventive (evidence-based) approach to quality general dental care. Med Princ Pract 2003; 12(Suppl 1): 12–21.
Espelid I, Tveit AB. Diagnostic quality and observer variation in radiographic diagnoses of approximal caries. Acta Odontol Scand 1986; 44: 39–46.
Espelid I, Tveit AB. Variation in diagnosis of secondary caries and defects in connection with amalgam fillings. Caries Res 1987; 21: 187.
Espelid I, Tveit AB, Fjelltveit A. Variations among dentists in radiographic detection of occlusal caries. Caries Res 1994; 28: 169–75.
Fejerskov O. Changing paradigms in concepts on dental caries: consequences for oral health care. Caries Res 2004; 38: 182–91.
Fejerskov O, Nyvad B. Is dental caries an infectious disease? Diagnostic and treatment consequences for the practitioner. In: Schou L, ed. Nordic Dentistry 2003 Yearbook. Copenhagen: Quintessence, 2003: 141–52.
Friedman JW, Atchison KA. The standard of care: an ethical responsibility of public health dentistry. J Public Health Dent 1993; 53: 165–9.
Gimmestad AL, Holst D, Fylkenes K. Changes in restorative caries treatment in 15-year-olds in Oslo, Norway, 1979-1996. Community Dent Oral Epidemiol 2003; 31: 246–51.
Goldstein GR, Preston JD. Therapy: anecdote, experience, or evidence? Dent Clin North Am 2002; 46: 21–8.
Gordon SM, Dionne RA. The integration of clinical research into dental therapeutics. Making treatment decisions. J Am Dent Assoc 2005; 136: 1701–8.
Grace M. The relevance of evidence. Quintessence Int 1998; 29: 802–5.
Grytten J. Models for financing dental services. A review. Community Dent Health 2005; 22: 75–85.
Hartshorne J, Hasegawa TK. Overservicing in dental practice – ethical perspectives. J S Afri Dent Assoc 2003; 58: 364–9.
Heidmann J, Helm S, Helm T, Poulsen S. Changes in prevalence of approximal caries in 17-year-olds and related restorative treatment strategies over a 6-year period. Community Dent Oral Epidemiol 1988; 16: 167–70.
Hume WR. Research, education, caries, and care – taming and turning the restorative tiger. J Dent Res 1992; 71: 1127.

Hyatt TP. Prophylactic odontotomy. The cutting into the tooth for the prevention of disease. *Dent Cosmos* 1923; **65**: 234–41.

Innes NPT, Evans DJP, Clarkson JE, Foley JI. Obtaining and evidence-base for clinical dentistry through clinical trials. *Prim Dent Care* 2005; **12**: 91–6.

Ismail AI, Bader JD. Evidence-based dentistry in clinical practice. *J Am Dent Assoc* 2004; **135**: 78–83.

Ismail AI, Birch S, Sohn W, Lepkowski JM, Belli RF. Utilities of dentin regeneration among insured and uninsured adults. *Community Dent Oral Epidemiol* 2004; **32**: 55–66.

Kay EJ, Blinkhorn AS. A qualitative investigation of factors governing dentists' treatment philosophies. *Br Dent J* 1996; **180**: 171–6.

Kay EJ, Locker D. Variations in restorative treatment decisions: an international comparison. *Community Dent Oral Epidemiol* 1996; **24**: 376–9.

Kay E, Nuttall N. Clinical decision making – an art or a science? Part I: an introduction. *Br Dent J* 1995a; **178**: 76–8.

Kay E, Nuttall N. Clinical decision making – an art or a science? Part II: making sense of treatment decisions. *Br Dent J* 1995b; **178**: 113–16.

Kay E, Nuttall N. Clinical decision making – an art or a science? Part III: to treat or not to treat? *Br Dent J* 1995c; **178**: 153–5.

Kay E, Nuttall N. Clinical decision making – an art or a science? Part IV: assessing risks and probabilities? *Br Dent J* 1995d; **178**: 190–3.

Kay E, Nuttall N. Clinical decision making – an art or a science? Part V: patient preferences and their influence on decision making. *Br Dent J* 1995e; **178**: 229–32.

Kay E, Nuttall N. Clinical decision making – an art or a science? Part VI: decision making in dental practice: a case study. *Br Dent J* 2006; **1995**: 269–73.

Kidd EAM. The operative management of caries. *Dent Update* 1998; **25**: 104–10.

Kidd EAM. How 'clean' must a cavity be before restoration? *Caries Res* 2004; **38**: 305–13.

Kidd EAM, Fejerskov O. What constitutes dental caries? Histopathology of carious enamel and dentin related to the action of cariogenic biofilms. *J Dent Res* 2004; **83**(Spec Issue C): C35–8.

Kim MY, Lin J, White R, Niederman R. Benchmarking the endodontic literature on MEDLINE. *J Endodont* 2001; **27**: 470–3.

Kress GC. Toward a definition of the appropriateness of treatment. *Public Health Rep* 1980; **95**: 564–71.

Lewis DW, Kay EJ, Main PA, Pharaoh MG, Csima A. Dentists' stated restorative treatment thresholds and their restorative and caries depth decisions. *J Publ Health Dent* 1996a; **56**: 176–81.

Lewis DW, Kay EJ, Main PA, Pharaoh MG, Csima A. Dentists' variability in restorative decisions, microscopic and radiographic caries depth. *Community Dent Oral Epidemiol* 1996b; **24**: 106–11.

Lo ECM, Schwarz E, Wong MCM. Arresting dentine caries in Chinese preschool children. *Int J Paediatr Dent* 1998; **8**: 253–60.

Manji F, Fejerskov O, Nagelkerke NJD, Baelum V. A random effects model for some epidemiological features of dental caries. *Community Dent Oral Epidemiol* 1991; **19**: 324–8.

Marinho VCC, Richards D, Niederman R. Variation, certainty, evidence, and change in dental education: employing evidence-based dentistry in dental education. *J Dent Educ* 2001; **65**: 449–55.

Mileman PA, van den Hout WB. Comparing the accuracy of Dutch dentists and dental students in the radiographic diagnosis of dentinal caries. *Dentomaxillofac Radiol* 2002; **31**: 7–14.

Mileman PA, van den Hout WB. Preferences for oral health states: effect on prescribing periapical radiographs. *Dentomaxillofac Radiol* 2003; **32**: 401–7.

Mileman P, Purdell-Lewis D, van der Weele L. Variation in radiographic caries diagnosis and treatment decisions among university teachers. *Community Dent Oral Epidemiol* 1982; **10**: 329–34.

Mjör IA. Clinical diagnosis of recurrent caries. *J Am Dent Assoc* 2005; **136**: 1426–33.

Mjör IA, Gordan VV. Failure, repair, refurbishing and longevity of restorations. *Oper Dent* 2002; **27**: 528–34.

Mjör IA, Toffenetti F. Secondary caries: a literature review with case reports. *Quintessence Int* 2000; **31**: 165–79.

Mjör IA, Reep RL, Kubilis PS, Mondragon BE. Change in size of replaced amalgam restorations: a methodological study. *Oper Dent* 1998; **23**: 272–7.

Mjör IA, Dahl JE, Moorhead JE. Age of restorations at replacement in permanent teeth in general dental practice. *Acta Odontol Scand* 2000; **58**: 97–101.

Moles DR, Downer MC. Optimum bitewing examination recall intervals assessed by computer simulation. *Community Dent Health* 2000; **17**: 14–19.

Neilson P. It works in my hands. Isn't that good enough? *Quintessence Int* 1998; **29**: 799–802.

Niederman R. The methods of evidence-based dentistry. *Quintessence Int* 1998; **29**: 811–17.

Niederman R, Leitch J. 'Know what' and 'know how': knowledge creation in clinical practice. *J Dent Res* 2006; **85**: 296–7.

Niederman R, Chen L, Murzyn L, Conway S. Benchmarking the dental randomised controlled literature on MEDLINE. *Evid Based Dent* 2002; **3**: 5–9.

Nishimura K, Rasool F, Ferguson MB, Sobel M, Niederman R. Benchmarking the clinical prosthetic dental literature on MEDLINE. *J Prosth Dent* 2002; **88**: 533–41.

Nyvad B. Diagnosis versus detection of caries. *Caries Res* 2004; **38**: 192–8.

Nyvad B, Fejerskov O. Active root surface caries converted into inactive caries as a response to oral hygiene. *Scand J Dent Res* 1986; **94**: 281–4.

Nyvad B, Fejerskov O. Assessing the stage of caries lesion activity on the basis of clinical and microbiological examination. *Community Dent Oral Epidemiol* 1997; **25**: 69–75.

Nyvad B, ten Cate JM, Fejerskov O. Arrest of root surface caries *in situ*. *J Dent Res* 1997; **76**: 1845–53.

Nyvad B, Machiulskiene V, Baelum V. Reliability of a new caries diagnostic system differentiating between active and inactive caries lesions. *Caries Res* 1999; **33**: 252–60.

Park J, Niederman R. Estimating MEDLINE's identification of randomized control trials in pediatric dentistry. *J Clin Pediatr Dent* 2002; **26**: 395–9.

Pitts N. Understanding the jigsaw of evidence-based dentistry. 1. Introduction, research and synthesis. *Evid Based Dent* 2004a; **5**: 2–4.

Pitts N. Understanding the jigsaw of evidence-based dentistry. 2. Dissemination of research results. *Evid Based Dent* 2004b; **5**: 33–5.

Pitts N. Understanding the jigsaw of evidence-based dentistry. 3. Implementation of research findings in clinical practice. *Evid Based Dent* 2004c; **5**: 60–4.

Plasschaert AJM, Holbrook WP, Delap E, Martinez C, Walmsley AD. Profile and competences for the European dentist. *Eur J Dent Educ* 2005; **9**: 98–107.

Raiffa H. *Decision analysis. Introductory lectures on choices under uncertainty.* New York: Random House, 1968: 1–309.

Renshaw J. After the first 125 years of the BDJ where might clinical dentistry be heading? *Br Dent J* 2005; **199**: 331–7.

Robbins JW. Evidence-based dentistry: what is it, and what does it have to do with practice? *Quintessence Int* 1998; **29**: 796–9.

Rushton VE, Horner K, Worthington HV. A two-centre study to determine dentists' agreement with current guidelines on the frequency of bitewing radiography. *Community Dent Oral Epidemiol* 1996; **24**: 175–81.

Russo SP, Fiorellini JP, Weber HP, Niederman R. Benchmarking the dental implant evidence on MEDLINE. *Int J Oral Maxillofac Implants* 2000; **15**: 792–800.

Rytömaa I, Järvinen V, Järvinen J. Variation in caries recording and restorative treatment plan among university teachers. *Community Dent Oral Epidemiol* 1979; **7**: 335–9.

Sackett DL, Rosenberg WMC, Gray JAM, Haynes RB, Richardson WS. Evidence based medicine: what it is and what it isn't. *Br Med J* 1996; **312**: 71–2.

van der Sanden WJM, Mettes DG, Plasschaert AJM, Grol RPTM, Mulder J, Verdonschot EH. Effectiveness of clinical practice guideline implementation on lower third molar management in improving clinical decision-making: a randomized controlled trial. *Eur J Oral Sci* 2005; **113**: 349–54.

Sheiham A. Minimal intervention in dental care. *Med Princ Pract* 2002; **11**(Suppl 1): 2–6.

Shugars DA, Bader JD. Cost implications of differences in dentists' restorative treatment decisions. *J Public Health Dent* 1996; **56**: 219–22.

Thylstrup A. Mechanical vs. disease-oriented treatment of dental caries: educational aspects. *J Dent Res* 1989; **68**: 1135.

Thylstrup A, Bille J, Qvist V. Radiographic and observed tissue changes in approximal carious lesions at the time of operative treatment. *Caries Res* 1986; **20**: 75–84.

Tinanoff N, Douglass JM. Clinical decision-making for caries management in primary teeth. *J Dent Educ* 2001; **65**: 1133–42.

Tveit AB, Espelid I. Variation in treatment decisions on replacement of amalgam fillings. *Caries Res* 1987; **21**: 187.

Wilson NA, Whitehead SA, Mjör IA, Wilson NHF. Reasons for the placement and replacement of crowns in general dental practice. *Prim Dent Care* 2003; **10**: 53–9.

Wright D, Batchelor PA. General dental practitioners' beliefs on the perceived effects of and their preferences for remuneration mechanisms. *Br Dent J* 2002; **192**: 46–9.

Yang S, Needleman H, Niederman R. A bibliometric analysis of the pediatric dental literature in MEDLINE. *Pediatr Dent* 2001; **23**: 415–18.

26

Promoting oral health in populations

E. Kay and R. Craven

Defining oral health and health education and promotion

Defining health has been likened to 'shovelling smoke' (Levin & Ziglio, 1997). It is even more difficult to define 'oral health' since, by doing so, we are limiting the concept of health to a single body part. Doing so flies in the face of rationality, as mouths, oral cavities and body parts cannot be 'healthy' or 'unhealthy'. Health is fundamentally an attribute of a human being, not of an anatomically defined orifice. Moreover, health seems to be a word which, 'means anything one chooses it to mean'. This problem will be explained further later in the chapter, but it is introduced here because, if the problem of defining oral health is not acknowledged, it is unlikely that we will be able to develop effective and viable ways of promoting it.

Indeed, the term oral health promotion also sets a semantic challenge and purists may view it as a discipline in its own right (Bunton & Macdonald, 1992). More helpfully, it can be seen as describing any activity that aims to improve the health of the mouths of the population. Broadly, these activities can be separated into two main areas: first the preventive approach, and secondly the educational approach. The former includes the ever-developing systems of therapeutics and psychology, which can be used to bring about reductions in measurable disease, and behavior change conducive to oral health. The latter is concerned with trying to help individuals to make informed choices, and adapting the environment so that the healthy choices become as easy to make as the unhealthy ones.

Returning to the issue of defining oral health, traditionally a medical model of oral health has been used, in which clinical measures are used to define the person's 'health' or lack of it. Using such a system means that 'oral health' is defined by the presence or absence of pathology. However, oral health does not actually fit well with the medical model of health and disease. This is partly because oral diseases are not usually life threatening, and more importantly because clinical assessments of oral health have only a weak relationship to the individual's perception of their own oral health or their oral health needs.

In the last decade a biopsychosocial model of oral health has become widely accepted (Tones & Green, 2005). This paradigm proposes that symptoms, diseases and disorders interact and interplay with both the psychology of the affected individual and the social system in which the symptoms, disease or disorder are found. For example, how an individual perceives their oral health, the type of person they are, their general well-being and their stress levels will affect the impact that a given level of pathology makes on them. In addition, the society in which the individual lives and their place within it will affect what they do about the symptoms.

Oral health promotion is therefore important because poor oral health can limit personal choices and social opportunities. That is, diseases and deviations from normal occurring in the mouth may diminish life satisfaction in the same way as diseases of other body systems.

In 1994 oral health was defined by the UK Department of Health as 'a standard of health of the oral and related tissues which enables an individual to speak and socialise without active disease, discomfort or embarrassment and which contributes to well being' (Cohen & Gibb, 1995). It is therefore now generally accepted that oral health, and the outcomes of oral health promotion and education, should be based on social, psychological, cultural and economic effects of oral pathologies and abnormalities. The multi-dimensional nature of oral health has therefore resulted in the development of three categories of oral health 'impacts' or potential 'outcome measures', these being:

- tooth loss and oral function (Manty & Vinton, 1951; Mersel & Mann, 1986; Agerberg, 1988; Aukes et al., 1988)
- facial pain and symptoms (Miller & Swallow, 1970; Miller et al, 1975; Locker & Gruska, 1987; Lipton et al, 1993)
- oral well-being/quality of life (Heyink & Schaub, 1986; Kiyal & Mulligan, 1987; Locker & Gruska, 1987; Reisine & Weber, 1989; Karuza et al., 1992).

Understanding the impact of oral health on both individuals and societies is implicit in the 'promotion' of oral health. Unless a benefit from oral health education and promotion can be demonstrated, resources will not be made available for such activities. If oral health promotion benefits individuals and societies in a desirable way, this needs to be identified and quantified so that the health gain from such activities can be clearly demonstrated to all (including clinicians and funders) (Kay, 2004).

In 1974, Lalonde, a Canadian Minister of Health, pointed out that lifestyle, behavior and environment probably contributed more to death and disease than most factors. This led to the development of the Ottawa Charter (Daly et al., 2002), which outlined five key activities as being 'health promoting'. These were:

- the creation of supportive environments
- building healthy public policy
- strengthening community action
- developing personal skills
- reorienting health services.

The World Health Organization (WHO, 1986) has defined health promotion as 'a unifying concept for those who recognize the need for change in the ways and conditions of living in order to promote health. Health promotion represents a mediating strategy between people and their environments, synthesizing personal choice and social responsibility in health to create a healthier future'.

Health promotion therefore has three key elements:

- addressing the determinants of health

- working with stakeholders across and between communities
- having a strategic approach.

A useful analogy when trying to clarify what health promotion achieves is McKinlay's 'Upstream–downstream' argument (McKinlay, 1975) (see Figs 28.4–28.6). He described trying to treat cardiovascular patients using an analogy whereby he was hauling drowning people from a river, but was so busy applying artificial respiration, that he could not walk upstream to find out who was pushing them in, or post warning signs ... All he could do was to work very hard at managing and trying to repair the damage done. The health promotion approach suggests that all health-care providers, including oral health personnel, take a walk 'upstream' and attempt to slow down or stop the development of damaging health outcomes by considering what might be done to reduce the number of people who end up with problems.

The point of oral health promotion (as opposed to oral health education) is that the factors affecting dental caries are influenced not only by individual action but also by complex social, cultural, economic and political factors.

The final section of this chapter will focus on practical tips for promoting oral health in a one-to-one setting, but for groups of people, five basic strategies are available: operative and non-operative treatment, changing behavior, education, empowerment and social change.

Changing behavior

Behavior change in an individual can and will reduce that person's risk of disease. However, although non-operative treatments are often effective on a one-to-one basis, only certain sectors of the population will be reached by such an approach, and the public health benefits of encouraging individuals to be responsible for their own health are limited.

Education

This approach seeks to offer individuals the ability to change their lifestyle, should they choose to do so. The educational approach aims to give information, and also offers personal and decision-making skills so that people's ability to make healthy choices is enhanced. It is a slightly less directive approach than behavior change (see above), in that it does not predetermine what choices the individual should make, but simply offers them the wherewithal to make decisions and act by their own choices.

Empowerment

This model of oral health promotion suggests that the priorities and concerns of individuals and communities, rather than the views of health professionals, should form the basis for action. Thus, by supporting and facilitating,

health promoters can help individuals and communities to take steps to protect or enhance their own health. Examples of this approach include counselling, which seeks to develop a person's understanding of their health priorities and challenges, and community development, wherein groups of people agree how they wish to change their environment to improve their health.

Social change

This approach recognizes that many of the answers to health problems lie within the economic and political arenas, and that the necessary changes require negotiation with politicians, advocacy and lobbying skills. Although not relevant to the clinical setting, it is important that dental care professionals recognize that, when they act in unison, they can present a powerful political voice. To give an example, the British Dental Association organized their members to lobby MPs with regard to the Water Act, and this united action helped to bring about the change in law which permitted fluoridation in the UK.

Often, the most effective strategy will be a combination of two or more approaches. By considering the needs of the individual or group concerned, the barriers that may prevent change (organizational, commercial, political), the communities' profile and way of working, market forces, the characteristics of individuals (see next section) and the research evidence (see subsequent section), the most appropriate and efficient combination of approaches can be decided upon.

Theories of health-related behavior

Health-related behaviors can be broadly divided into three types (Kasl & Cobb, 1996):

- behavior that aims to prevent disease (e.g. reducing intake of non-milk extrinsic sugars, brushing daily with a fluoride toothpaste)
- behavior that aims to seek a remedy (e.g. attending a dentist for check-ups and restorative care)
- behavior that helps an individual to feel better (e.g. taking antibiotics for a dental abscess).

In general, a health-related behavior is exactly what it says: any action taken by an individual that may affect his or her health status.

The recognition that an individual's behavior is one of the main determinants of their health was promulgated in 1979 by McKeown. While McKeown's thesis was supported by reference to lung cancer, coronary heart disease and cirrhosis of the liver, his arguments are just as relevant to dental disease. Theories of health behavior will be outlined below in relation to dental disease. Perhaps the easiest example to use when discussing oral health-related behavior is the sugar–caries relationship.

Observational studies across the globe have repeatedly shown there to be a relationship between the consumption of sugars and caries development (Bradford & Crabb, 1961; Takahashi, 1961; Harns, 1963; Fisher, 1968; Zitzow, 1979; Sreebny, 1982; Newbrun, 1989). The relationship has also been demonstrated in interventional studies in both humans (Gustafsson et al, 1954; Scheinin & Makinen, 1975; Anaise, 1978; Roberts & Roberts, 1979; Frencken et al, 1989; Rodrigues et al., 1999). and animals (Konig et al., 1968; Grenby et al., 1973; Shaw, 1979), and in in vitro experiments (Koulourides et al., 1976; Innfeld, 1977; Grenby et al., 1989). As a result, the following recommendations have been made:

- both the amount and the frequency of sugar consumption should be reduced, and where possible limited to mealtimes
- no more than 10% of the energy in an individual's diet should be provided by sugar.

Since this advice is quite clear-cut and relatively simple, it perhaps seems strange that caries lesions have not yet been eradicated via the sugar-reduction approach.

The theories outlined below demonstrate why changing a behavior, particularly a socially and culturally important one such as feeding behavior, is much more complicated than the sugar–caries evidence would imply.

Health locus of control

This theory suggests that people vary in relation to whether they feel that they control events (internal locus of control) or that events are not controllable by them (external locus of control). This concept can be directly applied to health issues (Wallston & Wallston, 1982). Thus a person may believe 'I am responsible for my health' or they may feel that 'my health is a matter of luck'. Alternatively, they may regard their health as something that someone else has control of: 'the dentist will make my teeth healthy'.

A person's health locus of control therefore predicts whether they are likely to make changes in their life to enhance their health, and also has a bearing on the style of communication with health professionals to which they react best. People with an external health locus of control (i.e. do not consider themselves responsible for their oral health) are unlikely to respond to exhortations from their dentist to eat less sugar or to brush more regularly.

Unrealistic optimism

The phenomenon of 'unrealistic optimism' was first described by Weinstein in 1983. Basically, this theory suggests that people, despite having been given information about health threats, continue to behave in an unhealthy manner. This is explained by the fact that people can tend to ignore their own risk-increasing behavior ('I eat a lot of sweets but that doesn't matter') and focus on their risk-reducing behaviour ('but I brush my teeth'). There is also a tendency for people to compare favorably their own behaviors with the behaviors of others. So, they will focus selectively on the times they do limit their sugar intake and ignore the times when they eat masses and, at the same time, will focus on how much *more* sugar others consume and ignore the times when they witness sugar limitation in others.

Stages of change model

This model of behavior change (Prochaska & Di Clemente, 1982) is also known as the transtheoretical model of behavior change. The theory suggests that there are five stages of behavior change, but that individuals may move back and forth between the stages. The stages are:

- precontemplation: not thinking about changing
- contemplation: beginning to think change may be a 'good thing'
- preparation: making small changes
- action: undertaking the new behavior
- maintenance: the new behavior becomes 'normal' to the individual.

To put this in context, a patient who has never considered their oral hygiene to be relevant to the number of fillings they had (precontemplation) may be informed by their dentist of the need to limit sugar intake (contemplation). They may go to purchase diet drinks and avoid the sweet shop (preparation) and after a second prompt from the dentist may begin to reduce the amount of sugar they eat (action). In time, the new low-sugar regimen becomes an established routine (maintenance).

Many patients move between the stages many times, sometimes relapsing completely, before the new behavior becomes a 'normal' part of their life.

The health belief model

The health belief model (HBM) has been developed over a number of years after its first introduction by Rosenstock in 1966. The model relies on belief in cognition, i.e. that individuals act in a rational and predictable way (which much evidence suggests is *not* the case). The HBM predicts that a set of perceptions held by an individual will influence their health-related behavior. The core beliefs that the model suggests are important are:

- a person's belief that they are susceptible to a health threat (e.g. my teeth are likely to decay)
- a person's belief that the disease will have severe implications (e.g. decayed teeth cause pain and make me ugly)
- a person's belief about the 'costs' of changing their behavior and the likelihood of disease (e.g. if I eat less sugar I will lose too much weight)
- a person's belief about the benefits of change (e.g. if I reduce my tooth decay I will save a lot of dental fees)

- cues to action which may be internal (e.g. the appearance of visible decay) or external (e.g. advice from a dentist).

If all of the above are in place, behavior is more likely to change. In addition, the individual actually needs to care about their oral health and must be confident that they can make the necessary changes (e.g. I am confident that I can reduce the amount of sugar I eat) (Becker & Rosenstock, 1987).

Theories of reasoned action and planned behavior

There has been a debate concerning the relationship between attitudes and behavior for many years, and the theory of reasoned action (TRA) has been central to that debate, particularly in relation to health behavior (Armitage & Conner, 2001).

TRA developed later into the theory of planned behavior (TPB). The TPB suggests that a person's beliefs lead to particular behavioral intentions. A 'behavioral intention' is a plan to act in a certain way, and these intentions are affected by the three beliefs held by the individual about the behavior in question. These are:

- their attitude towards the behavior (e.g. not eating sugar makes me feel good and will improve my dental health)
- their perceptions of social pressures with regard to the behavior. (e.g. people who I like will think I'm much better looking with clean nice teeth, and I want them to like me)
- their beliefs about whether they can successfully undertake the new behavior and that they can overcome both external and internal barriers (e.g. the dentist said my decay rate had slowed, and I will get used to less sugar).

All of these factors influence behavioral intentions which, in turn, influence behavior. However, the last factor (beliefs about successfully undertaking the behavior) can also influence behavior directly.

The health action process approach

The health action process approach (HAPA) (Schwarzer, 1992) is a fairly recent theoretical development. It draws on all the theories and models described above, to a greater or lesser extent. The newer elements that it emphasizes are the importance of time and of self-efficacy. The HAPA predicts actual behavior as well as behavioral intentions, and differs from the other models by distinguishing between the decision-making phase of taking up a new behavior and the action actually being taken.

According to the HAPA, an individual's decision to change a health-related behavior depends on three elements:

- self-efficacy (I am confident that I can give up sugar)
- outcome expectancies (giving up sugar will improve my oral health and people will be pleased about that)

- threat appraisal (if I don't give up sugar all my teeth will rot as I'm very prone to decay).

Of the above factors, self-efficacy (belief in one's own ability to enact the new behavior successfully) has been shown to be the most predictive of behavior change.

Conclusion

While all of the models described above have flaws, and none has been conclusively demonstrated to predict health behaviors reliably in all circumstances, all of them have some predictive and explanatory value. The importance of such models is that they provide information that can be useful in attempts to achieve change in health behaviors in both individuals and populations. Indeed, it is possible that if more interventions had been theory based, many more would have been successful, but guidelines as to how theory should best be translated into practice are not always available. A working knowledge of these theories at the very least provides a framework for developing the field of oral health promotion and placing it on a sound theoretical and conceptual basis.

Oral health education: does it work?

Evidence for effectiveness

It is accepted that all health interventions should be based on the best available evidence. This applies to promoting oral health as well as to clinical care. Several systematic reviews have examined the evidence about oral health promotion (Kay & Locker, 1996, 1998; Sprod *et al.*, 1996; Department of Human Services, 1999). The key findings were as follows:

- Mass-media campaigns can raise awareness of an issue, but have not been shown to be effective in increasing knowledge or changing behavior.
- All programs that have been effective against dental caries have included fluoride.
- One-to-one advice on oral hygiene has been shown to be effective, but the improvement tends not to be sustained.
- Dental/oral health education programs have been shown to improve knowledge and attitudes about oral health issues, but it is not generally possible to extrapolate from these to changes in behavior.
- Water fluoridation remains the most effective and cost-effective public-health measure for caries prevention.

Difficulties in assessing effectiveness

This is an area that is fraught with difficulty. Reviewers have bemoaned the poor quality of many evaluations. It is also striking that few studies of oral health promotion programs include a mention of any underpinning theoretical framework or model. Many studies have used measures that relate to the process of running the program or to outcomes that do not relate specifically to improvements in oral health, and reported behavior change is a common but flawed outcome measure. As in other aspects of evidence-based care, randomized controlled trials (RCTs) are seen as the optimal methodology for evaluating health interventions. While this will be appropriate to many interventions it works less well with others. For programs that work with people rather than do things to them, where programs evolve and adapt with time and where programs act in a complementary way, the RCT is unlikely to be an appropriate evaluation tool (Daly & Watt, 1998).

Alternative approaches will use qualitative methods (Nutbeam, 1998) and triangulation (drawing on evidence from different sources and possibly using different methods to draw conclusions about the same program) (Speller et al., 1997; Watt et al., 2004). A further difficulty with the evaluation of oral health promotion lies in the timescale for the carious process. Evaluators must wait at least 2–3 years before being able to assess the outcome of a caries prevention program if changes in disease are the outcomes of interest. Hence, it may be appropriate to use various proxies for impact on caries increment, e.g. the validated increased use of fluoride toothpaste of appropriate strength. Finally, there is the issue of transferability of results. Implementing an oral health education program is not like administering a drug. It is a human interaction and much will depend not just on content and process, but also on the details of how it is delivered, the personal style and enthusiasm of the educator, and possibly quite subtle aspects that may mean that a program may be successful in one situation but not in another.

Examples of oral health education programs

Many evaluations have measured the effect of school-based programs. Little impact on caries experience has been documented where the intervention was of dental health education alone and there was no use of fluoride in some form. A recent study in Belgium (Vanobbergen et al., 2004) evaluated a 6-year program of yearly 1 h sessions of health education starting at the age of 7 years, and showed fewer reports of toothache in the test group, but inconclusive results for plaque control and no reduction in caries increment. An Australian 2-year study compared the addition of a program of cleaning and health education to the standard preventive care delivered by the school dental service, and found no additional effect on first molars in children aged 6 years at the start of the study (Arrow, 2000), with around 20% of subjects in both groups developing new lesions in first permanent molars during the 2 years of the study. A Swedish study (Kallestal, 2005) compared various programs for high-risk 12-year-olds followed up over 5 years. The options compared advice alone with various applications of fluoride as varnish or prescription as lozenges, but no sig-

nificant differences were found between groups. The low caries increment may help to explain this, and the differences were largest for the groups where fluoride was used.

School-based programs of health education focussed principally on brushing have been tested in several studies (Ivanovic & Lekic, 1996; Redmond et al, 1999; Pine et al, 2000; Hawkins et al., 2001; Worthington et al., 2001). There is potential for reducing plaque levels in the short term and for up to 1 year. In a review of the effectiveness of oral health promotion on oral hygiene and gingival health, Watt and Marinho (2005) concluded that short-term reduction in plaque levels can be expected following health education programs, and may be sustained for up to 6 months. One recent study showed an effect on caries following a supervised school brushing scheme in an area of deprivation and using fluoride toothpaste at 1450 ppm F (Jackson et al., 2005).

Another supervised program of brushing combined with a home-based incentive scheme for 5-year-olds showed the differential effect of brushing frequency. Those reported to brush only once a day had 64% more caries than those who brushed twice a day. Although these are reported data and must be treated with some caution, they support other evidence on the impact of increased frequency of exposure to fluoride paste (Pine et al., 2000). However, another health education program in China focussed on brushing among primary school children and showed no effect on caries after 3 years (Petersen et al., 2004). It is difficult to interpret these results and this illustrates the problem of transferability (see above).

Examples of findings from other recent studies of health education in schools are listed below.

- Teaching brushing to small groups worked better than a whole class session approach for high-risk 5–6-year-olds in the USA (Hawkins et al., 2001).
- Use of lactobacillus counts for motivating 16–19-year-olds in 6-monthly advice sessions produced a reduction in proximal lesions, but the gain was small when compared with the costs (Nylander et al., 2001).
- Sugar-free chewing gum in a school-based program showed over 40% mean increment reduction in a high caries risk group of 6–7-year-olds (Peng et al., 2004).
- The addition to a health education program of 3-monthly cleaning and professional fluoride varnish application over a 2-year period gave a reduction in increment of early caries lesions (Zimmer et al., 2001).

The effectiveness of health education in nurseries and kindergartens has been reported in two recent papers. The effect of twice-daily brushing with 1100 ppm F toothpaste on school days combined with monthly health education to the children and 6-monthly health education to the parents was examined by Rong et al. (2003). After 2 years, the caries increment was significantly reduced, by 31%. A similar study, also in China, showed a reduction of 21% overall in caries increment through twice-daily brushing with 1100 ppm F paste and no other intervention (You et al., 2002). Given that fluoride toothpaste has not been available to the general public in China, it is very likely that the major impact in both these programs is that of fluoride rather than health education.

Attempts have been made to reach children at risk before the nursery/kindergarten stage. Some examples of interventions reported as successful are described below.

- A trial tested the effectiveness of a dental health educator within a general dental practice. A sample of children aged 1–6 years was seen every 4 months for a 2-year period for advice about brushing, fluoride toothpaste use and the control of sugar intake. At the end of the period the test group had 18% fewer primary teeth affected by decay, but the difference was insignificant (Blinkhorn et al., 2003). The children, although assessed as being at high risk of caries, were still regularly attending throughout the test period and so may not be representative of this group as a whole. The authors also expressed doubt as to whether the benefits of such a program justified the costs.
- The value of home visits was assessed in a 3-year study among a birth cohort of high-risk children in Leeds, UK. Visits commenced at 8 months. Significant differences were found between groups. Caries prevalence after 3 years was 4% in the test group and 33% in controls, but yearly visits were as effective as those at 3-monthly intervals (Kowash et al., 2000)
- One-to-one advice (from a lay person of similar background and culture) was combined with community-wide programs for the Vietnamese population in Vancouver, Canada (Harrison & Wong, 2003). At the end of the program the caries prevalence was 94% in the control group and 43% in the test group.
- A combination of community development projects was assessed in preventing early childhood caries (ECC) in preschool children in Glasgow (Blair et al., 2004). Reductions in caries increment were achieved of 46 and 37%, respectively, among 3–4 and 4–5-year-olds. The interventions included comprised:
  - nutrition projects in schools and nurseries: breakfast clubs, school fruit, snack and meal policies in nurseries
  - tooth-brushing schemes in nurseries, breakfast clubs and after-school care schemes
  - distribution of free fluoride toothpaste and brushes
  - health education by health visitors at surveillance checks, baby clubs and other community settings
  - opportunistic interventions at community health fairs, primary care settings, etc.

These were impressive results and further work is being done to develop and refine the program. As the authors

comment, it is not possible to tell which parts of the project were essential to its success.

- Advice was given at routine developmental checks by health visitors, covering issues of weaning, feeding and brushing with fluoride toothpaste, together with a pack of brush and paste and leaflets (Hamilton et al., 1999). This pilot program showed improvements in knowledge and reported behavior. This program has since been developed as the Brushing for Life program, implemented nationally in the UK in areas of high dental need. Further interventions with health visitor staff were added at the age of 18 months and 3 years. Evaluation of the full program is needed.
- Free fluoride toothpaste and advice leaflets were sent by post to the parents of children at high risk of caries in the UK. This began at the age of 12 months and continued until 5–6 years. A significant reduction of 16% in dmft was achieved where the toothpaste used was 1450 ppm F, but not for 440 ppm F (Davies et al., 2002).
- A similar program to the one described above was developed for delivering dental packs to parents of young children, aged 8–32 months, in deprived areas, and this achieved a reduction of 29% in the prevalence of ECC (Davies et al., 2005). Packs were distributed at designated doctors surgeries and clinics. Supplies of toothpaste (at 1450 ppm F) and brushes were delivered at intervals by post, plus a feeder cup, together with advice about infant feeding.
- Traditional health education (video and leaflet) was compared with the same intervention and an additional motivational interview plus a series of six follow-up telephone calls to parents of children aged 6–18 months in the USA (Weinstein et al., 2004). The motivational interview is a technique that has been used to change other behaviors, including alcohol and drug addiction. The interviewer explores reasons for change and encourages the client through the process, promoting a sense of their competency. A statistically significant improvement in caries increment was found at 1 year using the motivational interview when compared with controls (0.71 versus 1.91).

A few programs have aimed to reach mothers even before the birth of their children (Gomez et al., 2001; Zanata et al., 2003). A study in Brazil gave an intervention to pregnant women who had active caries. The interventions included oral hygiene instruction, oral hygiene self-care kits, the provision of restorative care with glass-ionomers and antimicrobial therapy to reduce transmission of cariogenic bacteria to the newborn. When assessed 2–5 years later, appreciable reductions were found in the prevalence and severity of caries in the children, compared with controls who did not receive the program.

Very little evidence is available comparing the costs and effectiveness of programs. The conclusions in those that have attempted this have been cautious about the validity of their results and in advocating widespread uptake of the dental health education programs tested (Davies *et al.*, 2003). This is an area where more work is needed. Those planning how to promote oral health have very little evidence with which to weigh one program against another and costs, which are a key element of these decisions, are unfortunately rarely researched.

One rare program aimed at older adults on low income living independently was recently carried out in Seattle, USA. The study tested several interventions over a 3-year period: usual care; 2 h of health education twice a year; health education plus weekly chlorhexidine rinses; as before plus twice-yearly fluoride varnish as before plus scaling and root planing at 6-monthly intervals. Those programs that included health education plus a weekly rinse of chlorhexidine (with or without 6-monthly fluoride varnish, and with or without 6-monthly scaling) had 27% and 23% reductions in coronal and root caries, respectively, when compared with those having health education alone or just their usual care (Powell *et al.*, 1999). Again, this is a key area for urgently needed research given the increase within industrialized countries in the numbers of older adults, many of them dentate and presenting with complex dental problems and deteriorating general health.

Advances in the research basis for oral health promotion have been made. A useful model and framework for health education evaluation has been developed giving possible methods for evaluation appropriate to the type of intervention. A range of outcome measures has also been developed as tools for evaluation (Nutbeam, 1998; Redmond *et al.*, 1999). A WHO-sponsored workshop reported on community-based oral heath promotion programs and gave comprehensive recommendations about the future for evaluation and research in health education. Among its recommendations was the idea of setting aside 10% of any budget for oral health-promotion programs to be used in the evaluation of their effectiveness (Petersen & Kwan, 2004).

Funding for the whole health-promotion endeavor is hardly proportional to its potential importance. One example quoted in the literature is that the total annual budget for health promotion in the UK National Health Service amounted to less than the budget for staff cars, traveling and subsistence in that year (Speller *et al.*, 1997). Given that health promotion is an easy target for budget cuts, it seems that these figures are unlikely to have improved.

Conclusions

- Fluoride remains the most potent preventive measure against caries.

- One-to-one tailored advice may be helpful for particular high-risk groups, e.g. new mothers of young children and members of minority ethnic groups.
- Combining population-based programs with more traditional health education may hold promise.
- School-based programs can improve oral hygiene in the short term, but the impact on caries is uncertain.
- More research is needed on improving the oral health of older adults.
- More research is required on the comparative costs of programs.
- Appropriate evaluation of health education needs more emphasis and proper funding.

Practical tips for influencing individual patients' behavior

This section attempts to translate the information from the previous sections into a set of practical tips for influencing patients' behavior (Fishbein, 1967) which dental care professionals can put to use in their surgeries to promote oral health. The information below results from a synthesis of the models described, plus elements from other theories and models, combined with many years of practical experience with patients. Although application of the techniques described below will not guarantee health in every single case, development of the skills that are outlined can result in the most amazing progress with some patients, which is one of the greatest successes a caring professional can achieve, i.e. turning a high disease risk patient into a low disease risk person.

Understanding the difficulties

It is important to recognize that people do not necessarily act in ways which fit with rationality, i.e. even when a person has a clear goal, and knows what action to take to reach that goal, they do not always succeed. Thus, it is essential that dental care professionals do not fall into the trap of assuming that if they merely inform their patients about what is helpful and what is harmful (e.g. a low-sugar diet, regular tooth brushing, appropriate attendance, completing courses of antibiotics), the patients will take action accordingly. One only has to watch the daily news to gather evidence that suggests that humans are not necessarily driven primarily by rationality. Dental teams must therefore lower their expectations and learn to support the process of behavior change, rather than thinking that lifestyle change is an instantaneous, information-based decision.

Information, awareness and knowledge are insufficient motivations to change the way in which people habitually behave (Fishbein & Azjen, 1975; Schwarzer *et al.*, 1994).

Exploring barriers to change

One of the first barriers experienced by people who are considering change is the attitudes of those around them. The beliefs and expectations of a person's peers have a very strong effect on a person's ability to see change through. So, recruiting people who support a behavior change (e.g. a child's parents, siblings, etc.) to express frequently to the individual concerned that they believe the new behavior to be 'a good thing' will be helpful. Other barriers to change are more easily dealt with. These tend to be structural barriers, such as time availability, an appropriate environment for the new behavior to take place, the right equipment and the necessary skills to undertake the actions required. So, a dental care professional who is expecting a patient to change should ensure first of all that the individual does have the time to take care of their personal health, and that they have the appropriate facilities (e.g. access to a bathroom, healthier foods available to them). Thus, the dental team who wish to support change in their patients must have a sensitive and respectful attitude to their patients' current lifestyle. Suggesting to someone that their current behavior is unacceptable, if they simply do not have the wherewithal to change, is unfair and probably counter-productive.

The process of change

Drawing on the stages of change model can offer helpful pointers as to how best to assist a person who is trying to make alterations to their lifestyle (Kay & Tinsley, 2004).

Long before a person takes action for the sake of their health, they will gather and absorb information (almost subconsciously) about the health threat. This may (or may not) stimulate them to think that perhaps they ought to do something about their current way of life. Once this happens, the individual will then be sensitized to listen assiduously to further information and may even ask for advice. If an individual is at this stage of change, immediate action should not be expected: the individual is going through the precontemplation and contemplation stages of the process of change. Although no change in behavior is yet witnessed, the person is moving towards change. The giving of information at this stage is important to the continuation of the process. Precontemplation and contemplation are lengthy stages in the process of change, and a host of other factors (some mentioned above) will influence whether or not the person concerned takes action as a result of the information they glean.

The preparation, action and maintenance stages of behavior change are also part of the process, rather than being ends in themselves.

Individuals who adopt new sets of behaviors sometimes take up the new actions fairly easily, but relapse (especially if the person's circumstances change) is common. It is important, when supporting patients' behavior changes, to expect relapses in behavior and to support the person rather than reprimand them for their relapses. For example, a patient might very successfully adopt a new oral hygiene regimen, then, when they go on holiday for a fortnight, the new pattern of behavior collapses. If at this point a patient is made to feel like a failure, they will become alienated and will return to the precontemplation stage of change, when what you want them to do is re-establish action; this requires support and reassurance that the relapse is not permanent.

Operant conditioning

The consequences of any given action determine the likelihood that that action will reoccur on a subsequent occasion. Thus, if something 'good' happens after a particular action has been taken, the action is more likely to happen again. Alternatively, if something unpleasant happens after a particular action, it is less likely to happen again.

Tooth brushing offers a helpful and practical example of how operant conditioning works. The action of brushing can be seen as offering a 'reward' or 'reinforcer' because it makes a person's mouth taste and feel good. However, should gingival bleeding occur each time the teeth are brushed, the consequences of the brushing action may be deemed to have elicited a 'punishment'. In the first case, brushing is more likely to happen on a subsequent occasion, and in the second example brushing becomes less likely. The consequences of an action can be enhanced by others. Praise and encouragement for an action can act as reinforcers. Using operant conditioning to encourage behavior change can be helpful, although dental 'rewards' (reduction in caries rates, tooth retention) are not powerful or immediate to most individuals. A personally relevant reinforcer must be stressed for each individual. For example, 'kissability' may act as a powerful incentive, particularly in those who are seeking to 'pair-bond'.

When seeking reinforcers for desired behaviors, the consideration of time is also crucial. The power of a consequence to act as a reward is directly related to how closely in time the consequence occurs after the action. For example, patients trying to limit their sugar consumption are being asked to forgo the immediately rewarding outcomes of satisfied hunger and sweet taste, for a gain which, although it may be important to them (healthy teeth), lies a very long and indeterminate amount of time in the future.

Thus, dental professionals must take care to specify appropriate and quick rewards if they wish to help to determine their patients' health. Immediate rewards from a desired behavior, e.g. kissability, feelings of self-control and short-term improvements in appearance, should be stressed, as these are more psychologically weighty than the long-term, more important consequences.

Cognitive dissonance

Dissonance is the feeling that people experience when they believe that a certain behavior is the best course of action, but then behave in a different way. It is the feeling of discomfort we feel when we are not doing as we feel we 'ought' (Elder *et al.*, 1999). For example, a mother who believes the recommendation that her child should eat fewer sweets will feel some sort of psychological discomfort when she gives some of the 'unhealthy' food to her infant. This is dissonance.

When an individual is feeling this way they need to relieve their dissonant position. Unfortunately, it is not always the behavior that changes to relieve the dissonance. It is also possible that the belief causing the dissonance may be altered. Thus, although the mother believes 'sweets are bad for my child's teeth', she may add provisos: 'but I don't give enough for it to matter' or 'but my daughter has got very strong teeth' or 'I'll brush them really well tonight' (see unrealistic optimism, earlier). Alternatively, and unfortunately, the mother may dismiss her original belief in order to relieve her sense of dissonance. 'That dentist is making things up.' Of course, she could alter her behavior and stop, or at least reduce the child's sweet consumption, but this may be difficult to do. Whether the belief or the behavior changes depends on the amount of reinforcement given to each. If the mother's peers (other mothers) encourage sweet-giving then it is unlikely to be the behavior that will alter. However, if the mother's family and friends all praised her frequently and supported the 'no sweets' regimen, then the mother would be more likely to alter her behavior, rather than her beliefs.

Consequences and antecedents to behavior

Every piece of behavior has a consequence. However, many behaviors also have antecedent circumstances, i.e. certain events often precede particular behaviors. Thus, the environment in which patients make decisions to change will influence what actions follow. Therefore, the circumstances and environment in which a new behavior is expected to take place are worthy of consideration.

The altering of the order of events can be a useful tip to pass on to patients. For example, if a female patient showers, washes her hair and applies make-up every morning, but is less than assiduous with her oral hygiene, a simple reordering of events may prove extremely helpful. Patients should be encouraged to make their habitual, everyday routines dependent on the successful completion of the new behavior; in this example, the woman could be advised not to allow herself to wash her hair or to apply make-up until her teeth have been adequately cleaned.

Self-efficacy and health locus of control

Both of these concepts were explained in an earlier section, but this section offers practical tips on how these theories can be used for patient benefit.

Most dentists and members of the dental team will have encountered a patient who seems to want to change their behavior, has the ability and knowledge to change their behavior, and also believes that the reward from the new behavior is highly worthwhile … and yet the patient still finds adopting and sustaining the new behavior extremely difficult. The concepts of self-efficacy and health locus of control are helpful in explaining why such a patient finds change so difficult.

Self-efficacy refers to one's belief in oneself, one's belief that one can do something if one puts one's mind to it. People who truly believe that they just cannot manage a new behavior pattern will not bother trying.

Therefore, if the dentist detects self-defeating beliefs in a patient, it is very important to identify something in their past when they have achieved something through being determined. Whether this is passing a driving test, coming top in an exam or running a marathon is immaterial – the issue is to point out to the person that their belief that they cannot stick to anything and achieve their goal is not true.

There are other patients who, although they seem to have great belief in their own ability to change, also seem to have an attitude of 'I couldn't be bothered'. Such individuals have a strong sense of self-efficacy and are confident that they can change. However, they do not do so because they are unconvinced that the outcomes will be worth the effort. That is, the person is making decisions about what to do based on their estimate of the likelihood of getting something 'good' or 'worthwhile'. So, a person with an external health locus of control, who believes that their health lies ultimately in the hands of fate, or a 'powerful other', will be unlikely to change their behavior for the sake of their health because they actually believe that it will not make any difference in the long run.

The dental team can help such patients by setting small, easily achievable goals (outcomes) and offering huge positive reinforcement for any achievement or progress towards behavior change. This will serve to point out to the person that what happens, at least to their mouths, is largely dependent on their own actions.

It should be clear from the above that offering patients a sense of 'control' in the surgery may be very important in relation to their ability to adopt self-care regimens. If dental practitioners take responsibility away from the patient and treat them as if they are merely the passive acceptors of dental care, then it is somewhat unfair and unreasonable to then send them away by telling them to take actions to care for themselves. Oral health is enhanced if, throughout the delivery of care in the surgery, careful attention is paid to maintaining the patient's sense of self-efficacy, and also internalizing their health locus of control.

Setting goals

The setting of clear goals is essential if behavior is to change, because throughout the process of behavior change, it is very important that all involved parties are very clear about what they are trying to achieve (Reisine & Litt, 1993). If the goals and end outcomes are not made clear, behavior change will not occur. Statements such as 'improve your diet' or 'you need to brush better' do not make anything clear. The patient is left not knowing exactly what it is they are supposed to do, or why they may want to do it.

When advising patients on behavior change the dentist needs to:

- give the patient a personally relevant reason for taking action, e.g. 'that is three fillings you have needed in the last year. I can tell you how to stop this white-spot lesion becoming a hole'
- make it clear what is to be achieved, e.g. 'limit sugar intake to mealtimes and completely stop taking any sweetened drinks'
- offer them a technique whereby the goal can be achieved, e.g. 'why not try using sweetener instead of sugar and eat your sweets at mealtimes?'

By making precise statements about why the person might want to change, by offering precise and achievable goals, and by describing exactly what changes to make, behavior change is more likely. All three steps are vital if patients are to benefit from the professionals' knowledge about the causes of oral diseases and their prevention.

Conclusions

This chapter has outlined the theory of oral health promotion and oral health education. The authors have attempted to explain not only how people behave and the consequences that their behavior has on their oral health, but have also tried to examine and interpret why people behave as they do. Such insights into the science of behavior are the key to promoting health, both within and outside surgery.

References

Agerberg G. Mandibular function and dysfunction in complete denture wearers – a literature review. *J Oral Rehabil* 1988; **15**: 237–49.

Anaise JZ. Prevalence of dental caries among workers in the sweets industry in Israel. *Community Dent Oral Epidemiol* 1978; **6**: 286–9.

Armitage CJ, Conner M. Efficacy of the Theory of Planned Behaviour: a meta-analytic review. *Br J Soc Psychol* 2001; **40**: 471–99.

Arrow P. Cost minimisation analysis of two occlusal caries preventive programmes. *Community Dent Health* 2000; **17**: 85–91.

Aukes J, Kayser A, Felling A. The subjective experience of mastication in subjects with shortened dental arches. *J Oral Rehabil* 1988; **15**: 321–4.

Becker MH, Rosenstock IM. Comparing social learning theory and the Health Belief Model. In: Ward WB, ed. *Advances in health education and promotion.* Greenwich: TAI Press, 1987; Vol. 2, pp. 245–9.

Blair Y, Macpherson LMD, McCall DR, McMahon AD, Stephen KW. Glasgow nursery-based caries experience before and after a community development-based oral health promotion programme's implementation. *Community Dent Health* 2004; **21**: 291–8.

Blinkhorn AS, Gratrix D, Holloway PJ, Wainwright-Stringer YM, Ward SJ, Worthington HV. A cluster randomised, controlled trial of the value of dental health educators in general dental practice. *Br Dent J* 2003; **195**: 395–400.

Bradford E, Crabb H. Carbohydrate restriction and caries incidence: a pilot study. *Br Dent J* 1961; **111**: 273–9.

Bunton R, Macdonald G, eds. *Health promotion: disciplines and diversity.* London: Routledge, 1992.

Cohen LK, Gibb H, eds. *Disease prevention and oral health promotion. socio-dental sciences in action.* London: Munksgaard, 1995.

Daly B, Watt RG. *Designing and evaluating effective oral health promotion.* London: OHERG, 1998.

Daly B, Watt R, Batchelor P, Treasure E. *Essential dental public health.* Oxford: Oxford University Press, 2002.

Davies GM, Worthington HV, Ellwood RP, *et al.* A randomised controlled trial of the effectiveness of providing free fluoride toothpaste from the age of 12 months on reducing caries in 5–6 year old children. *Community Dent Health* 2002; **19**: 131–6.

Davies GM, Worthington HV, Ellwood RP, *et al.* An assessment of the cost effectiveness of a postal toothpaste programme to prevent caries among five-year old children in the North West of England. *Community Dent Health* 2003; **20**: 201–10.

Davies GM, Duxbury JT, Boothman NJ, Davies RM, Blinkhorn AS. A staged intervention dental health promotion programme to reduce early childhood caries. *Community Dent Health* 2005; **22**: 118–22.

Department of Human Services. *Promoting Oral Health 2000–2004: strategic direction and framework for action.* Melbourne: Health Development Section, 1999.

Elder JP, Ayala GX, Harris S. Theories and intervention approaches to health behaviour in primary care. *Am J Prev Med* 1999; **17**: 275–84.

Fishbein M. Attitude and prediction of behaviour. In: Fishbein M, ed. *Readings in attitude theory and measurement.* New York: Wiley, 1967; pp. 477–92.

Fishbein M, Azjen I. *Belief, attitude, intention and behaviour: an introduction to theory and research.* Reading, MA: Addison-Wesley, 1975.

Fisher F. A field study of dental caries, periodontal disease and enamel defects in Tristan da Cunha. *Br Dent J* 1968; **125**: 447–53.

Frencken J, Rugarabamu P, Mulder J. The effects of sugar cane chewing on the development of dental caries. *J Dent Res* 1989; **68**: 1102–4.

Gomez SS, Weber AA, Emilson C. A prospective study of a caries prevention program in pregnant women and their children five and six years of age. *J Dent Child* 2001; **68**: 191–5.

Grenby T, Paterson F, Cawson R. Dental caries and plaque formation from diets containing sucrose and glucose in gnotobiotic rats infected with *Streptococcus* strain. *Br J Nutr* 1973; **29**: 221–8.

Grenby T, Phillips A, Saldanha M. The possible dental effects of children's risks: laboratory evaluation by two different methods. *Br Dent J* 1989; **166**: 157–62.

Gustafsson BE, Quensel CE, Lanke LS, *et al.* The Vipeholm dental caries study; the effect of different levels of carbohydrate intake on caries activity in 436 individuals observed for five years. *Acta Odontol Scand* 1954; **11**: 232–64.

Hamilton FA, Davis KE, Blinkhorn AS. An oral health promotion programme for nursing caries. *Int J Pediatr Dent* 1999; **9**: 195–200.

Harns R. Biology of the children of Hopewood House, Bowral, Australia. 4. Observations on dental-caries experience extending over five years (1957–1961). *J Dent Res* 1963; **42**: 1387–99.

Harrison RL, Wong T. An oral health promotion program for an urban minority population of preschool children. *Community Dent Health* 2003; **31**: 392–9.

Hawkins RJ, Zanetti DL, Main PA, *et al.* Toothbrushing competency among high-risk grade one students: an evaluation of two methods of dental health education. *J Public Health Dent* 2001; **61**: 197–292.

Heyink J, Schaub R. Denture problems and the quality of life in a Dutch elderly population. *Community Dent Oral Epidemiol* 1986; **14**: 193–4.

Innfeld T. Evaluation of the cariogenicity of confectionery by intra-oral wire-telemetry. *SSO Schweiz Monatsschr Zahnheilkd* 1977; **87**: 437–64.

Ivanovic M, Lekic P. Transient effect of a short-term educational programme without prophylaxis on control of plaque and gingival inflammation in school children. *J Clin Periodontol* 1996; **23**: 750–7.

Jackson RJ, Newman HN, Smart GJ, *et al.* The effects of a supervised toothbrushing programme on the caries increment of primary school children, initially aged 5–6 years. *Caries Res* 2005; **39**: 108–15.

Kallestal C. The effect of five years' implementation of caries-preventive methods in Swedish high-risk adolescents. *Caries Res* 2005; **39**: 20–6.

Karuza J, Miller WA, Lieberman D, Ledenyi L, Thines T. Oral status and resident well-being in a skilled nursing facility population. *Gerontologist* 1992; **32**: 104–12.

Kasl SV, Cobb S. Health behaviour, illness behaviour and sick role behaviour. *Arch Environ Health* 1996; **12**: 531–41.

Kay EJ, ed. *A guide to prevention in dentistry*. London: British Dental Journal Books, 2004.

Kay E, Locker D. Is dental health education effective? A systematic review of current evidence. *Community Dent Oral Epidemiol* 1996; **24**: 231–5.

Kay E, Locker D. A systematic review of the effectiveness of health promotion aimed at improving oral health. *Community Dent Health* 1998; **15**: 132–44.

Kay EJ, Tinsley SR. *Communication and the dental team*. Brackley: Stephen Hancocks, 2004.

Kiyal H, Mulligan K. Studies of the relationship between oral health and psychological well-being. *Gerodontics* 1987; **3**: 109–12.

Konig K, Schmid P, Schmid R. An apparatus for frequency controlled feeding of small rodents and its use in dental caries experiments. *Arch Oral Biol* 1968; **13**: 13–26.

Koulourides T, Bodden R, Keller S, *et al.* Cariogenicity of nine sugars tested with an intraoral device in man. *Caries Res* 1976; **10**: 427–41.

Kowash MB, Pinfield A, Smith J, Curzon ME. Effectiveness on oral health of a long-term health education programme for mothers with young children. *Br Dent J* 2000; **26**: 201–5.

Lalonde M. *A new perspective on the health of Canadians*. Ottawa: Health and Welfare, 1974.

Levin L, Ziglio E. Health promotion as an investment strategy: a perspective for the 21st century. In: Sidell M, Jones L, Katz J, Peberdy A, eds. *Debates and dilemmas in promoting health*. London: MacMillan, 1997.

Lipton JA, Ship J, Larach-Robinson D. Estimated prevalence and distribution of reported orofacial pain in the United States. *J Am Dent Assoc* 1993; **124**: 115–21.

Locker D, Gruska M. Prevalence of oral and facial pain and discomfort: preliminary results of a merit survey. *Community Dent Oral Epidemiol* 1987; **15**: 169–72.

McKeown T. *The role of medicine*. Oxford: Blackwell, 1979.

McKinlay JB. A case for refocusing upstream, the political economy of illness. In: Enelow A, Henderson J. *Applying behavioural science to cardiovascular risk*. Washington, DC: American Heart Association, 1975; pp. 7–17.

Manty R, Vinton P. A survey of cleaning ability of denture wearers. *J Dent Res* 1951; 30: 314–21.

Mersel A, Mann J. Denture quality: nutrition and socio-demographic factors. *Spec Care Dentist* 1986; **6**: 231–2.

Miller J, Swallow J. Dental pain and health. *Public Health London* 1970; **85**: 46–50.

Miller J, Elwood PC, Swallow JN. Dental pain: an incidence study. *Br Dent J* 1975; **139**: 327–8.

Newbrun E. *Cariology*, 3rd edn. Chicago, IL: Quintessence, 1989.

Nutbeam D. Evaluating health promotion – progress, problems and solutions. *Health Promot Int* 1998; **13**: 27–44.

Nylander A, Kumlin I, Martinsson M, Twetman S. Effect of a school-based preventive program with salivary lactobacillus counts as sugar-motivating tool on caries increment in adolescents. *Acta Odontol Scand* 2001; **59**: 88–92.

Peng B, Petersen PE, Bian Z, Tai B, Jiang H. Can school-based oral health education and a sugar-free chewing gum program improve oral health? Results from a two-year study in PR China. *Acta Odontol Scand* 2004; 62: 328–32.

Petersen PE, Kwan S. Evaluation of community-based oral health promotion and oral disease prevention – WHO recommendations for improved evidence in public health practice. *Community Dent Health* 2004; **21** (Suppl): 319–29.

Petersen PE, Peng B, Tai B, Bian Z, Fan M. Effect of a school-based oral health education programme in Wuhan City, People's Republic of China. *Int Dent J* 2004; **54**: 33–41.

Pine C M, McGoldrick PM, Burnside G, *et al.* An intervention programme to establish toothbrushing: understanding parents' beliefs and motivating children. *Int Dent J* 2000; (Suppl): 312–23.

Powell LV, Persson RE, Kiyak HA, Hujoel PP. Caries prevention in a community-dwelling older population. *Caries Res* 1999; **33**: 333–9.

Prochaska JO, Di Clemente CC. Transtheoretical therapy: toward a more integrative model of change. *Psychotherapy: Theory, Research and Practice* 1982; **19**: 276–88.

Redmond CA, Blinkhorn FA, Kay EJ, Davies RM, Worthington HV, Blinkhorn AS. A cluster randomized controlled trial testing the effectiveness of a school-based dental health education program for adolescents. *J Public Health Dent* 1999; **59**: 12–17.

Reisine S, Litt M. Social and psychological theories and their use for dental practice. *Int Dent J* 1993; **43** (Suppl 1): 279–87.

Reisine S, Weber J. The effects of tempero-mandibular joint disorders on patients' quality of life. *Community Dent Health* 1989; **6**: 257–70.

Roberts I, Roberts G. Relation between medicines sweetened with sucrose and dental disease. *BMJ* 1979; **ii**: 14–16.

Rodrigues C, Watt R, Sheiham A. The effects of dietary guidelines on sugar intake and dental caries in 3 year olds attending nurseries. *Health Promot Int* 1999; **14**: 329–35.

Rong WS, Bian JY, Wang WJ, Wang JD. Effectiveness of an oral health education and caries prevention program in kindergartens in China. *Community Dent Oral Epidemiol* 2003; **31**: 412–16.

Rosenstock IM. Why people use health services. *Milbank Mem Fund Q* 1966; **44**: 94–124.

Scheinin A, Makinen K. Turku sugar studies. *Acta Odontol Scand* 1975; **22** (Suppl): 1–349.

Schwarzer R. Self efficacy in the adoption and maintenance of health behaviours. In Schwarzer R, ed. *Self efficacy: thought control of action*. Washington, DC: Hemisphere, 1992: 217–43.

Schwarzer R, Jerusalem M, Hahn A. Unemployment, social support and health complaints: a longitudinal study of stress in East German refugees. *J Community Appl Soc Psychol* 1994; **4**: 31–45.

Shaw JH. Changing food habits and our need for evaluations of the cariogenic potential of foods and confections. *Pediatr Dent* 1979; **1**: 192–8.

Speller V, Learmouth A, Harrison D. The search for evidence of effective health promotion. *BMJ* 1997; **315**: 361–63.

Sprod A, Anderson R, Treasure E. *Effective oral health promotion. Literature review*. Cardiff: Health Promotion Wales, 1996.

Sreebny LM. The sugar–caries axis. *Int Dent J* 1982; **32**: 1–12.

Takahashi K. Statistical study on caries incidence in the first molar in relation to the amount of sugar consumption. *Bull Tokyo Dent Coll* 1961; **1**: 58–70.

Tones K, Green J. *Health promotion: planning and strategies*. London: Sage, 2005.

Vanobbergen J, Declerck D, Mwalili S, Martens L. The effectiveness of a 6-year oral health education programme for primary school children. *Community Dent Oral Epidemiol* 2004; **32**: 173–82.

Wallston KA, Wallston BS. Who is responsible for your health? The construct of health locus of control. In Sanders GS, Suls J, eds. *Social psychology of health and illness*. Hillsdale, NJ: Erlbaum, 1982; pp. 65–95.

Watt RG, Marinho VC. Does oral health promotion improve oral hygiene and gingival health? *Periodontology 2000* 2005; **37**: 35–47.

Watt RG, Harnett R, Daly B, *et al. Oral health promotion evaluation toolkit*. London: SHL, 2004.

Weinstein N. Reducing unrealistic optimism about illness susceptibility. *Health Psychol* 1983; **2**: 11–20.

Weinstein P, Harrison R, Benton T. Motivating parents to prevent caries in their young children: one year findings. *J Am Dent Assoc* 2004; **135**: 731–8.

World Health Organization. *The Ottawa Charter for Health Promotion. Health Promotion*, Vol. 1. iii–v. Geneva: WHO, 1986.

Worthington HV, Hill KB, Mooney J, Hamilton FA, Blinkhorn AS. A cluster randomized controlled trial of a dental health education program for 10-year old children. *J Public Health Dent* 2001; **61**: 22–7.

You BJ, Jian WW, Sheng RW, *et al.* Caries prevention in Chinese children with sodium fluoride dentifrice delivered through a kindergarten-based oral health program in China. *J Clin Dent* 2002; **13**: 179–84.

Zanata RL, Navarro MF, Pereira JC, Franco EB, Lauris JR, Barbosa SH. Effect of caries preventive measures directed to expectant mothers on caries experience in their children. *Braz Dent J* 2003; **14**: 75–81.

Zimmer S, Bizhang M, Seemann R, Witzke S, Roulet JF. The effect of a preventive program, including the application of low-concentration fluoride varnish, on caries control in high-risk children. *Clin Oral Investig* 2001; **5**: 40–4.

Zitzow R. The relationship of diet and dental caries in the Alaskan Eskimo population. *Alaska Med* 1979; **21**: 10–14.

27

Caries control for the individual patient

E.A.M. Kidd, B. Nyvad and I. Espelid

Introduction

How are current caries activity and risk of future caries progression assessed?

How is the information used to categorize patients into risk groups?

What non-operative treatments are available?

How is the individual helped to control disease progression?

When should the patient be recalled?

Caries control in children and adolescents

Caries control in patients with a dry mouth

Caries control in people who cannot care for themselves

Failure

References

Introduction

Evidence-based practice is the paradigm in all fields of medicine. This idea should also be part of our thinking in the dental community. Evidence-based practice may ensure that patients receive the best treatment available in a cost-effective manner. However, as discussed in Chapter 31, many of the diagnostic procedures and treatments that are used in daily practice today have not been evaluated properly in clinical trials. This also applies to non-operative programs aimed at the caries-active patient. Therefore, practitioners are sometimes inclined to adopt the treatment philosophy, 'what works in my hands is probably good for the patient'. In other cases the evidence exists but is not being implemented by the practitioner. Potential barriers could be that the knowledge and attitude of the practitioner, patient demands, the practice environment and the health-care system, including funding, block the implementation of new treatment routines.

The aim of this chapter is to gather the evidence presented in many of the previous chapters to give some practical guidelines for caries control for individual patients of all ages, from cradle to grave.

This chapter is divided into the following sections:

- How are current caries activity and risk of future caries progression assessed?
- How is the information used to categorize patients into risk groups?
- What non-operative treatments are available?
- How is the individual helped to control disease progression?
- When should the patient be recalled?
- Caries control in children and adolescents
- Caries control in patients with a dry mouth
- Caries control in people who cannot care for themselves.
- Failure.

How are current caries activity and risk of future caries progression assessed?

Remember that dentists treat patients, not just individual lesions. Assessment of the individual patient's current caries activity and risk of future caries progression is an important part of contemporary dental practice. The information is important for the following reasons.

- At the individual level, non-operative treatments should be focussed on those who need them the most.
- Dentists must identify which of the many risk factors involved and operating in concert play a particular role for the individual patient. This information is needed to ensure logical and effective management.
- Dental care neither begins nor ends with a single course of treatment, but is ongoing. When a course of dental

treatment is complete, dentist and patient must decide when it would be wise to monitor the effect of both non-operative and operative treatment. The initial risk assessment and the perceived response to a course of treatment will define this recall interval. The frequency of radiographic recall should also be based on this assessment.

- Patients should be made aware of their relative risk for developing new lesions and for progression of existing lesions. This knowledge may encourage them to keep appropriate recall appointments, to become involved in their own care and, if they pay for their own care, help them to budget for dental bills.
- Patients, as well as dental professionals, should be alert to possible changes in risk status.

How should the activity assessments be made?

The strongest evidence of caries activity is the presence of active carious lesions (cavitated and/or non-cavitated) at the time of examination (see Chapters 4 and 29). In this context it is important to note how many lesions are present and where the lesions are located. Furthermore, it may be informative to consider the recent caries activity of the patient, i.e. the number of new, progressing or filled lesions observed over the past 2–3 years.

There is no consensus as to how to define high caries activity as this is a relative judgment depending on the caries prevalence of the population. However, as a rule of thumb in most populations a yearly increment of two or more lesions, detected clinically and/or radiographically, would indicate a high rate of lesion progression. Multiple active lesions in regions of the mouth where the rate of flow of the salivary film is relatively rapid (lower incisors and buccal surfaces of upper molars) always suggest a high activity status.

When estimating the activity status due consideration should be given to the stage of development of the dentition. In children, occlusal surfaces of erupting permanent molars constitute a particular risk site. Adolescents may be more prone to caries development in approximal surfaces, especially the distal surface of second premolars and the mesial surface of second molars. In adults and elderly people, difficult-to-reach root surfaces may be the predominant risk sites, although coronal caries is also very important in this age group (Fejerskov & Nyvad, 1996; Thomson, 2004).

Identifying caries risk factors

Although it may only take a short time to obtain a subjective estimate of a patient's activity status, identifying the relevant risk factors may take a little longer. This is time well spent, however, because the patient may be able to modify some risk factors and thus slow down disease progression.

According to Beck (1998), a risk factor is defined as 'an environmental, behavioural, or biologic factor confirmed by temporal sequence, usually in longitudinal studies, which if present, directly increases the probability of a disease occurring, and if absent or removed, reduces the probability. Risk factors are part of the causal chain, or expose the host to the causal chain. Once disease occurs, removal of a risk factor may not result in a cure.' Important biological and environmental risk factors include salivary flow, level of oral hygiene, some dietary aspects and fluoride exposure, all of which are the determinants of the disease (see Chapter 1).

Identifying biological and environmental risk factors

When identifying the risk factors it is important to use a systematic approach, much like a detective; detectives look, listen, ask questions, listen again and collate the evidence. It is good practice to list the factors thought to be responsible for the individual's caries risk status (Table 27.1). This defines what should be modified for that particular individual. It may also define factors that cannot be modified, e.g. a dry mouth consequent to destruction of the salivary glands. Such a patient will always be a high caries risk.

Medical history

A proper way to start the detective work is to take a medical history. The importance of this cannot be overemphasized.

Complaints of a dry mouth (xerostomia) and reduced salivary output (salivary hypofunction) are common conditions, particularly in older populations. Persistent salivary hypofunction is likely to result in new and recurrent dental caries (see Chapter 11) and it can be really difficult to prevent this. Table 27.2 lists causes of dry mouth (for review see Ship, 2004).

Over 400 medications cause a side-effect of salivary gland hypofunction and 90% of the most commonly prescribed medications have been reported to cause dry mouth (Smith & Burtner, 1994). The intake of prescriptions increases with age and with increased intake of medications comes an increase in hyposalivation.

In addition, the systemic diseases for which these medications are taken may themselves contribute to the problem. These diseases tend to be more prevalent in older people, whose glands are more vulnerable to the deleterious

Table 27.1 Checklist of biological and environmental caries risk factors

Medical history
  Current and past diseases
  Current medications
  Xerostomia
Dental history
  Current activity state of caries lesions
  Past history of caries
Current oral hygiene practices and proficiency
Current exposure to topical fluorides from toothpastes, rinses or tablets
Current dietary pattern

Table 27.2 Causes of dry mouth

Medications	Antidepressants	Diuretics
	Antipsychotic drugs	Anti-parkinsonian drugs
	Tranquilizers	Appetite suppressants
	Hypnotics	Antinauseants
	Antihistamines	Antiemetics
	Anticholinergics	Muscle relaxants
	Antihypertensives	Expectorants
Systemic diseases or conditions	Sjögren's syndrome	Strokes
	Rheumatoid arthritis	Dehydration
	Diabetes	Hormonal changes
	HIV/AIDS	Pregnancy
	Scleroderma	Postmenopause
	Sarcoidosis	Neurological disease
	Lupus	Pancreatic disturbances
	Parkinson's disease	Liver disturbances
	Alzheimer's disease	Nutritional deficiencies
	Cystic fibrosis	Anorexia nervosa
	Asthma	Malnutrition
		Drug abuse
		Smoking
Head and neck radiotherapy		
Chemotherapy		

effects of the medications than are those of younger people (Ghezzi & Ship, 2003). The problems are thus compounded in elderly people, with estimates of the prevalence of xerostomia in adult free-living and nursing-home populations ranging from 16 to 72% (Thomson et al., 1999).

Sjögren's syndrome presents mainly in women during the fourth and fifth decades. It manifests in either primary or secondary form. Primary Sjögren's syndrome is characterized by dry mouth and eyes resulting from progressive loss of salivary and lacrimal function. Secondary Sjögren's syndrome involves one or both of these sites in the presence of another connective tissue disease such as rheumatoid arthritis, systemic sclerosis or lupus erythematous.

Patients with HIV/AIDS frequently experience salivary hypofunction from a lymphocytic destruction of the glands that results from medications.

Diabetes can also cause changes in salivary secretions, particularly where diabetes is poorly controlled. Salivary secretion will also be inhibited in Alzheimer's disease, Parkinson's disease, strokes, cystic fibrosis and dehydration.

All opiates reduce salivary secretion and their misuse is associated with high levels of caries (Scheutz, 1984). The management of opiate addiction can give rise to further oral health problems when methadone is used. Methadone itself causes a dry mouth and it can be prescribed in a sugary linctus form, although sugar-free versions are available and certainly preferable from a dental perspective. In addition, drug users may have a high level of sugar consumption (Molendijk et al., 1996) and a chaotic lifestyle that is hardly conducive to good oral hygiene or regular dental care. Alcoholics also fall into this group.

Radiation therapy, used in the treatment of head and neck cancers, causes permanent salivary gland hypofunction as a result of damage to, or loss of salivary acinar cells, and a persistent complaint of dry mouth. It is claimed there is only later recovery if the total dose to the salivary tissues is less than 25 Gy (Henson *et al.*, 1999).

Chemotherapy causes disturbances in salivary gland function, but the long-term impact on oral health is not clear. In the short term there may be decreased flow rate and increased numbers of organisms such as mutans streptococci and lactobacilli in saliva. In addition, there is an increased risk of oral candidiasis. Oral mucositis is a frequent, severe and sometimes a dose-limiting complication of cancer chemotherapy and radiotherapy (Jensen *et al.*, 2003).

In some of the cases of dry mouth described above, the patient will be very aware of this unpleasant symptom. Other patients may not complain, but dentists can often detect a dry mouth during the course of a clinical examination because the mouth mirror tends to stick to the mucosal surfaces or the saliva appears frothy. If a dry mouth is suspected, the diagnosis should be verified by measuring the stimulated and resting salivary flow rates (see Chapter 11).

Sometimes the medical history reveals a 'hidden' sugar exposure. Many medicines are produced in a sugar syrup form and some medicated pastilles are sugar based. Asthmatics often use inhalers, many of which contain lactose in the propellant, and asthma may itself result in a dry mouth. The dentist should always check the constituents of a drug to identify potential side-effects associated with caries.

Dental history

The patient's dental history will reveal additional important information. A history of multiple restorations that have to be frequently replaced may be an important indication of high caries risk. Sometimes the dental history will reveal changes in oral health, such as no dental problems for years and then a sudden deterioration leading to multiple restorations. In a case like this it will be important to identify the relevant change. The onset of a dry mouth is a good example of a change that increases the risk of dental caries (Bardow *et al.*, 2001).

Much of the information about caries risk emerges from asking the patient questions pertaining to the biological risk factors and listening carefully to their answers. For instance, it is always sensible to check the proficiency of oral hygiene and to ask how often teeth are cleaned, what brushes and interdental cleaning aids are used, which toothpaste is chosen and how it is cleared from the mouth (rinsing or spitting). The dentist should check that the paste contains fluoride by examining the contents listed on the tube. In some countries (e.g. Denmark) almost all toothpastes contain fluoride, while in others very little of the toothpaste is fluoridated. In other countries (e.g. the UK) most toothpastes are fluoridated but some products are fluoride free. The patient may also be asked whether they use any mouthrinses and it may be illuminating to ask why these mouthrinses are used. Sometimes it is because the patient perceives that they 'freshen' the breath. Since inadequate plaque control is a major cause of halitosis, this perception may subsequently be turned to advantage.

Questions about diet are obligatory when the patient presents with active carious lesions or a history of multiple restorations that are frequently replaced. Often a few simple questions will reveal an inappropriate dietary habit, such as frequent sipping of sugared coffee or tea, sugary soft drinks, pastilles and snacks (Fig. 27.1). In other cases it may be quite difficult to identify the nature of a caries-promoting diet, and only when using the imagination to conceive the patient's lifestyle is it possible to ask the right questions. In other cases a verbal enquiry does not suffice to reveal a suspected misuse of sugary foods and it may be necessary to ask the patient to fill in a diet sheet for further clarification.

In some countries microbiological or salivary chairside tests are recommended as an aid to predict the risk of caries. However, dental caries cannot be predicted with certainty (see Chapter 29). Neither microbiological, salivary nor dietary tests have been shown alone, or in combination, to be sufficiently accurate for the assessment of future caries risk at the individual level. The single best clinical predictor seems to be past caries experience, including the presence of non-cavitated carious lesions. There is also a well-documented association between the individual's past caries experience and the risk of developing root caries, showing that the principal biological factors associated with coronal and root caries are the same, despite the fact that the signs and the location of the lesions differ (Fejerskov & Nyvad, 1996).

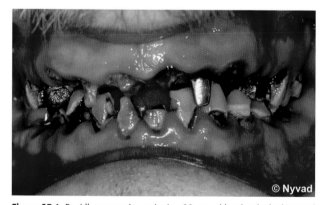

Figure 27.1 Rapidly progressing caries in a 28-year-old male who had ignored oral hygiene and who had been sipping sugared coffee regularly during the day for 5 years. The patient visited the dentist because it was difficult for him to get a new job.

Identifying social and demographic risk factors

Although not directly involved in the caries process, social factors can have an overriding influence on health and disease and on what lifestyle changes patients can make. How do dentists assess these important but sensitive issues? When dentist and patient first meet they know very little about each other, but a mutual summing up will begin.

The dental professional will notice such things as age, cleanliness, demeanor, disability, nationality, speech, dress, religion, educational status, employment status, and whether the patient is alone or accompanied. Some of these assessments are fraught with difficulty and jumping to conclusions can be very unwise. Poverty and educational status can have enormous implications and perhaps it is a pity that patients are seen in the surgery rather than in their homes. A hygienist whose job involved home visits in very poor areas once explained: 'You try giving oral hygiene instruction when 10 people share a tap that is three flights of stairs away and the family can't afford a toothbrush each, let alone expensive pastes and mouthrinses.'

How is the information used to categorize patients into risk groups?

What can and what cannot be modified by the patient?

For some patients the frequency of intake of a particular drink or food may be of overriding importance to their caries risk and modification of this factor may be essential to changing this risk. The role of the sweetened nursing bottle or dummy in nursing caries is a good example (Seow, 1998). In other patients the quality of the oral hygiene may need to be improved to change the risk status.

However, some factors that are highly relevant to a high caries activity cannot be modified. Some medications are only available in a sugar syrup base, although the dentist should always investigate whether there is an alternative formulation sweetened with an artificial sweetener. This can be done by reference to a drug formulary. If an alternative seems possible, the patient's general medical practitioner should be contacted. Other medications result in hyposalivation but may be essential for the patient's well-being. Again, reference to a formulary will show whether a particular medication has an effect on saliva flow.

A low salivary flow from glands damaged by radiotherapy for a head and neck malignancy is another example of a caries risk factor that cannot be modified. Hyposalivation as a result of Sjögren's syndrome is also permanent. Acknowledgment by both patient and dentist of factors that cannot be modified will be important so that alternate risk factors, such as plaque control and diet, can be controlled as far as possible.

Social and behavioral factors may be of overriding importance and dictate what dentist and patient can achieve. For instance, is the patient prepared to 'own the problem' and recognize his or her essential role in its solution? The answer to this question may lie in a patient's beliefs and educational background.

Sometimes the patient needs a carer to assist. Young children may be incapable of removing plaque and are not in control of their own diet. Similarly, a physically and/or mentally debilitated person is dependent on a carer for both plaque control and provision of food and drink. Old age may be relevant. While some old people are free living and independent, others are living in residential care because they cannot look after themselves. These residents may be physically and/or mentally impaired and many have a major caries problem (Simons et al., 1999a).

Money, or lack of it, can indirectly affect dental caries. Will the budget run to brushes, floss, artificial sweeteners, mouthwashes or even toothpaste? Can the patient spare the time to attend the surgery? For some patients even treatment that is free at the point of delivery is expensive if they lose earnings to keep an appointment.

Categorizing caries-activity status and caries-risk status

On the basis of the history and examination the patient may be allocated to one of the following caries activity and caries risk categories.

- *Caries inactive/caries controlled* (green): no (or maximally one) active lesion and no history of recent restorations.
- *Caries active but all relevant risk factors can potentially be changed* (e.g. plaque control, fluoride, diet) (orange): presence of active lesions and a yearly increment ≥2 new/progressing/filled lesions in the preceding 2–3 years. Caries control may be achieved through changes in the risk factors.
- *Caries active but some risk factors cannot be changed* (e.g. some dry mouths, some medications) *or risk factors cannot be identified* (red): presence of active lesions and a yearly increment ≥2 new/progressing/filled lesions in the preceding 2–3 years. This patient category will always be at high risk of caries, but it may be possible to control caries development by maximal control of the risk factors.

The dentist may wish to color code this concept of activity and risk status with green, orange and red stickers inserted in the notes. This visual representation is potentially helpful for all concerned. The aim is to help the patient to change the risk factors, e.g. to convert orange to green. However, some risk factors cannot easily be changed. To give an example, a patient with a dry mouth is always a caries risk (red). Nevertheless, caries activity can still be controlled with strenuous non-operative treatments.

What non-operative treatments are available?

This chapter will now describe the various non-operative treatments relevant to the caries process. Initially, a general approach to all age groups will be given. Subsequently, problems specific to children, patients with dry mouths and functionally dependent adults will be covered. In many of these the role of the dental team is to advise, educate and encourage behavioral change in the individual patient. Not too many changes should be attempted at one time. It is salutary to note here that the evidence that it is indeed possible to change behavior is lacking (Kay & Locker, 1998). This, however, in no way absolves the dental professional from trying to help a patient to prevent the progression of carious lesions. We, as individual dentists, do not expect carious lesions to form and progress in our own mouths. This would pertain even if we had a dry mouth and were therefore at high risk. It is only ethical to give patients the information we have and try to 'infect' them with some of our own enthusiasm for dental care.

The arrows in the non-operative quiver are:

- plaque control
- use of fluoride
- dietary modification.

The way in which each of these modalities is used will depend on the circumstances of the individual patient. Treatments with proven efficacy are highlighted here, but it is important to realize that there is no one protocol into which all patients can be fitted. It is quite intriguing that in Scandinavian countries different approaches to preventive treatment have produced similar good results. For instance, in Norway emphasis has been placed on fluoride tablets, in Sweden the major focus is diet, while in Denmark neither fluoride tablets nor diet has been particularly stressed, but rather the emphasis has been placed on oral hygiene with fluoride toothpaste.

In recent years computer programs have been designed to assist the dental practitioner in selecting individuals with a high caries risk and designing appropriate preventive protocols (Bratthal & Hänsel Petersen, 2005). It is tempting to feed relevant patient data into a computer and ask it to produce a feasible preventive program. However, this may create a false impression of objectivity when in fact the program can be no better than the data that were used to produce it.

Plaque control

Since carious lesions form as a result of the metabolic events in the dental plaque (see Chapter 1), good plaque control must be the cornerstone of preventive non-operative treatment. Teeth should be brushed regularly, at least once every day (Treasure *et al.*, 2001), with a fluoride-containing toothpaste (Marinho *et al.*, 2003a). The brushing interferes with the growth and ecology of the biofilm (see Chapter 10) and the fluoride application retards lesion progression (see Chapter 12). The time of day is not crucial, but it is advisable to establish a routine for tooth brushing at specified times of the day. If time is scarce, it is better to clean the teeth carefully once a day than to perform a careless job several times a day. The quality of cleaning, rather than the frequency, seems to be of prime importance (see Chapter 15). In any case, the patient's involvement and co-operation are essential. The patient should be shown the caries lesions, both clinically and on the radiograph. The patient may need a small mirror to see the diseased sites in the mouth. Disclosing solutions will demonstrate to the patient the direct relationship of the biofilm to the specific lesion.

Tooth brushing

Oral hygiene instruction should be both general to the whole mouth and site specific for a particular lesion. The patient should be advised to clean the diseased site(s) before cleaning the whole mouth, to ensure cleaning where it is most needed. A chart of plaque deposits and active lesions can be useful. The patient now has a picture of problem areas.

Having used a disclosing solution, the patient (or in the case of a small child, the parent) should be asked to brush. The following are worth noting.

- Can the patient remove the plaque? Is the brush reaching the salient area? Should it be angled differently? To give an example, perhaps half closing the mouth will allow access of the brush to the buccal surfaces of upper molar teeth.
- Would a different design of brush help? Perhaps the patient's brush is too big. Would an electric toothbrush help? Most modern powered toothbrushes have a small, circular head which performs oscillating, rotating or counter-rotational movements. Some models have timers that give useful feedback to the user on the time they have spent brushing. A recent review of evidence (Heanue *et al.*, 2003) concluded that powered toothbrushes with an oscillating/rotating movement were more effective in removing plaque and reducing gingivitis than manual brushes. It has also been reported that powered toothbrushes may improve compliance.
- Is thorough brushing in the surgery causing gingival bleeding? How does the patient react to this? Do they think they have been rough or can they appreciate that the gums are bleeding because they are inflamed? Can the patient distinguish healthy from bleeding gums? Do they appreciate that inflammation will resolve with good plaque control?
- Encourage the patient to feel the teeth with their tongue. Plaque-free teeth have a shiny feel, whereas plaque deposits feel furry to the tongue. Does the patient like the shiny feel of clean teeth? If they do, this may be a motivating factor to brush, but if they do not, motivating the patient to clean may be difficult.

It is surprising how difficult it is for most patients to comply with recommendations. Therefore, do not try to cover too much at one visit. Where a recall visit shows that brushing has not improved, the operator must try to decide where the problem lies. If the patient can remove plaque but does not, the problem is motivation, not manual dexterity. Most people can remove plaque but many do not!

Children need help with tooth brushing and this is of particular importance as teeth erupt. Eruption of permanent teeth can take 12–18 months and during this time the occlusal surface will be difficult to clean because it is below the occlusal plane. These erupting teeth should be brushed individually by the parent, who should stand behind the child, bringing the brush in at right angles to the arch.

Elderly people who are physically and mentally disabled may need a carer's help to clean their mouths. This matter must be handled with tact, as the person may not wish to admit they need help and the carer may find the task physically revolting. Mechanical toothbrushes may be easier for carers to handle than conventional brushes.

Interdental cleaning

Where active approximal lesions are present, either in enamel or on the root surface, an interdental cleaning aid will be needed. In young patients enamel lesions are best cleaned with dental floss or tape, whereas interdental brushes are preferred for cleaning larger interdental spaces and root surfaces. The operator will need to spend time showing a patient how to use these devices correctly. Many patients find this difficult, time consuming and tedious, and they cannot easily see the results of their efforts. Dentists can help in the following ways.

- They should give site-specific advice, by showing the patient the lesion(s) on the radiograph and teaching them where these sites are in the mouth. Ideally, every interdental space should be cleaned, but if this is not practical it may be more realistic to suggest cleaning the specific interdental spaces where the lesions are.
- Careful examination of the dental floss or interdental brush after use can show the patient that they have removed plaque. This is a potential motivating factor. The patient can see and smell that they have done something useful.
- Some patients may find it easier to use a special holder for the dental floss, particularly if their manual dexterity is poor. Alternatively, interdental brushes with a small diameter may be helpful.
- Patients should be taught the relevance of any bleeding during interdental cleaning. If this persists, either cleaning is inadequate and gingival inflammation has not resolved, or a cavity is present that the floss cannot reach.

Professional tooth cleaning

In caries-active patients who for some reason do not master plaque control themselves, and in patients with decreased salivary secretion (Table 27.2) (see also Chapter 11), it may be necessary to support the patient for a time with additional plaque control in the form of professional tooth cleaning. As described in Chapter 15, regular professional tooth cleaning has been shown to reduce dental caries by almost 100%. The clinical procedure is detailed below.

1. Disclose plaque.
2. Remove plaque with low-abrasive, fluoride-containing polishing paste (e.g. 0.1% NaF in silicon dioxide). A handpiece (rotating at up to 5000 rpm) is used, with pointed bristles for fissures and a soft rubber cup for free smooth surfaces. For proximal surfaces the paste is applied with a toothpick or an interdental brush, depending on the local anatomical conditions.
3. Disclose again and check that all plaque has been removed.
4. Apply topical fluoride (2% NaF) or fluoride varnish. Make sure that the fluoride application reaches the site(s) with active caries.
5. Control visits. The interval between appointments should be short at the beginning of the program (every 2–3 weeks), but may be extended when co-operation has improved and the patient has reached a satisfactory level of plaque control.

Use of fluoride

All patients should use fluoride toothpaste containing between 1000 and 1500 ppm F as a basic caries-control method. For practical purposes all individuals in the family may share the same brand of paste. However, children below the age of 7–8 years are recommended to use a smaller amount (pea size) (see also Chapter 18). Adult patients with risk factors that cannot be changed may benefit from a high-fluoride toothpaste.

In caries-active patients it is essential to intensify the fluoride therapy until the situation is under control. This could be achieved through the intensive use of fluoride toothpaste, fluoride-containing mouthwashes for home use, professional (operator-applied) topical applications or combinations of these methods (see Chapter 18). The choice of fluoride vehicle is not crucial as long as it is combined with improvement of the oral hygiene status (see Chapter 15). The important thing is that the patient accepts the mode of treatment and complies with the advice given.

Fluoride toothpaste has much to recommend it. It is cheap, requires minimal patient co-operation and enhances patients' appreciation of their own role in maintaining oral health. A recent systematic review (Marinho *et al.*, 2003a) concluded its use to be associated with a 24% reduction in caries in the permanent dentition of children and adolescents. Most of the evidence has been gathered in clinical trials lasting for 2–3 years. Thus, the benefits accrued through a lifetime experience may be substantially greater. Elevated intraoral concentrations of fluoride may be achieved by asking the patient to refrain from rinsing the mouth vigorously with water after brushing; however, the additional effect on caries control by abstaining from rinsing after toothbrushing is dubious (see Chapter 18). Therefore, the emphasis should be on the extreme importance of oral hygiene rather than the mechanism of clearing excess paste from the mouth. Fluoridated toothpastes may also be used therapeutically by asking the patient to apply the paste directly onto the clean active carious lesions with a finger or a brush, preferably immediately before going to bed, owing to decreased salivary secretion at night. This mode of application may ensure increased concentrations of fluoride for extended periods in the vicinity of the lesion.

Fluoride mouthwashes may benefit adults with active caries who are not able to clean their teeth adequately with a fluoride toothpaste, e.g. because of sensitive oral mucosa. The mouthwash (0.05 or 0.1% NaF) should be used for a full minute once or twice every day. Alternately, a 0.2% NaF solution may be used weekly. Fluoride mouthwashes are available over the counter in some countries, whereas in others they would have to be prescribed individually. It should be appreciated that the caries inhibition of fluoride mouthwashes is low (10–20%) when applied as an adjunct to unsupervised use of a fluoride dentifrice (Disney *et al.*, 1989).

Professional applications of high concentrations of fluoride, in the form of a 2% aqueous NaF or fluoride varnish (Duraphat/Fluor Protector) should follow professional plaque removal. These products should be applied on slightly dried teeth for 2–5 min. Their principal mode of action is to deposit calcium fluoride in active carious lesions, and this is a source of fluoride that is slowly released (see Chapters 12 and 18). The applications may be repeated every 2–3 months until caries activity is controlled. A recent systematic review (Marinho *et al.*, 2002) concluded that fluoride varnish reduced caries in the deciduous dentition by 33% and in the permanent dentition by 46% when compared with a placebo. The caries-inhibiting effect of professionally applied fluoride gel is likely to be lower (28%) (Marinho *et al.*, 2003b). Professional fluoride application is time consuming and therefore these methods may not be cost-effective unless used in individuals with a high caries activity.

In recent years a number of alternative *fluoride-containing products* have been launched as an aid to caries prevention, such as fluoride-containing chewing gum, fluoride-containing dental materials, and fluoridated toothpicks and dental floss. However, to the best of the authors' knowledge, none of these products has been tested in well-designed, large-scale clinical trials. Until proper documentation has been presented it would therefore be unwise to resort to these methods as the primary preventive strategy.

Dietary modification

No change in diet should be suggested for a caries-inactive patient, but the dentist should still make the patient aware of how a change in diet (e.g. frequent sugar attacks) may pose a problem if the oral hygiene is poor (see Chapter 15). Likewise, parents should be informed that nursing bottles and dummies may cause rampant caries (early childhood caries) if plaque control is inadequate (Seow, 1998). 'Sugar to mealtimes' or 'Saturday snacks' may be reasonable ways to proceed.

Changes in life may sometimes be accompanied by changes in diet, and where these changes are extreme they may have dental consequences. Thus, moving home, having a baby, unemployment, divorce, retirement and bereavement are times when a little advice on diet and caries may not go amiss.

Dietary analysis should always be carried out on patients with multiple active lesions. Sometimes a simple verbal analysis will suffice to identify a problem, while in other cases more elaborate analyses need to be performed.

There are two principal techniques for determining food intake. One, the 24 h recall system, records the dietary intake during the preceding 24 h. The other method is to obtain a 3–4 day written record, asking the patient to record food and liquid intake as it is consumed. Both methods rely on the patient's full co-operation as well as honesty. Furthermore, both forms of diet recording suffer from the disadvantage that the record may not be representative of the diet consumed over a much longer period, although it is this that is likely to have been responsible for the current caries and restoration status. Thus, a diet history is an unscientific tool that must be interpreted with caution.

Recording the diet

Figure 27.2 shows a suitable form for diet analysis. When this is given to the patient it should be explained that their help is needed to find the cause of their dental decay. Since this may be related to what they eat and drink, a record of this is needed, together with the time of eating. The patient should also be asked to include any medicine taken by mouth. This would allow the dentist to check whether it is sugar-syrup based or has a xerostomic effect. The patient should keep the diet sheet with them and fill it in at the time to avoid missing anything. Quantities of food consumed are not specifically requested, but it is important not to change anything just because a record is being kept.

Analysis of the dietary record

Once the patient returns the completed sheet, dentist and patient can begin to look at it together. The dentist should encourage the patient to identify the items that contain sugar; this will show whether the patient appreciates which items are potentially harmful. The effect of sugars on acid production in the biofilm should be explained in simple terms (see Chapters 10 and 11).

Then, the number of sugar attacks should be counted and this number recorded at the top of each day. Now the den-

	THURSDAY		FRIDAY		SATURDAY		SUNDAY	
	Time	Item	Time	Item	Time	Item	Time	Item
BEFORE BREAKFAST								
Breakfast								
MORNING								
Mid-day meal								
AFTERNOON								
Evening meal								
EVENING and NIGHT								

Figure 27.2 Diet analysis form.

tist can explain the relevance of frequency in a simple way. It would not be unreasonable to suggest that after a sugar attack the plaque may remain acidic for about 1 h; thus, nine attacks would equal 9 h of acid plaque. This is a simple explanation for someone with no knowledge of chemistry. With some patients it may be appropriate to draw and explain a Stephan curve (see Fig. 11.7). The method of delivering the message should be tailored to the educational level and understanding of the patient. Imagine explaining the problem to a biochemist or someone with no knowledge of chemistry.

Dietary advice

On the basis of the diet sheet, dentist and patient may be able to work out some realistic strategies for reducing the frequency of intake of sugar-containing foods and drinks. It is neither necessary nor possible to cut sugar completely out of the diet, but to restrict intake mainly to mealtimes may be a realistic and attainable goal.

The following suggestions may be useful.

- Try to confine sugar to main meals; eat and enjoy it.
- Substitute a savory snack for a sweet one. A list of sugar-free drinks, snacks and chewing gum is useful when discussing this with the patient.
- Substitute an artificial sweetener for sugar in tea and coffee.
- Water and milk are safe drinks between meals.

Age and diet

The attitude of the parents or carer is of great importance in achieving dietary change in children. The professional must be sensitive to possible feelings of guilt, anger and even denial when dietary problems that may be responsible for caries are discussed. In addition, the influence of social and cultural pressures may be considerable. In some cultures it is not the mother who determines what the family eats and drinks, although this may be person the professional meets.

Dietary preferences are likely to change with age. The teenage years can be a time of rebellion, and hygiene and

dietary practices may change, to the detriment of the dentition.

The dentist can only work with the young person, who may be fiercely resentful if a parent is involved. One of the useful things about caries is that the white-spot lesion is visible. Physicians trying to persuade young people to give up smoking may envy us this tangible sign of an ecological catastrophe!

Elderly and old people often revert to a soft diet because of a dry mouth or poor dental conditions. Studies have shown that the elderly occupants of residential homes may have multiple sugar attacks (Steele *et al.*, 1998) and it is very difficult to change this. Care staff are busy and often not dentally aware. Visitors often bring sweets as presents, and eating these may be one of the few pleasures left in life to care-home residents. In addition, poor nutrition and weight loss may be a consequence of illness and require frequent snacks, food enrichment and food supplements. These supplements are often high in sugar.

How is the individual helped to control disease progression?

The categories of caries risk that were defined earlier will now be considered individually. Each group will comprise a wide variety of individuals with different social backgrounds; thus, broad statements about management must still be tailored to the individual.

- *Caries inactive/caries controlled*: these patients only need encouragement to sustain careful oral hygiene with the use of fluoride toothpaste.
- *Caries active but all relevant risk factors can potentially be changed*: mechanical plaque control should be improved, and consideration given to supplementing fluoride toothpaste with chairside fluoride applications and/or mouthwashes. Where there are multiple active lesions,

the diet should also be investigated and advice given as to how it may be improved.

- *Caries active but some risk factors cannot be changed*: these cases are the most challenging. There is no standard preventive treatment that will meet the needs of all patients. In each particular case the preventive treatment must be designed individually, with due regard to the risk factors. All the caries control treatments, plaque control including professional tooth cleaning, use of fluoride, dietary modification and stimulation of salivary flow, may have a role to play. Patients with a dry mouth fall into this group and are discussed specifically in the following pages.

Caries-active patients for whom *the risk factors have not or cannot be identified* are frustrating because the dentist feels that he or she has missed something. The detective work should continue and the case be managed as in the preceding group.

When should the patient be recalled?

Setting the recall interval

Recalls should be scheduled according to current individual needs and based on an assessment of caries risk. Therefore, the recall interval may vary widely during the course of a treatment. Frequent automatic recalls, e.g. every 6 months, do not necessarily lead to better outcomes. Ironically enough, it has been shown that the more frequently the patient visits the dentist, the more fillings he or she accumulates (Sheiham *et al.*, 1985). These findings have been interpreted as indicating that while frequent dental visits may help to postpone tooth loss and to maintain dental function, they do not apparently help to prevent the onset of further disease. The following recommendations may be used as a guideline for setting the recall interval.

All caries-active patients should be recalled 2–3 weeks after the first instruction to check how they master plaque control and changes in lifestyle. If the dentist does not make a special effort to follow up on these matters before engaging in operative treatments, the patient may think that non-operative measures are not important. The atmosphere at this first control visit should be very positive, to encourage the patient to collaborate further. The patient should be shown what is good and what could be improved in the mouth, and helped with any modifications. Several control visits may be necessary before the risk factors are properly controlled.

Further recall will depend on the caries activity and risk status of the individual. A patient undergoing radiation may need to see the dentist every 2–3 weeks. A caries-active patient with a dry mouth might be seen every 2–3 months. A caries-active patient who has appeared to have mastered plaque control and dietary changes, and is using appropriate fluoride supplements, might be seen for a (first) recall in 6 months. A caries-inactive patient would have a longer recall interval of 1–2 years.

In younger patients the eruption status, particularly of the first and second molars, should influence recall. The occlusal surfaces of erupting molars are prone to plaque stagnation (Carvalho *et al.*, 1989) and it is probably wise to see such patients two to three times a year to check that plaque control is being maintained, in particular when there are signs of active caries. If proper plaque control cannot be achieved and active non-cavitated caries lesions are present in the fissures, a sealant should be applied (Weintraub, 2001).

Examining the mouth at recall

Clinical examination to determine current caries activity and risk status is very important. This examination should concentrate on plaque control and gingival health, which reflects plaque control. The whole dentition, as well as previously detected lesions, should be carefully examined for signs of caries arrest or progression. The patient should be both told and shown what has improved and what needs further improvement.

The decision to take new radiographs should be based on current caries activity as well as the depth of previously detected lesions (see Chapters 5 and 7). In caries-active patients where lesions have been managed with non-operative treatments, new bitewing radiographs, using film holders and beam-aiming devices, should be taken on the basis of individual needs. It is essential to obtain comparable radiographic views if lesions are to be monitored for progression or arrest.

Assessment of compliance at recall

Patient compliance seems to improve for a short period and then tends to relapse. In a review of methods of oral hygiene instruction and problems of compliance, it was concluded that relapse occurs irrespective of the method of oral hygiene instruction (Renvert & Glavind, 1998). This review cites several reasons why patients may fail to comply in the long term: unwillingness to perform oral self-care, poor understanding of recommendations, lack of motivation, poor dental health beliefs, unfavorable dental health values, stressful life events and low socioeconomic status.

However, an important factor in obtaining long-term results through oral hygiene instruction is regular recall visits (Renvert & Glavind, 1998). At these visits compliance with advice on plaque control, diet, fluoride use and saliva stimulation should be assessed by discussion. It is only human nature for the patient to try to please with these answers. Disclosing, recording of plaque and a follow-up diet sheet are a little more objective than simple discussion. In some cases it may be necessary to explain to the patient what the dentist sees as the consequences of poor compliance. The dentist must be honest and the conversation should be recorded in the notes.

Recording changes in oral health behavior and carious lesion activity at recall

Since knowledge of a patient's habits is so critical to management, a record of habits should be kept. This should include tooth brushing habits, use of interdental cleaning, use of topical fluorides and diet. A note should also be kept of any changes agreed with the patient or parent.

To maintain an overview of the non-operative treatments given and monitor their effects on caries lesion activity it may be helpful to record such variables in a sheet specifically designed for this purpose (Fig. 27.3). This may be particularly useful when treatment of the patient is shared between different people in the dental team. By doing so it will be easier not only to identify the specific points where additional focus is needed, but also to point out where the patient has already been successful in controlling lesion progression.

Resetting the recall interval

Based on the above, the interval to the next recall can be set. Where the reasons for the caries activity cannot be modified, or caries is active but the cause has not been established, recalls will be frequent. Conversely, if the clinical status is improving, the interval may be increased.

Caries control in children and adolescents

What is special about caries control in children and adolescents?

The cornerstones in caries control (plaque control, use of fluoride, proper diet) are the same for all ages, but up to the age of about 12 years it is the parents (or those who bring the child up) who play the most important role. When caries-control strategies are planned for children it should be remembered that caries in the child is the result of decisions taken by adults. There is a relationship between the parents' behavior and beliefs and the child's dental health at 7 years of age (Mattila *et al.* 2005). Indeed, parents' poor dental behavior could be considered a risk indicator for caries development in their children. Thus, a logical starting point in the discussion with parents of children with overt caries lesions might be their own dental health behaviors and attitudes.

The following may be relevant:

- Parents' knowledge on cause of caries, importance of diet and their child's eating habits.
- Do they supervise and help with tooth brushing?
- Is there a family crisis needing complex support from dental or other professionals?
- Is this a symptom of abuse or neglect needing intervention by social welfare workers or others? Untreated caries is more common among physically abused/neglected children (Olivan, 2003).

In contrast to the child, the growing adolescent comes to make their own choices and take responsibility. Early intervention to reinforce self-care for caries control is important because oral health behavior in young adults is often established in teenage years (Astrom, 2004).

A habit of tooth brushing twice daily at the age of 12 years may predict more stable oral hygiene practices through the adolescent years compared with those who brush less (Kuusela *et al*, 1988). A low tooth brushing frequency in teenagers may predict developing socioeconomic health differences in adulthood (Koivusilta *et al.*, 2003). Dietary habits are also often established in the mid-teens (Sweeting *et al.*, 1994). This indicates the importance of implementing training in tooth cleaning and having a conversation with the adolescent that includes aspects of dietary habits, during the recall visits.

Name: Jens Hansen ID: 210292-

Date	2006 02/02	02/16	03/19	05/07			
Instruction plaque control	+	+	+	+			
Dietary advice	+	+					
Professional fluorides	2% NaF			2% NaF			
Lesion assessment Activity: ● Active ○ Inactive Plaque: + Present - Absent							
⌈7 occ	●/+	●/+	●/−	○/−			
7⌉ occ	●/+	●/−	○/−	●/+			
7⌋ occ	●/+	○/−	○/−	○/−			
⌊7 occ	●/+	●/+	●/−	○/−			
5⌉ d	●/+	●/+	●/+	●/−			
⌈5 d	●/+	●/−	○/−	○/−			

Figure 27.3 Recording sheet used to monitor caries lesion activity and maintain an overview of the non-operative treatments given.

When to start caries control in children

Risk factors for caries control in young children have been reviewed by Harris *et al.* (2004). Oral hygiene and diet may interact such that good oral hygiene may balance the effect of a cariogenic diet (see Chapter 15). The role of oral hygiene was further emphasized by an epidemiological study of caries in children aged 3–4 years. Children were more likely to be caries free if teeth were brushed, twice per day, by an adult before the child was 1 year old. Indeed, the parents' perceived ability to implement regular tooth brushing was the most important predictor of whether children had caries, and this factor was also relevant in children from disadvantaged backgrounds (Pine *et al.* 2004).

Efforts to educate and encourage parents can start from pregnancy: it is never too early to point out they will be responsible for their infant's oral care. It is common that caregivers and their children first come into contact with dental professionals when the children are about 3 years old, but this may be too late: early childhood caries (ECC) is often defined as caries in children younger than 3 years. Home visits have been shown to be highly cost-effective in caries prevention in very young children in socially deprived areas (Kowash *et al.*, 2000, 2006). Trained personnel visited infants from 8 months of age, and their families, at 3-month intervals. They provided dental health education and short video demonstrations directed towards the child's needs. The dental health education was tailored to meet the mother's needs as well.

Early childhood caries

Children in the age group 12–30 months have a special caries pattern that differs from older children. Caries affects the maxillary primary incisors and first primary molars in a way that reflects the pattern of eruption. The longer the tooth has been present and exposed to the caries challenge, the more it will be affected. The upper incisors are most vulnerable, while the mandibular incisors are protected by the tongue and saliva from submandibular and sublingual glands. Common terms for rampant caries in infants or preschool children have been 'bottle caries' or 'nursing caries', but the terms ECC, and S-ECC in severe cases, are now more commonly used (De Grauwe *et al.*, 2004).

The lesions progress rapidly, they can be extensive and typically affect free smooth surfaces. Often the lesions cover many surfaces in each affected tooth (Fig. 27.4). In severe cases front teeth break down during eruption and parents may associate this with developmental defects rather than caries. The pulp may be involved and thus a need for extraction in these very young children is the result. Typical etiological factors are inadequate or missing dental hygiene combined with poor dietary habits, which may be frequent bottle feeding on demand (*ad libitum*), based on the infants'

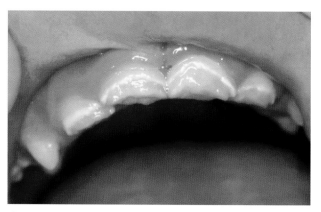

Figure 27.4 Caries has ruined the upper incisors in a 20-month-old child who sipped a bottle of sugar-containing liquid during the night. Note the whitish and chalky border of enamel, which indicates very high caries activity.

hunger cues and not on a scheduled basis. Sugared drinks during the day or night and nocturnal breast feeding after the age of 12 months are possible causes of ECC (van Palenstein Helderman *et al.*, 2006). Water should be the only drink offered to the child during the night.

The prevalence of ECC differs according to the group examined and a prevalence up to 85% has been reported for disadvantaged groups in developing countries (Carino *et al.*, 2003; Thitasomakul *et al.*, 2006). A strong association is found between socioeconomic status, ethnicity and prevalence of ECC in the Western world (Harris *et al.*, 2004; Skeie *et al.*, 2005).

Achieving behavior change (see Chapter 26)

It has been stated that behavior change is more likely when we 'hear' ourselves talk about the need to change rather than being told to change (Weinstein, 2002). Behavior change is rarely a discrete, single event: the patient or parent moves gradually from being disinterested (precontemplation stage) to considering a change (contemplation stage), to deciding and preparing to make a change (Zimmerman *et al.*, 2000).

So how should we talk with patients or parents? The motivational interviewing (MI) technique is one way of communicating that allows the exploration of an actual problem or topic in a supportive environment (Weinstein, 2002). The technique is not based on confrontation or 'finger pointing', but on the health professional asking open-ended questions. A condition of success is that the patient or parent talks. Key words in the interaction are rapport, empathy and trust. This rapport is often established as the health professional shows a genuine interest in the child. In a recent study (Weinstein *et al.*, 2004) in which MI was compared with traditional health education, MI was found to have a greater effect on children's dental health than traditional health education. Children aged 6–16 months were followed for 1 year. The participants (who were immigrants) were all at high risk of developing caries. The caries increment in the MI group was reduced by 68% compared with the control group (0.7 versus 1.9 new carious lesions). In this study the parents could choose from the following menu of caries-preventive options.

- Do not let anyone add anything sugary to your child's bottle.
- Clean your baby's teeth as soon they appear. Cleaning can be done with a small soft toothbrush or face cloth.
- Use a very small amount (smaller than a pea) of fluoride toothpaste.
- Hold your baby when feeding him or her, then lay the baby down to sleep; if the baby awakens, give him or her water, not milk or juice.
- Limit the time your child spends in sipping and snacking, because the longer he or she takes, the greater the chance of decay.
- Use a cup.
- Give no more than two or three snacks per day.
- Bring your child to the dental clinic at least twice a year so the dentist can protect the baby's teeth by painting a safe fluoride medicine on them.

Effective caries control in children

Brushing, by parents, using a small quantity of fluoride-containing toothpaste, is essential and should start as soon as teeth erupt. Pine *et al.* (2000) showed the benefit of twice-daily brushing in newly erupted first molar teeth compared with brushing once daily or less. This study also showed the importance of parental beliefs. If parents feel strongly that there is time to check their child's tooth brushing, the odds that their child actually brushes twice daily are about three times greater. Therefore, it is important to support the parents and convince them that their efforts make sense for the child's dental health and that they really contribute.

When the first primary molar erupts at 5–7 years of age it is important to inform the parents about the new challenge of keeping the tooth healthy. In the municipality of Nexö, Denmark, a program has been developed and evaluated which emphasizes mechanical plaque control (Ekstrand & Christiansen, 2005). Although the study was not a randomized controlled trial, the results indicate that a dedicated program focussing on plaque control, from 8 months of age, prevents caries. Erupting molars were considered a particular risk for caries development. The program is tailored towards the needs of each child and can be divided into three parts:

- education of the parents
- training in plaque control
- early non-operative intervention by the dental professional, including plaque removal, application of topical fluoride and use of sealants.

The number of visits is individualized for each child. The programme began in 1987, since when the reduction in caries among 15-year-olds has been greater in Nexö than in other municipalities serving as controls. Ekstrand and Christiansen (2005) could not explain this improvement by variables other than the specific preventive program in Nexö.

Orthodontic treatment

Children undergoing orthodontic treatment with fixed appliances have an additional risk for caries development (Fig. 27.5), especially where there is frequent consumption of sugar-containing soft drinks. Daily tooth brushing with fluoride-containing toothpaste, combined with use of a fluoride mouthrinse, is also the basic prevention method in this group. Individual preventive programs should be tailored for each patient. Patients with active caries are at special risk and consideration should be given to the use of professional tooth cleaning with fluoride applications during visits (Zimmer & Rottwinkel, 2004). It is also reasonable to suggest that orthodontic treatment is unwise in those where current caries status designates them as high risk.

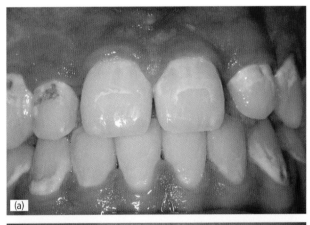

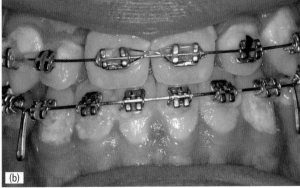

Figure 27.5 (a) Active caries with and without cavity formation caused by frequent snacking and poor oral hygiene in combination with fixed orthodontic treatment. (b) Excessive plaque formation seen at a previous visit before the appliance was removed.

Caries control in patients with a dry mouth

The numerous causes of dry mouth were detailed earlier. These patients are a particularly challenging group because their situation is often permanent. Thus, preventive measures may have to be intensified and continued throughout life (Joyston-Bechal, 1992) and despite these efforts, it is not always possible fully to control disease progression. However, some patients with moderately decreased salivary secretion (unstimulated flow between 0.2 and 0.3 ml/min) can possibly be managed by a combination of improved self-performed plaque control with fluoride toothpaste, and limiting sugar intakes.

Patients with dry mouth may find some toothpastes too astringent to be comfortable to use. A mild paste should be selected, preferably one without sodium lauryl sulfate. Where caries is active and difficult to control, a high-fluoride paste should be recommended (e.g. 2800–5000 ppm F) and in some countries this must be prescribed by a dentist. The patient should be warned that this paste should not be used by small children, for toxicological reasons.

Radiotherapy

Patients exposed to radiotherapy of the salivary glands inevitably develop ravaging dental caries (Fig. 27.6) unless stringent action is taken to protect the teeth (Fig. 27.7). Salivary flow decreases rapidly with irradiation and whether salivary flow returns has been related to the irradiation dose. Glands receiving over 26 Gy have little subsequent function and no significant recovery over time (Eisbruch et al., 1999). Thus, caries-preventive approaches must be instituted as soon as radiotherapy is begun. Since there is a dose–response relationship between the amount of radiation delivered to the oral tissues and the damage that eventually occurs, it is sensible for the dentist to request information about the total dose of irradiation that is planned for the patient. This information will allow the dentist to set the intensity of tooth cleanings, topical fluoride treatments, frequency of recall visits, etc.

Plaque control and fluoride

An effective approach consists of daily, self-applied 5 min topical applications with a 1% NaF gel in individually fitted trays (Dreitzen et al., 1977). In addition, patients should be instructed to remove all dye-disclosed dental plaque, by tooth brushing and using dental floss or interdental brushes, every day.

The main problem with the above treatment is compliance. Failure to comply strictly with the prescribed use of the fluoride gel invariably leads to rapid caries development. Therefore, preventive approaches that are easier to perform have been developed. Such treatments may include twice-daily mouthrinses with either fluoride (0.05% NaF) (Meyerowitz et al., 1991) or a combination of

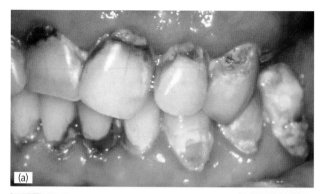

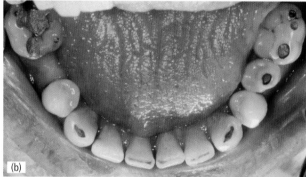

Figure 27.6 (a) The patient has been irradiated in the region of the salivary glands for the treatment of a malignant tumour. Heavy plaque deposits are obvious over the lesions (Kidd, 2005). (b) A typical pattern of caries attack on occlusal surfaces in a patient with a dry mouth, in this case caused by radiotherapy in the region of the salivary glands. The cusp tips and incisal edges are typically attacked because the dentin is often exposed by tooth wear in these areas. Plaque may stagnate in the concave areas (Kidd, 2005). (Reproduced with permission of Oxford University Press.)

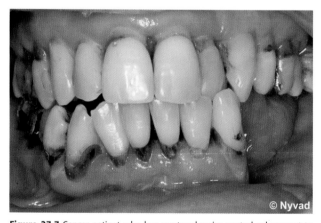

Figure 27.7 Cancer patient who has mastered caries control subsequent to resection of the left mandible and radiation therapy of the head and neck. The patient received regular professional tooth cleaning and topical fluoride therapy in conjunction with meticulous self-performed oral hygiene.

fluoride (0.05% NaF) and chlorhexidine-gluconate (0.2%) (Katz, 1982). The combined rinse could potentially be more effective than rinsing with fluoride solution alone because of simultaneous suppression of the oral microflora (see also Chapter 16). However, irrespective of the type of self-performed treatment, it is important to make the patient aware that meticulous daily plaque control is crucial to the outcome. If plaque control is insufficient the patient should also receive regular professional tooth cleaning, including topical application of fluoride, as detailed earlier in this chapter.

Dietary advice for patients with dry mouth

Diet analyses and advice are always important for patients with dry mouths because these patients are very likely to change their diet. Some foods are simply so dry that they are unusable by this group. Moreover, the diet sheet will often show that the patient takes frequent sips or drinks to lubricate the mouth. Plain water or milk should be used for this.

Conservative measures to relieve the symptoms

The following measures are helpful to relieve the discomfort that accompanies a severely dry mouth:

- sipping water frequently all day long
- restricting the intake of substances that exacerbate dryness, such as cigarettes, caffeine-containing drinks and alcohol
- avoiding astringent products such as alcohol-containing or strong mint-flavored mouthwashes, and strongly flavoured toothpastes
- coating the lips with lip salve or Vaseline
- humidifying the sleeping area.

Salivary stimulants

Salivary stimulants will only be helpful when there is some glandular activity present (Dodds *et al.*, 1991). The following agents have been used.

- Sugar-free gum: chewing can promote salivary flow; however, the caries-preventive effect of chewing sugar-free gum is relatively low and variable (Mäkinen *et al.*, 1995, Machiulskiene *et al.*, 2001). Medicated chewing gums containing chlorhexidine, fluoride, xylitol and/or carbamide have been recommended, but it is questionable whether the supplementation of gums with additives and sweeteners increases the caries-preventive effect over and above that of chewing per se (Machiulskiene *et al.*, 2001).
- Saliva-stimulating tablets, which are sucked (e.g. SST Sinclair, Salivin, Dentiplus): the tablets increase the secretion of saliva through physiological stimulation of the taste buds. The tablets contain sorbitol, xylitol, citric acid, citric acid salts, malic acid and a phosphate buffer so that they do not damage teeth.
- Proprietary lozenges (e.g. Salivix, Provalis) containing malic acid, gum Arabic, calcium lactate, sodium phosphate, lycasin and sorbitol: the manufacturers claim that the lozenge stimulates salivary flow and does not demineralize enamel, despite a pH of 4.0, because of the calcium lactate buffer present.

- The systemic use of pilocarpine hydrochloride has proved successful in stimulating saliva. The drug works by reproducing the effects of widespread stimulation of the parasympathetic nervous system and can have unpleasant side-effects.

Saliva substitutes

In the past, individuals with dry mouths have had to rely on frequent moistening with water. Several saliva substitutes are now available to make the patient feel more comfortable and to supply calcium, phosphate and fluoride ions to counteract demineralization. Saliva substitutes have been produced in the form of sprays, lozenges, or mouthwashes.

Sprays or mouthwashes to give viscosity

In Europe there are currently about 10 commercially available preparations, such as Luborant, Saliva Orthana, Glandosane, Saliveze, Xerostom, Salisynt and Proxident. They all try to mimic the inorganic composition of saliva by containing calcium, phosphate, magnesium and potassium. To provide viscosity either carboxymethyl cellulose or pig gastric mucosa-derived mucins are added to the product. A clinical trial comparing a mucin-based saliva substitute with a mucin-free placebo in patients with advanced malignant disease and dry mouth, found no difference in symptom relief between the two saliva substitutes (Brennen *et al.*, 2002). Some of these products contain fluoride (which is highly recommended) and as mucosal lubricants and protective components, olive oil and or betaine (a water-retaining osmoprotectant of skin and mucosal cells). The products should be directed towards the inside of the cheeks, lips and on the tongue, and not down the throat. It is recommended that the pH of the product is not less than 6.0. Clinical studies of the efficacy of these products are still limited.

Lozenges are only helpful if there is enough saliva present to dissolve them. Saliva Orthana is also available in the form of a lozenge. It does not contain fluoride, but is quite palatable.

Products containing antimicrobial proteins

Dentifrices, mouthrinses and gels are on the market in several countries containing antimicrobial proteins such as peroxidase, lysozyme and lactoferrins. The objective is to compensate for the lack of host-mediated protection derived from these proteins in those with normal salivary flow. Examples are the Biotene (Anglian) and BioXtra (Molar) product ranges. Clinical documentation of their efficacy is rather limited. Proteins for some products (toothpastes, mouthrinses, gels, chewing gums) are purified from cow's milk or colostrum because these milk proteins are structurally and catalytically almost identical to those in human saliva. Clinical experience of these products for severe xerostomia and cancer treatment has been positive (Tenovuo, 2004).

Viscous or ropy saliva

When saliva is present but is ropy, rinsing or gargling with a mouthwash made up by mixing half a teaspoonful of baking power with 1 liter of warm water will break up the mucus in the mouth and throat. This can help patients with mild mucositis due to radiotherapy.

Unfortunately, there has been no controlled study to date comparing the acceptability and effectiveness of these preparations, so no particular one can be recommended. Indeed, none of these agents is ideal and some patients still resort to filling a spray bottle with water to be used at frequent intervals. However, any preparation with an unbuffered, low pH should never be used for dentate patients. Ideally, the saliva substitute should contain fluoride and be supplemented by a daily fluoride mouthwash or a fluoride sucking tablet or chewing gum.

Caries control in people who cannot care for themselves

Dental problems in functionally dependent adults

Some individuals need help to do such basic things as wash and clean their teeth. Perhaps they are disabled by illness, which may be physical (e.g. cancer and its treatment, stroke) or neurological (e.g. dementias, Parkinson's disease, multiple sclerosis). Many of these conditions are associated with old age, but this is not invariably the case. These people are sometimes referred to as 'functionally dependent'. They may be living at home with assistance from carers, who may or may not be family members, or they may be in residential or nursing homes.

The oral health of elderly occupants of residential homes is particularly poor and surveys from the USA and Europe have shown a very high prevalence of coronal and root caries, poor oral hygiene, high plaque and gingival indices, high denture debris levels, denture stomatitis and angular cheilitis (Simons et al., 1999a). Many have difficulty eating and problems with taste. The majority receive medications known to produce a dry mouth and these medicines may be in the form of syrups containing sugar or tablets to be crushed and mixed with jam to make them palatable. The relationship between poor oral status and difficulties with oral hygiene has been established in a study that noted that clients who considered they needed help with cleaning had poorer oral health than those who did not. It was particularly telling to note that only 5% of those who requested help with oral hygiene reported help from their carers in cleaning their mouths (Simons et al., 2001).

It seems unacceptable that the mouth, one of the most personal and intimate parts of the body, should be neglected in this way. The poor oral status of institutionalized elderly people may contribute to the eating problems and low nutrient and vitamin C levels found in this group (Steele et al.,

1998). So, how may this group be helped with their mouths in general and caries in particular?

Oral health assessment and oral care plans

When clients are admitted to residential care an oral health assessment should be carried out (British Society for Disability and Oral Health). The oral assessment provides a mechanism to identify those who require help with daily oral hygiene and those who have oral and dental problems and therefore require help from a dental team.

On the basis of this assessment an oral care plan can be formulated which should be available for the carers to follow. Table 27.3 gives an example of an oral care plan. This plan is very client specific. Note that the carer is instructed to face the client when brushing her teeth. This is because she becomes distressed if eye contact is not maintained. It is easier to stand behind someone when brushing their teeth, but this is not appropriate for this client. It should be remembered that care assistants may know little about oral care, and mouth-care protocols (e.g. oral hygiene, care of dentures) should be written down and explained.

Unfortunately, carers may have difficulty with these suggestions. They may be busy, and have no experience of mouth care. They may find the task revolting, to the extent that some have said they would rather clean bottoms than mouths (Steele et al., 1998). For this reason alone, as well as cross infection control, gloves should be readily available. An oral health training program for carers would seem logical. However, when the effects of the delivery of such a program were studied, the results were disappointing. The program was well received and the carers' knowledge base was increased. However, this did not appear to result in a change in their behavior. The elderly residents noted no change in the help they received, their oral health did not improve and few of the carers originally trained were still working in the home after 1 year (Simons et al., 2002a). This study emphasizes the difficulties in improving oral care.

Some specific recommendations with respect to caries

Oral hygiene performed by carers, using a high-fluoride toothpaste, should be the bedrock of caries control.

Table 27.3 Oral care plan for Mrs Smith

1. Remove dentures each night and brush with large brush and gel provided. Brush over the sink, which should be filled with water.
2. Place dentures in pot overnight.
3. Brush teeth using electric toothbrush and paste provided.
4. Brush teeth with Mrs Smith facing you and maintain eye contact with Mrs Smith at all times. (Note: it is easier to stand on Mrs Smith's right, cradling her head with your left arm, but she is confused and she finds this distressing.)
5. Allow Mrs Smith to spit out, but not to rinse too vigorously.

A dry mouth is very common and in some clients it can be alleviated by chewing gum. Chewing promotes salivary flow and gums medicated with xylitol and xylitol/chlorohexidine have been shown to improve significantly perceived oral health and oral dryness (Simons et al., 1999b). In addition, these gums reduced plaque and gingival indices and alleviated denture sore mouth and angular cheilitis (Simons et al., 2002b). In these studies the gums were distributed and collected by carers twice daily after meals. The gums were called 'oral health gums' and the dentist was pleasantly surprised how well the gums were received and how the product did not stick to the clients' dentures.

It seems unlikely that diet can be modified. Poor nutrition and weight loss are a feature of many illnesses and require frequent snacks, food enrichment and food supplements, many of which are high in sugar. These problems are compounded by difficulty in swallowing and dry mouth. However, every attempt should be made to avoid sugar-based syrups by choosing medications sweetened with artificial sweeteners.

Failure

A few words on failure seem appropriate. Failure to obtain proper caries control may originate in a variety of factors, including dentists' knowledge and skills in performing non-operative interventions, as well as patients' motivation and diligence in complying with the recommended procedures. Dentists in some countries do not find non-operative caries treatments attractive to perform because there is no fee policy (whether state funded, insurance funded or private) that rewards such treatments. As regards the patients, it is the authors' subjective opinion that failure is usually the result of sociological rather than biological factors. In a review of the behavioral aspects of dental plaque-control measures, Schou (1998) states that socioeconomy and social class are strongly related to good oral hygiene behavior and a number of other health-related behaviors. People living in poor circumstances are more likely to have poor health behaviors (e.g. smoking, eating little fresh food, high intake of sweets), including poor oral hygiene. The dentist must remember that people have many problems that the dentist cannot solve. The non-operative techniques described in this chapter demand patient compliance. This is not always forthcoming but, in the final analysis, the teeth belong to the patient!

References

Astrom AN. Stability of oral health-related behavior in a Norwegian cohort between the ages of 15 and 23 years. *Community Dent Oral Epidemiol* 2004; **32**: 354–62.

Bardow A, Nyvad B, Nauntofte B. Relationship between medication intake, complaints of dry mouth, salivary flow rate and composition, and the rate of tooth demineralisation *in situ*. *Arch Oral Biol* 2001; **46**: 413–23.

Beck JD. Risk revisited. *Community Dent Oral Epidemiol* 1998; **26**: 220–5.

Bratthal D, Hänsel Petersen G. Cariogram – a multifactorial risk assessment model for a multifactorial disease. *Community Dent Oral Epidemiol* 2005; **33**: 256–64.

Brennen MT, Shariff G, Lockhart PB, Fox PC. Treatment of xerostomia: a systematic review of therapeutic trials. *Dent Clin N Am* 2002; **46**: 847–56.

British Society for Disability and Oral Health. *Guidelines for oral health care for people with a physical disability.* Available from URL: http://www.bsdh.org.uk

Carino KM, Shinada K, Kawaguchi Y. Early childhood caries in the northern Philippines. *Community Dent Oral Epidemiol* 2003; **31**: 81–9.

Carvalho JC, Ekstrand KR, Thylstrup A. Dental plaque and caries on occlusal surfaces of first permanent molars in relation to stage of eruption. *J Dent Res* 1989; **68**: 773–9.

De Grauwe A, Aps JK, Martens LC. Early childhood caries: what's in a name? *Eur J Paediatr Dent* 2004; **5**: 62–70.

Disney JA, Graves RC, Stamm JW, Bohannan HM, Abernathy JR. Comparative effects of a 4-year fluoride mouthrinse program on high and low caries forming grade 1 children. *Community Dent Oral Epidemiol* 1989; **17**: 139–43.

Dodds MWJ, Hsieh SC, Johnson DA. The effect of increased mastication by daily gum chewing on salivary gland output and dental plaque acidogenicity. *J Dent Res* 1991; **70**: 1474–8.

Dreitzen S, Brown LR, Daly TE, Drane JB. Prevention of xerostomia-related dental caries in irradiated cancer patients. *J Dent Res* 1977; **56**: 99–104.

Eisbruch A, Randall K, Ten Haken PHD, *et al.* Dose, volume and function relationships in parotid salivary glands following conformal and intensity-modulated irradiation of head and neck cancer. *Int J Radiat Oncol Biol Phys* 1999; **45**: 577–87.

Ekstrand KR, Christiansen ME. Outcomes of a non-operative caries treatment programme for children and adolescents. *Caries Res* 2005; **39**: 455–67.

Fejerskov O, Nyvad B. Dental caries in the aging individual. In: Holm-Pedersen P, Löe H, eds. *Textbook of geriatric dentistry.* Copenhagen: Munksgaard, 1996: 338–72.

Ghezzi EM, Ship J. Ageing and secretary reserve capacity of major salivary glands. *J Dent Res* 2003: **82**: 844–8.

Harris R, Nicoll AD, Adair PM, Pine CM. Risk factors for dental caries in young children: a systematic review of the literature. *Community Dent Health* 2004; **21**: 71–85.

Heanue M, Deacon SAA, Deery C. Manual versus powered toothbrushing for oral health (Cochrane Review). In: *Cochrane Library*, Issue 1. Oxford: Update Software, 2003.

Henson BS, Eisbruch A, D'Hondt E, Ship JA. Two year longitudinal study of parotid salivary flow rates in head and neck cancer patients receiving unilateral neck parotid-sparing radiotherapy treatment. *Oral Oncol* 1999; **35**: 234–41.

Jenson SB, Pederson AM, Reibal J, Nauntoste B. Xerostomia and hypofunction of the salivary glands in cancer therapy. *Support Care Cancer* 2003; **11**: 207–25.

Joyston-Bechal S. Prevention of dental disease following radiotherapy and chemotherapy. *Int Dent J* 1992; **42**: 47–53.

Katz S. The use of fluoride and chlorhexidine for the prevention of radiation caries. *J Am Dent Assoc* 1982; **104**: 164–70.

Kay E, Locker D. A systematic review of the effectiveness of health promotion aimed at improving oral health. *Community Dent Health* 1998; **15**: 132–44.

Kidd EAM. *Essentials of dental caries.* Oxford: Oxford University Press, 2005.

Koivusilta L, Honkala S, Honkala E, Rimpela A. Toothbrushing as part of the adolescent lifestyle predicts education level. *J Dent Res* 2003; **82**: 361–6.

Kowash MB, Pinfield A, Smith J, Curson MEJ. Effectiveness on oral health of a long term health education programme for mothers with young children. *Br Dent J* 2000; **188**: 201–5.

Kowash MB, Toumba KJ, Curzon ME. Cost-effectiveness of a long-term dental health education program for the prevention of early childhood caries. *Eur Arch Paediatr Dent* 2006; **7**: 130–5.

Kuusela S, Honkala E, Rimpela A, Karvonen S, Rimpela M. Trends in toothbrushing frequency among Finnish adolescents between 1977 and 1995. *Community Dent Health* 1998; **14**: 84–8.

Machiulskiene V, Nyvad B, Baelum V. Caries preventive effect of sugar-substituted chewing gum. *Community Dent Oral Epidemiol* 2001; **29**: 178–88.

Mäkinen KK, Benett CA, Hujoel PP, *et al.* Xylitol chewing gums and caries rates: a 40-month cohort study. *J Dent Res* 1995; **74**: 1904–13.

Marinho VCC, Higgins JPT, Logan S, Sheiham A. Fluoride varnishes for preventing dental caries in children and adolescents (Cochrane Review). In: *Cochrane Library*, Issue 3. Oxford: Update Software, 2002.

Marinho VCC, Higgins JPT, Sheiham A, Logan S. Fluoride toothpaste for preventing caries in children and adolescents (Cochrane Review). In: *Cochrane Library*, Issue I. Oxford: Software Update, 2003a.

Marinho VCC Higgins JPT, Logan S, Sheiham A. Fluoride gels for preventing dental caries in children and adolescents (Cochrane Review). In: *Cochrane Library*, Issue 1. Oxford: Update Software, 2003b.

Mattila ML, Rautava P, Ojanlatva A, *et al.* Will the role of family influence dental caries among seven-year-old children? *Acta Odontol Scand* 2005; **63**: 73–84.

Meyerowitz C, Featherstone JDB, Billings RJ, Eisenberg AD, Fu J, Shariati M. Use of an intra-oral model to evaluate 0.05% sodium fluoride mouthrinse in radiation-induced hyposalivation. *J Dent Res* 1991; **70**: 894–8.

Molendijk B, Ter Horst G, Kasbergen M, Truin GJ, Mulder J. Dental health in Dutch drug addicts. *Community Dent Oral Epidemiol* 1996; **24**: 117–19.

Olivan G. Untreated dental caries is common among 6 to 12-year-old physically abused/neglected children in Spain. *Eur J Public Health* 2003; **13**: 91–2.

van Palenstein Helderman WH, Soe W, van't Hof MA. Risk factors of early childhood caries in a Southeast Asian population. *J Dent Res* 2006; **85**: 85–8.

Pine CM, McGoldrick PM, Burnside G, *et al.* An intervention programme to establish regular toothbrushing: understanding parents' beliefs and motivating children. *Int Dent J* 2000; (Suppl): 312–23.

Pine CM, Adair PM, Nicoll AD, *et al.* International comparisons of health inequalities in childhood dental caries. *Community Dent Health* 2004; **21** (1 Suppl): 121–30.

Renvert S, Glavind L. Individualized instruction and compliance in oral hygiene practices: recommendations and means of delivery. In: Lang NP, Attström R, Löe H, eds. *Proceedings of the European Workshop on Mechanical Plaque Control*. Chicago, IL: Quintessence, 1998: 300–9.

Scheutz F. Five-year evaluation of a dental care delivery system for drug addicts in Denmark. *Community Dent Oral Epidermiol* 1984; **12**: 29–34.

Schou L. Behavioural aspects of dental plaque control measures: an oral health promotion perspective. In: Lang NP, Attström R, Löe H, eds. *Proceedings of the European Workshop on Mechanical Plaque Control*. Chicago, IL: Quintessence, 1998: 287–99.

Seow WK. Biological mechanisms of early childhood caries. *Community Dent Oral Epidemiol* 1998; **26** (Suppl 1): 8–27.

Sheiham A, Maizels J, Cushing A, Holmes J. Dental attendance and dental status. *Community Dent Oral Epidemiol* 1985; **13**: 304–9.

Ship JA. Xerostomia: aetiology, diagnosis, management and clinical implications. In: Edgar M, Davies C, O'Mullane D, eds. *Saliva and Oral Health*. London: BDJ Books, 2004: 50–70.

Simons D, Kidd EAM, Beighton D. Oral health of elderly occupants in residential homes. *Lancet* 1999a; **353**: 1761.

Simons D, Baker P, Knott D, *et al.* Attitudes of carers and elderly occupants of residential homes to antimicrobial chewing gum as an aid to oral health. *Br Dent J* 1999b; **187**: 612–15.

Simons D, Brailsford S, Kidd EAM, Beighton D. Relationship between oral hygiene practices and oral status in dentate elderly people living in residential homes. *Community Dent Oral Epidemiol* 2001; **29**: 464–70.

Simons D, Baker P, Jones B, Kidd EAM, Beighton D. An evaluation of an oral health training programme for carers of the elderly in residential homes. *Br Dent J* 2002a; **188**: 206–10.

Simons D, Brailsford S, Kidd EAM, Beighton D. The effect of medicated chewing gums on oral health in frail older people: a one-year clinical trial. *J Am Geriatr Soc* 2002b; **50**: 1348–53.

Skeie MS, Espelid I, Skaare AB, Gimmestad A. Caries patterns in an urban preschool population in Norway. *Eur J Paediatr Dent* 2005; **6**: 16–22.

Smith RG, Burtner AP. Oral side-effects of the most frequently prescribed drugs. *Spec Care Dent* 1994; **14**: 96–102.

Steele JG, Sheiham A, Marcenes W, Walls AWG. *National Diet and Nutrition Survey: people aged 65 years and over*, Vol. 2, *Report of the oral health survey*. London: The Stationery Office, 1998.

Sweeting H, Anderson A, West P. Socio-demographic correlates of dietary habits in mid to late adolescence. *Eur J Clin Nutr* 1994; **48**: 736–48.

Tenovuo J. Protective functions of saliva. In: Edgar M, Davies C, O'Mullane D, eds. *Saliva and oral health*. London: BDJ Books, 2004: 103–18.

Thitasomakul S, Thearmontree A, Piwat S, *et al.* A longidudinal study of early childhood caries in 9- to 18-month-old Thai infants. *Community Dent Oral Epidemiol* 2006; **34**: 429–36.

Thomson WM. Dental caries experience in older people over time: what can the large cohort studies tell us? *Br Dent J* 2004; **196**: 89–92.

Thomson WM, Chalmers JM, Spencer AJ, Ketabi M. The occurrence of xerostomia and salivary gland hypofunction in a population-based sample of older South Australians. *Spec Care Dent* 1999; **19**: 20–3.

Treasure E, Kelly M, Nuttall N, Nunn J, Bradnock G, White D. Factors associated with oral health: a multivariate analysis of results from the 1998 Adult Dental Health survey. *Br Dent J* 2001; **190**: 60–8.

Weinstein P. *Motivate your dental patients: a workbook*. Seattle, WA: University of Washington, 2002.

Weinstein P, Harrison R, Benton T. Motivating parents to prevent caries in theit young children: one-year findings. *J Am Dent Assoc* 2004; **135**: 731–8.

Weintraub JA. Pit and fissure sealants in high-caries-risk individuals. *J Dent Educ* 2001; **65**: 1084–90.

Zimmer BW, Rottwinkel Y. Assessing patient-specific decalcification risk in fixed orthodontic treatment and its impaction on prophylactic procedures. *Am J Orthod Dentofacial Orthop* 2004; **126**: 318–24.

Zimmerman GL, Olsen CG, Bosworth MF, A 'stages of change' approach to helping patients change behaviour. *Am Fam Physician* 2000; **61**: 1409–16.

28

Caries control for populations

V. Baelum, A. Sheiham and B. Burt

Introduction

The disease processes leading to dental caries must undergo lifelong control (Griffin *et al.*, 2005) in order to avoid the irreversible consequences of the later stages of caries development, namely cavity formation, restoration and the ensuing re-restorations, endodontic treatment, crown therapy, and possibly the ultimate loss of the tooth. Therefore, the word 'prevention' is used to mean preventing the occurrence of the irreversible caries signs and symptoms by controlling the caries process.

In this chapter, the authors argue the need to apply a common risk factor approach to prevention, for health promotion cannot be compartmentalized to specific parts of the body. Dental health is part of general health. Any attempt to improve dental health should be fully integrated into broadly based health-promoting strategies and actions. It is thus worth keeping in mind that caries, periodontitis, oral mucosal lesions, oral cancer, temporomandibular joint dysfunction and pain are related to diet, tobacco, alcohol and stress; and that trauma to teeth is related to accidents. Diet, alcohol, tobacco and stress are causes that are common to a number of chronic diseases such as cancer, heart diseases, diabetes and psychiatric diseases. It is therefore rational to use a common risk factor approach (Sheiham & Watt, 2000; Griffin *et al.*, 2005). This implies a new public health that is no longer oriented to single diseases, and preventive intervention approaches should no longer be organized around single clinical disease entities such as coronary heart disease, caries or cancer. Most behavioral and social risk factors transcend these particular diseases, and instead influence susceptibility to diseases in general. Moreover, decision makers and individuals will be more readily influenced by measures directed at the joint prevention of heart diseases, obesity, stroke, cancers, diabetes and dental caries than if disease-specific recommendations are made. Whenever possible, the strategies recommended for prevention and control of oral diseases, including dental caries, should therefore be part of a common risk factor approach to control the risks shared by a number of chronic diseases. Such strategies involve food and health policies to change unhealthy dietary practices, a community approach to improve general hygiene (including oral hygiene), smoking cessation policies and policies on reducing accidents. These strategies should supplement the more disease-specific policies, which in the case of dental caries involve rational use of fluorides and the availability of appropriate, acceptable and evidence-based dental health care.

The caries decline and changes in the practice of dentistry

The past decades have witnessed a tremendous decline in the age-specific prevalence and extent of dental caries in many populations (see Chapter 8). This decline is well documented for child populations in the high-income countries (Helm & Helm, 1990; Downer, 1992; Marthaler *et al.*, 1996; Davies *et al.*, 1997) and to a lesser extent in adult populations (Truin *et al.*, 1993; Marthaler *et al.*, 1996; Kalsbeek *et al.*, 1998; Eriksen, 1998). Caries levels are also dropping in some high-caries populations, such as those in several Eastern European countries (Marthaler *et al.*, 1996). Even though some believe that caries is generally increasing in Africa the available evidence suggests that the trend here is also downwards (Fejerskov *et al.*, 1994; Cleaton-Jones & Fatti, 1999).

This caries decline has been paralleled by important changes in the practice of dentistry. Where dental practice, as far as dental caries is concerned, only a few decades ago was almost entirely focussed on an operative treatment-oriented approach in the management of the most obvious cavities (Fejerskov & Kidd, 2003; Gimmestad *et al.*, 2003; Hudson, 2004) and their sequelae, contemporary dental practice devotes more efforts to early (precavitation stage) caries diagnosis, and to non-operative and preventive care for such early lesions (Elderton & Eddie, 1983, 1986; Brennan *et al.*, 1998; Brennan & Spencer, 2003a; Watt *et al.*, 2004). This trend for change seems particularly prominent in European dentistry, whereas US dentistry still tends to focus on restoring cavities (Ismail, 1997).

A key question is how this development should be interpreted. Has the caries decline been brought about by a change of focus in dental practice away from its 'drill, fill and bill' perspective (Anusavice, 2005) to a more preventive attitude to the management of caries? Or does the increased emphasis on early diagnosis and preventive care merely reflect a response to the presence of steadily fewer overt cavities from a dental profession that wishes to keep a full appointment book, to maintain income and its *raison d'être*? Indeed, some studies suggest that the latter mechanisms also operate (Grembowski & Milgrom, 1988; Grytten, 1991; Grembowski *et al.*, 1997; Brennan & Spencer, 2003b; Tickle *et al.*, 2003b).

It is very tempting for members of the dental profession to try to take all the credit for the caries decline. However, there are no reasons to do so, certainly as far as daily chairside preventive activities are concerned (Sheiham, 1997; Wang, 1998). The chairside preventive armamentarium available to dentists is relatively limited, encompassing oral hygiene instructions (Davies *et al.*, 2005), dietary advice (Lingström *et al.*, 2003; Watt *et al.*, 2003), pit and fissure sealants (Mejàre *et al.*, 2003; Locker *et al.*, 2003; Ahovuo-Saloranta *et al.*, 2004), and topical fluoride applications (Marinho *et al.*, 2002a, b, 2003c, d; Hawkins *et al.*, 2003; Seppä, 2004) given on an individual basis to people who for the most part appear in the dental office only once or twice a year. Even though the dentist may individualize the recall intervals and the contents and intensity of the preventive

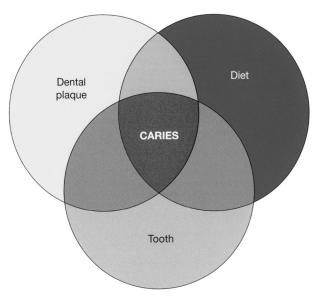

Figure 28.1 A popular, strictly biological view of the sufficient cause of caries, first described as Keyes' triad (Keyes, 1960). Later versions may incorporate time as a necessary component cause, but this is not needed when caries is viewed as a process.

chairside sessions to reflect the actual caries situation for the person in question (see Chapter 14), there is very limited evidence to suggest that annual or biannual recalls, even when they include oral hygiene instructions (Beirne *et al.*, 2005) (see Chapter 15) and individualized dietary counseling (Lingström *et al.*, 2003) (see Chapter 19), will affect caries development or progression. There is some evidence from clinical efficacy trials that the professional application of topical fluoride in the form of gels, mouthrinses or varnishes results in only small caries reductions on top of those found from fluoride toothpaste alone (Marinho *et al.*, 2004a). Indeed, analyses based on data from more than 15 000 children failed to demonstrate the expected negative association between the frequency of professional topical fluoride applications and the number of interproximal restorations placed (Eklund *et al.*, 2000). In addition, studies have indicated that the preventive care actually provided by general dental practitioners is ineffective in high-risk children (Tickle *et al.*, 2003b). Studies report that practitioners tend to provide prevention to asymptomatic patients in routine maintenance schedules rather than to patients at higher risk of caries (Eklund *et al.*, 2000; Brennan *et al.*, 2000; Brennan & Spencer, 2003b), and continue to perform early restorative intervention (Doméjean-Orliaguet *et al.*, 2004). This lends further support to the notion that the caries decline may not be attributable to the effects of the professional chairside preventive activities to the extent that dental professionals would like to believe. A study conducted in the Nordic countries has revealed considerable intercountry differences in the caries-preventive methods used by the dental professionals, while the caries

prevalence and severity was similar (Källestål *et al.*, 1999). Finally, ecological analyses indicate that social factors, rather than dental services, explain the major part of the geographical variation in caries experience (Nadanovsky & Sheiham, 1994), just as the contribution of dental services to the decline in dental caries is very much smaller than commonly thought (Nadanovsky & Sheiham, 1994, 1995). These analyses showed that dental services could explain only about 3% of the differences in the changes in caries levels among 12-year-olds across 18 countries. Most of the differences in the caries level changes were explained by broad socioeconomic factors, whether fluoridated toothpastes were included or not (Nadanovsky & Sheiham, 1995).

Why does caries occur?

Historically, the professional view on caries causation has been limited to a model consisting of the tooth, the dental plaque bacteria and sugars. Together, these three necessary component causes form the biologically sufficient cause of caries, formerly known as Keyes' triad (Keyes, 1960) (Fig. 28.1). From a theoretical standpoint, it is sufficient to block one of the component causes, e.g. the dental plaque bacteria or the intake of fermentable carbohydrates, to block the caries process. 'A clean tooth does not decay' has been a mantra for many preventive activities over the years. However, as the chairside caries-preventive activities, e.g. topical fluoride applications, oral hygiene instructions and dietary counseling, are specifically targeting each of these

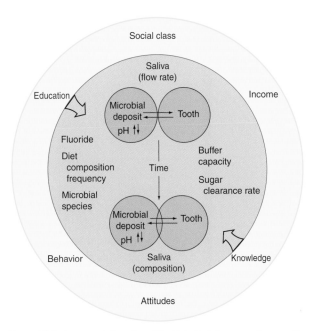

Figure 28.2 An expanded version of the biological view on caries causation (Fejerskov & Manji, 1990). The socioeconomic and behavioral factors included are not considered to play a direct biological causal role, but can be understood as determinants of the biological causes of caries.

three necessary component causes, one may ask why these chairside preventive efforts have had such limited success.

The answer is that dental researchers and clinicians alike have failed to grasp fully what caries causation is about. Even though more recent versions of the Keyes' triad have expanded the strictly biological causal model by adding more distant causes (Fejerskov & Manji, 1990) (Fig. 28.2), and despite the terms 'complex' and 'multifactorial' now being quoted in almost any statement pertaining to caries etiology, most still erroneously misunderstand the etiology of caries by considering it as a purely biological process (Holst *et al.*, 2001). This means that when dentists think about the causes of caries, they do not think beyond dental plaque bacteria and the dietary carbohydrates and sugars.

However, this viewpoint leads to self-delusion. For one thing, it ignores the causes of the causes (Holst, 2005). The biological model for caries causation does not provide answers to a number of pertinent questions, such as: why do some people eat highly 'cariogenic' diets while others don't? and why do some people maintain good oral hygiene while others don't? The second major limitation of the biological model for caries causation (Figs 28.1, 28.2) is that it understands causes as properties of individuals and ignores

structural and contextual causes (Fig. 28.3). Structural causes in relation to caries are those international, national, regional or local societal circumstances (e.g. industry, media, politics, economics, infrastructure) that affect the social context in which people live, e.g. the psychosocial environment, material wealth, workplace, home, and school (McMichael, 1995; Brunner & Marmot, 1999). The social context, in turn, shapes the behaviors, values and beliefs of individuals (Jarvis & Wardle, 1999; Chin *et al.*, 2000). Based on these findings it is clear that if one wants to change people's behaviors, a change is necessary in the environment that leads to the unwanted behaviors.

Dentists' chairside preventive activities are largely based on a somewhat naïve idea (Watt, 2002), the knowledge-attitude-behavior (KAB) model (Chin *et al.*, 2000). According to the KAB model, individuals behave rationally and always make choices that serve their best interests (Chin *et al.*, 2000). The idea is that knowledge provided to the individual (e.g. information about the unhealthy consequences of the current dietary and oral hygiene practices and advice/instructions for change) will bring about a change in the individual's values and beliefs and attitudes which, in turn, will result in the desired behavioral change (e.g.

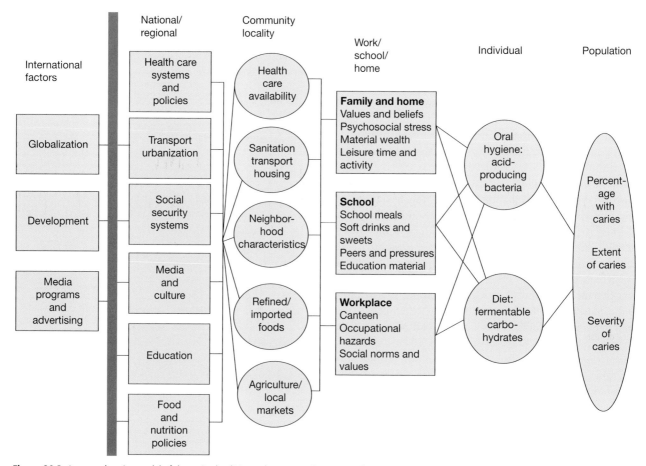

Figure 28.3 A comprehensive model of the societal policies and processes that may explain caries in populations. (Modified from Kumanyika *et al.*, 2002.)

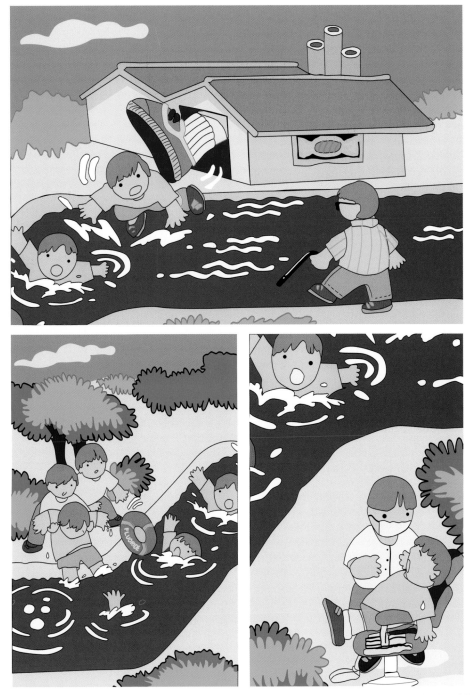

Figure 28.4 Upstream contextual and societal factors (e.g. the confectionary industry) push people into the caries river. Availability of lifebelts along the river (e.g. fluoride in the oral environment) may be helpful in rescuing victims, whereas downstream activities are restricted to victim rehabilitation (by means of restorations) by the dentist.

improved oral hygiene practices or healthier dietary habits). However, the available evidence generally suggests that the effects of such approaches, if at all demonstrable, are transient and of short duration (Kay & Locker, 1996; Watt & Marinho, 2005), and do not affect caries experience (Vanobbergen et al., 2004). The basic problem is that the approach fails to understand that individual behaviors are also shaped by contextual and societal factors that cannot be reduced to individual attributes (Chin et al., 2000; Holst, 2005).

There are numerous examples of the influences of such factors (Chin et al., 2000). In a dental context (Fig. 28.4), there are good reasons why the sweet shelves in the supermarkets are invariably placed near the checkout counter, where shoppers and their impatient children have to stand in line. There are also good reasons why soft-drink companies have entered into contracts with school districts in the USA that give the companies exclusive rights to stock their products in the schools' vending machines (Heller *et al.*, 2001). There are good reasons why a person, who lives in a social context where the tradition for oral hygiene procedures is limited and where toothache and tooth loss due to caries are seen as inevitable consequences of life, does not respond positively with the desired behavioral change when dental professionals give advice about the likely benefits of tooth brushing twice a day using fluoride toothpaste. Similarly, a person cannot be expected to stop smoking when everyone they live with, work with and spend their leisure time with smokes. Countless smokers will testify to the fact that the 'advice' typically given by the resourceful, to pull oneself together, rarely suffices to achieve permanent smoking cessation. It is not a trivial matter of providing more knowledge about caries and obesity, for a person used to frequent snacking, to cause him or her to abandon this habit when such snacking behavior is the norm in her social context, e.g. the family, workplace, or school. Similarly, it is much more difficult to convince young people that regular intake of large quantities of sugar-containing carbonated soft drinks is a bad idea from a caries and obesity perspective when multinational companies are allowed to use the youth culture media to portray this behavior as synonymous with success.

These arguments all point in one direction: if dental professionals really mean to bring about reductions in caries levels in the populations they serve, they need to comprehend the causes of caries beyond the strictly biological (Holst *et al.*, 2001; Newton & Bower, 2005; Holst, 2005).

Upstream or downstream: does it matter?

The failure of the present dominant dental approach to the prevention of caries in populations can be illustrated by an allegory. A doctor was standing by the side of a river and heard the cry of a drowning person, who had fallen off the bridge crossing the river (Fig. 28.5). He jumped in to rescue and to resuscitate him. Just as the rescued man was recovering on the river bank there were more cries from other drowning people. The rescuer jumped in again, brought some back and resuscitated them. The rescuer could not cope alone, so he fetched helpers and breathing machines. Still he could not cope. So they worked faster in teams, four-handed and six-handed, with more complex equipment and faster methods of resuscitation. So many people were drowning that some could not be rescued before permanent damage had occurred. How could he stop them from drowning? Swimming lessons were his solution. Health education. However, rescuing and swimming lesson activities kept the available doctors so busy that at no time did

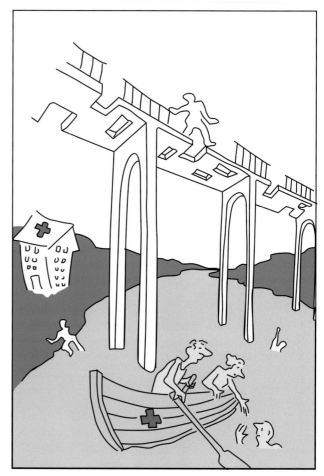

Figure 28.5 The downstream approach to the prevention of caries. Victims are pulled out of the river and resuscitated, when they flow by, but no attention is paid to the upstream reasons why people have fallen into the river.

they stop to consider why people who could not swim were in the river in the first place. Who was pushing them in upstream (Pearce, 1996; Watt, 2007)? Had the doctors had time to contemplate they would soon have realized by mere inspection of the bridge that simply providing the bridge with proper railings would have prevented many people from falling off the bridge (Fig. 28.6). Stopping people from falling off the bridge or making the river shallower, by health promotion, will prevent people from drowning even if they cannot swim. The dentists' concentration on the downstream victim rescue operation had completely distracted their attention from the upstream activities of the confectionery, food and drink companies who were 'pushing people into the water' (Fig. 28.4); just as it prevented dentists and their professional bodies from lobbying and putting pressure on politicians and other decision makers that unhealthy choices could be made more difficult (and healthy choices easier) if appropriate regulations were instigated. What this allegory suggests is that more efforts should be directed at making healthy choices the easier choices, and at controlling the activities of those pushing people into the

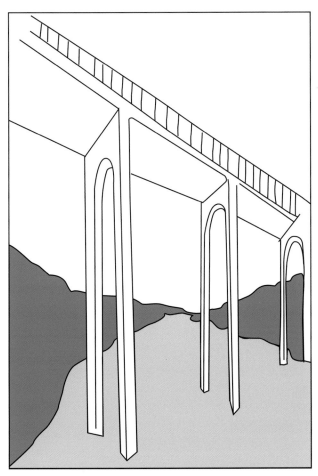

Figure 28.6 The upstream approach to the prevention of caries. The holes in the bridge have been mended, and proper railings have been added. Healthy choices have thus been made the easier choices.

water, i.e. a direct attack on the determinants of health. While dentists need not completely abandon their downstream activities in the form of evidence-based oral hygiene instructions, dietary counseling and topical fluoride applications, they should be aware of their limitations and realize that midstream activities, such as supportive health promotion, and upstream activities, such as appropriate regulations aiming at making healthier choices easier and unhealthy ones more difficult, carry much larger benefits for the population's health (Fig. 28.4).

Sick individuals or sick populations?

It is the centerpiece of appropriate clinical dentistry to ask not only 'what is the diagnosis, and which is the best treatment for this tooth?', but also 'why did this occur, and could it have been prevented?' (Rose, 1985). These questions arise out of the clinical dentists' natural concern for the patient, the sick individual. However, restricting oneself to this perspective is tantamount to not being able to see the forest for the trees.

The dental profession is also obliged to ask the question why some populations or groups have severe caries while in others caries is considerably less extensive. Figure 28.7 is just one of many possible illustrations that demonstrate the huge variation in the extent of caries recorded at the cavitation level across different populations. There was an eight-fold difference in the average number of decayed, missing, or filled primary teeth (dmft) among 5–7-year-old children between the most extensively affected European population (Albania; $dmft_{5-7} = 8.5$) and the least affected population (Spain; $dmft_{5-7} = 1.0$).

Considerable variation is also present for population groups within nations. Even though Denmark, according to Fig. 28.7, has lower caries levels than most countries (in this case dmft among 5–7-year-olds), there is considerable intra-country variation between the different Danish municipalities (Fig. 28.8). Within Denmark there is also an eight-fold difference in the average number of decayed, missing or filled permanent surfaces (DMFS) and a six-fold difference in the prevalence of caries at 15 years of age between the 'best' and the 'worst' Danish municipalities (Ekstrand *et al.*, 2003).

Figures 28.7 and 28.8 show caries data on an aggregate level; namely as mean dmf/DMF scores for populations or groups within populations. These statistics do not usually attract much attention from clinical dentists, whose main concern is caries in the individual patient. However, dentists are well aware that the caries experience of individuals may vary considerably among otherwise apparently similar individuals. An example of such within-group variation of dental caries is seen in Fig. 28.9, which contrasts the caries experience recorded at the cavitation level of 15-year-old Danish children from 'low' and 'high' caries municipalities. The distribution of DMFS is right-skewed in both the low and high caries groups, and the caries experience varies between children within each group. However, in the low caries municipalities about 60% of the 15-year-olds are caries free (40% have caries), compared with 17% of the children in the high caries municipalities (where 83% have caries). More than 25% of the 15-year-olds in the high caries municipalities had at least 10 DMFS, while only 0.5% of the children in the low caries municipalities had a DMFS of 10 or more.

It is quite understandable that the response of the dentists when faced with such distributions is to concentrate on the characteristics of the children who suffer extensive caries, i.e. those in the right-hand tail of the distributions. Hence, the answer to the clinical question – why do some patients get extensive caries while other patients who live in apparently similar social circumstances are caries free or suffer only the occasional lesion? – is based on an evaluation of differences in the characteristics of individuals and their families within the group.

However, the answer to the question why some municipalities or countries suffer extensive caries, while others

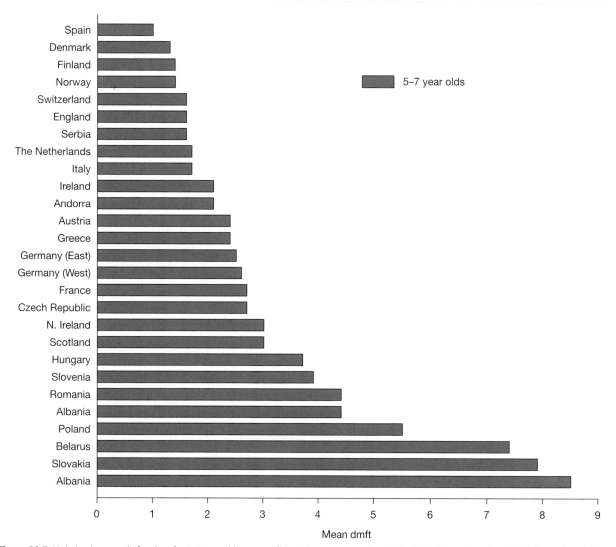

Figure 28.7 Variation in mean dmft values for 5–7-year-olds across different European countries, 1991–1995. (Data points from Marthaler *et al.*, 1996.)

have little, has to do with the determinants of the population mean (Rose, 1985). Unfortunately, these determinants are seldom of concern to the clinical dentist, because they are not found in the characteristics of the individual patients. Instead, they are to be found in factors that produce a shift in the whole distribution of caries. Several studies have shown that the distribution of caries in a population can be predicted by the mean DMFS or DMFT scores (Jarvinen, 1985; Batchelor & Sheiham, 2002). These results demonstrate that combating caries requires mass influences that act on the population as a whole; in other words, shifting the whole population's mean to the left.

The above illustrates a very important point that is not well understood: the causes of individual cases of caries are not always the same as the causes of the incidence of caries, in populations (Holst, 2005). The point is valid not only for

caries but applies to essentially all diseases afflicting humankind (Rose, 1985, 1992).

Options for change: which preventive strategy should be used?

So far, two fundamentally different approaches to prevention have been alluded to: the high-risk strategy and the population strategy. A third approach is used, namely the directed population strategy, also called geographic targeting, which is an amalgamation of the high-risk and the population strategies for prevention (Sheiham & Joffe, 1991). It was the British epidemiologist Geoffrey Rose (Rose, 1992) who first defined the strengths and weaknesses of the high-risk and population approaches to prevention of chronic diseases, including caries.

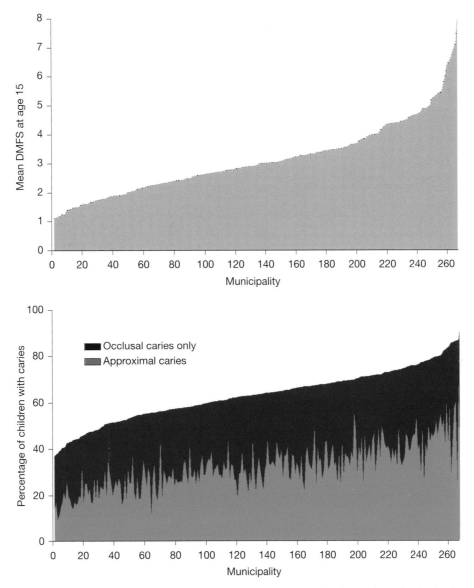

Figure 28.8 Variation across 267 different municipalities in the mean DMFS values (upper panel) and in the prevalence of occlusal and approximal caries (lower panel) among 15-year-old Danes in 2003. (Courtesy of Dr J. Heidmann.)

The high-risk approach

The high-risk approach to prevention is based on the concept that preventive efforts should be concentrated on that segment of the population that appears to have a high risk of disease. For dental caries this corresponds to a concentration of effort on those individuals who are at a high risk of ending up in the right-hand tail of the distribution of caries experience (Fig. 28.9), while little attention is paid to the majority of the population with small or negligible individual disease risks. To be able to target this right-hand tail it is necessary to be able to predict future caries development. This topic is discussed in Chapter 29, which concludes that

such prediction may be impossible. Even so, proponents of the high-risk strategy advocate this strategy on the basis of five principal arguments (Table 28.1).

- *Intervention is appropriate to the individual*: it makes sense to both dental professionals and patients at high risk and enhances motivation of both when dietary advice and oral hygiene instruction is given in response to unhealthy eating habits and poor oral hygiene conditions.
- *No intervention with those not at special risk*: if high risk of (extensive and severe) caries is confined to a minority, most people need not be troubled with preventive interventions as they have small risks. Urging preventive actions

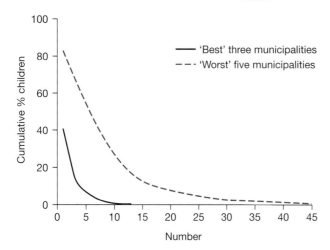

Figure 28.9 Variation in the DMFS counts between 15-year-old Danes in 2003 from two different municipalities with very different average caries levels. (Courtesy of Dr J. Heidmann.)

Table 28.1 Advantages and disadvantages of the high-risk strategy for prevention

Advantages	Disadvantages
Intervention is appropriate to the individual	Prevention is medicalized
No intervention with those not at special risk	Success palliative and temporary
Fits the ethos and organization of medical and dental care	Strategy behaviorally inadequate
Offers cost-effective use of resources Selectivity improves benefit–risk ratio	Limited by poor prediction Problems of feasibility and costs Contribution to overall control of disease may be disappointingly small

on the caries free who are unlikely to benefit makes little sense, and may actually constitute bad advice if it involves costs or other risks.

- *Fits the ethos and organization of health-care systems*: in dentistry, the link between curative and preventive actions has long been established. Decades ago people went to the dentist mainly in response to subjective complaints, e.g. toothache. Today, dental attendance patterns are largely preventive: people who do not have symptoms go to the dentist for check-ups because this is considered good preventive behavior, a notion which most dentists fully advocate.
- *Cost-effective use of resources*: resources for dental care are limited and some rationing is necessary. Priority should be given to those who are likely to benefit (the most) from the intervention.
- *Improved benefit–risk ratio*: if the risks of intervention are the same for everybody it follows that the benefit–risk ratio will be more favorable where the benefits are larger.

However, the high-risk strategy for prevention has important disadvantages:

- *Medicalization of prevention*: Rose explains this problem using an anecdote about a man who went to see his doctor because of a pain in his neck, but walked away from the doctor's office carrying the label 'hypertensive patient' and a prescription for antihypertensive drugs to be taken for the rest of his life (along with regular 'preventive' visits to the doctor). He went feeling 'normal' and left as a 'patient'. Hypertension is no more a disease than is dental plaque bacteria or bad dietary habits, yet this 'labeling' of a person as a patient will inevitably force him to think and act as a patient. This may result in anxiety, impaired self-confidence or altered self-image in normal people. Most practitioners will have met dental patients who are so downhearted by repetitive attempts to improve their oral hygiene that they actually ask us not to mention the problem anymore.
- *Palliative and temporary success*: the high-risk strategy is about protecting against the effects of exposure (as might be achieved by frequent topical fluoride applications), or about lowering the exposure (e.g. by improved oral hygiene or altered dietary practices) among the high-risk individuals. Neither of these two approaches deals with the basic reasons why people are exposed to the harmful determinants of caries. Their effects will therefore remain local, palliative and temporary. Here are some analogies: 'icebergs cannot be prevented by cutting off their tips, just as feeding the hungry does not tackle the causes of famine'.
- *Behaviorally inadequate*: along with most other lifestyle characteristics, people's oral hygiene practices and dietary habits are shaped and constrained by the norms prevailing in their surroundings, whether in society at large or in their homes and families. Trying to behave differently from one's family and friends is not an easy task, yet this stepping out of line is precisely what the high-risk approach to prevention is asking people with many problems to do.
- *Poor prediction*: application of the high-risk strategy to caries prevention necessitates identification of people at high risk of future caries development. As thoroughly discussed in Chapter 29, this may be a mission impossible.
- *Feasibility and cost problems*: the costs of screening for risk may be huge and the feasibility may be limited if the procedures used to assess risk are expensive and require special skills. In the case of dental caries this cost problem is prominent, and reinforced by the limitations of the candidate risk predictors (see Chapter 29).
- *Contribution to overall control of disease may be very small*: the contribution of a smaller number of people at high risk of the total caries experience may be negligible compared with the burden from the many people who

are at smaller risk. This paradox is perhaps best illustrated by the following example.

Figure 28.10a shows the risk of birth complications as a function of maternal age. The risk increases with age, markedly so from the age of 35 years, to reach a high of 80% at 45–49 years of age. If pregnant women aged 35 years and above are considered as the target 'high-risk' group for birth complications, then preventive intervention would be needed in a little less than 20% of all pregnant women (Fig. 28.10b). In view of the simple screening procedure (maternal age) this would be quite feasible. However, even if there existed a perfect intervention to prevent birth complications among these women, i.e. an intervention with 100% success, it would only be possible to prevent just under 23% of all cases of birth complications (Fig. 28.10c). This meager result arises from a combination of the smaller, but nevertheless non-zero, risk in the younger age groups and the fact that a majority of the births take place precisely in the age-groups with much smaller, non-zero risks.

For dental caries corroborating examples exist, and it has been shown that less than 6% of all new caries lesions developing over a 4-year period were found in those children who initially had been deemed at high risk, here defined as having a baseline DMFS of 7 or more (Batchelor & Sheiham, 2006). The vast majority of new lesions occurred in children who were caries free (DMFS = 0) at the beginning of the study. These observations clearly indicate that the high-risk strategy may be inappropriate for caries.

The population strategy for caries prevention

The population strategy for prevention is particularly useful with common diseases or diseases that have widespread causes. Dental caries is certainly a disease that fulfills both of these characteristics. The population strategy is based on the idea that the occurrence of disease reflects the make-up and circumstances of society as a whole. In previous sections, it has been repeatedly stressed that the nature of the direct biological causes of caries, dental plaque bacteria and fermentable carbohydrates, is dictated by oral hygiene practices and dietary habits. These behaviors are, in turn, socially determined, thus calling for actions at upstream levels beyond those of individual behaviors, i.e. in the social, economic, political and industrial fields.

Proponents of the high-risk strategy for prevention of caries have often focussed entirely on the conspicuous right-hand tail of the distribution of caries in the population (Fig. 28.9). Their objective is to truncate – to cut off the right-hand tail – this distribution by targeting the risk factors responsible for people being in the tail position. However, it is widely overlooked that a population-wide shift in the distribution of risk may exert a larger and longer lasting effect on the number of people falling in the right-hand tail of the distribution, because the shift of the

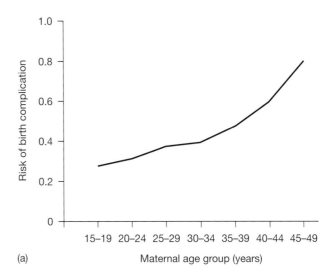

(a)

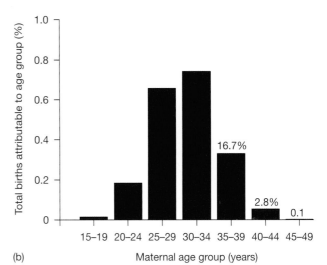

(b)

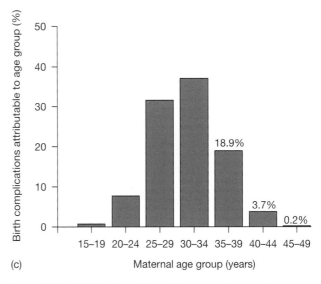

(c)

Figure 28.10 (a) Distribution of risk of birth complications as a function of maternal age. (b) Distribution of births according to maternal age. (c) Distribution of birth complications according to maternal age. (Data from Danmarks Statistik, 2003, www.dst.dk.)

whole population to the left pulls the right-hand tail with it. A population-based approach has the additional advantage of targeting also those many who have a smaller risk and who are responsible for most of the disease cases (see Fig. 28.10a–c).

This is illustrated in Fig. 28.11, using the aforementioned observations that the distribution of DMFS or DMFT counts can be predicted on the basis of knowledge of the population mean values (Jarvinen, 1985; Batchelor & Sheiham, 2002). The effect was calculated of a change in the mean DMFT values from 3.0 to 2.5 on the distribution of DMFT counts that would result from a hypothetical population-based preventive strategy in a population of 12-year-olds. Not only has this hypothetical intervention caused the prevalence of caries to decrease from 83% to 73%, but also the size of the 'high-risk' group has diminished. When an (arbitrary) cut-point of 5.0 DMFT is used to define 'high-risk' children, the 'high-risk' group has diminished from 26% to 14%, as a result of the population intervention. This has occurred as a result of a shift to the left in the whole distribution, indicating lower DMFT counts for all.

The population strategy for prevention has three key advantages (Table 28.2):

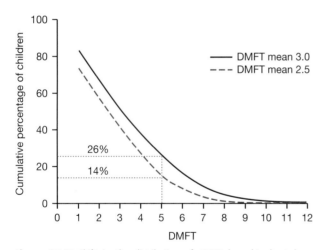

Figure 28.11 Shift in the distribution of DMFT brought about by a hypothetical population-based intervention that reduces the average DMFT from 3.0 to 2.5. The size of the high-risk group is diminished, no matter which DMFT threshold is used to define high risk.

Table 28.2 Advantages and disadvantages of the population strategy for prevention

Advantages	Disadvantages
Radical	Acceptability may be limited
Powerful	Not always feasible
Appropriate	Costs paid now; benefits come later

- *It is a radical approach,* because it confronts the determinants of disease at their roots, by tackling the social, economic, environmental and political circumstances that cause the biological disease determinants, i.e. the dental plaque bacteria and fermentable carbohydrates.
- *It is a potentially very powerful approach.* This is illustrated in Fig. 28.12, showing the effect of an achievable drop in the population distribution of the frequency of between-meal snacking from an average of seven to six between-meal snacks per week. Using the relationship between between-meal snacking and risk of caries lesion development in the next 3 months shown in Fig. 28.12, it

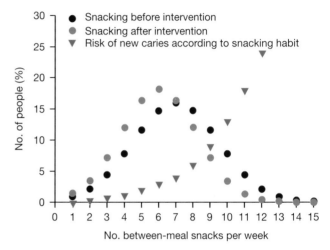

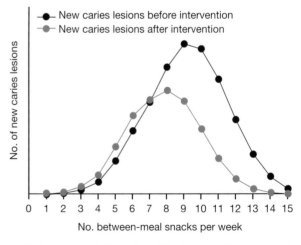

Figure 28.12 Upper panel: distribution of the frequency of between-meal snacking (per week) before and after a hypothetical intervention that reduces the average number of snackings per week from 7 to 6 (i.e. by 14%). Also given is the risk of new caries lesions according to snacking frequency. Lower panel: multiplication of the risk of caries for a given snacking level by the number of people who have that snacking habit results in two distributions of new caries lesions: one for the situation before the hypothetical intervention, and one for the situation after the intervention. The area under the curves represents the total number of new caries lesions that have developed. It can be shown that the area after intervention is 36% lower than the area before intervention, i.e. a 36% decrease in the number of new lesions.

may be calculated that the 14% decrease in between-meal snacking will result in a 36% decrease in the total number of new caries lesions that will develop within the next 3 months. Moreover, going back to the roots of disease has the advantage of potentially affecting a number of chronic diseases other than caries. Reducing between-meal snacking may not only prevent caries lesions developing, but also affect obesity. It is beyond doubt that population interventions aiming at changing people's dietary habits in a more healthy direction away from frequent intake of high-sugar, high-fat junk foods will not only affect dental caries, but also influence the much bigger cause of population ill-health: obesity, which predisposes to cardiovascular diseases, type II diabetes, some cancers, osteoarthritis and infertility. This is why the population strategy incorporates a common risk factor approach to prevention (Sheiham & Watt, 2000).

- *The population strategy for prevention is appropriate* because it acknowledges the social and contextual causes of disease (Holst *et al.*, 2001; Newton & Bower, 2005). In so doing it avoids the 'victim-blaming' (Chin *et al.*, 2000; Watt, 2007) that is inherent in the 'high-risk' strategy, where individuals in the tails of the risk distributions are specifically targeted as if they do not belong to the parent distribution. However, as Figs 28.9 and 28.12 clearly demonstrate, tails are intrinsic to distributions, and 'tail-cutting' exercises do not prevent the emergence of new cases, because the causes of the distribution have not been tackled and changed.

In view of these large advantages, why is it then so difficult to convince clinicians and policy makers about the population strategy for prevention (Rose, 1992)? There are major drawbacks (Table 28.2) to the population strategy:

- *Limited acceptability*: in general, knowledge does not cause those involved to act, unless the benefits of so doing are clearly visible, imminent and likely. People who eat 'cariogenic' diets will not stop this habit merely because they know about the possible consequences or are advised to do so. Faced with such advice they embark on trading-off of the personal gains against the losses associated with a change in dietary habits. Their values and perceptions are frequently different from those of the dentist. This touches on the problem of the preventive paradox (Rose, 1992): a preventive measure that may bring large benefits to the whole population may offer little benefit to each participating individual. The gains to be achieved for a person who reduces smoking from 10 to nine cigarettes per day are likely to be small compared with the benefits to society if smokers at large reduce smoking by this quantity. Moreover, health professionals, such as dentists, are usually dissuaded from embarking on general healthy-diet or antismoking campaigns because they perceive their success rate to be limited, and they lack the skills and

training to do so. Some reluctance to act at the political level with the aim of regulating behavior may also be noted, as there is much industrial lobbying against such action. Finally, the public may also resist such efforts, labeling them as part of the 'nanny state'.

- *Feasibility*: there are substantial political, economic and industrial barriers to the implementation of population preventive strategies. It is simply not in the interest of the confectionery industry to have campaigns running which aim at reducing the frequency of intake of cariogenic products in the population. Moreover, there is concern that the state may lose its revenue from sugar taxation, that confectionery industry employees may lose their jobs and that advertising agencies may experience reduced turnover, if such population strategies are implemented. It is no wonder, therefore, that many prefer to understand individual behaviors as based on conscious and fully informed choices reflecting individual values and preferences.

- *Costs now, benefits later*: it is a major barrier to the implementation of population-based preventive strategies that the costs of change, whether at the societal, industrial or individual level, must be paid now, whereas the benefits are deferred. However, the rapid and impressive caries declines that many populations have witnessed over the past few decades (see Chapter 8) testify to the responsiveness of caries to changes at the population level.

The directed population strategy

The directed population strategy combines the population and some elements of the high-risk preventive strategies in the sense that population-based methods are used to target sections of a population with a high proportion of high-risk subjects. Typically, they are populations living in geographically well-defined areas of a city (hence the alternative name of geographic targeting), known from other sources to harbor a large high-risk population (Burt, 2005). This strategy thus utilizes the aforementioned variation that exists within virtually all countries and was shown in Figs 28.8 and 28.9.

From a theoretical point of view, a well-conceived directed population strategy combines the advantages of the population strategy, i.e. it is radical, powerful and appropriate, with some of the advantages of the high-risk strategy, e.g. intervention only in groups at high risk and cost-effective use of resources. The directed population strategy does not screen individuals for risk. By targeting everybody in the area it also avoids the victim-blaming approach (Watt, 2007) inherent in the high-risk strategy. However, a major drawback is that the relatively higher cost-effectiveness of the approach may be obtained at the expense of introducing new inequities in access to health care (Tickle, 2002; Locker *et al.*, 2004). Those children with substantial dental health-care needs, who happen to reside in a location designated as 'low risk', are less likely to obtain the dental health-care benefits they really need. An additional problem lies in the fact that the geodemographic distribution of caries may undermine the practicality of the directed population strategy (Tickle *et al.*, 2003a), because the majority of the caries burden is not confined to just a small number of types of deprived areas.

A short history of caries-preventive strategies for populations

As described in detail in Chapter 18, the prominent role of fluoride in caries prevention originates with Dean's findings during the 1930s and early 1940s of an inverse relationship between the concentration of fluoride in the drinking waters and the prevalence of dental caries (Dean *et al.*, 1939, 1941, 1942). This observation very soon translated into public policies involving implementation of water fluoridation for caries-preventive purposes in some countries where fluoridation was technically possible (Chapter 18). As expected, large caries reductions were reported, typically ranging between 40 and 70% (Burt & Fejerskov, 1996). The percentage and actual reductions attributable to water fluoridation are much smaller now (McDonagh *et al.*, 2000a), partly because of the impact of fluoridated toothpaste, and partly because of the diminishing returns phenomenon. Water fluoridation has been of tremendous benefit as a population strategy for caries prevention in high-caries populations, e.g. most populations before the 1980s (Burt & Fejerskov, 1996). Indeed, the United States Centers for Disease Control and Prevention has listed water fluoridation among the top 10 public health achievements during the twentieth century (CDC, 1999).

This success led to the consideration of alternative means of providing fluoride exposure to populations at large. Such measures have included salt and milk fluoridation (Burt & Marthaler, 1996; Yeung *et al.*, 2005), and even sugar fluoridation (Mulyani & McIntyre, 2002). These means provide an illustration of the potential impact of engaging industry in producing more health-promoting products. Other fluoride programs aimed at populations at large include policies for the prescription of fluoride supplements (Hamasha *et al.*, 2005), typically in the form of tablets or drops, for children living in low-fluoride areas, and the implementation of fluoride rinsing programs (Marinho *et al.*, 2003a; Twetman *et al.*, 2004), typically delivered in school-based settings. Apart from the fluoride mouth-rinsing programs all the population strategies for caries prevention implemented from early on have involved the systemic intake of fluoride.

However, these population strategies for caries prevention using fluoride, many of which have been in widespread use since the 1950s, have increasingly been challenged (Disney *et al.*, 1990; Burt, 1999; McDonagh *et al.*, 2000b; Twetman *et al.*, 2004) on the grounds of an altered risk–benefit ratio. The general caries decline has resulted in a diminished effectiveness of these population prophylactic fluoride programs relative to earlier results (Hausen, 2004), while increasing concern has been voiced over the adverse effects of systemic fluoride ingestion, mainly dental fluorosis (Burt, 1999; McDonagh *et al.*, 2000b). This and the increasing awareness of the posteruptive cariostatic effect of fluoride have resulted in water fluoridation occasionally even being discontinued, without a resurgence of caries (Künzel & Fischer, 2000; Künzel *et al.*, 2000; Seppä *et al.*, 2000a, b 2002; Maupomé *et al.*, 2001). This is not so surprising because other substantial sources of fluorides exist, most notably fluoridated toothpastes (Twetman *et al.*, 2003; Marinho *et al.*, 2003b). Fluoridated toothpastes were first marketed in the USA in 1955 (Ellwood & Fejerskov, 2003) and they now dominate the toothpaste market in the high-income countries (Burt, 2002). While fluoridated toothpastes were not introduced in Denmark until 1964 (Helm & Helm, 1990), they nevertheless increased their market share to 80% in only 6 years (Helm & Helm, 1990). Today they account for more than 95% of all toothpaste sales in European countries (Arnadottir *et al.*, 2004). There is thus no doubt that fluoridated toothpastes are a crucially important vehicle for the delivery of the caries-preventive effects of fluoride to populations at large (Seppä, 2001).

Notwithstanding this trend towards more emphasis on the intraoral delivery of fluorides, a case may still be made for the use of water fluoridation in caries prevention (Burt, 2002; Tagliaferro *et al.*, 2004). For example, there are socioeconomic and behavioral aspects of caries prevention by means of fluoride supplements, topical fluorides and fluoridated toothpastes that may preclude socially and materially disadvantaged population groups from enjoying the benefits of intraoral delivery of fluorides. Poor and deprived people may simply not have the material and psychosocial resources necessary to buy toothbrushes and toothpastes and to access dental health care. It has thus been shown that the general trend for a caries decline is less marked among non-privileged children than among their more privileged counterparts (Van Nieuwenhuysen *et al.*, 2002), indicating an increased polarization of the caries occurrence attributable to social and material circumstances. As these groups are also commonly the groups that carry the more substantial part of the caries burden, water fluoridation may be a measure for reducing the social class disparities in dental caries (Burt, 2002; Tagliaferro *et al.*, 2004). It is a caries-preventive means for reducing socioeconomic disparities in caries occurrence (Riley *et al.*, 1999; Jones & Worthington, 1999, 2000), precisely because it is a classic population strategy.

Despite the logical and obvious advantages of using a population strategy, the high-risk strategies to caries prevention are recommended by a small number of cariologists and public health dentists because of the substantial decline in caries levels and the skewed distribution of caries in high-income nations (Burt, 1998). More children remain cavity free and the major proportion of the total caries burden is confined to a smaller proportion of children. This has led to the questioning of the cost-effectiveness of using population strategies for caries prevention (Burt, 1998). Instead, alternative approaches are suggested that specifically target those at high risk but, as outlined in this chapter and elsewhere, there are cogent arguments against using such approaches (Sheiham & Joffe, 1991; Hausen, 1997; Hausen et al., 2000; Batchelor & Sheiham, 2006).

High-risk approaches necessarily require methods to identify those subjects who are at high risk (Hausen, 1997; Burt, 2005). Even though the risk-prediction methods proposed are many and varied (Powell, 1998; Messer, 2000), it remains a fact that 'none of the reported measures for assessing caries risk was accurate enough to be relied on mechanically when targeting caries preventive measures' (Hausen, 1997). As discussed in Chapter 29, two additional requirements must be fulfilled for high-risk strategies: a sufficiently low occurrence of caries to justify the costs of screening for risk, and efficacious caries-preventive methods to offer to the high-risk subjects identified. As regards these requirements, there is good evidence that the high-risk strategy does not work in schoolchildren (Seppä et al., 1991; Hausen et al., 2000). There is some evidence that risk-based prevention involving basic prevention, sealants, chlorhexidine and fluoride varnishes at regular intervals may be effective (Pienihäkkinen et al., 2005), and under certain conditions also cost-reducing (Jokela & Pienihäkkinen, 2003), when instituted among very young (2–5-year-old) children. However, the results of a recent high-quality clinical trial of the caries reducing effect of a combination of oral hygiene, counseling, and non-invasive caries controlling measures given to children with active non-cavitated caries lesions has shown great promise (Hausen et al., 2007). This regimen proved able to reduce the DMFS increment among 11–12-year-old children by 44% over a 3½-year period.

In view of the difficulties it is perhaps not surprising that the cost-effectiveness of using a directed population strategy (geographic targeting) has received growing attention in recent years. The strategies evaluated for efficacy involve: supervised tooth brushing using fluoridated toothpaste among children attending schools in deprived areas (Curnow et al., 2002); fluoride varnishes given at different intervals to adolescents from socio-economically defined high-risk areas (Sköld et al., 2005); and provision of free fluoridated toothpaste and toothbrushes to children aged 1–5½ years residing in areas with different levels of material deprivation (Davies et al., 2003; Ellwood et al., 2004). While the results of the studies on the efficacy (Curnow et al., 2002; Ellwood et al., 2004; Sköld et al., 2005) and cost-effectiveness (Davies et al., 2003) appear promising, it remains to be elucidated how such strategies work when attempting to extend them to all high-risk areas in a country (Tickle et al., 2003a), and to what extent subjects with high preventive needs who happen to reside in low-risk areas are indeed precluded from enjoying the benefits of the caries-preventive programs (Tickle, 2002; Locker et al., 2004).

A wider perspective on prevention

Traditionally, the literature on prevention has used a distinction among primary, secondary and tertiary levels of prevention (Leavell & Clark, 1965). In this model, primary prevention encompasses activities undertaken to reduce the probability of disease occurrence (e.g. by vaccination campaigns). The term secondary prevention is used to describe activities that aim at early detection and treatment of disease (e.g. by means of screening for disease, such as the routine recall examination). Tertiary prevention covers activities that aim at preventing disease progression or recurrence. However, this model is entirely focussed on the expected outcomes of the preventive activities, and provides no guidance on the preventive strategies and the means and methods that may be employed. Prevention is therefore much better understood if an alternative scale of preventiveness is used, in which prevention is ranked in six levels (Table 28.3) that merge and overlap. This preventive model captures much better the causal chains that explain how environmental effects may shape or influence personal behaviors affecting the biological factors that promote the development and progression of diseases.

- *Prevention level 1*: the first level can be described as health promotional measures to make healthy choices the easy ones and unhealthy choices more difficult. Here, strategies seek to influence the material, social, economic and cultural circumstances that limit people's potential for behavioral change. The activities can be designed at several levels, including settings-based or structural levels. A settings-based approach, for example, would include activities at nurseries, schools, universities, workplaces and residential homes for older people (Anonymous, 1986). Structural approaches to prevention would include legislating against sugars in pediatric medicines, labeling of foods, regulations about school meals and advertising regulations. The overall objective is individual behavior change, but the point of attack shifts from the individual to the environments in which people live. The development of preventive programs that focus on settings or structural dimensions can influence the lives of more people and for longer periods than individually based interventions.
- *Prevention level 2*: the second level of prevention involves persuading people to change their behavior. This would include dissuading people from frequently ingesting so much refined sugar, and encouraging them to clean their teeth more effectively using fluoride toothpaste. Education and skill acquisition are key aspects, but it is well established that they often produce only limited or

Table 28.3 The six levels in preventive dentistry

Preventive level/target	Methods	Activities/actors
Preventive level 1: Environmental change	Economic change Social change Physical change	Health promotion Political system/the public
Preventive level 2: Behavioral change	Fluoride use Tooth cleaning Eating habits Use of dental services	Personal
Preventive level 3: Early diagnosis	Screening for early disease Dental check-ups Fluoride application Fissure sealing and simple restorations	Personal and clinical dental services
Preventive level 4: Preventive therapy	Oral hygiene Changing eating and drinking habits	Personal and clinical dental services
Preventive level 5: Rehabilitation therapy	Restorative treatment	Clinical dental services
Preventive level 6: Detection and prevention of impacts/disabilities/handicap	Restorative treatment of causes of sociodental impacts	Clinical dental services

temporary success regarding the desired behavioral changes (Kay & Locker, 1996). However, some evidence suggests that more success may be achieved by adopting a behavioral model that accommodates distinct stages of motivation for change, each of which may need different intervention approaches (Vallis *et al.*, 2003; Prochaska *et al.*, 2004).

- *Prevention level 3*: the third level is early or presymptomatic diagnosis of disease: screening for early signs of dental caries. Preventive visits to dentists or hygienists to see where there is disease – the dental check-up – is the most common preventive activity at this level. However, the evidence for the cost-effectiveness of such routine dental checks is equivocal (Davenport *et al.*, 2003a).
- *Prevention level 4*: the fourth level, closely related to the third, is preventive non-operative therapy. Here, efforts are made to arrest further lesion progression of early caries lesions by fluoride application combined with instruction on plaque control using fluoride toothpaste or use of fissure sealants and changing dietary habits. These preventive measures involve education. If the lesions have progressed beyond the point where arrest of further lesion development can be expected, operative procedures will be required.
- *Prevention level 5*: at the fifth level, preventive non-operative dentistry therefore merges with therapeutic or operative dentistry, because early treatment of the disease may alter the life history of the disease for the better.
- *Prevention level 6*: the sixth level is the detection and prevention of impacts, disability and handicap after disease has been halted. Replacement of missing teeth and treatment of discolored teeth are examples of prevention at this level.

Dental services are primarily preoccupied with activities characterizing the higher levels, e.g. levels 5 and 6 and levels 3 and 4. Levels 5 and 6 have a lower preventiveness rating and are predominantly palliative. The operative services rendered here do not prolong the survival of teeth significantly unless the dental disease rate of the individual has been changed. Even so, preventive levels 1 and 2 have been shown to be the main factors relating to the dramatic decline in caries in the past 30 years (Nadanovsky & Sheiham, 1995), and reductions in dental caries have been greatest in countries where general health has improved most (Nadanovsky & Sheiham, 1994, 1995).

Wanted: a population-based common risk factor approach to prevention

The discussion so far has essentially considered the pros and cons of different approaches to the prevention of a single disease, in this case dental caries. This focus on the prevention of single disease entities conforms to traditional dental thinking, which is largely concerned with responding to the dental needs of individuals, in particular their dental treatment needs. This organ-centered thinking is not unique to the oral cavity-focussed specialty named dentistry, but also pervades medicine with all its subspecialties, e.g. ear, nose and throat, dermatology, gastroenterology and hematology. However, the increasing realization that medical professionals need to address structural and contextual causes of diseases, rather than adhering to 'traditional' biological models for disease causation, implies that they need to adopt a different approach, and consider a whole range of diseases that have these causes in common.

When the traditional chairside preventive armamentarium, e.g. preventive check-ups, oral health education, oral hygiene instructions, dietary counseling, topical fluorides, and pit and fissure sealants (Marinho *et al.*, 2002a, b, 2003c, d; 2004b; Davenport *et al.*, 2003a, b; Källestål *et al.*, 2003; Lingström *et al.*, 2003; Mejàre *et al.*, 2003; Ahovuo-Saloranta *et al.*, 2004; Davies *et al.*, 2005; Beirne *et al.*, 2005), has been subjected to systematic reviews on their efficacy and cost-effectiveness, the results have all too often been disappointing. The reviews indicate that there is only very limited and usually poor-quality evidence for a beneficial effect of these methods. While absence of evidence cannot be taken to mean evidence of absence (Altman & Bland, 1995; Alderton, 2005), the time is ripe for acknowledging that interventions of demonstrated benefit should be of higher priority, and that it 'is no longer enough for us to faithfully believe that we are preventing disease, or promoting health, by suggesting that people reduce their sugar intake if there is no evidence that this is an effective activity' (Kay, 1998). The point made here is not to say that unlimited sugar intake would be acceptable, but to emphasize the urgent need for preventive measures for which there is evidence.

There are thus two important lessons to be learnt. Prevention must be applied using the common risk factor approach, just as a population-based approach to prevention must be emphasized. There is overwhelming evidence that the individualized approaches to behavioral changes, e.g. by dietary counseling or reinforcement of oral hygiene procedures in single patients in the dental office setting, are largely ineffective in bringing about permanent behavioral changes (Kay & Locker, 1996). That is why these behavioral changes are reinforced at regular intervals, often resulting in disappointment and frustration when the expected results do not come about (Kay, 1998). This limited effect is in stark contrast with the effects of institutional changes, e.g. by industry changing the composition of their products towards more health-sustaining components (fluoride in toothpastes, sugar-free confectionery, low-fat snacks, sugar-free soft drinks), or by government action (e.g. bans on smoking in public places, provision of free school meals, bans on the use of sugar in children's medicine, decreased consumption taxes on fruits and vegetables, restrictions on aggressive advertisements for unhealthy products). These changes have the potential to change norms and options permanently towards the healthier choices. When such changes have been widely implemented more resources will be available to devote to the smaller subgroups that continue to require intense and individualized prevention and treatment. It follows from this recommendation that the interventions needed must use multiple health-promotional approaches (e.g. education, social support, laws, incentives, behavior change) to change these determinants. Moreover, the interventions must take the long view of health outcomes, as changes often take many years to

become established. Finally, it is necessary that interventions involve a variety of sectors in a society that have not traditionally been associated with health-promotion efforts, including law, business, education, social services and the media (Anonymous, 1986). There is no doubt that population-based strategies are here to stay and proliferate. The exponential growth in the economic burden of the hitherto predominantly palliative approaches to population health problems will eventually force attention towards tackling the root causes of diseases, if we are to continue to cope with the cumulative effects of older populations presenting with many more preventable diseases.

Where does this leave the traditional dentist? Need for a new professionalism

Caries will probably continue to constitute a prevalent but not severe problem in most populations (see Chapter 8). The caries decline in children and young adults may represent a delay or slowing of caries development, rather than a permanent prevention of all future caries development, for the entire lifetime (Luan *et al.*, 2000; Hugoson *et al.*, 2000; Griffin *et al.*, 2005). Tooth extractions are no longer an acceptable solution to dental problems in many populations, and adult and elderly populations worldwide therefore retain increasingly more natural teeth (Kalsbeek *et al.*, 1998; Hugoson *et al.*, 2000, 2005; Fure, 2003; Petersen *et al.*, 2004) and experience reducing edentulism (Ahlqwist *et al.*, 1999; CDC, 2003; Hugoson *et al.*, 2005). Evidence also points to a decline in the propensity of dentists to carry out operative caries treatments in response to their clinical observations, indicating the use of more stringent criteria for operative treatment (Heidmann *et al.*, 1988; Gimmestad *et al.*, 2003). This would in itself contribute to a lower caries occurrence (Gimmestad *et al.*, 2003), partly by a reduction in the F component of the DMF index, and partly owing to the reduction in the D component resulting from the increased focus on non-operative treatment. The consequence of this development is a shift in the distribution of the caries burden, as illustrated for a Swedish population in Table 28.4. The table illustrates the marked change in the epidemiological characteristics of caries: the age at which people develop their (first) caries lesions is increasing, but people (at least in the high-income countries) live longer and retain many more teeth that may continue to be afflicted by caries (Schuller & Holst, 1998; Shay, 2004; Beltrán-Aguilar *et al.*, 2005). This results in an increasingly larger proportion of the total caries burden being found in the older sections of the population (Holst & Schuller, 2000; Beltrán-Aguilar *et al.*, 2005) (Table 28.4). Concomitant with these changes, changes are also seen in the distribution of caries across socioeconomic strata: the caries decline has resulted in an altered distribution of the total caries burden (Splieth *et al.*, 2004; Burt, 2005), such that the caries burden

Table 28.4 An example of the trends for change in caries, as observed in Sweden between 1973 and 2003: the total caries burden for ages 20–70 years declined (index 100 = 1973) to 98 in 1983, 95 in 1993 and 75 in 2003.

Age (years)		Examination year			
		1973	1983	1993	2003
20	Mean DFS[ab]	35.1	21.5	15.7	9.7
	% edentulous	–	–	–	–
	% of total caries burden in examination year[c]	16	10	8	5
30	Mean DFS[a]	48.4	40.7	23.3	14.0
	% edentulous	–	–	–	–
	% of total caries burden in examination year[c]	25	20	12	9
40	Mean DFS[a]	52.6	53.0	41.2	23.3
	% edentulous	1.0	–	–	–
	% of total caries burden in examination year[c]	18	28	21	16
50	Mean DFS[a]	50.5	53.6	55.2	34.9
	% edentulous	5.0	3.9	–	–
	% of total caries burden in examination year[c]	20	18	29	22
60	Mean DFS[a]	44.5	46.2	53.2	52.5
	% edentulous	20.0	14.3	9.8	3
	% of total caries burden in examination year[c]	14	16	16	32
70	Mean DFS[a]	41.0	39.1	52.4	51.0
	% edentulous	37.0	29.3	23	17
	% of total caries burden in examination year[c]	8	9	14	16

[a] In dentate people.

[b] Data for 1973, 1983 and 1993 from Hugoson et al. (2000); data for 2003: personal communication.

[c] Total burden for ages 20–70 years calculated by extrapolating finding to the actual Swedish population aged 20–70 years in each examination year, as reported in: http://www.scb.se/statistik/BE/BE0101/2005M05/Be0101Folkmangd1860-2004.xls

is increasingly polarized (Macek et al., 2004) towards less resourceful individuals from socially deprived areas or from lower socioeconomic population strata (Vargas et al., 1998; Jones & Worthington, 1999, 2000; Gillcrist et al., 2001; Mattila et al., 2005; Perinetti et al., 2005). A very strong argument for an intensified focus on caries prevention in populations is thus found in the problem of these health inequalities (Watt & Sheiham, 1999; Splieth et al., 2004; Brennan & Spencer, 2004), which traditional practice-based preventive dental services are not capable of reducing (Brennan et al., 2000; Ismail & Sohn, 2001; Tickle et al., 2002; Brennan & Spencer, 2005; Cabral et al., 2005), because people from lower socioeconomic strata may not go to the dentist until they are in pain. However, evidence suggests that the 'poor people–poor oral health' connection is less attributable to infrequent dental visiting and limited self-care than commonly thought (Sanders et al., 2006). This is precisely why tackling the social gradient in oral health also necessitates focus on the social environments in which health behaviors are developed and sustained.

Traditional dental thinking is largely concerned with responding to the needs of individuals, in particular their needs for treatment. This thinking has shaped dental ethics (responsibility for the dentally diseased person), the dental research questions (why do individuals get caries?) and the

organization of the dental health services (responding to individual demand). While this individual thinking has its roots in the history of dentistry and represents a long-standing tradition, it is increasingly at variance with scientific knowledge as well as the expectations of societies. It is thus gradually realized that traditional dental thinking does not lead to the eradication of a mass disease such as dental caries.

Dentistry is based on the implicit assumption that treatment of disease by dentists will achieve better oral health, and that resources will continue to be available to fund the dentists' efforts. However, in an era of evidence-based medicine and dentistry this assumption is no longer tenable. The major contribution to the reduction in caries falls outside conventional dental practice. This, and the relatively benign nature of caries (compared with many other threats to human health), makes it somewhat paradoxical that dental caries, unlike any other chronic human disease, requires 6- or 12-monthly surveillance and therapeutic interventions throughout life. Even though there is no evidence to support the necessity of routine 6-monthly check-ups for caries control (Davenport et al., 2003b), dental practitioners often continue to adhere to this regimen (Mettes et al., 2005), even for low-risk patients (Frame et al., 2000). The fact that caries persists as a public health problem despite such efforts from the dental health-care system strongly suggests that current approaches to caries prevention need to be reoriented. The population approach using a common risk factor approach is the orientation needed.

In addition to the traditional focus on symptomatic relief, society at large is increasingly expecting health-care systems (including the dental care systems) to engage in disease prevention, show solidarity with the weaker in society, acting against inequalities, and contributing to increasing the population's sense of security and quality of life and well-being (Holmstrup & Rossel, 2000; Benn, 2003). Dentistry has a long history of exercising paternalism and remains largely unregulated as to the appropriateness of the treatments provided (Friedman & Atchison, 1993; Hartshorne & Hasegawa, 2003), an approach that engenders public distrust (Ecenbarger, 1997). Society at large is therefore increasingly asking for accountability, transparency and sound professional standards (Cruess et al., 2000, 2002). In these respects the dental profession may have a long way to go.

The future of the traditional dentist is under scrutiny and criticism, owing to the increasing maintenance care caries burden (e.g. replacement of restorations, endodontic treatment) in the aging sections of many populations. Therefore, dentistry should engage in a new professionalism (Friedman & Atchison, 1993; Cruess et al., 2000, 2002; Holst et al., 2002). Even though traditional dental services may be necessary for some time, in the long run there will be a need for fewer and simpler procedures (Eklund, 1999), but of higher quality. Dentists will increasingly be expected to engage in advising patients about the risks to their dental or general health, and in the investigation and control of these risks. Dentists should continue to strive to influence the behavior of patients, and perform early diagnosis of incipient disease. The more crucial role of dentists in oral health promotion and caries prevention will be as health advocates. Health advocacy is the actions of health professionals and others with perceived expertise and authority in health issues to influence the decisions and actions of government, communities and individuals in a way that promotes health. Health advocacy involves a contribution to the education of the decision makers in government, communities and the media about health issues, as well as a contribution to the setting of political agendas aiming to improve the health of populations. Dentists must come out of their four-walled offices and use their new professionalism to engage in setting the public health agenda.

References

Ahlqwist M, Bengtsson C, Hakeberg M, Hägglin C. Dental status of women in a 24-year longitudinal and cross-sectional study. Results from a population of women in Göteborg. *Acta Odontol Scand* 1999; **57**: 162–7.

Ahovuo-Saloranta A, Hiiri A, Nordblad A, Worthington H, Mäkelä M. Pit and fissure sealants for preventing dental decay in the permanent teeth of children and adolescents [review]. *Cochrane Database of Systematic Reviews* 2004; Issue 3: Art. No: CD001830.pub2. DOI: 10.1002/14651858.CD001830.pub2.

Alderton P. Absence of evidence is not evidence of absence. *BMJ* 2005; **328**: 476–7.

Altman DG, Bland JM. Absence of evidence is not evidence of absence. *BMJ* 1995; **311**: 485.

Anonymous. Ottawa charter for health promotion. *Can J Publ Health* 1986; **77**: 425–30.

Anusavice KJ. Present and future approaches for the control of caries. *J Dent Educ* 2005; **69**: 538–54.

Arnadottir IB, Ketley CE, van Loveren C, et al. A European perspective on fluoride use in seven countries. *Community Dent Oral Epidemiol* 2004; **32** (Suppl 1): 69–73.

Batchelor P, Sheiham A. The limitations of a 'high-risk' approach for the prevention of dental caries. *Community Dent Oral Epidemiol* 2002; **30**: 302–12.

Batchelor P, Sheiham A. The distribution of burden of dental caries in schoolchildren: a critique of the high risk caries prevention strategy for populations. *BMC Oral Health* 2006; **6**: 3.

Beirne P, Forgie A, Clarkson JE, Worthington HV. Recall intervals for oral health in primary care patients [review]. *Cochrane Database of Systematic Reviews* 2005; Issue 2: Art. No.: CD004346.pub2. DOI: 10.1002/14651858.CD004346.pub2.

Beltrán-Aguilar ED, Barker LK, Canto MT, et al. Surveillance for dental caries, dental sealants, tooth retention, edentulism, and enamel fluorosis – United States 1988–1994 and 1999–2002. *MMWR Morb Mortal Wkly Rep* 2005; **54** (**no. SS-3**): 1–48.

Benn DK. Professional monopoly, social covenant, and access to oral health care in the United States. *J Dent Educ* 2003; **67**: 1080–90.

Brennan DS, Spencer AJ. Diagnostic and preventive service trends in private general practice: 1983–1984 to 1998–1999. *Aust Dent J* 2003a; **48**: 43–9.

Brennan DS, Spencer AJ. Provision of diagnostic and preventive services in general dental practice. *Community Dent Health* 2003b; **20**: 5–10.

Brennan DS, Spencer AJ. Changes in caries experience among Australian public dental patients between 1995/96 and 2001/02. *Aust N Z J Public Health* 2004; **28**: 542–8.

Brennan DS, Spencer AJ. The role of the dentist, practice and patient factors in the provision of dental services. *Community Dent Oral Epidemiol* 2005; **33**: 181–95.

Brennan D, Spencer AJ, Szuster F. Service provision trends between 1983–84 and 1993–94 in Australian private general practice. *Aust Dent J* 1998; **43**: 331–6.

Brennan DS, Spencer AJ, Szuster FSP. Service provision patterns by main diagnoses and characteristics of patients. *Community Dent Oral Epidemiol* 2000; **28**: 225–33.

Brunner E, Marmot M. Social organization, stress, and health. In: Marmot M, Wilkinson RG, eds. *Social determinants of health*. Oxford: Oxford University Press, 1999. 17–43.

Burt BA. Prevention policies in the light of the changed distribution of dental caries. *Acta Odontol Scand* 1998; **56**: 179–86.

Burt BA. The case for eliminating the use of dietary fluoride supplements for young children. *J Publ Health Dent* 1999; **59**: 269–74.

Burt BA. Fluoridation and social equity. *J Publ Health Dent* 2002; **62**: 195–200.

Burt BA. Concepts of risk in dental public health. *Community Dent Oral Epidemiol* 2005; **33**: 240–7.

Burt BA, Fejerskov O. Water fluoridation. In: Fejerskov O, Ekstrand J, Burt BA, eds. *Fluoride in dentistry*, 2nd edn. Copenhagen: Munksgaard, 1996: 275–90.

Burt BA, Marthaler TM. Fluoride tablets, salt fluoridation, and milk fluoridation. In: Fejerskov O, Ekstrand J, Burt BA, eds. *Fluoride in dentistry*, 2nd edn. Copenhagen: Munksgaard, 1996: 291–310.

Cabral ED, Caldas AF Jr, Cabral HAM. Influence of the patient's race on the dentist's decision to extract or retain a decayed tooth. *Community Dent Oral Epidemiol* 2005; **33**: 461–6.

Centers for Disease Control and Prevention (CDC). Ten great public health achievements – United States, 1900–1999. *MMWR Morb Mortal Wkly Rep* 1999; **48**: 241–3.

Centers for Disease Control and Prevention (CDC). Public health and aging: retention of natural teeth among older adults – United States 2002. *MMWR Morb Mortal Wkly Rep* 2003; **52**: 1226–9.

Chin NP, Monroe A, Fiscella K. Social determinants of (un)healthy behaviors. *Educ Health* 2000; **13**: 317–28.

Cleaton-Jones P, Fatti P. Dental caries trends in Africa. *Community Dent Oral Epidemiol* 1999; **27**: 316–20.

Cruess RL, Cruess SR, Johnston SE. Professionalism: an ideal to be sustained. *Lancet* 2000; **356**: 156–9.

Cruess SR, Johnston S, Cruess RL. Professionalism for medicine: opportunities and obligations. *Med J Aust* 2002; **177**: 208–11.

Curnow MMT, Pine CM, Burnside G, Nicholson JA, Chesters RK, Huntington E. A randomised controlled trial of the efficacy of supervised toothbrushing in high-caries-risk children. *Caries Res* 2002; **36**: 294–300.

Davenport C, Elley K, Salas C, *et al*. The clinical effectiveness and cost-effectiveness of routine dental checks: a systematic review and economic evaluation. *Health Technol Assess* 2003a; **7**(7).

Davenport CF, Elley KM, Fry-Smith A, Taylor-Weetman CL, Taylor RS. The effectiveness of routine dental checks: a systematic review of the evidence base. *Br Dent J* 2003b; **195**: 87–98.

Davies GM, Worthington HV, Ellwood RP, *et al*. An assessment of the cost effectiveness of a postal toothpaste programme to prevent caries among five-year-old children in the North West of England. *Community Dent Health* 2003; **20**: 207–10.

Davies MJ, Spencer AJ, Slade GD. Trends in dental caries experience of school children in Australia – 1977 to 1993. *Aust Dent J* 1997; **42**: 389–94.

Davies RM, Davies GM, Ellwood RP, Kay EJ. Prevention. Part 4: Toothbrushing: what advice should be given to patients? *Br Dent J* 2005; **195**: 135-41.

Dean HT, Jay P, Arnold FA Jr, McClure FJ, Elvove E. Domestic water and dental caries, including certain aspects of oral *L. acidophilus*. *Public Health Rep* 1939; **54**: 862–88.

Dean HT, Jay P, Arnold FA Jr, Elvove E. Domestic water and dental caries. II. A study of 2,832 white children aged 12–14 years, of eight suburban Chicago communities, including *L. acidophilus* studies of 1,761 children. *Public Health Rep* 1941; **56**: 761–92.

Dean HT, Arnold FA Jr, Elvove E. Domestic water and dental caries. V. Additional studies of the relation of fluoride domestic waters to dental caries experience in 4,425 white children aged 12–14 years of 13 cities in 4 states. *Public Health Rep* 1942; **57**: 1155–79.

Disney JA, Bohannan HM, Klein SP, Bell RM. A case study in contesting the conventional wisdom: school-based fluoride mouthrinse programs in the USA. *Community Dent Oral Epidemiol* 1990; **18**: 46–56.

Doméjean-Orliaguet S, Tubert-Jeannin S, Riordan PJ, Espelid I, Tveit AB. French dentists' restorative treatment decisions. *Oral Health Prev Dent* 2004; **2**: 125–31.

Downer MC. Time trends in caries experience of children in England and Wales. *Caries Res* 1992; **26**: 466–72.

Ecenbarger W. How honest are dentists? *Readers Digest* 1997; February: 50–6.

Eklund SA. Changing treatment patterns. *J Am Dent Assoc* 1999; **130**: 1707–12.

Eklund SA, Pittman JL, Heller KE. Professionally applied topical fluoride and restorative care in insured children. *J Public Health Dent* 2000; **60**: 33–8.

Ekstrand KR, Christiansen MEC, Qvist V. Influence of different variables on the inter-municipality variation in caries experience in Danish adolescents. *Caries Res* 2003; **37**: 130–41.

Elderton RJ, Eddie S. The changing pattern of treatment in the General Dental Service 1965–1981. Part 2 – Restorative treatment and implications for the future. *Br Dent J* 1983; **155**: 421–3.

Elderton RJ, Eddie S. Uptake of General Dental Service treatment in Great Britain 1965–1983 with special reference to radiography, prosthetics and the care of children. *Br Dent J* 1986; **161**: 93–8.

Ellwood R, Fejerskov O. Clinical use of fluoride. In: Fejerskov O, Kidd E, eds. *Dental caries: the disease and its clinical management*. Oxford: Blackwell Munksgaard, 2003: 189–222.

Ellwood RP, Davies GM, Worthington HV, Blinkhorn AS, Taylor GO, Davies RM. Relationship between area deprivation and the anticaries benefit of an oral health programme providing free fluoride toothpaste to young children. *Community Dent Oral Epidemiol* 2004; **32**: 159–65.

Eriksen HM. Has caries merely been postponed? *Acta Odontol Scand* 1998; **56**: 173–5.

Fejerskov O, Kidd EAM. Clinical cariology and operative dentistry in the twenty-first century. In: Fejerskov O, Kidd E, eds. *Dental caries. The disease and its clinical management*, 1st edn. Oxford: Blackwell Munksgaard, 2003: 3–6.

Fejerskov O, Manji F. Reactor paper: Risk assessment in dental caries. In: Bader JD, ed. *Risk assessment in dentistry*. Chapel Hill, NC: University of North Carolina Dental Ecology, 1990. 215–17.

Fejerskov O, Baelum V, Luan W-M, Manji F. Caries prevalence in Africa and the People's Republic of China. *Int Dent J* 1994; **44**: 425–33.

Frame PS, Sawai R, Bowen WH, Meyerowitz C. Preventive dentistry: practitioners' recommendations for low-risk patients compared with scientific evidence and practice guidelines. *Am J Prev Med* 2000; **18**: 159–62.

Friedman JW, Atchison KA. The standard of care: an ethical reponsibility of public health dentistry. *J Public Health Dent* 1993; **53**: 165–9.

Fure S. Ten-year incidence of tooth loss and dental caries in elderly Swedish individuals. *Caries Res* 2003; **37**: 462–9.

Gillcrist JA, Brumley DE, Blackford JU. Community socioeconomic status and children's dental health. *J Am Dent Assoc* 2001; **132**: 216–22.

Gimmestad AL, Holst D, Fylkenes K. Changes in restorative caries treatment in 15-year-olds in Oslo, Norway, 1979–1996. *Community Dent Oral Epidemiol* 2003; **31**: 246–51.

Grembowski D, Milgrom P. The influence of dentist supply on the relationship between fluoridation and restorative care among children. *Med Care* 1988; **26**: 907–17.

Grembowski D, Fiset L, Milgrom P, Conrad D, Spadafora A. Does fluoridation reduce the use of dental services among adults? *Med Care* 1997; **35**: 454–71.

Griffin SO, Griffin PM, Swann JL, Zlobin N. New coronal caries in older adults: implications for prevention. *J Dent Res* 2005; **84**: 715–20.

Grytten J. The effect of supplier inducement on Norwegian dental services; some empirical findings based on a theoretical model. *Community Dent Health* 1991; **8**: 221–31.

Hamasha AA, Levy SM, Broffitt B, Warren JJ. Patterns of dietary fluoride supplement use in children from birth to 96 months of age. *J Public Health Dent* 2005; **65**: 7–13.

Hartshorne J, Hasegawa TK. Overservicing in dental practice – ethical perspectives. *J S Afr Dent Assoc* 2003; **58**: 364–9.

Hausen H. Caries prediction – state of the art. *Community Dent Oral Epidemiol* 1997; **25**: 87–96.

Hausen H. How to improve the effectiveness of caries-preventive programs based on fluoride. *Caries Res* 2004; **38**: 263–7.

Hausen H, Kärkkäinen S, Seppä L. Application of the high-risk strategy to control dental caries. *Community Dent Oral Epidemiol* 2000; **28**: 26–34.

Hausen H, Seppä L, Poutanen R, Niinimaa A, Lahti S, Kärkkäinen S, Pietilä I. Noninvasive control of dental caries in children with active initial lesions. A randomized clinical trial. *Caries Res* 2007; **41**: 384–91.

Hawkins R, Locker D, Noble J, Kay EJ. Prevention. Part 7: Professionally applied topical fluorides for caries prevention. *Br Dent J* 2003; **195**: 313–17.

Heidmann J, Helm S, Helm T, Poulsen S. Changes in prevalence of approximal caries in 17-year-olds and related restorative treatment strategies over a 6-year period. *Community Dent Oral Epidemiol* 1988; **16**: 167–70.

Heller KE, Burt BA, Eklund SA. Sugared soda consumption and dental caries in the United States. *J Dent Res* 2001; **80**: 1949–53.

Helm S, Helm T. Caries among Danish schoolchildren in birth-cohorts 1950–78. *Community Dent Oral Epidemiol* 1990; **18**: 66–9.

Holmstrup P, Rossel P. Tandlægeetik i år 2000 – og fremover. *Odontologi 2000*. Copenhagen: Munksgaard, 2000: 23–38.

Holst D. Causes and prevention of dental caries: a perspective on cases and incidence. *Oral Health Prev Dent* 2005; **3**: 9–14.

Holst D, Schuller AA. Oral health changes in an adult Norwegian population: a cohort analytical approach. *Community Dent Oral Epidemiol* 2000; **28**: 102–11.

Holst D, Schuller AA, Aleksejuniene J, Eriksen HM. Caries in populations: a theoretical, causal approach. *Eur J Oral Sci* 2001; **109**: 143–8.

Holst D, Sheiham A, Petersen PE. Regulating entrepreneurial behaviour in oral health care services. In: Saltman RB, Busse R, Mossialos E, eds. *Regulating entrepreneurial behaviour in European health care systems*. Buckingham: Open University Press, 2002. 215–31.

Hudson P. Conservative treatment of the class I lesion. A new paradigm for dentistry. *J Am Dent Assoc* 2004; **135**: 760–4.

Hugoson A, Koch G, Slotte C, Bergendal T, Thorstensson B, Thorstensson H. Caries prevalence and distribution in 20–80-year-olds in Jönköping, Sweden, in 1973, 1983, and 1993. *Community Dent Oral Epidemiol* 2000; **28**: 90–6.

Hugoson A, Koch G, Göthberg C, *et al.* Oral health of individuals aged 3–80 years in Jönköping, Sweden during 30 years (1973-2003). II. Review of clinical and radiographic findings. *Swed Dent J* 2005; **29**: 139–55.

Ismail AI. Clinical diagnosis of precavitated carious lesions. *Community Dent Oral Epidemiol* 1997; **25**: 13–23.

Ismail AI, Sohn W. The impact of universal access to dental care on disparities in caries experience in children. *J Am Dent Assoc* 2001; **132**: 295–303.

Jarvinen S. Epidemiologic characteristics of dental caries: relation of DMFT and DMFS to proportion of children with DMF teeth. *Community Dent Oral Epidemiol* 1985; **13**: 235–7.

Jarvis MJ, Wardle J. Social patterning of individual health behaviours: the case of cigarette smoking. In: Marmot M, Wilkinson RG, eds. *Social determinants of health*. Oxford: Oxford University Press, 1999. 240–55.

Jokela J, Pienihäkkinen K. Economic evaluation of a risk-based caries prevention program in preschool children. *Acta Odontol Scand* 2003; **61**: 110–14.

Jones CM, Worthington H. The relationship between water fluoridation and socioeconomic deprivation on tooth decay in 5-year-old children. *Br Dent J* 1999; **186**: 397–400.

Jones CM, Worthington H. Water fluoridation, poverty and tooth decay in 12-year-old children. *J Dent* 2000; **28**: 389–93.

Källestål C, Wang NJ, Petersen PE, Arnadottir IB. Caries-preventive methods used for children and adolescents in Denmark, Iceland, Norway and Sweden. *Community Dent Oral Epidemiol* 1999; **27**: 144–51.

Källestål C, Norlund A, Söder B, *et al.* Economic evaluation of dental caries prevention: a systematic review. *Acta Odontol Scand* 2003; **61**: 341–6.

Kalsbeek H, Truin GJ, van Rossum GMJM, van Rijkom HM, Poorterman JHG, Verrips GH. Trends in caries prevalence in Dutch adults between 1983 and 1995. *Caries Res* 1998; **32**: 160–5.

Kay EJ. Caries prevention – based on evidence? Or an act of faith? *Br Dent J* 1998; **185**: 432–3.

Kay EJ, Locker D. Is dental health education effective? A systematic review of current evidence. *Community Dent Oral Epidemiol* 1996; **24**: 231–5.

Keyes PH. The infectious and transmissible nature of experimental dental caries. Findings and implications. *Arch Oral Biol* 1960; **1**: 304–20.

Kumanyika S, Jeffery RW, Morabia A, Ritenbaugh C, Antipatis VJ. Obesity prevention: the case for action. *Int J Obes* 2002; **26**: 425–36.

Künzel W, Fischer T. Caries prevalence after cessation of water fluoridation in La Salud, Cuba. *Caries Res* 2000; **34**: 20–5.

Künzel W, Fischer T, Lorenz R, Brühmann S. Decline of caries prevalence after the cessation of water fluoridation in the former East Germany. *Community Dent Oral Epidemiol* 2000; **28**: 382–9.

Leavell HR, Clark EG. *Preventive medicine for the doctor in his community; an epidemiologic approach*, 3rd edn. New York: McGraw-Hill, 1965.

Lingström P, Holm A-K, Mejare I, *et al.* Dietary factors in the prevention of dental caries: a systematic review. *Acta Odontol Scand* 2003; **61**: 331–40.

Locker D, Jokovic A, Kay EJ. Prevention. Part 8: The use of pit and fissure sealants in preventing caries in the permanent dentition of children. *Br Dent J* 2003; **195**: 375–8.

Locker D, Frosina C, Murray H, Wiebe D, Wiebe P. Identifying children with dental care needs: evaluation of a targetted school-based dental screening program. *J Public Health Dent* 2004; **64**: 63–70.

Luan W-M, Baelum V, Fejerskov O, Chen X. Ten-year incidence of dental caries in adult and elderly Chinese. *Caries Res* 2000; **34**: 205–13.

McDonagh M, Whiting P, Bradley M, *et al.* *A systematic review of public water fluoridation*. University of York: NHS Centre for Reviews and Dissemination, 2000a: 1–100.

McDonagh MS, Whiting PF, Wilson PM, *et al.* Systematic review of water fluoridation. *BMJ* 2000b; **321**: 855–9.

Macek MD, Heller KE, Selwitz RH, Manz MC. Is 75 percent of caries really found in 25 percent of the population? *J Public Health Dent* 2004; **64**: 20–5.

McMichael AJ. The health of persons, populations, and planets: epidemiology comes full circle. *Epidemiology* 1995; **6**: 633–6.

Marinho VCC, Higgins JPT, Logan S, Sheiham A. Fluoride gels for preventing dental caries in children and adolescents [review]. *Cochrane Database of Systematic Reviews* 2002a; Issue 1: Art. No.: CD002280. DOI: 10.1002/14651858.CD002280.

Marinho VCC, Higgins JPT, Logan S, Sheiham A. Fluoride varnishes for preventing dental caries in children and adolescents [review]. *Cochrane Database of Systematic Reviews* 2002b; Issue 1: Art. No.: CD002279. DOI: 10.1002/14651858.CD002279.

Marinho VCC, Higgins JPT, Logan S, Sheiham A. Fluoride mouthrinses for preventing dental caries in children and adolescents [review]. *Cochrane Database of Systematic Reviews* 2003a; Issue 3: Art. No.: CD002284. DOI: 10.1002/14651858.CD002284.

Marinho VCC, Higgins JPT, Logan S, Sheiham A. Fluoride toothpastes for preventing dental caries in children and adolescents [review]. *Cochrane Database of Systematic Reviews* 2003b; Issue 1: Art. No.: CD002278. DOI: 10.1002/14651858.CD002278.

Marinho VCC, Higgins JPT, Logan S, Sheiham A. Systematic review of controlled trials on the effectiveness of fluoride gels for the prevention of dental caries in children. *J Dent Educ* 2003c; **67**: 448–58.

Marinho VCC, Higgins JPT, Logan S, Sheiham A. Topical fluoride (toothpastes, mouthrinses, gels or varnishes) for preventing dental caries in children and adolescents [review]. *Cochrane Database of Systematic Reviews* 2003d; Issue 4: Art. No.: CD002782. DOI: 10.1002/14651858. CD002782.

Marinho VCC, Higgins JPT, Sheiham A, Logan S. Combinations of topical fluoride (toothpastes, mouthrinses, gels, varnishes) versus single topical fluoride for preventing dental caries in children and adolescents. *Cochrane Database of Systematic Reviews* 2004a; Issue 1: Art. No.: CD002781. DOI: 10.1002/14651858.CD002781.pub2.

Marinho VCC, Higgins JPT, Sheiham A, Logan S. One topical fluoride (toothpastes, or mouthrinses, or gels, or varnishes) versus another for preventing dental caries in children and adolescents. *Cochrane Database of Systematic Reviews* 2004b; Issue 1: Art. No.: CD002780. DOI: 10.1002/14651858.CD002780.pub2.

Marthaler TM, O'Mullane DM, Vrbic V. The prevalence of dental caries in Europe 1990–1995. *Caries Res* 1996; **30**: 237–55.

Mattila M-L, Rautava P, Aromaa M, *et al.* Behavioural and demographic factors during early childhood and poor dental health at 10 years of age. *Caries Res* 2005; **39**: 85–91.

Maupomé G, Clark DC, Levy SM, Berkowitz J. Patterns of dental caries following the cessation of water fluoridation. *Community Dent Oral Epidemiol* 2001; **29**: 37–47.

Mejàre I, Lingström P, Petersson LG, *et al.* Caries-preventive effect of fissure sealants: a systematic review. *Acta Odontol Scand* 2003; **61**: 321–30.

Messer LB. Assessing caries risk in children. *Aust Dent J* 2000; **45**: 10–16.

Mettes TG, Bruers JJM, van der Sanden WJM, *et al.* Routine oral examinations: differences in characteristics of Dutch general dental practitioners related to type of recall interval. *Community Dent Oral Epidemiol* 2005; **33**: 219–26.

Mulyani D, McIntyre J. Caries inhibitory effect of fluoridated sugar in a trial in Indonesia. *Aust Dent J* 2002; **47**: 314–20.

Nadanovsky P, Sheiham A. The relative contribution of dental services to the changes and geographical variations in caries status of 5- and 12-year-old children in England and Wales in the 1980s. *Community Dent Health* 1994; **11**: 215–23.

Nadanovsky P, Sheiham A. Relative contribution of dental services to the changes in caries levels of 12-year-olds children in 18 industrialized countries in the 1970s and early 1980s. *Community Dent Oral Epidemiol* 1995; **23**: 331–9.

Newton JT, Bower EJ. The social determinants of oral health: new approaches to conceptualizing and researching complex causal networks. *Community Dent Oral Epidemiol* 2005; **33**: 25–34.

Pearce N. Traditional epidemiology, modern epidemiology, and public health. *Am J Public Health* 1996; **86**: 678–83.

Perinetti G, Caputi S, Varvara G. Risk/prevention indicators for the prevalence of dental caries in schoolchildren: results from the Italian OHSAR survey. *Caries Res* 2005; **39**: 9–19.

Petersen PE, Kjoller M, Christensen LB, Krustrup U. Changing dentate status of adults, use of dental health services, and achievement of national dental health goals in Denmark by the year 2000. *J Public Health Dent* 2004; **64**: 127–35.

Pienihäkkinen K, Jokela J, Alanen P. Risk-based early prevention in comparison with routine prevention of dental caries: a 7-year follow-up of a controlled clinical trial; clinical and economic aspects. *BMC Oral Health* 2005; **5**: 2.

Powell LV. Caries prediction: a review of the literature. *Community Dent Oral Epidemiol* 1998; **26**: 361–71.

Prochaska JO, Velicer WF, Prochaska JM, Johnson JL. Size, consistency, and stability of stage effects for smoking cessation. *Addict Behav* 2004; **29**: 207–13.

Riley JC, Lennon MA, Ellwood RP. The effect of water fluoridation and social inequalities on dental caries in 5-year-old children. *Int J Epidemiol* 1999; **28**: 300–5.

Rose G. Sick individuals and sick populations. *Int J Epidemiol* 1985; **14**: 32–8.

Rose G. *The strategy of preventive medicine*. Oxford: Oxford University Press, 1992: 1–138.

Sanders AE, Spencer AJ, Slade GD. Evaluating the role of dental behaviour in oral health inequalities. *Community Dent Oral Epidemiol* 2006; **34**: 71–9.

Schuller AA, Holst D. Changes in the oral health status of adults from Trøndelag, Norway, 1973–1983–1994. *Community Dent Oral Epidemiol* 1998; **26**: 201–8.

Seppä L. The future of preventive programs in countries with different systems of dental care. *Caries Res* 2001; **35**(Suppl 1): 26–9.

Seppä L. Fluoride varnishes in caries prevention. *Med Princ Pract* 2004; **13**: 307–11.

Seppä L, Hausen H, Pollanen L, Karkkainen S, Helasharju K. Effect of intensified caries prevention on approximal caries in adolescents with high caries risk. *Caries Res* 1991; **25**: 392–5.

Seppä L, Kärkkäinen S, Hausen H. Caries in the primary dentition, after discontinuation of water fluoridation, among children receiving comprehensive dental care. *Community Dent Oral Epidemiol* 2000a; **28**: 281–8.

Seppä L, Kärkkäinen S, Hausen H. Caries trends 1992–1998 in two low-fluoride Finnish towns formerly with and without fluoridation. *Caries Res* 2000b; **34**: 462-8.

Seppä L, Hausen H, Kärkkäinen S, Larmas M. Caries occurrence in a fluoridated and a nonfluoridated town in Finland: a retrospective study using longitudinal data from public health records. *Caries Res* 2002; **36**: 308–14.

Shay K. The evolving impact of aging America on dental practice. *J Contemp Dent Pract* 2004; **5**: 101–10.

Sheiham A. Impact of dental treatment on the incidence of dental caries in children and adults. *Community Dent Oral Epidemiol* 1997; **25**: 104–12.

Sheiham A, Joffe M. Public dental health strategies for identifying and controlling dental caries in high and low risk populations. In: Johnson NW, ed. *Risk markers for oral diseases*. Vol. 1, *Dental caries. Markers of high and low risk groups and individuals*. Cambridge: Cambridge University Press, 1991: 445–81.

Sheiham A, Watt RG. The common risk factor approach: a rational basis for promoting oral health. *Community Dent Oral Epidemiol* 2000; **28**: 399–406.

Sköld UM, Petersson LG, Lith A, Birhhed D. Effect of school-based fluoride varnish programmes on approximal caries in adolescents from different caries risk areas. *Caries Res* 2005; **39**: 273–9.

Splieth CH, Nourallah AW, König KG. Caries prevention programs for groups: out of fashion or up to date? *Clin Oral Invest* 2004; **8**: 6–10.

Tagliaferro EPS, Cypriano S, Sousa MLR, Wada RS. Caries experience among schoolchildren in relation to community fluoridation status and town size. *Acta Odontol Scand* 2004; **62**: 124–8.

Tickle M. The 80:20 phenomenon: help or hindrance to planning caries prevention programmes? *Community Dent Health* 2002; **19**: 39–42.

Tickle M, Milsom KM, Blinkhorn AS. Inequalities in the dental treatment provided to children: an example from the UK. *Community Dent Oral Epidemiol* 2002; **30**: 335–41.

Tickle M, Milsom KM, Jenner TM, Blinkhorn AS. The geodemographic distribution of caries experience in neighboring fluoridated and non-fluoridated populations. *J Public Health Dent* 2003a; **63**: 92–8.

Tickle M, Milsom KM, King D, Blinkhorn AS. The influences on preventive care provided to children who frequently attend the UK General Dental Service. *Br Dent J* 2003b; **194**: 329–32.

Truin GJ, König KG, Kalsbeek H. Trends in dental caries in The Netherlands. *Adv Dent Res* 1993; **7**: 15–18.

Twetman S, Axelsson S, Dahlgren H, *et al.* Caries-preventive effect of fluoride toothpaste: a systematic review. *Acta Odontol Scand* 2003; **61**: 347–55.

Twetman S, Petersson LG, Axelsson S, *et al.* Caries-preventive effect of sodium fluoride mouthrinses: a systematic review of controlled clinical trials. *Acta Odontol Scand* 2004; **62**: 223–30.

Vallis M, Ruggiero L, Greene G, *et al.* Stages of change for health eating in diabetes. *Diabetes Care* 2003; **26**: 1468–74.

Van Nieuwenhuysen JP, Carvalho JC, D'Hoore W. Caries reduction in Belgian 12-year-old children related to socioeconomic status. *Acta Odontol Scand* 2002; **60**: 123–8.

Vanobbergen J, Declerck D, Mwalili S, Martens L. The effectiveness of a 6-year oral health education programme for primary schoolchildren. *Community Dent Oral Epidemiol* 2004; **32**: 173–82.

Vargas CM, Crall JJ, Schneider DA. Sociodemographic distribution of pediatric dental caries: NHANES III, 1988–1994. *J Am Dent Assoc* 1998; **129**: 1229–38.

Wang NJ. Preventive dental care of children and adolescents in the 1990s: Denmark, Iceland, Norway, and Sweden. *Acta Odontol Scand* 1998; **56**: 169–72.

Watt RG. Emerging theories into the social determinants of health: implications for oral health promotion. *Community Dent Oral Epidemiol* 2002; **30**: 241–7.

Watt RG. From victim blaming to upstream action: tackling the social determinants of oral health inequalities. *Community Dent Oral Epidemiol* 2007; **35**: 1–11.

Watt RG, Marinho VC. Does oral health promotion improve oral hygiene and gingival health? *Periodontol 2000* 2005; **37**: 35–47.

Watt R, Sheiham A. Inequalities in oral health: a review of the evidence and recommendations for action. *Br Dent J* 1999; **187**: 6–12.

Watt RG, McGlone P, Kay EJ. Prevention. Part 2: Dietary advice in the dental surgery. *Br Dent J* 2003; **195**: 27–31.

Watt RG, McGlone P, Evans D, *et al.* The prevalence and nature of recent self-reported changes in general dental practice in a sample of English general dental practitioners. *Br Dent J* 2004; **197**: 401–5.

Yeung CA, Hitchings JL, Macfarlane TV, Threlfall AG, Tickle M, Glenny AM. Fluoridated milk for preventing dental caries [review]. *Cochrane Database of Systematic Reviews* 2005; Issue 3: Art. No.: CD003876. DOI: 10.1002/14651858.CD003876.

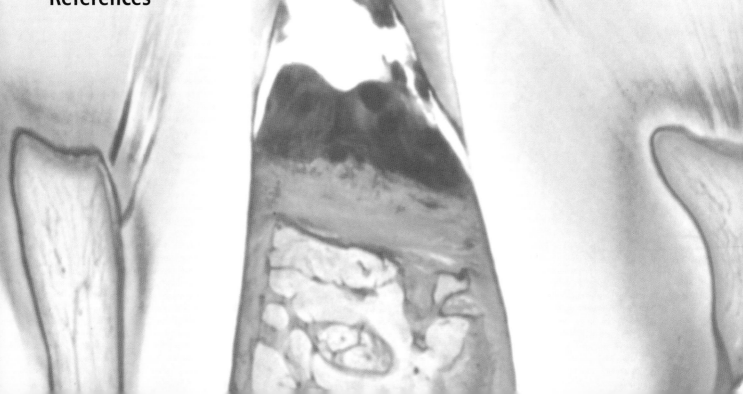

29

Caries prediction

H. Hausen

Introduction

The distribution of caries lesions is uneven among contemporary populations. Especially among children and adolescents in the industrialized countries, the majority often has little or no experience of cavitated caries and most of the cavities occur among a minority of the population. The shape of a typical current distribution of caries experience is shown in Fig. 29.1, in which the percentages of the 12-year-old residents of two Finnish towns, Jyväskylä and Kuopio, are presented according to the number of DMF (decayed, missing and filled) tooth surfaces. The polarization of the caries problem appears even more clearly in Fig. 29.2, where the cumulative percentage of DMF surfaces of the same individuals has been plotted against the cumulative percentage of children. It can be seen that the worst-off quarter of the children accounted for 70 and 80% of all DMF surfaces in Kuopio and Jyväskylä, respectively.

The dentists in the two towns would certainly have liked to detect in advance the individuals who now have ended up on the right-hand side of the caries distribution in Fig. 29.1 or the lower left-hand corner of the distribution in Fig. 29.2, and to have given them some individual protection so that they too could have joined the great majority with few or no cavities. This is the traditional and natural approach to prevention which Rose (1985) called the high-risk strategy. This approach is illustrated graphically in Fig. 29.3. If the high-risk susceptible individuals can be identified and offered effective individual protection, a truncation of the risk distribution will occur when the risk of the individuals on the right-hand side of the distribution is reduced to an acceptable level without affecting the risk of the remaining segment of the population.

There are three basic prerequisites for a successful application of the high-risk strategy to control dental caries. First, the occurrence of caries must be low enough to justify the

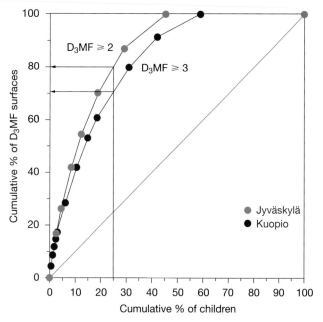

Figure 29.2 Cumulative percentage distribution of D_3MF surfaces in descending order plotted against the cumulative distribution of 12-year-olds in Kuopio and Jyväskylä in 1998. If all children had had the same number of DMF surfaces, the curves would have coincided with the diagonal.

effort and expense of identifying individuals who are believed to develop an unacceptably high number of cavities. Secondly, accurate, acceptable and feasible measures are needed for identifying the subjects with a high risk. Thirdly, effective and feasible preventive measures must be available for helping the high-risk individuals. In this chapter an attempt is made to address the second prerequisite: can we identify with sufficient accuracy the high caries risk-susceptible individuals who need individual protection to avoid having an unacceptably high number of new cavities?

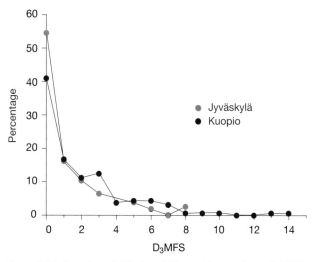

Figure 29.1 Percentage distribution of 12-year-olds according to D_3MFS in Kuopio (*n* = 161) and in Jyväskylä (*n* = 154) in 1998.

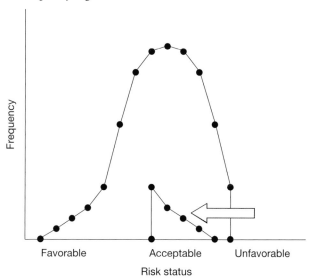

Figure 29.3 A graphical look at the high-risk strategy.

Clinicians assess risk, researchers predict

For the purposes of this chapter, caries risk is defined as the probability of an individual developing at least a certain number of caries lesions reaching a given stage of disease progression during a specified period. This is conditional on the exposure status remaining stable during the period at issue. So, in interpreting quantitative estimates of caries risk, a number of preconditions should be considered. Stating, for instance, 'this patient's caries risk is 30%' is highly uninformative. An informative statement could be: 'Given that no remarkable changes occur in the dental health behaviors and/or oral environment of this patient, there is a 30% probability that he will develop at least three new caries lesions reaching the dentin during the following 1-year period'.

When trying to identify the high-risk individuals, the clinical dentists are, at least implicitly, making conditional predictions such as, 'this patient will develop new cavities within the next 12 months unless something is done to prevent the lesions from developing'. Understandably, the dentist will be disappointed if this prediction comes true. To make these individual risk assessments clinicians need to know what happens to individuals with different levels of various risk factors with no individual protection offered to them. This information comes from prediction studies, in which predictions of the type 'this patient will develop at least one cavity within the next 12 months' are evaluated against the true course of events. Naturally, the researcher, who is trying to predict future caries development, and not to prevent it, will be disappointed if the prediction does not come true. Thus, the interests of the clinicians and researchers are different. The clinicians try to help their patients directly, while the researcher is trying to learn and develop measures that clinicians can use for taking care of their patients. This conflict of interest brings about a major problem with prediction studies: it is difficult, and ethically dubious, to keep the high-risk participants from receiving individual protection, but this may invalidate the results of a prediction study.

The course of a typical prediction study

In studies whose aim is to identify risk factors that compromise the population's health, the effect is typically expressed by using measures of association such as difference in mean values, correlation, risk difference, risk ratio or odds ratio. Significant associations have been found between caries experience and a number of factors, such as past caries experience, microbial counts and salivary parameters. However, even a fairly strong association does not necessarily imply that a factor could be used successfully for predicting future onset of caries lesions. The same holds for other diseases as well. For instance, the observed strong association between tobacco smoking and lung cancer justifies efforts to prevent lung cancer by means of reducing the exposure to tobacco smoke. Yet, information on smoking status cannot be used to predict the onset of lung cancer accurately, since the majority of smokers never contract the disease.

In prediction studies, the main question is how accurately the individuals studied can be classified into those having a high and those having a low risk. For evaluating the power of a potential predictor the same measures are used that are applied for assessing the accuracy of diagnostic tests, such as sensitivity and specificity. The predictors may be risk factors, i.e. factors for which a causal association with the outcome has been established, but they may also be risk markers or risk indicators, i.e. factors that are statistically associated with the outcome (here caries experience), but for which the relationship does not need to be a causal one.

Figure 29.4 shows the outline of a typical study for evaluating the predictive power of a risk marker of dental caries. At the beginning, the baseline caries status and the level of the selected predictor(s) are assessed. Caries recordings at the end of the follow-up period make it possible to assess the caries increment during the period. Prediction studies deal with two dichotomies: (i) the dichotomy between the individuals for whom we believe that the risk is high and the individuals for whom we consider a low risk, and (ii) for both groups, the dichotomy between the individuals for whom we observe a high true caries increment and the individuals among whom the observed true caries increment is low. Thus, group 'a' in Fig. 29.4 consists of correctly classified individuals, true positives, for whom it was believed that the risk is high and whose actual caries increment was high. Correspondingly, group 'd' represents correctly classified true negatives. For individuals falling into groups 'b' and 'c', a misclassification has occurred. For the false positives in group 'b', a high risk was assumed, but the true caries increment was low. Correspondingly, the false negatives in group 'c' were believed to have a low risk, but their actual caries increment was high.

The above design can be used for only one predictor at a time. In practice, several predictors are often considered in

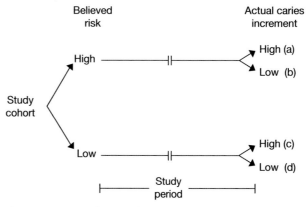

Figure 29.4 Outline of a typical follow-up study for evaluating the predictive power of a dichotomous marker of caries risk.

prediction studies. In the case of multiple predictors, each of them can be considered separately, which leads to predictor-specific numbers of true and false positives, and true and false negatives, respectively. Alternatively, the information on many predictors can be condensed into a single variable, on the level of which is based the prediction of high versus low risk. The techniques for this kind of condensing range from combinations of two variables, e.g. mutans streptococci count and lactobacilli count, to sophisticated regression-based multivariable models. Even single predictors are usually not natural dichotomies. For instance, salivary flow rate is a continuous variable and microbiological dip-slide tests can take several values. To be able to generate the four groups of interest, i.e. true and false positives and true and false negatives, the multiple-level predictors need to be artificially dichotomized. A threshold value is selected, above which the risk is considered high and below which the risk is believed to be low. The same is true for the outcome, i.e. true caries increment, which in the data collection is usually regarded as the number of new DMF teeth or surfaces, not as a high/low dichotomy. The dichotomization can be done using different threshold values. Each threshold level for believed high risk and for observed high true caries increment leads to a different distribution of the studied subjects among the four groups of interest (true and false positives, and true and false negatives). Thus, when evaluating the results of a prediction study it is important to take into consideration the threshold levels that have been used.

To estimate the accuracy of the classification (the four end groups in Fig. 29.4), the quantities a, b, c and d are organized in the form of a 2×2 table (Table 29.1), below which different measures of accuracy and their estimators have also been given. To obtain an idea about the accuracy of a prediction, it is not necessary to know the values of all of them. Since reports of caries prediction studies may include any of the measures in Table 29.1, however, brief definitions of each of them are given below.

Sensitivity and specificity

Sensitivity is the proportion of those who were believed to have a high risk among those whose actual caries increment during the follow-up was high. Specificity is the proportion of those who were believed to have a low risk among those whose actual caries increment was low. In Table 29.1, the above measures have been presented as proportions whose values range from 0 to 1. In the literature they are often expressed as percentages. Multiplying a proportion by 100 converts it to a percentage. It should be noted that the maximum sensitivity of 1 or 100% could easily be achieved by using a predictor with no predictive power at all, if the whole population will have a positive test result. This will, however, result in a specificity of 0. The situation will be reversed if all of the population will have a negative test result. Consequently, one should never look at the sensitiv-

Table 29.1 A 2×2 table for evaluating the accuracy of a dichotomous prediction and formulae for selected measures of accuracy

Believed risk	Actual caries increment		Total
	High	Low	
High	a	b	a + b
Low	c	d	c + d
	a + c	b + d	n

a: True positives (TP); b: false positives (FP); c: false negatives (FN); d: true negatives (TN).

Sensitivity (Se) = true-positive rate (TPR) = a/(a + c)
Specificity (Sp) = true-negative rate (TNR) = d/(b + d)

False-positive rate (FPR) = b/(b + d) = 1 − Sp
False-negative rate (FNR) = c/(a + c) = 1 − Sn

Positive predictive value (PV+) = a/(a + b)
Negative predictive value (PV−) = d/(c + d)

Crude hit rate = proportion of correctly classified (CHR) = (a + d)/n
Youden's index (J) = 1 − (FPR + FNR) = 1 − [(1 − Sp) + (1 − Se)]
Diagnostic odds ratio (DOR) = (a×d)/c×b)

Likelihood ratio+ (LR+) = Se/(1 − Sp)
Likelihood ratio− (LR−) = (1 − Se)/Sp

ity or specificity alone: both determine the power of a predictor. False-positive rate and false-negative rate carry exactly the same information as sensitivity and specificity, but they reveal proportions of misclassified subjects. False-positive rate is the proportion of those who were believed to have a high risk among those whose actual caries increment during the follow-up was low, and false-negative rate is the proportion of subjects who were believed to have a low risk among those whose actual caries increment was high. When using the percentage expressions, values of 1 in the formulae of Table 29.1 need to be replaced by 100.

Positive and negative predictive value

Positive predictive value is the proportion of those whose actual caries increment was high among those who were believed to have a high risk, and negative predictive value is the proportion of subjects whose actual caries increment was low among those for whom a low risk was predicted. The predictive value is not a property of the predictor alone. It is determined by the sensitivity and specificity of the predictor, but also by the occurrence of disease in the population being screened. Sensitivity and negative predictive value go together: given a constant occurrence of the disease, an increase in sensitivity brings about an increased negative predictive value, and vice versa. A similar association exists between specificity and positive predictive value. If the sensitivity and specificity remain the same, an increase in the occurrence of the disease (which may be achieved by applying the test to a high disease population) results in an increased positive predictive value and a decreased negative predictive value.

Crude hit rate, Youden's index and diagnostic odds ratio

Crude hit rate, Youden's index and the diagnostic odds ratio (Table 29.1) summarize the information regarding accuracy into a single numeric value. Crude hit rate or proportion of correctly classified subjects is easy to understand, and it has been used frequently in the dental literature. There are situations, however, in which this measure can give a heavily distorted impression of the accuracy of a classification. Therefore, it should never be relied on as the only measure in evaluating the predictive power of risk markers. For a look at the pitfalls related to this measure, see Weiss (1986). For those who prefer to look at a single numeric value only, Youden's index (J) is more advisable. If the prediction is invariably correct, i.e. the false-positive rate = 0 and at the same time the false-negative rate = 0, the index takes its maximum value J = 1. If a predictor has no predictive power, which is the case when the true-positive rate and the false-positive rate are equal, the index takes the value J = 0. Negative Youden's index values may be the consequence of misinterpretation of the test or due to chance if the sample is small. They should be interpreted as an indication of no predictive power. Diagnostic odds ratio (DOR) can take values between 0 and infinity. High DOR values indicate good predictive power. If DOR = 1, the predictor has no power at all. Values < 1 are equivalent to negative Youden's index values. Even though Youden's index and DOR are not likely to give a distorted picture of the predictive power of a test, they have the disadvantage of not carrying any information about the direction of the misclassifications. For a patient, however, the consequences of being a false positive are very different from those of being a false negative.

Likelihood ratio+ and likelihood ratio−

The remaining two measures, LR+ and LR−, can take any non-negative value. LR+ indicates how many times more likely a person who is believed to have a high risk, is to have a high caries increment than a low increment. LR− expresses the same ratio for a person who is believed to have a low risk. If the predictor does have some predictive power (TPR > FPR), the resulting value of LR+ is bigger and the value of LR− smaller than 1. These likelihood ratios have the valuable property that by using them one can calculate the post-test probability of having a high increment while taking into consideration the pretest probability.

Practical examples

Single dichotomous predictor

In the following, numerical examples are used to elucidate further the idea of assessing caries risk. As an example of the use of a single dichotomous predictor, data from a study by Alaluusua and Malmivirta (1994) are used, in which the presence of visible plaque on the labial surfaces of maxillary incisors at the age of 19 months was used as a marker of the risk of having signs of caries experience at the age of 36 months (Table 29.2). The risk was considered high if visible plaque was detected on the labial surfaces of all four incisors, and low otherwise. At the end of the follow-up, signs of caries were considered present if at least one lesion was found.

As can be seen from Table 29.2, 83% of subjects having caries at the end of the study were identified correctly (sensitivity), and among those for whom the risk was considered low, the assessment was correct for 92% (specificity). The percentages of false positives and negatives were 8 and 17, respectively. The observed positive predictive value reveals that 63% of the children for whom the risk was considered high actually developed caries during the follow-up. Correspondingly, 97% of the children who were regarded as having a low risk remained caries free until the end of the study (negative predictive value). The crude hit rate (91%) clearly gives a more optimistic picture of the performance of the predictor than does the Youden's index value (0.75), which is due to the fact that plaque and caries were detected in a minor proportion of the subjects (18 and 13%, respectively). The value of the DOR (60.83) is much bigger than the null value (1), indicating strong predictive power, but the actual performance of a predictor is perhaps easier to discern by looking at the Youden's index value, whose upper bound is 1. A child with visible plaque was 10.38 (LR+) and a child with no plaque 0.18 (LR−) times more likely to have than not to have caries at the end of the follow-up.

Table 29.2 Summary of the results of a study where visible plaque on the labial surfaces of maxillary incisors at the age of 19 months was used for predicting the onset of at least one caries lesion by the age of 36 months

Visible plaque at 19 months	Signs of caries at 36 months		Total
	Present	Absent	
Present	10[a]	6[b]	16
Absent	2[c]	73[d]	75
	12	79	91

Data from Alaluusua & Malmivirta (1994).
[a] TP; [b] FP; [c] FN; [d] TN.

Se = 10/12 = 0.83 = 83%
Sp = 73/79 = 0.92 = 92%

FPR = 6/79 = 0.08 = 8%
FNR = 2/12 = 0.17 = 17%

PV+ = 10/16 = 0.63 = 63%
PV− = 73/75 = 0.97 = 97%

CHR = 83/91 = 0.91 = 91%
J = 1− (0.08 + 0.17) = 0.75
DOR = (10×73)/(2 × 6) = 60.83

LR+ = 0.83/0.08 = 10.38
LR− = 0.17/0.92 = 0.18

Finally, the post-test probabilities of developing caries can be calculated for a child with and without visible plaque. For this purpose, a pretest probability is required. This is the average probability of a child who has not been tested developing caries within the period of interest. In everyday practice, a value obtained from the literature or a value based on personal clinical observations can be used. For the current example, let us use as the pretest probability the proportion of all children, irrespective of the presence of visible plaque, who developed at least one caries lesion ($12/91 = 0.13$, Table 29.2). As the next step, this quantity is converted to pretest odds using the formula odds $= p/(1 - p)$, where p stands for the probability. Thus, the pretest odds $= 0.13/(1-0.13) = 0.15$. Now the post-test odds can be calculated as a product of the pre-test odds and the likelihood ratios (LR+ and LR–). For a child with plaque, the post-test odds $= 0.15 \times 10.38 = 1.56$, and for a child without plaque $0.15 \times 0.18 = 0.03$. The post-test odds can be converted to a probability using the formula $p = $ odds$/($odds$ + 1)$. Thus, the post-test probability for a child with plaque developing caries is $1.56/(1.56 + 1) = 0.61 = 61\%$, and for a child with no plaque $0.03/(0.03 + 1) = 0.03 = 3\%$. One can skip the conversions between odds and probability values by using a handy nomogram that can be found as an annex of a related textbook (Sackett *et al.*, 2000). If the prediction is valuable, the post-test probability for a test-positive individual developing the problem of interest is clearly higher than the pretest probability, and the post-test probability for a test-negative individual is clearly lower. In this example, the resulting post-test probability for a child with plaque developing caries (61%) was much higher and the post-test probability for a child with no plaque (3%) was decisively lower than the pretest probability (13%). It may be concluded that among these toddlers the presence of visible plaque on the maxillary incisors was a fairly strong predictor of the subsequent occurrence of caries.

Several multiple-level predictors

The second example deals with several predictors. The subjects were initially 13-year-old children ($n = 384$) and they participated in a clinical trial comparing the effectiveness of an intensified and a basic prevention regimen among subjects who were believed to have a high risk for developing caries lesions (Hausen *et al.*, 2000). A low-risk comparison group (LRB) was also included. During the 3-year follow-up, the low-risk children received similar basic prevention that was given to the high-risk control group (HRB). By using data of these basic prevention groups it is possible to determine the power of different predictors for the risk of developing caries lesions without selective prevention interfering with the risk assessment. At baseline, the following salivary parameters were determined: salivary flow rate, mutans streptococci score, lactobacilli score and buffer capacity score (Dentocult SM Strip mutans®, Dentocult® LB,

Dentobuff® Strip; Orion Diagnostica, Helsinki, Finland). Teeth were examined clinically and radiographically. Caries lesions were graded as follows: D_{1i} = inactive lesion with no break in the continuity of enamel, D_{1a} = active lesion with no break in the continuity of enamel, D_2 = enamel lesion with loss of tooth substance, and D_3 = lesion with loss of tooth substance extending further than the enamel–dentin junction. In addition, the examiners estimated how many new fillings each child would need after 1 year if the level of prevention would remain as before. Risk of developing caries lesions was considered high if at least one of the following conditions was met:

- estimated number of new fillings needed after one year $\geqslant 2$
- salivary flow rate $\leqslant 0.7$ ml/min and buffer capacity score $= 1$
- two or more dentinal caries lesions
- one or more dentinal caries lesions on the approximal surfaces of incisors
- one dentinal caries lesion and lactobacilli score $\geqslant 3$ and mutans streptococci score $\geqslant 2$
- lactobacilli score $= 4$ and mutans streptococci score $= 3$.

Figure 29.5 shows the distribution of the believed high- and low-risk children (HRB and LRB, Hausen *et al.*, 2000) according to the number of new D_3MFS surfaces during the 3-year follow-up. On average, the high-risk individuals developed clearly more new D_3MF surfaces (5.1, SD 5.0) than did their low-risk counterparts (2.0, SD 2.4). The believed high-risk group included individuals who had no new lesions, however, and among the believed low-risk group there were subjects who developed up to 12 D_3MF

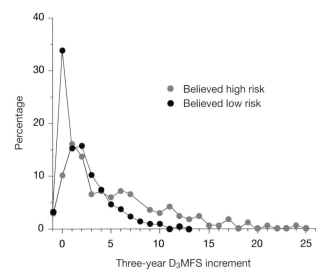

Figure 29.5 Percentage distribution by the number of new D_3MFS surfaces in a 3-year period among subjects for whom the risk of developing caries lesions was considered high and for whom it was considered low in a cohort of 384 initially 13-year-old children living in Vantaa. For the criteria of high and low risk, see text.

surfaces. So, at the individual level the risk assessment was far from being perfect.

The same data can be used to have a closer look at the performance of multiple-level predictors of future caries experience. The following predictors are used as educational examples: baseline DMFS score and salivary lactobacilli, mutans streptococci and buffer capacity score. Let us first consider baseline DMFS. The use of past caries experience as an indicator of future caries increment has been justly criticized by the argument that the aim should be to detect the high-risk susceptible individuals before there are any signs of past caries experience. The fact is, however, that past caries experience still remains the most powerful single predictor of future caries increment, and one could also argue that if some past caries experience were already visible, it would be a mistake not to use this information in assessing the risk of new cavities. The percentage distribution of the members of the study cohort according to the D_3MFS value at baseline is shown in Fig. 29.6. The shape of the distribution reveals that beyond perhaps the limit between no and at least one D_3MF surface there is no natural threshold, the level of which could be used for discriminating between subjects with a high and a low caries experience. To obtain an overall idea of the predictive power of D_3MFS, 10 different dichotomies were formed so that the selected threshold levels were distributed throughout the range of D_3MFS at baseline. The results appear in Table 29.3, where each row represents a 2 × 2 table like the one in Table 29.1. For the first row (Table 29.3), risk for new lesions was considered high if the baseline D_3MFS score was ⩾1 and low if D_3MFS score was = 0. Correspondingly, the last row represents a prediction where risk was considered high if the baseline D_3MFS value exceeded 13, and low if the value was 0–13. Throughout Table 29.3 the true 3-year D_3MFS increment

Table 29.3 Prediction of 3-year caries increment = 5 (n = 104) by baseline D_3MFS score in a cohort of 384 initially 13-year-old children living in Vantaa

Baseline D_3MFS score	TP	FP	FN	TN	Se (%)	Sp (%)	J	BHR (%)
⩾1	96	175	8	105	92	38	0.3	71
⩾2	86	130	18	150	83	54	0.4	56
⩾3	77	98	27	182	74	65	0.4	46
⩾4	66	74	38	206	63	74	0.4	36
⩾5	57	55	47	225	55	80	0.4	29
⩾6	46	41	58	239	44	85	0.3	23
⩾7	39	27	65	253	38	90	0.3	17
⩾8	33	22	71	258	32	92	0.3	14
⩾9	25	14	79	266	24	95	0.2	10
⩾14	10	1	94	279	10	100	0.1	3

TP: true positives; FP: false positives; FN: false negatives; TN: true negatives; Se: sensitivity; Sp: specificity; J: Youden's index; BHR: percentage of subjects believed to have a high risk.

was considered high if it was more than four surfaces (27% of the subjects), and low if it was 0–4 surfaces (73%). The last column (BHR) gives the percentage of subjects who were believed to have a high risk ('test-positives'). This is the percentage of subjects who should be treated as high-risk susceptible individuals if the given threshold level would actually be applied for picking up patients who need intensified individual protection against caries.

On the basis of the information in Table 29.3, how accurately can high future caries increment be predicted by using D_3MFS at the baseline as the predictor? The question is not easy to answer, since the distribution of the subjects, among the true positives, false positives, false negatives and true negatives, varies strongly among the different threshold levels of the predictor. The same is true for the percentage of subjects who are believed to have a high risk. From the practical point of view, it can be concluded that there is little sense in treating as high caries risk susceptible individuals a group of people whose size exceeds 40% of the target population. If the proportion of risk individuals in a population is close to half or more, this clearly implies that the occurrence of caries is not low enough to justify the effort and expense of identifying risk individuals. In such a situation the preventive efforts should rather be targeted to the whole population. This means that in the current cohort, threshold levels of baseline D_3MFS smaller than ⩾4 are unusable, irrespective of the accuracy of the classification. If the sensitivity value falls below 50% (which implies that the false-negative rate exceeds the true-positive rate), the predictor must not be relied on in picking up high-risk individuals. This leaves only two rows of Table 29.3 to look at (baseline DMFS ⩾4 and ⩾5), and it may be concluded that by aiming to pick up a manageable percentage of high-risk susceptible individuals (29–36%), applying baseline D_3MFS as a predictor of 5 or more D_3MF surfaces within a period of 3 years gives a sensitivity in the range of 55–63%,

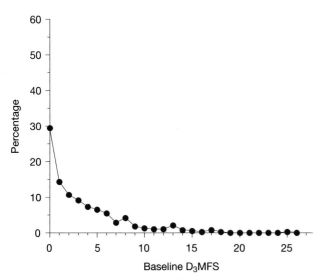

Figure 29.6 Percentage distribution of subjects according to D_3MFS scores at baseline in a cohort of 384 initially 13-year-old children living in Vantaa.

the corresponding specificity and Youden's index values being 85–80% and 0.4, respectively. This level of predictive power is consistent with the abundant literature. It must be noted, however, that a certain threshold level of D_3MFS results in different percentages of believed high-risk individuals in populations with different levels of caries occurrence.

For many people, diagrams are easier to interpret than tables with lots of figures. Receiver operating characteristic (ROC) curves are an alternative way of summarizing the predictive power of a multiple-level risk marker. In them, values of true-positive rate (sensitivity) at different levels of the predictor are plotted against the false-positive rate (1 – specificity, or 100 – specificity in the case of percentage values) at the respective levels. The curve for D_3MFS in Fig. 29.7 shows the results of Table 29.3 in such a form. The diagonal from the lower left-hand corner to the upper right-hand corner represents the curve for a risk marker with no predictive power (true-positive rate and false-positive rate are equal at all levels). The bigger the area under the curve, the more powerful the predictor. For a predictor that results in a perfect classification at all levels, the area covers the whole box. For a detailed introduction to the meaning of the area under an ROC curve, see Hanley and McNeil (1982). In the case of baseline D_3MFS (Fig. 29.7), the curve is clearly above the diagonal, which indicates that D_3MFS does have some predictive power. Adding D_{1a} and D_2 lesions to the baseline DMFS score increases its predictive power, as shown from the ROC curve for baseline $D_{1a23}MFS$ (Fig. 29.7). The fact

that the area above even this curve is fairly large reveals that the predictive power of past caries experience is far from being perfect. By looking at ROC curves one can quickly and easily obtain an overall picture of the performance of predictors. There is one major disadvantage, however: information about the percentages of individuals for whom high risk is suggested (BHR in Table 29.3) is not readily available from the curves.

The performance of the five-level salivary lactobacilli score has been summarized in Table 29.4, which is organized similarly to Table 29.3. From the point of view of a manageable percentage of believed high-risk individuals, only the last row (score = 4) is worth looking at. At this level, the sensitivity is so low that it would not make any sense to use lactobacilli score for identifying high caries risk susceptible individuals among a target population like the study cohort. The power of the remaining two predictors, i.e. salivary mutans streptococci and buffer capacity score, was even more modest. Therefore, the results regarding them are only given as ROC curves in Fig. 29.8, which also includes the curve for baseline $D_{1a23}MFS$ score for comparison. It can be concluded that among the four single predictors, the power of baseline $D_{1a23}MFS$ score was clearly highest. From the point of view of risk assessments in everyday practice, however, even its power must be considered modest.

Finally, an effort was made to find out whether combining the information of four predictors (Fig. 29.8), i.e. baseline $D_{1a23}MFS$ score and salivary lactobacilli, mutans streptococci and buffer capacity score, would lead to a more accurate prediction of 3-year D_3MFS increment than was achieved by regarding each of the predictors separately. For this purpose, a logistic regression model was constructed with all four predictors as independent variables. As the outcome, the logistic regression analysis produces for each individual a risk score whose values range from 0 to 1. By using these risk scores, the study cohort was divided into nine percentiles (Table 29.5). In risk percentile 10 (the first row of Table 29.5), the 90% of the study cohort with the highest scores were included in the predicted high-risk group, and the 10% with the lowest scores in the predicted low-risk group. In the last row, the situation is reversed.

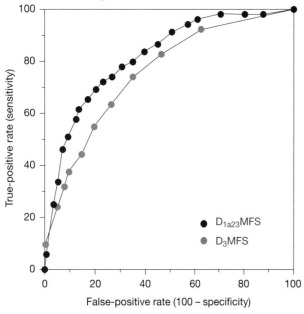

Figure 29.7 Receiver operating characteristic curves illustrating the relationship of the true- and false-positive rates at different threshold levels of baseline DMFS score. For D_3MFS, the figures are the same as in Table 29.3, where this score was used as a predictor of 3-year D_3MFS increment = 5.

Table 29.4 Prediction of 3-year caries increment = 5 ($n = 104$) by baseline lactobacilli (LB) score in a cohort of 384 initially 13-year-old children living in Vantaa

Baseline LB score	TP	FP	FN	TN	Se (%)	Sp (%)	J	BHR (%)
≥1	96	235	8	45	92	16	0.1	86
≥2	75	153	29	127	72	45	0.2	59
≥3	63	107	41	173	61	62	0.2	44
=4	27	47	77	233	26	83	0.1	19

For abbreviations, see Table 29.3.

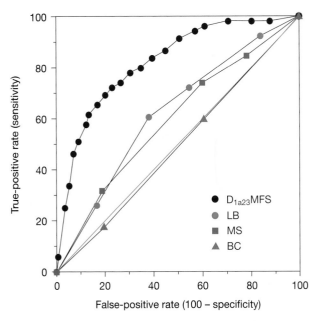

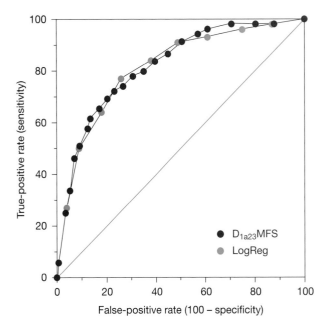

Figure 29.8 Receiver operating characteristic curves for baseline $D_{1a23}MFS$, salivary lactobacilli (LB), mutans streptococci (MS) and buffer capacity score (BC) in a cohort of 384 initially 13-year-old children living in Vantaa.

Figure 29.9 Receiver operating characteristic (ROC) curve for the logistic risk function (Table 29.5) including all four predictors (LogReg). The ROC curve for baseline $D_{1a23}MFS$ (Figs 29.7 and 29.8) has been repeated for comparison.

According to the latter threshold, the 10% of subjects with the highest scores were believed to have a high risk and the 90% with the lowest scores a low risk. As in the case of baseline D_3MFS (Table 29.3) the threshold levels were selected throughout the range of the risk scores to obtain an overall picture of the performance of the risk function. The predictive power of the risk function including all the four predictors was very similar to that of baseline $D_{1a23}MFS$ score alone. This can be seen clearly from Fig. 29.9, where the ROC curves of the logistic risk function and the baseline $D_{1a23}MFS$ score are presented together. It is apparent that

practically all the predictive power of the logistic regression function comes from the baseline $D_{1a23}MFS$ score. The remaining three predictors do not add anything to the accuracy of the prediction, even when regarded together.

So far, the evaluations of caries prediction have been based entirely on measures that are derived from the distribution of the study subjects among the true and false positives, and true and false negatives. This is consistent with the clinical decision problem: should the dentist treat the patient in front of him or her as a high caries susceptible risk individual or not? Keeping in mind the threshold for observed high caries increment, five or more lesions within 3 years, which was used throughout the latter example, one could argue that it is not a big issue to miss a few individuals whose true caries increment is just a little higher than the threshold level. Therefore, it is advisable to take a closer look at the severity of the misclassifications, especially among the false negatives. In Fig. 29.10, the percentage distribution of the study subjects according to the observed number of new D_3MF surfaces has been given separately for the subgroups whose baseline $D_{1a23}MFS$ score was 0–13, and >13. The latter group represents the individuals who would have been treated as high-risk susceptible individuals, if this particular threshold had been used for assessing high versus low risk for new cavities. As can be seen from Fig. 29.10, the false negatives that would erroneously have been treated as having low risk included individuals who developed up to 13 new D_3MF surfaces within 3 years. Errors are also likely to occur if the lack of signs of past caries is used for picking

Table 29.5 Prediction of 3-year caries increment = 5 ($n=104$) by a logistic risk function in a cohort of 384 initially 13-year-old children living in Vantaa

Risk percentile	TP	FP	FN	TN	Se (%)	Sp (%)	J	BHR (%)
10	102	244	2	36	98	13	0.1	90
20	100	210	4	70	96	25	0.2	81
30	97	172	7	108	93	39	0.3	70
40	95	136	9	144	91	51	0.4	60
50	87	106	17	174	84	62	0.5	50
60	80	74	24	206	77	74	0.5	40
70	67	50	37	230	64	82	0.5	30
80	52	25	52	255	50	91	0.4	20
90	28	11	76	269	27	96	0.2	10

Predictors included in the risk function: baseline DMFS, lactobacilli score (0–4), mutans streptococci score (0–3) and buffer capacity score (0–3). For abbreviations, see Table 29.3.

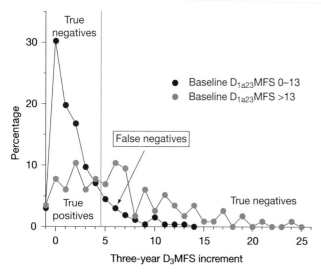

Figure 29.10 Percentage distribution of subjects according to 3-year D_3MFS increment among those whose baseline $D_{1a23}MFS$ score was 0–13 and = 14, respectively, in a cohort of 384 initially 13-year-old children living in Vantaa.

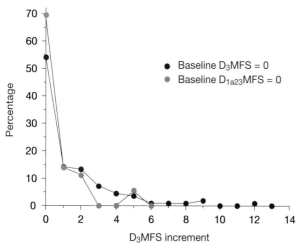

Figure 29.11 Percentage distribution of subjects with no baseline DMFS according to D_3MFS increment in a cohort of 384 initially 13-year-old children living in Vantaa.

up individuals with a low risk of developing new lesions. Figure 29.11 shows the percentage distribution of those individuals for whom baseline D_3MFS score was = 0 (29% of the cohort). Among them, the mean 3-year D_3MFS increment was 1.3 (SD 2.1), with the maximum value being 12. When $D_{1a23}MFS = 0$ was used as a screening criterion, the mean D_3MFS increment was 0.6 (SD 1.3) and the highest score was = 5 (Fig. 29.11). In the latter case, the error rate might have been tolerable. The small percentage of 'test positives' (9% of the cohort), however, calls into question the practical value of this screening criterion.

What level of accuracy would be sufficient in everyday practice?

A perfect predictor has a sensitivity of 100% and a specificity of 100%. Consequently, false-positive rate and false-negative rate take the value of 0%, positive predictive value = 100%, negative predictive value = 100% and Youden's index J = 1. A perfect accuracy means that the predicted high-risk group would consist of true high-risk individuals only and that only true low-risk individuals would be included in the predicted low-risk group. Unfortunately, no such predictor is available for the assessment of the risk of developing caries lesions. Errors must be accepted. However, there are no generally accepted rules as to what the acceptable error rate might be.

It has been suggested that in a risk model, the sum of sensitivity and specificity should be at least 160% before a caries risk marker can be considered a legitimate candidate for targeting individualized prevention (Kingman, 1990). This is in agreement with an alternative suggestion (Wilson & Ashley, 1989) according to which a sensitivity and specificity of 80% would be acceptable for practical use in the community. The corresponding Youden's index value is J = 0.6. Neither of these suggestions takes into account the fact that errors related to poor sensitivity have consequences that are different from those related to poor specificity. In other realms of medicine, such as prenatal diagnostics, utility gains and losses related to true and false positives and negatives are being used for evaluating the performance of tests and for setting their threshold values (for an example, see Felder & Robra, 2005). When waiting for corresponding developments in cariology we use the above suggestions (Wilson & Ashley, 1989; Kingman, 1990) as a benchmark in evaluating the performance of proposed markers for a high risk of developing caries lesions.

What would a combined sensitivity and specificity of 160% mean? If both the sensitivity and specificity were 80%, every fifth individual with a true high risk would remain undetected and thus would not receive the intensified protection against caries that he or she would have needed. Correspondingly, every fifth individual with a true low risk would erroneously be included in the high-risk group and receive preventive measures to no or little purpose. Thus, even the proposed level for an acceptable accuracy would result in a regrettably high rate of misclassifications.

What level of accuracy can be achieved?

Prediction of the onset of caries lesions has been a popular study subject. Even the number of related reviews is remarkable (Vanderas, 1986; Beck et al., 1988; Krasse, 1988; Seppä & Hausen, 1988a; Winter, 1988; Bader, 1990; Demers et al., 1990; Eriksen et al., 1991; Johnson, 1991; Stamm et al., 1991; Banting, 1993; van Houte, 1993; Moss & Zero, 1995; Tinanoff,

1995; Hausen, 1997; Kidd, 1998; Pitts, 1998; Powell, 1998a, b; Reich *et al.*, 1999; Messer, 2000). One major difficulty in reviewing the literature is that many study reports fail to provide full information on the distribution of subjects among the true and false positives and true and false negatives. In addition, they often fail to reveal the proportion of subjects who should be treated as high- and low-risk individuals if the proposed risk marker were to be used in everyday clinical practice.

In the following, excerpts from the vast literature will be highlighted to give an idea about the predictive power that can be achieved today. The possible usefulness of the predictors for purposes other than identifying high- and low-risk individuals will not be considered in this chapter.

Signs of past caries experience

Past caries experience summarizes the cumulative effect of all risk factors, known and unknown, to which an individual has been exposed. Therefore, it is not surprising that in studies comparing multiple predictors past caries experience has usually been the most powerful single predictor of future caries increment (Klock & Krasse, 1979; Honkala *et al.*, 1984; Wilson & Ashley, 1989; Alaluusua *et al.*, 1990; Russell *et al.*, 1991; Disney *et al.*, 1992; Alaluusua 1993; Mattiasson-Robertson & Twetman, 1993; Raitio *et al.*, 1996; van Palenstein Helderman *et al.*, 2001a). Exposure to risk factors and hence caries activity may vary over time, which reduces the predictive power of past caries experience. At a population level, however, there is a strong correlation between past caries experience and future caries increment (Demers *et al.*, 1990), which implies that a person who has had cavities is likely to develop them in the future. As a consequence, past caries experience is probably the most commonly used predictor for the risk of developing caries lesions. There are numerous reports about its predictive power in terms of sensitivity and specificity. The study by Alaluusua *et al.* (1990) is a typical example of a setting in which the past experience of cavitated caries has been used for prediction. In this study, the cut-off point for baseline DFS was selected so that 29% of the subjects were included in the predicted high-risk group. The observed sensitivity was 61% and specificity 82%. The proportions of false negatives and false positives were 39% and 18%, respectively. Results of prediction studies where site-specific past caries experience variables have been used instead of total DMFS scores have revealed that the condition of the most recently erupted or exposed tooth surface is the most appropriate measure of past caries experience (Powell, 1998b). Even for the most accurate risk functions using site-specific predictors (van Palenstein Helderman *et al.*, 2001b), however, the sum of sensitivity and specificity tends to remain below the benchmark of 160% (Kingman, 1990).

Active enamel caries lesions can be arrested so that a filling can be avoided. Therefore, early stages of caries lesions

would seem more attractive than advanced lesions or fillings as a measure of identifying high-risk individuals. According to some studies comparing the number of initial caries lesions and other caries scores, initial caries seems to correlate with subsequent caries increment more strongly than do FS or DS scores (Klock & Krasse, 1979; Seppä *et al.*, 1989). Sensitivity increased from 49 to 51% and specificity from 76 to 78% when initial caries score was added to FS and DS scores in a study (Seppä & Hausen, 1988b) where the participants were 11–13 years old at baseline and 5-year DMFS increment was used for validation. The proportion of test positives was 31% in both instances. Considering initial caries lesions, cavities and fillings (0 versus >0) resulted in a sensitivity of 62% and specificity of 82%, with the proportion of test positives being 44%, in another study where caries experience in the fissures of the permanent molars at the age of 7 years was used to predict the increment of DF surfaces (0 versus >0) between the ages of 7 and 11 years (van Palenstein Helderman *et al.*, 1989). When only cavities and fillings were used for prediction, sensitivity, specificity and proportion of test positives were 31%, 95% and 21%, respectively. These results are in line with those of the previous example (Fig. 29.7). It can be concluded that considering initial caries in addition to the more advanced lesions may increase the accuracy of prediction, but the improvement is not substantial.

Caries experience in the primary dentition has been used for the assessment of future caries in permanent dentition, with varying success (Poulsen & Holm, 1980; Alaluusua *et al.*, 1987; ter Pelkwijk *et al.*, 1990; Gray *et al.*, 1991; Raadal & Espelid, 1992; Vanobbergen *et al.*, 2001; Li & Wang, 2002). Despite major changes in the occurrence of caries during the past few decades, the predictive power of caries in the primary dentition has remained fairly stable (Helm & Helm, 1990). The value of dmft recorded at the age of 6 years seems to be a stronger predictor of caries increment between the ages of 7 and 13 years than is caries in permanent first molars (Seppä *et al.*, 1989). Relatively good results have been obtained by using information on the state of primary teeth and first molars in a statistical model (Helfenstein *et al.*, 1991; Steiner *et al.*, 1992; Imfeld *et al.*, 1995).

Most of the information about past caries experience as a predictor of risk has been obtained from studies conducted in children and adolescents. In adults and older people with a considerable proportion of the tooth surfaces filled, the DMF score might be a less powerful predictor for coronal caries than it is among young people. However, there is a well-documented association between the individual's past caries experience and the risk of developing root-surface caries (Vehkalahti, 1987; DePaola *et al.*, 1989; Locker *et al.*, 1989). Moreover, it has been shown in longitudinal studies that there is a positive correlation between baseline root-surface caries score and the individual's later root-surface caries experience (Ravald *et al.*, 1986; Leske & Ripa, 1989).

When considering the use of past caries experience in risk assessment, one must take into account the fact that an established high DMF score remains high independent of possible subsequent changes in caries risk. A person with a high DMF score may have little risk for further lesions if his or her oral conditions no longer favor demineralization. The opposite situation is also possible.

Microbiological tests

Use of microbiological tests is based on the principle that subjects carrying high numbers of cariogenic bacteria in saliva should be identified and treated before signs of clinical caries lesions develop. The assessment of microorganisms in saliva is based on the findings that there is an association between types and numbers of bacteria in dental plaque and those in saliva (Schaeken et al., 1987). Caution should be observed when interpreting the results of salivary microbiological tests, however, since the oral microflora is complex and the role of different bacteria in the caries process may not be fully understood (Beighton, 2005).

Salivary lactobacilli

The lactobacilli count of saliva is one of the oldest and most widely used tests of caries activity. Lactobacilli may not play a significant role in the initiation of a caries lesion, but a high level of lactobacilli in saliva is considered to be an indicator of high sugar consumption and thus also an indicator of an increased risk for developing cavities.

Salivary lactobacilli count has been found to correlate with the occurrence of caries. However, the use of the lactobacilli score as a screening test seems to be of limited value. Although repeated lactobacilli tests appeared to have a very good predictive power in the early study by Snyder (1942), in most later studies they have not proven as powerful in regard to the assessment of the risk for developing caries lesions (Crossner, 1981; Pienihäkkinen et al., 1987; Wilson & Ashley, 1989; Alaluusua et al., 1990; Ravald & Birkhed, 1991; Russell et al., 1991; Vehkalahti et al., 1996; van Palenstein Helderman et al., 2001a). Moreover, several studies suggest that in children and adolescents with today's low caries incidence the predictive power of microbiological tests has decreased further (Klock et al., 1989; Sullivan et al., 1989). A typical example is the study by Alaluusua et al. (1990), in which sensitivity was 55% and specificity 68% when 38% of the studied children were regarded as having a high caries risk on the basis of the level of lactobacilli in saliva. This is comparable to the predictive power of lactobacilli score in the previous example (Table 29.4, Fig. 29.8).

Salivary mutans streptococci

Numerous studies have shown an association between the number of caries lesions and the level of mutans streptococci in saliva or plaque in both children and adults (for reviews, see Beighton, 1991; Bratthall, 1991). The predictive power of the level of mutans streptococci in saliva, however, has consistently been modest (Söderholm & Birkhed, 1988; Sullivan & Schröder, 1989; Wilson & Ashley, 1989; Alaluusua et al., 1990; Ravald & Birkhed, 1991; Russell et al., 1991; Scheinin et al., 1992, 1994; Vehkalahti et al., 1996; van Palenstein Helderman et al., 2001a). The ROC curve in Fig. 29.8 gives a fairly good idea of the predictive potential of the salivary mutans streptococci test. At present, the test cannot be considered useful for the assessment of the risk of developing cavities. Preschool children, however, may be the exception. There is tentative evidence (Alaluusua & Renkonen, 1983; Köhler et al., 1988; Thibodeau & O'Sullivan, 1999; Seki et al., 2003; Pienihäkkinen et al., 2004) that the level of salivary mutans streptococci is a more accurate predictor of future caries among small children than it is in other age groups.

Mothers are the primary source of transmission of mutans streptococci to children, and infants with a high level of these bacteria are likely to have caries in primary molars (Köhler & Bratthall, 1978; Alaluusua & Renkonen, 1983). Prevention targeted to mothers with high salivary levels of mutans streptococci has resulted in a significant reduction in mutans streptococci and caries in their children (Köhler et al., 1983, 1984; Söderling et al., 2001). However, the usefulness of the level of salivary mutans streptococci in mothers for predicting the development of cavities in their children remains undetermined. In the study by Alaluusua and Malmivirta (1994), sensitivity was 54% and specificity 75% when an effort was made to identify 19-month-old high-risk individuals on the basis of mothers' salivary level of mutans streptococci, with the proportion of test-positives being 29%. The presence versus absence of caries at the age of 36 months was used for validation.

Salivary yeasts

The value of salivary yeasts in caries prediction has rarely been studied. Pienihäkkinen et al. (1987) evaluated the caries predictive value of salivary counts of lactobacilli and yeasts (Candida species) in 6–11-year-old children over a period of 3 years. The predictive power was in the same range as that of lactobacilli, which means that the level of salivary yeasts is a fairly weak predictor of future caries increment. The same was true when the level of yeasts in saliva was used to identify older adults with a high risk of root caries (Scheinin et al., 1994).

Other salivary factors

The role of saliva in caries development is well known. In the context of risk assessment, the two most commonly considered salivary factors are the flow rate and buffer capacity. Severe reduction in the flow rate of saliva is known to predispose teeth to caries attack (Ravald & Hamp, 1981; Powell et al., 1991). Thus, a patient whose salivation is compromised is in need of intensified protection against caries. Apart from true hyposalivation, however, the caries predictive power of salivary flow rate is modest. Buffer capacity has generally been thought to vary with caries activity. Although a negative correlation between buffering capacity of saliva and the occurrence of caries lesions has been found in some studies, the predictive power of buffer capacity is so low that it cannot be used for identifying high-risk individuals (Fig. 29.8). Other properties of saliva, such as pH, ammonia and protein concentrations, calcium and phosphorus concentrations and enzyme activity, seem to be of even less value for caries prediction (Pearce, 1991).

Dietary habits and oral hygiene

Although the relationship between sucrose and caries has been clearly established, the value of self-reported dietary habits for predicting the onset of caries lesions is unclear. Both a positive correlation and a lack of correlation between the intake of sucrose-containing foods and the occurrence of caries lesions have been reported. The vague correlations in industrialized countries may be due to the almost universal exposure to fluoride from different sources and the minor variation in the generally high sucrose intake in the studied groups. In addition, obtaining accurate information about dietary habits is difficult. Self-reported sucrose intake seems to have little value as a means of identifying high- and low-risk individuals.

A relationship between the presence of plaque and dental caries is also clearly established. It has been shown that professional plaque removal can result in a significant reduction in caries (Lindhe et al., 1975). However, the relationship between caries and the amount of plaque on teeth or the frequency of self-reported oral hygiene measures is vague (Bellini et al., 1981). Preschool children may be an exception, as shown in the study by Alaluusua and Malmivirta (1994), in which the presence of plaque on the labial surfaces of upper incisors at the age of 19 months was a powerful predictor of caries at the age of 36 months (Table 29.2). In another study among infants and toddlers (Wendt et al., 1994), however, the predictive power of oral hygiene was more modest.

High sucrose consumption and bad oral hygiene are often found in the same individual, and the effect of one of these two factors may vary with the degree of exposure to the other. In a study of 5–13-year-olds, the occurrence of caries lesions increased significantly with increasing sugar consumption only when oral hygiene was simultaneously poor (Kleemola-Kujala & Räsänen, 1982). In another study, 3-year-old children with clean teeth, irrespective of dietary habits, had a low caries experience (Schröder & Granath, 1983). Likewise, in adults and the elderly, only oral hygiene was associated with root caries experience, and was considered the only relevant predictor of risk of further lesion development (DePaola et al., 1989).

Social factors

There is no doubt that dietary and health habits are affected by income, education and social environment. It has been shown convincingly that in Western industrialized countries people whose socioeconomic status is low tend to have more caries lesions than do people with a high socioeconomic status (Hunt, 1990). In spite of the clear correlation between social status and caries, in the assessment of caries risk the reported sensitivities and specificities have been low (Hausen, 1997). It is helpful, however, to consider the social background of the patient as a natural part of the dental history when assessing his or her caries risk.

Joint predictive power of multiple predictors

The fact that the power of any single predictor has not been satisfactory has led to attempts to improve the accuracy of risk assessment by using screening criteria based on multiple factors. Combining the information of past caries experience and one microbial test makes a simple example of this approach. For instance, Alaluusua et al. (1990) formed a risk group using a high DFS score and high score of mutans streptococci. This resulted in a predicted high-risk group including 32% of the target population. The sensitivity was 71% and the specificity 81%. The observed accuracy was higher than that for DFS or mutans streptococci score alone, but even these figures cannot be considered satisfactory for targeting preventive measures.

When considering more than three predictors simultaneously, multivariable prediction models are generally used. The methods applicable in the assessment of caries risk include different regression techniques, discriminant analysis (Koch & Beck, 1990) and classification tree prediction models (Stewart & Stamm, 1991).

Perhaps the most extensive attempt to produce statistical models for the assessment of caries risk has been made by the Caries Risk Assessment Study of the University of North Carolina (Disney et al., 1992). With 25% of the target population in the predicted high-risk group, they aimed at a sensitivity of at least 75% and a specificity of 85%. The original data included 30 clinical, microbiological, sociodemographic and dental health behavioral factors. In the logistic regression model for the 5–6-year-olds, nearly 20 predictors were used. The sensitivity was 59%, the specificity 83–84% and the corresponding Youden's index value 0.42–0.43. With one exception, information based on clinical examinations provided the only statistically highly significant predictors, and the microbiological predictors contributed little to the power of the models.

The caries predictive power of recent multifactorial prediction models was reviewed by Powell (1998b). Among the 30 models for which sensitivity and specificity values were given, the average Youden's index value was 0.48 (SD 0.12). The corresponding sum of sensitivity and specificity is 148, which implies a simultaneous sensitivity and specificity of 74% if the false-negative rate and false-positive rate are equal. In general, the accuracy of multivariable approaches seems to be lower than what one would expect on the basis of the performance of individual predictors. The main part of the predictive power seems to originate from information related to past caries experience, with the status of the most recently exposed tooth surface being especially informative. The most powerful model, with a sensitivity of 87% and a specificity of 83% (Grindefjord *et al.*, 1995), dealt with the prediction of 2.5-year caries increment among initially 1-year-old children, which confirms the other findings that caries can be predicted more accurately in infancy than in older age groups. The fact that the importance of single predictors included in the models varied considerably according to the target population reveals that even the most sophisticated multifactorial models do not remove the inescapable uncertainty in the assessment of the risk of developing caries lesions.

How valuable are the proposed measures?

If one attempts to identify a manageable proportion of the individuals with the highest risk of developing cavities, the most powerful measures of risk assessment today result in sensitivities in the range of 70–80% and specificities of 80–90%. Even at this level of performance the rate of misclassifications, false negatives and false positives is too high. It can be concluded that the predictive power of even the best measures that are currently available is modest. In fact, none of the reported measures of assessing caries risk is accurate enough to be relied on mechanically when selecting patients for intensified caries prevention. Consequently, any screening program relying on methods that are available today fails to identify a considerable proportion of people with a true high risk, and/or suggests a high risk for an unacceptably high number of people with actual low risk.

The difficulty of predicting the onset of caries lesions is not unexpected. The multifactorial etiology of dental caries makes it likely that even the most sophisticated models using known risk factors and risk markers cannot predict future caries development very accurately. Moreover, even a perfect test is only capable of predicting a person's future caries experience if the conditions on which the prediction is based remain stable. In most industrialized countries, where virtually all the prediction studies have been conducted, the populations are exposed to a variety of professional prevention and treatment regimens as well as self-care which, if applied selectively, most probably reduce the observed power of such studies. Living conditions and oral health behavior may change over time, thus modifying a person's caries risk in either direction. For these reasons it is not likely that caries risk can be assessed accurately even

in the future. If accurate predictions were possible, that would imply that it is hard to affect an individual's established caries risk. This would be disappointing for all parties involved in the prevention of the development of caries lesions.

As no mechanical algorithms are applicable in deciding whether a person needs intensified caries prevention or not, a dental professional must make the decision for each individual. Clinical examination and proper dental history are the most important sources of information for the decision. In addition to the recorded information, the subjective judgment of an experienced clinician has been found to be important (Stewart & Stamm, 1991; Isokangas *et al.*, 1993; Alanen *et al.*, 1994). In the light of the current knowledge, the uncertainty related to the decision is not markedly reduced by information on additional factors, such as microbiological or salivary parameters. These factors may, however, be important for other purposes, e.g. for planning and implementing causal caries therapy for people with an established caries problem.

The purpose of this chapter has been to discuss whether sufficiently accurate measures for identifying the high caries risk susceptible individuals are available to justify the application of the high-risk strategy (Fig. 29.3) to control dental caries. The other basic requirements for the high-risk strategy that were mentioned at the beginning of the chapter were a low enough occurrence of dental caries to justify the effort and expense of identifying high-risk individuals, and the availability of effective measures to offer individual protection to them. At present, it may well be that none of these requirements is fully met. Despite the declining trends, dental caries still is a common disease. The experiences from the dental clinics reveal that the service system may be unable to offer proper individual protection to the most caries-prone individuals. There is even scientific evidence on the difficulty of reducing the risk of the high-risk individuals to an acceptable level (Seppä *et al.*, 1991; Hausen *et al.*, 2000; Källestål, 2005). Therefore, the prevention of the development of caries lesions should primarily be based on the whole population (Rose, 1985) or the targeted or directed population strategy (Watt, 2005). More reasons for caution with the high-risk strategy can be found in the classic paper by Rose (1985). Instead of being too concerned with predicting the future of their patients, clinical dentists should focus on giving due consideration to the control of caries lesions that their patients have at present. Appropriate treatment of progressing initial lesions, the precondition of which is proper self-care, also helps to prevent the onset of future cavities.

Background literature

Bader JD, ed. *Risk assessment in dentistry*. Chapel Hill, NC: University of North Carolina Dental Ecology, 1990.

Johnson NW, ed. *Risk markers for oral diseases*, Vol. 1, *Dental caries. Markers of high and low risk groups and individuals.* Cambridge: Cambridge University Press, 1991.

Stamm JW, Stewart PW, Bohannan HM, Disney JA, Graves RC, Abernathy JR. Risk assessment for oral diseases. *Adv Dent Res* 1991; **5**: 4–17.

References

Alaluusua S. Salivary counts of mutans streptococci and lactobacilli and past caries experience in caries prediction. *Caries Res* 1993; **27**: 68–71.

Alaluusua S, Malmivirta R. Early plaque accumulation – a sign for caries risk in young children. *Community Dent Oral Epidemiol* 1994; **22**: 273–6.

Alaluusua S, Renkonen O-V. *Streptococcus mutans* establishment and dental caries experience in children from 2 to 4 years old. *Scand J Dent Res* 1983; **91**: 453–7.

Alaluusua S, Kleemola-Kujala E, Nyström M, Evälahti M, Grönroos L. Caries in the primary teeth and salivary *Streptococcus mutans* and lactobacillus levels as indicators of caries in permanent teeth. *Pediatr Dent* 1987; **9**: 126–30.

Alaluusua S, Kleemola-Kujala E, Grönroos L, Evälahti M. Salivary caries-related tests as predictors of future caries increment in teenagers. A three-year longitudinal study. *Oral Microbiol Immunol* 1990; **5**: 77–81.

Alanen P, Hurskainen K, Isokangas P, et al. Clinicians' ability to identify caries risk subjects. *Community Dent Oral Epidemiol* 1994; **22**: 86–9.

Bader JD, ed. *Risk assessment in dentistry.* Chapel Hill, NC: University of North Carolina Dental Ecology, 1990.

Banting DW. Diagnosis and prediction of root caries. *Adv Dent Res* 1993; **7**: 80–6.

Beck JD, Kohout F, Hunt RJ. Identification of high caries risk adults: attitudes, social factors and diseases. *Int Dent J* 1988; **38**: 231–8.

Beighton D. The value of salivary bacterial counts in the prediction of caries activity. In: Johnson NW, ed. *Risk markers for oral diseases*, Vol. 1, *Dental caries. Markers of high and low risk groups and individuals.* Cambridge: Cambridge University Press, 1991: 313–26.

Beighton D. The complex oral microflora of high-risk individuals and groups and its role in the caries process. *Community Dent Oral Epidemiol* 2005; **33**: 248–55.

Bellini HT, Arneberg P, von der Fehr FR. Oral hygiene and caries. A review. *Acta Odontol Scand* 1981; **39**: 257–65.

Bratthall D. The global epidemiology of mutans streptococci. In: Johnson NW, ed. *Risk markers for oral diseases*, Vol. 1, *Dental caries. Markers of high and low risk groups and individuals.* Cambridge: Cambridge University Press, 1991: 287–312.

Crossner C-G. Salivary lactobacillus counts in the prediction of caries activity. *Community Dent Oral Epidemiol* 1981; **9**: 182–90.

Demers M, Brodeur J-M, Simard PL, Mouton C, Veilleux G, Frechette S. Caries predictors suitable for mass-screenings in children: a literature review. *Community Dent Health* 1990; **7**: 11–21.

DePaola PF, Soparkar PM, Tavares M, Kent RL. Clinical profiles of individuals with and without root surface caries. *Gerodontology* 1989; **8**: 9–15.

Disney JA, Graves RC, Stamm JW, Bohannan HM, Abernathy JR, Zack DD. The University of North Carolina Caries Risk Assessment study: further developments in caries risk prediction. *Community Dent Oral Epidemiol* 1992; **20**: 64–75.

Eriksen HM, Bjertness E. Concepts of health and disease and caries prediction: a literature review. *Scand J Dent Res* 1991; **99**: 476–83.

Felder S, Robra BP. A preference-based measure for test performance with an application to prenatal diagnostics. *Stat Med* 2005; **25**: 3696–706.

Gray MM, Marchment MD, Anderson RJ. The relationship between caries experience in the deciduous molars at 5 years and in first permanent molars of the same child at 7 years. *Community Dent Health* 1991; **8**: 3–7.

Grindefjord M, Dahllöf G, Nilsson B, Modéer T. Prediction of dental caries development in 1-year-old children. *Caries Res* 1995; **29**: 343–8.

Hanley JA, McNeil BJ. The meaning and use of the area under a receiver operating characteristic (ROC) curve. *Radiology* 1982; **143**: 29–36.

Hausen H. Caries prediction – state of the art. *Community Dent Oral Epidemiol* 1997; **25**: 87–96.

Hausen H, Kärkkäinen S, Seppä L. Application of the high-risk strategy to control dental caries. *Community Dent Oral Epidemiol* 2000; **28**: 26–34.

Helfenstein U, Steiner M, Marthaler TM. Caries prediction on the basis of past caries including precavity lesions. *Caries Res* 1991; **25**: 372–6.

Helm S, Helm T. Correlation between caries experience in primary and permanent dentition in birth-cohorts 1950–70. *Scand J Dent Res* 1990; **98**: 225–7.

Honkala E, Nyyssönen V, Kolmakow S, Lammi S. Factors predicting caries risk in children. *Scand J Dent Res* 1984; **92**: 134–40.

van Houte J. Microbiological predictors of caries risk. *Adv Dent Res* 1993; **7**: 87–96.

Hunt RJ. Behavioral and sociodemographic risk factors for caries. In: Bader JD, ed. *Risk assessment in dentistry.* Chapel Hill, NC: University of North Carolina Dental Ecology, 1990: 29–34.

Imfeld TN, Steiner M, Menghini GD, Marthaler TM. Prediction of future high caries increments for children in a school dental service and in private practice. *J Dent Educ* 1995; **59**: 941–4.

Isokangas P, Alanen P, Tiekso J. The clinician's ability to identify caries risk subjects without saliva tests – a pilot study. *Community Dent Oral Epidemiol* 1993; **21**: 8–10.

Johnson NW, ed. *Dental caries. Markers of high and low risk groups and individuals.* Cambridge: Cambridge University Press, 1991.

Källestål C. The effect of five years' implementation of caries-preventive methods in Swedish high-risk adolescents. *Caries Res* 2005; **39**: 20–6.

Kidd EA. Assessment of caries risk. *Dent Update* 1998; **25**: 385–90.

Kingman A. Statistical issues in risk models for caries. In: Bader JD, ed. *Risk assessment in dentistry.* Chapel Hill, NC: University of North Carolina Dental Ecology, 1990: 193–200.

Kleemola-Kujala E, Räsänen L. Relationship of oral hygiene and sugar consumption to risk of caries in children. *Community Dent Oral Epidemiol* 1982; **10**: 224–33.

Klock B, Krasse B. A comparison between different methods for prediction of caries activity. *Scand J Dent Res* 1979; **87**: 129–39.

Klock B, Emilson CG, Lind S-O, Gustavsdotter M, Olhede-Westerlund AM. Prediction of caries activity with today's low caries incidence. *Community Dent Oral Epidemiol* 1989; **17**: 285–8.

Koch GG, Beck JD. Statistical concepts: a matrix for identification of model types. In: Bader JD, ed. *Risk assessment in dentistry.* Chapel Hill, NC: University of North Carolina Dental Ecology, 1990: 174–92.

Köhler B, Bratthall D. Intrafamilial levels of *Streptococcus mutans* and some aspects of the bacterial transmission. *Scand J Dent Res* 1978; **86**: 35–42.

Köhler B, Bratthall D, Krasse B. Preventive measures in mothers influence the establishment of the bacterium *Streptococcus mutans* in their infants. *Arch Oral Biol* 1983; **28**: 225–31.

Köhler B, Andréen I, Jonsson B. The effect of caries-preventive measures in mothers on dental caries and the oral presence of the bacteria *Streptococcus mutans* and lactobacilli in their children. *Arch Oral Biol* 1984; **29**: 879–83.

Köhler B, Andréen I, Jonsson B. The earlier the colonization by mutans streptococci, the higher the caries prevalence at 4 years of age. *Oral Microbiol Immunol* 1988; **3**: 14–17.

Krasse B. Biological factors as indicators of future caries. *Int Dent J* 1988; **38**: 219–25.

Leske GS, Ripa LW. Three-year root caries increments: an analysis of teeth and surfaces at risk. *Gerodontology* 1989; **8**: 17–21.

Li Y, Wang W. Predicting caries in permanent teeth from caries in primary teeth: an eight-year cohort study. *Dent Res* 2002; **81**: 561–6.

Lindhe J, Axelsson P, Tollskog G. Effect of proper oral hygiene on gingivitis and dental caries in Swedish schoolchildren. *Community Dent Oral Epidemiol* 1975; **3**: 150–5.

Locker D, Slade GD, Leake JL. Prevalence of and factors associated with root decay in older adults in Canada. *J Dent Res* 1989; **68**: 768–72.

Mattiasson-Robertson A, Twetman S. Prediction of caries incidence in schoolchildren living in a high and a low fluoride area. *Community Dent Oral Epidemiol* 1993; **21**: 365–9.

Messer LB. Assessing caries risk in children. *Aust Dent J* 2000; **45**: 10–16.

Moss ME, Zero DT. An overview of caries risk assessment, and its potential utility. *J Dent Educ* 1995; **59**: 932–40.

van Palenstein Helderman WH, ter Pelkwijk L, van Dijk JWE. Caries in fissures of permanent first molars as a predictor for caries increment. *Community Dent Oral Epidemiol* 1989; **17**: 282–4.

van Palenstein Helderman WH, Mikx FH, van't Hof MA, Truin G, Kalsbeek H. The value of salivary bacterial counts as a supplement to past caries experienceas caries predictor in children. *Eur J Oral Sci* 2001a; **109**: 312–15.

van Palenstein Helderman WH, van't Hof MA, van Loveren C. Prognosis of caries increment with past caries experience variables. *Caries Res* 2001b; **35**: 186–92.

Pearce EIF. Salivary inorganic and physical factors in the aetiology of dental caries, and their role in prediction. In: Johnson NW, ed. *Risk markers for oral diseases*, Vol. 1, *Dental caries. Markers of high and low risk groups and individuals*. Cambridge: Cambridge University Press, 1991: 358–81.

ter Pelkwijk A, van Palenstein Helderman WH, van Dijk JWE. Caries experience in the deciduous dentition as predictor for caries in the permanent dentition. *Caries Res* 1990; **24**: 65–71.

Pienihäkkinen K, Scheinin A, Banoczy J. Screening of caries in children through salivary lactobacilli and yeasts. *Scand J Dent Res* 1987; **95**: 397–404.

Pienihäkkinen K, Jokela J, Alanen P. Assessment of caries risk in preschool children. *Caries Res* 2004; **38**: 156–62.

Pitts NB. Risk assessment and caries prediction. *J Dent Educ* 1998; **62**: 762–70.

Poulsen S, Holm A-K. The relation between dental caries in the primary and permanent dentition of the same individual. *J Public Health Dent* 1980; **40**: 17–25.

Powell LV. Caries risk assessment: relevance to the practitioner. *J Am Dent Assoc* 1998a; **129**: 349–53.

Powell LV. Caries prediction: a review of the literature. *Community Dent Oral Epidemiol* 1998b; **26**: 361–71.

Powell LV, Mancl LA, Senft GD. Exploration of prediction models for caries risk assessment of the geriatric population. *Community Dent Oral Epidemiol* 1991; **19**: 291–5.

Raadal M, Espelid I. Caries prevalence in primary teeth as a predictor of early fissure caries in permanent first molars. *Community Dent Oral Epidemiol* 1992; **20**: 30–4.

Raitio M, Pienihäkkinen K, Scheinin A. Assessment of single risk indicators in relation to caries increment in adolescents. *Acta Odontol Scand* 1996; **54**: 113–17.

Ravald N, Birkhed D. Factors associated with active and inactive root caries in patients with periodontal disease. *Caries Res* 1991; **25**: 377–84.

Ravald N, Hamp S-E. Prediction of root surface caries in patients treated for advanced periodontal disease. *J Clin Periodontol* 1981; **8**: 400–14.

Ravald N, Hamp S-E, Birkhed D. Long-term evaluation of root surface caries in periodontally treated patients. *J Clin Periodontol* 1986; **13**: 758–67.

Reich E, Lussi A, Newbrun E. Caries-risk assessment. *Int Dent J* 1999; **49**: 15–26.

Rose G. Sick individuals and sick populations. *Int J Epidemiol* 1985; **14**: 32–8.

Russell JI, MacFarlane TW, Aitchison TC, Stephen KW, Burchell CK. Prediction of caries increment in Scottish adolescents. *Community Dent Oral Epidemiol* 1991; **19**: 74–7.

Sackett DL, Strauss SE, Richardson WS, Rosenberg W, Haynes RB. *Evidence-based medicine. How to practice and teach EBM*, 2nd edn. New York: Churchill Livingstone, 2000.

Schaeken MJM, Creugers TJ, van der Hoeven JS. Relationship between dental plaque indices and bacteria in dental plaque and those in saliva. *J Dent Res* 1987; **66**: 1499–502.

Scheinin A, Pienihäkkinen K, Tiekso J, Holmberg S. Multifactorial modeling for root caries prediction. *Community Dent Oral Epidemiol* 1992; **20**: 35–7.

Scheinin A, Pienihäkkinen K, Tiekso J, Holmberg S, Fukuda M, Suzuki A. Multifactorial modeling for root caries prediction: 3-year follow-up results. *Community Dent Oral Epidemiol* 1994; **22**: 126–9.

Schröder U, Granath L. Dietary habits and oral hygiene as predictors of caries in 3-year-old children. *Community Dent Oral Epidemiol* 1983; **11**: 308–11.

Seki M, Karakama F, Terajima T, *et al.* Evaluation of mutans streptococci in plaque and saliva: correlation with caries development in preschool children. *J Dent* 2003; **31**: 283–90.

Seppä L, Hausen H. Die Identifizierung von Kariesrisikopatienten. Eine Übersicht. *Oralprophylaxe* 1988a; **10**: 96–107.

Seppä L, Hausen H. Frequency of initial caries lesions as predictor of future caries increment in children. *Scand J Dent Res* 1988b; **96**: 9–13.

Seppä L, Hausen H, Pöllänen L, Helasharju K, Kärkkäinen S. Past caries recordings made in public dental clinics as predictors of caries prevalence in early adolescence. *Community Dent Oral Epidemiol* 1989; **17**: 277–81.

Seppä L, Hausen H, Pöllänen L, Kärkkäinen S, Helasharju K. Effect of intensified caries prevention on approximal caries in adolescents with high caries risk. *Caries Res* 1991; 25: 392–5.

Snyder ML. Correlation and comparison of laboratory findings with the clinical evidence of caries activity in a group of sixty-six children. *J Am Dent Assoc* 1942; **29**: 2001–11.

Söderholm G, Birkhed D. Caries predicting factors in adult patients participating in a dental health program. *Community Dent Oral Epidemiol* 1988; **16**: 374–7.

Söderling E, Isokangas P, Pienihäkkinen K, Tenovuo J, Alanen P. Influence of maternal xylitol consumption on mother-child transmission of mutans streptococci: 6-year follow-up. *Caries Res* 2001; **35**: 173–7.

Stamm JW, Stewart PW, Bohannan HM, Disney JA, Graves RC, Abernathy JR. Risk assessment for oral diseases. *Adv Dent Res* 1991; **5**: 4–17.

Steiner M, Helfenstein U, Marthaler TM. Dental predictors of high caries increment in children. *J Dent Res* 1992; **71**: 1926–33.

Stewart PW, Stamm JW. Classification tree prediction models for dental caries from clinical, microbiological, and interview data. *J Dent Res* 1991; **70**: 1239–51.

Sullivan Å, Schröder U. Systematic analysis of gingival state and salivary variables as predictors of caries from 5 to 7 years of age. *Scand J Dent Res* 1997; **97**: 25–32.

Sullivan Å, Granath L, Widenheim J. Correlation between child caries incidence and *S. mutans*/lactobacilli in saliva after correction for confounding factors. *Community Dent Oral Epidemiol* 1989; **17**: 240–4.

Thibodeau EA, O'Sullivan DM. Salivary mutans streptococci and caries development in the primary and mixed dentitions of children. *Community Dent Oral Epidemiol* 1999; **27**: 406–12.

Tinanoff N. Dental caries risk assessment and prevention. *Dent Clin North Am* 1995; **39**: 709–19.

Vanderas AP. Bacteriologic and nonbacteriologic criteria for identifying individuals at high risk of developing dental caries: a review. *J Public Health Dent* 1986; **46**: 106–13.

Vanobbergen J, Martens L, Lesaffre E, Bogaerts K, Declerck D. The value of a baseline caries risk assessment model in the primary dentition for the prediction of caries incidence in the permanent dentition. *Caries Res* 2001; **35**: 442–50.

Vehkalahti MM. Relationship between root caries and coronal decay. *J Dent Res* 1987; **66**: 1608–10.

Vehkalahti M, Nikula-Sarakorpi E, Paunio I. Evaluation of salivary tests and dental status in the prediction of caries increment in caries-susceptible teenagers. *Caries Res* 1996; **30**: 22–8.

Watt RG. Strategies and approaches in oral disease prevention and health promotion. *Bull World Health Organ* 2005; **83**: 711–18.

Weiss NS. *Clinical epidemiology: the study of the outcome of illness*. New York: Oxford University Press, 1986.

Wendt LK, Hallonsten AL, Koch G, Birkhed D. Oral hygiene in relation to caries development and immigrant status in infants and toddlers. *Scand J Dent Res* 1994; **102**: 269–73.

Wilson RF, Ashley FP. Identification of caries risk in schoolchildren: salivary buffering capacity and bacterial counts, sugar intake and caries experience as predictors of 2-year and 3-year caries increment. *Br Dent J* 1989; **167**: 99–102.

Winter GB. Prediction of high caries risk – diet, hygiene and medication. *Int Dent J* 1988; **38**: 227–30.

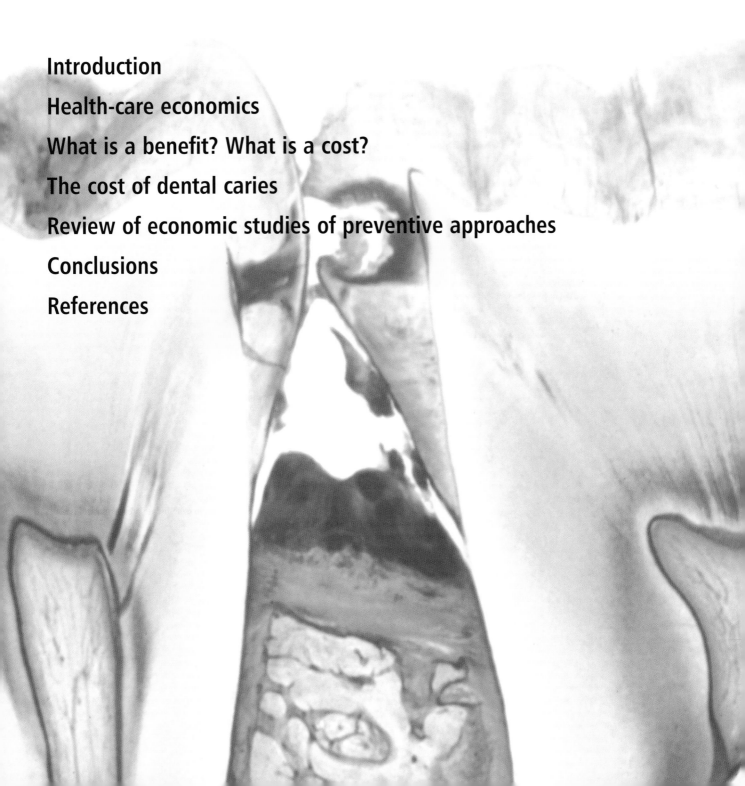

30

Preventing dental caries: what are the costs?

J. Feine, N. Jamal and S. Esfandiari

Introduction

In 2003, US$3.7 trillion was spent worldwide on health-care services (WHO, 2003a). In the USA alone, the total national general and oral health-care expenditures rose by 8% from 2003 to US$1.88 trillion in 2004 (Fig. 30.1). To put this amount into perspective, US citizens annually spend $6280 per capita on their health care, which works out to approximately $1 out of every $7 of the US final goods and services spent in the health-care industry. Over the past 40 years, as a proportion of the US gross domestic product, health-care spending increased from 5.2% in 1960 to 16.0% in 2003 (Centers for Medicare & Medicaid Services, 2006). These costs may in part be due to the fact that people are demanding more health services, visiting their physicians more frequently and utilizing new technologies (e.g. laser eye surgeries) to improve their health status. If this previous trend serves as a prediction of future health-care costs, the sustainability of providing quality health-care services in the USA is in question.

Health-care economics

The field of economics is concerned with the production, distribution and consumption of scarce goods and services in society. Economics does not provide a set of rigid guidelines that must be followed in the decision-making process, but rather, provides a set of principles that allow decisions to be based on the efficient allocation of resources. Considering the tremendous quantity of resources allocated to the health-care sector, the discipline of health-care economics was created to ensure that the maximum benefit can be derived from the resources available (Folland *et al.*, 2004).

The value of any health-care treatment is based primarily on its ability to improve the quality of life of the patient. However, the use of a given treatment cannot be considered without analyzing all of the financial and resource costs involved. Subsequently, economic assessment methods, such as cost-effectiveness analyses, are used to determine the efficient treatment action based on alternative treatments that meet a common objective (Drummond *et al.*, 1997). Considering that dental fees are most often incurred by the patient, economic comparisons among treatment options are of critical interest to patients and their oral health-care physicians. Economic assessments are also of value to third party payers such as dental insurance companies and to oral public health program managers, as these must decide which treatments should be supplied.

The demand for health-care services is rising in the face of resource limitations (Romanow, 2002). Thus, like any other good or service, there will never be a sufficient quantity of resources available to meet demand. This is the economic concept of scarcity, as these goods and services are in short supply and will always have a higher demand than what is available. Consequently, scarcity of financial, human and technological resources is the major cause of today's health problems. As a result, decisions must be made in the health-care sector for the allocation of the goods and services that will result in the maximum total benefit for the members in the community. This is the concept of economic efficiency (Drummond *et al.*, 1997).

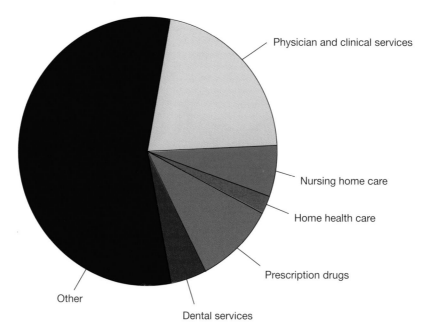

Figure 30.1 US national health expenditures in 2004. (Data obtained from the Centers for Medicare and Medicaid Services.) Total health expenditure in 2004: US$1.88 trillion; total oral health expenditure in 2004: US$81.5 billion.

What is a benefit? What is a cost?

The clear benefit of receiving oral health treatment is the improvement in the quality of life of the patient. The absence of pain or disability allows an individual to contribute fully to society's production of goods and services. The true cost of a resource (any amount of a good, service or time) is the benefit that would have been gained by its best alternative use. In economics, this is referred to as the opportunity cost of a resource. All goods, patient and clinician time, and clinician services involved in a treatment that have an alternative use have an opportunity cost that must be considered when making decisions about treatment options (Drummond *et al.*, 1997).

In health-cost analyses, it is critical to account for all resources required for a certain treatment. Ideally, the micro-costing method should be used to account for the enumeration and costs of resources used in a specific treatment. The microcosting approach can be applied to clinical policy analysis, because these systems provide detailed and accurate estimates of supplier and patient costs. This microcosting method accounts for all changes in resource use (e.g. labour and consumable supplies), other support services outside the health sector (e.g. voluntary services) and patient resources (e.g. prescription drugs and time lost from work for traveling, treatment and post-treatment care) (Fig. 30.2) (Gold *et al.*, 1996). Unfortunately, very few dental economic studies related to caries use the microcosting approach. These studies will be described in detail later in the chapter.

In the oral health system, the benefit gained from the prevention of dental caries is relative to the value one places on a healthy tooth. Unfortunately, many cost–benefit and cost-effectiveness studies often attach a financial value to a healthy tooth in terms of treatment costs averted. However, according to Mitchell and Murray (1989), it is 'virtually impossible' to place a financial sum on the benefit gained from a healthy unfilled tooth when comparing it to a healthy filled tooth, since future restoration and replacement needs are extremely difficult to measure.

The cost of dental caries

Restorative dentistry places a significant economic burden on industrialized countries, as 5–10% of public health spending is dedicated to oral health care. Oral diseases are the fourth most expensive disease to treat in industrialized nations (Petersen *et al.*, 2005). In the year 2000 alone, the European Union spent a total of €54 billion on oral health care (Widstrom & Eaton, 2004). In the USA, expenditure for oral health-care services, including the prevention and treatment of dental caries, reached an astounding $81.5 billion in 2004 (Fig. 30.1) (Centers for Medicare & Medicaid Services, 2006). Yet this tremendous cost severely underestimates the real amount spent on oral disorders each year. To the direct cost of $81.5 billion must be added the tens of billions of dollars required for direct medical care and indirect costs associated with severe early childhood caries, temporomandibular disorders, trigeminal neuralgia, cleft-lip and palate, oral and pharyngeal cancers, autoimmune diseases, and injuries to the head and face. The costs continue to accumulate when taking into account the resulting loss of productivity from the 164 million hours of work lost each year owing to dental diseases and dental visits (US Department of Health, 2000). Unfortunately, the dental literature does not provide specific estimates of the economic burden of dental caries in industrialized countries. However, it has been documented that preventive programs targeted at the reduction of dental caries have resulted in substantial savings of dental expenditure (Petersen *et al.*, 2005).

The total financial cost to restore all carious lesions in children of low-income nations is estimated to be

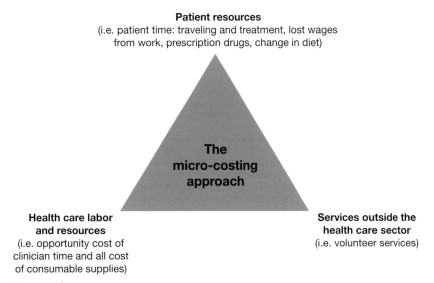

Patient resources
(i.e. patient time: traveling and treatment, lost wages
from work, prescription drugs, change in diet)

The micro-costing approach

**Health care labor
and resources**
(i.e. opportunity cost of
clinician time and all cost
of consumable supplies)

**Services outside the
health care sector**
(i.e. volunteer services)

Figure 30.2 The micro-costing approach.

US$861 million. This cumulative cost, when assessed on an individual country basis, dramatically exceeds the financial resources available for health care in the majority of developing nations. In fact, 75% of developing countries do not even have the financial capacity to provide essential health services (immunizations, nutrient supplementation and public health interventions), let alone the capability to provide restorative care. As a result, private households are often faced with the financial responsibility for their own oral and general health necessities (Yee & Sheiham, 2002). Considering that the average per capita health expenditures in the poorest nations are devastatingly low, ranging from US$4 in the Democratic Republic of the Congo to US$5 in Ethiopia and US$11 in Afghanistan, it is not surprising that 90% of dental caries remains untreated in low-income countries (Yee & Sheiham, 2002; WHO, 2006).

To develop a true taste of the financial implications of dental caries in developing countries, consider an example provided by Yee and Sheiham (2002). In Nepal, the direct cost of an amalgam restoration is US$4. At face value, this may seem like an insignificant amount of money. However, this cost does not take into account the indirect costs incurred by rural families such as travel arrangements (either bus fare or the possibility of walking for a few days to reach the closest dentist), meals while traveling, accommodation and the parent's opportunity cost of time away from work. When these costs are included, this simple amalgam restoration may end up costing US$12. To put this amount in perspective, one should consider that the average wage for a day's work in Nepal is only US$0.75. The household must now make a decision whether to provide food for a starving family for 2 weeks or to restore one carious tooth for one child. This example clearly demonstrates the enormous barriers faced by low-income countries to provide restorative treatments designed to improve the level of oral health of their citizens. This underscores the need to promote preventive strategies to alleviate the problem at the source, before it becomes a substantial financial and health-related issue.

In general, there is a lack of studies that fully assess the costs of prevention versus intervention of dental caries. After reading this chapter, it will be apparent that the costs of preventive measures are considerably lower than the least expensive dental filling. The authors share the common belief that most dental caries-preventive measures are cost-effective methods of eradicating tooth decay when compared to restorative dentistry approaches (Griffin *et al.*, 2001). Therefore, this chapter assesses the costs of dental caries-preventive measures.

Review of economic studies of preventive approaches

Eradicating dental caries requires a considerable amount of resource. Subsequently, the goal is to raise awareness of the total costs associated with this disease beyond just its restorative burden. This chapter may be used as a guide to review previous preventive initiatives in combating dental caries. However, it should not be used as a tool to compare different preventive measures, as most of the reviewed studies are conducted in different settings. The reader should bear in mind that the costs of preventive programs are primarily dependent on the availability of resources and existing infrastructure in a country. Costs must be analyzed for each individual program (Marino, 1995).

Fluoridation

As discussed in Chapter 18, there are various routes of delivery of fluoride compounds, including community water fluoridation, fluoride dentifrices, professionally applied topical fluorides, fluoride mouthrinses and fluoride supplements. According to the World Health Organization (WHO), long-term exposure to fluoride at an optimal concentration leads to a reduction in dental caries in all populations (WHO, 2003b). This section will not compare the effectiveness of the different treatment modalities, but rather will present the costs involved in implementing fluoride-delivery programs in different countries. The economic aspects of these different fluoride-delivery methods are critical from a public health perspective, as policy makers must determine the effective allocation of scarce resources, aiming for a result of the largest decline in dental caries.

Community water fluoridation

The effectiveness of community water fluoridation is well supported in the literature as a method to reduce tooth decay. However, the implementation of water fluoridation in communities is dependent on economic evaluations that consider the total resource costs and the resultant 'carious surfaces averted'. One must consider the opportunity costs of the resources involved in water fluoridation to determine whether the same resources could be used in other oral health-care programs to achieve a similar reduction in dental caries in the population. From the economic analyses conducted to date, the addition of fluoride compounds to a communal water supply has been demonstrated to be a cost-effective public health intervention in preventing dental caries (US Department of Health, 2000; Griffin *et al.*, 2001; O'Connell *et al.*, 2005). Community water fluoridation is one of the few public health initiatives that actually conserve more financial resources than they spend in operation costs (US Department of Health, 2001). Owing to the cost-effectiveness and overall benefit of water fluoridation, the Centers for Disease Control and Prevention (CDC) listed community water fluoridation as one of 10 major public health achievements of the twentieth century (Centers for Disease Control and Prevention, 1999).

There are many economic evaluations on the implementation of community water fluoridation systems in specific areas or districts. However, these studies were conducted in areas where the population primarily obtains their drinking water from a municipal water supply (i.e. tap water). There are many areas that do not have this privilege. As a result, the following economic studies assess the incremental cost of the fluoridation of community water supplies.

Community water fluoridation, as a method of fluoride delivery, has the potential to contribute to the cost-savings in a household. In fact, for 5-year-old children living in a fluoridated community, 45% less is spent on dental treatment than for their 5-year-old counterparts in a non-fluoridated community (Downer *et al.*, 1981). A long-term study demonstrated that the cost of dental treatment for 5-year-old children was 57% lower for those living in a fluoridated community than for those in a non-fluoridated community (Attwood & Blinkhorn, 1989).

The most comprehensive analysis of costs involved in initiating and monitoring a community water fluoridation system was conducted in 44 Florida communities between 1981 and 1989 (Ringelberg, *et al.*, 1992). This cost analysis accounted for the initial one-time costs, the opportunity cost of the capital investment and the annual operational costs of installing a water fluoridation system in a community. Initial one-time fixed costs included costs of the fluoridation equipment, installation, testing equipment, safety equipment and engineering consultant fees. Operational costs included the cost of the chemicals, maintenance costs of equipment, repair costs and labor costs. According to this study, the initiation and annual operation of community water fluoridation systems in 44 communities in Florida ranges from US$0.14 to US$5.93 per person, with a mean of $0.45 per person, serving a total population over 1.6 million people (1988 dollars) (Ringelberg, *et al.*, 1992). Although these costs were calculated in the late 1980s, technological advancements in fluoride delivery have not drastically altered the viability of the data for use in recent cost analyses (Griffin *et al.*, 2001; O'Connell *et al.*, 2005). Another cost analysis performed by Garcia (1989) concluded that the cost per person for water fluoridation ranges from US$0.21 for a population of 4.9 million people to $1.16 for a population of 498 people (1989 dollars). This results in a mean annual cost of $0.46 per person for the institution of community water fluoridation systems for a population serving over 7.5 million people (Garcia, 1989).

As the previous findings demonstrate, the annual cost per person of water fluoridation is largely dependent on the size of the population. Quite simply, larger populations can absorb the initial fixed-cost and operation costs as there are more people who will benefit from the fluoride delivery. Further, the costs of any system will vary depending on the system design, number of fluoride injection points in the water supply, amount and type of fluoride chemicals used (including transportation and storage), type of system feeder and monitoring equipment, natural fluoride level present

in the municipal water and expertise of personnel at the water plant (Ringelberg, 1992; US Department of Health, 2001).

The most recent economic evaluation of community water fluoridation was conducted in the state of Colorado in 2003. The authors concluded that current community water fluoridation projects in Colorado resulted in an annual saving of US$148.9 million or an average of US$60.78 per person (2003 dollars). Further, this study states that the implementation of 52 new fluoridation systems in areas currently without fluoridation would result in an additional annual saving of $46.6 million. For smaller communities, the annual cost per person for the supply of fluoride compounds in the municipal water is $2.66, while the cost per person in larger communities is $0.43 (2003 dollars). This study provides further evidence for the cost-effectiveness and substantial cost-savings associated with the adaptation of community water fluoridation (O'Connell *et al.*, 2005).

One aspect of community water fluoridation that underestimates the true benefit of its usage is the diffusion of fluoride compounds to non-fluoridated communities. This halo effect can be explained since some foods and beverages produced in fluoridated areas are consumed by individuals in non-fluoridated areas, who unknowingly receive the anticaries benefit of fluoride (Lewis & Banting, 1994; O'Connell *et al.*, 2005). However, if individuals in a non-fluoridated community are using fluoride dentifrices, fluoride mouthrinses or taking fluoride tablets, the halo effect of water fluoridation may result in a greater intake of fluoride compounds, potentially leading to dental fluorosis during tooth development. The relationship between the halo effect and dental fluorosis has yet to be comprehensively analyzed and is thus just considered to be speculative (Lewis & Banting, 1994). Nonetheless, dental fluorosis is neglected in many economic evaluations (Garcia, 1989; Griffin *et al.*, 2001; O'Connell *et al.*, 2005), but should be considered as a potential cost of fluoridation.

Fluoride dentifrices

Compared with other fluoride-delivery methods, fluoride dentifrices provide the greatest global benefit in reducing caries among children (Burt, 1998). Fluoridated toothpaste is the most common method of fluoride delivery, with over 500 million people worldwide benefiting from its use (WHO, 2003). In developed countries, fluoridated toothpaste is widely available and is no more expensive than a non-fluoridated toothpaste. Subsequently, those individuals who brush their teeth on a regular basis to maintain a healthy oral cavity need not pay an extra cost to receive the benefit of fluoride in their dentifrice (US Department of Health, 2001).

In the USA, the annual per capita cost of toothpaste ranges between US$6 and US$12 (Jones *et al.*, 2005). Consequently, fluoride dentifrices may not be available in developing countries for economic reasons. The WHO is calling for the development of affordable, fluoridated toothpastes that are available at a price accessible to populations with low socieconomic status (SES) in developing countries. In the Philippines, affordable fluoridated toothpastes have been developed and sold for as low as US$0.50 for a 100 ml tube (O. Fejerskov, personal communication). At such a low cost, a reduction in dental caries could be observed in all populations. A WHO study conducted in Indonesia demonstrated that low-cost fluoridated toothpastes can significantly reduce dental caries in an area with a high prevalence of tooth decay. Specific cost data were not given in this study. However, the authors noted that the cost of production of affordable toothpastes is primarily based on the choice and availability of raw materials (Adyatmaka et al., 1998; Jones et al., 2005).

It is widely believed that the decline in caries is mainly due to the availability of fluoridated toothpaste. Subsequently, through the use of fluoride dentifrices, restorative treatment costs have declined. A study conducted in Nepal determined that the potential restorative treatment costs saved for 6–18-year-olds as a result of the availability of fluoridated toothpaste could range from US$594 466 to $2 442 333 (2002 dollars) (Yee et al., 2004). However, the efficacy of fluoridated toothpaste is highly dependent on the population's use of the product.

Previous public health initiatives that incorporated the use of fluoridated toothpastes included supervised tooth brushing and a postal toothpaste program where children with low SES are given free fluoridated toothpaste and toothbrushes. Studies have determined that supervised tooth brushing is an effective method of reducing dental caries, but its cost-effectiveness in comparison to other public health initiatives is highly questionable (Manau et al., 1987; Al-Jundi et al., 2006). An economic evaluation of community prevention programs in Spain demonstrated that the annual cost of saving 1 DMFS with a supervised tooth-brushing method was US$8.80. Comparatively, the cost of saving 1 DMFS using community water fluoridation in the same area was $0.39 (Manau et al., 1987). In this context, community water fluoridation seems to be a more suitable, cost-effective alternative initiative to eradicate dental caries.

The cost-effectiveness of a program that provides free toothpaste and toothbrushes is also very debatable in comparison to other public health approaches. A UK study concluded that the total cost of running a postal toothpaste program for 5000 children was £27.93 per child and the cost saving of reducing the DMFT by 1 was £80.83 (Davies et al., 2003).

Previous fluoridated toothpaste public health measures, in comparison to other programs such as community water fluoridation, do not appear to be cost-effective methods of eradicating dental caries. However, the addition of fluoride to dentifrices in areas that frequently use non-fluoridated toothpastes is a low-cost initiative. Since fluoridated toothpastes are no more costly than non-fluoridated toothpastes, this initiative may be more cost-effective than community water fluoridation measures.

Professionally applied topical fluorides

Professionally applied topical fluorides (PATFs) such as fluoride varnishes, fluoride foams and fluoride gels are often used as preventive measures for individuals with a high risk for dental caries (Ripa, 1993). A study that assesses the economic viability of PATFs must account for the true cost of resources involved by incorporating the opportunity cost of labor (oral health professional), materials (e.g. fluoride, brush tips, styrofoam trays), and patients' time and resources. Clearly, the main cost incurred by the clinician in applying these fluoride modalities is the opportunity cost of their time. To reduce these costs, dental auxiliaries (where permitted by law) usually administer the fluoride treatment to the patients.

A recent Canadian study evaluated the costs of fluoride varnishes and fluoride foams in a public health dental clinic. Dental hygienists administered fluoride varnishes or fluoride foam (in mouthtrays) to children considered at high risk for dental caries. All costs for the dental hygienist's labor, fluoride foam sytrofoam trays, fluoride varnish, brush tips and cotton rolls were accounted for. Overall, fluoride varnish was less expensive than fluoride foam, with a cost of Can$3.69 and $4.11 per application, respectively (2004 dollars). In addition, compared with the fluoride foam, fluoride varnish had a shorter application time (5.81 versus 7.86 min) and was generally more acceptable to the children (Hawkins et al., 2004). Although the time and cost differences between fluoride foam and fluoride varnish were small, the results of this study have major implications for public health policy. Because public health programs treat thousands of patients, savings of Can$0.42 and 1.95 minutes of the hygienist's time per application using fluoride varnish instead of fluoride foam will add up to significant savings.

As a whole, the dental literature generally agrees that the use of PATFs should be targeted at populations with a high prevalence of dental caries, as low-risk children are unlikely to benefit from PATF treatments (Lewis & Ismail, 1995; van Rijkom et al., 1998; Seppä, 2001). The cost-effectiveness of PATFs is arguable, since costly professional time is required for treatment that is administered on an individual patient basis. Further, as multiple applications of PATFs are required each year, the economic feasibility of its use is questionable (Burt, 1998).

Fluoride mouthrinses

Economic assessments focussed on fluoride mouthrinses were carried out based on their use as a public health approach rather than in dental practices. Subsequently, this section will describe the costs involved in administering public health fluoride mouthrinse programs.

Public health mouthrinse programs are primarily school based and are targeted at reducing the prevalence of dental caries among elementary school children. The most recent publications discussed work in the USA in the 1980s, when approximately 3 million students took part in a school-based fluoride mouthrinsing program (US Department of Health, 2001).

Mouthrinsing programs are a labor-intensive public health initiative, since labor costs account for approximately 85% of the total costs of the program (Doherty & Martie, 1987). In a majority of the programs, teachers and volunteer workers are trained to administer and monitor weekly mouthrinsing among their students. However, in some cases, school mouthrinsing programs used the services of field workers, co-ordinators, consultants and clerical staff (Garcia, 1989). Garcia (1989) conducted a study examining the direct cost of school-based mouthrinsing programs serving over 1.25 million children in 11 states in the USA. These direct costs accounted for the cost of personnel, materials and supplies, but did not account for the cost of the teachers' and volunteers' time. According to this study, the annual cost of running a fluoride mouthrinsing program ranged from US$0.52 to $1.78 per child, with a mean value of $1.30 per child (1988 dollars), with the most costly programs using the highest number of personnel.

Another school-based mouthrinsing analysis of 14 different programs in the USA serving 75 000 students concluded that the total annual cost ranged between $2.35 and $8.05 per child (1978 dollars). This study fully accounted for all costs involved, such as paid labor, annual capital charges for equipment, the cost of supplies and the opportunity cost of resources donated, including volunteer time (Doherty et al., 1984). It should be noted that the costs of a school-based system will fluctuate depending on the size of the student population (a system supplying more students incurs higher costs) and the method in which the materials are dispensed (from a pump or using premixed fluoride solutions) (Doherty et al., 1984; Doherty & Martie, 1987; Garcia, 1989).

Since the decline in caries following the 1980s, current literature suggests that school-based fluoride mouthrinsing programs should only be implemented in a population with a high caries rate (Wei & Yiu, 1993; Adair, 1998; Burt, 1998). Further, it has been suggested that the cost-effectiveness of this strategy as a public health initiative to reduce dental caries cannot be supported when other methods, such as community water fluoridation or fluoride dentifrices, are available (Niessen & Douglass, 1984).

Fluoride supplements

The use of fluoride supplements as a method of reducing the prevalence and severity of caries in primary and perma-

nent dentition is supported in the literature (Widenheim & Birkhed, 1991; Brambilla; 2001). Dietary fluoride supplement delivery, like many other prevention strategies, has been studied predominantly in school-based program settings. However, there is a lack of recent publications on the cost-effectiveness of such programs, which may suggest that such programs have not been frequently implemented in the past decade.

The costs of instituting and operating fluoride supplement programs are very similar to those of fluoride mouthrinsing programs, with the main differences being the cost of the fluoride tablets. In five US states, the annual cost of running a dietary fluoride supplement program was, on average, US$2.53 per child (1988 dollars). This study underestimated the true costs involved, as the travel, administrative costs and opportunity costs of teacher or volunteer time were not taken into account (Garcia, 1989). A study conducted in 22 schools in Manchester, UK, determined that the total cost of establishing the program, the operational cost of the program for 3 years and the cost of the fluoride tablets was £4.39 per child. However, the benefit, calculated from the restorative treatment avoided due to the fluoride supplement, was £3.23. At face value, this program seems to have an unfavorable cost–benefit ratio. However, like many other studies, the monetary value placed on the treatment avoided does not take into account the full value of a healthy tooth or the relief of pain (O'Rourke et al., 1988).

In developed countries, where the population has access to fluoridated water or fluoride dentifrices, the marginal benefit gained from the use of fluoride supplements is minimal. Consequently, the financial resources devoted to fluoride supplements may be better allocated to other public health initiatives. In addition, the potential for low compliance deems fluoride supplements to be a poor public health initiative in comparison with other fluoride modalities (Riordan, 1999).

Pit and fissure sealants

The use of sealants is recognized as an effective measure in the prevention of pit and fissure caries (NIH, 1983). Accordingly, oral health physicians, patients, third party payers and public health policy makers are interested in the economic viability of the use of pit and fissure sealants in a clinical setting. The effectiveness of pit and fissure sealants in relation to other dental caries-preventive measures will not be discussed in this chapter. Rather, the total costs involved in the delivery of sealants will be reviewed.

An ideal microcosting approach to the placement of pit and fissure sealants would include the cost of the resin-based material, all brushes/applicators used, the opportunity cost of the operator's time, lost wages incurred by the parents and travel costs. Of the costs incurred by the dental professional, the main cost in sealant application is the opportunity cost of their time. Since pit and fissure sealants are applied to individual teeth by oral health-care professionals, they are considered to be a resource-expensive preventive measure. Undoubtedly, the cost-effectiveness of sealants would be improved through their application by trained dental auxiliaries instead of oral health physicians (Burt, 1984; Mitchell & Murray, 1989; Deery, 1999). Other factors that would enhance the cost-effectiveness of sealants include improved sealant retention rates, increased sealant resin durability and use with other caries-preventative measures such as water fluoridation or fluoride dentifrices. Lastly, the economic viability of pit and fissure sealants would be dramatically enhanced if sealants were only placed on teeth that are destined to become carious (Mitchell & Murray, 1989). However, a diagnostic tool that offers accurate caries risk-assessment information is not yet available (Kitchens, 2005).

Many studies have conflicting results and conclusions in the cost–benefit and cost-effectiveness of pit and fissure sealants as a method of caries prevention (Garcia, 1989; Ripa, 1993; Morgan et al., 1998; Crowley et al., 2000; Werner et al., 2000.). Most of these cost-effective studies were conducted in school-based programs. However, the financial costs of sealing teeth as part of community programs are often lower than those found in clinical settings. Unfortunately, these economic assessments do not aid general oral health-care practitioners in determining whether pit and fissure sealants are worth the true cost of placement. As a result, real-world pragmatic studies are required that fully account for all resource uses and the opportunity cost of the clinician's time.

There has been a shift in the recent literature of the economics of pit and fissure sealants towards sealant delivery based on risk development of dental caries (Griffin et al., 2002; Quinonez et al., 2005). Weintraub et al. (1993) concluded that universal delivery of pit and fissure sealants is cost-saving in children of low SES, compared with no application of sealants. Two theoretically based studies both demonstrate this and conclude that risk-based sealant delivery is less costly than sealing all teeth or sealing no teeth (Griffin et al., 2002; Qunionez et al., 2005).

Unfortunately, the recent attention paid to the harmful effects of bisphenol-A, a component used in sealant material, emphasizes the need to include the cost of potential negative general health outcomes of the sealants; that is, if public reaction is not so negative that it renders pit and fissure sealant treatment completely unacceptable.

Conclusions

This chapter provides cost information on the most common preventive measures used to eradicate dental caries. However, the reader must keep in mind that the cost analyses of the dental caries-preventive measures outlined in this chapter were conducted on different population groups, in different years, in different countries and with different population sizes. The costs of each preventive program must be assessed on an individual country basis to determine which preventive modality may be the most cost-effective for that country.

In today's society, an oral health discrepancy exists because a disproportionate number of children in low SES communities suffer from dental caries and experience higher unmet treatment needs than high-income children (Vargas et al., 1998). The low SES population is characterized by low dental-care utilization and lower tooth-brushing compliance rates than their higher SES counterparts (Addy et al., 1990). However, even when treatment needs are met for low SES children, differences in dental caries prevalence are still observed (Ismail & Sohn, 2001). Consequently, factors beyond the obvious financial disparities must account for the differences in dental utilization and caries experience among the SES categories. Rather than providing universal dental care, prevention-based, public health initiatives appear to be the solution to eliminating the SES oral health disparity. For example, water fluoridation would provide the cariostatic benefits of fluoride compounds and would be accessible to all who obtain their water from a municipal supply (Burt, 2002). For the most part, the dental literature suggests that water fluoridation decreases the SES differences in caries prevalence, but does not eliminate them completely (Carmichael et al., 1989; Jones & Worthington, 2000).

The preventive measures reviewed in this chapter may not be applicable to all communities. For instance, it is not possible to institute community water fluoridation systems in underprivileged areas that do not have access to public tap water. In areas where the implementation of water fluoridation systems is not feasible, fluoride dentifrices could be used as a strategy to reduce the inequities involved in the distribution of dental caries. After the introduction of fluoridated dentifrice school-based programs in Indonesia, DMFT rates significantly declined in all age groups. Overall, water fluoridation and use of fluoridated toothpastes are simple, equitable strategies that should reduce the dental caries disparity within a population. Considering that annual water fluoridation costs $0.43 per person and affordable fluoridated toothpastes cost approximately $0.50 per 100 ml tube, these strategies are very cost-effective public health approaches to reducing dental caries (O'Connell et al., 2005; O. Fejerskov, personal communication).

There is an urgent need for economic evaluations to compare the aforementioned dental caries-preventive strategies outlined in this chapter. This information would allow public health policy makers, clinicians and patients to determine the most suitable cost-effective methods available in eradicating this widespread disease. However, this task is easily stated but will be difficult to accomplish, as cost-effective initiatives in one locale may not be the same for another.

References

Adair SM. The role of fluoride mouthrinses in the control of dental caries: a brief review. *Pediatr Dent* 1998; **20**: 101–4.

Addy M, Dummer PM, Hunter ML, Kingdon A, Shaw WC. The effect of toothbrushing frequency, toothbrushing hand, sex and social class on the incidence of plaque, gingivitis and pocketing in adolescents: a longitudinal cohort study. *Community Dent Health* 1990; **7**: 237–47.

Adyatmaka A, Sutopo U, Carlsson P, Bratthall D, Pakhomo G. School based-primary preventive programme for children. Affordable toothpaste as a component in primary oral health care. Experience from a field trial in Kalimantan Barat, Indonesia. Geneva: World Health Organization, 1998.

Al-Jundi SH, Hammad M, Alwaeli H. The efficacy of a school-based caries preventive program: a 4-year study. *Int J Dent Hyg* 2006; **4**: 30–4.

Attwood D, Blinkhorn AS. Reassessment of the effect of fluoridation on cost of dental treatment among Scottish schoolchildren. *Community Dent Oral Epidemiol* 1989; **17**: 79–82.

Brambilla E. Fluoride – is it capable of fighting old and new dental diseases? An overview of existing fluoride compounds and their clinical applications. *Caries Res* 2001; **35**: 6–9.

Burt BA. Fissure sealants: clinical and economic factors. *J Dent Educ* 1984; **48**: 96–102.

Burt BA. Prevention policies in the light of the changed distribution of dental caries. *Acta Odontol Scand* 1998; **56**: 179–86.

Burt BA. Fluoridation and social equity. *J Public Health Dent* 2002; **62**: 195–200.

Carmichael CL, Rugg-Gunn AJ, Ferrell RS. The relationship between fluoridation, social class and caries experience in 5-year-old children in Newcastle and Northumberland in 1987. *Br Dent J* 1989; **16**: 57–61.

Centers for Disease Control and Prevention. Ten great public health achievements – United States, 1900–1999. *MMWR Morb Mortal Wkly Rep* 1999; **48**: 241–3.

Centers for Medicare and Medicaid Services, Office of the Actuary. *Historical national health expenditure data.* 2006. Available at http://www.cms.hhs.gov/NationalHealthExpendData/downloads/tables.pdf

Crowley SJ, Campain AC, Morgan MV. An economic evaluation of a publicly funded dental prevention programme in regional and rural Victoria: an extrapolated analysis. *Community Dent Health* 2000; **17**: 145–51.

Davies GM, Worthington HV, Ellwood RP, et al. An assessment of the cost effectiveness of a postal toothpaste programme to prevent caries among five-year-old children in the North West of England. *Community Dent Health* 2003; **20**: 207–10.

Deery C. The economic evaluation of pit and fissure sealants. *Int J Paediatr Dent* 1999; **9**: 235–41.

Doherty NJ, Martie CW. Analysis of the costs of school-based mouthrinsing programs. *Community Dent Oral Epidemiol* 1987; **15**: 67–9.

Doherty NJ, Brunelle JA, Miller AJ, Li SH. Costs of school-based mouthrinsing in 14 demonstration programs in USA. *Community Dent Oral Epidemiol* 1984; **12**: 35–8.

Downer MC, Blinkhorn AS, Attwood D. Effect of fluoridation on the cost of dental treatment among urban Scottish schoolchildren. *Community Dent Oral Epidemiol* 1981; **9**: 112–16.

Drummond MF, O'Brien B, Stoddart GL. Torrance GW. *Methods for the economic evaluation of health care programmes*, 2nd edn. New York: Oxford University Press, 1997.

Folland S, Goodman, AC, Stano M. *The economics of health and health care*, 4th edn. New Jersey: Pearson Prentice Hall, 2004.

Garcia AI. Caries incidence and costs of prevention programs. *J Public Health Dent* 1989; **49**: 259–71.

Gold MR, Siegel JE, Russell LB, Weinstein MC. *Cost-effectiveness in health and medicine.* New York: Oxford University Press, 1996.

Griffin SO, Jones K, Tomar SL. An economic evaluation of community water fluoridation. *J Public Health Dent* 2001; **61**: 78–86.

Griffin SO, Griffin PM, Gooch BF, Barker LK. Comparing the costs of three sealant delivery strategies. *J Dent Res* 2002; **81**: 641–5.

Hawkins R, Noble J, Locker D, et al. A comparison of the costs and patient acceptability of professionally applied topical fluoride foam and varnish. *J Public Health Dent* 2004; **64**: 106–10.

Ismail AI, Sohn W. The impact of universal access to dental care on disparities in caries experience in children. *J Am Dent Assoc* 2001; **132**: 295–303.

Jones CM, Worthington H. Water fluoridation, poverty and tooth decay in 12-year-old children. *J Dent* 2000; **28**: 389–93.

Jones S, Burt BA, Petersen PE, Lennon MA. The effective use of fluorides in public health. *Bull World Health Organ* 2005; **83**: 670–6.

Kitchens DH. The economics of pit and fissure sealants in preventive dentistry: a review. *J Contemp Dent Pract* 2005; **6**: 95–103.

Lewis DW, Banting DW. Water fluoridation: current effectiveness and dental fluorosis. *Community Dent Oral Epidemiol* 1994; **22**: 153–8.

Lewis DW, Ismail AI. Periodic health examination, 1995 update: 2. Prevention of dental caries. The Canadian Task Force on the Periodic Health Examination. *CMAJ* 1995; **152**: 836–46.

Manau C, Cuenca E, Martinez-Carretero J, Salleras L. Economic evaluation of community programs for the prevention of dental caries in Catalonia, Spain. *Community Dent Oral Epidemiol* 1987; **15**: 297–300.

Marino, R. Should we use milk fluoridation? A review. *Bull Pan Am Health Organ* 1995; **29**: 287–98.

Mitchell L, Murray JJ. Fissure sealants: a critique of their cost-effectiveness. *Community Dent Oral Epidemiol* 1989; **17**: 19–23.

Morgan MV, Crowley SJ, Wright C. Economic evaluation of a pit and fissure dental sealant and fluoride mouthrinsing program in two nonfluoridated regions of Victoria, Australia. *J Public Health Dent* 1998; **58**: 19–27.

National Institutes of Health. Dental sealants in the prevention of tooth decay. *NIH Consens Dev Conf Consens Statement* 1983 Dec. 5–7; **4**(11).

Niessen LC, Douglass CW. Theoretical considerations in applying benefit–cost and cost-effectiveness analyses to preventive dental programs. *J Public Health Dent* 1984; **44**: 156–68.

O'Connell JM, Brunson D, Anselmo T, Sullivan PW. Costs and savings associated with community water fluoridation programs in Colorado. *Prev Chronic Dis* 2005; **2** (Special No.): A06.

O'Rourke CA, Attrill M, Holloway PJ. Cost appraisal of a fluoride tablet programme to Manchester primary schoolchildren. *Community Dent Oral Epidemiol* 1988; **16**: 341–4.

Petersen PE, Bourgeois D, Ogawa H, Estupinan-Day S, Ndiaye C. The global burden of oral diseases and risks to oral health. *Bull World Health Organ* 2005; **83**: 661–9.

Quinonez RB, Downs SM, Shugars D, Christensen J, Vann WF Jr. Assessing cost-effectiveness of sealant placement in children. *J Public Health Dent* 2005; **65**: 82–9.

van Rijkom HM, Truin GJ, van 't Hof MA. A meta-analysis of clinical studies on the caries-inhibiting effect of fluoride gel treatment. *Caries Res* 1998; **32**: 83–92.

Ringelberg ML, Allen SJ, Brown LJ. Cost of fluoridation: 44 Florida communities. *J Public Health Dent* 1992; **52**: 75–80.

Riordan, PJ. Fluoride supplements for young children: an analysis of the literature focusing on the benefits and risks. *Community Dent Oral Epidemiol* 1999; **27**: 72–83.

Ripa LW. A half-century of community water fluoridation in the United States: review and commentary. *J Public Health Dent* 1993; **53**: 17–44.

Romanow, RJ. *Building on values – the future of health care in Canada.* Canada: Commission on the Future of Health Care, 2002.

Seppä L. The future of preventive programs in countries with different systems for dental care. *Caries Res* 2001; **35**: 26–9.

US Department of Health and Human Services. *Oral health in America. A report of the Surgeon General.* Rockville, MD: US Department of Health and Human Services, National Institutes of Health, National Institute of Dental and Craniofacial Research, 2000.

US Department of Health and Human Services. Centers for Disease Control and Prevention. Recommendations for using fluoride to prevent and control dental caries in the United States. *MMWR Morb Mortal Wkly Rep* 2001; **50**.

Vargas CM, Crall JJ, Schneider DA. Sociodemographic distribution of pediatric dental caries: NHANES III, 1988–1994. *J Am Dent Assoc* 1998; **129**: 1229–38.

Wei SH, Yiu CK. Mouthrinses: recent clinical findings and implications for use. *Int Dent J* 1993; **43**: 541–7.

Weintraub JA, Stearns SC, Burt BA, Beltran E, Eklund SA. A retrospective analysis of the cost-effectiveness of dental sealants in a children's health center. *Soc Sci Med* 1993; **36**: 1483–93.

Werner CW, Pereira AC, Eklund SA. Cost-effectiveness study of a school-based sealant program. *ASDC J Dent Child* 2000; **67**: 93–7.

Widenheim J, Birkhed D. Caries-preventive effect on primary and permanent teeth and cost-effectiveness of an NaF tablet preschool program. *Community Dent Oral Epidemiol* 1991; **19**: 88–92.

Widstrom E, Eaton KA. Oral healthcare systems in the extended European union. *Oral Health Prev Dent* 2004; **2**: 155–94.

World Health Organization. *National health accounts.* Geneva: WHO; 2003a. Available at http://www.who.int/nha/en/

World Health Organization. *World oral health report 2003.* Geneva: WHO; 2003b.

World Health Organization. *World health statistics 2006.* Geneva: WHO; 2006.

Yee R, Sheiham A. The burden of restorative dental treatment for children in Third World countries. *Int Dent J* 2002; **52**: 1–9.

Yee R, McDonald N, Walker D. A cost–benefit analysis of an advocacy project to fluoridate toothpastes in Nepal. *Community Dent Health* 2004; **21**: 265–70.

Part VII
Dentistry in the twenty-first century

31

Variation in clinical decision making related to caries

J.D. Bader and D.A. Shugars

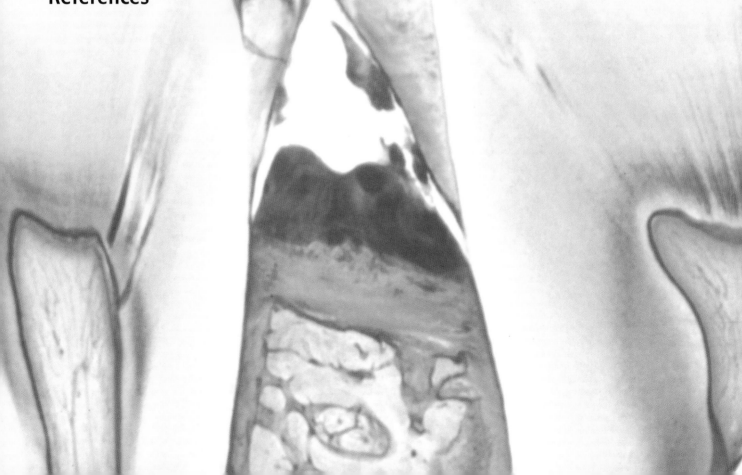

Introduction

Variation among clinicians in the detection and management of dental caries represents a substantial problem in dentistry. The problem arises because patients visiting different dentists are likely to receive different treatment for the same condition. Unless all possible treatments, from doing nothing to intervening surgically, have the same outcomes, some patients will not receive appropriate treatment. The extent of differences among dentists in detecting caries lesions and in deciding how to manage them is greater than generally appreciated by either the profession or the public, and the profession is currently in the earliest stages of recognizing and addressing the problem. This chapter is intended to contribute to that process. It first examines evidence describing the extent of variation in the detection of caries, and explores reasons for this variation. It then repeats this process for caries management decisions. The consequences of this variation are then discussed, and approaches to reduce the extent of such variation are suggested. The evidence presented in this chapter is not complete; it is not the result of systematic reviews on each of the topics addressed. Rather, it is a selected majority of studies on these topics that is intended to represent current understanding.

Variation in detection of caries lesions

Dentists do not agree

When two or more clinicians examine the same patient, they will often disagree on the caries status of specific tooth surfaces, i.e. the presence and stage of caries lesions. Table 31.1 summarizes several studies of agreement among dentists in detecting caries lesions. Such studies have been conducted over the past quarter-century as the profession has begun to recognize that dentists exhibit substantial variation when detecting caries lesions. In the table, the extent of variation is indicated either by the range of positive decisions among a group of dentists examining the same surfaces, teeth or subjects, or by an index of agreement among the dentists such as the kappa statistic or the intraclass correlation (ICC). Neither method is entirely satisfactory for describing the variation. The range of positive decisions relies on the outliers, or extremes of the distribution, and may not reflect the extent of agreement among the majority of examiners. However, these ranges do highlight the extreme nature of variation between at least some dentists. The kappa statistic and ICC do reflect the contributions of all dentists to the variation, but are less familiar and may be difficult for many to interpret. It has been suggested that kappa, which reflects agreement beyond chance, be interpreted as a set of categories of agreement, where values less than 0.00 represent a state of poor agreement, those from 0.00 to 0.20 represent slight agreement, from 0.21 to 0.40 is fair agreement, 0.41 to 0.60 is moderate agreement, 0.61 to 0.80 is substantial

agreement, and above 0.81 is almost perfect agreement (Landis & Koch, 1977). ICC values can be interpreted similarly.

Variation occurs among all dentists, not just a few outliers

All of the studies listed in Table 31.1 found variation in the detection of caries lesions, whether the diagnostic material was clinical inspection of patients, inspection of extracted teeth, inspection of radiographs or a combination of these methods. Among the studies reporting ranges for positive decisions, the magnitude of these ranges means that regardless of the number of dentists involved in the study, some dentists were reporting the presence of nearly three times as many lesions as other dentists examining the same patients or teeth. Because these extremes occurred even in studies comparing detection among small numbers of dentists, it appears that variation occurs across almost all dentists, rather then being the result of relatively rare outlier dentists. The kappa and ICC values generally reflect fair to moderate agreement, which supports the general interpretation of widespread variation, although one study did report substantial agreement in distinguishing between sound surfaces and carious surfaces radiographically.

Disagreement is irrespective of accuracy

From the limited results available, it would seem that agreement between dentists is stronger when detecting caries lesions radiographically than clinically, and that there is less variation in detecting dentinal caries lesions than caries lesions in enamel. However, these are extremely tentative observations, and variation is apparent in all diagnostic situations. It is important to realize that this discussion has not addressed the extent to which the identifications are correct. The accuracy of detection is not at issue here, simply the differences among examiners. While any efforts to reduce this variation will be based on the objective of improving the accuracy of dentists' caries detection, it is useful to examine the possible reasons for the observed variation without also introducing the issue of accuracy, i.e. why some dentists are more accurate than others, because it helps to focus the discussion on the reasons why such variation arises. There are several possible sources for this variation that should be considered.

Differences in detection methods

A principal source of variation among dentists in practice is not reflected in Table 31.1, where all examiners in a given study used the same method. The method used for detection of caries lesions is a substantial source of the variation seen among dental practitioners, where a wide variety of methods is in use. As noted in earlier chapters, each of these methods has its own established range of accuracy (i.e. the sensitivity and specificity values or area under the curve for

Table 31.1 Variation in dentists' caries detection decisions

Study	Diagnostic decision	Case type	No. of dentists	No. of decisions	Range of positive decisions	Interexaminer agreement
Rytömaa et al. (1979) Finland	Dentin caries, any surface	Clinical in vivo	12 faculty	NR[a]	33–82[b]	–
Mileman et al. (1982) Netherlands	Any proximal caries	Radiographs	42 faculty	300 surfaces	18–53%	–
Langlais et al. (1987) USA	Any dentin caries	Radiographs	34 faculty	182 teeth	–	0.57[c]
	Any enamel caries	Radiograph	34 faculty	182 teeth	–	0.34[c]
	Any caries	Radiographs	34 faculty	182 teeth	–	0.72[c]
Mileman & van den Weele (1990) Netherlands	Any dentin caries	Radiographs	276 clinicians	105 surfaces	7–50%	–
Noar & Smith (1990) UK	Proximal dentin caries	Radiograph	86 clinicians	48 teeth	15–75%	–
		Clinical in vitro	86 clinicians	48 teeth	6–69%	–
Lazarchik et al. (1995) USA	Any occlussal caries	Radiographs	15 faculty	100 teeth		0.53[c]
Rosen et al. (1996) Sweden	Sound/early/or coronal: 0.40[c]	Clinical in vivo	3 clinicians	1974 teeth	–	
	Cavitated status root: 0.37[c]			1752 teeth	–	
Thomas et al. (2000) USA	Occlusal dentin caries	Clinical in vitro	4 clinicians	100 teeth		0.54[d]
Ermis & Aydin (2004) Turkey	Secondary caries	Clinical and radiographs	3 clinicians	112 class I restorations	–	0.41[c]
Nuttall & Clarkson (2005) UK	Tooth with cavitated lesion	Clinical in vivo	10 clinicians	NR[a]	–	0.30[c]
Ekstrand et al. (2005) Denmark	Visual status	Clinical in vitro	3 clinicians	30 arrested	–	0.06–0.25[e]
	Tactile status	Clinical in vitro	3 clinicians	Enamel lesions	–	–0.08–0.26[e]
	Activity status	Clinical in vitro	3 clinicians			0.06–0.16[e]

[a] 10 patients, number of teeth/surfaces not reported.
[b] Number of surfaces with caries.
[c] Mean kappa statistic.
[d] Intraclass correlation coefficient.
[e] Range of kappa statistics.

the method, as reported by various investigators). Unless the method has perfect accuracy, i.e. sensitivity and specificity values are 100, some surfaces will be misidentified as being sound when a lesion is present, or vice versa. What is less widely appreciated, however, is that when two detection methods with the same accuracy are applied to the same surfaces, there can be substantial differences in the specific tooth surfaces identified as being carious. Figure 31.1 illustrates a situation where method A, with a sensitivity of 80 and a specificity of 80, and method B, with the same performance characteristics, each identifies 20 surfaces as being carious in a population of 40 surfaces with a true caries prevalence of 0.50. Only 12 of the 20 truly carious teeth are identified by both methods, and the four false positives that each method produces are completely different between the methods.

Multiple methods further complicate matters

Thus, as perhaps the most obvious explanation of variation between dentists, differences in the method that individual clinicians choose to use to detect caries lesions are likely to lead to differences in the surfaces identified, even when the methods used have equivalent accuracy. In addition, clinicians often use multiple methods for detection. Their application will lead to further differences in assessments of specific surfaces. Here, differences in which surfaces are subjected to the additional methods (all surfaces, or just those indicated by the first method as being carious), and how the results of multiple tests are combined to identify lesions (all test results positive, any test result positive, a majority of test results positive) will inevitably lead to differences in surfaces identified as having a lesion.

Differences in criteria for caries lesions for a given detection method

The examiner may be just as important as the method

As Table 31.1 shows, even when clinicians use the same detection method, there will be disagreements in the surfaces identified as being carious. The widespread nature of

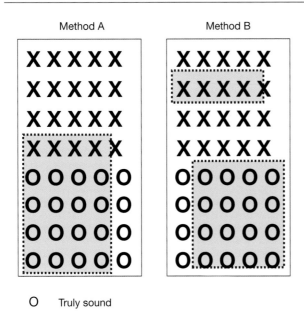

O	Truly sound
X	Truly caries
⫶⫶⫶	Caries identified by method

Figure 31.1 Teeth identified as carious by two methods, each with sensitivity = 0.80, specificity = 0.80.

this variation is illustrated by examining the findings of two systematic reviews of the performance of various caries diagnostic methods. In these reviews substantial variation was seen among the results of studies examining the accuracy of detection of a specific lesion type by a single diagnostic method (Bader et al., 2002; Bader & Shugars, 2004). Table 31.2 summarizes the ranges of sensitivities reported for a variety of methods and lesion types. The ranges shown

for most diagnostic applications are extreme, suggesting that who uses a diagnostic method may be just as important a factor in the sensitivity of the examination as what diagnostic method is used. The fact that sensitivity varies substantially even though the method used to detect caries is held constant demonstrates that other factors also contribute to the variation.

The criteria may be just as important as the method

A primary reason for the variation seen in the sensitivities reported by the various studies was identified in the systematic reviews as differences in the criteria used for determining the presence of disease. For example, a recent review identified 29 indices for the visual and visual–tactile identification and classification of coronal caries lesions (Ismail, 2004). Some of the criteria for a given caries status decision were similar or identical across most of the indices. Nevertheless, there were sufficient differences in how signs were described, and how signs were grouped together to denote a particular stage of disease to make it almost inevitable that assessments using one set of criteria would differ from those made with another set. Although a similar review has not been performed for radiological criteria for caries, it is apparent that the criteria that clinicians report using to identify caries lesions will differ owing to their beliefs about the extent to which radiographic images underestimate the extent of demineralization (Espelid et al., 1985).

Quantifying the results does not necessarily reduce differences

Table 31.2 shows that substantial variation in sensitivity was also present for laser fluorescence and electrical con-

Table 31.2 Range in sensitivity values among studies of caries detection methods, by method, tooth surface and type of caries

Method	Surface	Depth or characteristic	No. of studies	Range of sensitivity
Visual	Occlusal	Cavitated	4	0.31 to 0.91
		Dentin	12	0.12 to 0.95
		Enamel	3	0.10 to 0.72
		Any	5	0.27 to 0.89
Visual/tactile	Occlusal	Dentin	2	0.14 to 0.24
		Any	2	0.17 to 0.61
	Proximal	Cavitated	3	0.29 to 0.93
Radiographic	Occlusal	Dentin	27	0.14 to 0.93
		Enamel	4	0.17 to 0.25
		Any	7	0.12 to 0.79
	Proximal	cavitated	7	0.35 to 0.99
		Dentin	9	0.16 to 0.63
		Enamel	3	0.35 to 0.46
		Any	12	0.15 to 1.00
Laser fluorescence	Occlusal	Dentin	12	0.19 to 1.00
		Enamel	5	0.38 to 0.79
Electrical conductance	Occlusal	Dentin	15	0.58 to 0.97
		Any	8	0.61 to 0.92

Sources: two systematic reviews (Bader et al., 2002; Bader & Shugars, 2004).

ductance. These methods are considered to be more objective diagnostic methods in that the test returns a number that is associated with the likelihood of disease. However, even here differences in criteria play a role in variation. The reviews noted that the fluorescence and conductance studies used a variety of cut-points, or values at which a surface was designated as having an enamel lesion or a dentin lesion. Thus, in addition to differences in interpretation of subjective criteria, differences in the meaning assigned to a supposedly objective criterion, an electrical or digital measure, contribute to variation in the identification of caries lesions

Clinician error and clinician differences

Testing and training examiners may not eradicate differences

The contribution that clinician error makes to variation in caries identification has not been examined thoroughly, but its presence is suggested across all methods of caries identification through the existence of less than perfect intraexaminer and interexaminer reliability, or reproducibility, reported in assessments of diagnostic performance (Bader *et al.*, 2002; Bader & Shugars, 2004). In these assessments the method of detection and the criteria for detection are held constant and intensive training in use of the diagnostic

method and criteria is provided before the assessment. In addition, research subjects tend to be co-operative, radiographs are selected to be error free, and extracted teeth are easily accessible, dry and well-lit. Yet reliability in these assessments is seldom perfect. Examiners almost inevitably disagree among themselves, and/or within themselves upon a second application of the diagnostic method.

Examiners make mistakes

The reason for these persistent inconsistencies is usually explained as examiner error. In reported analyses of this error in clinical and radiographic examinations, no systematic sources of error were identified: the error was characterized as random error, where examiners simply 'missed' a lesion on one examination while they identified it on another (Poulsen *et al.*, 1980; Rosen *et al.*, 1996). This observation is supported by performance data for clinical and radiographic examinations. They typically present lower sensitivity and higher specificity values, suggesting that missing a lesion is a far more common occurrence than incorrectly identifying a sound surface as carious.

Multiple causes of examiner errors

Missed lesions, presumably due to a lack of clinician diligence or possibly skill in examining a tooth surface, is likely

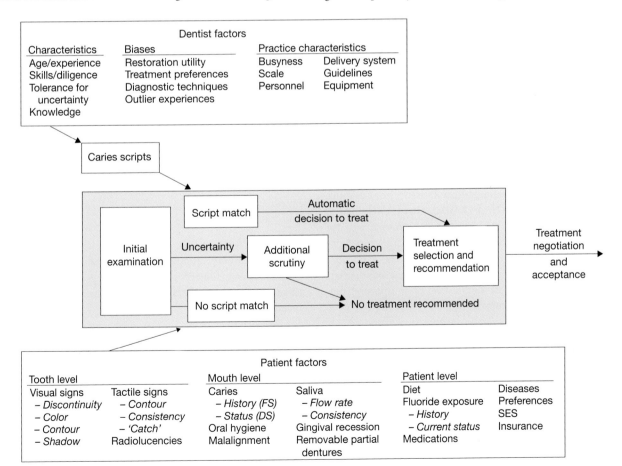

Figure 31.2 Conceptual model for dentists' caries-related treatment decisions. (From: Bader & Shugars, 1997.)

to represent only part of the variation thought to exist among clinicians in dental practice (as opposed to the variation seen in carefully controlled assessments of diagnostic methods). The effect of environmental variables such as

- clinician visual acuity
- use of magnification
- clinical examination
- view box illumination

have also been shown to affect diagnostic performance (Mileman *et al.*, 1984; Mann *et al.*, 1990; Forgie *et al.*, 2002). The effects of other environmental variables remain largely unexplored. A conceptual model (Fig. 31.2) of the restorative decision-making process hypothesized a variety of such environmental variables, and these will be discussed in a later section of this chapter (Bader & Shugars, 1997).

Examiners need frequent retraining

Individual differences in how clinicians interpret the subjective criteria that comprise most caries-detection criteria can clearly be a source of variation as well. The need to standardize dentist-examiners frequently is well known to researchers conducting longitudinal epidemiological caries examinations. Excellent agreement (kappa values above 0.80) between a gold standard, or reference examiner and other examiners usually can be achieved at the start of a study through an intense training session, typically involving paired or multiple examinations of more than 50 subjects over the course of a week. However, this level of agreement cannot be maintained without refresher standardization sessions on a semiannual or annual basis, depending on the examination cycle. Examiners drift, i.e. their interpretations of the examination criteria change over time, becoming dissimilar to those of the reference examiner. This is a natural phenomenon that occurs in the application of most subjective criteria, and the inevitable drifting necessitates restandardization to the reference examiner at frequent intervals. A similar drift is assumed to occur for clinicians in practice, but the opportunity for restandardization is rarely present after graduation from the educational program where the criteria were first learned, because except where patients are shared, dentists seldom find themselves in the position of comparing their caries-detection decisions with those of other dentists.

Dentists use patterns or 'scripts' to trigger restorative treatment

To complicate the issue further, there is some reason to suspect that dentists do not always identify caries using the process they were taught to use in most dental schools, namely, applying sequentially each criterion in a set of standardized criteria to each tooth surface. As usually taught, this 'search for signs' is the basis of most caries examination protocols, and when applied, it results in the informal or subjective determination of the probability that a lesion

exists on the surface in question. The search usually begins with a visual examination, but the results of this examination may prompt the collection of additional data from a more detailed visual examination and/or the use of ancillary diagnostic devices. It has been hypothesized that with experience, dentists adopt a more efficient version of this search process, based on pattern recognition. In this process each tooth or tooth surface, or its radiographic image, is scanned for similarity to one of a set of patterns or 'caries scripts' that signal to the dentist that restorative treatment is needed (Bader & Shugars, 1997; Baelum *et al.*, 2006).

From examination to treatment decision, omitting diagnosis

This process is outlined in Fig. 31.2. If the surface in question is an exact or a near exact match to one of many caries scripts maintained in a dentist's memory, the practitioner mentally designates the surface as in need of treatment, and often states that need in terms of exactly what treatment is recommended. Hence the fairly common observation of a dentist pointing to a radiolucency shown on the proximal surface of a bitewing radiograph, and stating 'that's a DO amalgam'. There has been no conscious diagnosis, just a match with an individualized, and often highly idiosyncratic pattern that the clinician recognizes as a clinical presentation that requires a particular restoration. In instances where the match is incomplete, i.e. some but not all features of the surface in question match determinative features of the script, a more careful inspection of the surface, and possibly ancillary detection methods may be used to gather additional information that can improve the match. Clearly, to the extent that this process operates, standardized caries detection criteria will have been subject to modification through clinicians' individual clinical experience and idiosyncrasies, as reflected in the caries scripts, with the result that the likelihood of agreement between any two dentists on the caries status of the surface will have been reduced.

Discussion

In this section an attempt has been made to demonstrate that there is extensive variation among clinicians in the identification of caries lesions. The variation occurs for several reasons:

- Clinicians use a variety of diagnostic methods that exhibit different levels of diagnostic performance.
- They apply different criteria for what constitutes a caries lesion even when using the same diagnostic method.
- Their interpretation of the same set of subjective criteria may vary, and their results may also vary owing to their diligence during examination, their visual acuity and examination conditions.
- Their level of suspicion, which may be related to their diligence, may vary depending on whether they have assessed

a patient's risk of caries, and the level of risk assigned to a patient.

- Their incorporation of their own personal experience and beliefs through the use of caries scripts may also contribute to differences in the classification of tooth surfaces.

A legitimate question may be: why has the dental profession tolerated this extensive variation in the detection of a widespread dental disease? While there is no simple answer to this question, it is instructive to mention some considerations related to how dentists practice that may help to explain why efforts to reduce this variation have not been in the forefront of improvements in dentistry.

It should be recognized that most dentists are comfortable with some degree of variation in caries detection because they experienced it during their clinical training, when their instructors disagreed. Most dental schools have not achieved standardization in caries detection among their staff, either because it has not been attempted, or because the attempts have been unsuccessful. This lack of concern in the face of differences in diagnostic performance stems in part from dentistry's roots in craftsmanship and its historical emphasis on technical excellence. In the not so distant past, the product was regarded by much of the profession as being far more important than the process, so that a dentist's worth was judged almost exclusively by the technical quality of his or her restorations. Diagnosis was simply a means of determining on which patients and teeth to bestow this technical excellence. Thus, diagnostic performance (accuracy) has been historically underemphasized in the profession compared with treatment performance. In addition, at least in the USA, there has been a historical tradition of not criticizing the diagnostic decisions and treatment of other clinicians (Bader & Shugars, 1995). The tradition seems to reflect the attitude of many clinicians that outcomes are dependent on circumstances not necessarily apparent at a later date, so that differences may not be the 'fault' of the clinician, and should not be criticized. This attitude would tend to reduce discomfort with disagreements about caries detection. Finally, it is not certain that the actual extent of the variation is recognized by most clinicians, because after their predoctoral dental education has been completed, they seldom have the opportunity to compare the results of their caries examinations with those of other dentists

Variation in caries management decisions

Variation among dentists in decisions associated with the management of caries is quite prevalent in dental practice. The variation is expressed principally through disagreement among dentists about whether restorative intervention is indicated following the detection of a lesion, but substantial variation may also occur in decisions about providing non-operative interventions and in the identification of people deemed to be at risk for dental caries.

Decisions about restorative interventions

Dentists do not agree when a restoration is required
The extent of disagreement among clinicians concerning decisions to intervene surgically by placing a restoration is summarized by the studies shown in Table 31.3. Similar to the examination of variation in caries detection, researchers began to assess variation in caries management decisions in the late 1970s, and these types of descriptive investigation have continued to appear since then. The studies in the table do not constitute an inclusive set of all such studies, but they do represent the majority of studies, and are those where the decision to intervene has been most clearly linked to the presence and extent of a caries lesion, rather than the condition of an existing restoration or any other reasons for restorative intervention. Remember that the variation reflected in this table is not a measure of what proportions of clinicians' treatment decisions are 'correct'. The included studies did not compare a clinician's decisions to a gold standard, simply to decisions of other clinicians.

Disagreements in selected treatment are substantial
Each of the studies of differences among clinicians' decisions to restore reflects substantial variation. When expressed as a range between the most frequent and least frequent rates, the ranges are generally near two-fold or greater and, with the exception of the study that included only three clinicians (Ermis & Aydin, 2004), seem not to be related to the number of clinicians providing treatment decisions. The kappa values and the ICC reflect moderate agreement levels over chance. Thus, the ranges found probably represent the general range of clinicians' decisions, rather than an abnormally wide range due to the inclusion of outliers. The variation is not clearly related to the method used to present the restorative decision, i.e. radiographs only, clinical examination only or both.

Variation is due to differences in detection and restorative treatment thresholds
It should be noted that these studies do not separate the variation due to differences in caries detection from the variation due to differences in what dentists think is the point in the development of a lesion where restoration is necessary. The variation due to detection of caries lesions is a part of the overall variation in decisions to restore teeth due to caries. The remainder of the variation occurs because dentists differ in their assessment of how advanced the caries process is, and in their restorative treatment thresholds, the point in the caries process where a dentist believes that restorative treatment is necessary. Several studies have asked dentists at what depth of caries penetration they typically decide that a restoration is required. The question is usually posed through a questionnaire or using line drawings of proximal lesions, with thresholds reported in terms of caries penetration into outer and inner halves, or outer,

Table 31.3 Variation in dentists' caries detection decisions

Study	Management decision	Case type	No. of dentists	No. of decisions	Range of positive decision	Interexaminer agreement
Rytömaa et al. (1979) Finland	Restoration indicated	Clinical *in vivo*	12 faculty	NR[a]	31–72[b]	–
Mileman et al. (1982) Netherlands	Restore proximal caries	Radiographs	42 faculty	300 surfaces	4–28%	–
Elderton & Nuttall (1983) UK	Restoration indicated	Clinical *in vivo* and radiographs	15 clinicians	NR[c]	20–153[b]	–
Mileman & van der Weele (1990) Netherlands	Restoration indicated	Radiographs	276 clinicians	105 surfaces	11–57%	–
Noar & Smith (1990) UK	Proximal restoration indicated	Clinical *in vitro* Radiograph	86 clinicians 86 clinicians	48 surfaces 48 surfaces	0–46% 6–50%	– –
Tveit & Espelid (1992) Norway	Replace proximal restoration	Clinical *in vitro* and radiographs	15 clinicians	77 surfaces	35–64%	–
Bader & Shugars (1995) USA	Restoration indicated	Clinical *in vivo* and radiographs	Mean of 6.7 clinicians	1187 teeth	–	0.53[d]
Lavonius et al. (1997) Finland	No treatment/restore/ seal occlusal surface	Clinical *in vitro*	10 clinicians	60 third molars	–	0.46[e]
Ermis & Aydin (2004) Turkey	Replace occlusive restoration	Clinical *in vivo*	3 clinicans	112 class I restorations	11–24%	0.46[e]

[a] Not reported, 10 subjects.
[b] Range of number of positive decisions.
[c] Not reported, 18 subjects.
[d] Intraclass correlation.
[e] Kappa statistic.

middle and inner thirds of enamel and dentin. Results of these types of studies demonstrate that there is variation in dentists' reports of the depth of penetration that signals the need for a restoration. For example, nine Canadian dentists felt it appropriate to intervene restoratively when caries reached the dento-enamel junction, three would restore enamel caries, and four would wait until caries had extended into the dentin (Lewis *et al.*, 1996). Perhaps more importantly, some of these studies also compared the dentists' stated restorative treatment thresholds with their recommendations for restorative treatment for several patient cases, presented as radiographs and a brief written description (Kay *et al.*, 1992; Mileman *et al.*, 1992; Lewis *et al.*, 1996). These studies determined that dentists do not adhere to their own stated thresholds when recommending treatment. It is not clear whether the differences were due to respondents' inaccuracy or inability to state the threshold clearly (Nuttall *et al.*, 1993), patient cases that contained features that caused dentists to depart from those thresholds, dentists' misinterpretation of caries penetration based on radiographs (Mileman *et al.*, 1992), or the fact that decisions to intervene restoratively are based on a complex set of factors, of which lesion depth is only one (Kay *et al.*, 1992). It may well be that dentists are not able to articulate

clearly the components of the particular caries script that signals the need for intervention.

Decisions about non-operative interventions

Little information is available on variation in non-operative interventions

The evidence describing variation in dentists' decisions about the non-operative management of patients with caries lesions, and those at elevated risk for such lesions, is less plentiful than for dentists' restorative decisions. The available studies have not compared dentists' non-operative treatment decisions for the same patients, so that the extent of agreement for individual patients for these types of caries-related treatment interventions is not known. What is available are studies describing dentists' 'practice patterns'. These patterns are determined either through asking dentists what they usually do with respect to non-operative caries interventions for their patients, or by examining dentists' treatment records to determine distributions of non-operative treatments. Similar to dentists' reports of treatment thresholds, information from dentist self-reports must be regarded with some caution, as dentists may tend to overestimate their frequency of use of non-operative interventions (Hassall & Mellor, 2001).

Patterns are often consistent within a practice

There is good evidence that, at least for children, a given general dentist will tend to provide the same non-operative treatment to every patient in his or her practice, which implies that the individual needs of children are not reflected in personalized treatment. Two-thirds of 1556 US dentists whose insurance claims were inspected provided fluoride treatments for more than 98% of children examined in their practices, while for an additional 20% of those dentists, no fluoride treatments were claimed (Eklund *et al.*, 2000). The recall intervals and non-operative treatment received by Finnish children with and without previous caries histories differed very little (Karkkainen *et al.*, 2001). More than two-thirds of Canadian dentists indicated that 6 months was the optimum recall interval for all child and adolescent patients, and fewer than 10% indicated that individual recall intervals should be determined for each patient (Main *et al.*, 1997). However, responses to a survey of US pediatric dentists indicated that they did take into account the severity of existing caries in deciding how to manage patients (Seale & Kendrick, 2001)

Practice patterns vary extensively between dentists

Even though individual general dentists may display practice patterns that seem relatively insensitive to individual children's non-operative treatment needs, these practice patterns can vary extensively among dentists. Differences have been reported in general dentists' use of various non-operative interventions, such as dietary advice, oral hygiene instruction, fluoride varnish, sealants and chlorhexidine rinses (Fiset & Grembowski, 1997; Fiset *et al.*, 2000; Eklund *et al.*, 2000; Hassall & Mellor, 2001). Some of these differences for more recently developed interventions have been ascribed to differences in the dentists' rates of adoption of innovation (Fiset & Grembowski, 1997; Fiset *et al.*, 2000).

Non-operative treatment for adults is rare

There is virtually no information describing dentists' use of non-operative treatment for adult patients. A test of performance measures in two public health clinics, two private dental practices, and two prepaid group dental practices, yielded six different estimates of the rate at which caries-active adults received any non-operative treatment that varied between 0 and 28% (Bader *et al.*, 1999b). Four of these rates were means, representing the treatment decisions of multiple dentists. These data suggest that decisions to provide non-operative treatment to adult patients who are presumably at elevated risk of caries vary among dentists, and among groups of dentists, although the variation occurs within a reduced range, as the provision of such treatment to adults is not common overall.

Dentists' assessment of caries risk status is also variable

Patient risk assessment has been advocated since the mid-1990s as a means of managing caries within dental practices

by directing non-operative treatment to those individuals who are most likely to experience caries activity (ADA, 1995; Pitts, 1998, NIH, 2001; Featherstone, 2004). Various assessment systems have been developed, but interrater reliability in categorizing patients using these systems has not been reported. Some systems are objective and use formulae for producing a risk score (van Palenstein Helderman *et al.*, 2001; Hänsel Petersson *et al.*, 2002), while others are essentially subjective assessments based on guidelines (Bader *et al.*, 2005). One pilot study of a subjective system that was tested in 16 private dental practices reported ranges for proportions of adult patients categorized at low, moderate and high risk for future caries. The range for high-risk classifications was from 0 to 16% of all patients classified, with a mean of 7%. For moderate risk, the range was much broader, from 8 to 61%, with a mean of 30% (Bader *et al.*, 2003). These mean proportions of patients classified at high and moderate risk are similar to the mean proportions classified at these risk levels from the only other two distributions that have been reported. Both of these other distributions also represent means of adult patients assessed by dentists in each of two prepaid group practices (Bader *et al.*, 2005). High-risk classifications were assigned to 4% and 11% of all patients, and moderate classifications accounted for 41% and 29%. No range of classification proportions reported by individual dentists was reported for either group practice. The guidelines for assessment were similar but not identical for all of these assessments. This very limited evidence corroborates the accuracy of caries risk assessments described in Chapter 29, and suggests that dentists' assessments of caries risk status will exhibit the same extensive variation found in their detection of lesions and in their management decisions.

Discussion

Variations can lead to accusations of dishonesty

A nationally circulated magazine in the USA published an article entitled 'How honest are dentists?' (Ecenbarger, 1997). The article reported the experiences of the author, who had visited 50 dentists across the country posing as a new patient seeking an examination and a treatment plan. The author received recommendations for treatment of between one and 28 teeth, with costs ranging from approximately $500 (the cost of one crown) to $29 850. The author questioned the honesty of dentists because they rendered such differing professional opinions. A representative of the American Dental Association (ADA) responded in the article by acknowledging that variation among dentists was to be expected because dentistry was both an art and a science, and by suggesting that second opinions were warranted if any doubts arose. Some letters appearing in professional journals questioned the accuracy of the author's methods, such as equating recommendations for 'basic' treatment with those for cosmetic treatment, but the majority railed at the author's conclusion that variation in diagnostic and treatment decisions raised issues of integrity.

Dentists acknowledge and accept the variation

This incident is instructive, in that it supports the suggestions in the previous section that dentists individually, and the profession as a whole, acknowledge that there is variation among dentists and that dentists do not realize how extensive the variation is. Clearly, the variation can lead to dramatic differences in the cost of treatment, and cost is an effective yardstick with which to capture the public's attention. Indeed, this should not have surprised the profession, as at least two similar cost analyses had already appeared in the professional literature (Elderton & Nuttall, 1983, Shugars & Bader, 1996). Despite the profession's apparent recognition of variation in treatment decisions, efforts to understand this variation as a first step towards reducing its magnitude have been limited. As the profession's public response to the 1997 article suggests, it has accepted the variation as an inevitable consequence of the subjective nature of treatment decisions required by practicing dentists.

Factors hypothesized to influence decision making

However, some assessments of the reasons for this variation have occurred. Figure 31.2 summarizes much of the findings of these assessments in the lists of 'dentist factors' and 'patient factors' that are hypothesized to influence the decision-making process. The model suggests that three types of patient factors:

- tooth level
- mouth or intraoral level
- patient level

influence treatment decisions. Tooth-level and mouth-level patient factors will be principal determinants of any treatment decision because they comprise most caries-detection criteria. What the model indicates is what was demonstrated in the previous section, i.e. that these factors can affect dentists differently, with the result that one dentist's treatment decision will differ from that of another dentist. Tooth- and mouth-level factors are posited to operate primarily through their incorporation into the caries scripts that drive treatment decisions. Because the caries scripts tend to be idiosyncratic, these factors will be important to some dentists, but not to others in making treatment decisions. Patient-level factors are more likely to play a role when the additional scrutiny pathway is activated, as the clinician gathers additional information in an attempt to improve an imperfect match with an existing script. This process is thought to be more consciously analytical and, hence, require the most information. Patient-level factors are also thought to be involved during the negotiation and acceptance process that occurs following the presentation of treatment recommendations.

The model also suggests that three types of dentist factors influence treatment decisions:

- personal characteristics
- biases
- practice characteristics.

The personal characteristics include skill/diligence, age/experience, knowledge and tolerance for uncertainty. As noted, there are suggestions that dentists' visual acuity may affect caries detection. In addition, dentists' tactile discrimination sensitivity (Dedmon, 1985; Pippin & Feil, 1992) may influence such detection, especially with respect to lesions associated with existing restorations. Dentist diligence is as yet unmeasured. Dentist age, and by extension, experience has been shown to influence treatment decisions, with older dentists typically being less aggressive (Bader & Shugars, 1992). Knowledge is a function of initial professional education and subsequent formal and informal learning. As used in the model, knowledge refers to accurate information describing the pathophysiology and epidemiology of dental caries and the outcomes of restorative and non-operative treatment for caries. Tolerance of uncertainty is assumed to play a yet-to-be elucidated role in treatment thresholds, perhaps increasing the probability for intervention among less tolerant dentists to lower the anxiety associated with doing nothing (Kahneman et al., 1982).

Dentists' opinions and preferences influence decisions

Dentists' biases are opinions and preferences that are obvious sources of subjectivity. The biases included in the model are their beliefs about treatment utilities, their treatment preferences, their use of diagnostic techniques and their 'outlier experiences'. Dentists' beliefs about the absolute and relative effectiveness of various non-operative and restorative interventions in terms of longevity and minimization of further disease will color treatment decisions. Treatment preferences, presumably based on the foregoing beliefs as well as convenience factors, personal experience and perceived skills, will also influence the decision. As previously discussed, the diagnostic techniques used will certainly influence the presentation of disease, and thus, its treatment. Outlier experiences which are unusual or unexpected outcomes of previous treatment decisions, often with serious consequences, can affect subsequent treatment decisions by being given greater consideration or weight by the dentist than their incidence would suggest they merit. Another bias that may operate is dentist belief about lesion activity. Some dentists do not attempt to differentiate lesions by activity status, while activity status is an important consideration in other dentists' treatment decisions. Because activity status is a subjective determination, consideration of this characteristic of a caries lesion will increase the likelihood of variation among dentists' treatment decisions.

Personal beliefs and opinions are favored in the absence of evidence

The relative paucity of evidence surrounding the prognosis of individual caries lesions with and without intervention is undoubtedly a major contributor to variation in both restorative and non-operative management decisions. Dentists' personal beliefs and opinions will dominate the model whenever sound information describing outcomes of alternative interventions for specific clinical situations is lacking. Unfortunately, long-term observational studies of the natural history of caries lesions in the absence of any intervention are scarce, as are evaluations of prognostic factors for successful non-operative treatments of specific lesions. In the absence of this type of information, dentists can and will substitute personal experience and opinion, both of which are subject to numerous biases.

Practice characteristics can influence treatment decisions

Finally, the model suggests that dentists' practice characteristics can influence treatment decisions. These relationships are generally assumed to be present, but they are currently incompletely documented and the method of influence is often not understood. These characteristics may affect the amount of time dentists spend with their patients, a dentist's willingness to undertake particular types of treatment, the scope of treatments that dentists are able to provide to their patients, or even the aggressiveness with which dentists conduct their examinations and recommend treatment of identified lesions. Differences in treatment services that patients receive, for example, have been found to be associated with reimbursement arrangements (Hazelkorn, 1985; Atchison & Schoen, 1990).

Possible reasons for underprovision of non-operative services

The model offers several explanations for the apparent underprovision of non-operative services to adults. For older dentists, knowledge factors may operate, in that dentists trained a generation ago were not always taught the importance of non-operative interventions for adult patients. Patient-level and practice-level factors may also operate, in that some financing schemes do not include adult non-operative treatment as a reimbursable expense. Finally, the model reflects observed dentist behavior during a dental examination, i.e. a tooth-by-tooth assessment of treatment needs, and suggests that for routine patient examinations, dentists do not consciously separate the detection of a caries lesion from the decision about the treatment of that lesion. Thus, the dentist's examination behavior naturally focusses on tooth-related restorative treatment for individual teeth. However, with the exception of dental sealants, non-operative interventions are usually applied to the entire dentition rather than a single tooth. There is no mechanism in the typical examination wherein the perceived need for non-operative treatment is intensified incrementally each time a caries-related restorative intervention is determined. As a result, it is more likely that a patient's non-operative needs will be overlooked.

The consequences of variation

Variation in decisions implies that some may be wrong

Variation among dentists in caries detection is a problem because it signals that some diagnoses will be incorrect, and that even given accurate detection, some management decisions will be likely to be inappropriate. Logically, if two dentists disagree on the presence of a lesion on a specific surface, one of those dentists will be wrong. The erroneous detection decision is very likely to lead to the provision of unnecessary treatment, or failure to provide needed treatment. Thus, the magnitude of the problem represented by variation in caries detection will depend on the outcomes associated with unnecessary treatment and the outcomes associated with the failure to provide needed treatment. In instances where caries has been detected, differences among dentists in decisions to intervene raise similar issues with respect to outcomes. Finally, even when dentists agree that caries is present and that intervention is necessary, differences in their decisions about what intervention to select will mean that some patients receive treatment that is, or may be, less appropriate than other patients. This occurs because the outcomes of the selected treatments will be different, and some may be less desirable than others. A brief consideration of what is meant by treatment outcomes should help to put these problems in perspective.

Treatment outcomes

Technical outcomes are frequently measured, but may be of minor importance

Treatment outcomes are events or conditions that are used as measures of the results of treatment. Traditionally, dentistry in general, and restorative dentistry in particular, has concerned itself with a small number of outcomes assessing a narrow range of clinical results, namely the 'quality' outcomes that dentists felt responsible for from a technical standpoint, such as smoothness of margins or adequacy of contours (Bader & Ismail, 1999). These outcomes are used to assess the quality or adequacy of restorations. However, there is very little evidence to suggest that these mechanical factors are important determinants of longer term, more global outcomes such as survival of the restoration, survival of the tooth or patient satisfaction (Bader & Shugars, 1995). These outcomes and others are likely to be of importance to patients and to those who pay for the treatment. Table 31.4 illustrates a classification system of oral health outcomes where the outcomes are grouped into four dimensions:

Table 31.4 Classification of outcomes of oral health care

Dimension	Examples
Biological:	
Physiological status	Salivary flow and consistency, demineralization, inflammation
Microbiological status	Oral microflora composition, presence of specific pathogens
Sensory status	Presence of pain, parethesia
Clinical:	
Survival status	Longevity/loss of tooth, pulp, tooth surface, restoration
Mechanical status	Smoothness of margins, conformation of contours
Diagnostic status	Presence of pathology, caries, periodontal disease
Functional status	Ability to chew, speak, swallow
Psychosocial:	
Satisfaction	Satisfaction with treatment, dentist, oral health
Perceptions	Aesthetics, oral health self-rating
Preferences	Values for health states and health events
Oral health-related quality of life	Ratings for how oral health affects life
Economic:	
Direct costs	Out-of-pocket payments, third party payments
Indirect costs	Time away from work, child-care payments

- biological
- clinical
- psychosocial
- economic (Bader & Ismail, 1999).

The examples listed in this table are intended to be illustrative, but not inclusive. The outcomes most familiar to clinical dentists are probably the mechanical outcomes, which are found within the clinical dimension, although clearly other outcomes in that dimension that address issues of survival, as well as outcomes in other dimensions that address satisfaction, sensation and cost may well be more important to patients.

Outcome information is sparse

Ideally, considerations of the outcomes associated with caries detection and management-related decisions should include as broad a selection of outcomes as possible. However, owing to its historically narrow focus, the profession's breadth of knowledge of outcomes of restorative treatment is extremely limited. Perhaps more surprisingly, the profession's depth of knowledge for even the most commonly considered outcomes is also quite shallow (Bader & Shugars, 1995; Bader & Ismail, 1999). For example, the incidence rate for pulp death following caries-related restorative treatment is thought to be quite low based on empirical observation. However, this outcome has not been determined accurately with prospective longitudinal studies either overall or by factors important to applying the information to individual patients, such as type of and size of restoration or patient age. A similar low rate was assumed to exist for crown restorations, but outcome studies subsequently demonstrated rates of more than 5% within 5 years (Martin & Bader, 1997) and 10 years (Kolker *et al.*, 2005). Thus, when seeking to quantify the extent to which variation can affect

outcomes, there is only a small palate of information with which to paint the picture. For example, it is not possible to state that an unnecessary restoration exposes the patient to an X% greater probability that the tooth will need additional restorative treatment in the next 10 years, or a Y% greater risk of loss of the tooth. Lack of this type of outcome information with which to quantify the risks of various treatment strategies makes it impossible to rank objectively the strategies in terms of the extent to which they minimize the risks that the dentists or patients most wish to avoid. A related problem is that determination of longer term outcomes of a given treatment requires time, and during that time, the standard treatment may change through the introduction of new materials or new methods. Thus, much of dentistry's treatment outcomes information will be outdated by the time it becomes available. Nevertheless, it is useful simply to identify the wide variety of outcomes that could potentially be affected by variation in dentists' detection and management decisions.

Outcomes affected by unnecessary treatment

Unnecessary operative treatment may be more detrimental than non-operative treatment

The short-term outcomes associated with unnecessary caries-related treatment will be the same as those associated with necessary treatment for dental caries, with the exception that no improvement in the patient disease status or disease risk status is gained as an outcome. The patient is exposed to the small, but not infinitesimal health risks associated with restorative dental treatment, spends time and perhaps money to receive the treatment, and perhaps suffers some small amount of physical or mental discomfort before, during or after the treatment. In the longer term, if the unnecessary treatment was non-operative in nature, no additional significant outcomes would be expected. If the intervention included placing a restoration, however, the probability increases that the tooth will require additional restorative treatment in the future, and that each succeeding restoration will result in the loss of additional tooth structure, increasing the risk of eventual tooth fracture (Elderton, 1990; Brantley *et al.*, 1995). However, the rapidity with which replacement takes place is not clear (Downer *et al.*, 1999), let alone the probability of other events in this cascade. An insufficient number of long-term observational studies of the natural history of restorations has been performed to permit a determination of how serious it is to place a restoration where none was needed. It is clear, however, that unnecessary restorative treatment does increase the likelihood of subsequent additional treatment for the same tooth, thus adversely affecting cost, convenience and satisfaction outcomes, as well as clinical outcomes associated with the long-term prognosis for the tooth.

Outcomes affected by failure to provide necessary treatment

Failure to provide non-operative treatment where such treatment would be appropriate will result in an increased probability of lesion development or progression. The outcomes associated with this unfortunate occurrence are the same as those discussed for unnecessary treatment. Although management is not 100% effective, i.e. some of the lesions that develop in the absence of non-operative treatment would have formed regardless of any prior intervention, others would have been prevented and, thus, can be considered as unnecessary. Assuming that these lesions eventually receive operative treatment, that treatment must also be considered as unnecessary because the lesions would not have arisen if the required non-operative treatment had been provided.

If, however, appropriate restorative treatment is not provided, then the outcomes are identical to the more general case of failure to provide necessary treatment. Here, outcomes will be dependent on the rapidity of progression or regression of the lesion, and the effect that the progression rate has on the likelihood that the lesion will be identified and treated before pulpal death or tooth loss occurs. With delayed intervention, the principal concern will be the increase in the probability of pulp death, and its attendant outcomes. Short of such catastrophic outcomes, delay may still affect the eventual size of the restoration and, hence, survival of the tooth over the longer term. Clearly, without intervention, some if not many lesions for which intervention is appropriate will progress to pupal death and eventual loss of the tooth. This process can involve discomfort, distress and functional impairment. Subsequent effects on functional, perceptual and preferential levels of outcomes must also be considered following tooth loss.

Outcomes affected by variation in treatment selection

Even when dentists agree that a non-operative intervention or a restorative intervention is necessary, differences among the interventions selected can influence outcomes. Again, because of incomplete information, it is difficult to quantify these differences. For example, with respect to non-operative interventions, fluoride varnishes and gels are both used in dental practice and fluoride mouthrinses are also recommended for home use, but there is conflicting evidence with respect to which intervention is more effective. A systematic review of studies that directly compared the three interventions found no conclusive evidence for differences between them (Marinho *et al.*, 2004), but when the studies comparing each intervention to a negative control are examined in other systematic reviews, the effectiveness estimates are different, albeit with overlapping confidence intervals. The prevented fraction for fluoride varnish was 46%, while for fluoride gel and mouthrinse it was 28% and 26%, respectively (Marinho *et al.*, 2002a, b, 2003). Similarly, when restorative interventions are selected, outcomes may vary among dentists owing to the specific nature of the intervention. For example, longevity is dependent on dentist-related factors such as restoration design and material, and operator skill.

Weighing the outcomes under uncertainty

The reason why the lack of broad and in-depth knowledge of the outcomes associated with caries detection and treatment is problematic can be illustrated by considering the management of 'suspicious areas', i.e. where a clinician is unsure about the presence of caries, typically on an occlusal surface. In such instances where the clinician estimates the probability of a lesion to be about 50%, the management decision is essentially a decision made under circumstances of uncertainty. Thus, the clinician must weigh or trade off the possible favorable and unfavorable outcomes associated with the treatment options. The options are to do nothing, to apply non-operative treatment or to initiate restorative treatment. Doing nothing, the classic 'watch', may an appropriate intervention if a lesion is present but inactive or slowly progressing. Here, delaying treatment to permit an assessment of change over time does not appreciably increase the risk of unsatisfactory outcomes such as marked progression, pulpal death, pain, tooth loss or associated increased costs of treatment. However, the lesion may be active and capable of rapid progression, in which instance a delay would increase the likelihood that one or more of these unfavorable outcomes may occur. Unfortunately, there is very little information available describing the actual clinical conditions and the outcomes associated with suspicious areas (Bader & Shugars, 2006). The meager evidence suggests that dentists' designations of suspicious areas are appropriate;

about 50% of these areas are, in fact, caries lesions that involve the dentin. However, estimates of the proportion of these suspicious areas that progress to demonstrable dentin caries over time range from 16% to 77% over 2 or more years (Hamilton *et al.*, 2002; Meiers & Jensen, 1984), offering clinicians little additional useful information upon which to base their management decisions.

Limited evidence on outcome of treatments

Non-operative treatment may be an appropriate intervention under some circumstances, because it offers the possibility of an additional favorable outcome, the cessation of demineralization, and possibly partial remineralization, depending on the non-operative therapy applied. Again, however, the available evidence describing outcomes of non-operative treatment for suspicious areas is quite limited (Bader & Shugars, 2006). No studies of the effects of fluorides or antimicrobial treatment on suspicious surfaces have been reported. One study of sealing over suspicious areas has appeared, which reported progression on two out of 17 surfaces after 5 years (Going *et al.*, 1978). A non-systematic review of the effects of sealing over frank caries lesions found either no progression or low rates of progression when sealants remained intact (Bader & Shugars, 2006). When sealants were not intact, however, progression was more frequent.

Outcomes of restorative treatment for suspicious areas also have not been explicitly studied. A systematic review of conservative restorative treatment in the form of preventive resin restorations, the type of restoration that would presumably be most frequently used for suspicious areas, found strong evidence for effectiveness, but again, only if the sealant remained intact (McComb, 2001).

Variation is inevitable with limited evidence to inform decisions

This, then, is the available scientific evidence to inform a clinician's decision concerning the management of a 'suspicious' area. It offers little in the way of strong indications for a decision one way or another. There is almost no information to describe the outcomes of chief clinical importance, and no information about other outcomes that may be relevant to patients. In the absence of this evidence, clinicians will make decisions, or will help patients to make decisions based only on their clinical experience and their own preferences and biases. There will be substantial variation in these decisions, and because of the lack of evidence, no one can say which decisions are appropriate, and which are inappropriate.

A long-term approach to reducing variation

The extensive variation among dentists' caries detection and management decisions documented in this chapter has been shown to arise through several causal mechanisms. To reduce the magnitude of this variation, which presumably will have the effect of reducing the amount of inappropriate care provided to dental patients, dentistry must adopt approaches that address most if not all of these mechanisms. Formal and informal regulatory methods exist that attempt to reduce some of the variation associated with treatment selection, including administrative regulations and reimbursement policies. These methods will not be discussed here because they do not address the causal mechanisms of variation. Rather, these methods tend to reduce variation by limiting dentists' and patients' options. Variation related to detection of caries lesions may be substantially reduced with the introduction and adoption of new technology that eliminates the need for subjectivity while increasing accuracy. A discussion of such developing technology is beyond the scope of this chapter, but it is instructive to realize that one of the first such emerging technologies has been shown to be less effective than more traditional methods (Bader & Shugars, 2004), a reminder that 'early adopters' should maintain their objectivity and demand sound studies demonstrating equivalence or superiority to existing methods. To a significant degree, the causal mechanisms of variation are related to a lack of current, accurate, specific knowledge, both that held by individual dentists and that available in the professional dental knowledge base. This section describes applications of a general approach known as evidence-based dentistry to address this lack of knowledge.

Evidence-based dentistry as a possible solution

Evidence-based dentistry has been defined as 'the judicious integration of systematic assessments of clinically relevant scientific evidence, relating to the patient's oral and medical condition and history, with the dentist's clinical expertise and the patient's treatment needs and practices' (ADA, 2003). Perhaps a more straightforward definition would be the application of the most current knowledge to patient care. What is 'new' about this concept is the emphasis it places on the direct incorporation into practice of systematic assessments of clinically relevant scientific evidence. From its earliest origins, dentistry has relied on 'experts' to inform and guide professional practice through their integration and communication of the professional knowledge base (Bader, 2004a). The amount and depth of information available to these experts have gradually increased in quantity and improved in accuracy as its basis has transitioned from individual clinical experience, through uncontrolled observation, case studies and series and prospective cohort studies, to randomized clinical trials (Bader, 2004a). However, despite this steady increase in quantity and quality of available information, the principal methods used to organize and disseminate that information to practitioners have changed very little. Dentistry still relies on the opinions of experts, in the form of journal articles, 'practice gurus' and continuing education presentations. The problem with this approach of experts filtering the primary scientific literature is that, just like clinicians, experts can and will disagree. The promise of evidence-based dentistry is the attention paid to objective collection, analysis and dissemination of all of the relevant information to answer specific clinical questions for practitioners. Not only will the existing knowledge be more effectively packaged for use in practice, but also gaps in knowledge will be more readily identified and, possibly, filled more quickly by new investigations. As has been demonstrated in preceding sections, both the existence of needed knowledge and its application are problems that plague the diagnosis, treatment and prevention of dental caries.

Systematic reviews

The process of systematic reviews

The collection and analysis of the scientific literature that characterizes evidence-based dentistry are accomplished through systematic reviews (Bader, 2004b; Ismail & Bader, 2004). Table 31.5 shows the steps in performing a systematic review, which is designed to answer a specific clinical question. The question is usually quite narrow in its scope, so that the answer can be applied directly to patients by practitioners. The first step in a systematic review is to structure the clinical question by specifying

- the population
- the intervention
- the comparison
- the outcome of interest.

Identifying these elements will increase the utility of the review to practitioners by indicating more directly those clinical situations to which the results of the review can be applied. Criteria for inclusion and exclusion are stated so that only high-quality, directly relevant studies are included in the review. A thorough search is then performed using several electronic and paper indices, as well as inspection of reference lists of relevant studies and searches of the gray literature (e.g. dissertations, conference reports, abstracts, unpublished studies). Each possibly relevant study identified by the search is examined by two reviewers, who independently apply the inclusion and exclusion criteria to determine whether it should be included in the review. If included, information describing the study's methods and results as well as an objective assessment of study quality are abstracted, again by two reviewers separately, and included in an evidence table. This evidence table then serves as the basis of a narrative review that presents the pertinent results from all included studies as well as classifying the strength of this available evidence. Where possible, given the nature of the available studies, a meta-analysis is also performed, which combines the results of the included studies statisti-

cally. Both the qualitative and quantitative summaries attempt to synthesize objectively the information in the evidence table to produce a clear, direct answer to the clinical question that initiated the review process, as well as a commentary on the quality of the research that answers the question (Bader 2004b). Each step of the review is itself reviewed by an expert advisory panel whose function is to provide oversight to refine each of these processes.

Eliminating bias

Systematic reviews minimize the biases that are inherent in the expert-based system of information collection, analysis and dissemination, as characterized by the traditional literature review. Bias can enter a traditional review through an unfocussed question, a less than thorough search of the literature, subjective inclusion of studies from among those identified by the search, a lack of consideration of the strengths and weaknesses of individual studies, and a subjective synthesis of results. While all of this sounds thoroughly academic, it is important to realize that dentistry is entering an era where better information about the outcomes of treatment will be demanded by purchasers of care, whether the purchaser be an individual patient, an insurance company or the purchaser of that insurance, or a governmental entity. Systematic reviews of the scientific evidence, as a principal element of evidence-based dentistry, will form an increasingly important means of summarizing and standardizing the current knowledge about the outcomes of detection and diagnostic decisions. The number of clinically relevant published systematic reviews is growing rapidly, and the reviews that constitute this growth have both clarified the effectiveness of many dental treatments by objectively quantifying the outcomes of that treatment, and exposed the relative paucity of high-quality studies of outcomes for many other dental treatments (Bader & Ismail, 2004).

Identifying gaps in knowledge; focussing subsequent research

Systematic reviews also identify the additional specific knowledge necessary to answer clinical questions satisfactorily. They do this both by noting instances where there is insufficient information to answer the specific clinical question posed by the review, and by identifying questions where the available research is of low quality. Low-quality research is typically defined as research where the design of the study and/or the methods used leave the results open to bias, i.e. an event, trend or predilection that distorts the results of a study. Results from studies open to bias must be considered equivocal, and are less useful in resolving clinical issues. The great hope, as yet unevaluated in any formal manner, is that the identification of questions for which systematic reviews reveal that there is no, or only low-quality research will lead to resolution of the problem through the initiation of new studies that address the needed questions and use designs

Table 31.5 Steps in performing a systematic review

1. **Formulate key clinical question**

   Population or patient type: persons for whom an answer is sought

   Intervention or exposure: treatment or clinical condition of interest

   Comparison: alternative treatment or control condition

   Outcome: measure(s) used to assess effects

2. **State inclusion and exclusion criteria**

   Key question PICO[a] elements

   Details of population/subject eligibility

   Details of treatment procedures

   Details of evaluation procedures

   Publication language(s)

   Publication dates

   Study design(s)

3. **Develop search strategy**

   Electronic indices: Medline, Embase, etc.

   Cochrane library

   Handsearching: current and non-indexed journals

   Reference listings

   Gray literature: theses, dissertations, conference reports, abstracts, unpublished

4. **Search and select studies**

   Application of inclusion and exclusion criteria

   Two reviewers independently list studies included and excluded

   Rules for resolving disagreements, calculation of agreement statistics

   Two stages: title/abstract, full paper

   Log of reasons for exclusion (at full-paper stage only)

5. **Extract data**

   Design evidence table: identify needed data elements, i.e. research design, subjects, methods, results, additional quality criteria

   Design abstraction form

   Two abstractors independently fill in abstraction forms

   Rules for resolving disagreements

6. **Analyze and present results**

   Evidence table(s)

   Quality of included studies

   Qualitative summary: designs, outcomes

   Quantitative summary: heterogeneity, meta-analysis, meta-regression, sensitivity analysis

7. **Interpret the review results**

   Limitations of the review

   Implications for needed research

   Implications for the clinician

   Strength of the evidence

[a] PICO is an acronym for population, intervention, comparison, outcome.

that minimize bias. While the health sciences have relied principally on individual investigators to develop new knowledge using this exact process informally, the formal assessment of needed knowledge presented in a systematic review is expected to focus investigators' efforts, resulting in more rapid and efficient acquisition of new information. This idealistic expectation may be facilitated by administrative interventions on the part of organizations that fund and/or pursue research that would demand that research proposals be accompanied by systematic reviews that demonstrate the need for and potential application of the proposed research.

Translation to practice

How do dentists acquire information?

Systematic reviews have the potential to resolve a major source of variation among dentists, inaccurate information. It is quite possible to read different traditional reviews of the literature and find that the reviewers reach entirely oppo-

site conclusions (see, for example, reviews assessing the clinical utility of caries dyes: van de Rijke, 1991; Ross, 1998; McComb, 2000; Young, 2002). This type of variation is less likely to occur when the reviews are systematic, because the opportunities for bias are strictly limited. However, as Figure 31.2 indicates, a simple lack of knowledge (and concomitant reliance on experience and opinion) is perhaps as potent a source of variation as possession of incorrect knowledge. As defined, practicing evidence-based dentistry requires dentists to 'judiciously integrate' the information in systematic reviews into their clinical decision making. However, the methods through which dentists are to acquire and learn this information are undefined. This process of acquisition and application of new knowledge and techniques, variously termed science transfer, adoption of innovation, dissemination of information, provider behavioral change and translation to practice, must operate across a large majority of clinicians if evidence-based dentistry is to reduce variation in clinicians' detection and treatment decisions.

Practice guidelines and evidence summaries

Two vehicles are most likely to become the principal methods of dissemination of scientific knowledge to practitioners in the future: evidence-based clinical practice guidelines and evidence summaries. An evidence-based clinical practice guideline is based on one or more systematic reviews, but it is usually developed by a panel of experts who examine and analyze the systematic reviews in an effort to understand all of the available information pertaining to the subject of the guideline (Field & Lohr, 1992). The guideline typically identifies a particular clinical situation, lays out the clinical decisions that are inherent in addressing the situation, summarizes the evidence informing those decisions, and usually describes a preferred course of action in the form of a highly summarized set of suggestions representing what a reasoned, well-informed clinician would do in the situation described by the guideline. An example could be a description of the recommended approach to treating 'suspicious areas', based on the available evidence. An evidence summary is essentially a highly condensed version of a systematic review, often accompanied by an expert clinician's commentary. Note that even in these evidence-based methods of translation to practice, the presence of the expert has been preserved, although the role of the expert has been changed from 'knowledge giver' to 'clinical consultant'.

Achieving behavior change among dentists

With evidence summaries and evidence-based clinical practice guidelines, accurate, unbiased information and associated clinical suggestions or commentary are made easily accessible to practitioners. However, printed materials alone have been shown to have only minor effects on physicians' practice behaviors (Freemantle et al., 2000). Achieving behavioral change among dentists to reduce variation will undoubtedly require more effective intervention techniques. Again, among physicians, there is evidence for the effectiveness of three intervention techniques:

- participatory workshops (Thomson O'Brien et al., 2001)
- audit and feedback (Jamtvedt et al., 2003)
- educational outreach (Thomson O'Brien et al., 2000).

The high cost of educational outreach interventions, where a consultant works directly with an individual dentist or dental practice to accomplish defined goals, probably renders this approach impractical for achieving mass change in dentistry. However, both participatory workshops and audit and feedback programs that are integrated into existing continuing dental education networks represent potentially effective methods for achieving practitioner behavioral change among large numbers of currently practicing dentists. This approach would require continuing education

providers consciously to adopt an evidence-based approach for all of their course presentations, including ensuring that presenters:

- design their courses around relevant clinical questions
- base their presentations on the results of systematic reviews
- structure the learning activities to include active participation.

Active participation would also furnish opportunities for participants to standardize caries detection decisions. Audit and feedback require practitioners to analyze their own treatment records to determine the distribution of short- and longer term outcomes in their practices associated with specific treatments. A practitioner's outcomes are compared to standards derived from systematic reviews or, if standards have not been promulgated, to the outcomes of their peers. These comparisons then serve as the focus for discussions of changes in practice procedures that may lead to improvements in the outcomes.

Practice guidelines and evidence summaries may gradually change practice and reduce variation

The growing presence of treatment guidelines and evidence summaries, and the anticipated inclusion of effective strategies for behavioral change in continuing education, will lead to gradual change in how dentists practice and concomitant reduction in variation among dentists and improvement in the outcomes of treatment. However, these types of intervention cannot promise rapid change. Human nature being what it is, rapid change is seldom achieved. Even the transition from 'wet fingers' to the universal use of gloves, a change made imperative by the spread of AIDS in the mid-1980s, was not accomplished easily, and practitioners' resistance was typically overcome only gradually (Brantley et al., 1986). The pace of change could be quickened by other types of intervention. For example, if the evidence for the effectiveness of non-operative intervention for caries-active adults were sufficiently strong, it is conceivable that governmental regulatory entities or payers might mandate the use of these interventions for such patients. At present, despite more than a decade of urging such interventions (ADA, 1995), there has been scant evidence of the effectiveness of any non-operative intervention among adults (NIH, 2001), or of the routine use of such interventions for patients thought to be at risk for caries development or progression (Bader et al., 2003).

Modifying caries scripts

It should also be noted that the application of evidence-based principles to dental practice will affect caries management decisions more than caries detection decisions. To the extent that Figure 31.2 is correct in suggesting that for experienced practitioners, caries detection is highly idiosyncratic, and represents the sum of a practitioner's experience, skill and diligence, many of the interventions described above may not be highly effective in influencing those decisions. Arguably, what might be the most effective 'evidence-based' approach to achieving change in caries detection decisions would be to demonstrate that an individual practitioner's decisions do not agree with those of the majority. This type of evidence could be generated by asking continuing education participants to complete a set of standardized visual detection exercises. Outliers in this exercise would be alerted to their status, and given the opportunity to review their personal detection criteria. The emphasis would be on attempting to modify the caries scripts that had been developed over the dentists' time in practice to reflect the most accurate set of criteria reported in the literature. Such an intervention might also entail evidence-based changes in dentists' examination procedures. However, it is unlikely that such an intervention would be a popular choice among current practitioners in the absence of incentives for change, and the effectiveness of such an intervention is also open to question.

Translation to education

Dental education should embrace these ideas

Another avenue for the eventual reduction of variation in dentists' caries detection and management decisions lies in changes in predoctoral dental education. As suggested in the introduction to this chapter, and demonstrated in Tables 31.1 and 31.2, the variation seen in dental practice is also evident in the microcosm of a dental faculty. By setting the example of good agreement among professionals based on the evidence, students will be more aware of instances of disagreement, and may take greater pains to scrutinize their own decisions in the light of what is known, rather than what they believe. For some educators, such an emphasis on the unbiased evidence as presented in systematic reviews will require the same types of behavioral change required of clinicians in full-time practice. However, such change can be accomplished more readily in a controlled environment with administrative oversight.

Faculty should review evidence and develop guidelines

The types of change that could be instituted include thorough departmental reviews of clinical curricula to ensure that what is taught clinically is supported by the available evidence. Where the evidence is lacking, a faculty might consider initiating the studies necessary to develop that evidence. Departments might consider developing evidence-based practice guidelines for application in the school's clinics as a means of accomplishing these goals. Likewise, all didactic presentations should also be based on the evidence, and this evidence should be accessible by students. As a reminder, when one claims that a position or a decision is based on the evidence, it implies that a thorough, unbiased search of the available evidence has been performed. All too

often an expert, such as a dental instructor, will offer a single citation as the evidence in support, with little or no consideration of what the totality of the evidence indicates.

Standardize faculty and students in caries detection

Another change in dental education that could promote an eventual reduction in variation in the detection of dental caries in dental practice would be to achieve better initial standardization of dental students. Within a single dental school, such standardization would first require the faculty who supervise these students to achieve and maintain standardization. An evidence-based single method or set of methods and procedures for caries detection would have to be adopted, together with their associated criteria. Frequent standardization sessions would be necessary to achieve and maintain a single standard for detection. However, the effort could pay dividends in that students would not only be in good agreement with other students and with the faculty in detection decisions, but also be more likely to seek out opportunities to maintain standardized status following graduation. In the longer term, the profession should become more concerned about variation in caries detection, presumably with a positive effect on agreement.

Develop single professional standards

Ideally, dental school faculties would also strive to reduce interprogram variation, essentially trying to achieve a single professional standard for caries detection. As with standardization within a single dental school, such a goal would require adoption of a single protocol for caries detection, and this requirement may make such a goal unachievable. Given this observation, and the previous acknowledgement that attempting to change caries detection behaviors among those already in practice is likely to be difficult, it may be that the best strategy for minimization of variation among practitioners is to concentrate efforts towards the development of completely objective detection techniques, so that the need for subjective interpretation is minimized.

Discussion

Evidence-based dentistry is not a panacea for the extensive variation that exists in caries-related treatment decisions. The purpose of presenting a discussion of evidence-based dentistry as a possible long-term approach for reducing variation in caries decision making is to drive home the realization that a principal underlying cause of this variation is a lack of knowledge. In some instances the needed knowledge does not exist, while in others it is available, but not being used by clinicians. Evidence-based dentistry, by making the linkage between clinical questions and the dental knowledge base explicit and specific, both reminds professionals of their obligation to continue to learn and provides them with objective summaries of all that is known about specific clinical decisions that they make routinely in their practices. To the extent that this linkage appears repeatedly in all professional contexts, the breadth, quality and utility of the information available to practitioners should improve. Immersion in evidence-based dentistry in predoctoral dental education, coupled with repeated exposure in all postdoctoral and continuing dental educational contacts as well as universally in the professional literature, could lessen the profession's widespread trust in and dependence on personal experience and unsupported expert opinion as the primary determinants for clinical decision making.

References

American Dental Association, Council of Access, Prevention, and Interprofessional Relations. Caries diagnosis and risk assessment: a review of professional strategies and management. *J Am Dent Assoc* 1995; **126** (Suppl):1–24S.

American Dental Association. *ADA policy on evidence-based dentistry.* 2003. Available from: http://www.ada.org/prof/resources/positions/statements/evidencebased.asp; accessed 23 January 2006.

Atchison K, Schoen M. A comparison of quality in a dual-choice dental plan: capitation versus fee-for-service. *J Public Health Dent* 1990; **50**: 186–93.

Bader J. The fourth phase. *J Evid Based Dent Pract* 2004a; **4**: 12–15.

Bader J. Systematic reviews and their implications for dental practice. *Texas Dent J* 2004b; **121**: 380–7.

Bader J, Ismail A. A primer on outcomes in dentistry. *J Public Health Dent* 1999; **59**: 131–5.

Bader J, Ismail A. Survey of systematic reviews in dentistry. *J Am Dent Assoc* 2004; **135**: 464–73.

Bader J, Shugars D. Understanding dentists' restorative treatment decisions. *J Public Health Dent* 1992; **52**: 102–10.

Bader J, Shugars D. Variation, treatment outcomes, and practice guidelines in dental practice. *J Dent Educ* 1995; **59**: 61–96.

Bader J, Shugars D. What do we know about how dentists make caries-related treatment decisions? *Community Dent Oral Epidemiol* 1997; **25**: 97–103.

Bader J, Shugars D. A systematic review of the performance of a laser fluorescence device for detecting caries. *J Am Dent Assoc* 2004; **135**: 1413–26.

Bader J, Shugars D. The evidence supporting alternative management strategies for early occlusal caries and suspected occlusal dentinal caries. *J Evid Based Dent Pract* 2006; **6**: 91–100.

Bader J, Shugars D, White B, Rindal D. Development of effectiveness of care and use of services measures for dental care plans. *J Public Health Dent* 1999a; **59**: 142–9.

Bader J, Shugars D, White B, Rindal D. Evaluation of audit-based performance measures for dental care plans. *J Public Health Dent* 1999b; **59**: 150–7.

Bader J, Shugars D, Bonito A. A systematic review of the performance of methods for identifying carious lesions. *J Public Health Dent* 2002; **62**: 201–13.

Bader J, Shugars D, Kennedy J, Hayden W, Baker S. A pilot study of risk-based prevention in private practice. *J Am Dent Assoc* 2003; **134**: 1195–202.

Bader J, Perrin N, Maupome G, Rindal B, Rush W. Validation of a simple approach to caries risk assessment. *J Public Health Dent* 2005; **65**: 76–81.

Baelum V, Heidmann J, Nyvad B. Dental caries paradigms in diagnosis and diagnostic research. *Eur J Oral Sci* 2006; **114**: 263–77.

Brantley C, Heymann H, Shugars D, Vann W. The effects of gloves on psychomotor skills acquisition among dental students. *J Dent Educ* 1986; **50**: 611–13.

Brantley C, Bader J, Shugars D, Nesbit S. Does the cycle of rerestoration lead to larger restorations? *J Am Dent Assoc* 1995; **126**: 1407–13.

Dedmon H. Ability to evaluate non-visible margins with an explorer. *Oper Dent* 1985; **10**: 6–11.

Downer M, Azli N, Bedi R, Moles D, Setchell D. How long do routine dental restorations last? A systematic review. *Br Dent J* 1999; **187**: 432–9.

Ecenbarger W. How honest are dentists? *Readers Digest* 1997; (February): 50–6.

Eklund S, Pittman J, Heller K. Professionally applied topical fluoride and restorative care in insured children. *J Public Health Dent* 2000; **60**: 33–8.

Ekstrand K, Ricketts D, Longbottom C, Pitts N. Visual and tactile assessment of arrested initial enamel carious lesions: an *in vivo* pilot study. *Caries Res* 2005; **39**: 173–7.

Elderton R. Clinical studies concerning re-restoration of teeth. *Adv Dent Res* 1990; **4**: 4–9.

Elderton R, Nuttall N. Variation among dentists in planning treatment. *Br Dent J* 1983; **154**: 201–6.

Ermis R, Aydin U. Examiner agreement in the replacement decision of class I amalgam restorations. *J Contemp Dent Pract* 2004; **5**: 1–8.

Espelid I, Tveit A, Haugejorden O, Riordan P. Variation in radiographic interpretation and restorative treatment decisions on approximal caries among dentists in Norway. *Community Dent Oral Epidemiol* 1985; **13**: 26–9.

Featherstone J. The caries balance: the basis for caries management by risk assessment. *Oral Health Prev Dent* 2004; **2** (Suppl 1): 259–64.

Field M, Lohr K, eds. *Guidelines for clinical practice; from development to use.* Washington, DC: National Academy Press, 1992.

Fiset L, Grembowski D. Adoption of innovative caries-control services in dental practice: a survey of Washington State dentists. *J Am Dent Assoc* 1997; **128**: 337–45.

Fiset L, Grembowski D, Del Aguila M. Third-party reimbursement and use of fluoride varnish in adults among general dentists in Washington State. *J Am Dent Assoc* 2000; **131**: 961–8.

Forgie A, Pine C, Pitts N. The use of magnification in a preventive approach to caries detection. *Quintessence Int* 2002; **33**: 13–16.

Freemantle N, Harvey E, Wolf F, Grimshaw J, Grilli R, Bero L. Printed educational materials: effects on professional practice and health care outcomes. *Cochrane Database Syst Rev* 2000; (Issue 2): CD000172.

Going R, Loesche W, Grainger D, Syed S. The viability of microorganisms in carious lesions five years after covering with a fissure sealant. *J Am Dent Assoc* 1978; **97**: 455–62.

Hamilton J, Dennison J, Stoffers K, Gregory W, Welch K. Early treatment of incipient carious lesions: a two-year clinical evaluation. *J Am Dent Assoc* 2002; **133**: 1643–51.

Hänsel Petersson G, Twetman S, Bratthall D. Evaluation of a computer program for caries risk assessment in schoolchildren. *Caries Res* 2002; **36**: 327–40.

Hassall D, Mellor A. An investigation into sealant restoration usage in general dental practice in England. *Br Dent J* 2001; **191**: 388–90.

Hazelkorn H. A comparison of dental treatment plans under different reimbursement systems. *J Public Health Policy* 1985; **6**: 223–35.

Ismail A. Visual and visuo-tactile detection of dental caries. *J Dent Res* 2004; **83** (Special No. C): C56–66.

Ismail A, Bader J. Evidence-based dentistry in clinical practice. *J Am Dent Assoc* 2004; **135**: 78–83.

Jamtvedt G, Young J, Kristoffersen D, Thomson O'Brien M, Oxman A. Audit and feedback: effects on professional practice and health care outcomes. *Cochrane Database Syst Rev* 2003; (Issue 3): CD000259.

Kahneman D Slovic P, Tversky A. *Judgment under uncertainty: heuristics and biases.* Cambridge: Cambridge University Press, 1982.

Karkkainen S, Seppa L, Hausen H. Dental check-up intervals and caries preventive measures received by adolescents in Finland. *Community Dent Health* 2001; **18**: 157–61.

Kay E, Nuttall N, Knill-Jones R. Restorative treatment thresholds and agreement in treatment decision-making. *Community Dent Oral Epidemiol* 1992; **20**: 265–8.

Kolker J, Damiano P, Caplan D, et al. Teeth with large amalgam restorations and crowns: factors affecting the receipt of subsequent treatment after 10 years. *J Am Dent Assoc* 2005; **36**: 738–48.

Landis J, Koch G. The measurement of observer agreement for categorical data. *Biometrics* 1977; **33**: 159–74.

Langlais R, Skoczylas L, Prihoda T, Langland O, Schiff T. Interpretation of bitewing radiographs: application of the kappa statistic to determine rater agreements. *Oral Surg Oral Med Oral Pathol* 1987; **64**: 751–6.

Lavonius E, Kerosuo E, Kallio P, Pietila I, Mjor I. Occlusal restorative decisions based on visual inspection – calibration and comparison of different methods. *Community Dent Oral Epidemiol* 1997; **25**: 156–9.

Lazarchik D, Firestone A, Heaven T, Filler S, Lussi A. Radiographic evaluation of occlusal caries: effect of training and experience. *Caries Res* 1995; **29**: 355–8.

Lewis D, Kay E, Main P, Pharoah M, Csima A. Dentists' stated restorative treatment thresholds and their restorative and caries depth decisions. *J Public Health Dent* 1996; **56**: 176–81.

McComb D. Caries-detector dyes – how accurate and useful are they? *J Can Dent Assoc* 2000; **66**: 195–8.

McComb D. Systematic review of conservative operative caries management strategies. *J Dent Educ* 2001; **65**: 1154–61.

Main P, Lewis D, Hawkins R. A survey of general dentists in Ontario, Part II: Knowledge and use of topical fluoride and dental prophylaxis practices. *J Can Dent Assoc* 1997; **63**: 607, 610–17.

Mann D, Makinson O, Pietrobon R. Operating illumination to differentiate dental hard tissues. *Quintessence Int* 1990; **21**: 741–7.

Marinho V, Higgins J, Logan S, Sheiham A. Fluoride varnishes for preventing dental caries in children and adolescents. *Cochrane Database Syst Rev* 2002a; (Issue 3): CD002279.

Marinho V, Higgins J, Logan S, Sheiham A. Fluoride gels for preventing dental caries in children and adolescents. *Cochrane Database Syst Rev* 2002b; (Issue 2): CD002280.

Marinho V, Higgins J, Logan S, Sheiham A. Fluoride mouthrinses for preventing dental caries in children and adolescents. *Cochrane Database Syst Rev* 2003; (Issue 3): CD002284.

Marinho V, Higgins J, Sheiham A, Logan S. One topical fluoride (toothpastes, or mouthrinses, or gels, or varnishes) versus another for preventing dental caries in children and adolescents. *Cochrane Database Syst Rev* 2004; (Issue 1): CD002780.

Martin J, Bader J. Five-year treatment outcomes for teeth with large amalgams and crowns. *Operat Dent* 1997; **22**: 72–8.

Meiers J, Jensen M. Management of the questionable carious fissure: invasive vs noninvasive techniques. *J Am Dent Assoc* 1984; **108**: 64–8.

Mileman P, van der Weele L. Accuracy in radiographic diagnosis: Dutch practitioners and dental caries. *J Dent* 1990; **18**: 130–6.

Mileman P, Purdell-Lewis D, van der Weele L. Variation in radiographic caries diagnosis and treatment decisions among university teachers. *Community Dent Oral Epidemiol* 1982; **10**: 329–34.

Mileman P, Purdell-Lewis D, van der Weele L, Leertouwer H. Diagnostic variation caused by differences in viewbox illumination and visual ability. *Dentomaxillofac Radiol* 1984; **13**: 51–8.

Mileman P, Mulder E, van der Weele L. Factors influencing the likelihood of successful decisions to treat dentin caries from bitewing radiographs. *Community Dent Oral Epidemiol* 1992; **20**: 175–80.

National Institutes of Health, Consensus Development Panel. Diagnosis and management of dental caries throught life. NIH Consensus Development Statement March 26–28, 2001. *J Dent Educ* 2001; **65**: 1162–8.

Noar S, Smith B. Diagnosis of caries and treatment decisions in approximal surfaces of posterior teeth *in vitro*. *J Oral Rehabil* 1990; **17**: 209–18.

Nuttall N, Clarkson J. Can dental epidemiological information be gathered during routine dental examinations by general dental practitioners? *Community Dent Health* 2005; **22**: 101–5.

Nuttall N, Pitts N, Fyffe H. Assessment of reports by dentists of their restorative treatment thresholds. *Community Dent Oral Epidemiol* 1993; **21**: 273–8.

van Palenstein Helderman W, Mulder J, van't Hof M, Truin G. Validation of a Swiss method of caries prediction in Dutch children. *Community Dent Oral Epidemiol* 2001; **29**: 341–5.

Pippin D, Feil P. Interrater agreement on subgingival calculus detection following scaling. *J Dent Educ* 1992; **56**: 322–6.

Pitts N. Risk assessment and caries prediction. *J Dent Educ* 1998; **62**: 762–70.

Poulsen S, Bille J, Rugg-Gunn A. Evaluation of a calibration trial to increase interexaminer reliability of radiographic diagnosis of approximal carious lesions. *Community Dent Oral Epidemiol* 1980; **8**: 135–8.

van de Rijke J. Use of dyes in cariology. *Inter Dent J* 1991; **41**: 111–16.

Rosen B, Birkhed D, Nilsson K, Olavi G, Egelberg J. Reproducibility of clinical caries diagnoses on coronal and root surfaces. *Caries Res* 1996; **30**: 1–7.

Ross G. Air abrasions and caries detection dues: The new standard of care. *Ont Dent* 1998; **75**: 43–5.

Rytömaa I, Jarvinen V, Jarvinen J. Variation in caries recording and restorative treatment plan among university teachers. *Community Dent Oral Epidemiol* 1979; **7**: 335–9.

Seale N, Kendrick A. A survey of pediatric dentists' management of dental caries in children three years of age or younger. *Pediatr Dent* 2001; **23**: 211–16.

Shugars D, Bader J. Cost implications of differences in dentists' restorative treatment decisions. *J Public Health Dent* 1996; **56**: 219–22.

Thomas C, Land M, Albin-Wilson S, Stewart G. Caries detection accuracy by multiple clinicians and techniques. *Gen Dent* 2000; **48**: 334–8.

Thomson O'Brien M, Oxman A, Davis D, Haynes R, Freemantle N, Harvey E. Educational outreach visits: effects on professional practice and health care outcomes. *Cochrane Database Syst Rev* 2000; (Issue 2): CD000409.

Thomson O'Brien M, Freemantle N, Oxman A, Wolf F, Davis D, Herrin J. Continuing education meetings and workshops: effects on professional practice and health care outcomes. *Cochrane Database Syst Rev* 2001; (Issue 1): CD003030.

Tveit A, Espelid I. Class II amalgams: interobserver variations in replacement decisions and diagnosis of caries and crevices. *Int Dent J* 1992; **42**: 12–18.

Young D. New caries detection technologies and modern caries management: merging the strategies. *Gen Dent* 2002; **50**: 320–31.

32

'for richer, for poorer, in sickness and in health ...' The role of dentistry in controlling caries and periodontitis globally

V. Baelum, W. van Palenstein Helderman, A. Hugoson, R. Yee and O. Fejerskov

Introduction

This last chapter attempts to assess the relative importance of the major oral diseases, dental caries and periodontal diseases, from a global perspective. It will explore the future role of dentistry through examples from different contemporary populations representing different oral health-care scenarios. The examples are intended to highlight the major challenges for the already existing and well-developed oral health-care services typical for the Western industrialized high-income countries; and for the often rudimentary oral health-care services that prevail in many low-income countries. By examining the occurrence, extent and severity of the two major oral diseases, dental caries and periodontitis, and their sequelae in different populations, some strategies are described that may be implemented to address these problems.

The oral disease profiles, as well as the already existing dental services and health-care systems, differ significantly between countries (Widström & Eaton, 2004) and continents. The origins of these differences are to be found in historical developments. Clinical dentistry, the way it is practiced today, has a long history (Fig. 32.1), and it is possible to identify distinct evolutionary phases that have fundamentally shaped the philosophies, the contents and the methods used in contemporary clinical dental practice.

Development of dentistry: the profession

The barber-surgeon phase

Oral problems, in the form of tooth decay, gum diseases, pain and abscesses are oral scourges known to have existed as long as humankind. For centuries, the treatments used to remedy these ailments consisted almost exclusively of tooth extractions. So-called barber-surgeons tried to meet the demands for relief of pain and discomfort of the populations mainly by extracting the troublesome teeth. In the resulting event of edentulism, this was sometimes remedied by dentures made from ivory, bone or natural teeth harvested from corpses. However, such dentures and other luxurious treatments, including gold foil for restorations, were reserved for the small élite of society. Overall, this phase was characterized by clinical dentistry evolving as a response to the imminent and tangible needs and wants of the most affluent sections of the populations.

In many ways, this phase bears a resemblance to the dental health services currently available in many low-income countries in Africa, Asia and South America, where in particular the rural populations do not have access to dental services rendered by trained dental personnel.

From barber-surgeons to dental surgeons

The birth of dentistry began in the second half of the eighteenth century. This was not a sudden event, but more a

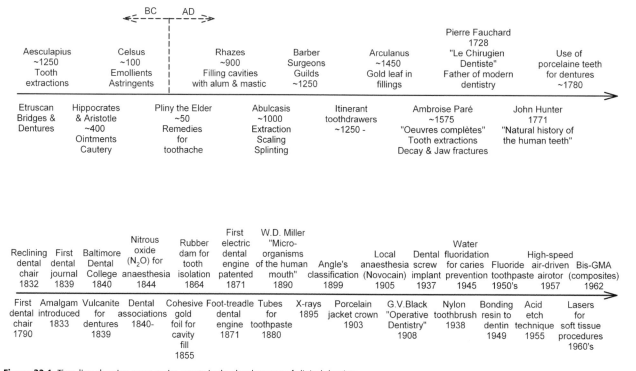

Figure 32.1 Time-line showing some major events in the development of clinical dentistry.

gradual crystallization into a separate discipline from a variety of different occupations. Many types of craftsmen provided dental treatment, which included leeching, cupping and tooth extractions, as a sideline to their main businesses, in which they may have worked as barbers, wigmakers, blacksmiths and apothecaries. Not surprisingly, tales of quackery and malpractice were countless.

The gradual emergence of dentistry in the eighteenth century is explained by a growing awareness of physical appearance. Traditionally, decayed and infected teeth were simply extracted, but people began to realize the cosmetic and social advantages of tooth replacements and restorations. The increased availability and consumption of sugar further added to the caries incidence and progression and thus further increased the demand for treatment for dental decay. Simultaneous with these developments, technical improvements gradually began to increase the appeal of dentistry to the public (Huisman, 2003).

The development of the armamentarium for the clinical dentist accelerated considerably around the middle of the nineteenth century. The emergence of the reclining dental chair, the first (private) dental college, amalgam, vulcanite for dentures and the dental engine (Gelbier, 2005b, c) (Fig. 32.1) marked important improvements, not only in the appeal of dentistry to the public, but also in the status of the so-called dental surgeons who began working exclusively on dental problems from small, home-based businesses. This phase, which lasted for most of the nineteenth century, seeded the bias of clinical dentistry towards mechanical repair and technical restorations as valuable responses to the destruction caused by caries and periodontal diseases.

Professionalization of dentistry

The next phase in the history of clinical dentistry began with the professional takeover from around the end of the nineteenth century. Dental societies and associations began to organize with a view to obtaining a registration of dental practitioners, and to controlling entry into the dental trade by means of licensing procedures (Fraundorf, 1984; Gelbier, 2005a). The further purpose of this registration was two-fold: to ensure the standards of care provided, and to raise and control the economic profitability of dental practice (Fraundorf, 1984) by control of the supply. As a result, the practice of dentistry became a legal issue in many countries, and acts were passed granting the titles of 'dentist', 'dental practitioner' or 'dental surgeon' only to those registered under these acts. However, this procedure still did not guarantee that title holders had any formal education in dentistry, and legislations were gradually tightened up so that licensing required a degree or a diploma from a dental school.

The focus on education and licensing resulted in the gradual evolvement of clinical dentistry from its cottage-industry roots. The contents gradually changed to comply with concepts and paradigms held by leading dental professionals, who wrote scores of 'scientific' articles, mainly of the 'In my opinion/experience' type. However, the bias towards mechanical repair and technical restoration remained deep-rooted, and the belief in treating caries and periodontal disease with metals continued (Niederman & Leitch, 2006). Undoubtedly, the meaning of professionalism was instilled in clinical dentistry during this phase and became embedded in the 'integrated infrastructure of education, licensing, boards, reimbursement, corporate insurance purchasing, and public perception' (Niederman & Leitch, 2006), which continues to prompt dentists to respond with technical solutions to biological problems.

Decades of the twentieth century had to pass before dentistry had fully gained its present status of a profession, which is 'united and self-regulating, with a well-established code of ethics and a strong sense of social purpose' (Gelbier, 2005a). Despite the stated commitment to a societal responsibility, it is clear that the dental profession most of all perceives itself as a 'free and liberal profession' (Widström, 2004). One result of this view is that the dental profession has remained somewhat detached from the developments in many countries towards increasing public involvement in the extent and type of health care provided to the populations at large (Wylie, 2002; Widström & Eaton, 2004). The dental profession seems more engaged in enforcing its statutory rights as a learned profession than in providing solutions to imminent problems regarding the availability of and access to dental services for underserved regions and population groups, of which the recent Alaska debate is just one example (American Dental Association, 2006; Alaska Native Tribal Health Consortium, 2006; Dentists in the United States Public Health Service, 2006).

Having said this, there have been notable exceptions. In Sweden, the quest for public oral health care was initiated by dental professionals in the first decade of the twentieth century. The dentists used ideas originating in the more prestigious field of medicine (the theory of focal infection; see below) to argue that tooth decay could be the port of entry for severe diseases, such as tuberculosis, which was a serious general health problem for the Swedish population at that time. They also presented calculations of the substantial losses in gross domestic product (GDP) resulting from people being absent from work owing to toothache. Finally, they sought to instill a notion of the importance of oral hygiene among the public as well as among the political decision makers. Thereby, they managed to engage politicians and other important decision makers in their campaign, and the first motion for a public oral health service aiming to benefit schoolchildren and military recruits was submitted to the Swedish parliament as early as 1904 (Lindblom, 2004). Although this motion did not immediately pass, a public dental health-care system gradually evolved, and a publicly funded epidemiological mapping of the oral health conditions among schoolchildren led to the presentation in 1914 of a proposal for the organization of a nationwide school dental health service in Sweden. Thereby, the foundation was laid for the subsequent gradual inclusion of small children, adults and elderly in the target group for the Swedish public dental health-care service (Lindblom, 2004), which is now widely known as *Folktandvården* (the Public Dental Service).

Development of dentistry: the disease concepts

The technical and professional developments in dentistry have been paralleled by a gradual evolution in the understanding of the causes and the natural history of the major dental diseases.

Dental caries

In the eighteenth century, at least two competing theories on the causes of dental caries could be identified. One theory, originating from the fourteenth century (Black, 1914a), the 'chemical theory of caries of the teeth', held that caries was caused by 'clinging particles of food', which decompose to acid, whereby the teeth are eaten away. This theory was contrasted by the widely held 'inflammatory theory of dental caries' (Hunter, 1771, 1778; Fox, 1806), according to which dental caries resulted from inflammation from within the dentin. However, in the mid-nineteenth century, studies of dental histology, enabled by technical developments in microscopy, soon led scientists such as John Tomes to refute the inflammatory caries theory in favor of the chemical theory. This refutation was strongly supported by

the microbiological works of W.D. Miller (1890), who identified a number of acid-producing bacteria residing in the oral cavity and in caries lesions. By the beginning of the twentieth century, the chemical dissolution theory on dental caries had completely supplanted the inflammatory caries theory (Black, 1914a).

It is noteworthy that G.V. Black (1914a) was very aware that 'decay of these [tooth surfaces] can be perfectly controlled by the use of the tooth brush and plain water by the patient, whenever the habit is sufficiently formed that it will not be neglected'. Even so, the principles used in caries treatment did not change much from the obsession with technical restorative treatment towards more focus on disease control and prevention by means of adequate oral hygiene procedures. However, G.V. Black himself may have been instrumental in preventing this change, when he instead focussed on the now notorious 'extension for prevention' principles for cavity preparation (Black, 1914b). Thereby, the foundation was laid for the unfortunate dichotomy, which still prevails in many places, between restorative dentistry on the one hand and cariology on the other. The bottom line was that a firm belief was instilled in the dental professional mindset, that caries control was chiefly a question of technical perfection and appropriate restorative materials.

Periodontal diseases

It was not until the writings by Pierre Fauchard (1969a, b) and John Hunter (1771, 1778) in the eighteenth century that proper schools of thought on the nature and causes of 'gum' diseases began to crystallize (Baelum, 1998). One school of thought held that periodontal diseases were systemic in

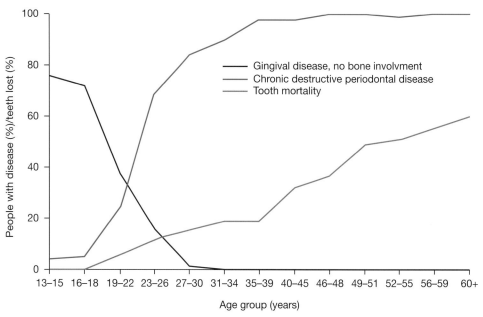

Figure 32.2 Results of an epidemiological study of the occurrence of gingival disease, destructive periodontal disease and tooth mortality in a representative sample of the population in Boston, USA. (Data from Marshall-Day *et al.*, 1955.)

nature, whereas the other implicated local factors in the disease causation. In the course of the nineteenth century, three new theories emerged: the school of atrophy, the school of occlusal traumatism and the school of infection. All these competing theories had different treatment implications, some of which still survive (e.g. occlusal therapy, scaling and root planing, surgical resection of diseased tissues).

Major changes in the disease concepts had to await developments in the middle of the twentieth century. Figure 32.2 presents the results of a cross-sectional epidemiological study of periodontal diseases carried out among a representative sample of teenagers, adults and elderly people in Boston, USA (Marshall-Day *et al.*, 1955). These results were interpreted as evidence for a sequence of events according to which gingivitis progresses to periodontitis which, in turn, progresses to tooth loss. Until a few decades ago it was a widely held belief that periodontal diseases are the major causes of tooth loss among adults and elderly people, that gingivitis inevitably progresses to periodontitis, and that the progression of periodontitis is linear and continuous.

However, these beliefs originated in unfortunate interpretations of cross-sectional epidemiological data, including those illustrated in Figure 32.2. Forgotten, or disregarded, was first of all the fact that the recording methods used precluded the recording of gingivitis as a separate disease entity. When both marginal gingivitis and bone loss was observed, the diagnosis would be periodontitis. If, therefore, the prevalence of periodontitis was observed to increase with age, the prevalence of gingivitis necessarily had to decline. The ensuing interpretation of these observations as evidence that gingivitis progresses to periodontitis thus reflected more the recording methods employed than the natural history of gingivitis and periodontitis.

A second problem lay in the interpretation of the observed tooth loss as being the inevitable result of periodontal destruction. Indeed, one may wonder why dental caries was not thought of as a cause of the observed tooth loss. The answer is that caries was considered a disease confined to childhood and adolescence, during which very few teeth were lost (Fig. 32.2). The idea that caries was restricted to the young originated in observations that the DMFT/S values did not increase much after people had entered their twenties. However, once a tooth or tooth surface has experienced a caries lesion, new caries lesions in that tooth or tooth surface can no longer add to the DMFT/S count. The apparent stability of the DMFT/S counts beyond certain ages may therefore merely show the inability of the DMF index to capture caries incidence and progression.

The now classical 'experimental gingivitis' study (Löe *et al.*, 1965) showed that when subjects abstained from all oral hygiene procedures for some time gingivitis would develop, but this gingivitis could be resolved by means of reinstitution of appropriate oral hygiene procedures. These results

firmly established the infectious disease paradigm for periodontal diseases, and provided the rationale for plaque control as a key element in their treatment. However, from today's perspective it is only fair to say that too much reliance was placed on the infectious disease paradigm thus established. It is now well known from experimental as well as observational studies that periodontal diseases should be understood as multifactorial diseases, the causes of which also include host-response factors as well as more distant factors, such as smoking and stress. It is also known now that there is no law of nature, which dictates that gingivitis will inevitably progress into periodontitis. The view of periodontitis progression as a linear and continuous process is no longer tenable, and tooth loss is therefore no longer regarded as an inescapable consequence of untreated periodontitis. As a result, it is gradually becoming apparent that the contribution of periodontitis to tooth mortality has been exaggerated in many populations.

Focal infection: a phobia in dentistry

Perhaps the most important concept introduced to clinical dentistry by means of the 'expert opinion' kind of sciences exercised in the late nineteenth and early twentieth century was the focal infection paradigm. This paradigm has exerted a profound and deleterious influence over clinical dentistry throughout the twentieth century.

The focal infection paradigm in dentistry originates in a strong belief in oral infectious foci as the causes of disease in other parts of the body (von Kaczorowski, 1886; Miller, 1890, 1891). This concept was vigorously promoted in dentistry, and it was recommended that all 'pulpless' teeth (teeth with apical periodontitis) and teeth with 'alveolar pyorrhea' (marginal periodontitis) be extracted (Price, 1925; Rosenow, 1926) to prevent serious systemic diseases. Rooted as they were in a barber-surgeon tradition, the dentists readily took the advice, and 'thousands of sound teeth have been needlessly sacrificed in this wave of extraction, in the vain hope of giving relief to suffering humanity' (Buckley, 1925) or in the vain hope of preventing systemic diseases. Some leading dental professionals went so far as to commend dentists for 'coming to realize that it is their positive duty to free the mouths of patients from infection, even though this requires the extraction of a number of teeth' (Black, 1918), concluding that this practice style 'is preventive dentistry that is worth while, for it is cutting off at the source much systemic disease' (Black, 1918).

Clinical dentistry's adherence to the focal infection paradigm in the first half of the twentieth century and the resulting 'mass dental extermination' (Burt, 1978) earned this period the label of the 'blood and vulcanite era' (Weintraub & Burt, 1985). The results in the form of high rates of edentulism may still be seen in some populations (Fig. 32.3). In addition to inflating the rates of edentulism in populations with access to dental services, the focal infection paradigm

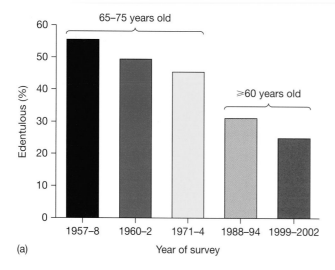

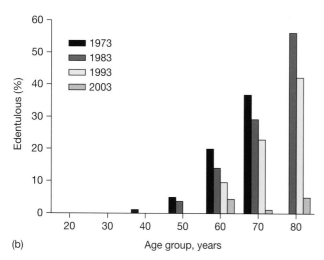

(a)

(b)

Figure 32.3 Trends in edentulism (a) over the past five decades in the USA (Weintraub & Burt, 1985; Beltrán-Aguilar *et al.*, 2005) and (b) over three decades in Sweden (Hugoson *et al.*, 2005b).

served to distort dentistry's perception of why teeth were lost (Baelum, 1998). As mentioned above, it remained a widely held concept in dentistry until the 1980s that periodontitis was the main cause of tooth loss in adults beyond the age of 35–40 years (Waerhaug, 1966; WHO, 1978). This interpretation was apparently further substantiated by the frequent observations that the prevalence of edentulism increased dramatically from this age, such that 40–50% of the elderly population would end their lives being edentulous (Fig. 32.3). Forgotten, or disregarded, was the fact that millions of teeth were extracted because the prevailing focal infection philosophy in dentistry dictated this; not because the caries status or the periodontal condition of the teeth per se required extraction (Burt, 1978). Unfortunately, this belief in periodontitis as a major cause of tooth loss among middle-aged and older adults came to distort the philosophies underpinning the treatment of periodontitis. It was gradually forgot-

ten that the real reason why so many periodontitis affected teeth were lost was the focal infection paradigm, and the belief was firmly established that periodontitis was a continuously progressing disease, which ultimately led to loss of the affected teeth. This resulted in the somewhat ironic situation that many teeth were deemed of periodontally 'dubious prognosis' (Hirschfeld & Wasserman, 1978), and subsequently extracted because of their perceived poor prognosis, i.e. out of fear that disease might overtake the dentist and his forceps. In particular, earlier studies on the effect of periodontal treatment used extractions of a substantial number of teeth during the initial, presurgical treatment phase (Lindhe & Nyman, 1975).

Development of dentistry: low-income countries

As already mentioned, the development of dentistry in low-income countries has followed a different path. In many countries in Africa, Latin America and Asia only a few dental professionals are available who have formal qualifications in dentistry. Moreover, the few dentists who exist in these countries tend to cluster in the major cities, where the possibilities for earning a decent income are greater (Manji & Sheiham, 1986). The rural populations, which, in these low-income countries, means the vast majority of the populations, are predominantly served by barber-surgeons, such as blacksmiths and traditional healers, who have acquired some manual skills that make them confident in performing extractions of teeth that cause pain or discomfort (Fig. 32.4). Dentistry, the way it is known to populations in the Western high-income countries, is reserved for the very

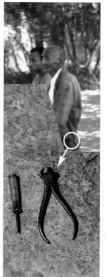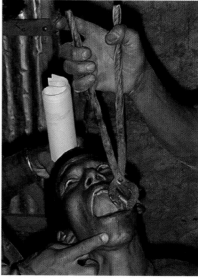

Figure 32.4 Clinical armamentarium of an elderly 'barber-surgeon' who was active among a rural Kenyan population in the late 1980s (left panel). The instruments in his pocket (circle) are shown. The right panel shows how tooth extractions are performed in Nepal.

few belonging to the political or business élite. This has a profound influence on the oral health conditions of these populations as they may be seen today. Edentulism is often virtually absent (Manji *et al.*, 1988) and dental restorations are extremely rare (Manji *et al.*, 1989) in populations whose access to dental care is limited to the local tooth-pullers. In some populations, a few local people possess additional skills and may provide people with rather unorthodox prosthetic solutions inserted on top of the root remnant meant for replacement (Baelum *et al.*, 1988b; Luan *et al.*, 1989a). The number of teeth present is generally higher than seen for populations in the high-income countries (Baelum & Fejerskov, 1986; Baelum *et al.*, 1988b, 2002; Manji *et al.*, 1988; Tirwomwe *et al.*, 1988; Luan *et al.*, 1989a; Matthesen *et al.*, 1990). Caries levels are lower than seen among most populations in the high-income countries (Tirwomwe *et al.*, 1988; Manji *et al.*, 1989; Luan *et al.*, 1989b, 2000; Fejerskov *et al.*, 1994). Most of the caries experience is made up of untreated caries, and there is therefore a considerable unmet demand for relief of pain services. Undoubtedly, gingivitis is much more prevalent and severe, and the oral hygiene situation worse, than generally seen in high-income countries; but there is no solid evidence to suggest that this has resulted in periodontitis being more prevalent or severe in the low-income populations (Baelum, 1998; Baelum & Scheutz, 2002; Lopez, 2003).

Planned dental services: wishful thinking or achievable goal?

During the 1960s and 1970s, the concept gradually evolved that the oral health situation of the world's populations should be described with a view to using the data for projecting the future needs for oral health care of the populations. The wider purpose was to allow oral health administrators to develop appropriate oral health-care programmes and plan the numbers and types of personnel needed. The World Health Organization (WHO) has been a major driving force in this process, and has issued manuals that describe in detail the methods recommended for such purposes (WHO, 1971, 1977, 1987, 1997).

Methods used to assess caries and periodontal status

The method currently recommended by the WHO (1997) for the recording of dental caries for planning purposes specifically states that the stages of caries lesion formation that precede cavitation be excluded on the grounds that 'they cannot be reliably diagnosed'. Teeth are recorded as sound, decayed (i.e. cavitated), filled or missing due to caries, and the components of the DMFT index are tabulated for the indicator age groups examined. The diagnostic criteria used thus confer a considerable risk that the data generated serve to favor the traditional expensive and resource-demanding

clinical drill and fill approach to the management of carious cavities, over a more disease-controlling approach focussed on the prevention of new caries lesion formation and the non-operative control of already existing non-cavitated lesions. It is also clear (see Chapters 4 and 9) that the caries recording methodology recommended by WHO (1997) results in serious underestimation of the prevalence and extent of dental caries in the populations.

The methods recommended by WHO for the recording of periodontal diseases have varied. In the first edition of the oral health survey manual (WHO, 1971), periodontal diseases were recorded using Russell's Periodontal Index (Russell, 1956), which amalgamates the signs of gingivitis with those of periodontitis (Baelum, 1998). However, since the 1987 edition of the manual (WHO, 1987) the recommended method has been based on the Community Periodontal Index of Treatment Needs (Ainamo *et al.*, 1982). Use of the CPITN and the CPI (CPITN without treatment needs) involves the scoring of each of 10 indicator teeth for the presence of pockets 6+ mm (code 4), pockets 4–5 mm (code 3), calculus (code 2) or bleeding on probing (code 1). The highest code is recorded for each tooth and subject, and 'code 0' indicates that the indicator tooth/subject is healthy. The use of the CPITN as a periodontal status measure has been much criticized (Holmgren, 1994; Baelum & Papapanou, 1996), which has resulted in attachment level measurements being added to the recommended WHO survey methodology (WHO, 1997).

Use of the data for planning purposes

Descriptive dental epidemiological studies of the prevalence and severity of dental caries and periodontal diseases have frequently been carried out for the stated purpose of facilitating the planning of oral health services for the population. The WHO Global Oral Data Bank contains the results of numerous such studies. However, the stated planning objective has rarely materialized. It is therefore erroneous to believe that the existing dental health-care services have been carefully planned with a view to combating dental caries and periodontal diseases as the key contributors to the global burden of oral diseases.

A number of barriers to planning and implementation may be identified, which include the following factors.

Available resources and priorities

It is extremely difficult to use oral health status data to estimate the magnitude of finances and workforce required to provide oral health services for the population, since other determinants play a decisive role, such as the available resources and the prioritization of goods and services. It is a historical fact that the oral health services in the Western industrialized countries have rarely developed as a result of a plan, but evolved gradually to meet the wants and demands of the population, given the available resources. In most of these countries, national oral health survey data on oral health status were not in existence before the 1980s. Despite the availability of national oral health data in the more recent decades, oral health services in these countries have evolved more as a result of political (a combination of people's and the dental profession's perception of what is needed) and economic circumstances than from accurate information on the prevalence and severity of oral diseases.

Epidemiological information on oral health status might be useful for planning oral health care for specific target groups and services, such as school dental services, provided sufficient resources are available. However, such information has a minor impact on the planning and implementation of national oral health services in resource-limited countries, where oral health services are still in their infancy. The reasons are obvious, as there are other needs and wants of these populations, which necessitate the prioritization of the scarce resources available for health care.

The costs of dental care

The classical restorative approach to dental treatment is an economic burden, even in the high-income industrialized countries where 5–10% of public health spending is used for oral health care. Oral disease is the fourth most expensive disease to treat in most industrialized countries (Petersen *et al.*, 2005). In the year 2000, the European Union spent a total of €54 billion on oral health care (Widström & Eaton, 2004) and in the USA the 2004 expenditure for oral health care was US$81.5 billion (Historical National Health Expenditure Data, 2006). These costs do not include the additional costs of dental care performed under the medical umbrella.

It is not surprising that these costs dramatically exceed the financial resources of low- and middle-income countries. A study performed in Kenya showed that the costs of treatment to control periodontal diseases in children on the basis of the CPITN (Ainamo *et al.*, 1982) data greatly exceeded the total national health-care budget (Manji & Sheiham, 1986). Another study of the total costs of restoring dental caries cavities of the child population in Nepal by amalgam restorations indicated that the costs would exceed the total health-care budget for children (Yee & Sheiham, 2002).

Moreover, the costs of traditional restorative dental care should be considered in the context of the costs of general health care. An essential general health-care package, which contains school health programs, expanded immunization, micronutrient supplementation and essential public health interventions, can eliminate about 30% of the burden of mortality and disability among the 0–14-year-old children in low-income countries at a cost of about US$4 per child. The cost of restoration of the permanent dentition of children of low-income countries using amalgam restorative dentistry costs almost the same as the essential health-care package! Moreover, 75% of the 48 low-income countries

cannot afford to fund an essential health package for children (Yee & Sheiham, 2002), and an additional budget for amalgam restorations therefore remains a naïve wish.

The lack of public funding of dental treatment in low-income countries leaves the burden of costs with the private households. As an example, the cost of a single surface restoration is about US$5 in Nepal. To this, one should add the cost of transportation for the Nepali village child to the dentist who practices in an urban clinic. The costs amount to US$14 and do not include lost wages of the accompanying parent. For an average Nepali who earns less than US$0.75 a day, this amount is equivalent to half a month's wage or enough food for a month. It is easy to understand that when having to choose between food for the family for 2 weeks and the restoration of one carious tooth in a child, the choice made does not necessarily favor the maintenance of good dental health.

Care index and gross domestic product

The above examples show that planning intervention strategies entirely on the basis of epidemiological data without considering the social, economic and political conditions is doomed to fail. In particular, the national economic conditions appear to be an important determinant of restorative care. Taking the care index ($F/DMFT \times 100\%$) for 34–44-year-olds as an indicator of the country's restorative care level, it appears that no country with a GDP below US$5000 has a care index higher than 30% (Brunton *et al.*, 2003), which further underpins that restorative treatment is unaffordable in low-income countries.

DMFT and CPI/CPITN data: reflect inefficient concepts

Epidemiological data in the form of decayed, missing and filled teeth (DMFT) and CPI/CPITN (WHO, 1997) data represent the professional health-care provider's normative assessment of dental treatment needs rather than the people's perceived needs and wants. These data ignore the pain and suffering of the people, just as they focus on the traditional very costly and inefficient chairside dentist-to-patient approach to oral health-care delivery.

As the DMFT data commonly collected for planning purposes take into account only the cavitated stages of caries lesion formation, they inevitably bias the oral health-care delivery towards ineffective and inefficient (see Chapters 20 and 28) operative repair approaches at the expense of control and prevention strategies. However, non-cavitated caries lesions are very amenable to treatment and control using non-operative (e.g. topical fluoride) or preventive means (e.g. improved daily oral hygiene procedures using fluoride toothpaste) (see Chapters 14–19), just as their occurrence can be controlled using population preventive strategies using common risk-factor approaches (see Chapter 28).

The use of the periodontal CPI data for oral health-care planning purposes hinges on the traditional view of the natural history of periodontal diseases detailed above: accumulation of plaque leads to the formation of gingivitis, which inevitably progresses to periodontitis and ultimately causes extensive tooth loss, unless the chain of events is broken at the very first step, plaque accumulation. This view dictates that all gingivitis should always be resolved, all calculus removed, and all deepened pockets eradicated to prevent tooth loss due to periodontal destruction. As previously mentioned, attempts to estimate treatment needs on the basis of CPI/CPITN data have resulted in absurdly large estimates for low-income (Manji & Sheiham, 1986) and middle-income (Songpaisan & Davies, 1989) countries, and even high-income countries may be hard pressed to meet the demands indicated by such estimates (Oliver et al., 1989, 1993). Moreover, it has proved unreasonable to expect that regular scaling and oral hygiene instructions will keep calculus deposits away for good (Songpaisan & Davies, 1989), just as many studies have indicated that the CPI data lead to a considerable overestimation of the treatment needs, particularly among younger age groups (Gjermo et al., 1983; Takahashi et al., 1988; Baelum et al., 1995).

DMFT and CPI/CPITN data: inadequate for decision makers

It is important to appreciate that no one outside the dental field is concerned with, let alone understands, the meaning of the DMFT and CPI/CPITN figures. If such data are included in health reports presenting morbidity and mortality data of general diseases, the usual reactions of health-care decision makers of middle- and low-income countries are: 'oral diseases are not a problem since they are not life threatening', or, 'our country has a low DMFT according to WHO, so a budget for oral health is not necessary and certainly not a priority'.

Health-care decision makers at the national and international level are frequently presented with DMFT and CPI estimates that have been produced by national dental institutes or international organizations for the purpose of advocating a particular policy change. However, decision makers are keener on independent and objective quantification estimates of the burden of a specific disease in order to make comparisons with similar measures of other diseases. This allows decision makers to prioritize health problems and decide how resources for health improvement should be allocated.

What is really required for planning is information that is easy to understand and represents people's real needs and wants. The options must be affordable and use appropriate technology, which can be easily integrated into the country's existing health structures, and not solutions based on technically oriented dental approaches. Preferably, the planning should be at the district level, since national poli-

cies based on national means have a tendency to exacerbate the differences between rich and poor (Lalloo et al., 1999). Some of the essential determinants for the formulation of a plan are:

- people's perceived needs and treatment demands
- people's knowledge and habits related to oral health
- existing health-care system and structures
- available human and financial resources.

Regrettably, these points are not adequately captured in the current WHO guidelines for the collection of information required for oral health-care planning (WHO, 1997).

The magnitude of disease burdens

Years lived with disability

Quantification of the disease burden requires a unit of measurement. In the past, mortality (crude death rate) was the dominant health outcome considered, but non-fatal health outcomes, which may have a considerable impact on the quality of life, are increasingly recognized as important measures. Years lived with disability (YLD) is considered a quantification with a value that nearly every society recognizes as legitimate. Of course, there are individual characteristics and cultural aspects that impact differently on the burden of a disability, just as the perception of pain and suffering may differ between communities and cultures.

Even so, YLD is used to indicate the burden of disease and injury. It represents the product of the weight (severity) of disability and the duration of disability of a population. YLD data are generated based on independent evaluations of a particular disease burden in the context of other disease burdens and this type of data is desired by health-care decision makers.

The burden of caries and periodontal diseases in the context of other diseases

Figure 32.5 shows the distribution of the YLD in thousands per million population for the different regions of the world according to the three major classes of diseases and injuries assessed in 1990 (Murray & Lopez, 1996). Sub-Saharan Africa has the highest total disease burden, closely followed by India. Both of these regions stand out as carrying a heavy disease burden owing to communicable diseases (infectious and parasitic diseases). This is in contrast with the established market economy countries, where non-communicable diseases (in particular psychiatric conditions) play a major role.

Figure 32.5 also shows that oral disease, which includes caries, periodontal diseases and edentulism, contributes relatively little to the total YLD per million population. The countries having the highest oral disease contribution to the total YLD per million population are found in the Middle Eastern crescent, closely followed by Latin America and the

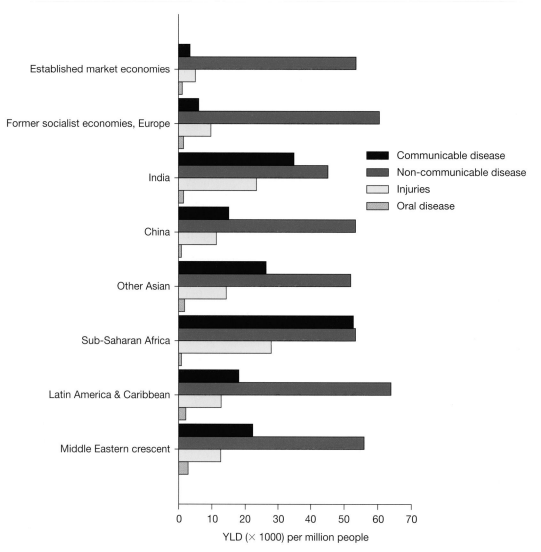

Figure 32.5 Distribution of the burden of disease measured as years lived with disability (YLD in thousands) per million people for different regions of the world.

Caribbean, and other Asian countries; whereas the lowest contributions are found in Sub-Saharan Africa and in China. Worldwide, caries, periodontal diseases and edentulism contribute 1.6% of the total YLD. This percentage is a worldwide average, and the proportional burden is different in various regions, ranging from 0.6% for the Sub-Saharan Africa to 3.0% for the Middle Eastern crescent countries. In Table 32.1, the relative YLD values for oral diseases are compared with those of some other common diseases with comparable YLD values.

Contribution of caries and periodontal diseases to tooth loss and edentulism

As seen in Table 32.2, dental caries seems to contribute about 10 times more to the YLD measure than do periodontal diseases. This is perhaps not so surprising, in view of pain being a comparatively frequent sequel to caries. While the presence of gingivitis may be noted as the occasional occur-

rence of bleeding gums it typically goes unnoticed, just as periodontitis does not cause symptoms until rather late in the disease process, when the teeth begin to appear elongated, drift or exhibit increased mobility. However, the 'dark horse' in the evaluation of the relative disease burden is tooth loss and edentulism. For the populations in the established market economies, the former socialist economies in Europe and the Middle Eastern crescent region, edentulism contributes as much as caries to the oral disease burden (Murray & Lopez, 1996). If periodontitis is the major cause of tooth loss and edentulism among adults in these populations, it might contribute as much to the oral disease burden as dental caries.

Although it used to be common wisdom that periodontitis is the major cause of tooth loss among adults and elderly, this belief does not hold. Undoubtedly, the very high rates of edentulism previously experienced in many established market economy countries are in part attribut-

Table 32.1 Percentage distribution of years lived with disability (YLDs) for oral diseases compared with some other common diseases in 1990 (Murray & Lopez, 1996)

World total	Established market economy countries	Sub-Saharan Africa	China and India	Latin American countries	Middle Eastern crescent
Oral diseases					
1.6	1.8	0.6	1.1	2.4	3.0
Diarrhoeal diseases					
1.0	0.4	1.1	1.3	1.3	1.0
Malaria					
0.8	0	4.0	0.3	0.2	0.4
Diabetes mellitus					
1.1	3.1	0.3	0.7	1.3	1.5
Tuberculosis					
0.9	0	1.1	1.0	0.4	0.5
All causes					
100	100	100	100	100	100

Table 32.2 Relative contribution of caries, periodontal diseases and edentulism to the oral disease burden for different regions of the world (Murray & Lopez, 1996)

	Established market economies	Former Socialist economies, Europe	India	China	Latin America and Caribbean	Sub-Saharan Africa	Middle Eastern crescent
Caries	46.7	50.5	64.3	58.4	89.8	73.9	50.4
Periodontal diseases	4.0	3.5	6.8	3.3	1.8	7.0	1.5
Edentulism	48.8	46.0	27.7	35.8	7.7	16.8	47.7

able to the focal infection paradigm (Weintraub & Burt, 1985), which influenced dentistry until the middle of the twentieth century. Moreover, non-dental factors, such as the accessibility, availability and costs of services, treatment philosophies and dentist and patient attitudes, have pronouncedly influenced the decision processes leading to tooth extractions (Baelum, 1998). Many of us know the tales of people in our not so distant ancestry who received their first set of full dentures as a present during their teenage years. At the time this was seen as a boon to the subject, using the logic that an extracted tooth cannot cause pain and suffering, or entail further expenses. In a Norwegian study of edentulism among the elderly (Rise & Helöe, 1978) it was observed that two-thirds of the edentulous had never had a filling prior to the full-mouth extraction. Similar observations have been made in other studies (Ettinger, 1971), indicating that restorative care was not even attempted before the full-mouth extraction. Figure 32.2 shows that modern elderly populations still continue to show evidence of these philosophies.

A large number of studies exist from different parts of the world where attempts have been made to assess the reasons for tooth loss (Ainamo et al., 1984; Cahen et al., 1985; Bailit et al., 1987; Manji et al., 1988; Chauncey et al., 1989; Corbet & Davies, 1991; Klock & Haugejorden, 1991; Reich & Hiller,

1993; Morita et al., 1994; Angelillo et al., 1996; Murray et al., 1996; Ong et al., 1996; Caldas, 2000; McCaul et al., 2001; Sanya et al., 2004; Oginni, 2005; Kida et al., 2006). Many of these studies have been carried out by asking dentists to record the reason whenever they extract a tooth. Thereby, the risk is great that the reasons given for the tooth extractions change from strictly disease-related causes to more technical reasons, such as pre-prosthetic considerations, or to reasons related to the dentist's evaluation of the prognosis of the tooth in question. Certainly, studies carried out in this way may report on a substantial proportion of teeth extracted owing to such non-disease causes (Ainamo et al., 1984; Bailit et al., 1987; Chauncey et al., 1989; Klock & Haugejorden, 1991; Reich & Hiller, 1993; McCaul et al., 2001). Even so, it is an almost unanimous finding in these studies that dental caries and its sequelae remain the most important reasons for tooth extractions. Other studies, usually carried out in low-income countries, are based on interviewing people about the reasons for their tooth losses (Manji et al., 1988; Kida et al., 2006) and these have also resulted in dental caries and its sequelae being the main culprit (Fig. 32.6). Therefore, it may be concluded that on a population basis, the burden of caries remains substantially larger than the burden of periodontitis. This situation may well change, however, if the caries decline continues. This

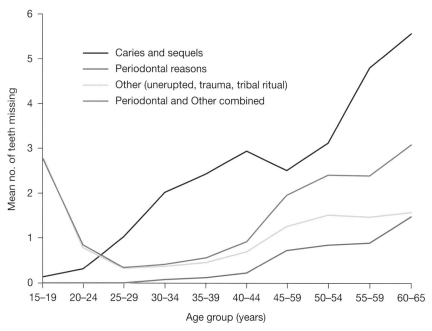

Figure 32.6 Age-specific reasons for tooth loss in an adult, rural Kenyan population (Manji *et al.*, 1988).

will increase tooth retention and may increase the relative importance of periodontitis as a cause of tooth loss.

The burden of periodontal diseases

Most people in the world have gingivitis (bleeding from the gingiva) and calculus (Petersen & Ogawa, 2005), but bleeding of the gingiva and the presence of calculus are not adequate indicators of periodontitis. Unfortunately, the diagnostic criteria for the presence of 'periodontitis' or 'severe periodontitis' are not well defined (Baelum & Lopez, 2003; Tonetti & Claffey, 2005), and this reduces considerably the possibilities for comparisons between populations or over time in the same population of the prevalence (percentage of people with), the extent (number of teeth affected) and the severity (depth of the lesions) of periodontitis (Baelum, 1998). Rather than reporting on distinct and well-defined diagnostic categories, epidemiological studies of periodontitis typically report on several different periodontal parameters, including radiographic bone height, probing pocket depth and clinical attachment level. Owing to the use of different examination methods, different criteria and diagnostic thresholds, extreme caution must be exercised when attempting to draw firm conclusions on the basis of comparing results of different studies.

Even so, some broad epidemiological patterns can be outlined. The prevalence of edentulism is often substantially higher, and the mean number of teeth retained therefore markedly lower, among populations in high-income countries compared with populations in low- and middle-income countries (Fig. 32.7). The oral hygiene conditions are typi-cally substantially better, and the levels of gingivitis there-fore lower, among populations in high-income countries compared with populations in low- and middle-income countries (Fig. 32.8).

The prevalence of periodontal attachment loss is high from an early age, and both the extent (the proportion of teeth affected) and the severity (the lesion depth) increase with increasing age, whether considering populations in the established market economies, Sub-Saharan Africa or China (Fig. 32.9). For any given age group, the distribution of the number of teeth affected follows a continuum, such that no sharp distinction exists between periodontal health and disease, or between mild, moderate and severe disease (Fig. 32.9). In other words, absence or low severity of clinical attachment loss merges imperceptibly into high severity of clinical attachment loss. Figure 32.10 also shows that the distribution of subjects according to the number of affected teeth is positively skewed towards a long right-hand tail. This distribution shape signals inequality in the distribution of the total disease burden, and it may be calculated that 48% of the total clinical attachment loss burden among the 20–29-year-old Chinese in Fig. 32.10 is carried by only 10% of the subjects, and that 22% of the subjects carry 75% of the total attachment loss burden.

Population control of periodontitis

Traditionally, the control of periodontal diseases, including periodontitis, has been almost entirely focussed on a classical chairside approach to combat the presumed local causal factor, the bacteria in the dental plaque deposits. Dental patients have been given instructions in proper oral hygiene

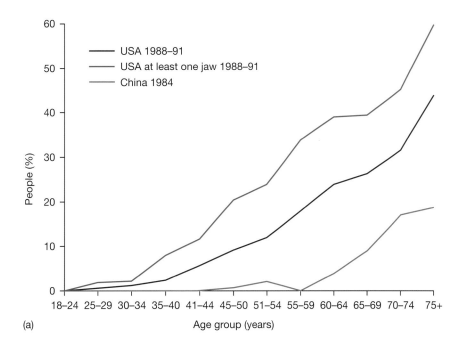

(a)

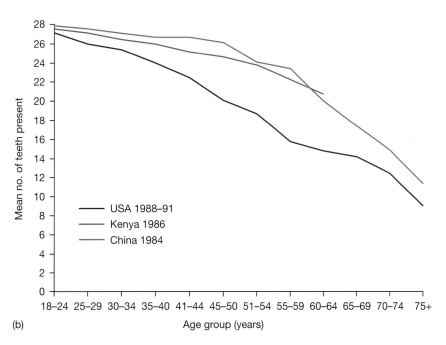

(b)

Figure 32.7 (a) Prevalence of edentulism according to age in the USA (Marcus *et al.*, 1996) and PR China (Luan *et al.*, 1989a), and (b) mean number of teeth retained in the total population according to age in the USA (Marcus *et al.*, 1996), Kenya (Manji *et al.*, 1988) and PR China (Luan *et al.*, 1989a). In Kenya, the prevalence of edentulism was negligible, less than 0.3%.

practices to achieve meticulous, self-performed plaque control, and for susceptible individuals, this has been combined with regular professional prophylaxis (supragingival and subgingival scaling and root planing). It has gradually become clear, however, that a chairside approach essentially devoted to the control of the supragingival and subgingival microbiota may be insufficient to control periodontitis

(American Academy of Periodontology, 2005), not least at population level. For many years, important factors have been discounted, which directly affect the host defense system, including stress (Genco *et al.*, 1999) and smoking (Tomar & Asma, 2000; Hujoel *et al.*, 2003). Smoking seems to be a major causal factor for periodontitis, and studies indicate that more than half of the periodontitis cases in

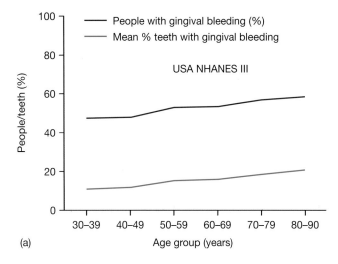

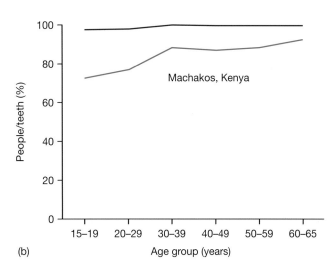

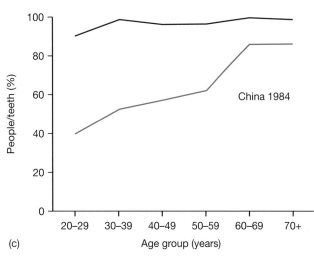

Figure 32.8 Prevalence of gingival bleeding, and the mean proportion of teeth with gingival bleeding, according to age in the USA (Albandar & Kingman, 1999), Kenya (Baelum *et al.*, 1988a) and PR China (unpublished data).

the USA may be attributable to this one factor alone (Tomar & Asma, 2000). Psychosocial stress resulting from poverty, malnutrition, unemployment, lack of control over one's situation and poor living conditions may affect the ability to adopt oral health-promoting habits, such as daily tooth brushing using fluoride toothpastes, and to abstain from deleterious habits, such as smoking and betel nut chewing. It is therefore not surprising that, as with many other diseases, a strong social gradient exists in the distribution of periodontitis within a given population (American Academy of Periodontology, 2005; Lopez *et al.*, 2006; Borrell *et al.*, 2006).

Clearly, in low- and middle-income countries both simple and more advanced periodontal treatment, which are based on the traditional professional chairside approaches adopted from high-income countries, are only attainable for the few élite. For the majority of these populations these forms of treatment are unaffordable. When attempts have been made to launch community oral health programs for deprived communities that follow these principles, the results have been disappointing. The oral health program launched in Thailand consisted of oral examinations, preventive advice and scaling (Anumanrajadhon *et al.*, 1996). Young people who had finished secondary school were trained during 2 weeks to become village scalers who used hand instruments for the removal of calculus. However, the programme had to be discontinued, because the village scalers became frustrated. One of the reasons was the villagers' lack of appreciation of the significance of periodontal diseases as an oral health problem and the resulting lack of demand for services (Anumanrajadhon *et al.*, 1996). Moreover, there is a lack of evidence to show that the removal of calculus is a prerequisite to prevent the onset of periodontitis. In fact, calculus removal is not indicated in the majority of individuals (Lembariti, 1994). Scaling is of little use in controlling the periodontal status if it is performed occasionally and without repeated oral hygiene instructions (Lembariti *et al.*, 1998), just as scaling may be iatrogenic if performed on shallow periodontal pockets (Frandsen, 1986). Hence, the most appropriate oral hygiene tool to control gingivitis and periodontitis is not the scaler but the toothbrush, and calculus removal is only indicated if otherwise compromising adequate oral hygiene procedures. Accordingly, the WHO now excludes scaling as part of the first phase of primary oral health care (Frencken *et al.*, 2002).

Needed: a whole-population approach to common risk factors

An advocacy process for better oral hygiene in communities with poor oral hygiene is a first priority. The strategy for periodontal health should be based on the whole-population approach and the tackling of the common risk

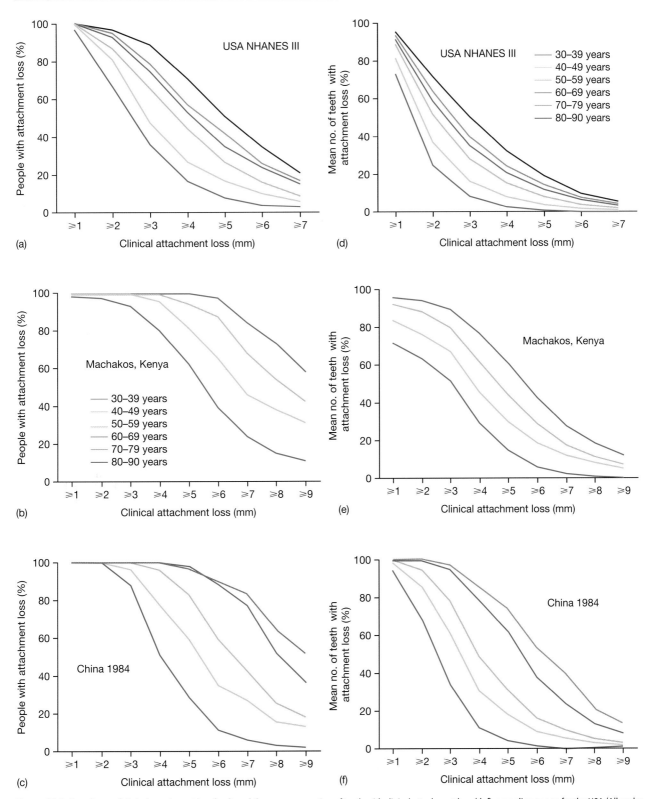

Figure 32.9 Prevalence of clinical attachment loss (a–c), and the mean proportion of teeth with clinical attachment loss (d–f), according to age for the USA (Albandar *et al.*, 1999), Kenya (Baelum *et al.*, 1988a) and PR China (unpublished data).

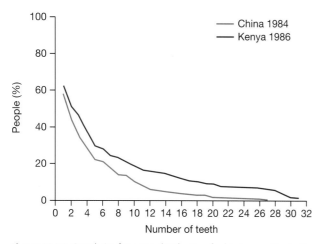

Figure 32.10 Cumulative frequency distribution of subjects according to the number of teeth with clinical attachment loss ⩾3 mm. Data are for 20–29-year-olds from Kenya and PR China.

factors (see Chapter 28). A small shift in the whole population brushing their teeth will have a major impact on the prevalence and incidence of gingivitis and periodontitis. By focussing action on the common underlying determinants of health (malnutrition, poor sanitation, poor hygiene, usage of tobacco products and alcohol) with the co-operation of governments and non-government agencies, a large number of diseases, including caries and periodontal diseases, may be controlled at a lower cost and greater efficiency and effectiveness than with a disease-specific approach (Sheiham & Watt, 2000). The public health goal for periodontal health should be to achieve an oral hygiene level and a smoking frequency compatible with the maintenance of a natural functional, acceptable dentition for a lifetime (Sheiham, 1996). Oral hygiene through self-care and abstention from tobacco use are the main community measures to control periodontal diseases. These measures can reduce both the prevalence of gingivitis and the incidence of periodontitis.

Dental caries: the major oral disease burden

Since dental caries and its sequelae are the main causes of oral pain, suffering, disability and tooth loss, the remaining part of this chapter will deal with the distribution of caries worldwide and the consequences of the varying socioeconomic conditions in different parts of the world for control and management.

Dental caries in the deciduous dentition before the age of 6 years

Caries may develop in the deciduous dentition before the end of the first year of an infant's life (Douglass *et al.*, 2001; Vachirarojpisan *et al.*, 2004). At this age, caries lesions may first be seen on the upper primary incisors, since these teeth are among the first teeth to erupt. If the cariogenic challenge continues to exist, other teeth will become affected accord-

ing to their eruption sequence. The lower anterior teeth usually remain unaffected, probably because the tongue prevents exposure of the lower anterior teeth to the cariogenic challenge and because of the protective mechanism of the sublingual and submandibular salivary gland secretion. A common characteristic of this early caries, which was described in the middle of the nineteenth century (Jacobi, 1862), is the rapidity with which cavities develop. In the first comprehensive description of early caries, this condition was termed 'nursing bottle mouth' (Fass, 1962) because an association was observed with the practice of providing infants with a nursing bottle of (sweetened) milk before putting them to sleep. Since then, early caries has been termed in various ways: 'night bottle mouth', 'nursing bottle caries', 'night bottle caries' and 'baby bottle tooth decay'. These names all suggest the inappropriate use of the nursing bottle as the primary cause of early caries. However, this form of caries has also been associated with sugary supplements during weaning and with the use of sweetened pacifiers to comfort the child; and early caries in infants has been reported in developing countries in communities where feeding bottles were rarely used (Matee *et al.*, 1994; van Palenstein Helderman *et al.*, 2006). The existing uncertainties regarding the many possible causes that may lead to early caries in infants living under different social, economic and cultural circumstances prompted a more neutral term to be assigned for this form of caries, 'early childhood caries (ECC)' (CDCP, 1994; American Academy of Pediatric Dentistry, 2005). ECC is a diagnosis used to describe the presence of at least one decayed (non-cavitated or cavitated lesion), missing (due to caries) or filled surface in any primary tooth (dmft > 0) in a child aged 71 months or less (i.e. before the age of 6 years) (American Academy of Pediatric Dentistry, 2005).

Prevalence of early childhood caries

When defined as at least one affected primary tooth in 1–3-year-old children, the prevalence of ECC ranges between 0 and 9% in Western developed countries (Milnes, 1996). In East and South Asia, in Western Pacific countries (Table 32.3) and in Brazil (Dini *et al.*, 2000) the prevalence may be much higher. However, reports indicate that minority groups in the Western world, such as Native American and Canadian populations, also have a high prevalence of ECC (Kelly & Bruerd, 1987; Albert *et al.*, 1988; Broderick *et al.*, 1989).

The fact that the prevalence of ECC may be so high in the first years of life while the prevalence of caries in the first years of the permanent dentition is so low in communities in Asia offers circumstantial evidence of unique risk factors prevailing in these communities. A prospective study among Chinese children found a correlation between caries in primary molars and caries in the permanent dentition, but no correlation between caries in the primary upper incisors and

Table 32.3 Prevalence of early childhood caries in 1–3-year-old infants in South and East Asia and in Western Pacific countries

Age (years)	Study	Country	% with cavities in anterior teeth
2–3	Majid et al., 1987	Malaysia	59
2	Hu & Liu, 1992	China, Chengdu	18
3			50
3	Douglass et al., 1994	China, Beijing	67
2	Du et al., 2000a	China Hubei	35
2	Hartono et al., 2002	Indonesia	48
3			78
2	Cariño et al., 2003	Philippines	59
3			85
1–1.5	Vachirarojpisan et al., 2004	Thailand	41
2	Van Palenstein Helderman et al., 2006	Myanmar	47

caries in the permanent dentition (Zhang & van Palenstein Helderman, 2006). This implies that specific cariogenic rearing practices exist that are responsible for caries in the primary upper incisors, but disappear later in life.

Indeed, a comprehensive review of the literature has demonstrated that ECC is associated with particular rearing practices. Hence, bottle feeding with sweetened milk or fruit juice, night-time bottle feeding, high consumption of sugary drinks or snacks, night-time meals or drinks, use of a sweetened comforter or pacifier (Harris et al., 2004), and breast feeding for over 1 year beyond tooth eruption (Valaitis et al., 2000) have been found to be associated with early childhood caries. The review also showed that the deleterious effects could to a certain extent be counterbalanced by early tooth brushing with fluoride toothpaste. As one would expect, the use of caries-promoting rearing practices was associated with sociodemographic factors such as family income, parental education, ethnicity, number of children per family, and rural or urban residence.

It is important to be aware that in deprived communities in East and South Asia and in Western Pacific countries, but possibly elsewhere as well, specific deeply entrenched culturally determined rearing practices exist that are quite different from those used in high-income industrialized countries. Prolonged breast feeding and the sharing of the mother's bed are common practices in rural areas throughout South and East Asia, the Western Pacific and in communities in Africa. In Myanmar, where infants share the bed with their mother, no association was found between breast-feeding duration and ECC, whereas a strong association was found with nocturnal breast feeding. None of the infants who were breast fed up to 1 year had ECC, just as daytime breast feeding after the age of 1 year was not associated with this form of caries. However, children who were breast fed more than twice at night after the age of 1 year had a much higher risk (odds ratio = 35) of having ECC. Finally, the use of caries-promoting supplementary food during the weaning period was also associated with caries in these infants (van Palenstein Helderman et al., 2006).

Malnutrition, enamel defects and early childhood caries

Over one-third of the world's children suffer from malnutrition and high rates of infection in early life (Onis et al., 2001), which results in a lower resistance to diseases and salivary gland hypofunction (Psoter et al., 2005), and predisposes to the development of enamel defects (Rugg-Gunn et al., 1998). In third world communities an association was found between enamel hypoplasia and ECC (Harris et al., 2004); and the presence of enamel defects and ECC have been found to be associated in infants in Guatemala, Tanzania, Australia, China, Thailand and Brazil (Infante & Gillespie, 1977; Matee et al., 1992, 1994; Pascoe & Seow, 1994; Kanchanakamol et al., 1996; Li et al., 1996; Oliveira et al., 2006).

Caries in the deciduous dentition of older children

The caries experience in the deciduous dentition is much higher in low- and middle-income countries than in high-income countries (Table 32.4). This high caries experience is to a certain extent attributable to the already high caries experience at preschool age, which is further enhanced by dietary habits that pose a risk for the teeth in the absence of adequate fluoride protection by means of daily tooth brushing with fluoride toothpaste. Worldwide, decayed deciduous teeth are not treated, whether restoratively or non-operatively, and even in high-income countries more than 70% of the cavitated caries lesions in the deciduous dentition remain unrestored (Fig. 32.11). In a wealthy country, such as the UK, only 12% of the carious cavities in 5-year olds were restored in 2003/04 (Pitts et al., 2005). Similarly, children with high levels of dental caries have problems accessing dental care in the USA (Seale & Casamassimo, 2003).

Effects of caries in the deciduous dentition and consequences for management

Children with caries and pain in the deciduous dentition may have problems with eating and sleeping and they have

Table 32.4 Average caries experience in the deciduous dentition of children aged 3–9 years in low-, middle- and high-income countries (Yee & Sheiham, 2002).

Category	n	dmft
Low-income African countries	7	3.1
Low-income Asian countries	5	4.1
Middle-income countries	16	4.3
High-income countries	5	1.6

n: number of surveys; d: cavitated; m: missing due to caries; f: filled; t: primary teeth.

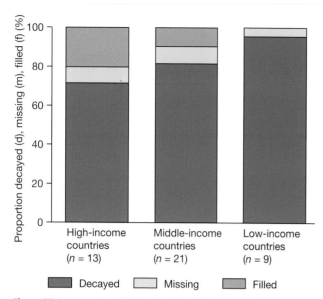

Figure 32.11 Proportional distribution of the dmft components in the primary dentition of children aged 4–9-years between 1990 and 2004 (WHO, 2006). d: cavitated, m: missing due to caries, f: filled, t: primary teeth.

a lower oral health-related quality of life than children without caries (Low *et al*., 1999; Filstrup *et al*., 2003). Toothache caused by caries in the deciduous dentition may impact on growth because it can alter eating and sleeping habits of the young child. Failure to thrive (FTT), characterized by poor weight gain in otherwise healthy children, may be associated with dental decay and toothache (Elice & Fields, 1990). Young children requiring multiple extractions were significantly lighter than control children (Miller *et al*., 1982) and children with one pulpally involved tooth were lower in weight than control children (Acs *et al*., 1992). Turkish children with ECC were significantly lighter and shorter than controls without caries (Ayhan *et al*., 1996). Subsequent dental rehabilitation in children with associated poor weight gain led to improvements in weight gain (Acs *et al*., 1992, 1999) and to significant improvements in the children's eating preferences, quality of food eaten, social behavior and sleeping habits as reported by their parents (Acs *et al*., 2001; Thomas & Primrosch, 2002; Filstrup *et al*., 2003).

Official guidelines in many countries still advocate a vigorous approach to restoring all cavitated caries lesions in primary teeth. These recommendations are based on the idea that untreated caries can lead to general health problems and poor well-being. However, the evidence in favor of such a vigorous restorative approach to carious cavities in primary teeth is weak. Two independent studies both reported that approximately 80% of the primary teeth with carious cavities exfoliate without causing pain (Levine *et al*., 2002; Tickle *et al*., 2002). In addition, no difference was found in the occurrence of pain, extractions due to pain or sepsis, or the prescription of antibiotics, in restored and unrestored carious molars. Since it seems that only a small percentage

of untreated carious primary teeth may result in pain and sepsis, a less interventionist approach may be more appropriate. Since dental pain impacts on children's quality of life and on their growth, treatment of painful carious cavities in primary teeth is necessary, but painless carious primary teeth that do not cause infection may be left unrestored, and a non-operative approach using topical fluoride applications and oral hygiene is preferable.

Carrying out restorative treatment in young children is not without difficulties or side-effects. Restorative treatment is no guarantee against pain and discomfort, and there is evidence suggesting that invasive dental procedures may cause dental fear and anxiety among young children (Milsom *et al*., 2003; Wogelius & Poulsen, 2005). Restorations carried out in primary teeth may not survive long (see Chapters 23 and 24), leading to a cycle of re-restorations; and the often uncooperative small children may be difficult to treat using operative approaches.

The observations of large variations in the restorative index, in England and Wales ranging from 4 to 43% (Pitts *et al*., 2005), may therefore be attributed to huge variations in general dental practitioners' philosophies, beliefs and attitudes towards the management and care of young children (Threlfall *et al*., 2005), because they weigh differently the various pros and cons of using restorative approaches to the management of caries in the deciduous dentition.

It is, moreover, a reality that a traditional dental professional approach focussed on restorations for the management of caries in young children is not feasible for the majority of the world's child populations, namely those living in low- and middle-income countries. Other management approaches have therefore been devised. Daily tooth brushing using a 1000 ppm fluoride toothpaste resulted in arrest of 45% of the caries on proximal surfaces of primary anterior teeth, but only 7% of the caries in primary molars (Lo *et al*., 1998) after 3 years among young Chinese kindergarten children. Some of the caries lesions even spontaneously arrested in the control group who did not brush their teeth with fluoride toothpaste. An additional arresting effect on caries in primary teeth has been reported using a silver diamine fluoride (SDF) paint (44 800 ppm F) on the caries lesions (Chu *et al*., 2002; Llodra *et al*., 2005). However, it remains to be established whether these extremely high fluoride concentrations are really needed to obtain caries-arresting effects above those achieved by means of tooth brushing with fluoride toothpaste, or by standard topical fluoride solutions.

In summary, the evidence for a vigorous restorative approach to the management of caries in the primary dentition is very weak. A large proportion of the carious primary teeth will remain symptom free and will exfoliate naturally. A small proportion of the caries lesions in the primary dentition arrest spontaneously. This process of arresting caries can be enhanced by daily tooth brushing with fluoride toothpaste, and an additional caries-arresting effect can be achieved with fluoride applications.

Dental caries in the permanent dentition of children

The caries experience, measured as the mean number of cavitated, filled and missing teeth, in the permanent dentition of 12-year-olds is higher in middle-income countries than in low- and high-income countries (Table 32.5). Children in low-income countries in general have a low caries experience because their eating and dietary habits are compatible with dental health. In high-income countries, the eating and dietary habits pose a much greater risk to the teeth, but regular oral hygiene with fluoride toothpaste counterbalances the cariogenic challenge. Although people in countries undergoing a period of economic transition, such as the former socialist economies of Europe, may change their dietary habits towards increased sugar consumption (Hobdell, 2001), and may not yet have adopted oral hygiene habits involving daily use of fluoride toothpaste, there is nonetheless evidence that the caries decline also manifests itself in these countries (see Chapters 8 and 28).

In low-income countries almost all caries in children remains untreated (Fig. 32.12). The proportion of the 'filled' component of the DMFT index in middle-income countries is only 20%, and in high-income countries just about 50% of the cavitated caries lesions are restored. This unexpectedly high figure of untreated cavitated caries in high-income countries is mainly due to minority groups who live under deprived conditions and who do not fully benefit from the existing oral health-care services.

Access to health and health services is a fundamental human right, which is equally valid for oral health and oral health care, since oral health is an integral part of general health (Liverpool Declaration, 2006). Unfortunately, these privileges have not been fully realized for children since untreated dental caries remains a global public health problem, especially in low- and middle-income countries and in deprived communities in high-income countries.

Dental caries in adults

The caries experience, measured as the mean number of DMF teeth or surfaces, is generally considerably higher in

Table 32.5 Average caries experience in the permanent dentition of 12-year-old children in low-, middle- and high-income countries (Yee & Sheiham, 2002).

Category	n	DMFT
Low-income countries	45	1.9
Middle-income countries	55	3.3
High-income countries	26	2.1

n: number of surveys; D: cavitated; M: missing due to caries; F: filled; T: permanent teeth.

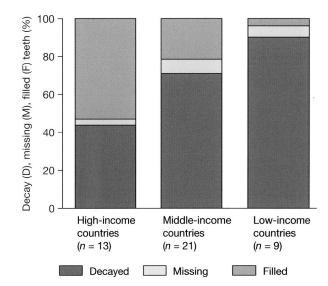

Figure 32.12 Proportional distribution of the DMFT components in the permanent dentition of children aged 11–14-years between 1991 and 2004 (WHO, 2006). D: cavitated, M: missing due to caries, F: filled, T: permanent teeth.

high-income countries than in low- and middle-income countries (Fig. 32.13). While Fig. 32.13 may seem to show that the caries experience of populations with different socioeconomic profiles tends to equalize among the oldest age groups, it should be noted that the figure concerns dentate persons only. As shown in Fig. 32.7, the prevalence of edentulism is much higher in the high-income (US) populations than among the middle-income (PR China) and low-income (Kenya) populations. If this is taken into account, the between-population contrasts in the caries experience are exacerbated, and the higher caries experience of the high-income countries will become more apparent.

Figure 32.13 shows an important feature of the caries experience measured by the DMF index. The figure shows that across populations with different socioeconomic profiles, there is a clear gradient in the composition of the DMF index from the high-income countries to the low-income countries. In the high-income countries restorations are the major contributor to the DF value, whereas restorations are extremely rare in the low-income countries, where the DF value is essentially identical to the D component counting untreated caries.

Even though the caries experience measured by the mean DMF count may indicate a relatively low caries experience, it should be borne in mind that caries is nonetheless a phenomenon that affects virtually everybody in a population. This is shown in Fig. 32.14, which concerns the adult Kenyan population shown in Fig. 32.13 to have a relatively low caries experience. Figure 32.14a shows the cumulative distribution of people according to the number of carious cavities, and Fig. 32.14b shows the distribution according to the total number of caries lesions (cavitated and non-cavitated) for

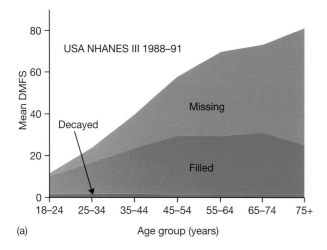

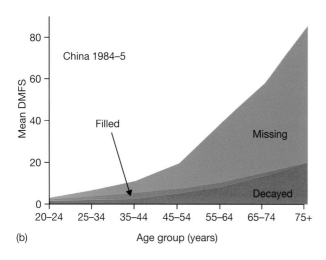

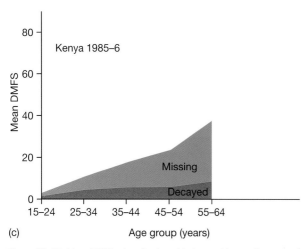

Figure 32.13 Mean DMFS values (cavitated lesions only) according to age for the dentate adult populations in (a) the USA (Winn *et al.*, 1996), (b) PR China (Luan *et al.*, 1989b) and (c) Kenya (Manji *et al.*, 1989). Third molars are excluded.

different age groups. The prevalence of carious cavities is quite high, ranging between 42 and 76%, and, depending on age, 10–50% of the adults present with at least five carious cavities (Fig. 32.14a). Even so, it is clear that the prevalence of caries approaches 100% when the non-cavitated caries lesions are also included in the caries experience of these adults (Fig. 33.14b). The shift of the curves towards the upper right-hand corner is, moreover, an illustration of the concomitant increase in the number of caries lesions. Hence, depending on age, 56–76% of the adult Kenyans present with five or more caries lesions (Fig. 32.14b).

Trends in the burden of oral diseases

As thoroughly discussed in previous chapters (see Chapters 8 and 28), caries has declined markedly over the past 50 years, and particularly so among children and young adults in high-income countries. The caries decline continues and gradually trickles into adult and middle-aged

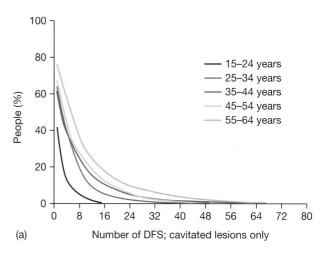

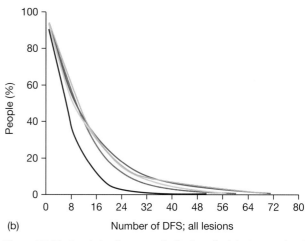

Figure 32.14 Cumulative frequency distribution of adult Kenyans (Manji *et al.*, 1989) according to (a) the number of cavitated caries lesions, and (b) the total number of caries lesions. Data are shown according to age.

groups. Unless counterbalanced by other developments this would imply that the total oral disease burden is rapidly declining. However, the caries decline among the younger population segments concurs with a pronounced improvement in tooth retention among the middle-aged and elderly population segments. The question is therefore whether we are just witnessing a redistribution of the oral disease burden. In other words: is the oral health burden just moving from the simpler problems seen among younger people to the more complicated needs of the now retained teeth among the old, whose oral health situation may be further aggravated by medications, and physical and cognitive impairment?

Fortunately, studies exist that can be used to glean information on the trends in the occurrence of oral diseases. The US National Health and Nutrition Examination Surveys, carried out at regular intervals, and the Norwegian Trøndelag surveys are pertinent examples of such studies. However, from the point of view of comprehensiveness in design and reporting, the most informative studies are the Swedish Jönköping studies (Hugoson *et al.*, 2005a, b). Briefly, in each of the years 1973, 1983, 1993 and 2003, random samples have been drawn of the 20-, 30-, 40-, 50-, 60-, 70- and 80-year-old residents in the town of Jönköping, Sweden. The selected subjects have undergone a very detailed clinical and radiographic examination using consistent methods and diagnostic criteria. Figure 32.15a shows that the prevalence of edentulism has decreased considerably since 1973. Although it is likely that bias has caused some underestimation of the prevalence of edentulism among the elderly in the 2003 survey, the data nonetheless indicate that edentulism is rapidly on its way out. Concomitant with this trend for change, there has been a considerable increase across all ages in the number of teeth retained among the dentate, amounting to an average of up to two teeth per decade (Fig. 32.15b).

Figure 32.16a shows that the mean DFT has declined among the younger adults and increased among the older age groups over the past three decades. This pattern is consistent with the caries decline gradually trickling into the younger adult groups and the increased retention of teeth in the older age groups. In each survey the 1943 generation presents as the cohort with the highest DFT experience. The mean number of endodontically treated teeth has declined in all younger age groups, and only increased among the very old (Fig. 32.16b). This is consistent with the 1923 generation being the cohort with the highest endodontic treatment experience. The mean number of teeth showing evidence of periapical destruction, whether this has undergone attempted treatment or not, shows a steady decline in all age groups since 1973 (Fig. 32.16c).

Figure 32.17a shows that the oral hygiene situation has improved in all age groups from 1973 to 2003, although the 1983 and 1993 situations appeared quite similar. The development in the oral hygiene situation was paralleled by the

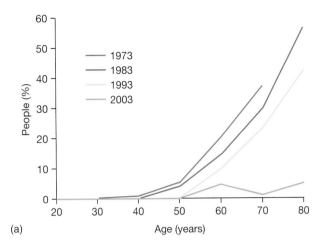

(a)

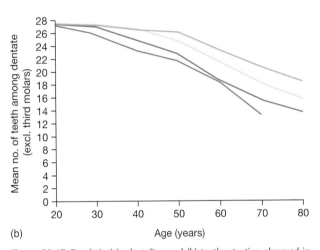

(b)

Figure 32.15 Trends in (a) edentulism and (b) tooth retention observed in Jönköping, Sweden, between 1973 and 2003 (Hugoson *et al.*, 2005b).

development in the gingivitis situation, and the proportion of surfaces that bleed upon probing has also declined in all age groups (Fig. 32.17b). The pocket prevalence increased slightly among the younger age groups from 1973 to 1983, but has since decreased below the 1973 level (Fig. 32.18a). In the older age groups the pocket prevalence has remained high at about 80% since 1973. The mean radiographic bone levels have improved since 1973, most pronouncedly among the older age groups (Fig. 32.18b).

In 1973, most people irrespective of age could be diagnosed with either gingivitis or mild periodontitis (Fig. 32.19a). The fraction having moderate or severe periodontitis was relatively small, and confined to the older ages; and the fraction diagnosed as periodontally healthy was also modest and confined to the younger age groups. The development from 1973 to 1983 indicates two apparently opposing phenomena: more healthy people across all ages, and more middle-aged and older people with moderate or severe periodontitis (Fig. 32.19b), at the expense of the fractions of people with gingivitis or mild periodontitis. This may be

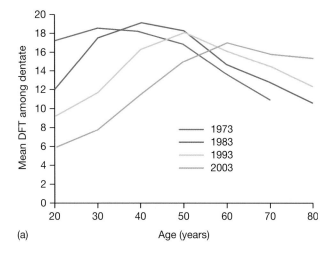

(a)

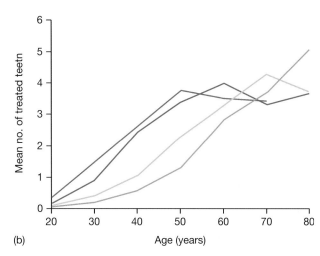

(b)

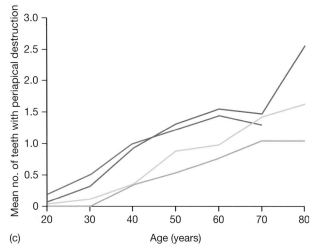

(c)

Figure 32.16 Trends in (a) caries experience measured as the mean number of DFT (cavitated and non-cavitated lesions) and (b) the caries-related treatment experience in the form of the mean number of endodontically treated teeth and (c) mean number of teeth showing periapical destruction among adults in Jönköping, Sweden, between 1973 and 2003 (Hugoson *et al*., 2005b).

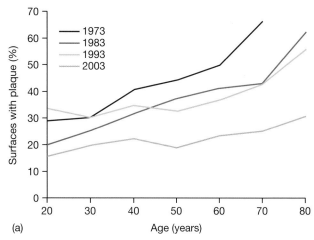

(a)

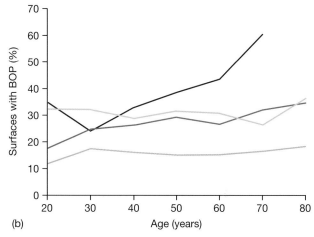

(b)

Figure 32.17 Trends in the (a) oral hygiene level, measured as percentage of surfaces with plaque, and (b) gingivitis, measured as percentage of surfaces with bleeding on probing, among adults in Jönköping, Sweden, between 1973 and 2003 (Hugoson *et al*., 2005b).

explained as resulting from the improved oral hygiene situation manifesting itself, concomitantly with a trend for increased retention of the periodontitis-affected teeth. This is likely to reflect a change in the treatment philosophies used by the dentists, as well as possibly a change in the public perception of the value of one's own teeth. The change from 1983 to 1993 is mainly an increase across all ages in the proportion of people who are deemed periodontally healthy or with gingivitis only (Fig. 32.19c), whereas the change from 1993 to 2003 indicates that the prevalence and severity of periodontitis are on the return (Fig. 32.19d).

The high-income countries are undergoing marked changes in the demographic profile of the populations towards a proportional increase in the aging population resulting from a combination of increased life expectancy and decreasing birth rates. It has therefore been speculated that the declining oral disease burden among the younger

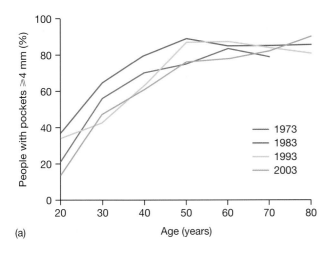

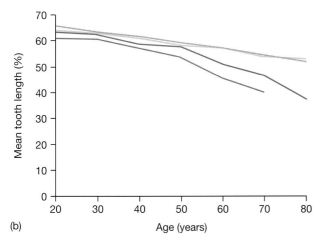

Figure 32.18 Trends in (a) the prevalence of periodontal pockets ≥4 mm, and (b) the mean periodontal bone level, among adults in Jönköping, Sweden, in the period between 1973 and 2003 (Hugoson *et al.*, 2005b).

age groups is compensated by many more middle-aged and elderly people retaining many more teeth that are either at risk of or present a definitive treatment need. However, by combining the Jönköping data with the actual demographic profile of the Swedish population in each of the four survey years, it can be shown that the increase in the number of elderly people and their increased tooth retention are insufficient to compensate for the decline in the oral disease burden among the younger generations.

Clearly, such marked changes call for considerations about the implications for the future need and demand for dental services. In 1990, a WHO expert committee (WHO, 1990) predicted that a dramatic decrease would occur in the moderate-technology tasks (restorations, prostheses, extractions), which for decades have been at the core of dentistry in the high-income countries. It was further predicted that although the demand for high-technology dentistry (defined as precision prosthetics, orthodontics, complex surgery and oral medicine, all based on comprehensive examination,

diagnosis and treatment planning) would increase and new high-tech procedures would be introduced, this would be insufficient to compensate for the decrease in the amount of core services for more than three or four decades (WHO, 1990). The Jönköping data indicate that these three to four decades may have already passed in Sweden.

Social gradients in oral disease burdens

In this chapter so far, broad generalizations have been made concerning high-, middle- and low-income countries. However, it is exceedingly important to bear in mind that 'low' groups exist within 'high' countries, and vice versa. There is thus a wealth of studies demonstrating a considerable social gradient in the occurrence and distribution of oral diseases. The affluent, well-educated and resource-rich population groups are generally both the healthiest and the most vigorous consumers of health-care services. In contrast, the socioeconomically disadvantaged groups carry the major disease burdens, but have *de facto* restricted access to the health-care services. Even in high-income, equity-and-equality-focussed countries such as Sweden, the major disease burdens still cluster in socioeconomically disadvantaged groups that may be difficult to reach (see Chapters 8 and 28).

Disease burdens: whose burdens?

The DMFT/DMFS value is often used to represent the dental health status of populations. However, it actually only provides information on caries and treatment experience and not on the health of the dentition. It does not provide information related to the quality of life or the perception of pain or discomfort of individuals or populations, nor does it say anything about the function of the oral cavity in terms of impairment, disability or handicap. The DMFT gives equal weight to all components of the index, and a DMFT value of 10 may indicate 10 filled teeth, which is not associated with disability or handicap, or 10 missing teeth, which may indeed be coupled with functional limitations. These extreme interpretations of DMFT are real and occur in high- and low-income countries. When the FS-T index, representing the number of functional (filled and sound) teeth, was compared with DMFT among 35–44-year olds on a country basis, the DMFT values were found to be higher in high-income than in low-income countries. However, the FS-T values would indicate that the dental health status was better in high-income countries than in low-income countries (Table 32.6), where the F-component is much lower and the D-component much higher.

Disease impacts

The reality is that caries does not impact on people unless it causes pain, discomfort, functional limitations, disability

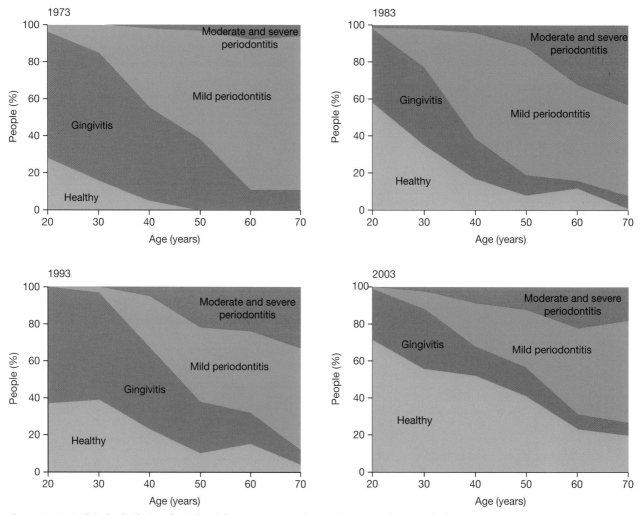

Figure 32.19 Trends in the distribution of periodontal diagnoses among adults in Jönköping, Sweden, for each of the years 1973, 1983, 1993 and 2003 (Hugoson *et al.*, 1998). Note how the fraction of subjects with a healthy periodontium increases from decade to decade, while the fraction of subjects with moderate to severe periodontitis shows a peak value in 1983 and has declined substantially since then.

or handicap. Hence, a key *raison d'être* for dentistry is to assist in the prevention of these conditions, and to provide relief when prevention has failed. In line with this, focus has increasingly been turning away from the traditional normative oral disease burden assessment towards assessments of how oral diseases and conditions impact on people's lives (Locker, 1989).

A large survey among Nepali schoolchildren, 9–11 years of age, indicated that 45% of the schoolchildren had suffered toothache, and 25% had suffered from toothache in the week before the survey. The most frequent impact on the quality of life was the inability of children to eat (62%), followed by the inability to sleep (13%) (Yee *et al.*, 2003). A cross-sectional study of 1126 Thai schoolchildren aged 11–12 years revealed that 90% had oral impacts, mostly due to dental pain (Gherunpong *et al.*, 2004). The most commonly reported impact was the inability to eat (73%). A survey among native American schoolchildren revealed

that 25% avoided laughing or smiling, and 20% avoided meeting other people because of the appearance of their teeth (Chen *et al.*, 1997). In Western Cape, South Africa, 88% of the children surveyed reported experiencing dental pain, with 70% suffering dental pain within the past 2 months (Naidoo *et al.*, 2001). Seventy per cent of the children missed school because of pain. Among 380 first grade Filipino schoolchildren, 82% had experienced toothache, 32% had suffered from toothache in the 4 weeks before the survey and 12% had experienced toothache in the past few days (B. Monse, personal communication, 2006).

In the USA, 3 days are lost per 100 youths aged 5–17-years owing to acute dental conditions, mostly dental caries (US Department of Health and Human Services, 2000). The problem is more extensive among children of the lower socioeconomic groups, who had 12 times as many missed school days because of dental problems compared with children from higher income families (Adams & Marano, 1995).

Table 32.6 Ranking of 35–44-year-olds in 30 countries, according to their DMFT (decayed, missing and filled teeth) counts, and their FS-T (filled and sound teeth) counts (Namal *et al.*, 2005.)

Country	DMFT rank	DMFT	FS-T	New rank
Afghanistan	1	8.3	19.9	16
Papua New Guinea	2	9.0	19.2	20
Georgia	3	9.2	19.5	18
Kiribati	4	9.2	19.4	19
Italy	5	9.4	23.8	4
Singapore	6	9.8	23.4	8
Uzbekistan	7	9.9	19.7	17
Malta	8	10.0	17.9	24
Sri Lanka	9	10.1	18.3	21
Vanuatu	10	10.1	18.1	23
Spain	11	10.9	20.0	15
Turkey	12	11.6	16.9	25
Algeria	13	11.8	18.1	22
Israel	14	12.1	23.5	7
Morocco	15	12.7	15.4	28
Malaysia	16	12.9	16.2	26
Madagascar	17	13.1	15.1	29
Panama	18	13.2	15.4	27
USA	19	13.3	23.1	9
Japan	20	13.7	24.2	2
France	21	14.6	23.8	5
Austria	22	14.7	25.6	1
Slovenia	23	14.7	21.9	11
Philippines	24	15.0	13.3	30
Germany	25	16.1	23.6	6
UK	26	16.6	21.3	12
Denmark	27	16.7	24.1	3
Netherlands	28	17.4	21.2	13
Norway	29	20.5	22.5	10
Australia	30	20.8	20.3	14

Note how countries change ranking depending on how the consequences of dental caries are regarded.

In a school survey of native American schoolchildren, one-third of children reported missing school because of dental pain (Chen *et al.*, 1997). Children with chronic dental pain were unable to focus and unable to complete school assignments, and this affected their school performance, negatively impacting their self-esteem (Schechter, 2000). The extent of the toothache problem can be judged by the fact that the Department of Education in the Philippines reported that the principal reason for absenteeism from schools is due to toothache (Araojo, 2003).

Quo vadis? Priorities in oral health care for low- and middle-income countries

Perceived oral health problems and treatment demands in underserved populations

A survey on perceived oral health-care needs in a low-income country revealed that perceived oral health problems were strongly related to pain and discomfort (Mosha & Scheutz, 1993). This is in line with the observation that relief of pain due to the sequelae of dental caries is the main reason for people to visit a dental clinic in low-income countries such as Sri Lanka (Warnakulasuriya, 1985; Ekanayake *et al.*, 2001), Tanzania (van Palenstein Helderman & Nathoo, 1990; Mandari & Matee, 2006), Cambodia (Todd & Durward, 1994), China (Du *et al.*, 2000b), Vietnam (van Palenstein Helderman *et al.*, 2000), Nigeria (Oginni, 2004) and Burkina Faso (Varenne *et al.*, 2005).

Lack of dental workforce

To meet the described perceived oral health problems and treatment demands, low- and middle-income countries are not only limited by lack of financial resources, but also constrained by the lack of a dental workforce. Nepal has one dentist per 80 000 people, Bangladesh one dentist per 70 000 people and Indonesia 1 dentist per 25 000 people (WHO, 2006). To this, one should add that the majority of dentists have their practice in the big cities, thus the dentist to population ratio in the rural areas where most people live is even more adverse (Manji & Sheiham, 1986). This is well illustrated in India, where the dentist to population ratio is 1:27 000, but in rural areas the ratio is 1:300 000 (Shah, 2001). In Africa the dentist to population ratio is 1:150 000, while most industrialized countries have a ratio of 1:2000 (Petersen, 2003).

The strategy traditionally used when human resources are lacking is to train more dentists. However, in the context of dental care in low- and middle-income countries this strategy is fallacious. At best, training more dentists merely means better access to services for the élite in urban centres and continued lack of care for the more populous rural population. At worst, it means training for the benefit of others, as many dentists in low-income countries emigrate for better paid jobs abroad.

Low impact of dentists on untreated caries

That training of more dentists in low- and middle-income countries is an erroneous approach is well illustrated with the situation in Syria, with a population of 17 million. Between 1985 and 1998, the number of dentists in Syria increased from about 2000 to 11 000, resulting in a dentist to population ratio of 1:1500. Even so, the care index (F/DMFT × 100%) of the child population remained unchanged, and that of adults increased only moderately from 17 to 33% (Beiruti & van Palenstein Helderman, 2004). Thus, the enormous increase in number of dentists in Syria had only a marginal impact on the care index of the population. The reason for the situation described is that the majority of the population in Syria cannot afford the restorative care provided by dentists. Another example is the Philippines, with a dentist to population ratio of 1:5000, which approaches that of high-income countries. Nevertheless, the care index of children is very low and

Table 32.7 Dentist: population ratio, mean DMFT counts (cavitated lesions only) and care index of 12–13-year olds of some Asian nations (WHO, 2006)

Country	Dentist: population ratio	Mean DMFT	Care index (F/DMFT×100%)
Nepal	1:80 000	0.5	5%
Pakistan	1:29 000	1.4	7%
Indonesia	1:25 000	2.2	5%
Sri Lanka	1:20 000	1.4	7%
Philippines	1:5000	4.6	3%

comparable to that of other Asian countries with a more adverse dentist to population ratio (Table 32.7).

In summary, Western-oriented dental care provided by dentists is too expensive and not affordable for the large majority of people in low- and middle-income countries.

Western-oriented dental care model inefficient

It is important to realize that not only is the Western-oriented dental care model too expensive for populations in low- and middle-income countries but it has also been shown in the past century to have limited impact on the incidence and distribution of disease in the population. A symposium on dental care in Scandinavia (Frandsen, 1982), a review of oral health-care delivery in Europe (Møller, 1987) and the WHO International Collaborative Study of Dental Manpower Systems in seven countries (Cohen, 1978) have all come to the conclusion that the dental services as seen in the Western-oriented dental care model have had a marginal effect in improving the oral health status of the population. Likewise, in an analysis of data on 12-year-old children in 18 industrialized countries, curative dental services only accounted for 3% of the variation in the decline in DMFT for 12-year-olds in the 1970s and 1980s (Nadanovsky & Sheiham, 1995).

Recommendations for priorities

Surveys have shown that most people in low- and middle-income countries do not practice habits conducive to oral health, just as their oral health knowledge is poor in Tanzania (Kabalo & Mosha, 1988), Bangladesh (van Palenstein Helderman et al., 1998), Indonesia (van Palenstein Helderman et al., 1997) and China (Peng et al., 1997; Petersen et al., 1997).

Taken together, these observations and the considerations about (i) the perceived oral health problems and treatment demands, (ii) the lack of oral health mindedness, (iii) the unaffordable Western-oriented dental care provided by dentists, and (iv) the fact that Western-oriented care by dentists has a limited impact on the oral health status of populations, calls for a completely different oral health-care strategy than the traditional Western one for low- and middle-income countries. This leaves decision makers with a dilemma, because the dental profession would undoubtedly recommend copying the Western-oriented dentistry

model. However, evidence from the high-income countries suggests that such copying may result in a long period during which these populations undergo a phase of 'mass dental extermination'. As long as the total treatment demand exceeds the capacity of the available dentists, these are more likely to resort to quick, cheap and radical solutions, such as tooth extractions, than to attempt to embark on the more expensive conservative procedures (Bouma et al., 1987).

A population-based strategy for health education and education for self-care based on a common risk-factor approach are much needed. As already mentioned in the context of controlling periodontal diseases, a whole-population approach for better oral hygiene within the frame of general hygiene programmes should be prioritized. Inclusion of fluoride for the control of caries in oral hygiene programs can be materialized by promoting the availability and affordability of fluoride toothpastes on the local market and the daily use of fluoride toothpaste through tooth brushing. The unmet perceived oral health problems and treatment demands should be addressed by the provision of basic relief of pain services.

This promotional and basic oral health-care program should be integrated in the primary health care (PHC) systems that exist in most low- and middle-income countries (van Palenstein Helderman et al., 1999). The philosophy of the PHC approach is to focus on the promotion of health by providing a supportive environment for community self-care and preventive action, and to provide basic curative care. These PHC systems aim to make essential care accessible at a cost that the country and community can afford. Thus, the PHC system is the appropriate place for basic oral health-care programmes. Health centres are the administrative and executive centres for PHC. The type of personnel required to provide basic oral health-care depends on the precise community needs, available human resources and local legislation. Personnel for oral health care must be appropriately trained and legally allowed to provide this type of care. Dentists are too expensive to provide basic care in the PHC system, but they are needed as district or regional supervisors of the system and they should serve as dentists in district or regional hospitals for referred cases from the PHC field. Guidelines are available for the delivery of basic oral emergency care regarding minimal equipment needed (Baart et al., 2005) and infection control (Yee, 2006).

A report was recently published, endorsed by WHO, which describes in greater detail the above strategy for oral health care in low- and middle-income countries and deprived communities in high-income countries (Frencken et al., 2002). The contents provide information on practical aspects and highlight the principles of the three components of the basic package of oral care: oral urgent treatment, affordable fluoride toothpaste and atraumatic restorative treatment (see Chapter 23). In countries with limited financial resources, the latter component may only be feasible in school dental services.

Quo vadis? Priorities for high-income countries

The dilemma for the high-income countries is also great, but of a fundamentally different nature. As shown in this and preceding chapters, the oral health and disease profiles in high-income populations have changed substantially within just a few decades. The dental treatment philosophies have changed as a result of application of present-day knowledge about oral diseases, and this has primarily led to increased tooth retention among the older age groups. However, the relative role of traditional chairside dentistry for the substantially lower oral disease incidence observed in children and adults until the fourth or fifth decade of life is questionable. The altering oral disease profiles leave the high-income countries with a structure and organization of their dental health-care systems which is increasingly out of touch with the distribution of oral disease and treatment needs. The dental profession continues to recommend people to adopt regular dental attendance patterns, arguing that such regular dental screening examinations are important for the prevention of oral diseases. There is an increasing tendency for these regular consumers of oral health care to be those least in need, as a substantial fraction of the younger population groups in high-income countries are increasingly unlikely ever to develop oral diseases. This trend for change will gradually also reach into the older age groups.

It is a historical fact that traditional chairside dentistry as known in the Western high-income countries has made little effort to reach socioeconomically disadvantaged groups, who carry the major oral disease burdens, and are too marginalized to contemplate dental visits as a part of their health behavior. Similarly, the needs and wants of the increasing numbers of disabled elderly people in old people's homes, who carry substantial disease burdens but are unlikely ever to appear in a dental clinic, do not receive much attention.

With few exceptions, dental services for the adult populations in the Western high-income countries are provided by private dentists who have freedom to establish themselves within the bounds set by the requirements for authorization as a dentist. In principle, private dentists work in a free competitive market, but research has shown that competition plays a limited role (Grytten & Sørensen, 2000). Patients have no information base that allows them to find the dentist who provides the best trade-off between price and quality of care. Dental services are experience goods, which means that to evaluate their quality they must be tried, and the dental fees often vary too little to make the effort of shopping around for a dentist worthwhile. Moreover, patient loyalty to the dentist is a characteristic that is further promoted by the dentists, who may react negatively to patients trying to shop around to find the best deal. Finally, there is a considerable asymmetry of information between dentists and patients. Patients have no basis for judging the appropriateness of the diagnostic procedures used, the diagnoses made or the treatments recommended, but have to rely on the advice given and recommendations made by the dentist. The large variation that has been documented (see Chapter 31) to exist between dentists in the diagnoses made and treatments recommended for the same patients is an illustration of the extent to which these factors allow the dentists to control the market for dental services. This control of the dental service market by the dentists manifests itself in supplier-induced demand and utilization of dental services. It is thus well known from several studies (Grytten, 1990, 1991, 1992, 2005; Grytten *et al.*, 1992; Wright & Batchelor, 2002) that dentists may use the frequency of preventive check-up visits and the amount of diagnostic and treatment procedures prescribed per patient to control the demand for and utilization of dental services, and hence their income. As long as this situation prevails, the deprived and underprivileged sections of the populations in the high-income countries are unlikely to enjoy the benefits of dental health care.

It is the present authors' view that appropriate solutions to these dilemmas may require a thorough rethinking of the role and organization of dentistry in the high-income countries. The rapidly changing disease profiles, not only in the oral health field, but also in general health, necessitate a higher degree of integration of the oral health-care services into the framework of the general health-care systems. The health-care services should increasingly make use of the fact that many risk factors for diseases are shared, and adopt a common risk factor strategy for prevention and control. The health-care services in the high-income countries should also take into account the increasing polarization of disease burdens. They should acknowledge, in content and in organization, that deprived and disabled population groups exist for whom self-care and health-care utilization are not merely a matter of individuals being willing to make the extra effort, and that contextual and structural factors effectively prevent these groups from making healthy choices.

The Nobel-prize winning German physicist Max Planck noted that a new concept 'does not triumph by convincing its opponents and make them see the light, but rather because its opponents eventually die, and a new generation grows up that is familiar with it'. The crucial question is, therefore, whether we, at this moment in time, have this new generation that understands and advocates the need for new strategies in oral health care.

References

Acs G, Lodolini G, Kaminsky S, Gisneros GJ. Effect of nursing caries on body weight in a pediatric population. *Pediatr Dent* 1992; **14**: 302–5.

Acs G, Shulman R, Ng MW, Chussid S. The effect of dental rehabilitation on the body weight of children with early childhood caries. *Pediatr Dent* 1999; **21**: 109–13.

Acs G, Pretzer S, Foley M, Ng MW. Perceived outcomes and parental satisfaction following dental rehabilitation under general anesthesia. *Pediatr Dent* 2001; **23**: 419–23.

Adams PF, Marano MA. *Current estimates for the National Health Interview Survey, 1994*. Vital and Health Statistics: Series 10, Data from the National Health Survey, No. 193. Hyattsville, MD: Department of Health and Human Services, National Center for Health Statistics, 1995.

Ainamo J, Barmes D, Beagrie G, Cutress T, Martin J. Development of the World Health Organization (WHO) Community Periodontal Index of Treatment Needs (CPITN). *Int Dent J* 1982; **32**: 281–91.

Ainamo J, Sarkki L, Kuhalampi ML, Palolampi L, Piirto O. The frequency of periodontal extractions in Finland. *Community Dent Health* 1984; **1**: 165–72.

Alaska Native Tribal Health Consortium. http://www.anthc.org/. Accessed 6 August 2006.

Albandar JM, Kingman A. Gingival recession, gingival bleeding, and dental calculus in adults 30 years of age and older in the United States, 1988–1994. *J Periodontol* 1999; **70**: 30–43.

Albandar JM, Brunelle JA, Kingman A. Destructive periodontal disease in adults 30 years of age and older in the United States, 1988–1994. *J Periodontol* 1999; **70**: 13–29.

Albert RJ, Cantin RY, Cross HG, Castaldi CR. Nursing caries in the Inuit children of the Keewatin. *J Can Dent Assoc* 1988; **54**: 751–8.

American Academy of Pediatric Dentistry. Policy on early childhood caries (ECC): classifications, consequences, and preventive strategies. *Pediatr Dent* 2005; **27**: 31–5.

American Academy of Periodontology. Epidemiology of periodontal diseases. Position paper. *J Periodontol* 2005; **76**: 1406–19.

American Dental Association. *Alaska Native Dental Health Initiative*. http://www.ada.org/public/media/presskits/alaska/index.asp. Accessed 6 August 2006.

Angelillo IF, Nobile CGA, Pavia M. Survey of reasons for extraction of permanent teeth in Italy. *Community Dent Oral Epidemiol* 1996; **24**: 336–40.

Anumanrajadhon T, Rajchagool S, Nitsiri P, *et al.* The community care model of the intercountry Centre for Oral Health at Chiangmai, Thailand. *Int Dent J* 1996; **46**:325–33.

Araojo JR. *Phillipine country report on school health promotion programme*. 2nd Asian Conference on Oral Health Promotion for School Children. Prospectus for our Future Generation. Ayyuthaya, Thailand: Thammasat University, 2003.

Ayhan H, Suskan E, Yidirim S. The effect of nursing or rampant caries on height, body weight and head circumference. *J Clin Pediatr Dent* 1996; **20**: 209–12.

Baart J, Bosgra J, van Palenstein Helderman WH. Basic oral emergency care by auxilliaries for under-served populations. *Developing Dentistry* 2005; **6**: FDI, Practical guide.

Baelum V. *The epidemiology of destructive periodontal disease. Causes, paradigms, problems, methods and empirical evidence*. Thesis, University of Aarhus, 1998.

Baelum V, Fejerskov O. Tooth loss as related to dental caries and periodontal breakdown in adult Tanzanians. *Community Dent Oral Epidemiol* 1986; **14**: 353–7.

Baelum V, Lopez R. Defining and classifying periodontitis: need for a paradigm shift? *Eur J Oral Sci* 2003; **111**: 2–6.

Baelum V, Papapanou PN. CPITN and the epidemiology of periodontal disease. *Community Dent Oral Epidemiol* 1996; **24**: 367–8.

Baelum V, Scheutz F. Periodontal diseases in Africa. *Periodontol 2000* 2002; **29**: 79–103.

Baelum V, Fejerskov O, Manji F. Periodontal diseases in adult Kenyans. *J Clin Periodontol* 1988a; **15**: 445–52.

Baelum V, Luan WM, Fejerskov O, Chen X. Tooth mortality and periodontal conditions in 60–80-year-old Chinese. *Scand J Dent Res* 1988b; **96**: 99–107.

Baelum V, Manji F, Wanzala P, Fejerskov O. Relationship between CPITN and periodontal attachment loss findings in an adult population. *J Clin Periodontol* 1995; **22**: 146–52.

Baelum V, Pongpaisal S, Pithpornchaiyakul W, *et al.* Determinants of dental status and caries among adults in southern Thailand. *Acta Odontol Scand* 2002; **60**: 80–6.

Bailit HL, Braun R, Maryniuk GA, Camp P. Is periodontal disease the primary cause of tooth extraction in adults? *J Am Dent Assoc* 1987; **114**: 40–5.

Beiruti N, van Palenstein Helderman WH. Oral health in Syria. *Int Dent J* 2004; **54** (Suppl 1): 383–8.

Beltrán-Aguilar ED, Barker LK, Canto MT, *et al.* Surveillance for dental caries, dental sealants, tooth retention, edentulism, and enamel fluorosis – United States 1988–1994 and 1999–2002. *MMWR Morb Mortal Wkly Rep* 2005; **54** (No. SS–3):1–48.

Black AD. Roentgenographic studies of tissues involved in chronic mouth infections. *Dent Summary* 1918; **38**: 924–32.

Black GV. *A work on operative dentistry*. Vol. 1. *Pathology of the dental hard tissues of the teeth*. Chicago, IL: Medico-Dental Publishing Co., 1914a.

Black GV. *A work on operative dentistry*, Vol. II, *The technical procedures in filling teeth*. 2nd edn. Chicago, IL: Medico-Dental Publishing Co., 1914b.

Borrell LN, Burt BA, Warren RC, Neighbors HW. The role of individual and neighborhood social factors on periodontitis: the third national health and nutrition examination survey. *J Periodontol* 2006; **77**: 444–53.

Bouma J, Schaub RMH, van de Poel ACM. Relative importance of periodontal disease for full mouth extractions in the Netherlands. *Community Dent Oral Epidemiol* 1987; **15**: 41–5.

Broderick E, Mabry J, Robertson D, Thompson J. Baby bottle tooth decay in Native American children in Head Start Centers. *Public Health Rep* 1989; **104**: 50–4.

Brunton PA, Vrihoef T, Wilson NHF. Restorative care and economic wealth: a global perspective. *Int Dent J* 2003; **53**: 97–9.

Buckley JP. Buckley–Price debate. Subject: Resolved, that practically all infected pulpless teeth should be removed. *J Am Dent Assoc* 1925; **12**: 1499–524.

Burt BA. Influences for change in the dental health status of populations: an historical perspective. *J Public Health Dent* 1978; **38**: 272–88.

Cahen PM, Frank RM, Turlot JC. A survey of the reasons for dental extractions in France. *J Dent Res* 1985; **64**: 1087–93.

Caldas AF. Reasons for tooth extraction in a Brazilian population. *Int Dent J* 2000; **50**: 267–73.

Cariño KMG, Shinada K, Kawaguchi Y. Early childhood caries in northern Phillipines. *Community Dent Oral Epidemiol* 2003; **31**: 81–9.

Centers for Disease Control and Prevention (CDCP) Conference. Atlanta, GA: Centers for Disease Control, 1994.

Chauncey HH, Glass RL, Alman JE. Dental caries. Principal cause of tooth extraction in a sample of US male adults. *Caries Res* 1989; **23**: 200–5.

Chen MS, Andersen RM, Barmes DE, Leclercq MH, Lyttle CS. *Comparing oral health care systems: a second international collaborative study*. Geneva: World Health Organization, 1997.

Chu CH, Lo ECM, Lin HC. Effectiveness of silver diamine fluoride and sodium fluoride varnish in arresting dentin caries in Chinese pre-school children. *J Dent Res* 2002; **81**: 767–70.

Cohen LK. Dental care in seven countries: the international collaborative study of dental manpower systems in relation to oral health status. In: Ingle JE, Blair P, eds. *International dental care delivery systems: issues in dental health policies*. Cambridge, MA: Ballinger, 1978: 201–14.

Corbet EF, Davies WIR. Reasons given for tooth extractions in Hong Kong. *Community Dent Health* 1991; **8**: 121–30.

Dentists in the United States Public Health Service. *Community Health Aide Program*. http://www.phs-dental.org/depac/newfile50.html. Accessed 6 August 2006.

Dini EL, Holt RD, Bedi R. Caries and its association with infant feeding and oral health-related behaviours in 3–4-year-old Brazilian children. *Community Dent Oral Epidemiol* 2000; **28**: 241–8.

Douglass JM, Yi W, Xue ZB, Tinanoff N. Dental caries in preschool Beijing and Connecticut children as described by a new caries analysis system. *Community Dent Oral Epidemiol* 1994; **22**: 94–9.

Douglass JM, Tinanoff N, Tang JM, Altman DS. Dental caries patterns and oral health behaviors in Arizona infants and toddlers. *Community Dent Oral Epidemiol* 2001; **29**: 14–22.

Du M, Bian Z, Guo L, Holt R, Champion J, Bedi R. Caries patterns and their relationship to infant feeding and socioeconomic status in 2–4-year-old Chinese children. *Int Dent J* 2000a; **50**: 385–9.

Du M, Petersen PE, Fan M, Bian Z, Tai B. Oral health services in PR China as evaluated by dentists and patients. *Int Dent J* 2000b; **50**: 250–6.

Ekanayake L, Weerasekare C, Ekanayake N. Needs and demands for dental care in patients attending the University Dental Hospital in Sri Lanka. *Int Dent J* 2001; **51**: 67–72.

Elice CE, Fields HW. Failure to thrive: review of the literature, case reports, and implications for dental treatment. *Pediatr Dent* 1990; **12**: 185–9.

Ettinger RL. An evaluation of the attitudes of a group of elderly edentulous patients to dentists, dentures, and dentistry. *Dent Pract Dent Rec* 1971; **22**: 85–91.

Fass EN. Is bottle feeding of milk a factor in dental caries? *J Dent Child* 1962; **29**: 245–51.

Fauchard P. *The surgeon dentist or treatise on the teeth*, Vol I. New York: Milford House, 1969a.

Fauchard P. *The surgeon dentist or treatise on the teeth*, Vol. II. New York: Milford House, 1969b.

Fejerskov O, Baelum V, Luan WM, Manji F. Caries prevalence in Africa and the People's Republic of China. *Int Dent J* 1994; **44**: 425–33.

Filstrup SL, Briskie D, de Fonseca M, Lawrence L, Wandera A, Inglehart MR. Early childhood caries and quality of life: child and parent perspectives. *Pediatr Dent* 2003; **25**: 431–40.

Fox J. *The history and treatment of the diseases of the teeth, the gums, and the alveolar processes, with the operations which they respectively require.* London: Thomas Cox, 1806.

Frandsen A. *Dental health care in Scandinavia.* Chicago, IL: Quintessence, 1982.

Frandsen A. Mechanical oral hygiene practices. In: Löe H, Kleinman DV, eds. *Dental plaque control measures and oral hygiene practices.* Oxford: IRL Press, 1986: 93–116.

Fraundorf KC. Organized dentistry and the pursuit of entry control. *J Health Polit Policy Law* 1984; **8**: 759–81.

Frencken JE, Holmgren CJ, van Palenstein Helderman WH. *Basic package of oral care.* Nijmegen: WHO Collaborating Centre for Oral Health Care Planning and Future Scenarios, 2002.

Gelbier S. 125 years of developments in dentistry, 1880–2005. Part 2: law and the dental profession. *Br Dent J* 2005a; **199**: 470–3.

Gelbier S. 125 years of developments in dentistry, 1880–2005. Part 3: Dental equipment and materials. *Br Dent J* 2005b; **199**: 536–9.

Gelbier S. 125 years of developments in dentistry, 1880–2005. Part 4: Clinical dentistry. *Br Dent J* 2005c; **199**: 536–9.

Genco RJ, Ho AW, Grossi SG, Dunford RG, Tedesco LA. Relationship of stress, distress and inadequate coping behaviors to periodontal disease. *J Periodontol* 1999; **70**: 711–23.

Gherunpong S, Tsakos G, Sheiham A. The prevalence and severity of oral impacts on daily performances in Thai primary school children. *Health Qual Life Outcomes* 2004; **2**: 57.

Gjermo P, Bellini HT, Marcos B. Application of the Community Periodontal Index of Treatment Needs (CPITN) in a population of young Brazilians. *Community Dent Oral Epidemiol* 1983; **11**: 342–6.

Grytten J. The effect of the price of dental services on their demand and utilisation in Norway. *Community Dent Health* 1990; **8**: 303–10.

Grytten J. The effect of supplier inducement on Norwegian dental services; some empirical findings based on a theoretical model. *Community Dent Health* 1991; **8**: 221–31.

Grytten J. Supplier inducement – its relative effect on demand and utilization. *Community Dent Oral Epidemiol* 1992; **20**: 6–9.

Grytten J. Models for financing dental services. A review. *Community Dent Health* 2005; **22**: 75–85.

Grytten J, Sørensen R. Competition and dental services. *Health Econ* 2000; **9**: 447–61.

Grytten J, Holst D, Grytten L. Supply decisions among dentists working within a fixed-fee system of dental care provision. *J Public Health Dent* 1992; **52**: 204–9.

Harris R, Nicoll AD, Adair PM, Pine CM. Risk factors for dental caries in young children: a systematic review of the literature. *Community Dent Health* 2004; **21** (Suppl 1): 71–85.

Hartono SWA, Lambri SE, van Palenstein Helderman WH. *Early childhood caries in breastfed infants in a rural area in West Java, Indonesia.* Nijmegen: WHO Collaborating Centre for Oral Health Planning and Future Scenarios, 2002.

Hirschfeld L, Wasserman B. A long-term survey of tooth loss in 600 treated periodontal patients. *J Periodontol* 1978; **49**: 225–37.

Historical National Health Expenditure Data. Centers for Medicare & Medicaid Services, Office of the Actuary. http://www.cms.hhs.gov/NationalHealthExpendData/downloads/tables.pdf. Accessed 1 August 2006.

Hobdell MH. Economic glabalization and oral health. *Oral Dis* 2001; **7**: 137–43.

Holmgren CJ. CPITN – interpretations and limitations. *Int Dent J* 1994; **44**: 533–46.

Hu D, Liu D. Trends of caries prevalence and experience in children in Chengdu City, West China, 1982–1990. *Community Dent Oral Epidemiol* 1992; **20**: 308–9.

Hugoson A, Norderyd O, Slotte C, Thorstensson H. Distribution of periodontal disease in a Swedish adult population 1973, 1983 and 1993. *J Clin Periodontol* 1998; **25**: 542–8.

Hugoson A, Koch G, Göthberg C, et al. Oral health of individuals aged 3–80 years in Jönköping, Sweden during 30 years (1973–2003). I. Review of findings on dental care habits and knowledge of oral health. *Swed Dent J* 2005a; **29**: 125–38.

Hugoson A, Koch G, Göthberg C, et al. Oral health of individuals aged 3–80 years in Jönköping, Sweden during 30 years (1973–2003). II. Review of clinical and radiographic findings. *Swed Dent J* 2005b; **29**: 139–55.

Huisman F. Itinerant dentists and patent remedies in the Dutch republic. In: Hillam EC, ed. *Dental practice in Europe at the end of the 18th century.* Amsterdam: Editions Rodopi, 2003.

Hujoel PP, Bergström J, del Aguila MA, DeRouen TA. A hidden periodontitis epidemic during the 20th century? *Community Dent Oral Epidemiol* 2003; **31**: 1–6.

Hunter J. *The natural history of the human teeth: explaining their structure, use, formation, growth, and diseases.* London: J. Johnson, 1771.

Hunter J. *A practical treatise on the diseases of the teeth; intended as a supplement to the natural history of those parts.* London: J. Johnson, 1778.

Infante PF, Gillespie GM. Enamel hypoplasia in relation to caries in Guatemalan children. *J Dent Res* 1977; **56**: 493–8.

Jacobi A. *The dentition and its derangements.* Course lectures. New York: New York Medical College, 1862.

Kabalo JM, Mosha HJ. Dental awareness among mothers attending MCH clinics in Bagamoyo District, Coast Region, Tanzania. *Afr Dent J* 1988; **2**: 65–8.

von Kaczorowski. Der ätiologische Zusammenhang zwischen Entzündung des Zahnfleisches und anderweitigen Krankheiten. *Dtsch Monatsschr Zahnheilkd* 1886; **4**: 115–17.

Kanchanakamol U, Tuongratanaphan S, Lertpoonvilaikul W, et al. Prevalence of developmental enamel defects and dental caries in rural pre-school Thai children. *Community Dent Health* 1996; **13**: 204–7.

Kelly M, Bruerd B. The prevalence of baby bottle tooth decay among two native American populations. *J Public Health Dent* 1987; **47**: 94–7.

Kida IA, Åstrøm AN, Strand GV, Masalu JR. Clinical and socio-behavioral correlates of tooth loss: a study of older adults in Tanzania. *BMC Oral Health* 2006; **6**: 5.

Klock KS, Haugejorden O. Primary reasons for extraction of permanent teeth in Norway: changes from 1968 to 1988. *Community Dent Oral Epidemiol* 1991; **19**: 336–41.

Lalloo R, Myburgh NG, Hobdell MH. Dental caries, socio-economic development and national oral health policies. *Int Dent J* 1999; **49**: 196–202.

Lembariti BS. *Periodontal diseases in Tanzania. A study on susceptibility and prevention programmes.* Dar es Salaam: University of Dar es Salaam, 1994.

Lembariti BS, Van der Weijden GA, van Palenstein Helderman WH. The effect of a single scaling with or without oral hygiene instruction on gingival bleeding and calculus formation. *J Clin Periodontol* 1998; **25**: 30–3.

Levine RS, Pitts NB, Nugent ZJ. The fate of 1,587 unrestored carious deciduous teeth: a retrospective general dental practice based study from northern England. *Br Dent J* 2002; **193**: 99–103.

Li Y, Navia JM, Bian JY. Caries experience in deciduous dentition of rural Chinese children 3–5 years old in relation to the presence or absence of enamel hypoplasia. *Caries Res* 1996; **30**: 8–15.

Lindblom C. *Waiting for dental care – how tooth decay became politics.* Stockholm: Carlssons Bokförlag, 2004.

Lindhe J, Nyman S. The effect of plaque control and surgical pocket elimination on the establishment and maintenance of periodontal health. A longitudinal study of periodontal therapy in cases of advanced disease. *J Clin Periodontol* 1975; **2**: 67–79.

Liverpool Declaration: Promoting oral health in the 21st century. A call for action. www.who.int/entity/oral_health/events/liverpool declaration. Accessed 1 August 2006.

Llodra JC, Rodriguez A, Ferrer B, Menardia V, Ramos T, Morato M. Efficacy of silver diamine fluoride for caries reduction in primary teeth and first permanent molars of schoolchildren: 36-month clinical trial. *J Dent Res* 2005; **84**: 721–4.

Lo ECM, Schwarz E, Wong MCM. Arresting dentine caries in Chinese preschool children. *Int J Paediatr Dent* 1998; **8**: 253–60.

Locker D. *An introduction to behavioural science and dentistry.* London: Routledge, 1989.

Löe H, Theilade E, Jensen SB. Experimental gingivitis in man. *J Periodontol* 1965; **36**: 177–87.

Lopez R. *Periodontitis in adolescents. Studies among Chilean high school students.* Thesis, University of Aarhus, 2003.

Lopez R, Fernandez O, Baelum V. Social gradients in periodontal diseases among adolescents. *Community Dent Oral Epidemiol* 2006; **34**: 184–96.

Low W, Tan S, Schwartz S. The effect of severe caries on the quality of life in young children. *Pediatr Dent* 1999; **21**: 325–6.

Luan WM, Baelum V, Chen X, Fejerskov O. Tooth mortality and prosthetic treatment patterns in urban and rural Chinese aged 20–80 years. *Community Dent Oral Epidemiol* 1989a; **17**: 221–6.

Luan WM, Baelum V, Chen X, Fejerskov O. Dental caries in adult and elderly Chinese. *J Dent Res* 1989b; **68**: 1771–6.

Luan WM, Baelum V, Fejerskov O, Chen X. Ten-year incidence of dental caries in adult and elderly Chinese. *Caries Res* 2000; **34**: 205–13.

McCaul LK, Jenkins WMM, Kay EJ. The reasons for the extraction of various tooth types in Scotland: a 15-year follow up. *J Dent* 2001; **29**: 401–7.

Majid ZA, Hussein NNN, Meon R. The oral health of pre-school children in a satellite town in Malaysia. *J Int Assoc Dent Child* 1987; **18**: 36–40.

Mandari GJ, Matee MI. Atraumatic restorative treatment (ART): the Tanzanian experience. *Int Dent J* 2006; **56**: 71–6.

Manji F, Sheiham A. CPITN findings and the manpower implications of periodontal treatment needs for Kenyan children. *Community Dent Health* 1986; **3**: 143–51.

Manji F, Baelum V, Fejerskov O. Tooth mortality in an adult rural population in Kenya. *J Dent Res* 1988; **67**: 496–500.

Manji F, Fejerskov O, Baelum V. Patterns of dental caries in an adult rural population. *Caries Res* 1989; **23**: 55–62.

Marcus SE, Drury TF, Brown LJ, Zion GR. Tooth retention and tooth loss in the permanent dentition of adults: United States, 1988–1991. *J Dent Res* 1996; **75**: 684–95.

Marshall-Day CD, Stephens RG, Quigley LF. Periodontal disease: prevalence and incidence. *J Periodontol* 1955; **26**: 185–203.

Matee MIN, Mikx FHM, Maselle SYM, van Palenstein Helderman WH. Rampant caries and linear hypoplasia. *Caries Res* 1992; **26**: 205–8.

Matee M, van't Hof M, Maselle SY, Mikx FHM, van Palenstein Helderman WH. Nursing caries, linear hypoplasia, and nursing and weaning habits in Tanzanian infants. *Community Dent Oral Epidemiol* 1994; **22**: 289–93.

Matthesen M, Baelum V, Aarslev I, Fejerskov O. Dental health of children and adults in Guinea-Bissau, West Africa, in 1986. *Community Dent Health* 1990; **7**: 123–33.

Miller J, Vaughan-Williams SE, Furlong R, Harrison L. Dental caries and children's weights. *J Epidemiol Community Health* 1982; **36**: 49–52.

Miller WD. *The micro-organisms of the human mouth. The local and general diseases which are caused by them.* Philadelphia, PA: S.S. White Dental Mfg. Co., 1890.

Miller WD. The human mouth as a focus of infection. *Dent Cosmos* 1891; **33**: 689–713.

Milnes AR. Description and epidemiology of nursing caries. *J Public Health Dent* 1996; **56**: 38–50.

Milsom KM, Tickle M, Humphris GM, Blinkhorn AS. The relationship between anxiety and dental treatment experience in 5-year-old children. *Br Dent J* 2003; **194**: 503–6.

Møller IJ. Oral health in Europe. In: Leparski E, ed. *The prevention of non-communicable diseases: experiences and prospects.* Copenhagen: WHO Regional Office for Europe, 1987: 79–102.

Morita M, Kimura T, Kanagae M, Ishikawa A, Watanabe T. Reasons for extraction of permanent teeth in Japan. *Community Dent Oral Epidemiol* 1994; **22**: 303–6.

Mosha HJ, Scheutz F. Perceived need and use of oral health services among adolescents and adults in Tanzania. *Community Dent Oral Epidemiol* 1993; **21**: 129–32.

Murray CJL, Lopez AD. *The global burden of disease. A comprehensive assessment of mortality and disability from diseases, injuries, and risk factors in 1880 and projected to 2020.* Cambridge, MA: Harvard University Press, 1996.

Murray H, Locker D, Kay EJ. Patterns of and reasons for tooth extractions in general dental practice in Ontario, Canada. *Community Dent Oral Epidemiol* 1996; **24**: 196–200.

Nadanovsky P, Sheiham A. Relative contribution of dental services to the changes in caries levels of 12-year-olds children in 18 industrialized countries in the 1970s and early 1980s. *Community Dent Oral Epidemiol* 1995; **23**: 331–9.

Naidoo S, Chikte UME, Sheiham A. Prevalence and impact of dental pain in 8–10-year-olds in the western Cape. *S Afr Dent J* 2001; **56**: 521–3.

Namal N, Vehid S, Sheiham A. Ranking countries by dental status using the DMFT and FS-T indices. *Int Dent J* 2005; **55**: 373–6.

Niederman R, Leitch J. 'Know what' and 'know how': knowledge creation in clinical practice. *J Dent Res* 2006; **85**: 296–7.

Oginni AO. Dental care needs and demands in patients attending the dental hospital of the Obafemi Awolowo University Teaching Hospital's Complex Ile-Ife, Nigeria. *Niger J Med* 2004; **13**: 339–44.

Oginni FO. Tooth loss in a sub-urban Nigerian population: causes and pattern of mortality revisited. *Int Dent J* 2005; **55**: 17–23.

Oliveira AFB, Chaves AMB, Rosenblatt A. The influence of enamel defects on the development of early childhood caries in a population with low socioeconomic status: a longitudinal study. *Caries Res* 2006; **40**: 296–302.

Oliver RC, Brown LJ, Löe H. An estimate of periodontal treatment needs in the US based on epidemiologic data. *J Periodontol* 1989; **60**: 371–80.

Oliver RC, Brown LJ, Löe H. Periodontal treatment needs. *Periodontol 2000* 1993; **2**: 150–60.

Ong G, Yeo J-F, Bhole S. A survey of reasons for extraction of permanent teeth in Singapore. *Community Dent Oral Epidemiol* 1996; **24**: 124–7.

Onis M, Monteiro C, Akre J, Clugston G. *The worldwide magnitude of protein-energy malnutrition: an overview from the WHO Global Database on child growth.* Geneva: World Health Organization, 2001.

van Palenstein Helderman WH, Nathoo ZAW. Dental treatment demands among patients in Tanzania. *Community Dent Oral Epidemiol* 1990; **18**: 85–7.

van Palenstein Helderman WH, Herowati T, Adyatmaka A, *et al.* Oral health awareness and behaviour as indicator for a community oral health programme in Cimareme, Bandung. *J PDG Indonesia* 1997; **46**: 17–21.

van Palenstein Helderman WH, Begum A, Joardar KMA. Awareness, knowledge and behaviour pertaining to oral health of a rural population in Sreepur. *J Oral Health Bangladesh* 1998; **4**: 4–7.

van Palenstein Helderman WH, Mikx F, Begum A, *et al.* Integrating oral health into primary health care – experiences in Bangladesh, Indonesia, Nepal and Tanzania. *Int Dent J* 1999; **49**: 240–8.

van Palenstein Helderman W, Mikx F, Truin GJ, Hoang TH, Pham HL. Workforce requirements for a primary oral health care system. *Int Dent J* 2000; **50**: 371–7.

van Palenstein Helderman WH, Soe W, Van't Hof MA. Risk factors of early childhood caries in a Southeast Asian population. *J Dent Res* 2006; **85**: 85–8.

Pascoe L, Seow WK. Enamel hypoplasia and dental caries in Australian aboriginal children: prevalence and correlation between the two diseases. *Pediatr Dent* 1994; **16**: 193–9.

Peng B, Petersen PE, Fan MW. Oral health status and oral health behaviour of 12-year-old urban schoolchildren in the People's Republic of China. *Community Dent Health* 1997; **14**: 238–44.

Petersen PE. The World Oral Health Report 2003: continuous improvement of oral health in the 21st century – the approach of the WHO Global Oral Health Programme. *Community Dent Oral Epidemiol* 2003; **31** (Suppl 1): 3–23.

Petersen PE, Ogawa H. Strenghtening the prevention of periodontal disease: the WHO approach. *J Periodontol* 2005; **76**: 2187–93.

Petersen PE, Peng B, Tai BJ. Oral health status and oral health behaviour of middle-aged and elderly people in PR China. *Int Dent J* 1997; **47**: 305–12.

Petersen PE, Bourgeois D, Ogawa H, Estupinan-Day S, Ndiaye C. The global burden of oral diseases and risks to oral health. *Bull World Health Org* 2005; **83**: 661–9.

Pitts NB, Boyles J, Nugent ZJ, Thomas N, Pine CM. The dental caries experience of 5-year-old children in England and Wales (2003/4) and in Scotland (2002/3). Surveys co-ordinated by the British Association for the Study of Community Dentistry. *Community Dent Health* 2005; **22**: 46–56.

Price WA. Buckley–Price debate. Subject: Resolved, that practically all infected pulpless teeth should be removed. *J Am Dent Assoc* 1925; **12**: 1468–99.

Psoter WJ, Reid BC, Katz RV. Malnutrition and dental caries: a review of the literature. *Caries Res* 2005; **39**: 441–7.

Reich E, Hiller K-A. Reasons for tooth extraction in the western states of Germany. *Community Dent Oral Epidemiol* 1993; **21**: 379–83.

Rise J, Helöe LA. Oral conditions and need for dental treatment in an elderly population in northern Norway. *Community Dent Oral Epidemiol* 1978; **6**: 6–11.

Rosenow EC. Oral sepsis in its relationship to focal infection and elective localization. In: *Transactions of the 7th International Dental Congress*, Vol. I. Philadelphia, PA: American Dental Association, 1926: 455–76.

Rugg-Gunn AJ, Al-Mohammadi SM, Butler TJ. Malnutrition and developmental defects of enamel in 2- to 6-year-old Saudi boys. *Caries Res* 1998; **32**: 181–92.

Russell AL. A system of classification and scoring for prevalence surveys of periodontal disease. *J Dent Res* 1956; **35**: 350–9.

Sanya BO, Ng'ang'a PM, Ng'ang'a RN. Causes and pattern of missing permanent teeth among Kenyans. *East Afr Med J* 2004; **81**: 322–5.

Schechter N. The impact of acute and chronic dental pain on child development. *J Southeastern Soc Pediatr Dent* 2000; **6**: 16–17.

Seale NS, Casamassimo PS. Access to dental care for children in the United States: a survey of general practitioners. *J Am Dent Assoc* 2003; **134**: 1630–40.

Shah N. Geriatric oral health issues in India. *Int Dent J* 2001; **51** (Suppl 3): 212–18.

Sheiham A. Oral health policy and prevention. In: Murray JJ, ed. *The prevention of oral diseases*. New York: Oxford University Press, 1996: 234–49.

Sheiham A, Watt RG. The common risk factor approach: a rational basis for promoting oral health. *Community Dent Oral Epidemiol* 2000; **28**: 399–406.

Songpaisan Y, Davies GN. Periodontal status and treatment needs in the Chiangmai/Lamphun provinces of Thailand. *Community Dent Oral Epidemiol* 1989; **17**: 196–9.

Takahashi Y, Kamijyo H, Kawanishi S, Takaesu Y. Presence and absence of bleeding in association with calculus in segments given code 2 in the Community Periodontal Index of Treatment Needs (CPITN). *Community Dent Oral Epidemiol* 1988; **16**: 109–11.

Thomas CW, Primrosch RE. Changes in incremental weight and well-being of children with rampant caries following complete dental rehabilitation. *Pediatr Dent* 2002; **24**: 109–13.

Threlfall AG, Pilkington L, Milsom KM, Blinkhorn AS, Tickle M. General dental practitioners' views on the use of stainless steel crowns to restore primary molars. *Br Dent J* 2005; **199**: 453–5.

Tickle M, Milsom K, King D, Kearney-Mitchell P, Blinkhorn A. The fate of the carious primary teeth of children who regularly attend the general dental service. *Br Dent J* 2002; **192**: 219–23.

Tirwomwe F, Ekoku Y, Manji F, Baelum V, Fejerskov O. *Oral health in Uganda. Results of the National Survey 1987*. Kampala/Nairobi: Ministry of Health Uganda/Kenya Medical Research Institute, 1988.

Todd R, Durward CS. Utilisation of dental services in Cambodia and the role of the traditional dentists. *Community Dent Health* 1994; **11**: 34–7.

Tomar SL, Asma S. Smoking-attributable periodontitis in the United States: findings from NHANES III. National Health and Nutrition Examination Survey. *J Periodontol* 2000; **71**: 743–51.

Tonetti MS, Claffey N. Advances in the progression of periodontitis and proposal of definitions of a periodontitis case and disease progression for use in risk factor research. *J Clin Periodontol* 2005; **32** (Suppl 6): 210–3.

US Department of Health and Human Services. *Oral health in America: a report of the Surgeon General*. Rockville, MD: US Department of Health and Human Services, National Institute of Dental and Craniofacial Research, National Institutes of Health, 2000.

Vachirarojpisan T, Shinada K, Kawaguchi Y, Laungwechakan P, Somkote T, Detsomboonrat P. Early childhood caries in children aged 6–19 months. *Community Dent Oral Epidemiol* 2004; **32**: 133–42.

Valaitis R, Hesch R, Passarelli C, Sheehan D, Sinton J. A systematic review of the relationship between breastfeeding and early childhood caries. *Can J Public Health* 2000; **91**: 411–17.

Varenne B, Msellati P, Zoungrana C, Fournet F, Salem G. Reasons for attending dental-care services in Ouagadougou, Burkina Faso. *Bull World Health Organ* 2005; **83**: 650–5.

Waerhaug J. Epidemiology of periodontal disease. In: Ramfjord SP, Kerr DA, Ash MM, eds. World Workshop in Periodontics. Ann Arbor, MI: University of Michigan, 1966: 179–222.

Warnakulasuriya S. Demand for dental care in Sri Lanka. *Community Dent Oral Epidemiol* 1985; **13**: 68–9.

Weintraub JA, Burt BA. Oral health status in the United States: tooth loss and edentulism. *J Dent Educ* 1985; **49**: 368–76.

Widström E. Prevention and dental health services. *Oral Health Prev Dent* 2004; **2**: 255–8.

Widström E, Eaton KA. Oral healthcare systems in the extended European Union. *Oral Health Prev Dent* 2004; **2**: 155–94.

Winn DM, Brunelle JA, Selwitz RH, *et al.* Coronal and root caries in the dentition of adults in the United States, 1988–1991. *J Dent Res* 1996; **75**: 642–51.

Wogelius P, Poulsen S. Associations between dental anxiety, dental treatment due to toothache, and missed dental appointments among six to eight-year-old Danish children: a cross-sectional study. *Acta Odontol Scand* 2005; **63**: 179–82.

World Health Organization. *Oral health surveys. Basic methods*, 1st edn. Geneva: WHO, 1971.

World Health Organization. *Oral health surveys. Basic methods*. 2nd edn. Geneva: WHO, 1977.

World Health Organization. *Epidemiology, etiology, and prevention of periodontal diseases*. Geneva: WHO, 1978.

World Health Organization. *Oral health surveys. Basic methods*. 3rd edn. Geneva: WHO, 1987.

World Health Organization. *Educational imperatives for oral health personnel: change or decay?* Technical Report Series, 794 edn. Geneva: WHO, 1990.

World Health Organization. Oral health surveys. Basic methods, 4th edn. Geneva: WHO, 1997.

World Health Organization. *WHO Oral Health Country/Area Profile Programme*. http://www.whocollab.od.mah.se. Accessed 1 August 2006.

Wright D, Batchelor PA. General dental practitioners' beliefs on the perceived effects of and their preferences for remuneration mechanisms. *Br Dent J* 2002; **192**: 46–9.

Wylie I. Repositioning dentistry. *Br Dent J* 2002; **193**: 124–5.

Yee R. Infection control for the delivery of basic oral emergency care. *Developing Dentistry* 2006; 7: FDI, Practical guide.

Yee R, Sheiham A. The burden of restorative dental treatment for children in Third World countries. *Int Dent J* 2002; **52**: 1–9.

Yee R, McDonald N, Walker D. An advocacy project to fluoridate toothpastes in Nepal. *Int Dent J* 2003; **53**: 220–30.

Zhang Q, van Palenstein Helderman WH. Caries experience variables as indicators in caries risk assessment in 6–7-year-old Chinese children. *J Dent* 2006; **34**: 676–81.

Index

Note: locators in *italics* denote tables and figures